Current Practice of Equine Surgery

Current Practice of Equine Surgery

Nathaniel A. White II, D.V.M., M.S.
Marion duPont Scott Equine Medical Center
Virginia-Maryland Regional College of Veterinary Medicine
Virginia Polytechnic Institute and State University
Leesburg, Virginia

James N. Moore, D.V.M., Ph.D.
College of Veterinary Medicine
University of Georgia
Athens, Georgia

J. B. Lippincott Company Philadelphia
Grand Rapids New York St. Louis San Francisco
London Sydney Tokyo

Acquisitions Editor: Nancy Mullins
Production: Bermedica Production, Ltd.
Project Coordinator: Lori J. Bainbridge
Compositor: Bi-Comp, Incorporated
Printer/Binder: Arcata Graphics Halliday

1 3 5 6 4 2

Library of Congress Cataloging-in-Publication Data

Current practice of equine surgery / [edited by] Nathaniel A. White, James N. Moore.
p. cm.
Includes bibliographical references.
ISBN 0-397-50937-5
1. Horses—Surgery. 2. Horses—Diseases. 3. White, N.A. (Nathaniel A.) 4. Moore, James N. (James Neil)
SF951.C92 1990 89-14412
636.1'0897—dc20 CIP

The authors and publisher have exerted every effort to ensure that drug selection and dosage set forth in this text are in accord with current recommendations and practice at the time of publication. However, in view of ongoing research, changes in government regulations, and the constant flow of information relating to drug therapy and drug reactions, the reader is urged to check the package insert for each drug for any change in indications and dosage and for added warnings and precautions. This is particularly important when the recommended agent is a new or infrequently employed drug.

To Leslie and Cynthia for their patience,
and
James and Elleen Moore for their continued support

Contributors

Stephen B. Adams, D.V.M., M.S.
Diplomate ACVS
Professor
Department of Veterinary Clinical Sciences
Purdue University
West Lafayette, Indiana

Douglas Allen, D.V.M., M.S.
Diplomate ACVS
Associate Professor
Department of Large Animal Medicine
University of Georgia
Athens, Georgia

Jennifer R. Allen, B.V.Sc.
Graduate Student
Department of Veterinary Clinical Medicine and Surgery
Washington State University
Pullman, Washington

Jörg A. Auer, Dr. Med. Vet., M.S.
Diplomate ACVS
Professor and Director
Large and Small Animal Surgical Clinic
University of Switzerland
Zurich, Switzerland

David D. Barbee, D.V.M., M.S.
Diplomate ACVR
Associate Professor
Department of Veterinary Clinical Medicine and Surgery
Washington State University
Pullman, Washington

William P. Barclay, D.V.M.
Diplomate ACVS
Illinois Equine Hospital
7 S 460 Donwood Drive
Naperville, Illinois

Alicia L. Bertone, D.V.M., Ph.D.
Diplomate ACVS
Assistant Professor
Department of Veterinary Clinical Sciences
The Ohio State University
Columbus, Ohio

Lawrence C. Booth, D.V.M., M.S.
Diplomate ACVS
Associate Professor
Department of Veterinary Clinical Sciences
Iowa State University
Ames, Iowa

Conrad H. Boulton, D.V.M.
Diplomate ACVS
Hospital Director and Surgeon
New England Equine Surgical Services
Concord, New Hampshire

Elizabeth P. Boulton, D.V.M.
Assistant Professor
University of New Hampshire
Durham, New Hampshire
Surgeon
New England Equine Surgical Services
Concord, New Hampshire

Karl Frederick Bowman, D.V.M., M.S.
Diplomate ACVS
Diplomate ABVP
Associate Professor, Equine Surgery
Department of Food Animal and Equine Medicine
North Carolina State University
Raleigh, North Carolina

Murray P. Brown, D.V.M., M.S.
Diplomate ACVS
Professor
Department of Large Animal Clinical Sciences
University of Florida
Gainesville, Florida

Robert W. Brusie, D.V.M.
Practitioner
Suwanee, Georgia

Charles A. Buffington, D.V.M., Ph.D.
Diplomate ACVN
Assistant Professor
Department of Veterinary Clinical Sciences
The Ohio State University
Columbus, Ohio

Michael F. Clem, D.V.M., M.S.
Diplomate ACVS
Supervisor of Experimental Surgery
Lab Animal Resources
University of Texas Health Sciences-San Antonio
San Antonio, Texas

Richard M. DeBowes, D.V.M., M.S.
Diplomate ACVS
Associate Professor
Department of Surgery and Medicine
Kansas State University
Manhattan, Kansas

Norm G. Ducharme, D.V.M., M.Sc.
Diplomate ACVS
Associate Professor
Department of Clinical Sciences
Cornell University
Ithaca, New York

Doris H. Dyson, D.V.M., D.V.Sc.
Diplomate ACVA
Associate Professor
Department of Clinical Studies
University of Guelph
Guelph, Ontario, Canada

Rolf M. Embertson, D.V.M.
Diplomate ACVS
Surgeon
Rood and Riddle Equine Hospital
Lexington, Kentucky

Gregory L. Ferraro, D.V.M.
Practitioner
Arcadia, California

Elwyn C. Firth, B.V.Sc., Ph.D.
Diplomate ACVS
Professor and Head
Department of Veterinary Surgery and
Companion Animal Health
Massey University
Palmerston North, New Zealand

Andrew T. Fischer, Jr., D.V.M.
Diplomate ACVS
Practitioner
Chino Valley Equine Hospital
Chino, California

David E. Freeman, M.V.B., M.R.C.V.S., Ph.D.
Diplomate ACVS
Assistant Professor of Surgery
Department of Clinical Studies-New Bolton Center
University of Pennsylvania
Kennett Square, Pennsylvania

Susan L. Fubini, D.V.M.
Diplomate ACVS
Assistant Professor
Department of Clinical Sciences
Cornell University
Ithaca, New York

Martin O. Furr, D.V.M.
Assistant Professor
Department of Large Animal Clinical Sciences
Virginia Polytechnic Institute and State University
Blacksburg, Virginia

Albert A. Gabel, D.V.M., M.S.
Diplomate ACVS
Professor Emeritus
Department of Veterinary Clinical Sciences
The Ohio State University
Columbus, Ohio

Richard P. Hackett, D.V.M., M.S.
Diplomate ACVS
Associate Professor
Department of Clinical Sciences
Cornell University
Ithaca, New York

Susan V. Hildebrand, D.V.M.
Diplomate ACVA
Associate Professor
Department of Surgery
University of California
Davis, California

Katrin Hinrichs, D.V.M., Ph.D.
Diplomate ACT
Assistant Professor
Department of Medicine
Tufts University
North Grafton, Massachusetts

Melissa Holland, D.V.M.
Diplomate ACVA
Assistant Professor
Department of Small Animal Clinical Sciences
Virginia Polytechnic Institute and
State University
Blacksburg, Virginia

Clifford M. Honnas, D.V.M.
Assistant Professor
Diplomate ACVS
Department of Large Animal Medicine and Surgery
Texas A & M University
College Station, Texas

Svend E. Kold, D.V.M., M.R.C.V.S.
Equine Clinical Unit
Animal Health Trust
Newmarket, Suffolk, England

Melinda K. Krpan, D.V.M., M.S.
Practitioner
Chino Hills Equine Hospital
Chino, California

Claire A. Latimer, D.V.M., M.S.
Diplomate ACVO
Veterinary Ophthalmologist
Lexington, Kentucky

William A. Lindsay, D.V.M.
Diplomate ACVS
Associate Professor
Department of Surgical Sciences
University of Wisconsin
Madison, Wisconsin

Michael A. Livesey, B.V.MS., M.Sc.
Associate Professor
Department of Clinical Studies
University of Guelph
Guelph, Ontario, Canada

K. C. Kent Lloyd, D.V.M.
Postdoctoral Fellow
Center for Ulcer Research and Education
University of California
Los Angeles, California

Mark D. Markel, D.V.M., Ph.D.
Diplomate ACVS
Research Associate
Orthopedic Biomechanics Laboratory
Mayo Clinic/Mayo Foundation
Rochester, Minnesota

Wayne N. McDonell, D.V.M., M.Sc., Ph.D.
Diplomate ACVA
Professor
Department of Clinical Studies
University of Guelph
Guelph, Ontario, Canada

C. Wayne McIlwraith, B.V.Sc., M.S., Ph.D., M.R.C.V.S.
Diplomate ACVS
Professor
Department of Clinical Sciences
Colorado State University
Fort Collins, Colorado

Dennis M. Meagher, D.V.M., Ph.D.
Diplomate ACVS
Professor
Department of Surgery
University of California
Davis, California

H. Carlton Newman, D.V.M.
Department of Companion Animal
and Special Species
North Carolina State University
Raleigh, North Carolina

Alan J. Nixon, B.V.Sc., M.S.
Diplomate ACVS
Assistant Professor
Department of Clinical Sciences
Cornell University
Ithaca, New York

David M. Nunamaker, V.M.D.
Diplomate ACVS
Jacques Jenny Professor of Orthopedic Surgery
Department of Clinical Studies-New Bolton Center
University of Pennsylvania
Kennett Square, Pennsylvania

James A. Orsini, D.V.M.
Diplomate ACVS
Assistant Professor of Surgery
Department of Clinical Studies-New Bolton Center
University of Pennsylvania
Kennett Square, Pennsylvania

John R. Pascoe, B.V.Sc., Ph.D.
Associate Professor
Department of Surgery
University of California
Davis, California

Peter J. Pascoe, B.V.Sc., D.V.A.
Diplomate ACVA
Associate Professor
Department of Surgery
University of California
Davis, California

W. L. Ragland, D.V.M., Ph.D.
Professor
Department of Pathology
University of Georgia
Athens, Georgia

Virginia B. Reef, D.V.M.
Diplomate ACVIM in Internal Medicine
Assistant Professor of Medicine
Department of Clinical Studies-New Bolton Center
University of Pennsylvania
Kennett Square, Pennsylvania

Eric L. Reinertson, D.V.M.
Associate Professor
Department of Veterinary Clinical Sciences
Iowa State University
Ames, Iowa

Dean W. Richardson, D.V.M.
Diplomate ACVS
Assistant Professor
Department of Clinical Studies-New Bolton Center
University of Pennsylvania
Kennett Square, Pennsylvania

Mark C. Rick, D.V.M.
Practitioner
Alamo Pintado Equine Clinic
Los Olivos, California

James T. Robertson, D.V.M.
Diplomate ACVS
Associate Professor
Department of Veterinary Clinical Sciences
The Ohio State University
Columbus, Ohio

Robert K. Schneider, D.V.M., M.S.
Diplomate ACVS
Assistant Professor
Department of Veterinary Clinical Sciences
The Ohio State University
Columbus, Ohio

Donnie E. Slone, Jr., D.V.M., M.S.
Diplomate ACVS
Head of Surgery
Peterson and Smith Equine Hospital
Ocala, Florida

Jack R. Snyder, D.V.M., Ph.D.
Diplomate ACVS
Assistant Professor
Department of Surgery
University of California
Davis, California

Ted S. Stashak, D.V.M., M.S.
Diplomate ACVS
Professor
Department of Clinical Sciences
Colorado State University
Fort Collins, Colorado

Robert R. Steckel, D.V.M., M.S.
Diplomate ACVS
Assistant Professor
Department of Surgery
Tufts University
North Grafton, Massachusetts

Eugene P. Steffey, V.M.D., Ph.D.
Diplomate ACVA
Professor
Department of Surgery
University of California
Davis, California

John A. Stick, D.V.M.
Diplomate ACVS
Professor
Department of Large Animal Clinical Sciences
Michigan State University
East Lansing, Michigan

Kenneth E. Sullins, D.V.M., M.S.
Diplomate ACVS
Associate Professor
Marion duPont Scott Equine Medical Center
Virginia Polytechnic Institute and
State University
Leesburg, Virginia

Lloyd P. Tate, Jr., V.M.D.
Diplomate ACVS
Associate Professor
Department of Food Animal and Equine Medicine
North Carolina State University
Raleigh, North Carolina

Walter R. Threlfall, D.V.M., M.S., Ph.D.
Diplomate ACT
Professor
Department of Veterinary Clinical Sciences
The Ohio State University
Columbus, Ohio

Cynthia M. Trim, B.V.Sc., M.R.C.V.S.
Diplomate ACVA
Professor
Department of Large Animal Medicine
University of Georgia
Athens, Georgia

Gayle W. Trotter, D.V.M., M.S.
Diplomate ACVS
Associate Professor
Department of Clinical Sciences
Colorado State University
Fort Collins, Colorado

Eric P. Tulleners, D.V.M.
Diplomate ACVS
Assistant Professor
Department of Clinical Studies-New Bolton Center
University of Pennsylvania
Kennett Square, Pennsylvania

Tracy A. Turner, D.V.M., M.S.
Diplomate ACVS
Practitioner, Surgeon
Rochester Equine Clinic
Rochester, New Hampshire

Anne Vachon, D.V.M., Ph.D.
Chino Valley Equine Hospital
Chino, California

Pamela C. Wagner, D.V.M., M.S.
Diplomate ACVS
Professor
Department of Large Animal Surgery
Oregon State University
Corvallis, Oregon

Jeffrey P. Watkins, D.V.M., M.S.
Diplomate ACVS
Associate Professor
Department of Large Animal Medicine and Surgery
Texas A & M University
College Station, Texas

Nathaniel A. White II, D.V.M., M.S.
Diplomate ACVS
Theodora Ayer Randolph Professor of Surgery
Marion duPont Scott Equine Medical Center
Virginia Polytechnic Institute and
State University
Leesburg, Virginia

Milton Wyman, D.V.M., M.Sc.
Diplomate ACVO
Professor
Associate Dean, Academic and Student Affairs
Department of Veterinary Clinical Sciences
The Ohio State University
Columbus, Ohio

John V. Yovich, B.V.MS., M.S., Ph.D.
Diplomate ACVS
Senior Lecturer in Equine Surgery
Murdoch University Veterinary Hospital
Murdoch University
Murdoch, Western Australia, Australia

Preface

Equine surgery has changed dramatically over the past two decades. This change has occurred in response to the increasing demand by an informed clientele for the best care possible for their horses and because of adaptation of both new diagnostic and surgical techniques from other disciplines. The resultant barrage of information in professional journals has created a new challenge in veterinary continuing education. In an effort to keep up with the rapid changes in equine surgery we have enlisted experts in various specialties of the profession to create *Current Practice of Equine Surgery.*

The goal of this text was to compile in one source the newest information on recent advances in equine surgery. It was our aim to provide the practitioner, veterinary student, and veterinarians in surgical training programs with a single reference source that would review specific surgical diseases, their diagnoses, the most current treatments, and expected prognoses. The vital roles of anesthesia and new technologic innovations dictated that these areas be included as individual sections in the text. In all sections we have encouraged the authors to include their personal experience and opinions in discussing their particular areas of expertise. Because some new information in this text may be controversial, we have included alternatives or divergent opinions where appropriate.

Current Practice of Equine Surgery is not designed to cover equine surgery in extreme depth. Consequently, the reader may find that other texts are required for the review of surgical anatomy, fundamental surgical techniques, and previously described diagnostic techniques. Furthermore, we recognize that there are individual topics that are not covered in this edition. It will be our aim to include as many new topics as possible as we update new advances in the practice of equine surgery in subsequent editions.

Nathaniel A. White II, DVM, MS
James N. Moore, DVM, PhD

Acknowledgments

Much of the work associated with this text was completed by the individual Section Editors. We were very pleased with the manner in which these individuals selected the contributors, guided the production of the chapters, and edited the final product. This text would have remained only an idea had not the section editors performed so masterfully. Finally, we are appreciative of the excellent work of Nancy Mullins, Alison Pierce, and others at J. B. Lippincott in preparation of this text.

Contents

Unit II Anesthesia
Section Editor: Peter J. Pascoe

Unit III Wound Healing
Section Editor: William A. Lindsay

Unit IV Neurology and Ophthalmology
Section Editor: Richard M. DeBowes

Unit VIIIA Developmental Musculoskeletal Disorders
Section Editor: Pamela C. Wagner

Unit VIIIB Traumatic Musculoskeletal Disorders
Section Editor: Pamela C. Wagner

Unit VIII C Septic Musculoskeletal Disorders
Section Editor: Pamela C. Wagner

Unit IX Fractures
Section Editor: Dean W. Richardson

Current Practice of Equine Surgery

UNIT I

New Surgical Technology

1
Operating Room Protocol

Robert W. Brusie

The risk of infection is related to the environment and the aseptic technique of the surgical team. Several studies in humans report risk of infection ranging from 1 to 5% for clean, from 3 to 11% for clean-contaminated, from 10 to 17% for contaminated, and over 27% for dirty wounds. Infection rates in dogs and cats from a teaching hospital were 2.5% for clean, 4.5% for clean-contaminated, 5.8% for contaminated, and 18.1% for dirty wounds. Wound infection rates for the horse have not been reported. In addition to wound contamination, host susceptibility and local wound pathophysiology must be considered in the biology of wound infection. In humans, a multivariate index of host susceptibility and wound contamination using four risk factors doubled the ability to predict the risk of surgical wound infection. These four risk factors were: (*a*) having an abdominal operation, (*b*) having an operation that lasts more than 2 hours, (*c*) having a contaminated or dirty operation by the traditional classification system, and (*d*) having more than three diagnoses.

The three sources of pathogens that infect surgical wounds are the hospital environment, personnel, and, most importantly, the patient. Wound susceptibility is primarily dependent on surgical technique and patient factors. These are interrelated as far as patient management is concerned but will be discussed separately.

CONTROL OF CONTAMINATION

Hospital Environment

Operating Room. The design of the operating room is important in reducing the number of pathogens to which the surgical wound is exposed. Walls and floors should be nonporous to facilitate complete removal of all debris. Horizontal surfaces such as cabinet tops should be avoided to prevent collection of dust and debris. Although floor drains in the operating room are not ideal, they are often included to facilitate cleaning. When used, floor drains should be placed away from the central surgical area and out of the flow of traffic. The operating room should be large enough to accommodate the patient and anesthetic, radiologic, and surgical equipment and still allow space for the non-scrubbed personnel to circulate.

Air in the operating room can be a source of pathogens. With increasing personnel activity, the contamination of air with dust, lint, respiratory droplets, and skin squamae increases. The ventilation system should provide at least 20 air changes (four changes should be fresh air) of highly filtered air (90% efficiency) per hour and maintain positive pressure within the operating room. Air contamination is further reduced by keeping doors closed, decreasing the number of personnel in the room, and increasing ventilation.

Instruments. Most surgical instruments can be sterilized with steam or ethylene oxide. A chemical indicator must be included in each pack to ensure that it has been exposed to the sterilization process. Chemical indicators, however, do not prove that sterilization has been achieved. Sterility should be evaluated periodically with biologic indicators such as *Bacillus stearothermophilus* for steam sterilizers and *Bacillus subtilis* var. *globigii* or var. *niger* for ethylene oxide sterilizers (Attest; 3M Medical Products Division).

Flash sterilization is performed on unwrapped metallic or porous items in emergency situations and on some specialty items such as rechargable batteries. Minimum exposure times and temperatures are defined for most items; however, some specialty items may require different exposure times as specified by the manufacturer. Implantable items should not be flash sterilized because of the reduction in the margin of safety for asepsis.

Sterilization problems arise with more sophisticated instruments such as arthroscopes, video cameras, and fiber optic equipment. Aeration time requirements of ethylene oxide sterilization preclude multiple daily use of these items. When rapid turnaround of steam-sensitive equipment is required, a high-level disinfectant or "cold sterilization" is commonly used. The product used should be registered as a high-level disinfectant with the Food and Drug Administration (FDA). The efficacy of these products decreases with contamination, dilution, and age. Disposal of the solution should be in accordance with the manufacturer's expiration date. A strict protocol should be established for preparing the instruments for cold sterilization. The instruments should be dismantled, cleaned, and dried before they are placed in the disinfectant. When removed from the disinfectant, the instruments should be aseptically submerged into sterile water, then rinsed with sterile water to remove all residual disinfectant and avoid chemical damage to the tissues of the user or patient.

The protocol followed at our hospital includes steam sterilization of all arthroscopic equipment (with the exception of the steam- and gas-sensitive items) after the last case of the day. For any given procedure the camera, light cable, and arthroscopes are placed into sterile trays containing 2% glutaraldehyde solution (Cidex; Surgikos, Inc.) when the patient is anesthetized. After the horse is positioned and the surgical site prepared and draped, the surgeon or scrubbed assistant removes the equipment from the solution and rinses it with sterile water. Between successive cases, the entire set is processed in the same disinfectant. The time the instruments are placed in the disinfectant is recorded to ensure at least 15 minutes' submersion time. The activated solution is stored in covered containers between uses and is discarded after 14 days (manufacturer's recommendation). The use of 2% glutaraldehyde as the disinfectant is effective, as evidenced by a report of five infections in 12,505 human arthroscopic cases.

Personnel

Everyone in the surgical suite should wear caps, masks, and scrub suits worn only in the clean area of the hospital. Lab coats or coveralls should be worn for preparation of the patient and taken off prior to entering the operating room. The use of shoe covers is advocated; however, their effectiveness in reducing floor contamination or reducing surgical wound infections has not been shown. Tacky or antiseptic mats at the entrance to the operating room may be used; however, these have not been shown to reduce the risk of infection.

Potential contamination of the wound from the hands of the surgical team is reduced by scrubbing. A 10-minute scrub has been advocated; however, recent studies have shown that a scrub lasting for 5 minutes does not increase the infection rate.

Because standard woven cotton gowns provide an ineffective barrier against penetration by microorganisms when compared with nonwoven disposable fabrics, many hospitals now use disposable gowns exclusively. Using a disposable gown and drape system, overall infection rates were significantly lower as compared to a cotton gown and drape system. When used, cotton surgical gowns should be made of Quarpel-treated, tightly woven cotton. This material has a limited number of launderings (about 75) before losing its effectiveness as an aseptic barrier.

The Patient

The patient is a major source of pathogens that infect the surgical wound. Preoperatively, the patient should be evaluated for signs of remote infections, which should be eliminated prior to performing elective procedures. The risk of surgical wound infection in humans has been shown to be decreased with shorter preoperative hospitalization; however, this has not been evaluated in the horse.

The preoperative preparation of the patient includes hair removal, scrubbing, and the sterile preparation of the skin. Hair removal should be performed with clippers immediately preoperatively and with care taken to avoid abrading the skin. In human studies, shaving with a razor causes injury to the skin, which increases the risk of infection. Therefore, when shaving is performed, it should be done immediately before the scrub by a skilled person using a safety razor. The equine surgeon may encounter dermatitis caused by counterirritants at the proposed incision site. This could allow colonization with pathogenic bacteria and alter local wound defense mechanisms. If the procedure is elective, the surgery should be postponed until the skin has healed.

The purpose of the surgical scrub is to remove dirt, debris, and superficial flora. This is followed by application of an antimicrobial agent to kill or inhibit the more adherent deep, resident flora. Several studies in humans indicate the most effective method of reducing bacterial numbers and slowing the rate of recolonization is to use an FDA-approved scrub (such as povidone-iodine or chlorhexidine) followed by an alcohol wipe, then application of a plastic adhesive drape containing a slow-release iodophor.

The protocol at our hospital is to clip the site before entering the induction stall. Once the patient is positioned in the operating room, the immediate area of the proposed incision site is shaved with a disposable safety razor. A 10-minute povidone-iodine scrub is performed, followed by a 3-minute alcohol paint by a gloved technician. The surgeon blots the area dry with a sterile towel, and an iodophor-containing adhesive drape is applied.

Various types of surgical drapes are available. As mentioned above, the effectiveness of conventional cotton fabric drapes as barriers to bacteria is questionable. Many hospitals are using nonwoven disposable drapes, which are effective barriers to bacteria even when the drapes are wet. Disposable drapes are available in a variety of sizes. Thus, it is possible to cover the entire patient with a single drape, thereby decreasing time required for draping and eliminating drape separation. Sterile adhesive strips are applied around the periphery of the fenestration, which effectively seals the surgical area from the rest of the patient.

SURGICAL TECHNIQUE

The single most important factor in preventing surgical wound infection is surgical technique. Infection and complication rates increase with wound exposure time, tissue trauma, and foreign material left in the wound.

Surgical time is minimized by having a thorough knowledge of the surgical anatomy, a preconceived plan, and the ability to adapt the plan to the situation. The surgeon must perform the operation expediently and at the same time handle tissue gently.

Tissue devitalization is reduced by preventing desiccation with adequate lavage during the procedure. The use of lavage/suction rather than sponging with dry gauze reduces tissue trauma. Electrocautery should be limited to pinpoint coagulation of vessels through mosquito hemostatic forceps. Charred tissue remnants following electrocautery can cause a foreign body reaction. Although blunt dissection may lead to less bleeding at the time of surgery, careful, sharp dissection is less traumatic.

The presence of foreign material in the wound greatly reduces the wound's ability to resist infection. Glove powder (corn starch) has been shown to cause intraabdominal granulomas and adhesion formation. Washing the gloves for 30 seconds in 1 L of sterile water reduces the starch content by approximately 90%. Essentially all of the starch can be removed by washing gloves with povidone-iodine scrub for 30 seconds followed by a 30-second rinse with sterile water. Effective glove washing is complete when an audible sticking sound is made when the thumb and index finger are pressed together, and then separated.

Hemoglobin within the wound increases susceptibility to infection. In addition to ensuring adequate hemostasis, blood within the wound should be removed before closure. It is preferable to lavage and adequately clean each successive layer before closure. The addition of antibiotics to lavage solutions has been shown

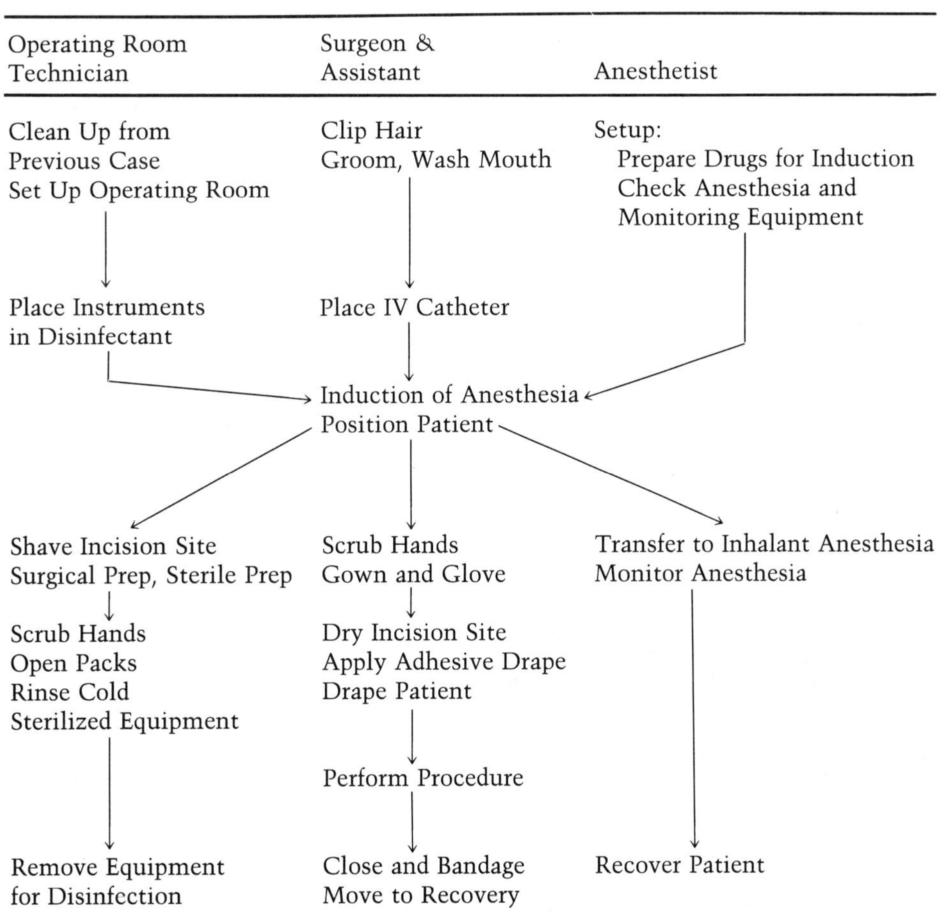

Figure 1–1. Task-oriented operating room procedure.

to be of some benefit. Thorough lavage using an isotonic balanced electrolyte solution throughout the entire surgical procedure prevents tissue desiccation, removes blood and debris, and dilutes the contaminating load of bacteria.

Every attempt should be made to eliminate dead space during closure of the wound to prevent collection of blood and tissue fluids, which serve as an excellent growth medium for bacteria. When fluid accumulates in a wound, it loses the ability to support opsonization of bacteria for phagocytosis and killing by neutrophils. If complete elimination of dead space cannot be performed, drains must be utilized. If asepsis is expected, drains should be of the closed suction type, and should not exit the skin through the primary skin incision. Drain management is extremely important to prevent ascending infections; the personnel performing primary care of the drain should be trained in aseptic technique. The amount of fluids produced by the wound should be monitored so the drain can be removed as soon as possible.

Anesthesia time should be minimized to reduce secondary complications. This is facilitated by the coordination of the surgical team, especially on the more frequently performed procedures. An example would be a routine arthroscopic surgery where setup of the operating room occurs simultaneously with preparation of the patient for anesthesia, and the preparation of the surgical field occurs simultaneously with the surgeon scrubbing. Everyone has a task from the beginning to the end of the procedure (Fig. 1–1).

Recently, the use of staples for skin closure has gained popularity because the time required for skin closure is reduced. There are several types of staples available (Chapter 2). Some will tend to invert or evert the skin, leading to a less desirable closure. The surgeon should try several types and be critical of the ability of the staple to adequately appose the skin.

If possible, a sterile, nonocclusive bandage should be applied to the wound so fluid will wick away from the incision. Serum and other fluids from the incision make an excellent growth medium for bacteria. Unless saturation of the bandage occurs, the bandage should stay in place for at least 24 hours postoperatively to allow a fibrin seal to form in the incision. If the bandage must be changed, it should be replaced with a sterile bandage using aseptic technique.

If an incision is made in an area that cannot be bandaged, a sterile stent bandage may be sutured over the incision. This bandage protects the wound from the environment and supplies pressure to decrease dead space and edema formation at the incision site.

BIBLIOGRAPHY

AORN Recommended Practices Subcommittee: Basic aseptic technic. *AORN J* 1987;45:784–789.

Cruse PJE, Foord R: The epidemiology of wound infection: A ten year prospective study of 62,939 wounds. *Surg Clin North Am* 1980;60:27–40.

Fraser I: Simple and effective method of removing starch powder from surgical gloves. *Br Med J* 1982;284:1835.

Gardner JS: CDC guideline for prevention of surgical wound infections, 1985. *Infect Control* 1986;7:193–200.

Maki DG, Hassemer CA: Flash sterilization: Carefully measured haste. *Infect Control* 1987;8:307–310.

Proposed recommended practices. Aseptic barrier materials for surgical gowns and drapes. *AORN J* 1986;44:612–616.

Proposed recommended practices. Preoperative skin preparation. *AORN J* 1987;46:719–724.

Recommended practices: Sterilization and disinfection. *AORN J* 1987;45:440–460.

Rogers DM, Blouin GS, O'Leary JP: Povidone-iodine wound irrigation and wound sepsis. *Surg Gynecol Obstet* 1983;157:426–430.

Vasseur PB, Levy J, Dowd E, et al: Surgical wound infection rates in dogs and cats: Data from a teaching hospital. *Vet Surg* 1988;17:60–64.

2 Surgical Stapling Devices and Their Applications

Kenneth E. Sullins

Surgical stapling devices have become common in equine abdominal surgery. Although reliable equipment has been available for some time, improvements in recent years have simplified operation of the instruments. Until quite recently, United States Surgical Corp. has been the most familiar manufacturer. Development of disposable instruments followed more recently by a Premium line of instruments have made use of their system more convenient, with reduced risk of malfunction or misuse. At the present time, similar instruments are available from Ethicon Inc. and 3M Company.

The basic wound created by a staple instrument consists of inverted or everted layers of tissue secured by staggered double rows of B-shaped stainless steel wire staples. Absorbable Lactomer staples are now available for the Premium TA-55. This material is almost identical to polyglactin 910 or polyglycolic acid suture material. Absorbable staples do not bend to form a "B," but instead have a fastener that snaps over the legs of the staple. Complaints of dyspareunia following hysterectomy in women and postoperative interference with computed tomography from steel staples were motivations for developing this staple. Resorption of staples is desirable in the urinary tract, since calculi can form around stainless steel staples. Stainless steel staples occasionally migrate from the original site of intestinal anastomosis, which is not usually a problem; however, in some areas random migration of staples is not acceptable.

During the first few days after surgery the bursting pressure of stapled anastomoses is generally equal to or stronger than that of sutured anastomoses. Since staple-inverted tissue does not undergo necrosis, as occurs following sutured inversion, it is reasonable that fibrin would not play as significant a role in maintaining anastomotic integrity, and that the strength of the anastomosis would be maintained during this period of enhanced fibrinolysis. As the fibroproliferative phase of intestinal healing is entered, no difference in wound strength is observed between stapled and sutured anastomoses.

LINEAR STAPLERS

Instruments that apply a linear-double-staggered row of staples are used to join two surfaces aligned in the way one would align sheets of paper for an office stapler. After the instrument in discharged and the staples are in place, the tissue is transected along the margin of the cartridge with a scalpel, producing an even everted tissue edge (Fig. 2–1). Multiple applications of linear staplers are permissible for bowel that is too wide for a single TA-90 cartridge. Care must be taken to ensure that the serial staple rows overlap at their junctions. Since everted patterns are predisposed to adhesion formation, the use of linear stapling instruments should be limited to areas where luminal patency is not desired. Adhesions (usually omental) to blind stumps have not presented significant problems, and contraction of such a site is inconsequential.

Linear staplers offer the advantages of faster, cleaner resection of tissue than open-ended suturing; however, if thickened tissue produces resistance in closure or discharge of the instrument, the staple rows should not be relied upon and should be inverted with two rows of suture. Although successful single-suture-row inversions have been performed, they should be generally considered inadequate. Inversion of the staple row obstructs perfusion to tissue in the staple line, causing it to slough, leaving only a single suture line. In this situation the staples should be considered to be only a means to increase speed and reduce contamination, the suture pattern being the primary means of closure. With severely thickened tissue, dehiscence can occur before completion of the suture inversion.

Procedures for which the linear staplers have been found most useful include creation of stumps in the ileum prior to ileocecostomy, amputation of the large colon after anastomosing the dorsal and ventral colons, and ovariectomy. The instrument can also be used for biopsy or resection of semisolid or solid organs such as the lung or liver. Stapled end-to-end small intestinal anastomoses are not recommended in horses.

Modifications of some of these instruments are available in configurations that compress the tissue for more effective hemostasis such as the V-TA-30 from United States Surgical Corp.

ANASTOMOSIS INSTRUMENTS

The anastomosis instrument creates an anastomosis consisting of four staggered staple rows and transects the interposed tissue, leaving two staple rows on either side. It can be applied across a hollow or parenchymatous organ to secure both sides of the apposed tissue and transect the tissue, such as for resecting a segment of small intestine and leaving two secure blind ends (Fig. 2–2). The most common application is via two stab incisions in two hollow organs to create an inverted side-to-side anastomosis. The instruments can be reloaded and reapplied in the same or the opposite direction if longer anastomoses are desired. The stab incisions admitting the instruments into the lumens should be closed by inverting sutures. Longitudinal apposition of this portal extends the circumference of the anastomosis approximately 2 cm.

Suture reinforcement of the stapled anastomosis is necessary at each end of the staple rows adjacent to the instrument insertion sites, and at the junction of the two applications (if performed) on the opposite side of the bowel from the instrument portals. As described for

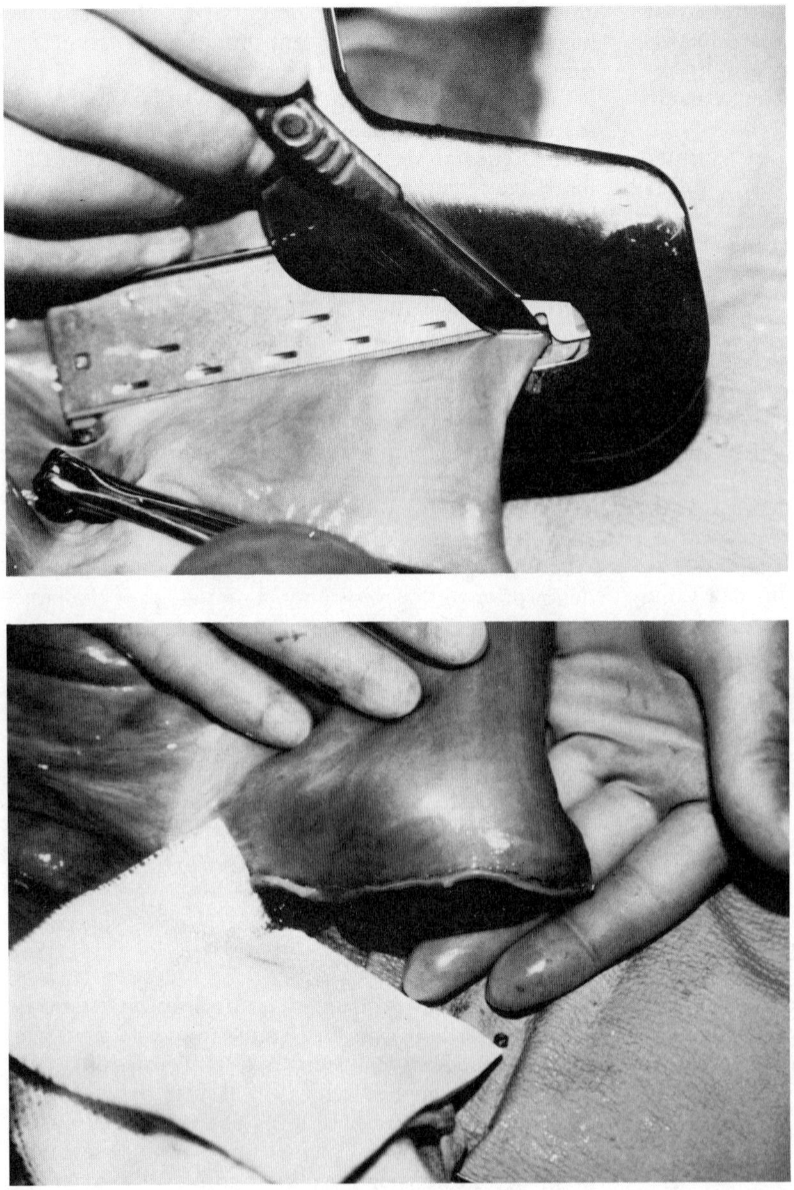

B

Figure 2–1. Linear stapler applied to bowel with scalpel ready to transect discard segment (*A*). Remaining stump after removal of segment and instrument is shown (*B*).

the linear staplers, sequential application of the instrument requires overlapping of the staple rows. Since visualization of the staple row opposite stab incisions is almost impossible, a defect frequently results at the junction of staple applications. This complication has been reported to be more prevalent when small intestine is joined midway between the mesenteric and antimesenteric borders rather than at the antimesenteric borders. When inspection of the opposite side of the anastomosis is not possible, the reinforcing suture should be applied before the staples are placed. If any difficulty is encountered in closing or discharging the instrument, the entire anastomosis should be oversewn. It should be noted that this staple instrument is least amenable to application on thickened tissue. Salvaging a sutured, double-inverted, side-to-side anastomosis from a disrupted staple application is much more difficult than suturing the anastomosis from the beginning. If the tissue is thick enough to be of concern, the instrument should not be used.

Procedures most suited for use of the anastomosis instruments include jejuno(ileo)cecostomy, ileocolostomy, anastomosis of the dorsal and ventral colons, gastrojejunostomy, functional end-to-end (side-to-side)

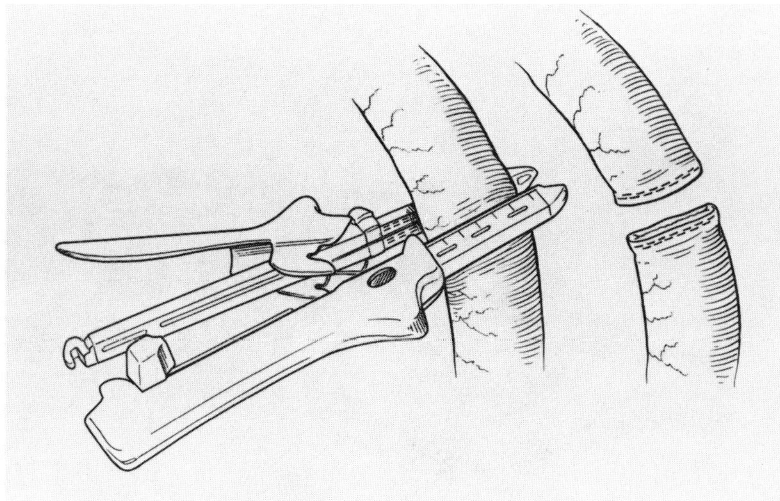

Figure 2–2. Gastrointestinal anastomosis application across small intestine to be transected with creation of two blind stumps. (Reprinted with permission from Sullins KE: Use of staples in gastrointestinal surgery, in White NA [ed], *Equine Acute Abdomen*. Philadelphia, Lea & Febiger, in press.)

small bowel anastomosis, and division of appropriately sized small bowel segments leaving two stapled stumps. Specifics of these procedures are described in the chapters in Unit VI (Gastrointestinal Tract).

The instruments available apply a 5-cm line of staples and are manufactured by all three American companies mentioned above. All three companies also have cartridges that can apply the four rows of staples with or without dividing the tissue. A 10-cm instrument has recently become available from United States Surgical Corp.

CIRCULAR STAPLING DEVICES

Circular stapling devices apply circular, double-staggered staple rows, creating a circular, inverted, end-to-end anastomosis of tubular organs (Fig. 2–3) or an end-to-side anastomosis of tubular to larger organs. The resulting anastomosis is inverted and secured by two rows of staples. Three sizes of anvils are available—25, 28, and 31 mm in outside diameter—producing inverted anastomoses with 15-, 18-, and 21-mm lumens, respectively.

The main disadvantage of the circular devices is that access to the anastomotic site usually must be via an incision in bowel that must remain in situ, and the diameter of the anvil dictates that a sizeable incision must be created. Depending upon the situation, modified end-to-side methods can be devised in which the instrument is inserted and withdrawn through tissue that is to be resected, making its use more reasonable. Because of diameter limitations of currently available equipment, the potential clinical applications appear to be limited to foals. The propensity of the foal to form peritoneal adhesions must be considered when creating additional tissue invasion required for this technique.

If the anvil is positioned after the shaft is inserted either through a linear staple line or through a small stab incision, the necessity for a purse-string suture in that half of the anastomosis is precluded. This method is especially useful for sites such as the stomach, where the tissue is so thick that the purse string draws in excessive tissue for the instrument, or in human colorectal surgery, where the rectal stump lies within the pelvic canal. A new disposable instrument model with a completely detachable anvil is available from United States Surgical Corp. This feature facilitates placement in difficult sites.

One of these instruments has been evaluated for end-to-end jejunal anastomosis in adult ponies (150 to 220 kg). All ponies did well in the postoperative period. Moderate omental and rare mesenteric or enterotomy adhesions were present but none produced any clinically apparent effect.

These instruments are available from United States Surgical Corp. (the end-to-end anastomosis [EEA] instrument), Ethicon Inc. (the intraluminal stapler [ILS]), and 3M Company. Their application in equine surgery is limited by the narrow diameter of anastomosis possible with currently available instruments.

VASCULAR LIGATION AND SEPARATION

Vascular ligation instruments are designed for application to vascular bundles that can be compressed to dimensions of 0.75 mm × 5 or 7 mm. Designed for efficient ligation and division of vascular pedicles, the instruments should be applied only after isolation of

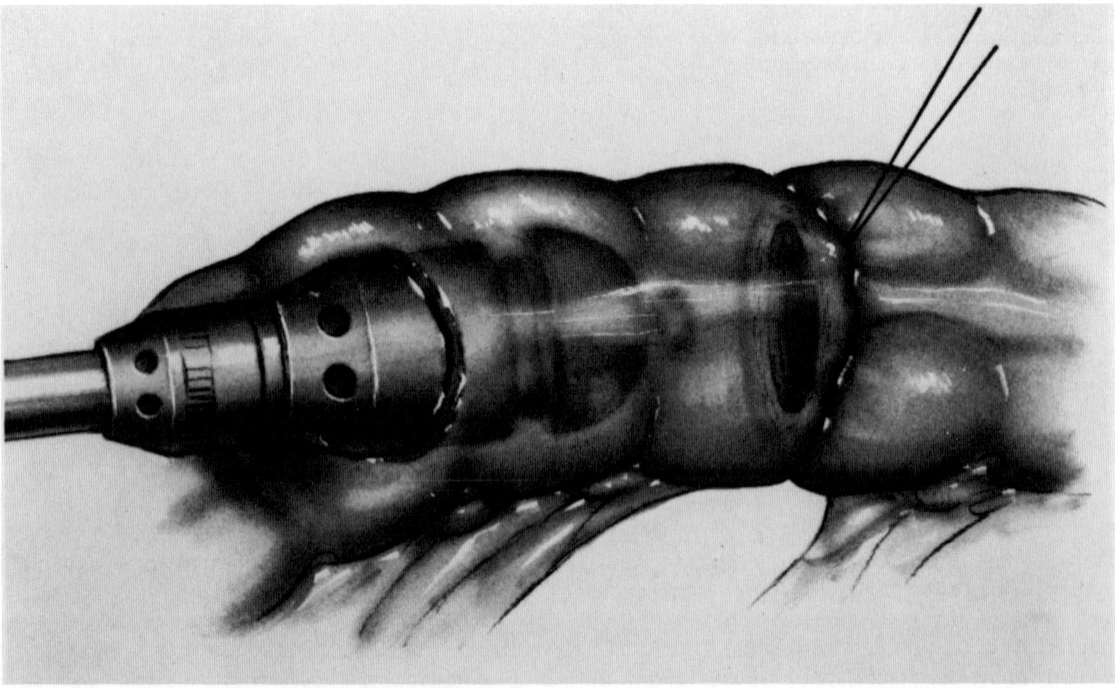

Figure 2–3. Pattern of anastomosis produced by circular stapling device (EEA). Note necessity of separate entry site for instrument. (Reprinted with permission from *Atlas of Surgical Stapling.* Norwalk, CT, United States Surgical Corp., 1980.)

the vascular tissue from mesentery and fat. The diameter restrictions recommended by the manufacturer should be closely heeded or postoperative hemorrhage can result. Although secure when properly applied, the vascular staple should not be relied upon as the only ligature in the adult horse; rather, it can serve as the second ligature distal to a suture ligature.

United States Surgical Corp. produces an instrument (LDS-2) that, when appropriately applied to a vessel, staples across the wall at two sites and cuts in between the staples (Fig. 2–4). Two sizes of cartridges are available for the pistol-grip application unit.

PRECAUTIONS AND COMPLICATIONS

When using linear staplers, it is possible to crush tissue that is thicker than that for which the particular instrument was designed. This will result in leakage from necrosis of tissue along the staple line. If difficulty is experienced during application of the instrument or firing the staples, the staple line should be oversewn with suture. One layer is sufficient for inverted staple lines; however, everted stumps should be completely inverted with two inverting suture lines. It is possible for the linear stapler cartridges to close in malalignment. In this instance, the staples will not fit the grooves in the anvil and will not close properly. Immediate leakage and separation are the most prominent features of this complication. A new staple row placed adjacent to the malformed row will correct the problem.

Stenosis or stricture of stapled anastomoses has been described most commonly when ingesta does not pass freely through the site (i.e., where there is another option for flow of ingesta, such as a gastrojejunostomy or colostomy). Direct healing of the exposed tissue edges across the stoma has been observed under these circumstances. One potential reason is that the undisturbed stoma allows the exposed tissue margins to heal together. The exposed viable edges of tissue also form more granulation tissue than a suture-inverted anastomosis. If the site is not challenged by the flow of ingesta, it is understandable that partial stenosis could occur. I have performed gastrojejunostomies, jejunojejunostomies, and ileo(jejuno)cecostomies without stricture. Jejunojejunostomies are most frequently performed to bypass an abnormal segment of bowel. Al-

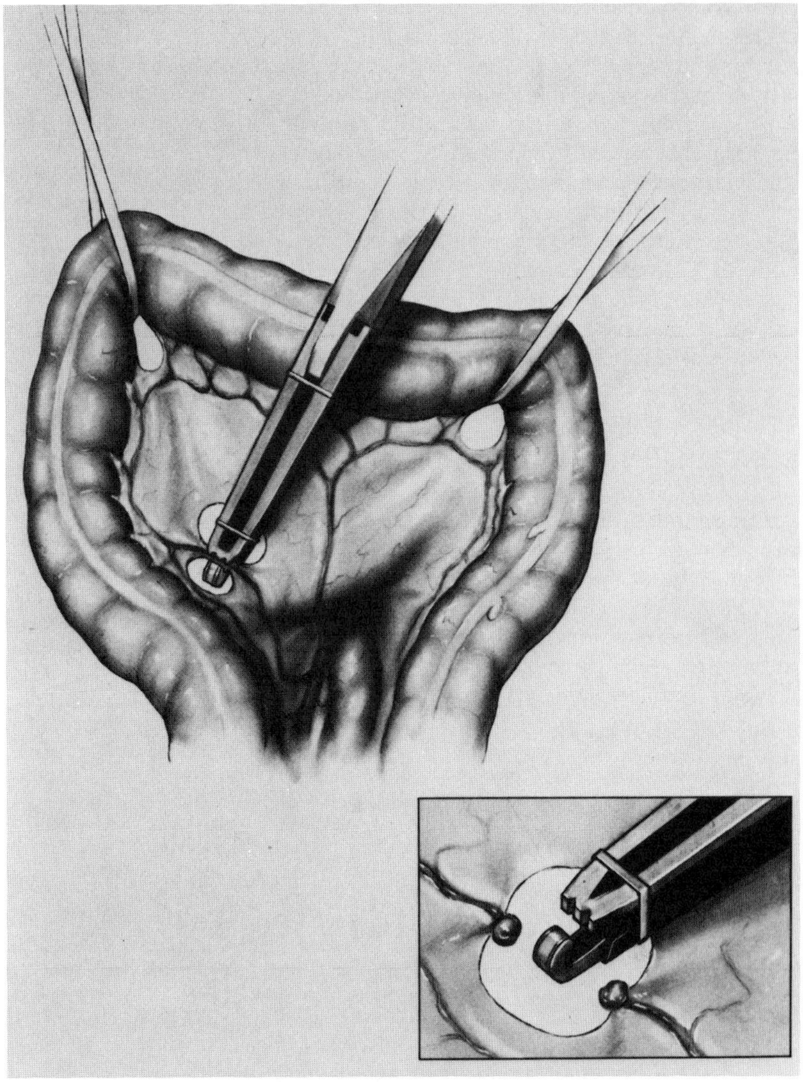

Figure 2–4. Pattern of occulsion and transection of vessel produced by LDS-2 instrument. (Reprinted by permission from *Atlas of Surgical Stapling.* Norwalk, CT, United States Surgical Corp., 1980.)

though a normal loop of bowel can pass between the anastomosis and the root of the mesentery to become strangulated, there is little that can be done for prevention. The surgeon should be aware of the potential complication and use the procedure only when absolutely necessary.

Separation of muscular and submucosal layers of anastomosed bowel has been observed several weeks to months after surgery. Only the mucosa and serosa, with a thin layer of interposed collagen, remained to preserve integrity of the bowel. This may be an incidental finding or can cause perforation. In these instances, the full thickness of the submucosal and muscular layers did not heal together in close apposition. Since there is minimal reaction at the stapled anastomosis, once the staples migrate from the site there is little fibrous tissue to bridge between the separated layers.

Staple lines should not be placed across hollow viscera for permanent closure unless the tissue is transected at the same time. It has been shown that these staples will displace and patency can become reestablished. This has been termed "in-continuity stapling." The lack of inflammation and interposition of normal mucosal surfaces seem to prevent permanent healing of the apposed tissues. Additionally, if the aboral segment is occluded and not completely patent on its aboral (opposite) end, a blind pouch syndrome or impaction can ensue. This is especially significant in conditions involving the distal ileum in the horse.

Upon completion of the staple placement, all staple lines should be closely inspected for hemorrhage. Since sizeable vessels can remain patent, hemorrhage can persist and become clinically significant. Inverted staple lines are the most vulnerable because inspection is difficult. Cautery or a small transmural ligature is indicated when such a bleeder is detected. The stomach and the colon have large vessels that cause this complication most often.

CONCLUSION

For those unfamiliar with stapling, the initial cost per case may seem high; however, considering time savings and patient benefit, the contribution to the overall cost of an acute abdomen case is small. The instruments can often be permanently loaned with a minimum purchase of cartridges. With experience, we continue to find new applications that benefit both horse and surgeon.

BIBLIOGRAPHY

Bertone AL, Stashak TS, Sullins KE, Ralston SL: Experimental large colon resection at the ceco-colic ligament in the horse. *Vet Surg* 1987;16:5–12.

Blackwell RB: Jejunocecostomy in the horse: A comparison of two techniques. *Proc 1st Equine Colic Res Symp Univ GA* 1982;288–289.

Craig DR, Pankowski RL, Car BD, Hackett RP, Erb HN: Ileocolostomy: A technique for surgical management of equine cecal impaction. *Vet Surg* 1987;16:451–455.

Mackey VS, Pascoe JR, Peterson PR: A potential technique error in stapled side-to-side anastomosis of the small intestine of the horse. *Vet Surg* 1987;16:189–192.

Orsini JA, Donawick WJ: Surgical treatment of gastroduodenal obstruction in foals. *Vet Surg* 1986;15:205–213.

Ramey DW: Healing in the small colon of the pony: Stapling vs suturing. *Proc 2nd Equine Colic Res Symp, Vet Learn Sys* 1985;2:166–167.

Steckel RR, Jann HW, Kaplan D, Jakowski RM, Schwartz A: Experimental evaluation of absorbable copolymer staples for hysterectomy. *Obstet Gynecol* 1986;68:404–410.

Sullins KE, Stashak TS, Mero KN: Evaluation of intestinal staples for end-to-end anastomosis of the small intestine in the horse. *Vet Surg* 1985;14:87–92.

Sullins KE, Stashak TS: Evaluation of two techniques for large intestinal resection and anastomosis in the horse. *J Inv Surg* 1989;2:115–124.

3 Cryosurgical Applications

Michael F. Clem
Richard M. DeBowes

MECHANISMS OF CRYONECROSIS

Cryonecrosis is the destruction of cells or tissues by freezing. Exposure of cells or tissues to temperatures below −20 °C results in cell death occurring in three general phases. These phases have been temporally characterized as the immediate, delayed, and late phases.

The *immediate phase* of cryonecrosis includes those events that occur during the freeze-thaw cycle. Cytolysis results from ice crystal formation, increased solute concentrations (hypertonicity), and membrane alterations. Protein denaturation and thermal shock obstruct biochemical function.

Rapid freezing has been shown to be more destructive than slow freezing as a result of autolysis from the formation of intracellular ice crystals. During slow thawing small ice crystals undergo a process of recrystallization. As this occurs, the crystals enlarge, increasing the severity of cellular damage. Thus, the goal of the procedure is to utilize rapid freezing and slow thawing to maximize cellular death. In other cryogen applications where cell destruction should be minimized (such as freeze branding), slower freezing and rapid thawing are indicated.

Vascular stasis during the hours following freezing results from endothelial damage in the frozen tissue and is responsible for the *delayed phase* of cryonecrosis. Thrombosis and ischemia produce cell death beyond direct cryogenic damage. In the *late phase* of cryonecrosis, there is evidence to support the development of an enhanced immune response to tissue that has been frozen. This enhanced response results from increased tumor-specific immunity by both humoral and cell-mediated mechanisms. This is most applicable to the cryosurgical treatment of neoplastic lesions. Clinical reports suggest that cryosurgical removal of isolated equine sarcoids has resulted in regression of distant lesions; this evidence must be viewed in light of the fact that sarcoids may undergo spontaneous remission.

CRYOGENS

The cryogen can be any substance capable of producing extremely low temperatures. The goal in cryosurgery is to rapidly reduce tissue temperatures to −20 °C. In practice, liquid nitrogen, nitrous oxide, or carbon dioxide are most commonly used. A variety of other cryogens include freon, liquid oxygen, liquid propane, and liquid air.

Liquid nitrogen has a variety of favorable characteristics, including a significantly lower boiling point than other agents. It is odorless, colorless, nontoxic, biologically inert, and relatively inexpensive. With a few precautions, it can be safely stored and utilized for application by a variety of methods. One disadvantage of liquid nitrogen is its short storage life; even when it is stored in a vacuum-insulated Dewar flask, one may anticipate an 8% daily loss.

Nitrous oxide acts as a cryoprobe coolant by the Joule-Thomson expansion principle; cooling is produced when a compressed gas is released through a small orifice into an area of reduced pressure. Probe temperatures of −89 °C can be attained, but these provide relatively slow cooling when compared to liquid nitrogen at −196 °C. The use of nitrous oxide is restricted to superficial lesions or small tumors. One advantage is its ease of storage as a compressed gas. Exposure to high levels of nitrous oxide may be hazardous, and appropriate ventilation must be maintained. Additionally, nitrous oxide is capable of supporting combustion.

Carbon dioxide may be used as a cryogen in either its solid or its gaseous forms. Solid carbon dioxide (dry ice) maintains a temperature of −79 °C, and carbon dioxide gas cooling by the Joule-Thomson effect reaches a temperature of approximately −75 °C. Either is cold enough to produce tissue necrosis, but not as deeply or as rapidly as liquid nitrogen.

Based upon the temperatures that can be achieved by the various cryogens, liquid nitrogen produces maximum tissue destruction. Carbon dioxide and nitrous oxide are useful in applications requiring only superficial freezing, more controlled freezing, or cryoadhesion. Any cryogen should be used only with appropriate equipment and knowledge of its method(s) of application.

METHODS OF APPLICATION

Direct application of the cryogen by spraying or pouring is the simplest method. Spray applicators are available to provide controlled tissue application and rapid freezing of large masses of tissue. A simple homemade spray applicator is shown in Figure 3–1. Liquid nitrogen may also be poured into core biopsy cavities or onto lesions contained within an insulating vessel on the surface of the area to be frozen. While direct application provides the most rapid and extensive areas of freeze, it also requires the most care to avoid excessive or inadvertent freezing of normal tissue.

Cryosurgical probes may be classified as solid or circulating. Solid probes are usually constructed of brass or copper and are precooled by immersion in liquid nitrogen before being applied to the tissue. They are not continuously cooled, as are circulating probes, and warming of the probe by tissue limits the area that may be frozen in a single application. Circulating probes are generally of the Joule-Thomson type, and are available for use with the commonly used cryogens. Circulating probes continue to be cooled during the freezing process, maintaining a more constant probe temperature.

Probes come in a variety of sizes. Lesions that are too large to be frozen by a single application may require debulking or multiple applications. Rigid probes allow compression of the target tissue, which can be used to reduce thickness and speed freezing by reducing perfusion. Highly vascular tissue is relatively cryoprotected by the "heat sink" effect of warm blood flow.

MONITORING

During cryogen application, several methods of monitoring the freeze should be employed. Palpation and visualization can provide an estimate of the amount and depth of tissue frozen. In many practice situations this method works well in relatively nonvital areas with experience. Electronic thermocouples are available for more precise monitoring and are recommended where excessive cryonecrosis would cause more severe consequences. These instruments accurately determine tissue temperatures at the base and periphery of the lesion. The probe should not come into excessive contact with normal tissue because freezing tempera-

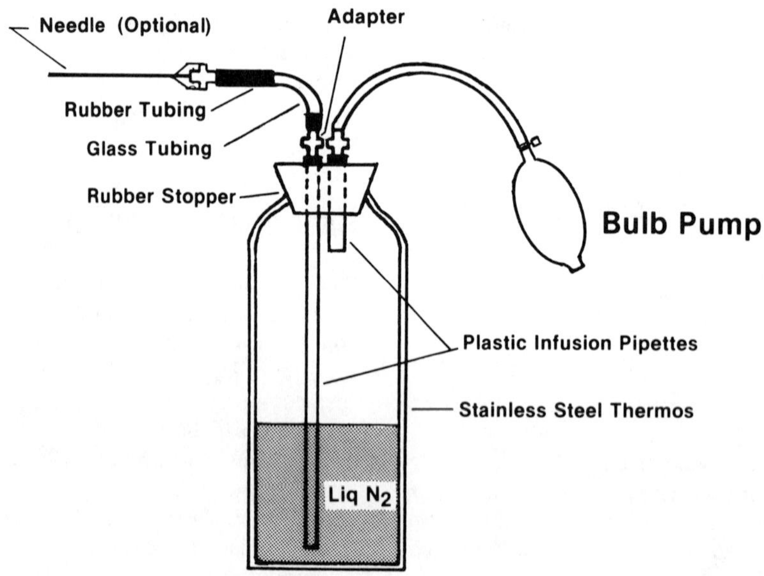

Figure 3–1. A diagram of a thermos bottle used to make a pressurized system to spray liquid nitrogen directly on the site to be frozen in cryosurgery.

tures may be transmitted along the metal probe. Inaccurate readings may be obtained when the probe is placed adjacent to large blood vessels, and monitoring should be supplemented by palpation and visualization.

BASIC TECHNIQUES

Adequate restraint will vary with patient demeanor, lesion location, positioning requirements, duration of procedure, and operator comfort and safety. Tranquilization of the horse is adequate for most procedures, but general anesthesia may be beneficial or required in specific instances. Although cryonecrosis may destroy sensory nerve endings, resulting in a relatively "painfree" postoperative lesion, pain is associated with the act of freezing. Local or regional anesthesia may be necessary.

Although cryogens are bactericidal, aseptic preparation should be performed to reduce bacterial populations in the area of postoperative necrosis. Hair should be clipped to expose the periphery of the lesion, but the clip should not have wide margins. Hair is an insulator and will protect surrounding tissue from inadvertent freezing. Other insulators, such as Styrofoam, may be placed adjacent to the lesion to protect surrounding normal tissue. Petroleum jelly applied over normal tissue will facilitate runoff and furnish insulation. Normal tissue that is inadvertently frozen should be rapidly thawed to minimize freeze injury.

A double freeze-thaw cycle produces the most consistent tissue destruction. When minimal scar formation is desired, such as with eyelid lesions, single freezes have been recommended. Tissue should be frozen to a temperature of −20 to −30 °C or until the palpable ice ball extends beyond the periphery of the lesion. This temperature should be maintained for 1 minute prior to thawing at room temperature. Dense tissues are more difficult to freeze and may require repeated applications to reach the optimal destructive temperature. Caution should be exercised to avoid overfreezing when the temperature begins to fall rapidly between applications.

POSTOPERATIVE APPEARANCE

The tissue changes occurring following cryosurgery are predictable and should be communicated to the client. During the first 3 to 4 hours after freezing, swelling and edema form and persist for 24 to 48 hours, followed by eschar formation. Hemorrhage may occur if biopsy or debulking procedures were performed. Bandaging may be beneficial during the initial stages of healing. The eschar falls away in 10 to 14 days, revealing granulation tissue that is left to heal by second intention. Cryosurgical wounds heal more by the formation of fibrous scar tissue and less by contraction than other wounds. A hairless, depigmented scar forms as a result of the cryosensitivity of melanocytes, hair follicles, and glandular structures.

SPECIFIC INDICATIONS

Equine Sarcoid

Cryosurgery is considered to be one of the most effective treatments to prevent recurrence of sarcoid tumors (see Chapter 24). Some reports indicate that an active late phase of cryonecrosis enhances immunologic response to remaining tumor cells. Multiple lesions may regress following cryosurgical removal of only a few. An overall success rate of 70 to 80% following cryosurgery indicates a significant benefit over the 50 to 60% recurrence rate reported with surgical excision. Success of sarcoid removal was found to be higher after three rather than two freeze-thaw cycles. It may be necessary to repeat cryosurgical removal to attain a higher rate of success. Large lesions should be surgically debulked before freezing. If hemorrhage is anticipated, debulking can be performed the day before cyrosurgery and the lesion bandaged if possible. In the periorbital region care should be taken to avoid excessive freezing and the complications of eyelid scarring. When treating lesions on the lower limb, freezing of the underlying periosteum and bone should be avoided. Since sarcoids are skin lesions, retention of subcutaneous mobility is a good indicator of sparing of the deeper tissue. With sarcoid recurrence following cryosurgery, the area may be refrozen or frozen in conjunction with other types of therapy.

Squamous Cell Carcinoma

Cryosurgery has been used extensively to treat squamous cell carcinomas in cattle, with 70 to 90% success. Similar results have been obtained in a limited number of equine cases. Since this tumor most frequently occurs in or around the orbit, care must be taken to avoid freezing adjacent structures, and probe applications are recommended. Penile and preputial lesions are also amenable to cryosurgical removal. These tumors may not be confined to the skin, making judgment of depth more difficult. Temperature probes can often be placed in "normal-feeling" deeper tissue. The prognosis for complete resolution is diminished for locally invasive tumors or in the presence of metastasis to regional lymph nodes.

Melanoma

Melanocytes are very cryosensitive; however, extensive reports of cryotherapy for melanomas in the horse are lacking. Cryosurgery in the management of oral melanomas in small animals has proven to be only palliative. However, oral melanomas in small animals are usually malignant in contrast to the cutaneous tumors seen in gray horses.

Mast Cell Tumors

Although mast cell tumors are relatively uncommon in the horse, they are mentioned here because experience in small animal patients suggests that they are not amenable to cryosurgical removal. Attempted cryosurgical removal has been associated with an unacceptable release of histamine in small animal patients.

Other tumors of small animals in which cryosurgical removal is reported to be contraindicated include osteosarcoma, urinary bladder neoplasia, nasal tumors, and prostatic neoplasia.

Ocular Conditions

Many of the neoplastic conditions that involve the eye or eyelids have been discussed above. With specific regard to tumors of the globe, cryosurgery may be utilized even in the face of the formation of an intraocular ice ball. The operator should be familiar with ancillary ocular therapeutics and other methods of treatment prior to utilizing cryosurgery on ocular lesions.

Other ophthalmic applications of cryosurgery include cryoextraction of the anterior capsule or lens, cyclocryosurgery in glaucoma (see Chapter 34), and selected techniques for corneal, iridic, and retinal disease. Equipment required for intraocular cryosurgery is specialized and usually utilizes nitrous oxide, carbon dioxide, or freon in a circulating probe design. Before attempting these techniques, the reader is referred to other texts for complete description of these methods and potential complications. Advanced training with these techniques is suggested.

Cryoneurectomy

Cryosurgery has the ability to destroy sensory nerves and has been used percutaneously or as an adjunct to surgical palmar digital neurectomy in the horse (Chapter 26). The freeze temperature will determine the extent of damage to the nerve and sheath. Temporary anesthesia occurs at −5 to −10 °C, whereas Schwann cell death at −20 to −25 °C causes nerve necrosis. With percutaneous cryoneurectomy, the anesthesia obtained is of short duration when compared to surgical techniques (47.5 versus 156 days for percutaneous versus surgically exposed cryoneurectomy). The incidence of development of neuromas-in-continuity after cryosurgical manipulation of the nerve did not appear to be significantly lower than that associated with other techniques. Percutaneous cryoneurectomy was also noted to result in the formation of a depigmented scar at the neurectomy site. The percutaneous method can only be recommended when transient anesthesia of the heel area is desired.

Upper Respiratory Tract

Ethmoid hematomas have been successfully treated by surgical excision/debulking followed by cryogen application to the base of the mass. The recurrence rate following cryogen application appears to be lower than with excision alone, and the procedure is associated with less hemorrhage than usually observed, with excision. In applying the cryoprobe or cryogen to the area of the involved frontal or maxillary sinus, thermocouples should be placed near the cribriform plate and orbit to monitor the depth of freezing and thereby prevent cryonecrosis of the rostral cerebral cortex or globe. When possible, cryoprobe application to the base of the excised and electrocoagulated lesion is recommended.

Horses with pharyngeal lymphoid hyperplasia or pharyngitis have been treated by cryogen application via either endoscopic visualization or laryngotomy. This technique is usually reserved for horses that have failed to respond to more conventional methods of therapy. A potential complication of laryngeal obstruction from swelling exists and should be monitored.

Orthopedic Applications

Only a limited number of orthopedic applications (those involving cryonecrosis of bone) have been reported in the veterinary literature. The potential to destroy the cellular elements of bone without disrupting the inorganic matrix is attractive in cases of osseous neoplasia. However, freeze injury to bone is reported to reduce osseous strength by 70% and could predispose to pathologic fracture. Frozen bone is slowly replaced by creeping substitution, resulting in a reduction in strength of the bone for several months. Additionally, achieving temperatures sufficient to produce cryonecrosis is difficult in all but the most superficial layers of the bone.

The use of point freezing by cryoprobe application ("freeze firing") has been described in the treatment of dorsal metacarpal disease (bucked shins, dorsal cortical fractures). The results of this treatment modality are questionable, and the potential for significantly weakening the third metacarpal bone should prompt a concurrent prolonged rest period, which in many cases might alleviate the problem. Often the depth and tissue temperature of the freeze are not known and therefore its effectiveness is based on clinical experiences. Other conditions that have been treated with reported success are osteitis of the small metacarpal/metatarsal bones (splints), plantar desmitis (curb), and cunean bursitis. There is a lack of controlled evidence reported to support use of these counterirritant applications.

Exuberant Granulation

Cryosurgical removal of exuberant granulation tissue has been shown to be effective, but comparison to simple excision would suggest that excision provides for more cosmetic end results and more rapid healing (0.56 mm/day by excision versus 0.44 mm/day with cryosurgery). The use of cryosurgery for management of wound healing is therefore not recommended.

BIBLIOGRAPHY

Fretz PB, Martin GS, Jacobs KA, McIlwraith CW: Treatment of exuberant granulation tissue in the horse. Evaluation of four methods. *Vet Surg* 1983;12(3):137–140.

Genetzky RM, Biwer RD, Myers RK: Equine sarcoids: Causes, diagnosis, and treatment. *Comp Cont Educ Pract Vet* 1983;5(8):416–420.

Harling DE, Pfeiffer RL, Cook CS: Excision and cryosurgical treatment of five cases of squamous cell carcinoma in the horse. *Eq Vet J* 1983;Suppl. 2:105–109.

Hoyt RF, Seim HB: Veterinary cryosurgery: Mechanisms of cell death, cryosurgical instrumentation, and cryogens. Part I. *Comp Cont Educ Prac Vet* 1981;3(5):426–436.

Munroe GA: Cryosurgery in the horse. *Eq Vet J* 1986;18(1):14–17.

Schneider RK, Mayhew IG, Clarke GL: Effects of cryotherapy on the palmar and plantar digital nerves in the horse. *Am J Vet Res* 1985;46(1):7–12.

Vestre WA: Cryosurgical techniques in veterinary ophthalmology. *Comp Cont Educ Prac Vet* 1984;6(6):481–487.

4
Advances in Arthroscopy

C. Wayne McIlwraith

In the past 10 years, arthroscopy in the horse has gone from being a diagnostic technique used by a few to the accepted way of performing the majority of joint surgery. During that time, prospective and retrospective data have substantiated the value of the technique in the treatment of various disorders of equine joints that would have previously been treated by arthrotomy.

As previously cited in earlier articles, arthroscopy provides considerably more information than recognized with our conventional diagnostic techniques of clinical and radiographic examinations and synovial fluid analysis. To permit full appreciation of this information, the anatomy of the individual joints has had to be relearned. Synovial plicae and other soft tissue features that were not known before have been recognized in various joints. Various degrees of damage to the medial palmar intercarpal ligament (which runs from the fossa of the third carpal bone to the caudal aspect of the radial carpal bone) have been recognized in horses with radiographic signs that were not commensurate with the degree of clinical compromise. Fragmentation of articular cartilage and bone at the distal aspect of the patella is another condition of significance that has been documented. Recognition of synovial disease (synovial proliferation, fibrosis, and adhesion) and different degrees of cartilage damage (fibrillation, eburnation) can be recognized arthroscopically (Fig. 4–1).

ARTHROSCOPIC SURGERY OF THE CARPAL JOINTS

Osteochondral chip fragments of the carpal joints were the first problems treated clinically using arthroscopic surgery and served somewhat as the showpiece for the technique. It is to be expected that most of the clinical data available document the value of this technique. The technique and results of arthroscopic surgery for the removal of osteochondral fragments from 1,000 carpal joints in 591 horses have been reported. Of the 591 horses, 580 were racehorses (including 349 Quarter Horses and 220 Thoroughbreds). The distal aspect of the radial carpal bone was the most commonly affected site, followed by the proximal aspect of the intermediate carpal bone and distolateral aspect of the radius. More than one carpal joint was simultaneously operated in 58.9% of the Quarter Horses and in 37.4% of the Thoroughbreds. Marked differences were noted in the amount of damage recorded at arthroscopy compared with what was observed on radiographic examination. The amount of discrepancy between radiographic and arthroscopic findings varied between sites. In most instances, the correlation in terms of fragment size and extent of damage was good with fractures off the distal intermediate carpal bone, proximal third carpal bone, and distolateral or distomedial radius. However, the extent of damage on the opposing articular cartilage surface has varied, particularly with the third carpal bone lesions. Major discrepancies between radiographic and arthroscopic findings were found on the distal radial carpal bone, proximal intermediate carpal bone, and, to a lesser extent, proximal radial carpal bone. In the distal radial carpal bone fractures, where radiography revealed a single chip, arthroscopy com-

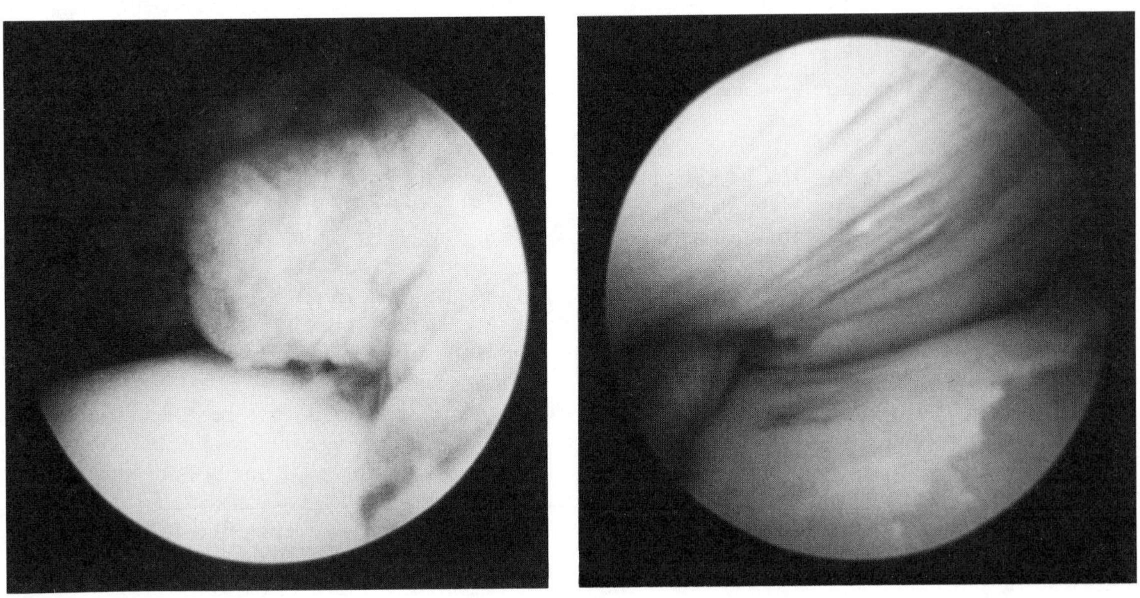

A B

Figure 4–1. A. Proliferative synovitis in the tarsocrural joint characterized by replacement of normal filamentous villus structure with thickened and clubbed synovial villi. **B.** Visualization of both full-thickness cartilage erosion on the lower surface and partial-thickness linear erosions on the opposing upper surface of this carpal joint.

monly revealed multiple fragments along the distal dorsal aspect of the radial carpal bone, with soft degenerative bone. There was also commonly a distinct fragment off the dorsolateral corner of the radial carpal bone that was not evident radiographically. In addition to this bone loss, there was often severe loss of articular cartilage over the surface of the radial carpal bone.

Based on this prospective study, arthroscopic surgery was considered to be an effective technique for removing the osteochondral fragments as well as for treating other lesions. The overall functional ability and the cosmetic appearance of the limbs were excellent. There was no postoperative intraarticular infection. Postsurgical follow-up information was obtained for 445 racehorses. After surgery, 303 (68.1%) raced at a level equal to or better than their preinjury level, 49 (11.0%) had decreased performance or still had problems referable to the carpus, 23 (5.2%) were retired without returning to training, 28 (6.3%) sustained another chip fracture, 32 (7.2%) developed other problems, and 10 (2.2%) sustained collapsing slab fractures while racing. For the purpose of evaluating the effect of varying articular cartilage damage on prognosis, four categories of articular cartilage damage were made. In grade I damage, there was minimal articular cartilage fibrillation or fragmentation at the edge of the defect left by the fragment and extending no more than 5 mm from the fracture line. In grade II damage, the articular cartilage damage extended for more than 5 mm from the osteochondral defect and included up to 30% of the articular surface of that bone. In grade III damage, there was a loss of 50% of the articular cartilage from the visible articular surface of the affected carpal bone. In grade IV damage, there was severe loss of bone associated with the fracture. Grade IV usually involved distal radial carpal bone fragments. When these four categories of articular damage were correlated to prognosis, performance in the two most severely affected groups was significantly inferior. One hundred thirty-three of 187 horses with grade I damage (71.1%), 108 of 144 with grade II damage (75.0%), 41 of 77 with grade III damage (53.2%), and 20 of 37 horses with grade IV damage (54.1%) returned to racing at a level equal to or better than their preinjury level. The success rate in horses with grade I and grade II lesions was significantly greater than in horses with grade III and grade IV lesions ($P < .01$).

The results of surgery were also assessed in relation to the location of the lesion. Only horses with a single site involved (or the same site bilaterally) were included. This study involved 187 Quarter Horses and 133 Thoroughbreds. The worst postoperative results were associated with third carpal bone fragments in Quarter Horses and distal radial carpal and third carpal bone fragments in Thoroughbreds. This was the only site where the results were significantly inferior. There was no significant difference between the other sites when they were compared. When results were assessed relative to the joint involved, with middle carpal joint involvement, 63.3% of the Quarter Horses and 66.2% of the Thoroughbreds returned successfully to racing. With antebrachiocarpal joint involvement 82.7% of the Quarter Horses and 65.5% of the Thoroughbreds successfully returned to racing.

The amount of débridement to be performed on articular cartilage defects and the relevance of this to prognosis continues to be somewhat controversial. Based on follow-up arthroscopy on joints that have been previously operated and the defects debrided, the author's observation has been that healing of defects as implied in earlier work does not occur. Although granulation tissue and fibrous tissue probably form within these defects postsurgically, such tissues cannot sustain the forces that develop when the horse goes back into training and racing, and the surgeon should consider these defects as permanent. It is therefore considered that a conservative approach to débridement is necessary, particularly in consideration of partial-thickness lesions. On the other hand, the results in the quoted prospective study would imply that up to a certain amount of articular cartilage loss is well tolerated by the horse.

Compared with the benefits from arthrotomy, it was considered that the benefits from arthroscopic surgery in the treatment of osteochondral chip fragments in the carpus included: (*a*) increased diagnostic accuracy (and therefore more definitive treatment of the condition); (*b*) less tissue damage and improved cosmetic appearance of the joint; (*c*) more complete irrigation and elimination of debris from the joint; (*d*) decreased postoperative pain; (*e*) the ability to operate multiple joints concurrently; and (*f*) improved performance after surgery. These advantages have been recorded for other conditions as well. Although the author considers earlier return to training and racing as another advantage, the prospective data generated thus far have not been sufficient to make a statistically accurate statement.

Arthroscopic surgery has been documented with a series of clinical cases as an accepted technique for fixation of routine slab fractures of the third carpal bone. With the exception of severely collapsing slab fractures within the carpus, the author now operates all carpal slab fractures arthroscopically. The defect in the fracture line is débrided and flushed and needles are placed for radiographic identification of the ideal placement and angle of the screw. How much advantage this arthroscopic technique provides is still uncertain. It is recognized that a longer time for healing must be allowed.

ARTHROSCOPIC SURGERY IN THE FETLOCK JOINTS

The most common condition operated arthroscopically within the fetlock joint is that of osteochondral fragments off the dorsoproximal aspect of the proximal phalanx. Most of these problems occur in the forelimbs. Results from this surgery have been documented previously, and since then considerably more cases have been added. In the earlier reported series, 74 fetlock joints in 63 horses were operated, for a total of 87 fractures during a 2-year period. The dorsomedial proximal aspect of the proximal phalanx of the forelimb was the most commonly involved site (59 fragments), followed by the dorsolateral proximal aspect (26 fragments), and two fractures occurred in the fetlock joint of the right hind limb. At surgery, 82 fragments were removed and 15 fragments that had healed and were embedded in the joint capsule were not removed. Of the fragments removed, 15 were fixed firmly to the proximal phalanx, 63 were easily removable by arthroscopic instrumentation (but had soft tissue attachments to the proximal phalanx), and 4 were floating free within the joint. Arthroscopic surgery allowed excellent visualization and appreciation of the attachment of fragments in this stage of healing. Horses returned to full race training at an average of 11.5 weeks after surgery (range 6 to 24 weeks).

Thirty-eight of the 46 horses (82.6%) having an adequate postoperative follow-up returned to athletic performance at least equal to that before fetlock injury. Using these relatively strict criteria for success, it was considered that these figures documented the value of arthroscopic surgery in the treatment of this condition. Rest has been previously recommended as the initial therapy because in some horses the fracture would heal and not result in permanent lameness. Removal via a dorsal arthrotomy had also been reported to result in periarticular bone growth, decreased range of joint motion, osteoarthritis, and persistent lameness when the horse was trained. It was found in the above-mentioned study that loose fragments often were found when operating on horses in which the fracture had been documented by radiography several months before surgery. This was considered to indicate that bony healing of osteochondral fractures of the proximal phalanx cannot always be anticipated. In addition, where firm bony healing of the fragment developed, the fragments were sometimes found in a displaced position in the fracture bed. For these reasons, it was considered that satisfactory healing with conservative therapy is not routinely predictable. Many horses in this series had been rested for 3 or more months after the fracture occurred but later became lame in training because of fetlock pain. Subsequent arthroscopic surgery with fragment removal relieved the lameness, indicating that not all horses are treated successfully with rest alone and that the length of time that the fracture has been present should not necessarily dictate the decision to operate. In the series of arthroscopic cases, enlargement of the fetlock joint or decreased range of joint motion was not observed after arthroscopic surgery. With fetlock arthrotomy, decreased range of motion secondary to fibrosis at the surgical site, joint capsule thickening, and adhesions of the joint capsule close to the articular edge of the proximal phalanx had been reported.

Arthroscopic surgery has also been used for treating horses with chronic proliferative (villonodular) synovitis. These cases include horses that are diagnosed as having the problem presurgically in addition to cases in which an enlarged synovial pad is found at arthroscopic examination when operating for a proximal phalanx chip fragment.

Palmar/plantar proximal phalanx fragments are now being operated arthroscopically with success. This involves both arthroscopic and instrument portals in the palmar or plantar recess of the fetlock joint. The most recent development with arthroscopic surgery in the fetlock joint is the removal of both apical and abaxial fragments from the sesamoid bone. These also involve arthroscopic and instrument portals through the palmar or plantar recess of the fetlock joint and the use of a specially curved osteotome for separation of the fragment from the suspensory ligament. A similar approach can also be used for the removal of basal sesamoid fragments.

ARTHROSCOPIC SURGERY OF THE TARSOCRURAL JOINT

Arthroscopic surgery has achieved considerable use in the tarsocrural joint, primarily because of osteochondritis dissecans. Indeed, in Europe, this joint is arguably the most commonly operated because of the significance of this problem and the lower incidence of traumatic osteochondral fragments in the carpus and the fetlock. Arthroscopic surgery has proved very valuable in the treatment of osteochondritis dissecans of the tarsocrural joint. Based on a series of over 250 cases, the usefulness of surgery in the treatment of osteochondritis dissecans is gratifying. The most common location of lesions is the distal intermediate ridge of the tibia. The lesion also occurs frequently on the lateral trochlear ridge of the talus, less commonly on the medial malleolus of the tibia, and least commonly on the medial trochlear ridge of the talus. Fragments of the lateral malleolus of the tibia also occur but are considered to be traumatic. It has also been recognized that arthroscopic surgery is not the appropriate method of treatment for lateral malleolar fractures because only a small part of the fragment is actually intraarticular.

Arthroscopy has also been used in the treatment of traumatic fragmentation and degenerative joint disease within the tarsocrural joint. These cases are relatively uncommon. Osteomyelitis lesions in foals on the proximal-most aspect of the trochlear ridges of the talus are operated using an approach through the plantar pouches of the tarsocrural joint. Flexion of the joint allows exposure of these lesions.

ARTHROSCOPIC SURGERY OF THE FEMOROPATELLAR AND FEMOROTIBIAL JOINTS

Osteochondritis dissecans is the most common indication for arthroscopic surgery in the femoropatellar joint. The results of this surgery in 40 joints in 24 horses were documented in the literature in early 1985. In this series, lesions were bilateral in 16 horses and unilateral in eight horses. Both diagnostic examination and the surgical treatment were performed through a single arthroscopic portal, but five different instrument portal locations and six instrument approaches were used in the treatment of these cases. Lesions were localized to the lateral trochlear ridge of the femur in 31 affected joints, medial trochlear ridge in 2 joints, lateral and medial trochlear ridge together in 2 joints, lateral trochlear ridge plus patella in 4 joints, and patella alone in 1 joint. The lesions consisted of subchondral defects containing chondral or osteochondral flaps or fragments; all were seen as dimpling, cracking, fibrillation, or erosion of articular cartilage, or intact cartilage over a subchondral defect. Loose bodies were found in three joints, and there was a poor correlation between radiographic and arthroscopic findings. The arthroscopic surgical manipulations included removal of flaps, fragments, and undermined articular cartilage and débridement of the subchondral defect. Immediate clinical improvement after surgery was evident in the 22 horses that survived. Long-term follow-up in 10 racehorses revealed that 2 have raced successfully, 2 were "ready to race," 3 were training sound, and 2 were sound at pasture (still in convalescence); one horse had been reoperated for another fragment. Of six horses used for show or pleasure, three were being shown sound, one was sound for pleasure, and two were training sound. The remaining six horses were convalescing. Since that time, additional follow-up has been documented. In additional cases, the same methods of treatment have been used and the same lesions found. Considerably more cases have been documented in follow-up. It has been shown that the prognosis for athletic soundness in racehorses is good.

It has been very impressive to the author that when horses are operated at a relatively young age, those with pathologic change extending the entire length of the lateral trochlear ridge of the femur (from the patella to the distal extremity of the trochlear ridge) have been able to race successfully. Arthroscopic surgery has proved to be particularly valuable in the femoropatellar joint. Rather than just providing advantages over the arthrotomy technique, it has allowed a predictable method of treatment, whereas arthrotomy was associated with considerable surgical morbidity.

Other conditions are now treated in the femoropatellar joint using arthroscopic surgery. Fragmentation of the distal patella (chondromalacia) has been seen and operated by the author. Most instances of this condition were seen following patellar desmotomy, but the association between upward fixation of the patella, medial patellar desmotomy, and the development of this condition is still uncertain. The clinical signs are consistent with gonitis, and radiographically fragmentation or lucency at the apex of the patella is seen. Arthroscopically there is fragmentation of articular cartilage and bone, and reasonably good results have been associated with débridement of these lesions.

Arthroscopic surgery has also been used in the treatment of osteochondral fractures of the patella within the femoropatellar joint. Skyline views of the patella are sometimes necessary to demonstrate these fragments. They can be removed arthroscopically.

Diagnostic arthroscopy of the femorotibial joints is now being performed, but the most caudal aspects of the joint are inaccessible to arthroscopic visualization at this stage. Surgical arthroscopy has also been performed within this joint in the treatment of subchondral cystic lesions. A cranial or lateral arthroscopic portal is used. Because the defect associated with the subchondral cyst is usually on the medial side of the medial condyle of the femur, the instrument portal comes from this direction. Additional clinical cases are required to document the overall success rate of arthroscopic surgery compared to that of arthrotomy in the treatment of this condition.

ARTHROSCOPIC SURGERY OF THE SHOULDER

Techniques for treating osteochondritis dissecans in the shoulder joint have been developed over the past 5 years. The surgery can be difficult, particularly in a large horse. Two different techniques have been reported in the literature and the results using one technique were reported in a prospective study. In this study, osteochondritis dissecans and subchondral cystic lesions of the humeral head and glenoid in 13 shoulders of 11 horses were operated. Nine horses were sound, five of them athletically sound, after 5 to 20 months.

At this stage additional clinical cases with follow-up are required to document the prognostic limitations according to size and location of lesions. However, it is believed that arthroscopic surgery does provide a means of achieving athletic soundness in many horses with this disease, whereas athletic soundness was never documented with conservative therapy previously. A technique of arthrotomy and its successful use has also been documented. It is not known whether arthroscopic surgery offers advantages in terms of results, but it is certainly recognized that the technique offers advantages in complete visualization of the joint. Presumably, this means more effective treatment of the condition.

THE USE OF ARTHROSCOPIC SURGERY IN OTHER JOINTS

Arthroscopic surgery has been used to remove osteochondral fragments from the distal proximal interphalangeal and distal interphalangeal joints. It is anticipated that other techniques will be developed. The author believes it can be stated at this stage that the overall number of joints operated with arthroscopic surgery will not increase that much. On the other hand, the continued improvement in technology will cause techniques to be changed and, it is hoped, more effective surgery to be performed. Recent developments in motorized equipment will probably cause further research in the use of synovectomy. At the present time, the use of synovectomy using motorized equipment is minimal, and most cartilage débridement is performed with hand tools.

BIBLIOGRAPHY

Bertone AL, McIlwraith CW, Powers BE, Trotter GW, Stashak TS: Arthroscopic surgery for the treatment of osteochondrosis in the equine shoulder joint. *Vet Surg* 1987;16:303–311.

Lewis RB: Treatment of subchondral bone cysts of the medial condyle of the femur using arthroscopic surgery, in *Proceedings of the American Association of Equine Practitioners.* 1987. pp 887–893.

McIlwraith CW: *Diagnostic and surgical arthroscopy in the horse.* Lenexa, KS, Veterinary Medicine Publishing Company, 1984.

McIlwraith CW, Martin GS: Arthroscopic surgery for the treatment of osteochondritis dissecans in the equine femoropatellar joint. *Vet Surg* 1985;14:105–116.

McIlwraith CW, Yovich JV, Martin GS: Arthroscopic surgery for the treatment of osteochondral chip fractures in the equine carpus. *J Am Vet Med Assoc* 1987;191:531–540.

Nickels FA, Sande R: Radiographic and arthroscopic findings in the equine stifle. *J Am Vet Med Assoc.* 1982;181:918–924.

Richardson DW: Technique for arthroscopic repair of third carpal bone slab fractures in horses. *J Am Vet Med Assoc* 1986;188:288–291.

Selway SJ: Arthroscopic surgery: The carpal and fetlock joints, in *Proceedings of the American Association of Equine Practitioners*, 1983. pp 95–102.

Yovich JV, McIlwraith CW: Arthroscopic surgery for osteochondral fractures of the proximal phalanx of the metacarpophalangeal and metatarsophalangeal (fetlock) joints in horses. *J Am Vet Med Assoc* 1986;188:273–279.

5 Principles of Antibiotic Prophylaxis

Murray P. Brown

Antibiotic prophylaxis in surgery may be defined as the administration of antibiotics to surgical patients that do not have evidence of established infection. The purpose of antibiotic prophylaxis is to reduce postsurgical infection rates below those observed if prophylaxis is *not* used. This practice has been routine since antibiotics became readily available and is a topic of much controversy and confusion. It is commonly believed that antibiotics usually will do some good and probably will not do any harm ("can't hurt, might help"), and therefore they are often used when not needed at all.

SHOULD ANTIBIOTIC PROPHYLAXIS BE USED?

There are a number of questions that the surgeon should ask with regard to antibiotic prophylaxis. What is the incidence of infection without prophylaxis? How is infection defined? How reliable is the microbiology laboratory? What are the consequences of infection? Are there unexploited alternatives to antibiotic prophylaxis that might more effectively reduce infection? Which antibiotic should be used and how? What is the likelihood of preventing infection? What are the undesirable effects? Is the blood supply to the surgical site adequate? What is the immune status of the host? The answers to these questions may not be immediately obvious, but it is hoped that their careful consideration will reduce unnecessary or ineffective antibiotic prophylaxis. Some surgeons may have very low infection rates without prophylaxis for a specific procedure for which others may find prophylaxis to have a demonstrable effect. Still other surgeons may have unacceptably high infection rates even with the appropriate use of prophylaxis. Those clinicians who have regular open rounds discussion of cases with peers are encouraged to take advantage of this forum to discuss antibiotic usage on individual cases.

Factors Related to Surgical Infection

A reliable microbiology laboratory is an important aid in both the prevention and the treatment of surgical infections. Microbiology reports should be interpreted carefully and unexpected results should be discussed with laboratory personnel rather than accepted without question. Open communication between the clinician and the microbiologist will maximize the information obtained when a sample is submitted for culture.

A wound can be considered infected if purulent material drains from it, even if bacterial culture is negative or not taken. Skin suture abscesses are not equivalent to an infected wound. Positive culture is not necessarily an indication of infection and infected wounds do not necessarily yield positive cultures. On the other hand, deep-seated wound infections may not drain purulent material, and it may be difficult to obtain material from them for culture. It may be practical to consider a wound infected if the attending veterinarian believes it to be.

Several basic assumptions must be made when antibiotic prophylaxis is used. It is assumed that one or more pathogenic bacteria will contaminate the surgical wound and that growth of these bacteria will be inhibited by the antibiotic selected. It is also assumed that effective concentrations of the drug will be reached at the surgical wound at the dose given. It is assumed that the therapeutic effect will not be markedly reduced by the presence of local wound factors such as fibrin, cellular debris, and decreased pH; these factors do tend to reduce antimicrobial activity but are usually associated with inflammation and infection. In studies done by Burke in guinea pigs, wounds made and inoculated with *Staphylococcus aureus* 1 to 2 hours before intravenous administration of antibiotics resulted in lesions similar to the *untreated* inoculated control incisions. When antibiotics were given before the incisions were made, the resulting lesions were indistinguishable from the *uninoculated* control incisions. Therefore, to be effective, the antibiotic must be given before bacterial contamination of tissues.

There are two general sources of bacterial contamination of a surgical wound: *exogenous*, from the surgical team or the environment through a break in asepsis, and *endogenous*, from the patient's skin and respiratory, gastrointestinal, or urogenital tract. As an aid in predicting the likelihood and degree of contamination during surgery, surgical procedures have been classified as clean, clean-contaminated, contaminated, or dirty. *Clean* wounds are made under ideal operating conditions with no break in aseptic technique and are closed primarily. No inflammation is evident and viscera are not entered. Antibiotics are not indicated unless a foreign body has been implanted. *Clean-contaminated* procedures include clean wounds with a minor break in asepsis or controlled entry into viscera. If prophylactic antibiotics are used, they should be present at the time of contamination. *Contaminated* procedures have a major break in asepsis, such as fresh traumatic wounds and gross contamination from viscera. Antibiotic prophylaxis is appropriate. *Dirty* wounds may contain devitalized tissue and foreign bodies; they are clinically infected and therefore antibiotic usage is therapeutic, not prophylactic. The presence of antibiotics may also protect those previously uninfected tissues that are invaded during dirty surgical procedures.

Potential Advantages of Antibiotic Prophylaxis

There are several potential advantages of antibiotic prophylaxis. These include prevention of infection and therefore, decreased length of hospitalization and cost. If these were achieved, it is possible that total antibiotic usage could be decreased and the development of bacterial resistance would be reduced. Unfortunately, these objectives often are not achieved and it is obvious that antibiotics have failed to eliminate bacterial infection as a cause of sickness and death in horses.

Potential Disadvantages of Antibiotic Prophylaxis

On the other hand, there are several potential disadvantages of antibiotic prophylaxis. Antibiotic "coverage" may cause relaxation of strict adherence to aseptic technique. Reduction of infection rates may not occur and resistant strains of bacteria may develop. Resistance to antibiotics tends to rise as antibiotic consumption rises and vice versa. Toxic reactions, both allergic and metabolic, have been recognized in horses following antibiotic administration. According to Yourtee and Root, complex interactions occur between antibiotics and the immune system. Many antibiotics cause a decrease in neutrophil function, including chemotaxis, phagocytosis, chemiluminescence, and microbicidal activity. Superinfections may occur, and colitis resulting from oxytetracycline administration to horses has been reported. Although it is unlikely that oral penicillin would be used for surgical prophylaxis, enteric salmonellosis has been associated with its use in horses. This is probably a result of alterations in gut flora caused by the high dosages required to achieve therapeutic concentrations. Antibiotics may mask localized infections, which should be drained and débrided. Myositis, phlebitis, or fever and depression may result from parenteral administration of antibiotics. Occasionally, horses (particularly foals) treated with procaine penicillin G will develop fever of unknown origin and often the body temperature will return to normal within 24 hours of discontinuation of the drug.

Unnecessary antibiotic usage means unnecessary expense. If the infection rate for a specific surgical procedure is 10% without antibiotic prophylaxis, then routine use of prophylaxis would unnecessarily expose 9 out of 10 horses to antibiotics. In such an example, total hospital usage of the antibiotic would be markedly increased, thereby increasing the likelihood that resistant organisms will develop. Obviously, the consequences of surgical infection will be considered in the decision to use antibiotic prophylaxis. If wound infection will result in complete surgical failure or even death, then the surgeon will be under greater pressure to use antibiotics.

Antibiotic prophylaxis is most likely to succeed if a single effective drug is used to prevent implantation of a specific organism, or eradicate it after it has become established but not clinically evident. Prophylaxis is doomed to failure if the intent is to prevent colonization or infection by any and all organisms from any source. Choice of the wrong antibiotic, inadequate dosage, or incorrect timing will also cause failure. There is much misunderstanding about the term "broad-spectrum antibiotics," and some consider their use to be a convenient way to ensure sterility of the surgical wound. It should never be assumed that all endogenous and exogenous flora will be sensitive to a broad-spectrum drug. In some circumstances, the drug may eliminate primarily nonpathogens, leaving resistant organisms to colonize the wound. In reports from some human hospitals, infection rates have fallen remarkably, with no apparent detrimental effect on the final outcome of infections, when all prophylactic and therapeutic antibiotic use was discontinued.

Other Considerations

Several factors are frequently overlooked in antibiotic prophylaxis. Some knowledge of the potential pathogens in a given surgical procedure is essential. The choice of antibiotic will obviously depend on this knowledge. For example, anaerobes as well as gram-negative and gram-positive aerobes should be anticipated during contaminated surgery of the equine intestinal tract. Pathogens most commonly involved in equine orthopedic infections include Enterobacteriaceae, *Streptococcus* spp, *Staphylococcus* spp, and *Pseudomonas* spp. Fecal and soil contamination associated with the environment of horses may account for the predominance of gram-negative organisms in wound infections. A combination of drugs should be used, if necessary, to provide coverage against anticipated pathogens. The toxicity of a drug should also be considered. For example, aminoglycosides may potentiate the neuromuscular blockade and cardiovascular depression caused by general anesthesia and, therefore, caution is advised if they are used in anesthetized horses. Intravenous administration of sodium ampicillin to anesthetized horses has been associated with hypotension. The topical, rather than systemic, use of some antibiotics during surgery may be effective and may reduce the toxicity of these drugs, but this approach remains controversial. Postoperatively, aminoglycosides may inhibit gut motility and may also contribute to nephrotoxicity in animals that are hypovolemic and are concurrently receiving other potentially nephrotoxic agents such as nonsteroidal anti-inflammatory drugs. In these instances the benefits of antibiotic use are weighed against the possible disadvantages.

Timing and Duration

Antibiotics should be given immediately preoperatively to ensure effective tissue concentrations at the time of contamination. They should not be started the day before surgery because nonpathogens may be eliminated, thus encouraging colonization of the wound by pathogens. Most parenterally administered antibiotics will achieve maximum body fluid and tissue concentrations within the first 1 to 2 hours, and therefore timing of administration should be carefully planned. Commencement of antibiotic prophylaxis *after* surgery is of *no value*. In humans, there is no conclusive evidence to support continuation of antibiotic prophylaxis beyond 3 to 6 hours after the surgical procedure. In a study of six prophylactic regimens, antibiotic courses of less than 2 days were found to be as effective as those lasting 5 days. Since primary contamination occurs at surgery, administration of prophylactic antibiotics longer than 2 to 3 days postoperatively constitutes therapy for "possible" infection and therefore cannot be justified. In our hospital, pharmacy charges frequently constitute a large portion of the final bill, and thus from an economic standpoint as well, unnecessarily prolonged use of expensive antibiotics such as aminoglycosides and cephalosporins should be criticized. Prolonged prophylaxis may in fact exceed the cost of treating an actual infection. Perhaps the term "short-course perioperative antibiotic prophylaxis" should be used to serve as a reminder of principles and limitations. Unfortunately, the duration of antibiotic administration is often ultimately determined by the length of hospitalization, rather than by a conscious decision by the clinician to terminate therapy. Prophylactic antibiotics should be discontinued without exception no later than 3 days after surgery. If there is fever or any other sign of sepsis at this time, the antibiotic should be discontinued and the patient reevaluated because the initial antibiotic may be ineffective. If possible, a sample for Gram's stain and culture should be obtained. Resist the temptation to blindly continue to use the most "powerful" (often the most expensive) antibiotic available. Clinicians often use these drugs out of fear of failure to give the horse what is thought to be the very best drug. It must be remembered that continuation of ineffective antibiotic therapy is worse than no antibiotic therapy at all.

Route of Administration

The intravenous or intramuscular route of administration should be used because of the unpredictability of absorption of orally administered drugs in horses. Cephalosporins are eliminated extremely rapidly when given intravenously to horses and therefore the intramuscular route should be considered. Although standard dosages of drugs are usually used, some advocate higher (e.g., double doses) if single injections of nontoxic antibiotics are used.

CONCLUSIONS

Antibiotic prophylaxis is a two-edged sword in which the disadvantages must be weighed against the advantages. It should not substitute for good surgical technique, including surgical site preparation, minimum surgical time and trauma, hemostasis, and obliteration of dead space. Until the incidence of infection in equine surgery is established, no specific recommendation for antibiotic prophylaxis can be given.

BIBLIOGRAPHY

Brown MP: Antibiotics and the surgical colic, in *Proceedings of the 1st Equine Colic Research Symposium*. University of Georgia, 1982, p 281.

Burke JF: The effective period of preventive antibiotic action in experimental incisions and dermal lesions. *Surgery* 1961;50:161.

Casewell MW: Prophylactic antimicrobial drug therapy, in Gruneburg RN (ed), *Current Status of Modern Therapy*. Baltimore, University Park Press, 1980, vol 4, pp. 33–62.

Di Piro JT, Record KE, Schanzenbach KS, Bivins BA: Antimicrobial prophylaxis in surgery: Part I. *Am J Hosp Pharm* 1981;38:320–334.

Simmons BP: Guideline for prevention of surgical wound infections, in *Antibiotic Prophlaxis in Surgery: A comprehensive Review*. Philadelphia: JB Lippincott Co, 1984, pp 157–176.

Van Scoy RE, Wilkowske CJ: Prophylactic use of antimicrobial agents. *Mayo Clin Proc* 1983;58:241–245.

Snyder JR, Pascoe JR, Hirsh DC: Antimicrobial susceptibility of microorganisms isolated from equine orthopedic patients. *Vet Surg* 1987;16:197–201.

Yourtee EL, Root RK: Effect of antibiotics on phagocyte-microbe interactions, in Root RK, Sande MA (eds), *New Dimensions in Antimicrobial Therapy*. New York: Churchill Livingstone, 1984, pp 243–275.

6
Immunotherapy

W. L. Ragland

Equine sarcoids have been reported to occur in horses, donkeys, and mules throughout the world. Sarcoids are by far the most common tumor of the horse. Sarcoids occur most frequently on the head, legs, and penis, and often are multiple. On the head and legs, they usually develop in areas subjected to trauma, such as lacerations on the legs and head abrasions from poorly fitted tack. I have been able to identify six cases in which tumor formation was preceded by trauma to the skin followed by uneventful recovery 3 to 8 months prior to development of tumor. Uneventful, prior injury also has been recognized in many cases of dermatofibrosarcoma protuberans in humans. This tumor is biologically and histopathologically similar to equine sarcoid except that it sometimes metastasizes. Metastasis of sarcoids has never been reported even though the tumors are locally aggressive and frequently are multiple. Although the two tumors resemble each other, a common cause has not been established. Presently there is no acknowledged etiologic agent for equine sarcoid.

Sarcoids may be verrucous (warty) or fibroblastic in appearance. Acanthosis and epithelial hyperplasia are usually but not always present, and are prominent in the verrucous sarcoids. Some sarcoids are a mixture of verrucous and fibroblastic types from their onset. As verrucous sarcoids expand, they become vulnerable to trauma and excoriation of the epithelial component. The fibroblastic component becomes ulcerated and infected, transforming the tumor to one of the fibroblastic type. Fibroblastic sarcoids may become quite large and pedunculated, but even verrucous sarcoids protected from trauma by their location may become pedunculated. Although clinical diagnosis from gross appearance and location of the tumor usually is accurate, definitive diagnosis can be made only by histopathologic examination of a biopsy taken from the margin of tumor that includes adjacent skin. It is especially important that biopsies be taken at the margin of fibroblastic sarcoids because this may be the only place where the epithelial component of the tumor can be identified.

Although early attempts at immunotherapy with autogenous vaccines were disappointing, mycobacterial immunotherapy, which enhances a number of immune functions by stimulating a cascade of cytokines involved in immune responses, has proven to be very efficacious. At first, Bacille Calmette-Guérin (BCG) vaccine (Glaxo Laboratories, Ltd.) was used for immunotherapy of equine sarcoid by intralesional inoculation, but it was later learned to be capable of causing severe anaphylactic reactions, some of which were fatal. Horses have since been premedicated with nonsteroidal anti-inflammatory drugs by most practitioners to avoid the anaphylactic reactions. Deproteinized mycobacterial cell walls do not produce positive skin sensitivity tests to tuberculosis, as does the BCG vaccine. The mycobacterial cell walls are much less likely to cause anaphylactic reactions, none of which have been fatal. It should not be surprising that they have replaced BCG vaccine in immunotherapy since they were first used to treat equine sarcoids at Colorado State University. Deproteinized mycobacterial cell walls are available in two forms. One is provided as a ready-to-use emulsion in multiple-dose vials (Regressin, Vetrepharm, Inc.) and the other is provided as a single dose in lyophylized form (Ribi-gen, Ribi ImmunoChem Research, Inc.). The lyophylized material must be vigorously mixed with a diluent for about 5 minutes just prior to use. Both products are infiltrated throughout the tumor and adjacent tissue to activate antitumor cell-mediated responses.

Large tumors should be surgically "debulked" prior to immunotherapy for better results. Treatment may be repeated once or more if necessary at 2- to 3-week intervals. Necrotic tumor tissue resulting from attack by stimulated killer cells will be resorbed or it will drain to the surface of the skin. Large tumors, even when they have been reduced in size by surgical "debulking," may drain considerably and be unsightly for a time. Infection is rare, and when the necrotic tissue has drained or been absorbed healing is surprisingly rapid, leaving only a small scar. Furthermore, it is not necessary to infiltrate every tumor when there are multiple sarcoids on the horse.

Cryotherapy may be as effective as immunotherapy for small sarcoids, but immunotherapy is superior for large sarcoids, often yielding rapid and dramatic results. Cryotherapy should be given greater consideration when sarcoids are located on the limbs because these tumors appear to be less responsive to immunotherapy than those located elsewhere on the body. Lavach et al. have reported that each of 32 horses that were treated for periocular sarcoid with a deproteinized cell wall fraction went into remission and that none of them has had a recurrence. Immunotherapy is unquestionably the treatment of choice for periocular sarcoids.

Hoffman et al. reported the successful treatment of three sarcoids with hyperthermia induced by radio frequency current produced with a Thermoprobe instrument (Hach Company). The only problem with this technique appears to be the initial cost of the equipment. It also is unlikely that 100% remission would be obtained in a larger series of cases. A modality of therapy that has not been reported but that should be tried is immunotherapy with mycobacterial cell walls followed by hyperthermia. Immunotherapy has been demonstrated to enhance the susceptibility of tumor cells to hyperthermia. In a report by Witt, this combination provided results superior to either therapy alone for treatment of squamous cell carcinoma of the eye in cattle.

Mycobacterial cell wall immunotherapy has been exceptionally effective in removing sarcoids and has been effective against canine mammary tumors and perianal gland tumors as well as rodent ulcers in cats and ocular carcinoma in cattle, but it has been disappointing for melanoma in horses and humans and has been ineffective against squamous cell carcinomas in horses, mammary tumors in cats, and liposarcoma in dogs. Efficacy correlates with antigenicity of the tumor. If a tumor is bordered by, and infiltrated with, lymphocytes and macrophages, immunotherapy may be worth trying. If the tumor is not, the owners should be advised not to attempt immunotherapy.

Introduction of additional immunotherapeutics is to be expected. Their major emphasis will be for treatment of infectious diseases, in spite of recent disappointments with interferon and *C. parvum* extracts for shipping fever in cattle. Another mycobacterial product for treating viral respiratory infections in horses (Equimune, Vetrepharm, Inc.) already has been approved in Canada and is under review in the United States. Various combinations of interferons and lymphokines have shown promise as therapeutic agents for influenzal and herpetic infections, and they are under development for human use by several pharmaceutical houses. Eventually, they may be developed for veterinary use. Meanwhile, products such as deproteinized mycobacterial cell walls will be useful therapeutics for infectious as well as neoplastic diseases.

BIBLIOGRAPHY

Hoffman KD, Kainer RA, Shideler RK: Radio-frequency current-induced hyperthermia for the treatment of equine sarcoid. *Equine Pract* 1983;5:24–31.

Klein WR, Bras GE, Misdorp W, Steerenberg PA, deJong WH, Tiesjema RH, Kersjes AW, Ruitenberg EJ: Equine sarcoid: BCG immunotherapy compared to cryosurgery in a prospective randomized clinical trial. *Cancer Immunol Immunother* 1986;21:133–140.

Lavach JD, Severin GA, Lueker D: Immunotherapy of periocular sarcoids in horses. *Vet Clin North Am Large Animal Pract* 1984;6:513–518.

Leneau H, Steinmeyer P, Ragland WI: Immunotherapy of equine infectious rhinopneumonitis, in Proceedings AAEP Ann Conven 1986; pp 615–816.

Ragland WL, Keown GH, Spencer GR: Equine sarcoid. *Equine Vet J* 1970;2:2–11.

Taylor HB, Helwig EB. Dermatofibrosarcoma protuberans. A study of 115 cases. *Cancer* 1962;15:717–725.

Witt RP: Treating ocular carcinoma in cattle. *Vet Med/Small Animal Clin* 1984;79:1087–1089.

7
Applications of Laser Surgery

Lloyd P. Tate, Jr.
H. Carlton Newman

HISTORY OF LASERS

For centuries, men of medicine and science have speculated on the healing properties of light. In the 1800s, Newton theorized that light consisted of waves of particles, and postulated that these particles contained energy. Later these particles came to be known as photons. In 1850, Maxwell devised a set of equations to prove that these photons traveled at a constant speed that later was recognized as the speed of light. Max Planck postulated the concept of quantum mechanics, in which light was conceived as a quanta or photon having a specific wavelength, frequency, and quantity of energy. In 1914, Neil Bohr introduced the concept of spontaneous emission of photons from an atomic system that had its own characteristic energy level.

In 1917, Einstein predicted that it would be possible to bring about repeated and continuous excitation and decay of electrons. The process of raising and lowering their ground state would produce the release of massive amounts of concentrated energy. This concept is referred to as stimulated emission. Actual construction of a device to produce stimulated emission of light did not occur until 1958, when Schawlow and Townes constructed a resonant cavity consisting of a box with mirrors at each end. The device contained energized ammonia gas. Photons traveling between the two mirrors would interact with already energized photons, resulting in additional release of photons. With each additional pass between the mirrors the photon mass gained additional energy, until it could break or pass through the semipermeable mirrors as a burst of coherent light. In 1960, Theodore Maiman produced a pure-red beam of monochromatic light of a single frequency. This is a laser, an acronym for light amplification by stimulated emission of radiation.

PROPERTIES AND COMPONENTS OF A LASER

Light is a form of electromagnetic radiation that can be defined by amplitude, wavelength, frequency, and velocity. Light produced from the sun or an incandescent light source is an example of spontaneous emission. Stimulated emission is not found to occur in nature. The photons of light produced from a laser source are dependent solely upon the makeup of that system and are defined by the laser medium. Thus, all light produced by the laser medium will have identical wavelength and frequency and is therefore referred to as coherent light. Laser mediums may be gases, crystals, or metals, each producing its own specific coherent form of electromagnetic radiation "light" when energized by an external force. The term "pumping" refers to the process of stimulating electrons within a medium to raise their energy level from a ground state to an excited state. Pumping can be effected by mechanical means, by high-voltage electricity, and by high-intensity light (as by another laser), and is solely a means of energizing the medium to produce coherent light. To concentrate the photons within the medium, a third component consisting of reflecting surfaces is required. The mirrors are situated at either end of the laser medium and contain a semitransparent area or shutter for release of the collimated beam. As pumping of the medium excites the atoms and photons are emitted, they travel at an axis parallel to the medium, being reflected back and forth through the medium by the mirrors. When more atoms in the medium are in an excited state than in the ground state, this is referred to as a population inversion. As the photons continue to increase in number and gain energy, a "photon cascade" occurs. When there is an increase in photon energy, it is called "gain." The coherent beam produced is of the same wavelength and is spatially and temporally in phase. In addition to coherence, two other characteristics of laser light are referred to as collimation and monochromicity. These three combined characteristics are critical to the transmission and focusing of the laser beam (Fig. 7–1).

The laser beam can be focused to a single point image at the focal length of a lens system. Manipulation of the focal distance allows control of the laser with respect to interaction with tissue. When the laser is applied at the focal length of a lens system, a point image is created with very concentrated light used for cutting or vaporization. Manipulating the focal point above or below the tissue surface creates a divergent effect, resulting in less concentrated light that is useful for coagulation.

It becomes obvious that in addition to wavelength, the effect of a laser on tissue is also dependent on its power. Power is measured in watts, and when time is added, the term "joule" is an expression of power or "power density" (watts/second). Focal spot size (area) is responsible for the concentration of energy within an area, known as "energy density" and expressed as joules/square centimeter. The advantage of a small spot size is concentration of energy and reduced time to cause lateral thermal effect, meaning that fewer cells will experience thermal death at the margins of the paraincisional line.

There are two parameters that determine the laser's effectiveness as a surgical tool: the wavelength and its power time performance or energy density. The actual thermal effect of the laser's beam on tissue, therefore, is determined by the energy concentration delivered to the tissue and the absorption characteristics of that tissue. When rapid incision is required by the laser, a small spot size is advantageous because it will concentrate a high number of joules into the cells, leading to rapid vaporization and incision.

Modern lasers can deliver their beam in a continuous mode, a chopped mode, or a super-pulse mode. The advantages of the chopped and super-pulse modes over

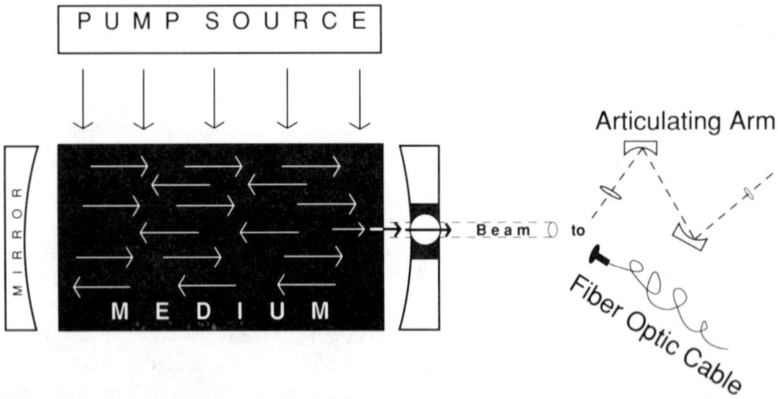

Figure 7–1. Schematic of a laser: the medium determines the frequency of the wavelength produced. The beam emitted is a specific wavelength that, when directed through an articulating arm or fiberoptics, may be focused on the target tissue.

the continuous mode are related to penetration for incisional depth and marginal thermal damage. Lasers that are chopped (meaning their irradiation cycles are delivered on and off at a very rapid interval) produce less lateral thermal damage than do those that operate in continuous mode. The chopped mode allows cells lateral to the incision to dissipate heat between bursts of irradiation. The super-pulse mode delivers the laser beam of irradiation to the target tissue infinitely faster than the chopped mode, and causes less lateral destruction of cells and a smoother incision in tissue.

TISSUE INTERACTION

The effectiveness of a laser is determined by the tissue—laser irradiation interaction that occurs. Laser irradiation interacts with biological tissues in four ways: (*a*) reflection, (*b*) transmission, (*c*) scattering, and (*d*) absorption.

The form of action that dominates laser-tissue interaction is dependent upon the frequency of electromagnetic irradiation, power density, and the mode. Each particular tissue has its own inherent response to exposure to a particular laser's irradiation. Absorption is the most critical interreaction because of the associated conversion of energy to heat. At 60 and 70 °C, denaturation of protein occurs that leads to coagulation necrosis. At 100 °C water within biological tissue boils, causing cells to explode. Absorption in tissue of laser energy used for surgical procedures produces necrosis, hemostasis, lymphostasis, vaporization (cutting), and membrane disruption. Depending on the laser's individual characteristics, one or more of these processes will dominate the laser-tissue interreaction.

SAFETY

Scattering and reflection of the surgical laser beam may be hazardous to patients, operators, and bystanders; safety precautions are required. All lasers are classified by the Bureau of Radiological Health and the Food and Drug Administration by accessibility to their radiation and power. All surgical lasers are in the Class IV category, which is the most hazardous category, in that burns can result from deflected or reflected laser beams. It is imperative that all personnel within the surgical area be aware of the importance of laser safety and be knowledgeable of the inner workings of the device and the wavelength produced.

Adequate protection must be provided for the patient, operator, personnel, and bystanders. To avoid fires, drapes around a surgical area should be covered with sterile, moistened towels or reflective material such as crinkled aluminum foil. When endotracheal tubes are used, they should be made of substances that will reflect or not interreact with the laser beam, or be covered with a reflective material to prevent ignition of oxygen. This is of particular importance when performing laser procedures within the respiratory tract, since combustion in the upper airway is usually fatal. Surgical instruments should be anodized to decrease the likelihood of the laser beam reflecting or scattering onto adjacent tissues. Depending on the wavelength of the laser irradiation being used, glasses or goggles designed to filter out damaging photons should be worn to prevent irreversible eye damage. Signs should be posted outside the operating theater and the doors locked during laser surgery. Most laser machines are equipped with electronic interlocks, which will disable the machine if the door is inadvertently opened. Other windows or doors should also be covered with protective shades, and signs placed on them when a laser is being used.

Laser surgery is based on heat production, which produces smoke that may be offensive to the operating personnel and irritating to both bystanders and patient. It is advisable that evacuation of the smoke be performed by various trapping mechanisms. One must consider that smoke is an irritant and that it may contain carcinogens, but this has never been proven.

SURGICAL LASERS

Carbon Dioxide Laser

The carbon dioxide (CO_2) laser produces a beam of electroirradiation in the far infrared range (10,600 nm). This beam of electromagnetic radiation is conducted through an articulating arm on the machine to the target tissue. Within the articulating arm are a series of mirrors and a focusing lens. By choosing various focusing lenses, the CO_2 laser can be adapted for use with an operating microscope. Surgeons may use the CO_2 laser in the focused or defocused mode. The CO_2 laser is an excellent tool for incisions and hemostasis. It can coagulate vessels up to 0.5 mm in diameter. In addition to sealing small vessels, the CO_2 laser seals lymphatics, a potential mechanism for spread of cancer cells.

This laser is used primarily for lesions that lie in a direct line of sight. Although attempts to produce flexible fibers to carry the CO_2 beam of electromagnetic irradiation are being made, these are hindered by extensive attenuation of power, and a short life span as a result of heat dissipation. Water is the primary mechanism through which the irradiation of CO_2 laser energy is absorbed. When using the CO_2 laser, the temperature of water is raised to a superheated steam state within cells, and the cell membranes virtually explode. This vaporizes the tissue, and cellular particles are pyrolyzed into plumes of steam and smoke. The water in adjacent tissues serves as a heat sink, limiting the thermal damage to adjacent tissue.

At the point of surgical interface, the zone of devitalized tissue produced by the CO_2 laser is more extensive than that produced by a scalpel but much smaller than that produced by electrosurgical cutting. Studies have demonstrated that there is a delay in the healing of skin wounds similar to that produced by electrosurgery. Therefore, the actual skin incision is often initially performed with a scalpel. It has been shown from surgery on humans that incisions made with the CO_2 laser are associated with less postoperative pain than are incisions made with a scalpel. This may be due to sealing of small transsected nerves by the laser during incision.

In veterinary medicine, the CO_2 laser is used for removal of skin lesions that require sealing of small vessels and sterilization of infected areas. Photovaporization of small tumors and photoablation procedures of any diffuse epithelial surface can be efficiently performed. The handling of tissue in a bloodless operating field is easily appreciated. The non-touch technique with the CO_2 laser effectively results in a "what you see is what you get" situation.

Nd:YAG Laser

The neodymium-yttrium-aluminum-garnet (Nd:YAG) laser is extremely useful for photovaporization and resection of diseased tissue by a noninvasive application through fiberoptic transmission (Fig. 7–2). The wavelength of electromagnetic irradiation for this laser is 1,060 nm, which allows transmission through fibers constructed of glass quartz. In contrast to the CO_2 laser, protein is the central tissue absorption mechanism. The photons produced by this laser penetrate the cell surface and are absorbed by protein, yielding additional scattering of radiation in forward, lateral, and backward planes. This produces diffuse tissue heating that leads to latent thermal necrosis of tissue surrounding the beam of electromagnetic radiation. The Nd:YAG laser does have the advantage of being able to coagulate vessels up to 4 mm in diameter. The laser beam is not readily absorbed by hemoglobin, melanin, or water, which allows its application in blood or fluid-filled body cavities. In contrast, the CO_2 laser is totally inefficient in fluid media or in blood. The Nd:YAG, despite its disadvantage of high potential for scattered radiation, has found many surgical applications because it can be transmitted through fiberoptics and has a high coagulation potential. It is effective in photovaporization of tissue where penetration is desired, even in high-density tissue.

In a recent innovation, a synthetic sapphire tip is attached to the distal end of the fiber in order to concentrate the heat at low power settings to provide surgical incision. These synthetic sapphires substantially reduce the power setting required, and surgery may be conducted with less than 15 watts of Nd:YAG energy. This is often referred to as the laser scalpel, in contrast to bare YAG fiber surgery. The distal tip of the sapphire must remain in constant contact with tissue when the laser is activated, or the sapphire will be destroyed by the heat produced. The synthetic sapphire has found application in both transendoscopic and hand-held techniques, particularly in performing tedious resection with coagulation in human surgery. These forms of cutting are referred

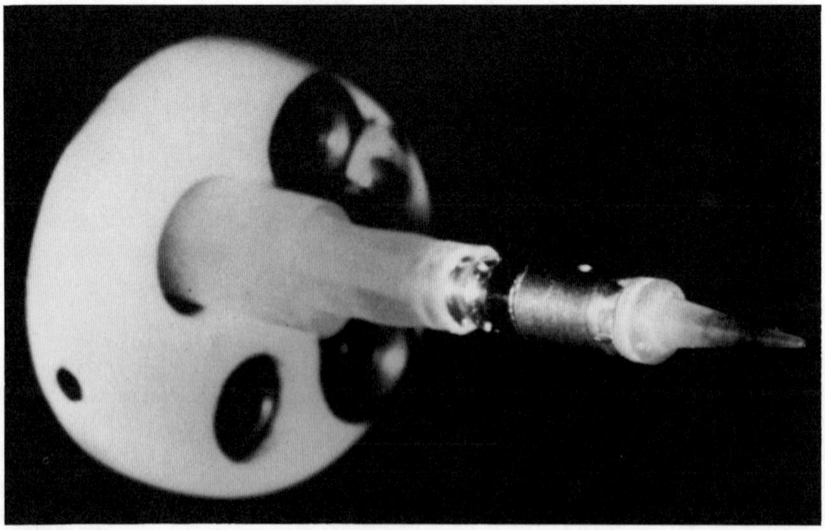

Figure 7–2. Distal end of a dual-lumen endoscope showing the synthetic sapphire tip on the laser fiber. This tip is used for contact cutting of tissue.

to as contact versus bare-fiber photofulguration, or noncut contact application.

APPLICATIONS

CO_2 Laser

In large animals, use of the CO_2 laser is restricted to superficial lesions. Various skin tumors such as sarcoids and squamous cell carcinoma may be ablated with this laser after infusion of local anesthetic under their base. Generally, the CO_2 laser is not used as a scalpel for resection, but is used in the defocused mode to ablate the base of the lesion. Pedunculated tumors should be cut either by scalpel or laser until the remainder of the lesion is parallel with the adjacent skin edges. The base is then ablated with the laser (tissue shaving) until tumor tissue has been vaporized and only normal parent tissue remains. The wounds are generally left to heal by second intention. This technique is favored over freezing, particularly in the area of the ear. The defocused beam allows precisional shaving of tissue, avoiding injury to adjacent structures such as the ear cartilage or cornea of the eye, where it is difficult to judge the amount of damage caused by freezing techniques. In addition to a nontouch technique, there is less swelling than that produced by freezing. Squamous cell carcinoma of the eye is another example of tissue that is an excellent candidate for CO_2 ablation. Tumors on the eyelids or nictitating membranes can be removed without general anesthesia. The laser can be used in the focused or defocused mode, and generally between 10 and 20 watts of power are required. With limbal or corneal invasion by squamous cell carcinoma, general anesthesia is required. The CO_2 laser, at lower power settings between 3 and 8 watts, can be used to vaporize the tumor. Practice and precision are required when working around the eye, particularly when the cornea is involved, in order not to damage this vital structure.

The CO_2 laser is also beneficial in preparing granulation tissue for pinched graft replacement of dermis. At high-wattage output settings, between 15 and 25 watts, the laser is initially applied in the focused mode to resect large portions of exuberant granulation tissue, or in the defocused mode on selectively trimmed surfaces. The CO_2 laser has proven to be excellent in the defocused mode for flattening roughened granulation tissue, or lowering the granulation tissue bed to just beneath the skin surface level in preparation for grafting. Use of the CO_2 laser in this fashion produces carbonized tissue, which may be flushed from the surface with isotonic fluids. Control of hemorrhage, sterilization of tissue, and a "no-touch" technique are the direct benefits of using the CO_2 laser over trimming with a scalpel. Furthermore, the recipient pockets for pinch grafts can easily be created with the CO_2 laser. The power setting used is between 7 and 15 watts. The laser is applied in the focused mode at an angle of 45 to 60 degrees to the tissue surface in a downward direction. Pockets 2 to 4 mm in diameter and 3 to 4 mm in depth are created. Precision is increased and less lateral damage of tissue will occur if the laser is placed in the chopped or super-pulse mode. Carbonized tissue is flushed from the pockets and the wound bandaged for 12 to 24 hours. Skin grafts are then placed into each of the pockets, and the wound again bandaged. The delay between pocket creation and graft placement is important to allow early capillary growth to begin, so an early host-graft vascular anastomosis can occur.

Transendoscopic Application of Nd:YAG Laser

Transendoscopic Nd:YAG application requires mild sedation and analgesia. The target tissue may be sprayed with topical anesthetic such as mepivacaine or lidocaine. Pain control and sedation can be accomplished by administration of xylazine (1.1 mg/kg intravenously [IV]) followed by butorphanol tartrate (0.044 mg/kg IV). The selection of endoscopic equipment is crucial for transendoscopic application of the laser. At least one 2-mm biopsy channel and sufficient length of the fiber bundle of the endoscope to reach the proposed target tissue are required. A second biopsy channel is preferred, but not essential. The second biopsy channel can be used for additional instrumentation or for evacuation of smoke.

Smoke may be irritating to mucous membrane or to small bronchioles. Removal of smoke produced from the lasing procedure is accomplished by suction or mechanical filtration devices. If standard suction is used, an in-line filter is necessary to prevent smoke particles and debris from soiling equipment and tubing. The quality of endoscopic viewing is quickly decreased by smoke production and interferes with completion of a transendoscopic laser procedure. When a second biopsy channel is not present, an additional tube should be placed beside the endoscope for smoke evacuation.

Eye protection is essential during the transendoscopic Nd:YAG application to prevent reflected irradiation from irreversibly damaging the retina of the surgeon's eye. This can be accomplished with designated eye goggles, or with a filter cap placed over the viewing port of the endoscope. Additional safety in viewing the target tissue can be obtained by coupling the endoscope to a video camera. Video viewing is preferable because magnification of the target tissue increases the precision of directing the laser. Video endoscopes can be used for transendoscoipic laser surgery but must be specially designed to prevent damage by the laser to the video camera located in the distal end of the endoscope.

Whenever lasing procedures are being performed, it is also essential to pass the laser fiber at least 1 cm past the distal port of the biopsy channel to prevent heat or hot material from damaging the operating end of the endoscope. Endoscopes that have a darkened surface at the distal end are more likely to be damaged than those that are constructed of metal or lighter colored materials. Several endoscopes are currently available that contain a special channel for pulsating flushing of lesions. This is advantageous during laser procedures in that it can provide cooling by water pulsation, or water pulsation may be used to débride carbonization from tissue that is being lased.

Specific Equine Applications

Ethmoid Hematoma and Other Nasopharyngeal Masses. In all cases, radiographic evaluation of the nasal passages, pharynx, and maxillary and frontal sinuses should be conducted. Lesions that are entirely within the nasal cavity, arising out of the normally visible turbinate area, are ideal for transendoscopic ablation with the Nd:YAG laser. Direct irradiation by applying the endoscope through the affected nostril should be done first. The beam of infrared radiation is directed at the center of the lesion, and vaporization is extended to the margins of the visible mass. To produce as much destruction as possible, the laser should be set at 100 watts of output in a continuous application mode. Ethmoid hematomas or other masses that do not occlude the nasal passage or the nasopharynx can be obliterated by this approach (Fig. 7–3).

Lesions that do occlude the nasal passage or nasopharynx should be approached both directly as described and through the contralateral nasal passage. To approach a mass through the unaffected nasal passage, the distal end of the endoscope is placed in the area of the epiglottis, and then flexed or flipped back on itself (180 degrees) toward the nasal passages. The operator must adjust to maneuvering the endoscope in this configuration to apply the laser irradiation. This configuration is beneficial because it decreases the possibility of irradiating the endoscope and damaging its fiberoptic bundles. Because it is difficult to feed the laser fiber through the distal portion of the biopsy channel when the endoscope is flexed 180 degrees, the laser fiber should be in position prior to performing this procedure. The purpose of this procedure is to apply laser irradiation to the mass just below the dorsal edge of the nasal pharynx. Multiple applications are routinely required to sever the stalk of the mass. A larger mass increases the necessity for multiple irradiations. Generally, a mass may be irradiated on an every-other-day basis until a snare can be applied through the direct approach to remove the coagulated mass. Laser irradiation is continued until the turbinate area is easily identified. After ablation of the mass and visualization of the remaining turbinates is accomplished, laser application should be halted for 4 to 7 days to allow sloughing of abnormal tissue. If abnormal tissue persists, it should be ablated.

Ethmoid hematomas that have a small sinus component can be approached through a trephination hole, made under local anesthesia. Tumors possessing a small sinus component can be irradiated while

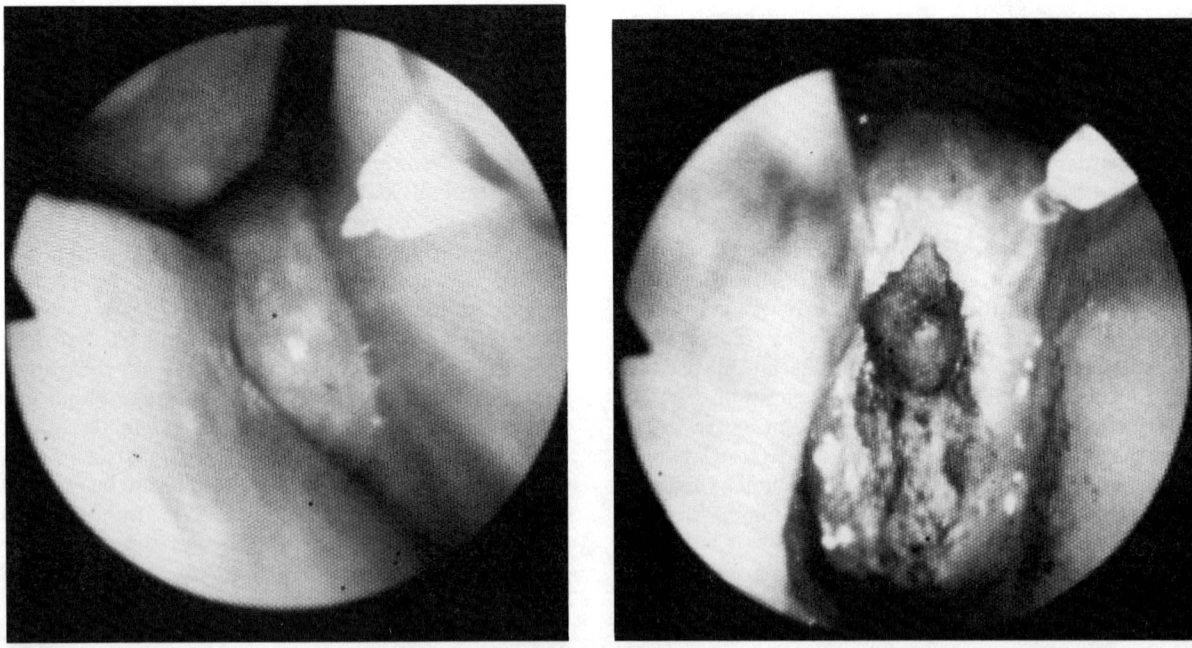

A B

Figure 7–3. A. End-on view of ethmoid hematoma with bare laser fiber present in the upper right-hand corner directed at the center of the mass. **B.** Photofulguration of ethmoid hematoma. Note cavitation starting at the center and working toward the margins.

transnasal irradiation of the adjacent portion is being conducted. Hemorrhage is usually minimal, but, if encountered, the laser may be applied to coagulate the injured vessel.

Tumors of the Dorsopharyngeal Recess. Ablation of tumors of the dorsopharyngeal recess and dorsal pharynx requires direct application of the laser. The power setting selected is 100 watts in a continuous mode. Vaporization should begin in the center of the mass and gradually work to the margins. Multiple applications may be required depending upon the size and density of the tumor. Applications past the margins of the tumor are not necessary because 4 to 6 mm of tissue will slough as a result of scattered irradiation and the latent thermal effect of the laser.

Dorsopharyngeal Cysts and Subepiglottic Cysts. Dorsopharyngeal cysts and subepiglottic cysts are approached directly at a midrange setting of the laser at 50 to 60 watts in a continuous mode. The visible surfaces of the cyst should be blanched with the laser at this setting. The Nd:YAG infrared irradiation is absorbed by protein, and extensive amounts of absorption occur in the fluid contained within the cyst. This is converted to heat and results in sclerosis of the inner cyst membrane. After the visible surface of the cysts has blanched, the laser should be set at a continuous mode of 100 watts of output and a 10- to 15-mm hole cut into the cyst and fluid allowed to evacuate. The laser may then be applied to the margins of the evacuated cyst in order to assure total ablation has occurred and to decrease the possibility of recurrence.

Soft Palate Displacement. Correction of soft palate displacement by resection of a portion of the free border of the palate can be performed with bare-fiber noncontact application or contact application using a wedge or conical-pointed sapphire tip attached to the distal end of the laser fiber. Free-fiber or noncontact application is performed at a 100-watt output, whereas contact application uses 10 to 14 watts of output. To perform partial resection, the soft palate must be displaced above the epiglottis. In a horse in which intermittent dorsal displacement of the soft palate occurs, one may be able to produce continuous displacement after administration of xylazine and butorphanol tartrate. The incision, made in the soft palate, should not exceed 1.5 cm in length, and is produced in a semicircular pattern. Frequently, a 1-cm incision allows correction of dorsal displacement of the soft palate. During the corrective procedure, the horse should be encouraged to swallow and try to reposition the epiglottis in its normal position.

Entrapment of the Epiglottis. Correction of entrapment of the epiglottis is routinely performed from the caudal border to the tip using the free-fiber technique. The tissue is initially blanched for the length of the entrapment at a width of 1 cm at a 50- to 60-watts power range setting. Relief of the entrapment is then made at 100 watts of output. The incision begins at the free border of the entrapment and progressed toward the tip. Once the cut is complete, residual tissue strands may be separated by encouraging the horse to swallow. Contact lasing with the use of a synthetic sapphire tip proceeds in a similar fashion, but incision begins at the tip of the epiglottis and progresses toward the rima glottis until correction is achieved.

Entrapments that are complicated by adhesions to the epiglottis will probably be uncorrectable by this technique unless the restricting tissue can be vaporized. Protrusion of the tip of the epiglottis through an entrapment should be correctable by transendoscopic laser technique. Particular care must be taken not to damage the epiglottis.

Guttural Pouch Application. The Nd:YAG is suitable for correction of guttural pouch tympanites, and may be used in assisting resolution of a mycotic or diphtheritic lesion on or near the internal carotid artery. Free-fiber or contact application can be used in this area. Smoke evacuation is essential to maintaining good visibility.

In correction of unilateral guttural pouch tympanites, a catheter is first placed in the abnormal guttural pouch through the pharyngeal opening. The distal end of the catheter is bent to approximately 60 degrees prior to insertion. The endoscope containing the laser fiber is inserted into the adjacent guttural pouch through the opposite pharyngeal opening. The catheter is rotated until the catheter tip can be seen pushing on the mucous membrane separating the two guttural pouches. The laser is set at 100 watts in a continuous mode for free-fiber application, and a hole more than 2 cm in diameter is created.

For guttural pouch mycotic lesions, balloon catheterization of the internal carotid artery is performed prior to laser ablation of an erosive lesion. Vaporization is performed with a blunt-ended sapphire tip or free-fiber ablation at low wattage settings, between 20 and 30 watts of output. Care must be taken not to incise or damage the cervical sympathetic ganglion or other vital vascular structures. For best results, the laser is applied multiple times with a delay of 3 to 4 days between applications to ensure sloughing of infected tissue. General flushing of the guttural pouch and suction evacuation of fluid contained within it using endoscopic technique is conducted frequently to ensure removal of tissue debris.

Laser Ventriculectomy. The Nd:YAG laser may be used to ablate the mucosal lining of the left laryngeal ventricle after surgical laryngoplasty has been performed. With the assistance of xylazine-butorphanol sedation, the endoscope is passed through the right nostril until the distal tip lies on the epiglottis. The laser fiber is then advanced into the ventricle, and the mucous membrane lining of the ventricle is ablated at a 100-watt power setting. Ablation should be continued until mucous membrane surfaces are blanched and swollen. This indicates that sufficient laser energy has been applied. After ablation, the animal should receive 30 days' stall rest before being placed in an exercise program. The damaged mucous membrane generally seals the ventricle completely by second-intention healing. The advantage to this technique is the reduced risk of the laryngotomy and of adjacent laryngoplasty incision infection. It is important in performing a ventriculectomy to actually situate the fiber in the ventricle in order to achieve total ablation and avoid additional scatter irradiation that could lead to laryngeal edema.

Arytenoidectomy. Transendoscopic laser arytenoidectomy is limited to the corniculate process of the arytenoid cartilage. Currently available Nd:YAG lasers do not produce sufficient energy to ablate the thickness of the body of the arytenoid cartilage. Theoretically, failed laryngoplasties should be more amenable than arytenoid chondritis to laser "partial" arytenoidectomy, because of minimal cartilage thickness. Also the body of the arytenoid cartilage would be stabilized in a failed laryngoplasty as a result of the previous surgical placement of the prosthesis, which would not be present in cases of chondritis.

Ablation of the corniculate process is performed by lasing the corniculate process on the midline in a dorsal-to-ventral or ventral-to-dorsal-pattern. The cartilage portion will necrose and slough in 10 days to 2 weeks as a result of the latent thermal necrosis that occurs with the Nd:YAG laser. Healing is by second intention and requires 8 to 12 weeks from the time of the initial lasing procedure. Repeat applications may be necessary for some cartilage obliteration or for control of granulation tissue. All forms of arytenoidectomy (partial) are controversial with respect to providing additional airway diameter, and studies in exercise physiology will eventually determine which procedure improves exercise tolerance.

BIBLIOGRAPHY

Freitas L, Chapman GA, Sielczak M, et al: Laser smoke effect on the bronchial system. *Lasers Surg Med* 1987;7:283–288.

Iwasaki M, Sasako M, Toshiro K, et al: Nd:YAG laser for general surgery. *Lasers Med Surg* 1985;5:429–438.

Joffe SN: *Neodymium YAG Laser in Medicine and Surgery.* New York, Elsevier Science Publishing Co, Inc, 1983, pp 1–80.

Kaplan I: *Laser Surgery II,* Jerusalem, Jerusalem Academic Press, 1978, pp. 133–222.

Ratz JL: *Lasers in Cutaneous Medicine and Surgery.* Chicago, Yearbook Medical Publishers, Inc, 1986, pp 1–28.

Tate LP, Newman HC, Cullen JM, Sweeney CL: Nd:YAG laser surgery in the equine larynx. A pilot study. *Lasers Surg Med* 1986;6:473–476.

Tate LP Jr, Newman HC, Sweeney CL, Fetrow J, Rader MBA: An overview of endoscopic laser surgery 3 clinical cases in the standing animal. *Proc AAEP* 1986;32:385–396.

8
Advances in Wound Management

Ted S. Stashak

Wound healing classically has been divided into four separate phases: inflammatory, débridement, repair, and maturation.

Inflammatory Phase

The inflammatory phase can be subdivided, but not separated into vascular and cellular reactions. The duration of this phase is dependent on many factors, including the degree of trauma, nature of injury, whether or not foreign substances remain, and if infection develops.

Vascular and Cellular Reactions Resulting in Localization of the Inflammatory Response. Serving to limit the amount of hemorrhage into the wound and subsequent blood loss after injury, small vessels adjacent to and within the wound become constricted, presumably under the influence of catecholamines. Coinciding with this initial vascular reaction, leukocytes in adjacent vessels begin to adhere to the endothelium of the small venules. Within 5 to 10 minutes, an active vasodilatation (primarily of these small venules) occurs, resulting in a leakage of blood and plasma into the wound. The term "active" is used because the endothelial cells separate under the influence of histamine-2, serotonin, the kinins, and prostaglandin E. Leukocytes passing through spaces created by separated endothelial cells within the vessel walls (diapedesis) begin to concentrate at the site of injury. With conversion of fibrinogen to fibrin and the production of a water-insoluble glycoprotein (fibronectin) comes the formation of a fibrocellular clot that fills and binds the wound together, providing early tensile strength. In this anoxic environment, the polymorphonuclear leukocytes die and release enzymes that contribute to the inflammatory response. Additionally, the plugging of the damaged lymphatics, which prevents drainage of fluids, results in localization of the inflammatory response characterized by swelling, redness, and heat, and in some cases pain due to pressure and chemical stimulation. The fibrocellular clot is also responsible for maintaining internal hemostasis as well as providing a scaffold for future repair. When the fibrocellular clot dehydrates to form a scab, it acts like a bandage, protecting the wound from external contamination. Even though the scab performs an important function, it is not required for wound healing to occur. In fact, some wounds heal more rapidly when kept moist under a bandage without scab formation (refer to Table 8.1 for an outline of vascular reactions, cellular movements, and localization of response).

Débridement Phase

During the débridement phase, the neutrophils and monocytes that were chemotactically stimulated by leukotaxine and a lymph node promoting factor to migrate into the wound now begin the cleanup process. The primary functions of the neutrophil include the ingestion of microorganisms by phagocytosis. The subsequent release of lysosomal enzymes contributes to the inflammatory response and aids the mononuclear cells in further breakdown of dead tissue. In the absence of infection, healing can progress without the polymorphonuclear cell. This has been documented through studies using antineutrophil serum in labora-

TABLE 8–1. VASCULAR, CELLULAR, AND LOCALIZATION FACTORS IN THE INFLAMMATORY PHASE OF WOUND HEALING

INJURY
Physical
Chemical
Surgical
Infection
↓
INFLAMMATION
Dose response
Basic responses are the same

VASCULAR	CELLULAR	LOCALIZATION
Vascular reaction	Leukocytes move by diapedesis from small venules	Fragile lymphatics increase damage
Vasoconstriction	Concentration at site of injury as cell aggregation centers	Fibrin plugs the lymphatics, resulting in reduced drainage
Vasodilatation leading to fluid leakage	PMNs + monocytes	Leakage of fluid from vessels leads to classic signs of inflammation
Endothelial cell separation	PMNs die → lyse → sterile pus	Fibronectin binds cells, fibrin, and collagen together
Leukocytes become sticky		

PMNs, polymorphonuclear leukocytes.

tory animals used for investigation of wound healing.

Conversely, monocytes are necessary for wound healing to progress. They become macrophages when they enter the wound and phagocytize dead tissue and extraneous debris. In addition to becoming macrophages, monocytes also coalesce to form multinucleate giant cells or transform into histiocytes or epithelioid cells. A very important function of the monocyte is to attract fibroblasts into the wound and perhaps stimulate them to undergo maturation for collagen synthesis. In experimental models where antimonocyte serum plus cortisone was used, it was noted that wound healing was delayed. There were fewer fibroblasts in the wound, and they were relatively immature and disoriented and exhibited a delay in the formation of ground substance and the production of tropocollagen.

The duration of this phase is obviously dependent upon the amount of debris and the degree of contamination. Consequently, surgical débridement, good hemostasis, and adequate drainage of the infected wound are paramount to the healing of a wound.

Repair Phase

The repair process involves epithelialization of the wound surface, migration of fibroblasts necessary for collagen formation, formation of granulation tissue, and wound contraction. This phase usually begins within the first 12 hours after wounding and proceeds after barriers such as blood clots, necrotic tissue, debris, and infection have been removed.

Epithelialization. The first sign of repair, epithelialization, is recognized about 12 hours postwounding by a flattening of the rete pegs of the epidermis. The flattening forces adjacent cells toward the wound edges. Simultaneously, basal cells of the epidermis begin to separate, duplicate, and migrate toward regions of cell deficit. Generally, epithelial cells continue to migrate on the surface of a wound until like cells are contacted. Factors that may arrest epithelialization prematurely include infection, excessive production of granulation tissue, repeated dressing changes, extreme hypothermia, desiccation of the wound surface, and reduction in oxygen tension. In the incised sutured wound, epithelial cells cover the wound in 12 to 24 hours. However, in the full-thickness open wound a granulating bed must be formed before epithelialization can occur. In this situation, there is usually a lag phase of 4 to 5 days before the epithelial cells begin to migrate. It may take several weeks to months for large defects to become completely covered. The rate of epithelialization varies with the region of the body. In the horse, 400-mm^2 defects in the flank epithelialize at a rate of 0.2 mm/

day, whereas similar defects on the lower limb epithelialize at 0.09 mm/day.

When several layers of epithelial cells cover the wound, cell differentiation and keratinization begin. Eventually these cells are laid down on a smooth surface of connective tissue that forms a loose bond, making it easy to knock or strip off the epithelial cells. This surface lacks adnexal structures and normal skin and is referred to as scar tissue epithelium.

Fibroplasia. Fibroblasts originating from undifferentiated mesenchymal cells in nearby connective tissue move into the wound by advancing along the previously formed fibrin lattice within the clot. They begin secreting a protein polysaccharide and glycoprotein, which are necessary components of the ground substance. This ground substance reaches its greatest development at about 3 to 5 days and is thought to be necessary for the collagen deposition that follows. Collagen is synthesized by the fibroblasts predominantly from hydroxyproline and hydroxylysine. The formation of collagen begins on about the fourth or fifth day and is initiated by extrusion of the tropocollagen molecule into the extracellular spaces. As these immature fibrils are produced, they begin to bind together to form a mature collagen fiber. As collagen content increases, the ground substance decreases.

It is generally accepted that the early rise in tensile strength is a result of collagen formation, whereas later gains in strength result from maturation of the scar. The major gain in tensile strength occurs from 5 to 15 days, after which much slower increases are observed. Only 80% of the original tensile strength may be reached at 1 year.

Granulation Tissue. Granulation tissue begins to appear in the wound about 3 to 6 days after injury. The granular appearance is a result of proliferating capillaries that form vascular loops. These loops grow behind the fibroblasts and form multiple anastomoses. Vascular endothelial cells that migrate into the wound contain plasminogen activators responsible for lysis of the fibrin network. As the capillaries develop, so do the lymphatics, but at a slower rate. Granulation tissue formation in an open wound is beneficial for several reasons: (*a*) it provides a surface for epithelial cells to migrate over, (*b*) it is resistant to infection, (*c*) the process of wound contraction is centered around its development, and (*d*) it carries the fibroblast responsible for collagen formation.

Studies on wound healing have shown that the horse is capable of collagen formation as early as the first day after wounding. More typically this capability is reached about the third or fourth day. These investigators also noted an increased formation of collagen and collagenase in horses' wounds when they were compared to similar wounds in the rat. They concluded that healing in the horse is prompt and excessive, tending toward abnormal repair.

Wound Contraction. Wound contraction is a process whereby an open skin wound reduces in size by centripetal movement of the full thickness of skin. This movement may begin between the third and fourth day and appears to be independent of the epithelialization process that is occurring at the same time. Skin movement is thought to result from the contractile properties of a modified fibroblast (myofibroblast) found in granulation tissue adjacent to the edge of the wound. These cells have good cell-to-cell and cell-to-stroma contact, plus they possess many properties of smooth muscle, including the ability to contract. As these cells contract, they draw the surrounding full thickness of skin toward the center of the wound. In doing so, the surrounding skin becomes temporarily stretched and thinned. Gradually, new collagen is added to the dermis and new cells are added to the epithelium. This process restores skin thickness and reduces tension, and is referred to as intussusceptive growth.

Wound contraction works best in regions where the skin is relatively loose. In these areas, wound contraction is usually sufficient to bring about complete closure of the wound with minimal scar formation. In areas where skin is under tension, contraction may not reach an ideal conclusion and as a result a wider scar is formed. This occurs in situations where contraction forces equilibrate with skin tension forces before wound edges are apposed. The rate of wound contraction also varies with the lesion location. In the horse, 400-mm^2 defects on the flank contract at a rate of 0.8 to 1 mm/day, whereas similar wounds on the lower limb contract at a rate of 0.2 mm/day.

Maturation Phase

The maturation phase is characterized by a reduction in fibroblast numbers with an equilibration of collagen production and collagen lysis. Functionally oriented collagen fibers begin to predominate as nonfunctional ones disappear. Despite the reduction in fibroblasts, blood vessels, and collagen fibrils, the tensile strength of the wound increases. This increase in wound tensile strength results from the alignment of collagen along lines of tension, intramolecular crosslinking assisted by lysyl oxidase, and the formation of more contact bundles. The junction between adjacent collagen bundles becomes less distinct as the fibers interlock. Even though the scar increases in tensile strength over a prolonged period of time, it still remains 15 to 20% weaker than the surrounding tissue.

SELECTED FACTORS THAT AFFECT WOUND HEALING

Malnutrition and Protein Deficiency

Recent evidence indicates that wound healing is impaired in human patients with mild to moderate short- or long-term protein-energy malnutrition. It appears that the direction the patient is moving metabolically (positive or negative) at the time of injury or surgery is most important, since the adverse effect of protein-energy malnutrition occurs well in advance of the external evidence of weight loss. The impairment in wound healing is easily reversed by providing adequate nutrition. Although this has not been proven in large animal species, it would seem logical there would be a similar effect. Therefore, it is recommended that animals be offered balanced nutrition in adequate amounts prior to elective surgery and/or after wounding and emergency surgery.

Hypoproteinemia alone adversely affects wound healing primarily by altering fibroplasia, neoangiogenesis, wound remodeling, and wound tensile strength. Consequently, the repair phase of healing is prolonged. The impairment in wound healing from hypoproteinemia is seen well in advance of alterations in the plasma protein levels. As an example, albumin fractions are depleted shortly after withdrawal of protein from the diet. Even though the alteration in wound healing is not well correlated to plasma protein levels, when plasma protein levels fall to 6 g/dL healing is retarded. Below 5.5 g/dL a 70% incidence of wound disruption is expected, and below 2 g/dL wound healing is disrupted, edema occurs, and death ensues. Since fats can be synthesized from carbohydrates and carbohydrates can be synthesized from protein, but protein can only be fabricated from protein or its digestive by-products (amino acids and peptides), a protein-rich-diet is required to counteract the adverse effects on wound healing. Feeding D,L-methionine to protein-deficient animals reverses the retardation in wound healing. The D,L-methionine is converted to cysteine, which may serve as an important cofactor in collagen synthesis and may also be involved in the disulfide crosslinking as collagen matures. Experimentally it has been shown that animals placed on high-protein diets have a more rapid gain in tensile strength with less edema formation when compared to animals on protein deficient diets.

Nonsteroidal Anti-Inflammatory Drugs

Since inflammation is a part of the wound-healing process, it is logical that anti-inflammatory drugs such as phenylbutazone, aspirin, indomethacin, and flunixin meglumine would have an effect on wound healing. In an incisional healing study done on horses, oxyphenbutazone administered at a loading dose of 12 mg/kg (2 days) and a maintenance dose of 6 mg/kg (5 days) significantly reduced inflammation and granulation tissue formation. It is theorized that phenylbutazone acts by decreasing capillary permeability, which in turn alters early fluid and cellular responses in wound healing processes. Aspirin and indomethacin inhibit the formation of prostaglandins. However, excessive amounts of these drugs are required to alter wound healing, because when they are used at recommended dosages no alteration in the quality of wound healing has been observed. In contrast, in an abdominal incisional study done on ponies, flunixin meglumine administered intravenously at 1.1 mg/kg 12 hours preoperatively and every 12 hours postoperatively for 7 days resulted in reduced tensile strength of 7-day-old skin and linea alba wounds when compared to untreated controls. It had no effect on jejunal wound strength but appeared to enhance colon healing strength. Histologic examination revealed poorer tissue continuity and greater inflammatory response in the treated group. Most surgeons find these drugs useful because they diminish pain from inflammation, improve overall well-being, and encourage ambulation, resulting in increased circulation especially in the distal limbs.

Corticosteroids

Corticosteroids, when given in moderate to large amounts within the first 5 days after injury, significantly retard wound healing. However, even though wound healing is retarded it occurs eventually. Corticosteroids retard healing by stabilizing the lysosomal membrane, which in turn prevents the release of enzymes that are responsible for initiating the inflammatory response. They also suppress fibroplasia, ground substance formation, collagen formation, capillary proliferation, and granulation tissue formation. Additionally, corticosteroids retard wound contraction, delay the gain in tensile strength, and may also retard epithelialization. Corticosteroids are most effective in delaying healing when they are administered before inflammation begins.

The anti-inflammatory effects of corticosteroids can be counteracted by the topical application or systemic administration of vitamin A. Vitamin A acts as a lysosomal labilizer that antagonizes the stabilizing effect of corticosteroids. This antagonism counteracts the corticosteroid's effect on inflammation and tensile strength.

Trauma

Excessive trauma, within the wound or from other sites of involvement (e.g., multiple lacerations or fractures) prolongs the early phase of healing, decreases the gain in tensile strength, makes the wound more susceptible to infection, and can result in excessive scar production. When the effects of simultaneous trauma from either fractures or muscle contusions made elsewhere on the body were examined, a delay in wound tensile strength was observed for as long as 15 days post-trauma. A delay in gain of wound tensile strength was also observed at the other sites when a second wound was made within 14 days of the first wound, and the degree and loss of wound tensile strength was proportional to the degree of trauma. Whether excessive trauma is associated with one wound or multiple wounds, the decrease in healing and reduction in gain in wound tensile strength appears to be a result of reduced capillary perfusion.

Surgeons can reduce local tissue trauma by using scalpel dissection rather than scissors, which crush tissue, or blunt dissection, which tears tissue. Furthermore, tissue trauma can be reduced by débriding the wound completely, reducing surgery time, using isotonic/isosmolar lavage solutions, maintaining hemostasis, reducing fluid accumulation in tissues, and apposing tissues with the proper tension with nonreactive suture material. For the traumatic wound, proper cleaning, thorough débridement, and protection are most important to the outcome. The use of systemic antibiotics to reduce the chances of infection and treatment with nonsteroidal anti-inflammatory drugs to reduce the swelling and pain are also important. With multiple lacerations, a reduced healing ability is expected.

Infection

Although virulence plays a role, generally speaking wound infection results when the number of organisms reaches a concentration of 10^6 organisms/g of tissue or 10^6 organisms/mL of fluid. At this concentration, the organisms exceed the capabilities of the host's defenses. Contaminated wounds with lesser concentrations of organisms may become infected when: (*a*) foreign bodies are present; (*b*) excessive necrotic tissue is left in the wound; (*c*) there is excessive bleeding (the ferric ion may also increase virulence and is necessary for replication); (*d*) local tissue defenses are impaired, as in the case of burn patients or patients on immunosuppressive drugs; or (*e*) the vascular supply is altered. High doses of local irradiation, particularly within the first 4 to 48 hours after wounding, make the contaminated wound more susceptible to infection. Foreign bodies such as organic material (common in the grossly contaminated wound), bone sequestra, suture material, glove powder, or bone plates and screws promote infection by providing protective surface areas for bacteria to grow. Importantly, the lower the initial inoculum of organisms, the longer it takes to reach the point of clinical infection and the greater the chances that host defenses will curtail the formation of active infection.

Infection delays healing by mechanically separating the wound edges with exudate, by reducing the vascular supply (a result of mechanical pressure and a tendency to form microthrombi and small vessels adjacent to the wound), and by increasing cellular responses, which in turn result in prolongation of the inflammatory and débridement phases of wound healing. Bacteria also produce enzymes that digest collagen.

Wound Lavage and Antiseptics

Since bacteria adhere to the wound surface by an electrostatic charge, lavage solutions are most effective when delivered by a fluid jet impacting on the wound with at least 7 psi. This pulsatile pressure can be achieved by forcefully expressing lavage solutions from a 35-mL syringe through an 18-gauge needle, or by using a spray bottle or a "Water Pik." Seven psi cannot be achieved by gravity flow or lavage with a bulb syringe.

Povidone-Iodine Solution (Betadine). Povidone-iodine solutions are commonly used to lavage wounds because of their broad antimicrobial spectrum. The free iodine, which gives the solution its antimicrobial activity, is complexed with polyvinylpyrrolidone (a polymer similar to dextran) to increase its stability and to reduce its irritating effect and staining properties. Unfortunately, this complexing tightly binds the iodine, which reduces the free iodine available for antimicrobial activity. Diluting the solution, however, uncouples this bond, making more free iodine available for antimicrobial activity. Dilutions (0.1% to 1.0%) have been shown to be more potent and more rapidly bactericidal in vitro than commercial 10% povidone-iodine solution preparations. In another in vitro study, 0.1% was not bactericidal. In a human study, an increased incidence of infection was noticed in wounds sprayed with 5% povidone-iodine solutions when compared to controls sprayed with sterile saline. When the povidone-iodine was diluted to 1%, the opposite was true. It was shown that the 5% povidone-iodine solution inhibited leukocyte migration into the wound, thus decreasing the ability to ward off infection.

In vitro studies with povidone-iodine solutions have documented the dose-dependent inhibition of neutrophil migration, monocyte function, and fibroblasticidal effects. Whereas concentrations greater than 0.05% inhibited neutrophil migration, concentrations between 0.005% and 0.03% stimulated neutrophil migration. Monocytes continue to be viable at povidone-iodine concentrations of 0.005%, yet this concentration is still effective as an antimicrobial. A 1% povidone-iodine solution killed fibroblasts but a 0.001% solution killed bacteria without harming fibroblasts. Concentrations of povidone iodine greater than 0.2% were cytotoxic to the equine neutrophil; below this concentration no effect was seen. The cytotoxic effects of povidone-iodine are all likely to be due to the free iodine, but the pH and osmolality may also play a role.

Although the bactericidal activity of povidone-iodine is maintained in vitro in concentrations down to 0.005%, large numbers of neutrophils (10^7/mL), such as would be found in an infected wound, inhibited the antimicrobial effect of povidone-iodine at 0.05% but not at 0.1%. Because of these studies, it appears that povidone-iodine solutions between 0.1 and 0.2% concentrations are best for wound lavage in the horse.

Chlorhexidine Diacetate Solution (Nolvasan). Chlorhexidine diacetate solutions, like povidone-iodine solutions, have a wide antimicrobial spectrum and are commonly used as lavage solutions, particularly in small animal species. In dogs chlorhexidine (0.05, or 0.5, or 1%) has been shown to be superior to povidone-iodine (0.05, 0.25, or 0.5%) in preventing infection in wounds contaminated with *Staphylococcus aureus.* When applied to the intact skin, its antimicrobial effect is immediate followed by a lasting residual effect, a result of binding to the protein in the stratum corneum. Systemic absorption, toxicosis or inactivation by organic material does not appear to be a problem. When injected in equine joints, a 0.5% chlorhexidine solution caused severe joint pain, lameness, limb edema and increased synovial protein concentration and a neutrophilic synovitis. These results would indicate that prolonged tissue contact with 0.5% chlorhexidine solution may be harmful, but additional studies are needed. Currently, 0.05% chlorhexidine solutions are recommended for use in wound lavage.

Hydrogen Peroxide. Although hydrogen peroxide is a commonly used wound irrigant with an impressive foaming action, it has little value as an antiseptic but is an effective sporocide. Three percent hydrogen peroxide is damaging to tissues, and in fact its cytotoxic effect on fibroblasts exceeds its bactericidal activity. Additionally, there is evidence that it causes thrombosis in the microvasculature adjacent to the wound margins. Because of this, hydrogen peroxide is not recommended for wound lavage.

Acetic Acid Solution. Although I have not used acetic acid solutions for wound lavage or under a dressing, 0.5 or 0.25% solutions are reported to be most effective against *Pseudomonas* organisms. Acetic acid solution effectively changes the pH of a wound, rendering it less acceptable for bacterial growth. However, its antimicrobial spectrum is not broad and its cellular toxicity is reported to exceed its bactericidal effect. Because it retards epithelialization and fibroblasts, acetic acid solution is regarded as unsuitable for wound care.

Suturing Techniques and Materials

Suturing, as well as the material selected, has an influence on wound healing. When simple interrupted sutures were compared to simple continuous sutures, the simple interrupted sutured wounds had less edema and an increased microcirculation (assessed by fluorescein dye) and a 30 to 50% greater tensile strength after 10 days. These results support the use of interrupted sutures rather than continuous sutures in situations in which impaired healing is anticipated and excessive tension is present. Since each passage of a suture through tissue creates a small wound, those patterns with a single passage, such as the simple interrupted pattern, create less inflammation than those patterns requiring a greater number of penetrations (e.g., vertical mattress and far-near-near-far suture).

When the biomechanical effects of fascial closure (tight versus loose apposition) were examined, wounds loosely approximated were stronger at 7 days after operation than wounds secured tightly with sutures. Consequently, it is recommended that wound edges just be apposed and overreduction of tissues be avoided. When excessive tension is present the use of tension suturing techniques is warranted.

Generally, the synthetic absorbable and nonabsorbable sutures cause less reaction than natural products (surgical gut, cotton, linen, and silk). A monofilament design suture has less reactivity compared to twisted and braided sutures. Polydioxanone (PDS; Ethicon, Inc) and polytrimethylene carbonate (Maxon; Davis and Geck) are relatively new monofilament synthetic absorbable sutures. They are reported to be stronger and less reactive than their braided synthetic counterparts, polyglycolic acid (Dexon; Davis and Geck) and polyglactin 910 (Vicryl; Ethicon, Inc). Although knot security is supposed to be improved and the tissue drag reduced, their handling qualities are generally less desirable.

Hematoma and Seroma

Collection of blood or serum within the tissues can delay healing by mechanically separating the wound. If the expanding fluid pressure is sufficient, it can also alter the local vascular dynamics enough to reduce the blood supply. Additionally, these fluids provide an excellent nutrient environment for bacterial growth. While hemoglobin inhibits local tissue defenses, iron is necessary for bacterial replication and the ferric ion may play a role in increasing virulence.

Hematomas, superficial or deep, can develop after blunt trauma, such as a kick from another horse, or if hemostasis has been less than ideal during a surgical procedure. A serous-like fluid can develop as a sequela to excessive accumulation of blood within the tissues, from excessive movement (e.g., grid flank incision in the horse), if a large dead space remains, or if reactive suture material such as surgical gut is used for closure. Meticulous hemostasis, elimination of dead space, proper drainage procedures, and appropriate bandaging techniques will often alleviate this problem.

Movement

Movement of one portion of the wound with respect to the other can disrupt neovascularization, cell migration, and the formation of early stromal elements within the wound. This results in prolonged wound healing, plus it promotes excessive scar tissue formation. Good suturing techniques, plus the use of appropriate bandaging and splinting techniques, can reduce the detrimental effects of movement. This is of particular concern with tendon lacerations in horses.

Bandaging and Dressing

Generally, bandaging is considered beneficial for the following reasons: (*a*) the wound is protected from further contamination; (*b*) the pressure reduces edema; (*c*) exudate is absorbed; (*d*) bandages increase temperature and reduce CO_2 loss from the wound surface, thus reducing pH; and (*e*) bandages can immobilize a part to reduce trauma (e.g., a wound on the dorsal surface of the hock). When discussing the effect of wound dressings on wound healing, one must consider the type of dressing.

Adherent dressings such as open mesh gauze, which allow newly formed cells to adhere and migrate into the dressing and absorb exudate, are beneficial when applied during the débridement phase and deleterious when used during the repair phase of wound healing. They aid the débridement of wounds by removing the absorbed exudate and necrotic tissue fragments. During the repair phase they tear loose the newly formed epithelial cells that are migrating across the wound bed and disrupt angiogenesis in the newly formed granulation tissue bed.

Nonadherent dressings (Telfa and petrolatum-impregnated gauze), either occlusive or semiocclusive, are most beneficial when applied to the wound during the repair phase. Depending on the type, they have been shown to enhance epithelialization and wound contraction. In humans, it was noticed that sutured wounds covered with nonadherent dressings had an epithelial covering in 24 hours, whereas similar wounds that were not bandaged did not have epithelial coverings for 72 hours. The composition of the nonocclusive dressing may also play a role. Several studies have documented slower epithelialization rates in wounds covered with USP petrolatum and white soft paraffin dressings. When the effects of petrolatum dressings, cotton nonadherent dressings, and rayon polyethylene dressings on wound healing were compared, a greater rate of wound contraction was observed at 7 days with petrolatum-impregnated dressings compared to others, but a decreased epithelialization rate between 7 and 21 days was seen compared to other dressings. The open mesh of the commercial petrolatum dressing allowed better absorption of the exudate and bacteria into the secondary overlying bandage. Biologic dressings such as porcine xenografts, even though they have reported benefits, are not used frequently because of the difficulty in obtaining them and the exorbitant cost.

Hydrophilic dressings such as copolymer flakes and dextranomer beads stimulate the diffusion of wound fluids through the tissue, from inside to outside, to bathe it; the fluids are then absorbed into the dressing. Through this process, tenacious coagulums on the wound surface are diluted and drawn into the dressings. Although not considered a substitute for débridement of wounds, hydrophilic dressings enable surface debris to be cleared and absorbed. Even though these dressings appear to have merit, they have not received wide acceptance in wound care in equine practice. Additionally a polyurethane foam dressing (Epi-lock; Calgon Vestal Laboratories) designed specifically to provide a moist healing environment is available. Though I have not had experience with this dressing, it is reported to enhance epithelialization and wound débridement.

Clinically, adherent dressings should only be used in the very early phases of wound healing when débridement is needed. If the wound requires little débridement but exudate and bacteria are present, the petrolatum semiocclusive dressings appear to be most beneficial. These dressings not only absorb the exudate and bacteria into the secondary bandage but may improve the rate of granulation tissue formation and subsequent wound contraction. After a healthy granulation tissue bed is formed, the use of other nonadherent semiocclusive dressings, such as Telfa (Kendall Company), is recommended.

Magnetic Fields

The use of magnetic dressings in the treatment of equine soft tissue injuries has become quite popular in Europe. Although they have been reported to increase circulation, reduce tissue inflammation, increase collagen synthesis, and suppress collagen lysis and keloid formation, the evidence of the effectiveness is largely speculative. When the effect of an Energy-Pak dressing that delivers 400 gauss with a maximum penetration depth of 7 mm on skin wound healing in rats was evaluated, no statistical difference was found between control (untreated) and treated (Energy-Pak) wounds, although a trend toward increased collagen synthesis in treated wounds was observed. Presently it is difficult to recommend the use of the magnetic field dressing until further work indicates a clearer benefit.

Blood Supply and Oxygen Tension

It is well recognized that healing wounds depend on adequate microcirculation to supply nutrients and oxygen for healing. Alteration in the microcirculation can occur from (*a*) applications of bandages or casts too tightly, (*b*) seroma formation, (*c*) tying sutures too tight, (*d*) local trauma, and (*e*) the use of local anesthetics with vasoconstrictive agents. Oxygen is required for cell migration, multiplication, and protein synthesis in healing wounds. Additionally, oxygen is required by the fibroblast for synthesis of collagen and the hydroxylation of protein, hydroxyproline, and lysine. Thus, the migration and synthetic capabilities of the wound fibroblast depend largely on the rate at which revascularization occurs. Since maintenance of the appropriate oxygen tension is the responsibility of the microvasculature, anything that impairs blood flow and subsequent delivery of oxygen will retard wound healing. Even though there is experimental evidence indicating that increased oxygen and hyperbaric oxygen (oxygen delivered under pressure) will accelerate wound healing, the clinical application in veterinary medicine has yet to be realized.

Temperature and pH

Wounds heal faster at higher temperatures and lower pH. Healing is accelerated at ambient temperatures of 30 °C compared to more normal room temperatures of 18 to 20 °C. Lower temperatures ranging from 12 to 20 °C reduce tensile strength in wounds by about 20%, whereas alternating warm and cold temperatures appear to delay wound healing. The application of warm hydrotherapy will accelerate wound healing. The inhibitory effect that lower temperatures have on wound healing appears to be a result of reflex vasoconstriction with subsequent reduction of local blood flow. Elevations in local wound temperatures by application of moist heat above 60 °C result in thermal injury to cells. On the other hand, moist heat at 49 °C applied to a recently incised wound appears to be optimum for acceleration of hemostasis. Warm water hydrotherapy presumably accelerates wound healing by increasing the blood flow.

When the effect of full-thickness skin burns and freeze-induced injury on wound healing was compared, it was noted that freeze-induced wounds did not contract, whereas the burn-created wounds contracted to one-third of their original diameter in 21 days. Evidently, slow removal and tissue replacement of the residual frozen tissue matrix reduce contraction. Histologically, the burn wound contained three times the amount of collagen found in normal skin and the freeze-injured skin contained only 1.75 times the amount of collagen seen in normal skin. The conclusion was that freeze-induced wounds healed more cosmetically than burn-injured wounds.

Acidification of a wound promotes healing by increasing the release of oxygen from hemoglobin. Alkalinity may result from loss of CO_2 from the wound or from urease-producing bacteria in the wound. Bandaging may be beneficial in that it increases the wound surface temperature and decreases the loss of carbon dioxide.

TREATMENT OF EXUBERANT GRANULATION TISSUE

Treatment of excessive granulation tissue has largely been by personal preference, including excision, cautery, cryotherapy, cast and bandage application, corticosteroids, counterirritation, and cytotoxic drugs. A few studies in the horse have documented the effect of different treatments on the formation of granulation tissue. In experiments using ponies as a model wounds on the dorsal surface of the fetlock left open to heal by second-intention healing and treated with casts and bandages produced more exuberant granulation tissue than wounds left uncovered with no treatment and wounds treated with cryotherapy. Although the wounds took longer to heal and excessive granulation tissue had to be removed, the cosmetic end result in wounds treated with bandage or cast was superior to those receiving no treatment and cryotherapy. The no treatment and cryotherapy groups developed more dermal fibrosis but healed more rapidly. The clinical significance of this trial remains uncertain, although it has provided valuable information regarding what can be expected with these four treatments on wounds left open to heal by second intention in these specific regions. It also gives the veterinarian some basic information as to the best approach for a given case where economic factors may be a consideration. Still of concern is the fact that ponies were used for the model of healing because they may not provide objective information about wound healing in mature horses.

The use of topically applied *N*-butyl cyanoacrylate in the treatment of open limb wounds in the horse has been evaluated. Although it was concluded to be cost effective and an efficient protective barrier to contaminants that suppressed the formation of exuberant granulation tissue, it has not been widely accepted as an approach to treatment at this writing, but can be considered as an alternative to treatment.

RECONSTRUCTIVE SURGERY

Tissue Expansion

Several new methods of tissue expansion to cover large, full-thickness skin defects in the horse are available. A "mesh expansion" method for mobilizing adjacent tissues to cover full-thickness skin defects has been evaluated experimentally and in clinical cases. Using this method the wound edges are undermined deep within the subcutaneous tissues, after which 10- to 15-mm tension-relieving incisions are strategically made in the undermined skin adjacent to the wound edge. As the skin is drawn over the wound the tension-relieving incisions expand as would occur with a mesh skin graft and the tension required for suture closure is reduced. Fifteen-millimeter long incisions are recommended when the skin is thickened and fibrotic (see Chapter 21).

A new technique that expands the normal tissues adjacent to the wound by stretching them two- to threefold is being evaluated. This is accomplished by inserting a temporary Silastic rubber expander in the subcutaneous tissues adjacent to the wound. Attached to the expander by a tube is a self-sealing injection dome that is implanted conveniently nearby yet remote to the Silastic expander. Tissue expansion is accomplished by injecting sterile saline into the injection dome until the skin becomes taut. Similar injections are carried out twice weekly until sufficient skin expansion has occurred to permit closure of the wound. Once expansion is sufficient, the expander and injection dome are removed and the expanded skin is undermined to cover the defect. Initially the expanded skin is thinner than normal, but this is short lived. Slow expansion of the skin is required to prevent necrosis. Generally the skin can be expanded to three times its original surface area. This technique is particularly attractive because normal skin with the same hair color and texture directly adjacent to the wound is utilized to cover the defect. Although this technique appears very exciting, more experience will be required before its full benefit and limitations will be appreciated.

Free Skin Flaps Using Microvascular Anastomosis

Large wounds, particularly those over the dorsal surface of the tarsus, remain difficult to treat by reconstructive surgical means. Recently a free skin flap technique using microvascular anastomosis was evaluated. Even though a large flank flap based on the caudal branch of the deep circumflex artery and vein was identified, attempts at transfer of the flap from the flank to the hock region using microvascular anastomosis to the tibial artery and vein resulted in failure in nine horses. Failure in these cases was due to a "no-reflow" phenomenon within the skin flap. More work needs to be done before the benefits of this approach can be realized.

A portion of this material was adapted from Stashak TS: *Wound Management and Reconstructive Surgery* Philadelphia, Lea & Febiger, in press.

BIBLIOGRAPHY

Amber EL, Swaim SF: An update on common wound antiseptics. *Aust Vet Pract* 1984;14:29–33.

Austad ED, Rose GL: A self-inflating tissue expander. *Plast Reconst Surg* 1982;70:588–592.

Bertone AL, Sullins KE, Stashak TS, Norrdin RW: Effect of wound location and the use of topical collagen gel on exuberant granulation tissue formation and wound healing in the horse and pony. *Am J Vet Res* 1985;46:1438.

Blackford J, Shires M, Gable D, Geiser D, et al: The use of *N*-butyl cyanoacrylate in the treatment of open leg wounds in the horse, in *Proceedings of the American Association of Equine Practitioners*, 1986, pp 349–355.

Chvapil M, Pfister T, Escalada S, Ludwig J. Peacock EE: Dynamics of the healing of skin wounds in the horse and compared with the rat. *Exp Molec Pathol* 1979;30:349–359.

Fretz PB, Martin GS, Jacobs KA, McIlwraith CW: Treatment of exuberant granulation tissue in the horse: Evaluation of four methods. *Vet Surg* 1983;12:137.

Geronemus RG, Mertz PM, Eaglstein WH: Wound healing: the effects of topical antimicrobial agents. *Arch Dermatol* 1979;115–1311–1314.

Leaper DJ, Foster ME, Brennan SS, Davies PW: Do magnetic fields influence soft tissue wound healing? A preliminary communication. *Equine Vet J* 1985;17:178.

Lee AH, Swaim SF, McGuire JA, et al: Effects of nonadherent dressing materials on the healing of open wounds in dogs. *J Am Vet Med Assoc* 1987;190:416–422.

Peacock EE Jr: *Wound Repair*. ed. 3. Philadelphia, WB Saunders Co, 1984; pp 122–136.

Schneiter HL, McClure JR, Cho DY, Crawford MP: The effects of flunixin meglumine on early wound healing of abdominal incisions in ponies. *Vet Surg* 1987;101(Abstr #79).

Speer DP: The influence of suture techniques on early wound healing. *J Surg Res* 1979;27:385–391.

9 Computed Tomography and Gamma Scintigraphy

David D. Barbee
Jennifer R. Allen

Technologic advances in diagnostic imaging over the last decade have revolutionized certain aspects of human medicine. Adaptation of some of these procedures for use in the horse has begun. One implication of technologic proliferation is that the clinician is confronted with more choices, and decisions about the most appropriate studies in an individual case are becoming more complex. The goal must be to obtain the maximum information with the least invasion at the lowest possible cost. This chapter outlines the indications, benefits, limitations, and cost of two contemporary imaging modalities: computed tomography and gamma scintigraphy.

COMPUTED TOMOGRAPHY

Computed tomography (CT) is so named because it uses a computer to reconstruct tomograms ("slice" or layer images). The term "computerized axial tomography" or "CAT scanning" is outdated because imaging is no longer restricted to the axial plane. To date, most applications of CT in veterinary medicine have involved small animals. However, with some modification of existing equipment CT scanning has been found feasible and valuable as a routine procedure in an equine referral center.

Principles

The CT scanner contains an x-ray tube and a series of radiation detectors that rotate under computer control around a circular aperture containing the patient. The percentage transmission of the highly collimated x-ray beam is measured at each degree of arc during rotation. These data are mathematically convolved by the computer to generate a cross-sectional image, in which each "pixel" or dot is assigned a number corresponding to its radiographic density. The result is displayed as a black-and-white image on a video monitor. It is also permanently stored as a numeric array on magnetic tape, allowing recall at any time for viewing or further manipulation under software control. A complete CT study consists of a sequential series of cross-sectional images taken at intervals (usually every 0.5 to 1.0 cm) through the region of interest.

Technical Advantages

The versatility of CT is difficult to appreciate from still photographs, because images on a CT video screen are normally viewed interactively. Computed tomography has a dynamic range of 2,000 density gradations. The viewer selects the level ("center") and range ("window") of densities displayed at any one time. Thus, it is possible to "remove" all soft tissue and examine bony structures in detail (Fig. 9–1A). Conversely, selecting a low center and narrow window allows detailed visualization of soft tissue components *in the same image* (Fig. 9–1B).

The digital nature of the CT image affords several further advantages. First, object sizes and distances are measured accurately and precisely, avoiding the problems of magnification and parallax errors encountered in conventional radiography. This feature has extensive utility in planning surgical approaches and repair methods. Second, quantitative density measurements may be obtained for any point or user-defined region of interest. In human medicine, such measurements have had clinical applications ranging from tumor identification to evaluation of osteoporosis. Third, software capabilities in image reformatting are impressive. These range from simple magnification and smoothing routines to generation of images in any desired plane by

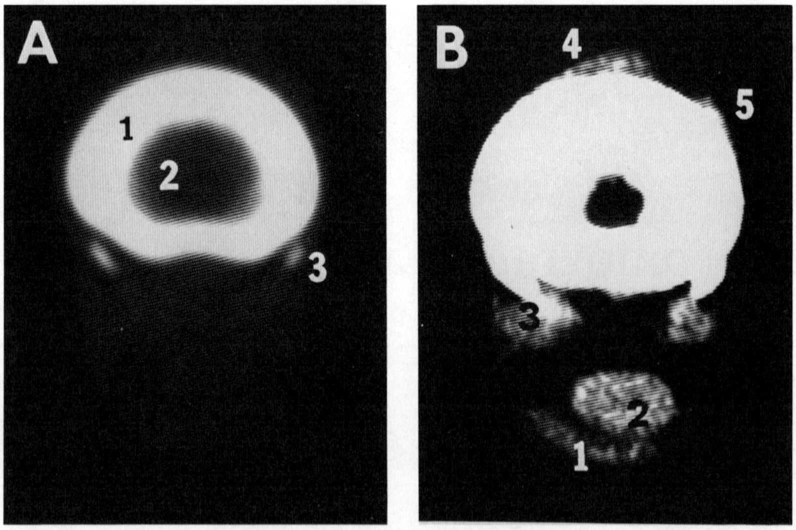

Figure 9–1. Two photographs of a single CT image from the distal metacarpal region of a normal horse. **A.** Viewed with window and center set to display bone and reject soft tissue. *1*, cortex and *2*, medulla of third metacarpal; *3*, fourth metacarpal. **B.** The same image viewed at a "tendon" setting. Material more dense than tendon (i.e., bone) appears white; material less dense than tendon (e.g., skin, loose connective tissue, blood vessels) is black. *1*, superficial and *2*, deep digital flexor tendons; *3*, branch of suspensory ligament; *4*, common and *5*, lateral digital extensor tendons. These photographs represent just two points from a continuum of density display combinations.

reprocessing of primary data. For example, it is possible to reformat a series of axial images into a longitudinal or oblique projection, at any time after the original scan. The most sophisticated software also yields three-dimensional image production.

Clinical Applications

Computed tomography is used routinely in a broad spectrum of human clinical problems, including abdominal, thoracic, and orthopedic disorders as well as central nervous system imaging. In the adult horse, physical limitations of scanner design currently restrict its use to the limbs, head, and neck. Thoracic and abdominal scanning are possible in foals and small ponies. General anesthesia is mandatory. However, anesthesia time is highly dependent on the type of scanner. Older models require from 45 minutes to 2 hours for a complete study. With newer equipment now available, image generation is 10 to 12 times faster, so positioning and preparation are likely to be the rate-limiting steps.

Skull. The osseous and dental structures of the equine skull are ideal candidates for CT imaging. Interpretation of conventional radiographs of this region is often hampered by anatomic complexity, superposition, and overlap. These problems are greatly simplified by cross-sectional anatomic representation on CT. The paranasal sinuses and individual tooth root structures can be examined thoroughly. The contents and morphology of the oral and nasal cavities, pharynx, larynx, guttural pouches, hyoid apparatus, temporomandibular joints, and the orbital, petrous temporal, and ethmoid regions are visualized in detail not obtainable with conventional techniques (Fig. 9–2).

Computed tomography is the technique of choice in diagnosis of disease of the equine sinuses and tooth root structures. It has also proven valuable in evaluation of cranial trauma, stylohyoid fractures, ethmoid hematomas, and neoplasia affecting the skull and for pre- and postoperative assessment of upper airway obstructions, including nasal septal deviations and malformations. In human medicine, this modality also has a prominent role in otolaryngologic imaging. For example, staging of human laryngeal neoplasia relies heavily on CT. Similar use in the horse depends on the type of scanner available. The lower resolution inherent with older machines hampers their capacity for detailed imaging of laryngeal structures. However, third- and fourth-generation scanners can be expected to contribute to evaluation of structural disorders of the larynx such as chondritis, malformations, and cysts. Computed tomography is not appropriate for diagnosis of functional complaints such as laryngeal hemiplegia or soft palate displacement.

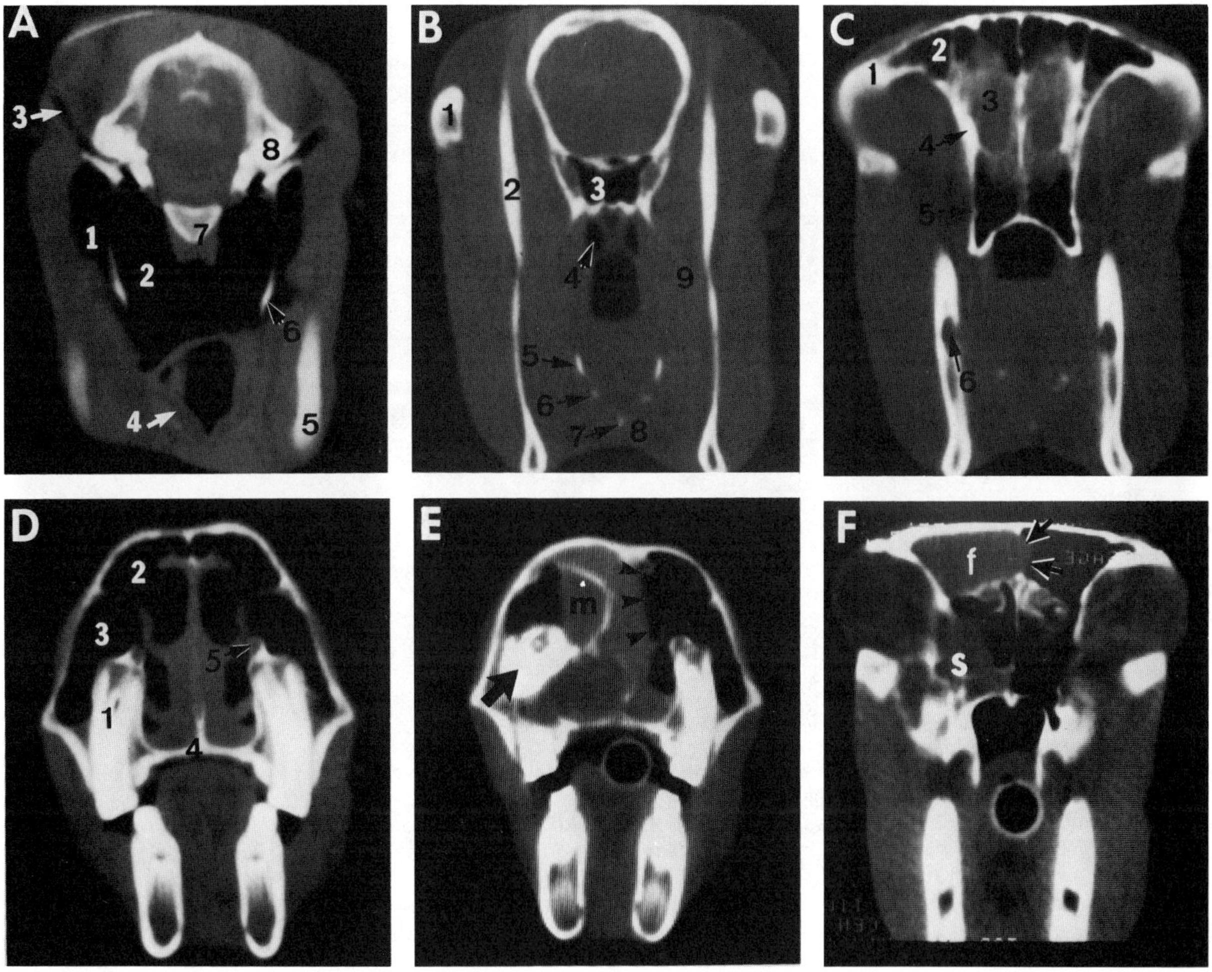

Figure 9–2. CT images of equine skull from a normal animal (**A** through **D**) and a clinical case (**E** and **F**). **A.** Plane through the temporohyoid articulation. *1*, lateral and *2*, medial compartments of guttural pouch; *3*, auditory canal; *4*, vocal fold, *5*, angle of mandible; *6*, stylohyoid bone; *7*, basilar part of occipital bone; *8*, petrous temporal bone. **B.** Plane just rostral to the temporomandibular articulation. *1*, zygomatic arch; *2*, vertical ramus of mandible; *3*, sphenoidal sinus; *4*, pharyngeal opening of guttural pouch; *5*, stylohyoid bone; *6*, thyrohyoid bone; *7*, lingual process of hyoid bone; *8*, omohyoideus muscle; *9*, medial pterygoid muscle. **C.** Plane through the ethmoid. *1*, supraorbital process; *2*, frontal sinus; *3*, lateral mass of ethmoid; *4*, orbital part of frontal bone; *5*, perpendicular part of palatine bone; *6*, mandibular canal. **D.** Plane through second molar (*1*). *2*, turbinate part of frontal sinus; *3*, maxillary sinus; *4*, hard palate; *5*, infraorbital canal. **E.** Image from the same level as **D**, from a 2-year-old gelding with dentigerous cyst of the root of the second molar (*arrow*). Note the fluid line in the maxillary sinus (*m*) (the horse was scanned in lateral recumbency), and the bulging of the nasal septum from the affected side (*arrowheads*). **F.** Image from the same animal as **E**, at a level similar to that shown in the normal horse in **C**. Note the fluid accumulation in the frontal (*f*) and sphenopalatine (*s*) sinuses and distortion of the median septum (*arrows*).

Limbs. Equine orthopedics is a second field in which CT has demonstrated considerable clinical utility. Visualization of regions of interest without superposition of adjacent structures is particularly useful in areas of complex anatomy, such as the carpus (Fig. 9–3), tarsus, and foot (Fig. 9–4). For example, neither the palmar surfaces of the carpal bones nor the intracarpal articulations are seen distinctly on conventional radiographs. Lesions in these areas that escape conventional radiographic detection can be clearly displayed on CT

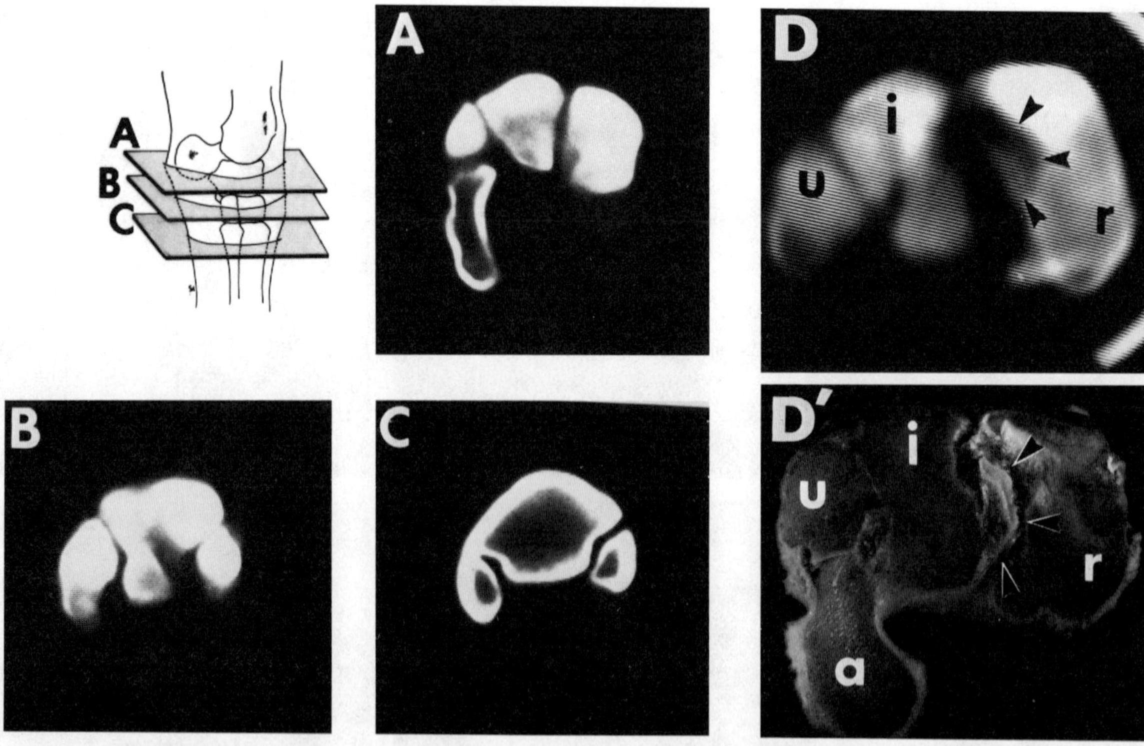

Figure 9–3. CT images of equine carpi. **A** through **C**. Images from normal horse through proximal row, distal row, and proximal metacarpus, respectively. Line drawing indicates the plane of each slice. **D**. Clinical case, image level approximately midway between **A** and **B**. Note the fracture of the axial aspect of the distal radial carpal bone (*arrows*). This fracture was not detected on conventional radiographic examination. *i*, intermediate, *r*, radial, and *u*, ulnar carpal bones. **D′**. Gross pathologic cross-section of the same carpus as **D**. The fracture fragment is denoted by *arrowheads*. The gross section is slightly proximal to the CT image and is somewhat oblique, hence the accessory carpal bone is visible (*a*) *i*, intermediate, *r*, radial, and *u*, ulnar carpal bones.

(Fig. 9–3). Similarly, erosive and cystic lesions in the palmar metacarpal region and proximal sesamoid bones have been diagnosed by CT after negative radiographic examinations. Although the ability of CT to diagnose lameness in the absence of radiographic abnormalities can be spectacular, a CT study is also indicated in many cases *after* conventional radiography has demonstrated osseous lesions. This practice permits more thorough assessment prior to surgery, reduces the risk of overlooking secondary lesions, and

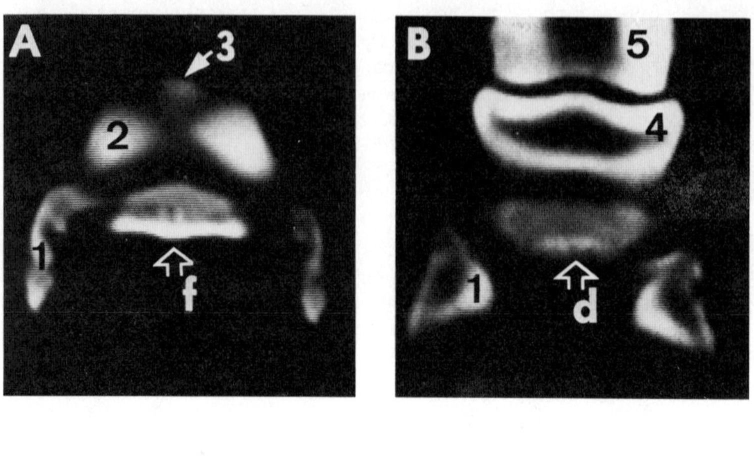

Figure 9–4. Two CT views of the navicular region of a normal horse. The plane of the scan was parallel to the coronary band in **A** and parallel to the longitudinal axis of the pastern in **B**. *Open arrows* indicate the silhouetted flexor surface (*f*) and distal border (*d*) of the navicular bone. *1*, wing of distal phalanx; *2*, condyle of middle phalanx; *3*, extensor process of distal phalanx; *4*, palmar aspect of proximal middle phalanx; *5*, palmar aspect of distal proximal phalanx.

allows more informed planning of the operative procedure.

Preliminary experience has shown that the sensitive density discrimination of CT gives good visualization of some soft tissue lesions in the limbs. For example, in villonodular synovitis the nodular mass is readily distinguished from accompanying synovial fluid distention of the joint capsule and subcutaneous edema can be differentiated from distention of tendon sheaths. However, conclusions regarding the clinical contribution of CT in horses with lameness of purely soft tissue origin must await controlled analysis of a larger number of cases. As yet no study has compared objectively the relative merits of CT and ultrasonography in equine tendon injuries.

Central Nervous System. The central nervous system (CNS) of the horse has long been a frustration to radiologists. Techniques of the "pre-CT" era such as pneumoencephalography and cerebral angiography were not often feasible in this species. Without the capacity for antemortem imaging, equine neurosurgery has lagged far behind developments in the human field.

Computed tomography now affords a means of noninvasive visualization of the CNS in live horses. Space-occupying lesions may be detected directly if they are associated with altered tissue density, or indirectly through displacement of the cerebral ventricles. The same iodinated contrast agents used for intravenous pyelography and cystography are routinely used for CT studies of the CNS. These agents do not cross the normal blood-brain barrier. They do, however, diffuse into CNS parenchyma, where there is disruption or increased permeability of the barrier, thereby outlining areas of inflammation, hemorrhage, or neoplasia.

Elaborate surgical intervention techniques for disorders affecting the equine brain are yet to be developed. However, the diagnostic means are now available for planning simple procedures such as treatment of abscesses or subdural hematomas. Experience in one case of CT-guided surgical drainage of a strangles-associated cerebral abscess indicates that this procedure can be feasible and clinically justified. For imaging of the equine spinal cord, CT does not replace myelography but it can be a useful adjunct to conventional techniques. In addition, the cross-sectional anatomic display provides valuable information for evaluating disorders of the vertebral column.

Limitations

Time, cost, and anesthetic risk are three factors to be considered. While economic constraints may be a limiting factor, expense is unlikely to preclude use of CT in most performance horses. Scan time is reduced substantially by modern equipment and goal-directed studies. Under optimal conditions, it is possible that CT could precede surgery within the same episode of anesthesia.

The quality and diagnostic value of a scan are influenced by a number of factors, including technical characteristics of the scanner and experience of the operator. As a rough guide, resolving power in the longitudinal plane is 0.5 to 1.0 cm for second-generation and 1 to 2 mm for fourth-generation scanners (resolution in the transverse plane is less than 0.2 mm for both types). Selection of the scan plane is therefore important, particularly in orthopedic applications (see Fig. 9–4). Small lesions may escape detection, especially if inappropriately positioned with respect to the chosen plane(s). Finally, CT is not free from artifacts. Interpretation requires some technologic understanding as well as familiarity with cross-sectional anatomy.

Summary

In summary, despite physical and technical constraints, CT offers a number of advantages over conventional radiography and greatly expands imaging horizons for the clinician. Its clinical utility is becoming increasingly evident and makes this modality a valuable adjunct to current diagnostic procedures.

GAMMA SCINTIGRAPHY

Nuclear medicine, also known as gamma scanning or gamma scintigraphy, is a well-established diagnostic modality in the health care of humans. This technology also offers benefits to the equine specialist. While the complex regulations covering the veterinary use of radioactive materials preclude significant use in private clinics, many veterinary colleges and some large equine care centers provide nuclear medicine services. Therefore, this section will provide the indications and rationale for using gamma scanning on a referral basis.

Technology

The technique consists of tagging a radioactive isotope to a physiologically active substance, injecting it intravenously, and using a gamma camera to detect the emitted radiation and visualize distribution in the patient's body. While several radioactive isotopes are used in human studies, the majority of equine studies are done with 99-metastable technetium (^{99m}Tc). This isotope has a 6-hour half-life, resulting in decay to background in 60 hours. Consequently, the patient can be released 3 days after the scan. As gamma camera technology has improved, the sensitivity of the scanners has increased to where a horse may be scanned standing, instead of requiring a general anesthetic. Each image may require from 10 to 120 seconds to acquire. Many scanners provide sophisticated computer analysis of the image, as well as dynamic measurements.

Studies

Bone Scan. The most common nuclear study in the horse is the bone scan. Usually ^{99m}Tc is tagged to a phosphate-containing molecule, such as medroic acid, which has affinity for areas of osteolytic and osteoblastic activity. The resulting images show a grey skeleton with a faint ghost of soft tissues. Active areas called "hot spots" are seen as darker grey to black regions. The anatomic resolution is inferior to radiographs, but the sensitivity is greater, allowing detection of lesions below the radiographic detection limit. Active areas may indicate normal physiologic activity, as is seen in growth plates, or abnormal activity, including arthritis, osteomyelitis, fractures, and tumors. The primary indication for a bone scan is occult lameness that has resisted diagnosis by other techniques. "Saucer" fractures, distal phalangeal fractures, and navicular conditions have been reported as examples of cases in which nuclear medicine aids diagnosis. A fracture may not be seen radiographically for nearly 2 weeks, but a negative bone scan 3 days after trauma is considered justification to remove fracture from the differential diagnosis list. A bone scan may be used to evaluate viability of a slow-healing fracture. Normal repair will be "hot," whereas devitalized bone or sequestra are "cold." Also, skeletal surveys in which radiography is too costly for examination of the entire animal may be done by nuclear means. Figure 9–5 is an example of a bone scan of a saucer fracture.

Kidney Scan. Prior to the application of diagnostic ultrasound, scintigraphy was the only way to image the kidneys of the adult horse. This procedure uses ^{99m}Tc tagged to a compound excreted by the kidneys, such as gluceptate. The normal kidney and urine-filled bladder image a dark black as a result of the intense concentration of the agent. Renal masses show as "cold spots" or filling defects. Total loss of renal function is suspected when no kidney image is seen. Besides static imaging of the kidneys, contemporary scanners are capable of computing glomerular filtration rates as a dynamic study. Figure 9–6 shows a kidney scan.

Blood Flow. Blood flow studies may be performed on either the pulmonary or the systemic circulation. Pulmonary blood flow information is critical in the diagnosis of pulmonary emboli and may be valuable in the

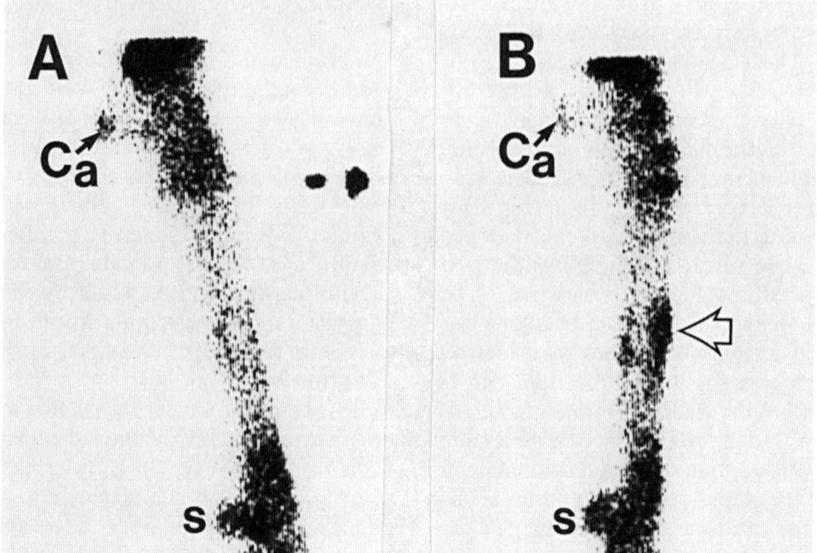

Figure 9–5. Bone scan of a 2-year-old thoroughbred with a 3-month history of right foreleg lameness. The scan was performed 2 hours after injection of 100 mCi ^{99m}Tc tagged to medronic acid. **A.** Lateral view, normal left foreleg. C_a, accessory carpal bone; *S*, proximal sesamoid bone (dorsal surface is to viewer's right). **B**. Lateral view, right foreleg (printed backward for comparison). C_a, accessory carpal bone; *S*, proximal sesamoid bone; *open arrow* indicates region of increased isotope uptake in dorsal aspect of metacarpal III from healing dorsal cortical stress fracture.

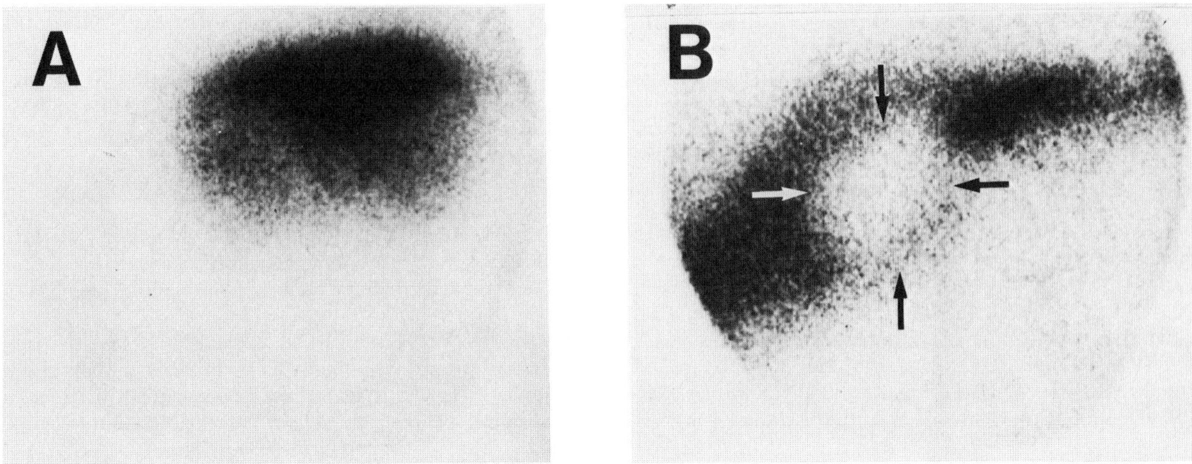

Figure 9–6. Renal scan of 14-year-old Thoroughbred mare performed with 115 mCi ^{99m}Tc tagged to gluceptate. Lateral views. **A**. Left side, cranial to viewer's right. Normal left kidney image. **B**. Right side, cranial to viewer's left. Right kidney not seen; in fact, *arrows* point to an area of decreased radiation. Postmortem examination revealed a large calculus occupying most of the right kidney.

study of exercise-induced pulmonary hemorrhage. Regional blood flow studies may be used to evaluate vascular supply to a traumatized limb or to localize arteriovenous malformations. A subspecialty of nuclear medicine is nuclear cardiology. Measurement of cardiac parameters by this essentially noninvasive method offers promise in exercise physiology and sports medicine, as well as clinical cardiology.

Brain Scan. Gamma scintigraphic scans of the brain often use the same agent as renal studies. In the brain scan, the compound cannot cross the intact blood-brain barrier. Therefore the normal study is "cold," showing a light grey from overlying muscles and little or no radiation detected from within the calvarium. Any condition that breaks that barrier allows agent to leak into the brain, causing "hot spots." Differential diagnoses include hemorrhage, infection, and tumors. In animals, CT scanning appears to be more effective in CNS diseases.

Other Studies. Additional organ systems may be examined, for example, the liver and thyroid glands. Fibrinogen has been tagged to seek thromboembolic lesions. Current research involving monoclonal antibodies as scanning agents may provide additional capabilities in the future.

Contraindications

Nuclear studies involve exposure to gamma radiation for both the patient and the operator. The dose to the patient is usually comparable with that from a major radiographic study, although the dose to localized regions, such as the kidneys during a renal scan, may be higher. Most state regulatory agencies demand that veterinarians hold scintigraphy patients until the isotope has delayed to background or normal levels of radioactivity. With ^{99m}Tc this means confining the patient for 60 hours after administration of the scanning agent. The exposure to operators can be minimized by proper technique. The term "nuclear" has adverse connotations to some clients, yet they seldom object to scintigraphy. The scanning agents used are essentially innocuous, with reactions being very rare.

Summary

In summary, gamma scanning is a valuable technique, especially in problem lamenesses. Progressive practitioners must understand the indications for these studies in order to obtain them in appropriate cases.

BIBLIOGRAPHY

Allen JR, Barbee DD, Boulton CR, Major MD, Crisman MV, Murnane RD: Brain abscess in a horse: Diagnosis by computed tomography and successful surgical treatment. *Equine Vet J* 1987;19:552–555.

Ambrose J: Computerized transverse axial scanning (tomography): Part 2. Clinical application. *Br J Radiol* 1973;46:1023.

Barbee DD, Allen JR, Gavin PR: Computed tomography in horses: Technique. *Vet Radiol* 1986;28:144–151.

Barbee DD, Allen JR, Grant BD, Riggs MW, Crawley GR, Sande RD: Detection by computed tomography of occult osteochondral defects in the fetlock of a horse. *Equine Vet J* 1987;19:556–558.

Collier MA, Rendano VT, Kallfelz FA: Repair of a delayed-union stress fracture of the dorsal cortex of a metacarpal bone in a horse. *J Am Vet Med Assoc* 1985;187:1040–1043.

Devous MD Sr, Twardock AR: Techniques and applications of nuclear medicine in the diagnosis of equine lameness. *J Am Vet Med Assoc* 1984;184:318–325.

Hornof WJ, Koblik PD, O'Brien TR: Use of nuclear scintigraphy to characterize an intrathoracic mass in a foal. *J Am Vet Med Assoc* 1982;180:1319–1322.

Kapoor W, Hemmer K, Herbert D, Karpf M: Abdominal computed tomography. Comparison of the usefulness of goal-directed Vs non-goal-directed studies. *Arch Intern Med* 1983;143:249–251.

Markel MD, Snyder JR, Hornof WJ, Meagher DM: Nuclear scintigraphic evaluation of third metacarpal and metatarsal bone fractures in three horses. *J Am Vet Med Assoc* 1987;191:75–77.

Potter GD: CT of the ear, nose and throat. *Radiol Clin North Am* 1984;22:1–280.

Stover SM, Hornof WJ, Richardson GL, Meagher DM: Bone scintigraphy as an aid in the diagnosis of occult distal tarsal bone trauma in three horses. *J Am Vet Med Assoc* 1986;188:624–628.

Theodorakis MC, Hillidge CJ, Allhands RA: External scintigraphy in evaluating delivery techniques of sodium cromolyn-[^{99m}Tc] diethylenetriaminepentacetic acid aerosol in the lungs of the horse. *J Pharm Sci* 1983;72:580–581.

10
Suture Materials

Robert R. Steckel

All sutures, whether absorbed from the wound site or permanent, are foreign bodies and cause a local inflammatory response. The magnitude of that response is determined by variables such as the size of the suture, the external physical and chemical properties of the suture, local trauma due to the type of needle used, and the manner in which the suture is placed. Suturing of the wound edges causes additional local trauma at the point where the needle and suture pass through tissue, resulting in a mild additional inflammatory response.

Controlled experiments and prospective clinical trials have shown that wound closure materials behave in a predictable manner based upon their physical and chemical characteristics. Physically, all braided or woven sutures cause more tissue trauma as a result of drag from their rough outer surfaces. In contrast, the smooth outer surface of a monofilament suture causes a negligible inflammatory reaction. Braided or woven materials also possess the undesirable property of capillarity. Tissue fluid "wicks" along the fibers of these materials and may cause bacteria to gain entrance after the wound has been closed. When different sutures were placed in fresh wounds and then purposely infected, two results were consistently observed. First, the presence of any type of suture in the wound resulted in a more severe infection than control wounds with no sutures present. Second, the braided or woven suture materials, regardless of their chemical makeup, caused a more severe infectious process than did the monofilament materials. This result held true in both acute and chronic studies, using the same number of infective microorganisms, comparing the same set of suture materials.

Chemically, absorbable sutures differ in the mechanism of their degradation in tissue. Catgut is a foreign protein that elicits a host immunologic cellular response in addition to the trauma of suture placement. Collagenase produced by phagocytic cells during the degradation of surgical gut is overall more inflammatory than the nonenzymatic hydrolysis of absorbable polymer sutures. In one study polyglactin apparently evoked a more intense early inflammatory response than surgical gut; however, additional histologic observations revealed that the intense reaction to polyglactin was short lived. Most investigators report the overall chemical reaction to absorbable polymer sutures to be mild when compared to catgut.

Synthetic nonabsorbable sutures react chemically similar to the absorbable polymer sutures. Physically, the same criteria regarding a rough or smooth outer surface apply. Stainless steel, although the most inert material chemically, can cause excess trauma during placement because of its stiffness and difficult knot tying, resulting in more nonchemical inflammation than nylon or polypropylene. The latter two materials are true monofilaments and both offer the same advantages of a smooth outer surface and noncapillarity, while possessing better handling properties than stainless steel. All three sutures have been proven, with very minor differences, to be chemically inert over prolonged periods of time in tissue. The most popular braided nonabsorbable suture, dacron, is also chemically inert, but possesses the inferior properties of a rough outer surface and capillarity characteristic of the absorbable multifilaments.

The type of needle used to suture wound edges has a slight influence on the healing surgical wound. In general, tapered-point needles cause less cellular destruction during passage through tissue than do cutting-point needles. Special thin-shanked needles are manufactured for bowel, bladder, and vessel suturing to reduce the size of the penetration hole, resulting in less leakage around the suture. The use of cutting-point needles should be restricted to dense collagenous tissue, such as the dermis. Unlike published information regarding the use of cutting needles in other species, the sheer density of some fascial sheets in horses (e.g., the prepubic tendon) requires a large cutting-point needle. Aside from these special areas, the tapered-point needle should be employed for most soft tissue suturing.

All the previously mentioned variables can affect the wound healing process after suturing. The concept of increased inflammation causing increased scarring and a stronger wound closure has been disproven. The optimum situation for normal wound healing is for the surgeon to use no larger a suture than necessary, and to be as atraumatic as possible.

The physiologic status of the patient and/or preexisting local inflammation or infection can adversely affect the wound healing process. Braided suture with its high capillarity, placed in a contaminated wound, often overwhelms the ability of the phagocytic cells to eliminate bacteria trapped in the interstices of the material, and local infection results. Smooth-surfaced monofilament sutures have been shown histologically to be preferable in the presence of local infection. When the surgical patient is in normal systemic health and the intended surgical site is not affected by abnormal local physiology, or excessive intraoperative bacterial contamination does not occur, all the currently available wound closure materials will perform acceptably. A horse in circulatory shock as a result of a strangulating gastrointestinal insult will have impaired ability to mount a normal inflammatory response, and the likelihood of local or generalized infection from contaminated intestinal surgery increases. The wound closure material proven to incite the least local inflammatory response, or with the least potential to induce local infection, should be chosen for both bowel and abdominal wound closures.

ABSORBABLE SUTURES

By definition, an absorbable suture is one that is eventually degraded after being placed in tissue. Ideally, the material holds the wound edges in firm apposition until the collagen gel secreted by fibroblasts begins to organize and gain tensile strength. Sutures that lose a significant portion of their initial tensile strength within 60 days after implantation are classified as absorbable, even though the "skeleton" of the material may remain in the tissue for a considerably longer period of time. Table 10.1 compares the relative degradation rates of the absorbable materials.

Surgical Gut

Catgut (Chromic Gut; Ethicon, Inc) is processed collagen from the submucosa of ovine or the serosa of bovine intestine. Plain catgut causes an intense inflammatory reaction and its use in general surgery is usually limited to vessel ligation. The addition of chromium salts hardens the raw material, increases its tensile strength, decreases its ability to initiate inflammation, and, depending on the amount of chromium salts added, delays its degradation. Catgut is one of the older suture materials available. Although newer synthetic materials are generally preferable because of their reduced inflammatory response, some surgeons still believe that surgical gut has its place in selected procedures because of its favorable handling characteristics and good knot security. The increased inflammatory reaction, however, can adversely affect wound healing and predispose to dehiscence if excessive swelling and edema result. If catgut is placed in a wound where excess tissue fluid is produced, it becomes slippery, and the knots can untie. Surgical gut has "withstood the test of time," but there are several absorbable sutures that are superior from a biologic standpoint for general equine surgery.

Absorbable Polymer Sutures

Three synthetic absorbable polymer sutures that offer distinct advantages over catgut are currently available for general wound closure. Polyglycolic acid (Dexon; Davis and Geck, Inc), polyglactin 910 (Vicryl; Ethicon, Inc), and polydioxanone (PDS, Ethicon, Inc) are all degraded by nonenzymatic hydrolysis. In other words, they simply dissolve. The polymers are first divided into monomers by water cleavage of ester bonds, then the individual monomers are metabolized to carbon

TABLE 10–1. LIST OF CURRENTLY USED ABSORABLE SUTURE MATERIALS FOR EQUINE PROCEDURES*

Suture Material	Physical Configuration	Tensile Strength Retention (days)	Degradation (days)
Plain catgut	Processed collagen	7–10	70
Chromic catgut	Tanned collagen	21–28	90
Polyglycolic acid	Braided	70% at 7 20% at 14	40–60
Polyglactin 910	Braided	60% at 14 30% at 21	60–90
Polydioxanone	Monofilament	70% at 14 50% at 28	210

* Information excerpted from the *Wound Closure Manual.* Somerville, NJ, Ethicon, Inc, 1985.

dioxide and water. This degradation process results in a substantially reduced inflammatory process because it is nonantigenic, and requires no cellular response.

Polyglycolic acid is a repeating homopolymer of glycolic acid. Polyglactin 910 is composed of glycolic and lactic acids in a 9:1 ratio. After breakage of the ester bonds, both glycolide and lactide enter the Krebs cycle, yielding carbon dioxide and water. Virtually no residue is left in tissue. Polydioxanone is similarly degraded, albeit at a much slower rate than the above two materials. The physical characteristics of these three sutures differ in that both polyglycolic acid and polyglactin 910 are braided multifilaments. They are limp and easily handled intraoperatively, but have the disadvantage of poor knot security. In contrast, polydioxanone is an absorbable monofilament that unlike the two previous sutures, has excellent knot security. This material lacks pliability, however, and can be difficult to handle in confined surgical openings. The larger sizes are brittle and occasionally fracture if mishandled.

Recently two new sutures have been made available and appear to be applicable for use in equine surgery. Polydioxanone has been modified to improve its handling characteristics (PDS II, Ethicon, Inc.). Polyglyconate is an entirely new absorbable monofilament which is eliminated from tissue by simple hydrolysis (Maxon, Davis and Geck, Inc.). Polyglyconate has superior tensile strength initially, but loses its strength twice as fast as polydioxanone. Both sutures possess excellent knot security while retaining desirable handling characteristics.

NONABSORBABLE SUTURES

A nonabsorbable suture is one that loses little to none of its original tensile strength after implantation in tissue for 60 days. Nonabsorbable sutures are indicated in procedures in which the normal healing process is slow (e.g., tendon reconstruction) or for use in the skin, where the suture will be removed. Older nonabsorbable materials like silk or cotton are no longer recommended for routine use because they cause an intense inflammatory response. None of the currently used nonabsorbable sutures are natural fibers. Nonabsorbable sutures are available in both multifilament and monofilament configurations. Table 10.2 lists the tensile strength properties of the commonly used nonabsorable sutures.

Nonabsorbable Multifilaments

Polyester fiber is a polymer of polyethylene trephthalate. These fibers are braided into one of the strongest sutures available (Mersilene; Ethicon, Inc), which has excellent handling characteristics and causes only a mild tissue reaction. Tensile strength loss over time is negligible. As previously stated, braided materials cause more tissue reaction as a result of their rough outer surface and resultant increased drag during placement. Various inert coatings such as Teflon (Tevdek; Deknatel) or polybutilate (Ethibond; Ethicon, Inc) have been added to the external surface of the suture to decrease drag and improve intraoperative handling. Un-

TABLE 10–2. LIST OF CURRENTLY USED NONABSORABLE SUTURE MATERIALS FOR EQUINE PROCEDURES*

Suture Material	Physical Configuration	Comparative Tensile Strength: Size 2-0 (Knot Pull Pounds)	Chemical Reaction
Polyester	Braided	6.0	Minimal
Nylon	Monofilament	6.5	None
	Twisted		
	Braided	4.8	
Polypropylene	Monofilament	5.7	None
Stainless steel	Monofilament or	13.1	Low
	twisted	10.7	

* Information excerpted from the *Wound Closure Manual*. Somerville, NJ, Ethicon, Inc, 1985.

fortunately, the low-friction coatings also reduce knot security, the largest disadvantage of these sutures.

A nonabsorbable braided suture is a liability in the presence of local infection. Bacteria become entrapped between the fibers, inaccessible to phagocytic cells. A suture sinus persists until the material is surgically removed. In spite of this potential complication, polyester suture has been used for years in equine surgery with overall good results. In such procedures as prosthetic laryngoplasty, the favorable handling characteristics counterbalance the undesirable physical properties.

Nylon suture is available as a multifilament, either twisted (Supramid; S. Jackson, Inc) or braided (Nurolon; Ethicon, Inc). The polyamide polymer of the individual fibers remains the same in both configurations. The twisted material is coated with a thin plastic sheath. Twisted multifilament nylon (Vetafil; S. Jackson, Inc.) has been and continues to be one of the most popular sutures for skin closure in all of veterinary surgery because of its low cost. Although the primary chemical makeup is only slightly reactive in tissue, the multifilament physical configuration harbors contamination. One possible mechanism of increased tissue inflammation is breakup of the plastic coating when tying this suture under tension (e.g., during closure of the linea alba). The equine surgeon should confine use of twisted nylon to closure of the skin. Braided nylon, while popular for use in human neurosurgery, has never gained wide usage in veterinary surgery.

Nonabsorbable Monofilaments

Monofilament nylon (Ethilon; Ethicon, Inc), as mentioned previously, is a polyamide polymer. Monofilament polypropylene (Prolene; Ethicon, Inc) is a homopolymer of polypropylene. Stainless steel wire (Steel Suture; Ethicon, Inc) is an iron alloy of chromium and nickel. All three sutures have been used extensively in veterinary surgery and have proven to be reliable, noninflammatory materials over a wide variety of applications. The major advantages of these sutures are their tensile strength, noninflammatory chemical composition, and smooth outer surface. The latter two properties make them the preferred materials in systemically compromised equine patients, or in any procedure in which the local wound environment may predispose to postoperative infection.

In equine patients, stainless steel suture sizes needed to close most wounds preclude safe intraoperative handling. One disadvantage of buried stainless steel suture is the potential for metal fatigue and initiation of a sinus tract months to years after the surgical procedure.

Monofilament nylon and monofilament polypropylene are used extensively in equine surgery. The advantages of their inert chemical nature and smooth outer surface are offset by their stiffness and overall poor knot security. Nylon is worse than polypropylene in both categories. Again, in contrast to polypropylene, nylon does undergo slow degradation in tissue, losing 30% of its original tensile strength over a 2-year period. In most instances this loss of strength is clinically unimportant. Both materials have a definite advantage for general wound closure in that any localized suppurative process postoperatively is self-limiting.

CLINICAL APPLICATION

The choice of suture material depends on the tissue strength requirement and suture reactivity. Table 10.3 lists the recommended suture type and size for routine

TABLE 10–3. RECOMMENDED SUTURE TYPE AND SIZE FOR SPECIFIC TISSUES IN EQUINE PROCEDURES

Tissue	Suture	Size
Linea alba	PDS or polyglactin	# 1–2
Subcutaneous tissue	PDS or polyglactin	# 000–0
Skin	Nylon or polypropylene	# 000–0
Vessel ligation	PDS or catgut	# 000–0
Intestine	PDS or polyglactin	# 000–00
Mesentery	Catgut or polyglactin	# 00
Bladder	PDS or polyglactin	# 00
Uterus	Polyglactin or PDS	# 00–1
Muscle fascia	Polyglactin or PDS	# 00–1
Joint capsule	PDS or polyglactin	# 00–0
Tendon repair	Nylon or PDS	# 1–2
Infected linea alba	Stainless steel or nylon	# 1–2
Laryngeal prosthesis	Coated polyester	# 5
Esophagus	PDS	# 00
Vaginal reconstruction	PDS or catgut	# 0
Inguinal ring	PDS or catgut	# 0–2

equine procedures, although this will vary among surgeons.

Fascial Closure

The adage of "surgeon's preference" is most applicable in the discussion of fascial closure. All of the sutures previously discussed, with the exception of stainless steel, have been employed extensively for fascial closure in the horse. Prior to the advent of the absorbable polymers, catgut was the mainstay of joint capsule, ligament, and muscle fascial closure. The absorbable polymer sutures are preferred, but the nonabsorbable synthetics may be used if the procedure has been clean and the patient is in good systemic health. The suture size depends on the particular structure being sutured, but sizes 3-0 through 1 are common.

Tendon Reconstruction

Severed flexor tendons pose a serious threat to the orthopedic soundness, and ultimately the life, of the equine patient. Recent research has shown the nonabsorbable monofilament sutures, in sizes 1 or 2, to be preferred. Since the wound environment is often not clean, braided suture of any kind is inappropriate for tendon reconstruction. The author has employed polydioxanone with good success as a substitute for nylon or polypropylene in selected cases where suture longevity was not required.

Bowel Closure

Traditional human surgical textbooks describing intestinal anastomotic techniques frequently cite the use of silk. The undesirable properties of this multifilament nonabsorbable material have caused silk to be largely replaced by absorbable sutures. Again, catgut was employed for years prior to the development of newer materials, but it is not recommended because of its rapid degradation and possible serosal inflammation. Virtually all the synthetic absorbable sutures, as well as monofilament nylon and polypropylene, may be used for general bowel closure or anastomosis in small suture sizes (2-0 or 3-0).

Linea Alba

All the discussed materials, including stainless steel, may be employed in the larger sizes, size 2 being minimum for adult horse breeds. Braided polyester is the only material available larger than USP size 2. Its use for linea alba closure, however, has not been popular over the years because of the frequent occurrence of suture sinus formation. With advances in equine abdominal surgery, original fears of incisional dehiscence continue to subside, as evidenced by the transition from various mattress suture patterns. Simple interrupted closure of the linea alba is probably the most commonly used pattern today. Continuous closure of the linea alba is being used more often. The continuous pattern has been shown to be stronger with in vitro testing when polyglactin 910 suture was used. The question remains whether the model sufficiently reproduces the clinical situation. One recent report indicates that a continuous linea alba closure compares favorably with interrupted patterns, and it can be employed to reduce operating time in physiologically compromised equine patients.

Subcutaneous Tissue

Ideally, if the deeper tissues are securely apposed, the subcutaneous reconstruction should substantially support skin apposition and eliminate dead space. All the previously mentioned materials, with the exception of stainless steel, can be employed in small suture sizes (3-0 to 0). Since the suture size is small, the stiff handling characteristics of the monofilaments are not a problem. There is little indication for nonabsorbable material, so again the synthetic absorbables are recommended.

Skin Closure

The nonabsorbable monofilaments are preferred for skin closure. Either nylon or polypropylene is commercially available in a wide variety of sizes, usually 4-0 through 2, prepackaged with swaged-on cutting needles. Polydioxanone, although absorbable, is also available prepackaged with cutting needles, and may be used for skin closure, since its degradation is sufficiently slow. Twisted nylon, as mentioned previously, still has a secure place in general equine surgery as a result of its low cost and favorable handling characteristics. Since skin sutures are typically removed during the proliferative phase of healing, it is hard to discriminate between these four materials for routine elective skin closure. For wound management where contaminating bacteria are invariably present in high numbers, the inert monofilament sutures, nylon and polypropylene, are preferred.

The author wishes to thank Ms. Barbara Matlaga, Ethicon Incorporated, Somerville, NJ and Dr. John Briddell, Pitman-Moore Incorporated, Washington Crossing, NJ for providing the illustrative material and statistical information about suture material, respectively.

BIBLIOGRAPHY

Jochen RF: Suture materials for large animal surgery, in Jennings PB (ed): *The Practice of Large Animal Surgery.* Philadelphia, WB Saunders Co, 1984, pp 1221–1233.

Looysen BS, DeBowes RM, Clem MF, Lundin CS, Leipold HW: Comparison of simple interrupted and continuous suture patterns for closure of the equine linea alba. *Vet Surg* 1988;17:36.

Nixon AJ, Stashak TS, Smith FW, Norrin RW: Comparison of carbon fibre and nylon suture for repair of transected flexor tendons in the horse. *Equire Vet J* 1984;16:93–102.

Schumacher J, Hanselka D, Adams G, Taylor TS: Stainless steel closure of the equine linea alba. *Equine Prac* 1981;3:47–53.

Stashak TS, Yturraspe DJ: Considerations for selection of suture materials. *Vet Surg* 1978;7:48–55.

Tate LP, Koch DB, Sembrat RF, Boles CL: Tracheal reconstruction by end- to-end anastomosis in the horse. *J Am Vet Med Assoc* 1981;178:253–258.

Tullners EP, Donawick WJ: Secondary closure of infected abdominal incisions in cattle and horses. *J Am Vet Med Assoc* 1983;182:1377–1379.

Varma S. Johnson LW, Ferguson HL, Lumb WV: Tissue reaction to suture materials in infected surgical wounds—A histopathologic evaluation. *Am J Vet Res* 1981;42:563–570.

Varma S, Lumb WV, Johnson LW, Ferguson HL: Further studies with polyglycolic acid (Dexon) and other sutures in infected experimental wounds. *Am J Vet Res* 1981;42:571–574.

UNIT II

Anesthesia

11
Preanesthetic Medication and Chemical Restraint

Melissa Holland

GENERAL CONSIDERATIONS

Preanesthetic agents currently recommended for use in horses fall into one of four principle categories: tranquilizers, sedative-hypnotics, opiate agonists and agonist-antagonists, and anticholinergics. The ideal preanesthetic medication would provide reliable patient cooperation, predictable analgesia, and good muscle relaxation with minimal adverse cardiopulmonary effects. Since no such agent has been developed, it is often necessary to use various combinations from the aforementioned categories to provide safe and effective preanesthetic sedation and/or standing chemical restraint in the equine species.

Drugs used to produce sedation or general anesthesia through variable degrees of central nervous system (CNS) depression also possess an array of other pharmacodynamic effects. The degree to which these effects will be manifest will depend on the patient's physical status, history of previous drug exposure, and individual temperament. All of these considerations will dictate agent selection and dose requirement. Tables 11–1 and 11–2 list the agents discussed in this review along with recommended dosage guidelines for the healthy elective equine patient. Not included, but of equal importance, are such preoperative adjunctive therapies as intravenous fluid replacement or supplementation and administration of nonsteroidal anti-inflammatory drugs and antimicrobials.

A precise description of all possible drug interactions is beyond the scope of this review; however, two potential such interactions deserve mention. These involve

TABLE 11–1. INTRAVENOUS DOSAGES OF DRUGS COMMONLY USED FOR PREANESTHETIC MEDICATION AND STANDING CHEMICAL RESTRAINT IN THE HORSE

Agent	Preanesthetic Dosage (mg/kg)	Restraint Dosage (mg/kg)	Comments
Tranquilizers:			
Acetylpromazine	0.03–0.05	0.05–0.08	Degree of sedation does not increase greatly with further increases in dose.
Sedative-hypnotics:			
Chloral Hydrate	15	30	Ataxia with higher doses.
Diazepam	0.04–0.1		Should not be used alone for sedation. Ataxia at higher doses.
Xylazine	0.3–0.6	0.1–1.1	1.1 mg/kg IV should be used prior to induction of general anesthesia with ketamine alone.
Detomidine	0.01–0.02	0.01–0.04	Prolongs the duration of ketamine anesthesia slightly when compared with xylazine.

TABLE 11–2. USEFUL DRUG COMBINATIONS FOR CHEMICAL RESTRAINT IN THE HORSE

Combination	Intravenous Dose (mg/kg)	Comments
Acetylpromazine- xylazine	0.02 0.6	Higher doses may produce profound hypotension (see Muir, 1981).
Xylazine- butorphanol	0.3–1.1 0.02–0.2	Various doses and methods of administration are recommended to achieve desired degree of sedation and analgesia. 1.1 mg/kg xylazine and 0.1 mg/kg butorphanol may be optimum (see Robertson and Muir, 1983) for surgical intervention in the standing patient.
Xylazine- morphine	0.3–1.1 0.3–0.6	Morphine should not be used alone in the horse without concomitant administration of a sedative to avoid excitement and undesirable motor activity.
Acetylpromazine- butorphanol	0.03 0.02–0.04	Excellent results as a preanesthetic medication.
Acetylpromazine- chloral hydrate	0.03 20.0	Excellent results as a preanesthetic medication.
Acetylpromazine- pentazocine	0.03–0.06 0.5	(See Riebold et al., 1982).
Acetylpromazine- pentazocine- chloral hydrate	0.03–0.06 0.3 12–25	Used along with appropriate local anesthetic technique for such procedures as castration and perineal laceration repair.
Detomidine- butorphanol	0.01–0.02 0.05–0.1	Ataxia is worse at the higher doses of these drugs.
Detomidine- morphine	0.01–0.02 0.3–0.6	Despite the longer activity of detomidine, morphine excitement may occur 2–4 hours after administration.

(*a*) the concurrent administration of phenylbutazone and barbiturates, and (*b*) the use of certain antibiotics prior to general anesthesia in which a potent inhalational anesthetic will be employed. The administration of the nonsteroidal anti-inflammatory drug phenylbutazone is common during the perianesthetic period. Phenylbutazone is highly protein bound, and, if it is given in the presence of an anesthetic agent with similar protein-binding characteristics (i.e., a thiobarbiturate), the anesthetic dose requirement of the barbiturate could be reduced. This reduction would be due to the availability of a higher unbound, and therefore, active drug fraction. Titration of anesthetic drugs to effect is recommended in these patients.

Aminoglycoside antibiotics interfere with neuromuscular transmission, enhance the blockade produced by neuromuscular blocking agents, and may also potentiate the muscle relaxation properties of the inhalational anesthetics. Neomycin is most often associated with acute muscular paralysis and apnea resulting from neuromuscular blockade. This effect can also be caused by kanamycin, amikacin, gentamicin, and tobramycin, in decreasing order of potency. In humans, most episodes of unexpected neuromuscular blockade have occurred in association with anesthesia or the administration of neuromuscular blocking agents. Furthermore, any patient that depends on hypoxemia for ventilatory drive should be carefully monitored for signs of respiratory depression when an aminoglycoside is used in the presence of an inhalational anesthetic. Finally, halothane anesthesia has been shown to prolong plasma half-life and clearance of gentamicin by approximately 50%, suggesting that a lesser dosage for gentamicin is necessary if this antibiotic is given in the perioperative period. This information has implications not only for neuromuscular function, but for renal function as well. Since gentamicin may cause proximal renal tubular damage even in unanesthetized patients, particular care should attend its use in patients whose renal blood flow and renal function may be adversely affected during general anesthesia.

Parasympatholytic agents (atropine, glycopyrrolate [Robinol-V]) are not required as preanesthetic medication in the horse and may in fact be detrimental. These agents decrease gastrointestinal motility and may lead to intestinal distention and ileus. Unlike other species, horses do not salivate excessively, and pulmonary secretion and laryngospasm do not significantly affect endotracheal intubation. Pupillary dilation may persist when atropine has been administered and horses may have difficulty walking after anesthesia because their depth perception has been altered. Therefore, the use of anticholinergics as routine premedicants is not necessary in the horse, and these agents are best reserved for the treatment of intraoperative bradycardia at recommended dosages of 0.01 mg/kg intravenously (IV) of atropine, or 0.006 mg/kg IV of glycopyrrolate.

TRANQUILIZERS

General Considerations

The major tranquilizers employed in equine practice are the phenothiazines. Acetylpromazine (Prom-Ace, Acepromazine) is the most popular agent of this group of drugs. Acetylpromazine may be used alone as the sole preanesthetic medication or in combination with other agents to produce a response ranging from mild tranquilization for minor procedures to potent neuroleptanalgesia for standing laparotomy. Phenothiazine derivatives exert a wide variety of actions on both the central and peripheral nervous systems, including antidopaminergic, anticholinergic, antiadrenergic, and antiganglionic activity. Generalized CNS depression leads to clinical behavior characterized by quieting, calming, indifference, and reduced motor activity.

Acetylpromazine causes no significant changes in heart rate or cardiac output and possesses antiarrhythmic activity. A reduction in hematocrit has also been reported consistently in horses given this agent. The most important cardiovascular effect of acetylpromazine is to produce arterial hypotension, primarily via peripheral α-adrenergic blockade and resultant vasodilatation. The use of acetylpromazine in situations in which exogenous or endogenous catecholamine levels are elevated as a result of excitement or fear could result in a dramatic fall in arterial blood pressure. This reaction is secondary to massive vasodilation caused by β-adrenergic receptor stimulation without concomitant vasoconstriction (α-adrenergic blockade). Most horses exhibiting this adverse reaction will respond to intravenous fluid administration at a rate of 16 to 22 mL/kg of balanced electrolyte solution given as a bolus. The use of α-adrenergic agonists (other than epinephrine) may also be considered. Contraindications to the use of acetylpromazine include major blood loss or marked dehydration (e.g., gastrointestinal disorders, profuse sweating).

Acetylpromazine demonstrates a number of other notable effects. Decreases in body temperature may be noted in foals or emaciated horses as a result of vasodilatation and resultant heat loss to the environment. Mild diuresis due primarily to decreased release of antidiuretic hormone accompanies the use of acetylpromazine. However, if arterial hypotension occurs, decreases in glomerular filtration rate and urine production might be expected to occur. Long-term paraphimosis has been reported following acetylpromazine administration. This effect appears to be dose related and occurs more frequently in stallions than in geldings. Although the incidence and duration of penile prolapse is greater at higher doses (>0.4 mg/kg IV), this effect has occurred at doses as low as 0.01 mg/kg IV. The author routinely uses a dose of 0.03 to 0.04 mg/kg IV in both stallions and geldings as preanesthetic medication and in neuroleptanalgesic combinations, with no long-term penile prolapse.

Clinical Use

Acetylpromazine may be used alone or in combination with a number of sedative-hypnotic drugs and opioid agonists and agonist-antagonists. Combinations commonly used or reported are given in Table 11–2. Acetylpromazine probably provides minimal if any analgesia and, therefore, some other agent possessing analgesic properties must be included if a surgical manipulation is to be performed. Xylazine (Rompun) (a sedative-hypnotic) and acetylpromazine are often combined when profound sedation and minor analgesia are desired. Some caution should attend use of this combination since the decrease in arterial blood pressure caused by acetylpromazine and the bradycardia and reduction in cardiac output produced by xylazine may lead to life-threatening hypotension in some individuals depending on dose given, degree of sympathetic stimulation, and preexisting circulatory volume.

SEDATIVE HYPNOTICS

General Considerations

Sedative-hypnotic drugs produce generalized CNS depression resulting clinically in a range of activity from mild, arousable sedation and muscle relaxation with decreased motor activity to total unconsciousness or coma. The effect depends on the agent and dose administered. This drug class includes barbiturates, chloral, and thiazine derivatives. Benzodiazepines have been variously classified as anxiolytics, minor tranquilizers, and sedative-hypnotics, and will be included with the sedative-hypnotics for the purposes of this discussion. The most commonly used agents in equine practice are xylazine, diazepam (Valium, Diazepam), chloral hydrate in its various forms, and detomidine (Dormosedan).

As a general rule, the agents in this classification do not produce analgesia until unconsciousness occurs. Exceptions to this generalization are xylazine and detomidine, which provide excellent analgesia for superficial and visceral pain at commonly administered sedative doses. Xylazine and detomidine are α_2-adrenergic agonists and are widely used to control pain associated with gastrointestinal disease, as preanesthetic sedatives, and as adjuncts to other analgesics for standing surgical procedures. Experimentally α_2-agonists are superior to opioid and other nonopioid analgesics for the relief of visceral pain. In contrast, sedative doses of other sedative-hypnotic agents may increase the patient's response to painful stimuli. Autonomic nervous system function is generally depressed by sedative-hypnotics. Again xylazine and detomidine are the exceptions to this generalization, having parasympathomimetic and sympathomimetic activity. Their α_2-adrenergic activity leads to a centrally mediated increase in vagal tone and baroreceptor activity.

Sedative-hypnotic agents produce a dose-dependent respiratory depression. Sedative doses of chloral hydrate produce minimal alteration in ventilatory function; however, at anesthetic doses respiratory depression is a significant complication. Because of this agent's narrow margin of safety at anesthetic dosages and its lack of analgesic activity at subanesthetic doses, its use should be confined to preanesthetic sedation or as an adjunct to opioid analgesia. The benzodiazepines (diazepam) have minimal effects on ventilation at routine dosages, whereas xylazine and detomidine may produce a decrease in respiratory rate and tidal volume. Upper airway obstruction due to laryngeal muscle relaxation and suppression of the cough reflex is associated with use of xylazine, and may increase the risk of aspiration and obstruction after upper airway surgery.

At sedative doses, chloral hydrate produces minimal change in arterial blood pressure and cardiac output, but first-, second-, and third-degree atrioventricular block may occur. Since xylazine, detomidine, and chloral hydrate are noted for producing similar bradyarrhythmias, their concomitant use should be avoided. The parasympathomimetic activity of xylazine and chloral hydrate may be countered with parasympatholytics (atropine, glycopyrrolate), but atropine does not reverse the initial bradycardia produced by detomidine. In addition to bradycardia, xylazine causes a decrease in cardiac output and an initial peripheral vasoconstriction as a result of its α-adrenergic activity, and may increase myocardial sensitivity to catecholamines in the presence of halothane. Arterial blood pressure initially increases, then decreases. Detomidine appears to have similar cardiovascular effects, although the initial hypertension is not followed by hypotension in the standing horse. Diazepam displays little adverse affect on cardiovascular function even at doses that produce recumbency.

The intravenous administration of xylazine in clinically recommended doses has been reported to produce ileus in horses lasting for up to 45 minutes. Results of a recent study indicated that xylazine administered intravenously either as a single 1.1-mg/kg dose, or repeatedly at the same dose, increases intestinal vascular resistance, motility, and oxygen consumption. Bowel viability may therefore be compromised by the simultaneous increase in oxygen demand and reduction in intestinal blood flow and oxygen delivery. Xylazine is a consistently effective analgesic for experimentally induced visceral pain, and is often used clinically for this purpose. However, in the light of this new evidence, the dose and frequency of administration may be of major clinical significance for postoperative intestinal viability. Detomidine is even more effective as an analgesic for visceral pain, and although its effects on the equine gastrointestinal system have not been investigated, it is likely that they will be similar to those of xylazine.

Sedative-hypnotics have various effects on the genitourinary system. Relaxation and temporary prolapse of the penis can probably be attributed to generalized CNS depression, and decreased uterine contractions may be associated with the use of xylazine. These agents cross the placental barrier, and the use of chloral hydrate in the mare is contraindicated at parturition because of the potent respiratory effect on the fetus. Xylazine at a dose of 1.1 mg/kg IV causes diuresis, decreased urine osmolality, decreased plasma antidiuretic hormone concentration, hyperglycemia, and hypoinsulinemia. Recently, an α_2-mediated reduction in antidiuretic hormone production or release has been postulated as the mechanism for xylazine-induced diuresis and decreased urine osmolality.

Clinical Use

In recent years, the clinical use of chloral hydrate has become less popular for sedation in the horse. Included among the reasons for this are (*a*) inability to produce clinically obvious sedation without significant cardiopulmonary depression and ataxia, (*b*) prolonged onset and duration of action, (*c*) lack of analgesia at subanesthetic doses, (*d*) lack of commercially available parenteral preparations, and (*e*) tissue necrosis if accidentally administered extravascularly. Despite these disadvantages, when properly used, chloral hydrate is still one of the safest and least expensive agents available for producing mild preanesthetic sedation in the horse. In combination with opioid analgesics, chloral hydrate is also useful for standing chemical restraint for minor surgical procedures such as castration and repair of lacerations.

Diazepam possesses excellent muscle relaxant properties but poor sedative characteristics when given alone to horses. At doses that do produce sedation (>0.15 mg/kg IV), ataxia may be a significant problem. This agent's primary use is as an adjunct to preanesthetic sedation or tranquilization, and to provide or augment muscle relaxation. The author has found diazepam at a dose of 0.02 to 0.04 mg/kg IV to be useful for augmenting xylazine's muscle relaxation when ketamine (Vetalar, Ketaset) is to be used as the induction agent.

Xylazine has proven useful as a preanesthetic medication when used alone or in combination with an opioid analgesic, an anesthetic, or a tranquilizer for more profound hypnosis or surgical anesthesia. Its onset, duration of action, and clinical effects are very predictable in most equine patients, and there are few absolute contraindications. Because xylazine is a potent sedative-hypnotic, other anesthetic agents must be carefully administered in order to avoid adverse cardiopulmonary effects. The judicious postanesthetic use of xylazine in small incremental doses of 0.1 to 0.3 mg/kg IV has been advocated to prevent a violent recovery and potential injury to the horse. The use of xylazine has been associated with an incidence of unpredictable hind limb movement and the occurrence of well directed kicks from an apparently well-sedated patient.

Detomidine is more useful as an analgesic and as an agent for standing chemical restraint than as a preanesthetic drug. It is much more potent than xylazine and will provide adequate restraint for minor procedures at doses as low as 10 μg/kg. At this dose, the sedation appears within 2 minutes and reaches a maximum level around 5 minutes with a duration of 20 to 30 minutes. At 20 μg/kg the sedation lasts for 50 to 60 minutes and at 80 μg/kg the effects last 3 to 4 hours. Detomidine would normally be given by intravenous injection, but the intramuscular route is effective, with the onset of action being delayed by 4 or 5 minutes. The analgesic effects of the drug are more profound than with xylazine, but there appears to be the same increased sensitivity to stimulus on the hind legs with low doses of detomidine (10 μg/kg). At doses above 20 μg/kg, the analgesia over the hind end of the horse is more consistent but shorter in duration than for the front legs. Side effects noted with this drug include sweating and piloerection. When used as a preanesthetic agent for induction with ketamine, detomidine can be given at a dose of 20 μg/kg 2 to 3 minutes before the ketamine. If the patient is going to be induced with a barbiturate, the detomidine can be given 15 to 20 minutes before induction. Compared with xylazine, detomidine combined with ketamine or barbiturate increases the time to recumbency and prolongs the time to recovery (induction to sternal recumbency takes about 25 minutes, with the horse standing by 30 minutes).

OPIOID AGONISTS AND MIXED AGONIST-ANTAGONISTS

General Considerations

Opioids act by reversibly combining with one or more specific opioid and nonopioid receptor sites in the brain and/or spinal cord, clinically producing sedation, euphoria, analgesia, excitement, and dysphoria. Commonly used agents in this group include morphine, a pure agonist, and butorphanol (Torbugesic) and pentazocine (Talwin-V), mixed agonist-antagonists. A number of other agents comprise this group; however, this discussion will be confined to these three, since they have proven most useful for the equine species.

In general, the ability of a given opioid to produce sedation and analgesia or excitement and dysphoria is dependent on the opioid receptor(s) for which the drug has affinity, the dose administered, the species, and the severity of pain that may be present. Excitement and inappropriate motor activity are undesirable conditions in the equine patient for which sedation, analgesia, and immobilization are needed. Recent evidence suggests that 0.22 mg/kg IV of butorphanol produces effective visceral analgesia in healthy horses; however, the same dose also commonly leads to excitatory behavior and ataxia in horses and ponies. To alleviate this effect butorphanol and other opioid agents are usually combined with a tranquilizer or sedative to produce neuroleptanalgesia. To further complicate the clinical picture, most opioids do not depress responses to tactile, visual, or auditory stimuli. Consequently, the use of these agents in a horse that is not in pain may lead to undesirable behavioral changes and increased motor activity. Conversely, administration of an opioid to a horse already experiencing pain usually results in a calming effect, with reduction in the behavioral activity that was previously indicative of pain.

Routinely recommended dosages of butorphanol, morphine, or pentazocine do not produce significant adverse cardiovascular effects. The vagally mediated bradycardia reported in other species is infrequent in the horse, probably because of the apparent increased susceptibility of the horse to the CNS excitatory properties of these agents. Therapeutic doses of opioids, when given to horses previously administered tranquilizers, sedatives, or anesthetics (inhalant or parenteral), usually produce clinically insignificant reductions in cardiac output, heart rate, and arterial blood pressure.

Opioids are potent depressants of all functions of ventilatory drive. The degree of respiratory depression produced is agent and dose dependent and may be evident at doses that do not result in obvious CNS depression. Opioid agonist-antagonists as a group demonstrate a ceiling effect on depression of respiratory function. Reductions in minute ventilation and response to increases in arterial P_{CO_2} are dose dependent to a point, beyond which no further depression of ventilatory function occurs regardless of dose. Pure agonists such as morphine do not exhibit this ceiling effect.

Clinical Use

In the horse, opioid agonists and agonist-antagonists are recommended for the alleviation of pain. Morphine is reportedly better for superficial than visceral analgesia in this species. Butorphanol provides visceral analgesia that is superior to that of morphine or pentazocine, and in combination with xylazine (1.1 mg/kg IV) produces a synergistic analgesic effect. A combination of 0.1 mg/kg IV of butorphanol and 1.1 mg/kg IV of xylazine given together produces optimal analgesia without ataxia for flank laparotomy. Butorphanol, morphine, and pentazocine have been used alone and with xylazine for the alleviation of gastrointestinal pain. While these agents often do provide excellent visceral analgesia in the horse with colic, their judicious use is cautioned in situations in which the cause of pain has not been adequately delineated and the masking of important clinical signs could delay appropriate surgical intervention.

BIBLIOGRAPHY

Greene SA, Thurmon JC, Benson GJ, Tranquilli WJ: Antidiuretic hormone prevents xylazine induced diuresis in mares. *Vet Surg* 1986;15:459.

Lindberg LA (ed): Sedative and analgesic effects of detomidine in horses and cattle. *Acta Vet Scand* 1986;82:1–208.

Muir WW: Drugs used to produce standing chemical restraint in horses. *Vet Clin North Am Large Animal Pract* 1981;3:17–44.

Riebold TW, Goble DO, Geiser DR: Anesthetic drugs, in Riebold TW (ed): *Large Animal Anesthesia, Principles and Techniques.* Ames, Iowa State University Press, 1982, pp 9–16.

Robertson JT, Muir WW: A new analgesic drug combination in the horse. *Am J Vet Res* 1983;44:1667–1669.

Robertson JT, Muir WW: Cardiopulmonary effects of butorphanol tartrate in horses. *Am J Vet Res* 1981;42:41–44.

Smith CM, Steffey EP, Baggot JD, Dunlop CI, Farver TB: Effects of halothane anesthesia on the clearance of gentamicin sulfate in horses. *Am J Vet Res* 1988;49:19–22.

Stick JA, Chou CC, Derksen FJ, Arden WA: Effects of xylazine on equine intestinal vascular resistance, motility, compliance, and oxygen consumption. *Am J Vet Res* 1987;48:198–203.

12 Induction and Recovery Techniques

Peter J. Pascoe

Before anesthetizing any horse, one needs to have the animal prepared and the equipment available for the procedure. Preparation of the animal for an elective procedure should include 18 hours of preoperative starvation. A horse that is anesthetized with a full intestine is much more likely to become hypoxemic during the period of recumbency. A thorough physical examination should be performed so that there are no surprises once the animal is anesthetized. A practical preanesthetic checklist is provided in Chapter 16. The horse's mouth should be washed out before the procedure, especially if an endotracheal tube is to be used. Having prepared the patient and set up for the surgical procedure, anesthesia can now be induced. The main factor in this process is safety, both for the patient and for the people who are assisting with this maneuver.

OUTDOOR SITE

When dealing with the outdoor environment, one is subject to the whims of the elements. Since an anesthetized animal has usually lost its ability to thermoregulate, its body temperature will drift toward the ambient temperature. This is not normally a problem for a short procedure, but in areas of extreme climate one should try to protect the animal. In a cold environment place a layer of straw on the ground to help insulate the horse from the cold earth and use a blanket over the animal during the surgery. In a hot climate the provision of shade and a cold water spray will aid in controlling body temperature.

The site chosen for induction of anesthesia should be large enough that the horse can stagger a few paces and not come into contact with any sharp objects. In a grassy paddock the area should be inspected carefully to make sure that there are no dangers hidden by the grass. It is also important that the surroundings be quiet, as noisy environment will stimulate the horse and make it more difficult to obtain a smooth induction and recovery. Because the horse is going to fall to the ground, the landing should be as soft as possible. In areas where the ground is hard, it is a good idea to make a straw mattress for the horse to lie on as it goes down. Padded blankets attached to the horse have been used by some individuals as an alternative to padding the ground. These blankets will protect the horse as it goes down and will also provide some insulation in a cold environment.

The horse's halter should be strong and snug enough that it will not slip off. The lead shank should be made of a soft, thick cotton rope so that it can be held with little risk of a rope burn to the handler. Such an item is relatively inexpensive and should be part of the veterinarian's anesthesia kit. The strong halter and the rope enable the person holding the animal to control the head and lessen the risk of injury during induction. Padded head protectors are also available. These protectors should not be relied upon to hold the horse's head because they are difficult to adjust to a snug fit.

The method used for holding the horse will depend on the location and to some extent the drugs used. With thiobarbiturate inductions, in particular, horses have a tendency to drop their hind quarters first, pulling the forequarters and head over backward. The person controlling the head needs to be aware of this tendency and should be strong enough to prevent it. If it is necessary to make the horse land on a particular spot, up to six people may be needed to support the horse during the induction. One person should be on the head, one on each shoulder and hip and one on the tail. After the anesthetic has been administered, these assistants attempt to support the horse so that it sinks to the ground. If little help is available and the paddock is soft and even, the only support needed is the person on the head collar. A person holding the tail may be able to prevent the horse's rump from hitting the ground hard and may also be able to control whether the horse falls onto its right or left side. Turning the head to one side or the other just prior to the horse going down will help cause the horse to fall in the opposite direction. Once the horse is recumbent, the eyes should be covered to protect them from dust and strong sunlight.

For the recovery, the horse should be stimulated as little as possible so that it arouses quietly. One wants the horse to attempt to stand only when it is competent to do so, and excessive prodding may force it into a premature and stormy recovery. The footing must be good so that the horse does not slip as it tries to get up. One of the biggest advantages of anesthetizing horses outside is that the footing is usually secure. The individual holding the lead shank should stand close to the dorsal part of the head. When the horse gets up, it is going to become sternal first and then move forward. Standing in front of the horse or by the feet can be dangerous because the animal may push the person over as it gets up. After the horse stands, it is often necessary to support the horse at the head and tail briefly until it regains its balance. Excessive lifting of the head during this period may cause the horse to lose its balance.

INDOOR ARENA

From some points of view, an indoor arena provides an ideal environment for equine anesthesia. The ground is soft, the footing is excellent, the ambient temperature is not extreme, and there is plenty of space for the recovery. However, it is also a very dusty place and so it does not provide an ideal surgical environment. Most of the comments applicable to an outside induction apply to an indoor arena. There is a choice between inducing anesthesia with the horse against a wall at the side of the arena or in the middle of the area. If a wall is chosen, it must extend the full height of the horse so that there is no risk of the animal falling or rearing over the wall. It is also important to protect the horse's eyes because dust from the arena may be very irritating. This can be accomplished by placing a clean cloth underneath the head and folding it over the upper eye. If the horse is positioned in dorsal recumbency a cloth is placed under the head and wrapped up over the mandible.

INDOOR STALL

Because of current management practices for racehorses, it is often necessary to carry out surgery in a box stall. These are often very small (e.g., 10 × 10 ft), so it is essential that the induction be as smooth as possible. To accomplish this the horse must be well tranquilized and the area should be quiet. The stall must be inspected to make sure that there are no hidden hazards for the animal. For example, does the wall of the stall come all the way to the ground? A horse could get its foot caught under a wall that does not reach the ground and fracture its leg during induction or recovery. There should be no fixed objects attached to the wall that could injure the horse or the people involved in anesthetizing the horse. Ideally the stall should have plain bare walls that extend from the floor to a height of at least 8 feet. The bedding should be clean but not too voluminous. A dusty environment will increase the risk of contamination of the surgical site and so straw is preferable to either shavings or peat. However, it is better not to lay a fresh bed of straw immediately prior to the surgery because this will also raise the level of dust.

Under these circumstances, it is essential that the anesthetic induction provide a very controlled transfer of the animal from vertical to horizontal. Only two people should be present in the stall at the time of induction, one holding the head and the other to support the side of the horse. With more people present, there is an increased risk of personnel injury if the horse falls away from the wall. Usually the horse will be positioned with its tail in the corner and the side that is to be operated upon against the wall. The induction then proceeds and the horse crumples gently to the ground and falls outward so its feet are pointing toward that wall.

In a small box stall the horse should be left to recover on its own. It is too dangerous to be in such a small space with a horse that may be incoordinated as it attempts to rise. The footing must be good and the horse must be positioned so that it has enough space to move forward as it stands up. The environment should be kept as quiet as possible during this recovery.

CLINIC

The induction and recovery area at a clinic can be very simple (e.g., a single tilt table) or it can involve a very sophisticated design to ensure personnel and patient safety, optimum surgical conditions, and a one-way traffic flow. The process of taking a 450-kg animal from vertical to horizontal, preparing it for surgery, operating, and then providing a safe environment for recovery is fraught with problems. This section will review some of the standard approaches to these problems.

One Room for Induction, Surgery, and Recovery

The single-room arrangement has the advantage that the horse does not need to be moved. Whenever the animal is moved, there is a risk of injury to personnel (e.g., back injury) and to the patient (e.g., falling off a table). Moving the horse is also a significant risk relative to the anesthetic since it is difficult to monitor the animal while it is being moved and alterations may occur in the equipment that could endanger the patient. For example, a flow meter could be turned off, the endotracheal tube could be kinked, or a catheter could be dislodged. From the surgical perspective, this system has the serious disadvantage that it is going to be hard to provide a clean environment. The flooring in such a unit must provide a good grip for the horse during recovery and by definition such a surface cannot be totally smooth and cleanable. The horse may urinate and defecate during recovery and the combination of a rough floor with this gross contamination provides a poor surgical environment. If the surgeries are not to be performed on the floor, then a hydraulic table sunk into the floor or a hoist that can pick the horse up and place it on a table is needed. The latter would be preferable since the table could be stored in a clean place between surgeries. However, these tables are often very heavy and do not move very well on a rough floor. The other major disadvantage with this system is that one has to wait for the horse to recover before carrying out the next surgery.

A variation on this theme is the tilt table used for induction, surgery, and recovery. Under the right conditions this can work very well, but the disadvantages with respect to surgical sterility apply as above. One also has to wait for the animal to recover and it seems that horses take longer to get up from a tilt table than they do when placed in a recovery stall. The induction and recovery periods carry some risks in that the horse must be brought into a metal stall and strapped to the table before the induction. This requires careful handling and heavy sedation of the patient. Most tilt tables have inadequate padding for a prolonged surgery and so the risk of myositis is increased. This can be overcome by the addition of a thick foam pad or a waterbed mattress. However, it is hard to preplace these before induction and so they must be added after the horse is on the table. This can be achieved with the help of several assistants, or a ceiling hoist mounted above the table can be used to reposition the animal. Horses can be placed in dorsal recumbency on a tilt table, but usually the surgeon only has access to one side of the horse.

Induction and Surgery in the Same Room with a Separate Recovery Stall

This system requires transport of the animal to the recovery stall but there is less risk to the horse because it is in a light plane of anesthesia. It also means that the floor for the surgery can be kept cleaner since it does not have to be as rough because the horse is not going to recover in this area. Nevertheless, the floor must be padded so that the horse does not injure itself as it goes down and the walls should be free of any major projections. The surgical site also has to be prepared in this area, which means that it is not as clean as it could be. This system was used successfully for many years at the Ontario Veterinary College.

The recovery stall either has to be big enough to allow people to stay with the horse or small enough so that the horse does not injure itself during recovery. A small stall should be 12 by 12 ft with the corners cut off so that the animal cannot get itself stuck in a corner. A small room allows the horse to rise but prevents it from gaining a lot of momentum as it staggers in this limited space. In a bigger stall the horse can get up a lot of speed as it is falling and staggering and it is therefore more likely to injure itself. If someone is going to stay with the horse, the room should be at least 16 by 14 feet. In either case the room should have escape doors that will allow personnel to get out quickly and easily but prevent the horse from escaping at the same time. Less satisfactory methods include the provision of a bar at about a height of 7 feet above the ground or strong vertical ropes on the walls with the ends at a reachable height. These devices allow one to pull oneself up and out of the way of the horse. If a horse is to be recovered with people attempting to control the animal, it is essential to limit the number of people in the stall. If more than three individuals are present, the risks of injury rise dramatically. To control the horse, the neck should be held in extension. The handler(s) should lean over the horse from the dorsal part of the neck and hold the head and neck down as long as possible. Holding the nose up with the neck on the floor or mat keeps the horse from using its head to attain momentum.

The walls of the recovery room should be smooth and free from any projections. Any power points, gas outlets, air vents, or rings should be recessed into the wall so that they can be covered with padding. The room should be padded to a height of 7 to 8 ft. The padding can be fixed and sealed to the wall or it can be loose padding that is hung from the wall. The latter is cheaper and easier to replace, but care must be taken to ensure that the horse does not get stuck behind or entangled in such loose padding.

The floor is probably the most critical feature of a recovery stall. It must be soft enough so that the horse does not injure itself if it falls. It must also have excellent traction so that the horse can get a good footing and not slip, and this grip must be maintained even when the floor gets wet. On top of this it must be possible to hose the floor down to get it as clean as possible. Additionally, it has to be very durable to cope with the abuse associated with equine recoveries. A floor consisting of 2 in of dense foam rubber covered with a rough sheet of rubber with grit bonded into this material provides most of the desired features. However, it is still rough and can be difficult to clean. Many clinics are now using vinyl-covered thick foam pads (10 to 12 in thick) for recovering horses and report good results with this material. The pads are soft and the horses appear to stay down longer on these pads compared with a standard recovery room floor. Thus once the horse attempts to stand it is usually awake enough to make a substantial effort with less ataxia. These pads provide good traction because the horse's feet sink into the pad and do not slide even when the pads are wet.

Combined Induction and Recovery Room with a Separate Surgery

This system is also commonly used but it suffers from the same problem as the first type. That is, one has to wait for one horse to recover before the next procedure can be started. A common design feature with this setup is to have a table or trolley as part of the induction/recovery room floor. The horse is induced and either falls onto or is moved onto a section of the floor that can then be wheeled into the surgery. This achieves the aim of separating the surgery from the preparation and recovery area and should therefore provide cleaner surgical conditions. It introduces a new problem in that either the floor of the recovery room has to be at a different level than the surgery or the table has to be on a hoist that can be lowered into the ground. If the induction/recovery area is raised above the surgery, one may have to use a ramp to get the horse into the room. This can be a problem with some animals. The other factor is that the drainage from the room is going to be down into the surgery, with a clear risk of contaminating the "clean" room. These problems can be avoided by using a pit for the table, but this increases construction costs because of the hoist and the fact that the pit has to be drained as well. This system also requires that the horse be moved and so it carries the risks associated with transport.

Separate Induction, Surgery, and Recovery Rooms

This is the most costly system to set up because it requires the most floor space. The main advantages associated with this system are that it makes the preparation area cleaner and more convenient and induction of the next case is possible as soon as the first animal goes into the recovery stall. This unidirectional flow is only an advantage in a busy clinic where one is attempting to do several surgeries in a day. The induction area presents the same problem as noted above in that either the floor must be higher than the surgery or a pit must be used to contain the table. One cheaper alternative to these approaches is to use a beam and hoist in the ceiling. Once the horse has been anesthetized, it is picked up and placed on the table. This can be done by using either hobbles or a net that is applied to the horse prior to induction. With this latter technique, the net is attached to the horse and provides excellent support for the torso as the animal is picked up, and it avoids the tension on the legs associated with the use of hobbles.

The induction room needs to have a method for restraining the horse well and must have enough space for the horse to be positioned and prepared for surgery. It should also be possible to drop the horse in such a way that it can be positioned in right lateral, left lateral, or dorsal recumbency. Figure 12–1 shows the induction stall at the Ontario Veterinary College, and shows the half-doors used to assist with the restraint of the animal. Once the animal is in this position, anesthesia can be induced quietly and safely. The pit in the floor holds a surgery table that can then be raised to floor level once the horse has been allowed to roll out on to the table. The pit is 2.5 ft from the wall, and this has worked very well for putting horses in lateral recumbency, but the animal must be pushed back toward the wall if it is going to be rolled into dorsal recumbency. One other problem to account for is that the door into the surgery should be wide enough to take the table and its leg supports. At some other institutions there has been a further separation in that the induction room leads into a preparation room and then on into the surgery. This has the advantage of separating the raised floor of the induction area from the surgical suite.

GENERAL TECHNIQUES FOR POSTANESTHETIC RECOVERY

If a horse is to be anesthetized for longer than about half an hour, its halter should be removed and should not be put back on the animal until the horse has stood up. This is to reduce the risk of nerve damage from the pressure of the straps. If someone is to be present to

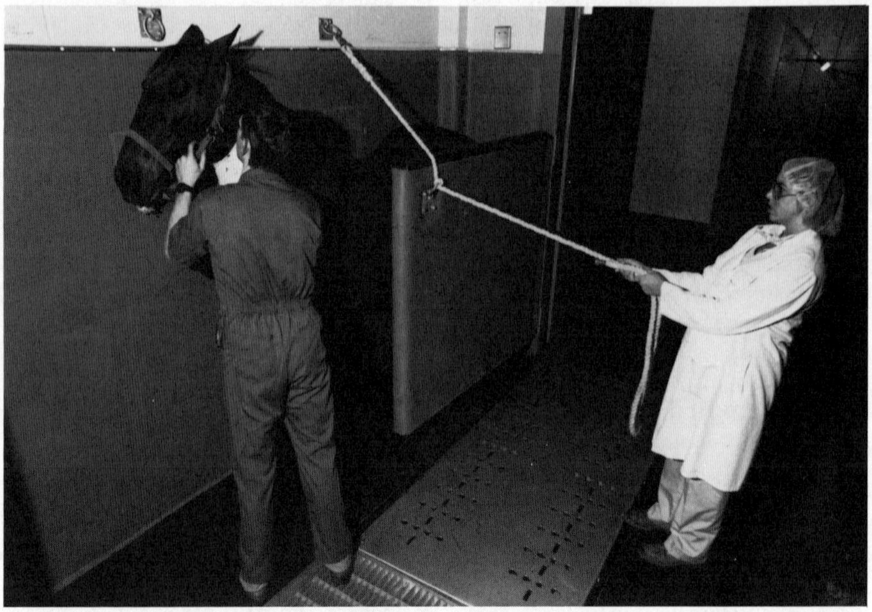

Figure 12–1. An induction stall showing the half-door used to restrain the horse and the pit containing the surgical table. A thick rubber mat is placed over this while the horse is being led into the induction room. The induction drugs are given and the animal collapses gently to the ground between the door and the wall. The table can then be lowered so that a 12-in thick pad can be placed on the table. The half-door is allowed to swing out and the horse then rolls out onto the pad. The table is then raised to floor level so it can be wheeled into the surgery.

assist the horse during recovery, then a padded head collar can be applied and used to assist in controlling the animal. This type of head collar reduces the risk of injury to the patient.

Oxygen supplementation during the recovery period has been the subject of much controversy. Accepted dogma stated that this was useful in increasing the arterial oxygen tension (P_aO_2) and this in turn would benefit the animal, leading to less disorientation during recovery. Some horses suffer from a partial upper airway obstruction during recovery; this can be reduced by passing a nasotracheal tube and fixing it in place during the recovery. In severe cases it is also possible to leave the endotracheal tube in place and tape it so that it comes out of the side of the mouth. If it is possible to measure P_aO_2 or arterial oxygen saturation after the animal has been on room air for a few minutes, it is then feasible to treat only those animals with low values. If this is not possible then it is better to treat all animals.

Oxygen supplementation should be given using a long tube (4 ft) that is passed through the larynx and down toward the carina (tubes that only supply gas to the nose will not make a large difference in the inspired oxygen tension). An oxygen flow rate of 15 L/min is used in an average-sized horse, and will raise the inspired oxygen to 30 to 50%. In animals that have a normal amount of venous admixture occurring in the lungs (20 to 30% is common following anesthesia), this supplementation will increase the P_aO_2. In animals in which the degree of venous admixture approaches 50%, this supplementation will not significantly change P_aO_2 unless an oxygen demand valve is used. This device will deliver a rapid flow of oxygen to the horse until the back pressure from the lung exceeds the preset value on the valve (usually 25 cm H_2O).

CONCLUSION

As can be seen from the above discussion, there are advantages and disadvantages with any of the induction-surgery-recovery layouts described. The anesthesiologist would prefer that the patient be induced and operated upon in one place, whereas the surgeon would like to have the clipping and preparation areas separate from the surgical suite. Everyone wants to minimize the amount of lifting and carrying that has to be performed to get the horse through the surgery. The safety of the patient and the personnel must be a prime consideration in the design. The type of facility used will depend largely on the funds available, the expected numbers and breeds of horses that are seen by the clinic, and the personnel available to assist with the procedures.

BIBLIOGRAPHY

American Association of Equine Practitioners: *Elements of an Equine Hospital,* Veterinary Economics Magazine, 1979.

Boss RL: Organization and implementation of anesthesia, surgery and intensive care in an equine practice, in *Proceedings of the American Association of Equine Practitioners.* 1985; pp 731–736.

Flynn DV: Soft mattresses in recovery, in *Proceedings of the American Association of Equine Practitioners.* 1976, pp 53–60.

Hall LW: Anesthesia of the horse, in Hall LW, Clarke KW (eds): *Veterinary Anaesthesia.* London, Balliere Tindall, 1983, pp 203–244.

Knapp JE, Anderson R: Large animal surgery, in *The Floor Plan Book of Veterinary Hospital Design.* Lenexa, Veterinary Medicine Publishing Company, 1986, pp 41b-47b.

Taylor PM: Anaesthesia, in Hickman J (ed): *Equine Surgery and Medicine.* London, Academic Press, 1985, pp 1–104.

13 Intravenous Anesthesia: Induction and Maintenance

Cynthia M. Trim

Intravenously administered anesthetic drugs may be given as a single injection to produce short-lived anesthesia for a minor procedure or to allow endotracheal intubation preparatory to maintaining anesthesia with an inhalation agent. Injectable drugs may also be given in increments to prolong anesthesia in an anesthetized horse. Greater knowledge of the physiologic responses of horses to anesthesia and the availability of new drugs have resulted in potentially safer general anesthesia. However, some problems still exist as a consequence of the horse's size and temperament. Specific management techniques must be used to prevent hypoxia and to minimize the risk of injury during recovery from anesthesia.

Oxygenation

Pressure of the abdominal organs on the diaphragm in an anesthetized horse dramatically decreases the volume of the lung when compared to that of the conscious animal. Addition of anesthetic-induced depression of ventilation and decreased cardiac output results in decreased arterial oxygen tension (P_aO_2). The risk of hypoxia increases with time because alveolar collapse progresses as the duration of anesthesia increases. Many drug combinations used to produce anesthesia result in respiratory rates not very different from values in awake horses. It should be remembered that low oxygen tensions may develop at these rates.

A variety of methods have been used to improve arterial oxygenation. Decreasing the volume of gastrointestinal contents diminishes the degree of lung collapse. One recommendation is to withhold hay and grain for 18 hours before anesthesia; water is allowed. Despite this preparation, ventilation during anesthesia may be inadequate. Supplementing the horse's inspired air with oxygen may prevent hypoxia. Oxygen may be delivered from an oxygen cylinder and flow meter via rubber tubing inserted up the nose or via an endotracheal tube. Oxygenation will be increased when the distal end of the oxygen delivery tube is passed deep into the trachea. An oxygen flow of 15 L/min should maintain normal arterial oxygenation in an adult horse provided that its respiratory rate is not depressed. Alternatively, a demand valve may be attached to an endotracheal tube and, drawing oxygen from an oxygen cylinder, used to artificially ventilate the anesthetized horse with a mixture of air and oxygen. The valve may be triggered by the patient's spontaneous respiratory movements or may be triggered manually.

Artificial ventilation can be accomplished in foals by attaching a resuscitator (Ambu) bag to an endotracheal tube. The inspired air can be enriched with oxygen by attaching an oxygen supply to the bag. Portable anesthesia machines are available (Summit Hill Laboratories) and can be used even though anesthesia is maintained with injectable drugs. Adequate arterial oxygen tensions should be achieved when the horse breathes 100% oxygen via an endotracheal tube attached to an anesthesia machine. An advantage of this system is that the contents of a small oxygen cylinder (E tank) should last 2 hours, compared with 10 minutes when using a demand valve.

Recovery from Anesthesia

Muscle weakness during recovery from anesthesia can cause horses to lose balance and fall, or make an uncoordinated movement, such that injury occurs. The goal for the recovery should be to have a tranquil horse with good muscle tone, so that the horse has no difficulty in standing up. The degree of sedation and muscle tone will be influenced by the type and amount of anesthetic drugs used. Thiobarbiturates are detoxified slowly; therefore, multiple dosing results in a slow decline in blood concentration and persistent muscle weakness. Redistribution and elimination of ketamine is more rapid in horses, and muscle weakness after several small supplementary dosages is not much greater than after a single dose.

Antagonists of anesthetic drugs have been used to enhance the speed of recovery, decrease the time to standing, and treat excessive central nervous system depression or cardiopulmonary collapse. The opiate antagonist naloxone (P/M Naloxone) will reverse the effects of pentazocine (Talwin-V) or butorphanol (Torbugesic). Diprenorphine (Revivon) is marketed specifically to reverse effects of etorphine (Large Animal Immobilon), and its administration is rapidly followed by the horse standing up. Doxapram (Dopram) is a respiratory stimulant that may be used in an emergency situation and will also partially counteract the effects of xylazine (Rompun) and other central nervous system depressant drugs. Yohimbine, a central α_2-adrenergic receptor blocking drug, has been used to reverse sedation caused by xylazine. Intravenous administration of yohimbine to ponies sedated with xylazine and anesthetized with thiopental caused them to regain their feet in a third less time than ponies that had not received yohimbine. Administration of yohimbine to horses anesthetized with xylazine and ketamine resulted in a shorter time to standing, but the emergence from anesthesia was described as rough, with repeated attempts to rise, head weaving, ataxia, and hypersensitivity to sound stimuli. Administration of 4-aminopyridine (4-AP), a drug with a central stimulatory effect, significantly decreased the time to standing in horses similarly anesthetized, and the recovery from anesthesia was fairly smooth. Yohimbine and 4-AP are still under experimental investigation. More potent and specific α_2-adrenergic antagonists, with fewer side effects than yohimbine, are being developed.

PREANESTHETIC SEDATION

A tranquilizer or sedative is almost always administered to horses before anesthesia to facilitate an excitement-free, relaxed induction. The drugs that are used have been described in detail in Chapter 11. It should be remembered that the degree of preanesthetic sedation produced should be considered when calculating the dosage of anesthetic drugs.

DOSAGE OF ANESTHETIC DRUGS

The dosages given in this section are to be used as a guideline and should be modified according to the individual patient. In general, a higher drug dose rate will be needed to cause anesthesia in an excited, anxious, or untrained horse than in a calm pleasure horse. This should be taken into account when calculating the dose of drug to be administered. However, administration of larger doses of anesthetic drugs may result in greater respiratory and cardiovascular depression and decrease the likelihood of a smooth recovery. Consequently, to minimize the effect of excitement and anxiety on drug requirements, a horse that is to be anesthetized should be handled quietly and efficiently. When the horse has been transported to an unfamiliar environment, a smoother anesthetic period is often obtained if the horse is allowed to remain overnight before anesthesia is administered.

The age of the patient should be considered when calculating drug doses. Generally, the young horse (<3 years) will need a higher dose than the adult, and an old horse (15 years and above) will need a lower dose.

Dose rate is also modified by body size of the patient; small horses require a higher dose rate than the average 450-kg (1,000-lb) horse, and horses over 550 kg require a lower dose rate. The decrease in dose rate is particularly apparent in adult draft horses and may be partly related to their smaller blood volume (72 mL/kg) compared with that of hot-blooded horses (100 mL/kg).

Some veterinarians have reported inadequate anesthesia produced in ponies, donkeys, and mules, particularly with the xylazine and ketamine combination. The author has had good results in these animals with the suggested dose rate of xylazine 1.1 mg/kg, and ketamine 2.2 mg/kg, but others have recommended that the initial dose rate of both drugs be increased 10 to 33%.

THIOPENTAL OR THIAMYLAL

Clinical Effects

Anesthesia with thiopental sodium (Pentothal) or thiamylal sodium (Bio-Tal, Surital) is usually preceded by administration of acetylpromazine (Prom-Ace, Acepromazine) or xylazine to facilitate a smooth induction of anesthesia and smooth recovery. The horse should become recumbent approximately 30 seconds after intravenous injection of thiobarbiturate, and anesthesia will last up to 15 minutes.

Arterial blood pressure is decreased significantly for the first 1 to 2 minutes after injection of the thiobarbiturate and then increases toward the normal resting value. Heart rate is significantly increased initially and progressively decreases to a normal rate after 15 minutes. Cardiac output is decreased. Apnea may be present for 20 seconds immediately after the horse becomes recumbent. The respiratory rate may be normal during anesthesia or assume a cluster breathing pattern involving runs of 2 to 6 rapid breaths separated by pauses. The P_aO_2 is usually low when the horse breathes air.

Administration

Acetylpromazine, 0.04 mg/kg or xylazine 0.6 to 1.1 mg/kg are commonly used intravenously to provide preanesthetic sedation. The degree of sedation predetermines the dose rate of thiobarbiturate. Thiopental 10 mg/kg may be injected after acetylpromazine tranquilization, whereas after xylazine 1.1 mg/kg a thiopental dose of 5.5 to 6.6 mg/kg is more appropriate. Thiamylal is a more potent drug than thiopental and the dose rate varies from 7.5 mg/kg in mildly sedated horses to 4.4 mg/kg in horses sedated with xylazine 1.1 mg/kg. A 5 or 10% solution of thiobarbiturate provides a convenient volume of drug for injection, but either concentration will cause tissue damage if accidentally injected outside the vein. When this happens, several milliliters of lidocaine, 2% without epinephrine, and 100 to 200 ml of saline should be infiltrated in the area in an attempt to decrease the degree of damage.

Horses that are anxious or have been excited may require a higher dose rate to produce anesthesia. In contrast, horses with low plasma proteins or who are ill will require less drug. Administration of thiopental or thiamylal to foals less than 8 weeks of age may result in a prolonged effect. Other drugs produce a better quality of anesthesia in foals.

Additional barbiturate may be administered to prolong anesthesia. An initial supplemental dose of 0.44 mg/kg should be injected and then further drug given to effect. Several supplementations will more often cause a poor recovery from anesthesia.

Recovery

Horses will usually stand about 30 minutes after a single injection of thiobarbiturate. Standing may be smooth and accomplished with ease. More frequently, horses stand after one or more unsuccessful attempts accompanied by muscle weakness and ataxia. In a prospective clinical trial, ponies were sedated with xylazine 1.1 mg/kg and anesthetized with either thiopental 5.5 mg/kg or ketamine 2.2 mg/kg. The quality of recovery from thiopental anesthesia varied equally between good and poor, whereas recovery from ketamine anesthesia was more frequently good to excellent, with few poor recoveries.

Modifications

The dose rate of barbiturate may be decreased when it is administered with guaifenesin. This combination results in less cardiovascular depression and a better recovery from anesthesia than administration of the barbiturate alone.

A technique that has been used in the past to improve muscle relaxation and provide a smoother induction of anesthesia has been to inject succinylcholine immediately after the injection of barbiturate. Succinylcholine must not be used in horses that have been treated with an organophosphate compound within 2 weeks because prolonged apnea may occur.

THIOPENTAL OR THIAMYLAL AND GUAIFENESIN

Clinical Effects

Guaifenesin (Gecolate) (also known as glyceryl guaiacolate or guaiacol glycerine ether) is a muscle-relaxing drug that is thought to act on the polysynaptic pathways in the spinal cord. There is evidence that guaifenesin may cause sedation and this may be due to action on the reticular formation of the brainstem. Because guaifenesin does not cause anesthesia, it should not be used alone in a healthy horse to provide immobilization or for a procedure that would be expected to cause pain. Instead, guaifenesin should be included in an anesthetic protocol to provide muscle relaxation and a smooth transition from the standing position to recumbency. Use of guaifenesin also allows a reduction in the dosage of anesthetic drugs.

Administration of guaifenesin or guaifenesin and thiobarbiturate to healthy sedated horses results in significantly increased heart rates for 5 to 10 minutes. Arterial blood pressure is significantly decreased. Respiratory rate is increased and the tidal volume decreased after infusion of guaifenesin. The arterial carbon dioxide tension (P_aCO_2) may be normal or increased. The P_aO_2 is usually decreased.

There have been concerns that guaifenesin may cause hemolysis. However, in vitro and in vivo studies of 5 or 10% solutions in water or in 5% dextrose did not produce evidence of hemolysis. Another study of various solutions demonstrated no changes in blood red cell count and hemoglobin concentration, or in urine hemoglobin concentration after administration of 10 or 15% solutions. Evidence of hemolysis was present after infusion of a 20% solution.

Administration

Healthy horses are sedated first, for example, by intravenous injection of acetylpromazine 0.04 mg/kg or xylazine 0.6 mg/kg. The thiopental or thiamylal and guaifenesin may be administered together or separately. Two grams of thiopental or thiamylal and 50 g of guaifenesin are usually sufficient to cause anesthesia in a 450-kg horse. They may be mixed together and infused at dose rates of up to 4.4 mg/kg thiobarbiturate and 110 mg/kg guaifenesin. The horse will assume recumbency when half the dose has been administered and then the remainder should be given until the desired relaxation has been obtained. Alternatively, the drugs may be administered separately. The guaifenesin should be infused until the horse appears to be heavily sedated (about 50 mg/kg), at which point the barbiturate should be injected as a bolus. Additional guaifenesin should be administered when the horse is recumbent. It should be remembered that the maximum effect of guaifenesin develops several minutes after administration has ceased. Excessive administration is accompanied by hypotension, respiratory depression, and rigidity of the limbs. The advantage of administering both guaifenesin and a barbiturate simultaneously is that the dosage can be tailored more closely to individual requirement and the infusion stopped when adequate anesthesia has been obtained. The disadvantage is that the onset of anesthesia is relatively slow and a period of incoordination may result. Incoordination should be avoided when the calculated dose of barbiturate is administered as a bolus.

Horses that are excited or have an athletic, lean body conformation may require a higher dosage of drugs to cause anesthesia. In horses weighing more than 550 kg, and particularly in adult draft horses, an equivalent effect is achieved with lower dosages of drugs. A survey of records at the University of Georgia revealed that healthy adult draft horses sedated with xylazine 0.35 to 0.5 mg/kg, required 15 to 20% less than the calculated dose of thiobarbiturate and guaifenesin. Depressed or ill horses will also require a lower dose rate to cause anesthesia. Immobilization of severely ill patients for endotracheal intubation before inhalation anesthesia may be accomplished with a lower ratio of barbiturate to guaifenesin, or even with guaifenesin alone.

Guaifenesin is most commonly used as a 5 or 10% solution in North America and as a 15% solution in European countries. In North America, guaifenesin is available as a powder that must be dissolved in water or 5% dextrose solution, or may be purchased as a sterile prepared 5% solution of guaifenesin and dextrose. Guaifenesin may be administered by gravity flow through a large-bore rubber infusion set and a large needle or catheter (10 to 14 gauge for an adult horse) or through an intravenous fluid infusion set after the bottle has been pressurized. Solutions of 7.5% and greater are irritant to tissues and will cause tissue necrosis when they are injected perivascularly. Use of an indwelling catheter is recommended to limit the risk of perivascular injection. Vascular thrombosis has been reported after infusion of 20% guaifenesin.

Monitoring

The palpebral reflex should be weak and the eyeball should be eccentrically placed in the socket (usually rolled rostroventral) during a moderate depth of anesthesia. The size of the pupil should be that of a relaxed conscious horse. Muscle relaxation should be present and the swallowing reflex should be absent when endotracheal intubation is attempted. The heart rate is normally increased immediately after induction of anesthesia to about 55 to 60 beats/min in an adult horse. The arterial blood pressure may be in the range of 120/85 to 85/55 mm Hg. Peripheral pulses may be easy to palpate as a result of vasodilation despite low blood pressure. The mucous membranes should be pale to bright pink and the capillary refill time should be from 1 to 1.5 seconds. The respiratory rate should be about 10 breaths/min but arterial oxygenation may be low.

Supplementation

Signs indicating the need for additional anesthetic drug are an increase in arterial pressure, a strong palpebral reflex, and the appearance of nystagmus. Incremental dosages of 30 to 50 mL guaifenesin-thiobarbiturate mixture (10% guaifenesin, 0.4% thiobarbiturate) will be needed approximately every 10 minutes to prolong anesthesia in adult horses, although this should be assessed on an individual basis. Administration of more than twice the initial dose may be followed by weakness and ataxia during recovery from anesthesia. Addition of local anesthesia may be necessary to provide analgesia for some procedures.

Recovery

Horses commonly stand approximately 50 minutes after the initial administration of thiobarbiturate and guaifenesin, or 30 minutes after the last supplemental dose. The responses of male and female ponies to guaifenesin administration have been compared. No difference was discovered in the dosage required for recumbency and relaxation, but a pronounced sex difference in the duration of effect was observed, with the duration in stallions being 1.5 times that in mares.

Modifications

Other drugs may be used in addition to acetylpromazine or xylazine to provide greater sedation before infusion of thiopental or thiamylal and guaifenesin. Xylazine 0.3 to 0.6 mg/kg may be combined with acetylpromazine 0.02 to 0.04 mg/kg, or either drug may be combined with an opioid drug, such as pentazocine 0.3 mg/kg or butorphanol 0.02 mg/kg. When drug combinations are used for sedation, less than the calculated dose rate of barbiturate and guaifenesin will be necessary to cause anesthesia. The initial concentration of inhalation agent administered should also be decreased to avoid overdosage or hypotension.

THIOPENTAL OR THIAMYLAL AND CHLORAL HYDRATE

A technique that has been used in the past involves tranquilization of the horse with acetylpromazine, heavy sedation induced by intravenous infusion of chloral hydrate, up to 50 mg/kg, and anesthesia induced by a bolus injection of thiamylal 4.4 mg/kg. Chloral hydrate significantly decreases arterial pressure and cardiac output. There is little information published about the cardiovascular effects of thiamylal with chloral hydrate. Recovery is prolonged when compared with barbiturate or barbiturate and guaifenesin anesthesia and is accompanied by muscle weakness.

METHOHEXITAL

Methohexital (Brevital) is an ultra–short-acting barbiturate used in a fashion similar to thiopental or thiamylal. Changes in heart rate, blood pressure, respiratory rate, and P_aO_2 are similar to those following administration of thiobarbiturate. Methohexital has two main differences from thiopental. First, it is more potent than thiopental and the dose rate to cause anesthesia is approximately half that of thiopental. Second, methohexital is more rapidly redistributed to the tissues and is rapidly detoxified in the liver. Both of these facts contribute to a faster recovery from anesthesia. The quality of recovery may be poor, with the horse making repeated attempts to stand, when methohexital has been used as the sole anesthetic agent. Methohexital may be administered with guaifenesin and anesthesia maintained with an inhalation agent. Recovery is then determined by the inhalation agent administered, with no residual effect from the methohexital.

KETAMINE

The first reports of use of ketamine (Vetalar, Ketaset) with xylazine for anesthesia in horses were in 1977. Although ketamine is used frequently for anesthesia in horses and is available for equine anesthesia in the United Kingdom, it is not licensed by the Food and Drug Administration (FDA) for use in horses in the United States.

Clinical Effects

Ketamine is a dissociative anesthetic that induces anesthesia by interrupting the flow of information from the unconscious to the conscious parts of the brain. Ketamine is 45 to 60% bound to plasma proteins, and that percentage is relatively independent of the concentration of ketamine in the plasma. Anesthesia is induced at a plasma concentration of about 1 μg/ml.

Ketamine causes excitement in horses when administered alone. Consequently, healthy horses are usually sedated first with xylazine. In one detailed investigation, xylazine 1.1 mg/kg administered intravenously to horses resulted in a 37% decrease in heart rate and no change in arterial blood pressure. Second-degree heart block was observed with various frequencies after xylazine administration in all horses. The cardiac output was decreased by 29%. Ketamine 2.2 mg/kg was administered 3 to 5 minutes later. The heart rate had returned to within 16% of the prexylazine value and the arterial blood pressure had increased above that value after 5 minutes of recumbency. The cardiac output remained decreased by 23%. The respiratory rate was decreased slightly during anesthesia and the arterial P_{CO_2} was mildly increased. The P_aO_2 decreased to 74 ± 15 mm Hg by 5 minutes after ketamine administration. When xylazine and ketamine were administered simultaneously, the hemodynamic pattern was similar, although the heart rate and cardiac output were not as depressed. It was noted that induction of anesthesia was accompanied by a brief period of excitement and extensor rigidity, which had not occurred when the injections of xylazine and ketamine were separated by a few minutes.

Ketamine administered alone or with xylazine in other species results in increased intraocular pressure, and its administration is contraindicated in a patient with a ruptured or damaged cornea. No increase in intraocular pressure was measured in healthy horses after xylazine and ketamine administration when combined with an auriculopalpebral nerve block.

Administration

Commonly, horses are sedated with xylazine 1.1 mg/kg injected intravenously and anesthesia is induced by intravenous injection of ketamine 2.2 mg/kg 3 to 5 minutes later. Recumbency is assumed about 60 seconds after the injection of ketamine. Horses may become excited before becoming recumbent when the xylazine and ketamine are given in quick succession. For induction of anesthesia to be smooth, the sedative effect of xylazine should be pronounced before the ketamine is injected. If the horse is not sedate, additional xylazine should be given, or an additional drug as suggested in the modifications section. It may be safer to postpone the procedure to another day if sedation is still not evident. Waiting longer than 10 minutes after xylazine administration before injection of ketamine may result in insufficient sedation remaining to promote smooth anesthesia.

The duration of anesthesia varies between 7 and 20 minutes. The shorter time is most likely to occur in horses that are anxious or excited before xylazine administration.

Xylazine and ketamine provide satisfactory anesthesia with a rapid recovery in foals. In healthy foals that are 1 to 4 months old this may result in a short duration of anesthesia, or they may require a dose that is one-third to one-half greater than that used in adults to achieve adequate anesthesia. A dose rate two-thirds the usual calculated dose is often satisfactory in foals less than 2 weeks of age.

Monitoring

During xylazine and ketamine anesthesia, the palpebral reflex should be vigorous, the pupils may be dilated, and the eyeball should be situated centrally or rolled slightly ventrally in the orbit. Low-amplitude nystagmus is often present. The arterial blood pressure is frequently high immediately after induction of anesthesia, with the systolic pressure exceeding 140 mm Hg and the diastolic pressure exceeding 100 mm Hg. The heart rate should be in the normal range. The peripheral pulses may be difficult to palpate, despite hypertension, because vasoconstriction is present. The respiratory rate should be about 12 breaths/min. The breathing pattern during the early part of anesthesia in some horses is characterized by runs of 6 or 8 breaths, with increasing and then decreasing tidal volume, separated by 10 seconds of apnea.

Supplementation

Anesthesia may be prolonged by the administration of additional xylazine and ketamine. Xylazine 0.3 mg/kg given with ketamine 0.7 mg/kg (one third of the initial dose) will provide an additional 10 to 20 minutes of anesthesia. Although the additional anesthesia time produced varies between individuals, it is consistent in each horse. Signs indicating returning consciousness and the need for additional drug are an increase in amplitude of nystagmus and a more vigorous palpebral reflex. The horse may also sigh. The ear may move shortly before the horse moves its legs. Blood pressure will decrease toward normal as the effect of ketamine wanes, but may increase again after a supplementary dosage has been injected.

Xylazine and ketamine are considered to provide analgesia, but horses anesthetized with this combination may respond with purposeful movement during castration or surgery of the limbs. Inclusion of local anesthesia by infiltration of lidocaine around the spermatic cord or by use of limb nerve blocks will ensure analgesia and prolong the duration of useful anesthesia.

Alternatively, guaifenesin may be administered with the xylazine and ketamine to improve muscle relaxation, or anesthesia may be maintained with halothane, isoflurane, or enflurane, in oxygen.

Recovery

The average time to standing after a single administration of xylazine and ketamine is about 30 minutes. Horses usually regain their feet at the first attempt. Clinical recovery of horses from ketamine is almost entirely due to extensive extravascular distribution of the drug. The biologic half-life of ketamine in horses is 45 to 60 minutes, and 90% of a dose has been eliminated in 1.6 hours. Data on the metabolism of ketamine in horses indicate that hepatic or renal impairment is less likely to influence the duration of anesthesia from ketamine than in other species.

Modifications

The suggested dose rates of xylazine and ketamine may not provide anesthesia in young or excited horses. Both inadequate anesthesia and complete failure to produce anesthesia after injection of ketamine have been reported. In most cases, the horse was anxious or excited before drug administration. Other drugs may be included with the basic xylazine and ketamine combination to increase the predictability of anesthesia, improve muscle relaxation, or increase the duration of anesthesia. Intravenous drugs that can be included with the xylazine are butorphanol 0.02 mg/kg, diazepam (Valium, Diazepam) 0.05 to 0.1 mg/kg, or acetylpromazine 0.02 to 0.04 mg/kg. Diazepam has the advantage of causing the least effect on blood pressure and ventilation. Detomidine (Dormosedan) 20 μg/kg may be substituted for xylazine. Guaifenesin may also be included in the anesthetic protocol, as described below.

KETAMINE AND GUAIFENESIN

Clinical Effects

Administration of guaifenesin with ketamine improves the predictability and quality of anesthesia by adding muscle relaxation. Less guaifenesin is used with ketamine than with thiopental or thiamylal, and the dosage of ketamine may be decreased when used with guaifenesin. The heart rate is similar to that obtained during xylazine and ketamine anesthesia and the arterial blood pressure is lower. A 40% decrease in cardiac output was measured during experimental investigation of this drug combination in horses.

Administration

Xylazine should be administered for sedation, 0.6 to 1.1 mg/kg intravenously or 2.2 mg/kg intramuscularly. The lower dose of xylazine is often sufficient and the horse is easier to manage because it is less ataxic during infusion of the guaifenesin. The rest of the xylazine dose may be administered after the horse is recumbent if additional muscle relaxation is needed. Guaifenesin should be infused up to 55 mg/kg and then ketamine 1.7 to 2.2 mg/kg injected intravenously as a bolus. Anesthesia should last for 20 minutes and the horse should stand about 40 minutes after the ketamine was injected.

Monitoring

The heart rate is normally 30 to 40 beats/min and the blood pressure is between 130/90 and 110/80 mm Hg. The respiratory rate is usually 10 to 14 breaths/min. Arterial P_{CO_2} usually remains in the normal range, but the P_{aO_2} may be decreased.

Supplementation

Anesthesia may be prolonged by xylazine 0.2 to 0.3 mg/kg, ketamine 0.6 to 0.7 mg/kg, and additional guaifenesin (30 to 50 ml 10% guaifenesin). The delayed onset of effect should be taken into account during administration. These drugs will prolong anesthesia by approximately 10 minutes. Alternatively, these supplementary drugs may be administered as a continuous infusion. Xylazine 500 mg and ketamine 1,000 mg, should be added to a solution containing 50 g of guaifenesin. When 1 L of 5% guaifenesin has been used, the infusion rate is 2.75 mL/kg/hr. Most horses have a severe decrease in arterial oxygenation by 1 hour of anesthesia with this drug combination. Anesthesia should not be further prolonged without use of endotracheal intubation and administration of oxygen. Supplementation of the inspired air with oxygen may be necessary and advisable after only 40 minutes of anesthesia. As with any anesthesia, the adequacy of cardiovascular function should be monitored. Recovery from anesthesia should be smooth but may reflect the temperament of the patient. Muscle weakness during recovery from anesthesia is increased by increasing the dosage of guaifenesin.

ETORPHINE-ACETYLPROMAZINE

A fixed-dose combination of the opiate etorphine and the tranquilizer acetylpromazine is available in the United Kingdom (Large Animal Immobilon). Although horses become recumbent, this combination produces a state of neuroleptanalgesia rather than general anesthesia. Etorphine is extremely potent and small doses can be fatal to people. Care must be taken to ensure that a contaminated needle does not accidentally penetrate human skin. Naloxone should be immediately available in case of an accident.

Intravenous injection of Immobilon is followed by recumbency usually within 60 seconds. Stiffness, marked muscle fasciculations, and coarse tremors are obvious. The heart rate increases up to 4 times the resting value by 5 minutes after injection, and remains significantly elevated until administration of the antagonist. Arterial blood pressure is also significantly increased after injection of Immobilon, but this decreases to the preinjection value by 15 minutes, and may further decrease after injection of the antagonist. Cardiac output is increased. In consideration of these hemodynamic effects, it has been suggested that the use of Immobilon be avoided in horses with a recent history of epistaxis. Moderate to severe hypercarbia and hypoxemia have been reported to occur during immobilization with Immobilon.

The hematocrit increases considerably after administration of Immobilon and is a further manifestation of increased sympathetic activity. A significant increase in plasma lactate concentration occurs, which may be the result of vasoconstriction, muscle activity, or hypoxemia.

Diprenorphine is used to terminate anesthesia, and horses should stand within 2 minutes of its administration. Enterohepatic recycling of etorphine has been described, resulting in excitement, compulsive walking, or immobilization several hours later. This effect occurs particularly in donkeys. These signs can be reversed by administration of an additional dose of antagonist. Administration at the time of the initial intravenous injection of antagonist of an additional one-third dose subcutaneously may prevent the effect of recycled etorphine by sustaining the plasma concentration of antagonist.

PROPOFOL

Propofol (Diprivan) is a nonbarbiturate drug that is being evaluated for use in animals and humans. Injection of propofol results in rapid induction of anesthesia. Investigations in ponies have determined that sedation is necessary before injection of propofol to produce an adequate effect for endotracheal intubation. Propofol caused a significant decrease in arterial pressure and a 60% decrease in cardiac output in one pony. The respiratory rates decreased and $Pa{CO_2}$ was increased.

Administration of xylazine 0.5 mg/kg followed in 4 minutes by propofol 2 mg/kg resulted in 10 minutes of light anesthesia and recovery in 20 to 40 minutes. Recovery time was shorter, 12 to 23 minutes, when acetylpromazine was used for sedation. Recovery from anesthesia was described as quiet and smooth. Anesthesia was prolonged in some ponies by continuous intravenous infusion of propofol 0.15 to 0.2 mg/kg/min, after which recovery occurred in 20 to 30 minutes. Further investigation of this drug is needed before it is used in general practice.

TABLE 13–1. SUMMARY OF SOME INJECTABLE DRUG COMBINATIONS AND SUGGESTED DOSAGES FOR GENERAL ANESTHESIA IN HEALTHY HORSES

Combination No.	Premedication		Anesthesia	
	Drug(s)	Dosage (mg/kg)	Drug(s)	Dosage (mg/kg)
1	Xylazine	0.6	Guaifenesin	110
			Thiobarbiturate*	4.4
2	Acetylpromazine	0.04	Guaifenesin	110
			Thiobarbiturate*	4.4
3	Xylazine†	1.1	Ketamine	2.2
4	Xylazine	0.6–1.1	Guaifenesin	50–55
			Ketamine	1.7
5	Xylazine	1.1		
	Butorphanol	0.02	Ketamine	2.2

* Thiopental or thiamylal. Increased dosage may be necessary for anxious patients; decrease dose by 15 to 20% for draft horses greater than 550 kg.

† Ensure good sedation before injecting ketamine.

CONCLUSION

Prolongation of anesthesia with injectable drugs is largely limited because progressive lung collapse and respiratory depression result in inadequate arterial oxygenation. Increased drug administration also increases the risk of a weak, incoordinated recovery. There is a wide variation in individual responses to anesthetic drugs, and the responses are influenced by the drug combination used. The risk of complications increases when injectable drugs are administered without oxygen supplementation to maintain a depth of anesthesia adequate for surgery longer than 45 minutes.

The injectable drug combinations listed in Table 13–1 can all be used for induction of anesthesia before use of an inhalation anesthetic agent. The initial vaporizer setting may be partly influenced by the drug combinations used. Anesthesia induced by guaifenesin and thiopental or thiamylal lasts longer than that induced by ketamine. Therefore, the initial vaporizer setting may need to be higher to provide anesthesia when ketamine has been used than after guaifenesin-thiobarbiturate. Insufficient uptake of halothane after using xylazine and ketamine for induction of anesthesia will be obvious when, after approximately 20 minutes, the horse starts to move as a result of rapid redistribution of the ketamine. In contrast, the initial vaporizer setting may have to be quite low to avoid overdose when heavy preanesthetic sedation was produced by a combination of drugs, such as xylazine and butorphanol or acetylpromazine and xylazine, or another opiate-sedative combination.

BIBLIOGRAPHY

Grandy JL, McDonell WN: Evaluation of concentrated solutions of guaifenesin for equine anesthesia. *J Am Vet Med Assoc* 1980;176:619–622.

Greene SA, Thurmon JC, Tranquilli WJ, Benson GJ: Cardiopulmonary effects of continuous intravenous infusion of guaifenesin, ketamine, and xylazine in ponies. *Am J Vet Res* 1986;47:2364–2367.

Hsu WH, McGruder JP, Zheng-Xing L: The effect of yohimbine on xylazine/thiopental anesthesia in ponies. *Vet Med* 1985;80:69–72.

Lees P, Hillidge CJ: Neuroleptoanalgesia and cardiovascular function in the horse. Equine Vet J 1975; 7:184–191.

Muir WW, Skarda RT, Milne DW: Evaluation of xylazine and ketamine hydrochloride for anesthesia in horses. *Am J Vet Res* 1977;38:195–201.

Muir WW, Skarda RT, Sheehan W: Evaluation of xylazine, guaifenesin, and ketamine hydrochloride for restraint in horses. *Am J Vet Res* 1978;39:1274–1278.

Nolan AM, Hall LW: Total intravenous anaesthesia in the horse with propofol. *Equine Vet J* 1985;17:394–398.

Watkins SB, Watney GCG, Hall LW, Houlton JEF: A clinical trial of three anaesthetic regimes for the castration of ponies. *Vet Rec* 1987;120:274–276.

14 Inhalation Anesthesia

Eugene P. Steffey

For various reasons, the number of inhaled anesthetic agents used in the anesthetic management of horses is limited compared to choices for human patients. Two agents are of particular importance and are emphasized in this review. Halothane (Fluothane) is the inhaled anesthetic most commonly administered to horses and has been almost the only agent used for the last three decades. Isoflurane (AErrane, Forane) was recently approved for equine use. In North America, isoflurane is now the most widely used potent inhaled anesthetic with human patients. Two other agents, nitrous oxide (N_2O) and the chemical isomer of isoflurane, enflurane (Ethrane), are used only sparingly in horses and therefore receive no more than casual attention in this review. Other agents, such as diethylether, chloroform, and methoxyflurane (Metofane), are of historic interest but, because of space limitations, are not covered here.

HALOTHANE

Halothane is a colorless, nonexplosive, nonflammable, volatile liquid. Since it is unstable, it requires the addition of thymol and must be stored in tinted bottles to prolong its shelf life. Because of halothane's relatively high vapor pressure (Table 14–1), its delivery from a precision vaporizer positioned outside the breathing circuit is advised.

TABLE 14–1. PROPERTIES OF INHALATION ANESTHETICS

Agent	Vapor Pressure (mm Hg at 20 °C)	Approximate Saturated Vapor Concentration (% at 20 °C)	Solubility (Partition) Coefficients (at 37 °C)		MAC for Horses	Useful Vaporizer Setting or Delivered Concentrations (vol %)	
			Blood/Gas	Oil/Gas		Induction	Maintenance
Halothane	243	32	2.3	244	0.9	3–5	1–3
Isoflurane	240	32	1.4	98	1.3	3–5	1.5–3.5
Enflurane	172	23	1.9	98	2.1	4–7	2.5–5
Nitrous oxide	—	100	0.47	1.4	205	60*	≤50*

* Inspired concentration.

The potency of inhalation anesthetics is best expressed as the minimum alveolar concentration (MAC) of anesthetic that prevents purposeful movement in response to a noxious stimulation. The MAC for an inhaled anesthetic represents the alveolar concentration that prevents 50% of normal, otherwise unmedicated horses from moving in response to a stimulus such as skin incision. The MAC for halothane in horses is 0.9%. At this point, it is important to stress that the concentration described is alveolar, and not that set on the vaporizer. The vaporizer dial setting will usually be two to five times greater than the actual alveolar concentration, especially during the early phases of anesthesia, and will depend, at least in part, upon characteristics of the anesthetic delivery equipment in use.

The rate of change of anesthetic level with inhalation agents depends on factors that include the inspired anesthetic concentration, the volume of lung ventilation, the solubility of anesthetic in blood, and the volume of blood clearing the agent from the lungs. Of these, agent solubility is particularly important. Halothane is the most soluble of the agents reviewed (Table 14–1). Accordingly, compared to the other agents a proportionally larger volume of halothane must enter the blood stream to induce or "deepen" anesthesia. Thus, induction of halothane anesthesia is rapid but not as fast as with the other volatile agents discussed here. Conversely, because blood retains more anesthetic as solubility increases, emergence from anesthesia is delayed.

Inhaled anesthetics are metabolized to some degree. Results of investigations with laboratory animals and humans suggest that about 10 to 20% of administered halothane is biotransformed by the microsomal fraction of the liver and perhaps other organs. This level of halothane metabolism is large in comparison to other contemporary inhaled anesthetics used for equine anesthesia. The major metabolite is trifluoroacetic acid, which is eliminated in urine. Other metabolites occurring in small amounts are chloride, bromide, and fluoride. At least in laboratory animals, induction of the hepatic drug-metabolizing enzyme system by various agents (e.g., barbiturates) increases halothane metabolism.

Cardiovascular Effects

Halothane is a potent depressor of blood circulation. In unmedicated, normal horses studied under laboratory conditions, halothane decreased arterial blood pressure in a dose-dependent fashion because cardiac output was reduced (Fig. 14–1).

Halothane is a direct myocardial depressant and decreases stroke volume. The reduction in stroke volume is the major factor causing cardiac output to decrease, since heart rate is little affected by doses of up to at least twice MAC.

Dysrhythmias are not common during halothane anesthetic management of horses. However, halothane increases the heart's sensitivity to the dysrhythmogenic effects of epinephrine and other sympathomimetic amines. As a result, local infiltration of epinephrine, desired for some surgical procedures, or systemic injection of vasoactive drugs may cause dysrhythmias, especially of ventricular origin.

Respiratory Effects

Depressed ventilation, as evidenced by an elevated arterial carbon dioxide partial pressure (P_aCO_2), is dose related to halothane (Fig. 14–2). A P_aCO_2 of at least 55 mm Hg (normal P_aCO_2 in awake horses is about 40 to 45 mm Hg) is common even in lightly anesthetized, spontaneously breathing horses. Respiratory frequency and tidal volume are both depressed. The magnitude of elevation of P_aCO_2 in horses is greater than that seen in other species during halothane anesthesia but is no worse, and may be less, than that caused by isoflurane and enflurane. Surgical stimulation may improve ventilation and return P_aCO_2 toward normal, especially at halothane doses of 1.5 times MAC or less.

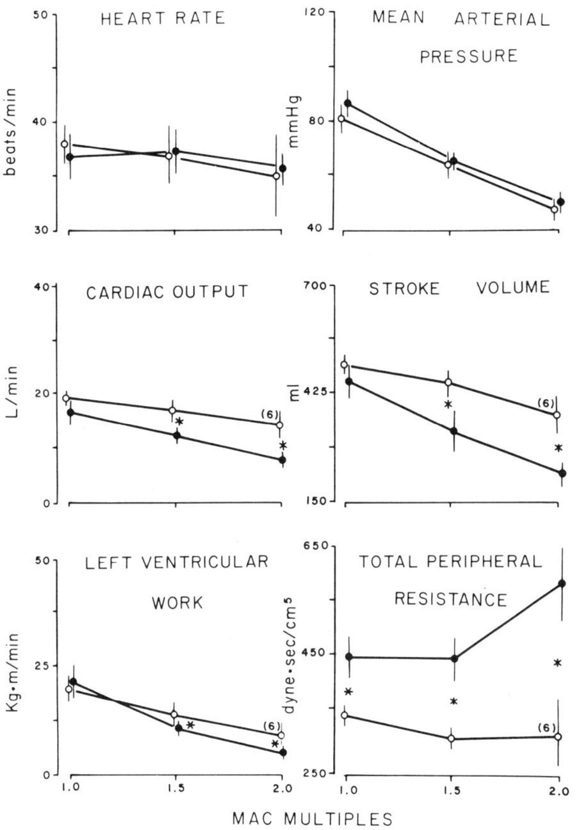

Figure 14–1. Halothane (●) and isoflurane (○) anesthesia compared in the same mechanically ventilated horses. Results are expressed as $\bar{X} \pm 1$ SEM and * indicates significant differences ($P < 0.05$) between the two groups at a similar multiple of MAC. MAC is the minimal alveolar concentration of anesthetic and equals, in horses, 0.9% and 1.3% for halothane and isoflurane, respectively. (Data are adapted from studies reported by the author in *Am J Vet Res* 1980;41:821–825.)

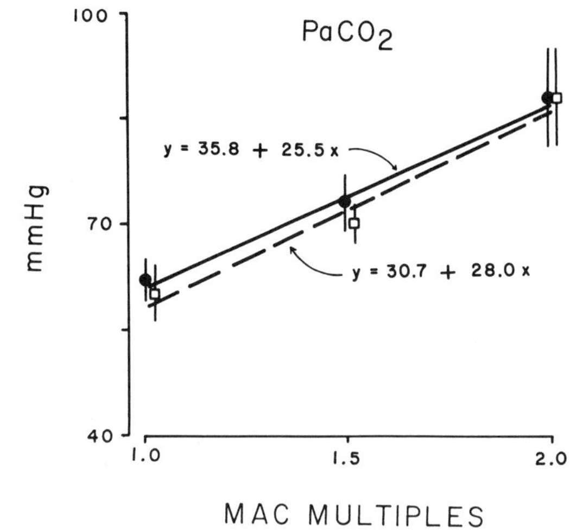

Figure 14–2. P_aCO_2 in spontaneously breathing horses anesthetized with halothane (●) or isoflurane (□) in oxygen. Results are expressed as $\bar{X} \pm 1$ SEM and the line of best fit for each anesthetic agent. MAC is the minimal alveolar concentration for each anesthetic and, in horses, equals 0.9% and 1.3% for halothane and isoflurane, respectively. (Data are from studies reported by the author in *Am J Vet Res* 1977;38:1037–1039.)

Other Effects

Halothane, like most inhaled anesthetics, causes a dose-dependent depression of hepatic and renal function that can be exaggerated by decreased organ blood flow. Function usually returns to normal or a compensatory increase occurs at the termination of anesthesia unless conditions were severe enough to cause direct toxicity (see below).

Malignant hyperthermia is a potentially life-threatening myopathy most commonly reported in susceptible swine and human patients. Its occurrence has been rarely reported in the horse. The syndrome is discussed in greater detail in Chapter 19.

ISOFLURANE

Isoflurane is a nonflammable, potent, fluorinated methylethyl ether recently approved for use in horses. It is a volatile anesthetic with many physical, pharmacologic, and clinical properties qualitatively similar to those of halothane (Table 14–1). It is stable without a preservative.

Isoflurane is less potent (MAC is greater) than halothane. It is the least metabolized of the fluorinated volatile anesthetics, and its blood solubility is also the lowest of the potent inhaled agents (Table 14–1). Low blood solubility permits more rapid induction/adjustment of anesthesia and also accounts for a more rapid elimination from the body at the conclusion of anesthesia. These anesthetic induction/recovery characteristics offer some advantage over halothane for the anesthetic management of foals. Conversely, there is a perception among at least some veterinarians that recovery of adult horses from isoflurane anesthesia is more commonly "rougher" and abrupt in comparison to that following halothane.

Cardiovascular Effects

As with halothane, cardiovascular depression associated with isoflurane is dose related (Fig. 14–1). Arterial blood pressure is reduced from awake levels and decreases as the dose of isoflurane increases. The magnitude of arterial pressure during isoflurane anesthesia is similar to that seen at comparable levels of halothane anesthesia.

As during halothane anesthesia, a decrease in cardiac output occurs and is dose related. However, cardiac output is better maintained during isoflurane anesthesia (especially in conjunction with controlled mechanical ventilation) because the decrease in stroke volume is not as marked as it is with halothane. During spontaneous ventilation, the heart rate also tends to be higher with isoflurane.

Results from initial studies with isoflurane anesthesia in horses indicate cardiac rhythm remains stable. Based on studies of other species, dysrhythmias caused by epinephrine and other vasoactive drugs are less likely to occur during anesthesia with isoflurane compared with halothane.

Respiratory Effects

Like halothane, isoflurane causes hypoventilation (Fig. 14–2). The elevation in P_aCO_2 is at least as large as that seen for a comparable alveolar dose of halothane. During isoflurane anesthesia, the horse's respiratory frequency is usually less, but tidal volume greater, than during halothane anesthesia.

Other Effects

Hematologic and biochemical tests of blood from a limited number of horses indicate no greater insult from isoflurane anesthesia than halothane anesthesia. In theory, the likelihood of toxicity with isoflurane should be among the lowest for potent inhaled anesthetics since there is minimal biotransformation of isoflurane. To date, clinical experience with horses supports this notion.

SELDOM USED INHALATION ANESTHETICS

Enflurane

Enflurane is a nonflammable, fluorinated methylethyl ether and chemical isomer of isoflurane. It was released for human patient use in 1972 and studied for use in horses. However, because of its emerging disadvantages and the relative safety of halothane and isoflurane, enflurane never gained widespread acceptance or federal approval for veterinary use. It is less volatile and less potent as an anesthetic than both halothane and isoflurane (Table 14–1). Its blood solubility is greater than that of isoflurane and offers only slight improvement over halothane. The extent of its biotransformation is also intermediate to both halothane (most) and isoflurane (least). As with isoflurane, free fluoride ion is a by-product of metabolism.

Circulatory and respiratory depression due to enflurane parallel alveolar dose and are similar to that with halothane. In horses large tidal volumes and low respiratory frequencies are even more characteristic of enflurane than isoflurane.

A major disadvantage accompanying the use of enflurane at moderate doses is its potential for causing abnormal muscle twitching and seizure-like activity, especially in unpremedicated horses. It offers no apparent advantages over halothane and isoflurane for equine anesthesia.

Nitrous Oxide

Nitrous oxide is a colorless, odorless gas that is nonflammable but supports combustion. It is marketed in blue cylinders as a liquid under pressure. Because it is relatively insoluble in blood (Table 14–1), the alveolar tension of N_2O rises rapidly. Nitrous oxide is far from a complete anesthetic in normal horses, but it may contribute to the production of anesthesia. Its limited anesthetic potency (high MAC; Table 14–1) requires high concentrations and concurrent use of other anesthetic drugs (e.g., halothane or isoflurane). Unfortunately, these high concentrations limit inspired oxygen levels. This is especially undesirable in the horse because of its greater tendency to develop hypoxemia during general anesthesia and recumbency.

Nitrous oxide reduces the requirement for other potent inhaled anesthetics. The magnitude of reduction is N_2O-dose dependent. For example, in normal horses 25% N_2O produces an average reduction in halothane requirement of about 12%.

Cardiovascular Effects. Nitrous oxide has minimal direct effects (mostly depressant) on cardiovascular function. The changes induced by N_2O in the presence of other inhaled anesthetics are usually limited and depend greatly on N_2O and other volatile anesthetic concentrations. Few studies of N_2O action in horses are available. Work to date indicates that circulatory changes associated with a halothane–N_2O (50%, inspired)–oxygen combination are qualitatively similar to those with equipotent halothane-oxygen anesthesia. However, the magnitude of circulatory depression is quantitatively less (i.e., cardiac output and arterial blood pressure are greater). The cardiovascular sparing effects are most apparent with light planes of anesthesia and disappear as N_2O dose decreases or halothane dose (and therefore anesthetic level) increases. Sympathetic nervous system activation may accompany N_2O administration and account for at least some of this cardiovascular sparing effect.

Nitrous oxide does not, per se, sensitize the myocardium to epinephrine-induced dysrhythmias, but adding N_2O to halothane anesthesia may further lower the threshold at which dysrhythmias occur.

Respiratory Effects. Nitrous oxide is generally regarded as a respiratory depressant, but the magnitude of direct effects is at best slight. Of greater concern in the horse is the influence of N_2O on reducing the inspired and arterial oxygen partial pressure. There is usually a large alveolar-to-arterial oxygen partial pressure difference in anesthetized horses that often exceeds in magnitude that measured in other commonly anesthetized mammals. It is therefore mandatory to use high oxygen concentrations in anesthetized horses, which limits the usefulness of N_2O. If N_2O is used in the anesthetic management of horses, an inspired N_2O concentration no greater than 50% for maintenance of anesthesia is recommended. It is important to note that the inspired concentration of N_2O may not be (and frequently is not) the same as the concentration that is calculated by comparing gas (oxygen and N_2O) flow meter settings. Differences between set and actual concentrations inspired by the horse usually exist and relate to accuracy of flow meters, absolute gas flow, size of the breathing circuit, size of the patient, and duration and characteristics of exposure to N_2O. Accordingly, at the very least, the use of an oxygen analyzer to accurately determine the inspired oxygen concentration is essential. Some quantitative monitoring of the adequacy of arterial oxygenation (e.g., analysis of arterial oxygen tension or saturation) is also desirable, especially considering the anesthetized horse's unpredictable alveolar-to-arterial oxygen partial pressure gradient.

Other Effects. For various reasons noted above, a potent inhaled anesthetic (e.g., halothane) is usually administered along with N_2O. During the early moments of anesthesia, there is a large volume uptake of N_2O from the lungs, which in turn influences the alveolar concentration of the second, simultaneously administered anesthetic. This rapid exit of N_2O from the lungs facilitates the blood uptake of the second gas beyond that which would have occurred if the second gas had been administered without N_2O and speeds inhalation anesthetic induction. This phenomenon is known as the second gas effect. Its value in equine anesthesia is largely related to induction of general anesthesia in foals via mask.

Horses have voluminous digestive tracts in which there is a continuous production of gas. Accordingly, the tendency of N_2O to enter and expand gas pockets is of major importance in anesthetized horses. The intestinal volume expansion and abdominal distention accompanying prolonged exposure (>2 hours) to N_2O increases the risk of life-threatening ventilatory depression.

An additional factor that warrants clinical consideration is diffusion hypoxia, a condition related to the outpouring of the large volume of N_2O into the alveoli from blood at the end of anesthesia. At this time, the quantity of other gases in the alveoli, notably oxygen is diluted. The dilution of oxygen, especially if already reduced by nitrogen (i.e., air breathing), may lead to hypoxemia. This combination can be minimized or prevented by increasing the oxygen flow rate to 8 to 10 L/min and keeping the horse on this system for at least 15 minutes before initiating air breathing.

TOXICITY OF INHALED ANESTHETICS

Most inhaled anesthetics are excreted primarily via the lungs and the expired breath. It is now recognized that these anesthetics are also biodegraded to varying degrees in the liver and to a lesser extent in the kidneys, lungs, and gastrointestinal tract. Current opinion, in most cases, is that direct toxicity associated with inhaled anesthetics is attributable to certain metabolites of the parent agent. Adverse responses may occur in patients or in personnel who are chronically, environmentally exposed to low-level concentrations of these anesthetics.

At least in human patients, the most notable organ toxicities manifested postoperatively are halothane-associated hepatic dysfunction and fluorinated anesthetic–induced nephrotoxicity. The exact mechanism responsible for halothane-associated hepatic dysfunction is unknown but presumed to be related in part to the extent that halothane is metabolized in vivo. Perhaps more important to the production of toxicity, especially hepatic necrosis, is the chance combination of events that may or may not depend upon alterations of the halothane molecule. Such events may include reduced hepatic blood flow, hypoxemia, and exposure to other drugs.

Results of several studies of normal horses indicate that halothane anesthesia is associated with transient alterations in liver function. The greatest organ dysfunction is reflected after prolonged (3 to 4 hours or more) anesthesia. Multiple exposures to halothane anesthesia of short duration (1 hour or less) are less stressful to the normal horse than prolonged exposure, but they are more insulting than a single short halothane anesthesia. To date results of toxicity studies of isoflurane in horses suggest that this agent presents no greater hazard to horses than does halothane.

In human patients and certain strains of laboratory rats, inorganic fluoride–induced nephrotoxicity is characterized by an inability to concentrate urine. The resulting polyuria leads to dehydration, increased serum osmolality, and hypernatremia. Enflurane and isoflurane are both fluorinated anesthetics metabolized in part to organic fluoride, but the resulting serum levels are low, especially with isoflurane. Results from studies of isoflurane-anesthetized adult horses and foals indicate the risk of fluoride-related renal toxicity is probably nonexistent.

Operating room personnel may be chronically exposed to trace concentrations of inhaled anesthetics. This is of concern because of evidence that long-term exposure to low levels of anesthetic gases may cause an increased incidence of spontaneous abortion, fetal malformation, and perhaps malignancies in female operating room personnel. Headaches and impaired cognitive and motor skills may also occur during exposure. Although a firm cause-effect relationship has not been established in humans, results of experiments with animals are suggestive. Accordingly, individual clinical practice should be evaluated and efforts made to protect operating room personnel against contamination by escaping anesthetic gases and vapors.

Broad recommendations include educating personnel about potential hazards, appropriate equipment maintenance to reduce gas leakage, and the use of anesthetic scavenging systems. Scavenging systems capture and dispose of waste gases and are especially important in small operating rooms with limited air exchanges when anesthetic gas flows are far in excess of patient requirements. The National Institute of Occupational Safety and Health (NIOSH) proposed operating room atmospheric concentrations of less than 5 parts per million (ppm) for volatile anesthetics and 25 ppm for N_2O.

DELIVERY OF INHALATION ANESTHETICS

General anesthesia is accomplished by attaining an adequate partial pressure of anesthetic in the brain. The partial pressure of anesthetic in the brain is controlled in part by altering the composition of the inhaled gas mixture. In so doing, an anesthetic pressure gradient is created between the inspired gas and the blood bathing the brain. Anesthetic molecules then move, like respiratory gases (oxygen, CO_2), according to the direction of the pressure gradient. Components of the inhaled gas mixture are usually expressed in terms of concentration (e.g., 2% halothane, 50% N_2O, 50% oxygen) and are best precisely controlled with appropriate equipment, which includes gas flow meter(s), precision anesthetic vaporizer, and breathing circuit. An understanding of the performance of this equipment is necessary, and this information is detailed in textbooks of veterinary anesthesia.

At least in North America, the circle system is the most commonly used patient breathing circuit for horses. In this system, anesthetic gases and oxygen circulate in one direction. The system is constructed of large-bore tubing of variable length, includes a gas reservoir bag 20 L or more in volume, and chemically neutralizes metabolically produced CO_2 exhaled into the circuit by the patient. Its internal gas volume may be more than 40 L.

Of particular importance to the clinical conduct of general anesthesia in horses is the time delay for equilibration between the gas (oxygen and anesthetic) flowing into the circle system and the gas actually inspired by the horse. Two principle dangers result: first, delivery of reduced and possibly inadequate quantities of oxygen, and, second, unknown and/or insufficient (or excessive) concentrations of anesthetic. This commonly occurs when low flow rates of delivered fresh gas (<4 L/min) and large-volume breathing circuits (30 to 40 L) are used—circumstances typical of contemporary anesthetic management of horses. To avoid these problems I attempt to balance clinical and economic needs by first using a delivered fresh gas flow rate of 8 to 10 L/min and then after 10 to 15 minutes reducing the total gas flow to a maintenance flow of 3 to 6 L/min.

BIBLIOGRAPHY

Eger EI II (ed): *Nitrous Oxide/N_2O*. New York, Elsevier, 1985.

Lumb WV, Jones EW: *Veterinary Anesthesia*, ed 2. Philadelphia, Lea & Febiger, 1984.

Short CE (ed): *Principles and Practice of Veterinary Anesthesia*. Baltimore, Williams & Wilkins, 1987.

Steffey EP, Dunlop CI, Farver TB, Woliner MJ, Schultz LJ: Cardiovascular and respiratory measurements in awake and isoflurane-anesthetized horses. *Am J Vet Res* 1987;48:7–12.

Steffey EP, Howland D Jr: Cardiovascular effects of halothane in the horse. *Am J Vet Res* 1978;39:611–615.

Steffey EP, Howland D Jr: Comparison of circulatory and respiratory effects of isoflurane and halothane anesthesia in horses. *Am J Vet Res* 1980;41:821–825.

Steffey EP, Howland D Jr: Potency of halothane-N_2O in the horse. *Am J Vet Res* 1979;40:372–376.

Steffey EP, Howland D Jr: Rate of change of halothane concentration in a large animal circle anesthetic system. *Am J Vet Res* 1977;38:1993–1996.

Steffey EP, Howland D Jr, Giri S, Eger EI II: Enflurane, halothane and isoflurane potency in horses. *Am J Vet Res* 1977;38:1037–1039.

15
Positive Pressure Ventilation

Eugene P. Steffey

Lung ventilation is the mass movement of gas into and out of the lung. Of particular importance to the vitality of the animal is the adequacy of alveolar ventilation, or the volume of inspired gas (e.g., per breath tidal volume; per unit time-minute volume) required to maintain normal arterial carbon dioxide and oxygen partial pressures (P_aCO_2, P_aO_2). Normal blood gases for healthy, unanesthetized horses breathing air or 100% oxygen at sea level are indicated in Table 15–1.

Ventilation is normally accomplished by the respiratory muscles working collectively to establish a pressure gradient between the atmosphere and the alveoli. In most terrestrial mammals the respiratory muscles are normally active only during inspiration. Expiration is passive and is the result of elastic recoil of the lungs and thoracic cage components. The equine species differs in that there usually are passive and active phases to both inspiration and expiration.

General anesthesia interferes with ventilation and gas exchange. This qualitative effect of anesthesia has no species bounds. However, the magnitude of effect is not the same for all animals. The results of investigations have repeatedly verified that anesthetized horses are especially susceptible to respiratory system depression imposed by general anesthesia (Table 15–2).

Body posture, the specific anesthetic agent used, and the level of anesthesia (i.e., depression of central nervous system sensors) further influence the magnitude of changes in P_aO_2 and P_aCO_2 in horses. For example, for a similar magnitude of ventilation (i.e., P_aCO_2) and level of anesthesia, P_aO_2 is usually greater when horses are positioned in a lateral posture than when they are placed in a dorsal posture. Isoflurane may be a more pronounced respiratory depressant in some horses than halothane. Finally, ventilatory adequacy is usually optimal when the anesthetic dose is at the lowest level compatible with surgical requirements.

TABLE 15–1. TYPICAL P_{aO_2} AND P_{aCO_2} OF HEALTHY, AWAKE, UNSEDATED DOGS, HORSES, AND HUMANS

	Air breathing	Oxygen breathing
P_aO_2 (mm Hg)	80–100	>450
P_aCO_2 (mm Hg)	38–45	38–45

MECHANICAL VENTILATION

Because of the marked ventilatory depression imposed by general anesthesia and recumbency, mechanical ventilation is commonly used to normalize (or reduce) P_aCO_2, respiratory acidosis, and the work of breathing. Normalization of P_aO_2 is also desirable but may be more complicated since optimal blood oxygenation is subject to manipulation of other factors (Table 15–3).

During anesthetic management of horses, mechanical ventilation can be provided by intermittent manual compression of the anesthetic machine rebreathing bag or, more commonly in adult horses, by mechanical devices. These methods produce intermittent expansion of the lungs by forcing fresh gas into the airway (i.e., intermittent positive pressure ventilation or IPPV) and allowing spontaneous expiration.

Mechanical devices for IPPV of horses include resuscitators and ventilators. Portable self-inflating bags (suitable only for foals under about 125 kg) and gas-powered demand valves are classified as resuscitators and are suitable for field or hospital use. These resuscitators are especially useful during general anesthesia provided solely by injectable agents or during the immediate postanesthetic recovery period. Although not absolutely necessary, tracheal intubation is desirable with both methods. Ventilators are highly automated and usually used as an integral part of the inhalation anesthetic delivery apparatus. While units manufactured for anesthetic management of humans usually suffice for foals, modified ventilators are needed to meet the increased breathing volume and gas flow requirements of adult horses.

Ventilators for use in equine anesthesia are either pressure or time cycled; that is, inspiratory gas flow continues until either a specific preset inspiratory pressure (e.g., Bird ventilator) or time (e.g., North America Dräger ventilator) is reached. Ventilators used to mechanically ventilate anesthetized horses are usually double-circuit devices. The gas supply powering the ventilator is used to compress an anesthetic breathing bag or bellows suspended in a drum. This arrangement permits some units to operate in a manner similar to a volume-preset (or limited) ventilator.

TABLE 15–2. TYPICAL P_{aO_2} AND P_{aCO_2} OF HEALTHY HALOTHANE-ANESTHETIZED, SPONTANEOUSLY BREATHING MAMMALS AT SEA LEVEL*

	Light Anesthesia			Deep Anesthesia		
	Dog	Horse	Human	Dog	Horse	Human
P_{aO_2} (mm Hg)	>450	300–400	>450	>400	200–300	>400
P_{aCO_2} (mm Hg)	42–47	55–65	42–47	50–55	>70	50–55

* Inspired oxygen is 95% or greater. The dog and horse are positioned in lateral recumbency and the human is supine. Positioning horses in a dorsal posture further reduces P_{aO_2}—typically, on average, by 50 to 100 mm Hg.

MODES OF VENTILATION

Spontaneous, Assisted, and Controlled

Mechanical ventilation may be used to assist (assisted ventilation) or replace (controlled ventilation) the horse's natural ability to breathe (spontaneous ventilation). Assisted ventilation implies that the animal initiates a breath and "signals" the ventilator to deliver a prescribed volume of gas. Since respiratory frequency and respiratory minute volume are determined by the horse, hypercapnia (i.e., a P_aCO_2 above normal) usually accompanies assisted ventilation.

Controlled IPPV is usually desired since this form of ventilation provides maximal control over the magnitude of P_aCO_2 (Table 15–4) and conserves at least most of the energy cost of breathing. Controlled ventilation is necessary either when spontaneous ventilation ceases unexpectedly or when it is a planned result of the use of neuromuscular blocking drugs such as succinylcholine, pancuronium, or atracurium.

Intermittent positive pressure ventilation may cause clinically important depression of cardiovascular function. A rise in pleural pressure that is proportional to the rise in airway pressure accounts for decreases in thoracic venous return and cardiac output. Depression of cardiac output is usually manifested clinically as a reduction in systemic arterial blood pressure. The magnitude of circulatory depression accompanying IPPV may be increased further by anesthetic drugs and in patients with naturally occurring preexisting compromise of cardiovascular function (e.g., hypovolemia). Indeed, the magnitude of circulatory depression imposed by IPPV provides us with a clinical indication of the horse's functional cardiovascular reserves. For example, while monitoring arterial blood pressure directly via an arterial catheter, it is common to note a sinusoidal rise and fall in systolic arterial blood pressure of about 5 to 10 mm Hg, 1 to 3 heart beats after peak inspiratory pressure. The magnitude of this change is increased in endotoxemia, hypovolemia, or abdominal distention. In addition, a net decrease in blood pressure usually persists throughout the application of IPPV (Fig. 15–1). Accordingly, close monitoring of arterial blood pressure has become an essential part of patient management during IPPV.

TABLE 15–3. FIVE IMPORTANT FACTORS INFLUENCING THE MAGNITUDE OF OXYGENATION OF ARTERIAL BLOOD

1. Partial pressure of inspired oxygen
2. Magnitude of alveolar ventilation
3. Magnitude of alveolar-pulmonary capillary diffusion limitations
4. Magnitude of alveolar ventilation and pulmonary capillary perfusion balance
5. Magnitude of arteriovenous shunt

As previously noted, the magnitude of P_aCO_2 is best controlled by controlled ventilation. However, of the three forms of ventilation discussed here, controlled ventilation is also the most depressing to cardiovascular function (Fig. 15–2). The decrease in cardiac output may substantially reduce oxygen transport to tissues in spite of any improvements in arterial oxygenation due to IPPV.

Spontaneous ventilation is associated with the most marked elevation in P_aCO_2 and respiratory acidosis, but also allows the best circulatory system performance in anesthetized horses (Fig. 15–1). In addition to the absence of IPPV-induced mechanical depression, the greater cardiovascular performance may be related to the elevated P_aCO_2. Elevation of P_aCO_2 is known to evoke sympathoadrenal responses that result in increased cardiac output and arterial blood pressure.

In some clinical circumstances assisted ventilation may provide an attractive alternative to the other methods of ventilation since there is less cardiovascular depression with assisted than with controlled ventilation. Furthermore, P_aCO_2 may be slightly less than during spontaneous ventilation. However, it is important to recognize that some presently available equine

TABLE 15–4. PATIENT AND ANESTHETIST CONTROL OF VENTILATION AND P_{aCO_2}

Mode of Ventilation	Frequency of Ventilation per Minute	×	Volume per Breath	=	Volume per Minute	∝*	P_{aCO_2}
Spontaneous	Patient		Patient		Patient		Patient
Assisted	Patient		Anesthetist		Patient		Patient
Controlled	Anesthetist		Anesthetist		Anesthetist		Anesthetist

* ∝, proportional.

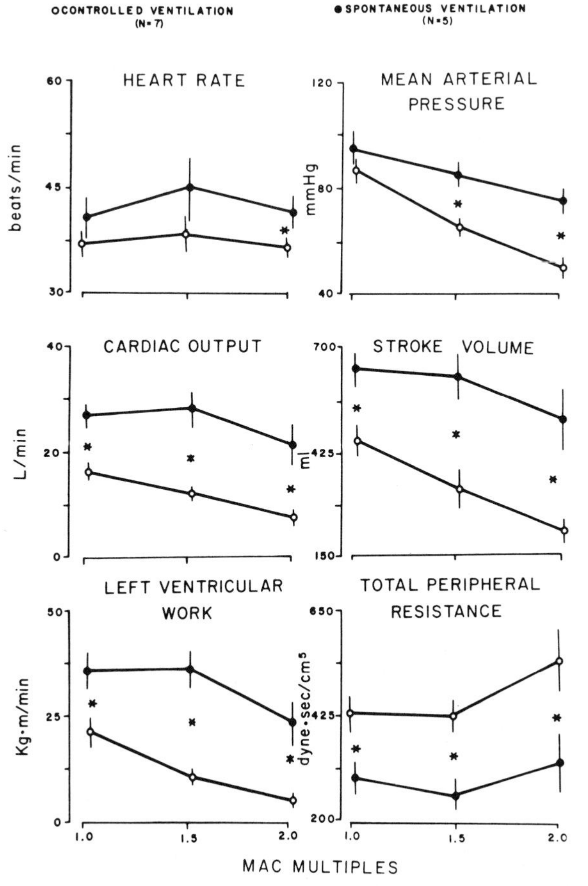

Figure 15–1. Halothane anesthesia in the same horses during spontaneous and controlled ventilation. P_{aCO_2} was 30 to 40 mm Hg during conditions of controlled ventilation and varied during spontaneous ventilation. The results are given as the $\bar{X} \pm 1$ SEM. Significant differences ($p < 0.05$) between results during controlled and spontaneous ventilation are indicated by *. MAC is the minimal alveolar concentration (0.9% halothane for horses). (Data are adapted from studies reported by the author in *Am J Vet Res* 1980;41:821–825.)

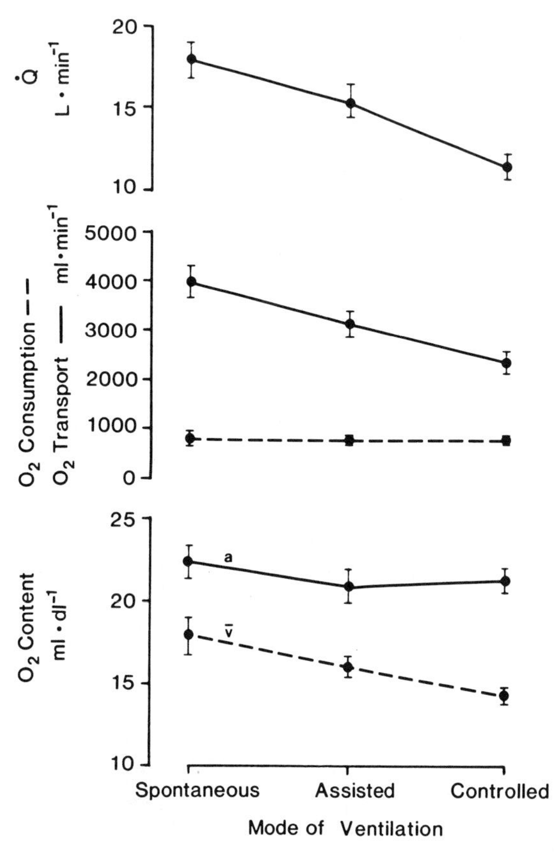

Figure 15–2. Cardiac output ($\dot{Q}$), oxygen transport, oxygen consumption, and oxygen content of arterial (a) and mixed venous ($\bar{v}$) blood during spontaneous, assisted, and controlled ventilation. Points represent $\bar{x} \pm 1$ SME. (From Hodgson DS, Steffey EP, Grandy JL, Woliner MJ: Effects of spontaneous, assisted and controlled ventilatory modes in halothane-anesthetized geldings. *Am J Vet Res* 1986;47:992–996.)

ventilators are not capable of providing an assisted mode of ventilation.

High-Frequency Positive Pressure Ventilation

High-frequency positive pressure ventilation is an alternative mode of controlled ventilation that is being investigated for use with equine patients. Characteristics of high-frequency ventilation include a very small tidal volume and high frequency of breathing (up to 600 breaths/min). The small tidal volume results in a low mean positive airway pressure throughout the respiratory cycle and thereby minimizes the insult of mechanical ventilation to cardiovascular function. Presently, high-frequency ventilation is not used clinically in the anesthetic management of horses and therefore will not be discussed further at this time.

Positive End-Expiratory Pressure

Generally, positive pressure ventilation refers to the inspiratory phase of ventilation. However, positive end-expiratory pressure (PEEP) is sometimes applied to human patients to increase P_{aO_2}. PEEP is produced by applying a resistance in components of the breathing circuit and this serves to prevent or retard full expiration. The goal is to "fine tune" the amount of PEEP that maximally improves P_{aO_2} without substantially reducing cardiac output or causing pressure-related trauma to the lungs. It is presumed that PEEP improves P_{aO_2} by minimizing the collapse of small airways and alveoli. As a result, the matching of ventilation to perfusion is improved. Laboratory investigation of the use of PEEP in anesthetized horses has failed to demonstrate any benefits. Indeed, in the horse, PEEP may increase P_{aCO_2} and decrease P_{aO_2} more than normally occurs during general anesthesia in the horse. Accordingly, there is no reason at present to consider the use of PEEP in the anesthetic management of horses.

CONCLUSION

There is no single specific ventilatory pattern that provides an optimal P_{aO_2} and P_{aCO_2} for all patients. A decision on the most appropriate approach is based on the means of mechanical ventilation available, the experience of the anesthetist, and details of the patient's specific needs. In managing horses, actual ventilator settings are usually based on a balance of fulfilling gas-exchange needs versus minimizing depression of cardiovascular function (i.e., optimizing tissue delivery of oxygen and removal of CO_2). Commonly used guidelines for controlled ventilation of otherwise healthy adult horses scheduled for elective surgery are given in Table 15–5. Guidelines for the initiation of ventilation are given in Chapter 16.

TABLE 15–5. GUIDELINES FOR CONTROLLED IPPV OF HEALTHY, ANESTHETIZED ADULT HORSES BREATHING OXYGEN

Respiratory frequency	6–10 breaths/min
Tidal volume	10–15 mL/kg*
Inspiratory: expiratory time ratio	1:2 or less
Peak inspiratory airway pressure	16–22 cm H_2O†
Peak inspiratory gas flow	>250 L/min
P_{aO_2}	>350 mm Hg
P_{aCO_2}	40–50 mm Hg
Systolic arterial blood pressure	>90 mm Hg‡

* Can be estimated from gas reservoir excursion during inspiration or expiration.

† Measured from the endotracheal tube lumen. Location of measurement will influence acceptable limits. For a given setting, pressures determined closer to the ventilator may need to be proportionally greater than those measured from the endotracheal tube.

‡ Referenced at approximately the aortic valve.

BIBLIOGRAPHY

Beadle RE, Robinson NE, Soronson PR: Cardiopulmonary effects of positive end-expiratory pressure in anesthetized horses. *Am J Vet Res* 1975;36:1435–1438.

Hall LW, Clarke KW: *Veterinary Anaesthesia.* London, Bailliere Tindall, 1983, pp 141–156.

Hodgson DS, Steffey EP, Grandy JL, Woliner MJ: Effects of spontaneous, assisted and controlled ventilatory modes in halothane-anesthetized geldings. *Am J Vet Res* 1986;47: 992–996.

Riebold TW, Evans AT, Robinson NE: Evaluation of the demand value for resuscitation of horses. *J Am Vet Med Assoc* 1980;176:623–626.

Steffey EP: Mechanical ventilation of the anesthetized horse. *Vet Clin NA* 1981;3:59–77.

Steffey EP, Berry JD: Flow rates from an intermittent positive pressure breathing—anesthetic delivery apparatus for horses. *Am J Vet Res* 1977;38:685–687.

Steffey EP, Wheat JD, Meagher DM, Norrie RD, McKee J, Brown M, Arnold J: Body position and mode of ventilation influences arterial pH, oxygen and carbon dioxide tensions in halothane-anesthetized horses. *Am J Vet Res* 1977;38: 379–382.

16
Monitoring the Anesthetized Horse

Wayne N. McDonell
Doris H. Dyson

Physiologic monitoring during general anesthesia is most logically an extension of the assessment carried out preoperatively. A practical preanesthetic evaluation checklist is presented in Table 16–1. Additional

TABLE 16–1. EQUINE PREANESTHETIC ASSESSMENT CHECKLIST

History	Clinical Examination	Laboratory Evaluation
Previous cardiovascular, respiratory, or renal problems?	Respiratory rate and character.	Hematocrit and total protein (minimum with all cases).
Previous neuromuscular problems (especially exertional rhabdomyolysis)? Family history of same?	State of hydration; evidence of nasal discharge, cough, pharyngeal lymph node enlargement?	Complete blood count and blood profile (prudent for elective anesthesia in a referral surgery setting, but rarely instructive).
Length of time out of training?	Pulse rate, intensity and regularity.	Creatine kinase and aspartate transferase evaluations should be carried out for elective procedures whenever there is a history of exertional rhabdomyolysis or postanesthetic myositis. These determinations may eventually prove to be of value as a general screening procedure.
Previous anesthetics? Adverse response?	Bilateral jugular vein patency?	Electrocardiographic (ECG) examination should be carried out whenever heartbeats are dropped in an irregular fashion, or if jugular fibrillation waves are noted (possible atrial fibrillation). A preanesthetic ECG should also be obtained whenever the regular dropped beat associated with a second-degree atrioventricular heart block does not disappear after mild exercise, or after administration of a phenothiazine tranquilizer as part of the premedication regimen.
Other drugs administered within past 48 hours, especially antibiotics, anti-inflammatory and analgesic agents?	Mucous membrane color and capillary refill time.	Electrolyte (Na^+, K^+, Cl^-), acid-base, and arterial blood gas analysis are desirable in critically ill animals, especially those with respiratory, gastrointestinal, or renal disorders.
	Auscultation of heart and lungs.	

tests, such as echocardiography and thoracic radiography, may be indicated in selected cases.

GENERAL RECOMMENDATIONS FOR MONITORING

Good clinical observation and judgment are absolute prerequisites to monitoring during anesthesia, along with some standard record or chart on which the observations are recorded. Aside from the medicolegal requirement of having an anesthetic record, changes in recorded values over time are often very instructive. Unfortunately, even the skilled anesthetist cannot properly evaluate all of the important parameters in the horse without the assistance of some equipment aids. This is particularly so in the case of blood pressure, temperature, and electrocardiographic (ECG) determinations. Cardiopulmonary insufficiency in the horse is usually first demonstrated by hypotension, rather than by the occurrence of apnea or arrhythmias. There is no question that the first monitoring aid beyond the clinical senses should be some method to objectively evaluate blood pressure. When mechanical/electrical monitoring devices are used, they should be used routinely, not just for the problem case, and should be kept in good repair. Routine periodic calibration of these devices is very important.

Although the depth of anesthesia has classically been divided into well-defined stages and planes, this categorization is not well suited to modern anesthetic agents and techniques. Most practicing anesthetists tend to categorize the depth of anesthesia into three simple catagories: (*a*) too light (usually associated with movement or the threat of imminent movement); (*b*) just right (for the particular animal and diagnostic/surgical procedure involved); and (*c*) too deep (associated with unacceptable cardiopulmonary depression, or the threat of same). The clinically perceived (and actual) level of central nervous system depression produced by a given dose of an anesthetic is affected by the premedication used, the age and temperament of the animal, the health of the horse, and the level of surgical stimulus. It is probably best to assess the information derived from as many of the sources listed below as possible when deciding upon the depth of anesthesia. With the inhalant anesthetics, the vaporizer setting, fresh gas flow, response to surgery, ocular signs, and blood pressure are especially useful. Previous actual experience with the drug(s) employed and with the typical equine response is an important factor in this judgment, and in providing relatively risk-free equine anesthesia.

IMPORTANT ASPECTS TO MONITOR

Respiratory Rate, Depth, and Rhythm

The respiratory rate, depth, and rhythm are most easily assessed by observation of thoracic and abdominal wall movement, and, during inhalational anesthesia, by excursions of the rebreathing bag. A brief period of apnea (up to 45 seconds) often occurs as a horse becomes recumbent subsequent to induction with a thiobarbiturate or ketamine. Thereafter, if anesthesia is light, breathing may be irregular and the animal may hold its breath, especially after endotracheal intubation. Larger doses of ketamine and barbiturates are often associated with prolonged periods of apnea or very shallow respiration, especially when the muscle relaxant succinylcholine is incorporated as one of the induction drugs. The occurrence of apnea and/or breath holding may be minimized by using guaifenesin as part of the induction, along with reduced doses of thiobarbiturate or ketamine, and by ensuring that the initial inspired concentration of isoflurane or halothane is kept below 2%. At stable, surgical levels of anesthesia respiration is regular and even at a rate of 4 to 12 breaths/min. An increasing respiratory rate, an irregular breathing pattern, and periodic large forceful tidal volumes may all signal that anesthesia is too light. Some horses will take several breaths in rapid succession and then breath hold for 60 to 90 seconds. This periodic apnea can occur at surgical levels of anesthesia and is most commonly associated with the use of ketamine. Such signs should not be confused with the slow periodic "gasping" breath that is characteristic of anoxia of the respiratory center. The latter situation can occur in response to severe hypotension, after cardiac arrest, or as a consequence of inadequate oxygen supply (airway obstruction, failure of equipment, etc.). It is usually accompanied by obvious ocular signs (absence of corneal reflex, pupillary dilatation) related to depression of the central nervous system.

Increasing depth of anesthesia is often associated with a progressive reduction in tidal volume, rather than a reduction in respiratory rate. Similar reductions of tidal volume may occur during lighter planes of anesthesia when lung volume is restricted or movement of the chest wall is limited by obesity, abdominal tympany, or neuromuscular blockade. A decrease in tidal volume is difficult to specifically quantitate by observation of the rebreathing bag, but the experienced anesthetist usually has no trouble in deciding that respirations are too shallow or too infrequent. The treatment is to decrease the anesthetic concentration or to institute intermittent positive pressure ventilation (IPPV).

Pulse Intensity and Rate

Digital palpation of the pulse rate and intensity is very useful and convenient. The facial, transverse facial, and great metatarsal arteries are readily accessible; the common digital and digital arteries are also palpable, but less so, especially when the systemic blood pressure is decreased. Tachycardia, bradycardia, and irregular heart rates are immediately obvious from palpation of the pulse, and should raise questions about the source of the problem and possible treatment. In the normal adult horse, heart rates may increase to 55 or 65 beats/min at the time of induction, but heart rates during maintenance anesthesia rarely exceed 50 beats/min unless the animal is too lightly anesthetized, hypoxic, hypercarbic, hypovolemic, or displaying the type of circulatory shock seen with an acute abdomen. Xylazine always tends to lower heart rate in the horse, and large doses may produce serious bradycardia (heart rate less than 25 beats/min), requiring treatment (see Chapter 11).

Pulse intensity is a subjective evaluation and is primarily determined by the systolic-to-diastolic blood pressure difference. Therefore, it is best not to equate pulse quality with any numeric estimate of either systolic or mean blood pressure. Nevertheless, if an anesthetist routinely palpates the pulse at a particular site, it will not be long before an appreciation is gained of a "good strong pulse," one that is "decreased in intensity," and one that is "inadequate." This progression correlates well with the depth of anesthesia in normal animals. It is common to observe a decrease in pulse intensity that is out of proportion to the depth of anesthesia during the first 20 to 30 minutes of inhalant general anesthesia or subsequent to a change in body position. These decreases in pulse intensity are reflective of arterial hypotension, and the patient may require supportive therapy with fluid or catecholamine administration (methoxamine, phenylephrine, dopamine, dobutamine).

Mucous Membranes

A reasonable appreciation of the adequacy of peripheral tissue perfusion can be gained by observing the rate of capillary refill after digital pressure is applied to the gingival mucous membranes (near the incisor teeth). In a normal animal refill of the blanched area is very brisk (less than 1.5 seconds) during light halothane anesthesia, and becomes progressively sluggish as the depth of anesthesia increases. Prolonged capillary refill times are usually associated with low cardiac outputs and low arterial blood pressures.

Gingival mucous membrane color is not as easy to interpret in the horse as in some other species. Cyanosis may reflect systemic hypoxia, or it may be reflective of the sluggish peripheral circulation seen in dehydrated, toxic animals. Pale mucous membranes may reflect anemia or peripheral vasoconstriction. The latter occurs after xylazine or ketamine administration for the duration of their influence, during light levels of general anesthesia with an inhalant agent, or in response to hypovolemia. Flushed, overly pink mucous membranes may indicate underventilation and carbon dioxide retention, and brick red or purplish mucous membranes are often associated with endotoxemia. Despite these limitations, the presence of pink mucous membranes and a brisk refill time provides considerable reassurance that other vital tissues are being adequately perfused.

Ocular Signs and Response to Surgery

Careful observation of the eye often provides useful clues as to the depth of anesthesia in the horse. If xylazine-ketamine or thiobarbiturate-guaifenesin combinations are used at the usual doses for anesthesia induction, most animals will show some spontaneous eye movement (nystagmus, blinking) shortly after induction. The eyelids are open, the eye is central and well lubricated, and the horse blinks when the dorsal or ventral eyelashes are lightly brushed (palpebral reflex). As the transfer is made to an anesthetic level of halothane or isoflurane, or if anesthesia is deepened with a thiobarbiturate, the eyelids gradually close, nystagmus stops, and the eyeball may show some rostral rotation so that the lateral sclera becomes visible. The palpebral reflex is weak but present, the cornea is moist, and the corneal reflex is vigorous. This latter reflex should only be elicited by careful pressure with a smooth, blunt object (not a fingertip!). If a palpebral reflex is present, there is no need to check for a corneal reflex. Overly deep anesthesia is associated with a loss of the palpebral reflex, a weak (or absent) corneal reflex, a dry, lusterless cornea, and a centrally fixed eyeball. Too light anesthesia may be associated with the obvious production of tears, nystagmus, and/or spontaneous blinking.

A number of practical factors influence ocular signs of anesthesia in the horse. The palpebral reflex appears to fatigue in animals if tested repeatedly. It is common to lose the palpebral reflex in the uppermost eye when a horse is in lateral recumbency and the reflex has been tested frequently, whereas the lowermost, previously untested eyelids will respond quite vigorously. The level of surgical stimulus can have a very marked influence on the eye reflexes. Horses that seem to be adequately anesthetized may suddenly show a vigorous palpebral reflex, caudal rotation of the eyeball, and even nystagmus when the skin or a joint capsule is incised. The authors believe this is related to a change in the level of central nervous system depression in response to sensory input, rather than an "error" in the eye reflex. Xylazine-ketamine anesthesia without subsequent inhalational anesthesia is characterized by the horse having an open eye, blinking, and a brisk palpebral reflex. When 50% nitrous oxide–oxygen anesthesia is used with halothane, it is possible to maintain more vigorous eye reflexes without having the horse move during orthopedic operations. It is not clear, however, whether this observation is related to lower halothane blood levels or to the effects of nitrous oxide on the reflexes.

All of the general anesthetics in present-day use produce dose-related cardiopulmonary depression, and it is therefore advisable to keep the horse in as light a level of anesthesia as possible. Ideally the horse should show some response to strong surgical stimulus, such as a slight change in eye reflexes, a modest increase in blood pressure, or an increase in respiration. The most common mistake the novice makes when anesthetizing horses is to keep the animal in an excessively deep level of anesthesia because of the fear of sudden violent movement. In actual fact, a horse lightly anesthetized with an inhalant agent very rarely goes from the point of appearing to be asleep (based on eye reflexes, respiration, and circulatory signs) to the point of violent movement, irrespective of the amount of surgical stimulus. Instead, the horse will slowly stretch the hind or forelegs if in dorsal recumbency, or show slow rhythmic movements of the upper forelimb if it is in lateral recumbency. These movements are easily controlled, and may be rapidly reversed by administering an intravenous supplement to the anesthetic. Our current practice is to use an intravenous bolus dose of ketamine (0.2 mg/kg) to provide this rapid, immediate supplementation. The inspired concentration of inhalant anesthetic can then be adjusted upward over the next 5 to 10 minutes, if necessary.

There are two surgical situations where it is desirable to maintain the anesthetic depth somewhat deeper to ensure safety of the equipment and operators. One of these is arthroscopy and the other is in the case of surgery of the head (especially the eye), wherein the surgical draping interferes with observation of the ocular signs of anesthesia. In the latter instance it is hard to determine lightening levels of anesthesia before movement occurs (see Chapter 17).

Blood Pressure

Objective measurement of arterial blood pressure is particularly useful as a monitoring procedure. It can be done inexpensively in a practice or field setting with a minimum of equipment, and is recommended as a routine procedure during all but the shortest (those less than 10 to 15 minutes) anesthetic periods. Either direct or indirect methods may be employed.

Indirect Measurement. The most practical indirect method for blood pressure measurement employs an inflatable occlusive cuff placed around an extremity (usually the base of the tail or hind limb just below the hock), and an ultrasonic Doppler probe (Parks 811; Parks Medical Electronics, Inc). The Doppler unit provides an audible indication of the return of blood flow (systolic pressure) through an artery as the proximal occlusive cuff is slowly deflated (Fig. 16–1). Pressure in the occlusive cuff is measured with a hand-held aneroid manometer (Tycos; American Hospital Supply Corp).

For an average-sized horse, the cuff width should be 9 cm (0.35 times the tail circumference) when the tail is used. The cuff should be applied snugly, but not tightly, as close to the origin of the tail as possible. The ventral midline of the tail just distal to the cuff should be cleaned of any debris or hair before the Doppler crystal is applied. A liberal amount of ultrasound gel (not ECG paste) should be applied to both the crystal and tail to ensure that contact is good with no residual air pockets. With the cuff deflated and the Doppler unit switched on, the crystal is positioned to provide a clearly audible sound with each heartbeat. The crystal is then fixed in place snugly, but not too tightly, with adhesive tape. A second strip of tape should be placed distally around the probe lead to keep the crystal aligned and immobile throughout the anesthetic period.

No adjustment need be made for systolic blood pressure determined at the tail with the horse in lateral recumbency. The readings will be somewhat higher (15 to 18 mm Hg) than the true systolic blood pressure when an average-sized horse is in dorsal recumbency, reflecting the hydrostatic pressure difference between the heart and tail. Indirect Doppler systolic blood pressure measurements are primarily useful to establish trends during anesthesia, rather than absolute pressure measurements. Although some authors have satisfactorily recorded systolic blood pressures down to 40 mm Hg, in routine clinical use the system is often unreliable when systolic blood pressure falls below 60 mm Hg.

Direct Measurement. With a little practice, the facial, transverse facial, and great metatarsal arteries are all easily palpated and catheterized. An 18- to 20-gauge, 32- to 44-mm arterial catheter should be used after aseptic preparation of the site and puncture of the skin with a 14- to 16-gauge needle. Once inserted, the arterial catheter is connected to a three-way stopcock,

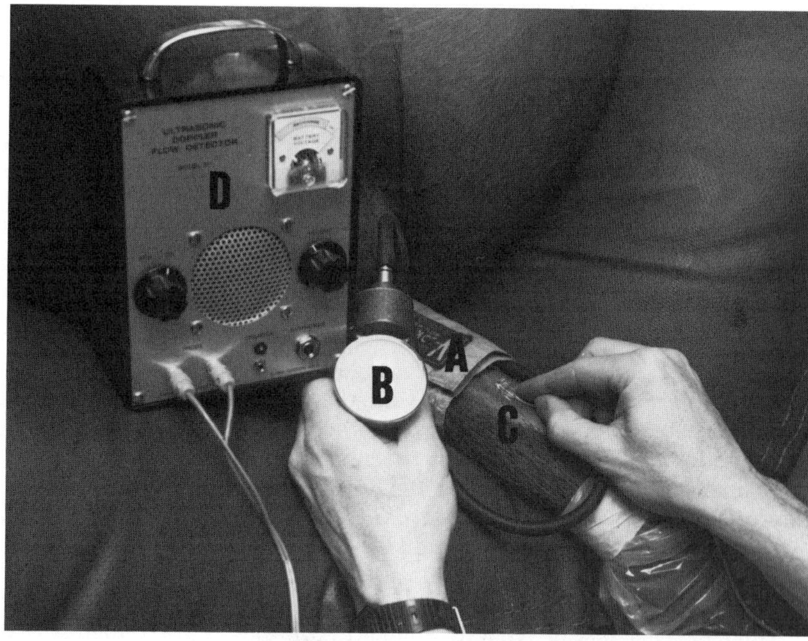

Figure 16–1. Ultrasonic Doppler system applied to the tail for indirect measurement of systolic blood pressure showing the inflatable cuff (*A*), aneroid manometer (*B*), crystal location (*C*), and monitor (*D*).

flushed with heparinized saline (5,000 units in 500 mL) and fixed securely in place. This is best done with one or two sutures. Alternatively, the catheter can be glued in place with a cyanoacrylate glue. Although there are theoretical possible complications to peripheral arterial catheterization, the authors have not encountered any significant problems as a consequence of routinely using such catheters in over 500 animals per year.

Once an arterial catheter is in place, it is possible to measure mean arterial blood pressure if a long extension line is half filled with heparinized saline and the air-filled end is connected to a hand-held aneroid manometer. This system is not particularly satisfactory for routine clinical use because retrograde flow of blood into the catheter and tubing will clot unless the system is frequently and carefully flushed, and any moisture reaching the aneroid will soon ruin the unit. An inexpensive commercial system (Pressureveil; Concept, Inc) eliminates the latter problem by providing a diaphragm to prevent fluid-air contact (Fig. 16–2). When combined with a continuous flushing device (Intraflow; Sorenson Research Co) providing a slow, continuous flush with heparinized saline from a pressurized bag, this system will permit long-term measurement of mean blood pressure. The fluid-air interface should be positioned at heart level. Similar systems can be constructed using a syringe barrel, rubber finger cot, rubber stopper, and extension tubing. Recent studies have confirmed the reliability of mean blood pressure measurements made with such simple methods when compared to the values obtained from

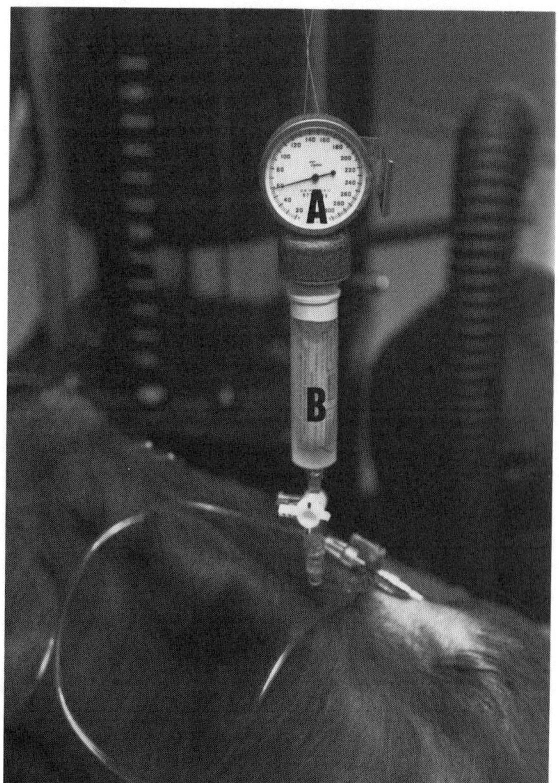

Figure 16–2. Inexpensive commercial system for direct measurement of mean blood pressure showing the aneroid manometer (*A*) and air-fluid diaphragm (*B*).

more sophisticated transducer/amplifier/recorder systems.

Because of their great convenience, more sophisticated multichannel monitor systems (Physio-Control VSM-1; Physio-Control Corp) are of immense value if the case load is high. These monitors usually provide an oscilloscopic trace of the ECG and digital information on body temperature and heart rate at the same time. The equipment is expensive, but modern portable monitors are durable and could certainly be considered as a good long-term equipment investment in many practices.

During inhalational anesthesia, changes in blood pressure correlate reasonably well with the depth of anesthesia. Low blood pressure may be produced by a decrease in peripheral resistance, a fall in cardiac output, or both. In the anesthetized horse, most hypotensive states are associated with decreases in cardiac output as a consequence of myocardial depression (anesthetic level, endotoxemia, acidosis), arrhythmias (bradycardia, sinus arrest, atrioventricular block, ventricular tachycardia), or reduced venous return (positional changes, abdominal tympany, hypovolemia).

Systolic blood pressures of 80 to 120 mm Hg are typical in anesthetized horses. A systolic pressure below 80 mm Hg is a cause for concern and for careful evaluation of the anesthetic depth and overall status of the horse. A systolic pressure below 60 to 65 mm Hg requires immediate corrective action. The equivalent values for mean blood pressure are 65 to 90 mm Hg as the typical levels, less than 60 to 65 mm Hg as the level at which there is cause for concern, and less than 50 to 55 mm Hg as the mean pressure requiring immediate restorative action (see Chapter 18). While higher blood pressures may be occasionally associated with hypercapnia, they usually indicate that the horse is too lightly anesthetized.

Electrocardiography

Continuous ECG monitoring provides an immediate measure of heart rate and will greatly facilitate the diagnosis of pulse deficits due to second- or third-degree atrioventricular heart blocks. It also will provide evidence of hyperkalemia (increased amplitude of T waves, a marked decrease in P wave amplitude, widening of QRS complexes, and irregular ventricular rate), and in some instances an early indication of myocardial anoxia (ST segment shift, increased amplitude and/or shift in polarity of T waves). The ECG is of immense value in deciding upon the correct emergency therapy when there is no detectable pulse. In the horse, acute circulatory failure is often characterized by an extremely low cardiac output and undetectable blood pressure in association with a weakly contracting myocardium. The treatment for this type of circulatory failure is different than for asystole or fibrillation (see Chapter 18). There is poor correlation between anesthetic depth and heart rate or any progressive change in the ECG complex. The horse is far less prone than many other species to the development of premature ventricular complexes, ventricular tachycardia leading to fibrillation, and atrial flutter or fibrillation.

The most practical way of displaying the ECG is with an oscilloscope. Usually some variation of the orthogonal Y lead is used with the RA (white) lead positioned on the withers or manubrium, the LA (black) lead on the sternum or xiphisternum, and the LL (red) lead on the lateral neck or shoulder. These lead positions are convenient to use and give easily recognizable P, QRS, and T wave complexes. It is best to use alligator clips and ECG electrode paste, and to consistently use the same lead placement.

Body Temperature

An inexpensive thermistor probe (Yellow Springs Instrument Co) can be easily placed in the nasopharynx and will provide continuous information on the core body temperature.

Serious hypothermia is not common even during prolonged anesthesia with extensive tissue exposure. The main value of temperature determination lies in the early detection of a rare generalized hypermetabolic state associated with generalized myositis. Body temperatures of 36 to 37.5 °C are typical during anesthesia, and any elevation above 38 °C should be viewed with suspicion and the possibility of malignant hyperthermia considered.

End-Tidal and Blood Gas Determinations

Infrared gas analyzers can be used to continuously monitor end-tidal carbon dioxide (CO_2) concentrations. These analyzers are reliable and provide a reasonable indication of arterial CO_2 levels. In the horse a significant (and variable) arterial-to–end-tidal CO_2 gradient of about 10 to 20 mm Hg is observed because of ventilation-perfusion disturbances that accompany anesthesia. The gradient varies slightly with time and body position. Infrared gas analyzers are expensive, and it is doubtful if their clinical usefulness warrants the expense unless the equipment can measure more than CO_2.

If the equipment to carry out the analysis is readily available and an arterial catheter is already in place for blood pressure measurements, routine blood gas analysis is very feasible and desirable. The results must be available within minutes to be of value. Serial blood gas, hematocrit, and total protein determinations are especially helpful in monitoring the critically ill animal. Unfortunately, blood gas analyzers are very expensive, but should be considered in hospitals that have a large number of critically ill animals needing surgery.

In the spontaneously breathing horse arterial carbon dioxide tension (P_aco_2) levels of 45 to 60 mm Hg are typical, and are well tolerated. When P_aco_2 levels exceed 60 to 65 mm Hg and/or the pH is less than 7.20, IPPV should be instituted. This situation is common when the duration of anesthesia exceeds 60 minutes. Arterial oxygen tensions (P_ao_2) are usually in the range of 150 to 400 mm Hg, with the lower values seen in aged or dorsally recumbent horses. With abdominal tympany, lung disease, excessive size, or low cardiac output, dangerously low P_ao_2 levels (less than 70 mm Hg) may occur even when 100% oxygen is being administered. IPPV should be instituted if the P_ao_2 falls below 100 mm Hg even if the P_aco_2 is within normal limits. From a practitioner's viewpoint, it would probably make more sense to invest in a good equine ventilator, to use 100% oxygen as the carrier gas for anesthesia, and to routinely ventilate all horses under general anesthesia lasting longer than 60 minutes so as to maintain eucapnea, rather than to purchase a blood gas analyzer (see Chapter 15).

Anesthetic Concentration

Until recently it has been impractical to accurately measure the end-tidal (alveolar) anesthetic gas concentration other than in a research setting. This is unfortunate because the vaporizer setting does not correspond to the actual inspired (or alveolar) concentration of the inhaled anesthetic when low fresh gas flows (6 to 8 L/min) are used in a large animal anesthetic circuit. The anesthetist learns by experience, however, that a particular vaporizer setting (e.g., 2, 3, or 4%) is generally required depending upon the duration of anesthesia, the supplemental drugs used, and the fresh gas flow.

The newer generation of anesthetic gas monitors (PB 252 Anesthesia Gas Monitor; Puritan-Bennett Corp) are capable of simultaneously measuring inspired oxygen and end-tidal CO_2 concentrations, as well as the anesthetic gas concentration (halothane, isoflurane, ethrane). These analyzers are expensive, but they may well find general clinical acceptance because of their compactness and capacity for multiple gas analysis.

Other

In the horse, central venous pressure measurements are variable and difficult to interpret during general anesthesia. Consequently, the measurement is not widely used.

Urine output provides a useful indication of renal perfusion and perhaps should be monitored more frequently. Most anesthetists rely upon arterial blood pressure measurements and the capillary refill time to provide an indication of organ perfusion, and use that information to deduce whether there is adequate renal perfusion. Urinary catheter insertion obviously carries some risk of inducing cystitis or urethritis. During a typical equine anesthetic, if the mean blood pressure is over 70 mm Hg, urine output is dependent upon the amount of xylazine used in the premedication and the volume of fluid administered.

When muscle relaxants are used, clinical monitoring of neuromuscular blockade is facilitated by use of a peripheral nerve stimulator on the facial or superficial peroneal nerves (see Chapter 17). Muscle pH, muscle temperature, and electroencephalographic monitoring have been attempted in research settings, but are not used in routine clinical anesthetics.

BIBLIOGRAPHY

Glazier DB, Littledike ET, Evans RD: Electrocardiographic changes in induced hyperkalemia in ponies. *Am J Vet Res* 1982;43:1934–1937.

Haskins SC: Monitoring the anesthetized patient, in Short CE (ed): *Principles and Practice of Veterinary Anesthesia.* Baltimore, Williams & Wilkins, 1987, pp 455–477.

Hubbell JAE, Robertson JT, Muir WW, Gabel AA: Perianesthetic considerations in the horse. *Compend Contin Educ Pract Vet* 1984;6:S401–S414.

Kvart C: An ultrasonic method for indirect blood measurement in the horse. *J Equine Med Surg* 1979;3:15–23.

Moens Y, DeMoor A: Use of infra-red carbon dioxide analysis during general anesthesia in the horse. *Equine Vet J* 1981; 13:229–234.

17
Muscle Relaxants

Susan V. Hildebrand

Muscle relaxants fall into three general categories, depending on their site of action:

1. *Centrally Acting:* These relaxants act on the central nervous system. Guaifenesin is an example of a centrally acting muscle relaxant that is used extensively in equine anesthesia (see Chapter 13). Despite its extensive use, however, there are still unanswered questions and controversy related to its activity. Nonetheless, guaifenesin continues to be a safe and reliable adjunct to general anesthesia. Since this chapter is intended to review new techniques in equine anesthesia, guaifenesin will not be addressed.
2. *Neuromuscular Transmission Blockers:* The second category of muscle relaxants are those that act at the neuromuscular junction. Neuromuscular blocking agents have been used as adjuncts to anesthesia for humans since the 1950s. Indeed, many advances in human anesthesia and surgery have resulted from the anesthesiologist's ability to produce profound muscle relaxation without cardiovascular compromise. Recent research and clinical studies indicate that equine anesthesia and surgery can similarly benefit from the use of neuromuscular blocking agents.
3. *Direct Acting:* The third category of relaxant acts directly on the muscle cell membrane. An example of a direct-acting relaxant is dantrolene sodium. Dantrolene has been used in the treatment of neurogenic muscle spasticity, and has been developed to prevent and treat malignant hyperthermia, a genetic muscle disorder best recognized in humans and swine. Dantrolene has also been used in the treatment of equine exercise- and anesthetic-related myopathy (see Chapter 19).

Muscle Relaxants as Adjuncts to Anesthesia

What improvements can muscle relaxants offer in anesthesia? In humans, a major function of a relaxant is to aid tracheal intubation. Other advantages include better surgical exposure, easier reduction of fractures, and provision of a motionless surgical field. Dose requirements of other anesthetic agents that can seriously depress cardiovascular and respiratory function are reduced, when muscle relaxants are used. This contributes to a smoother, more stable anesthesia. Furthermore, relaxation facilitates mechanical ventilation. Horses are relatively easy to intubate; thus the first-cited reason for the use of relaxants probably does not apply to horses. The remaining advantages of relaxants would be welcome in equine anesthesia.

MUSCLE RELAXANTS THAT ACT ON THE NEUROMUSCULAR JUNCTION

Neuromuscular Transmission Physiology

A brief review of normal neuromuscular transmission will facilitate the understanding of how the neuromuscular blocking agents and their antagonists work, and how to monitor their activity. Figure 17–1 illustrates structures and events at the neuromuscular junction. It is at this junction that the myelinated motor nerve loses its myelin sheath and multiple branches terminate at the synaptic cleft between the motor nerve ending and the motor end-plate on the muscle. In the terminal portion of the motor nerve branch, the neurotransmitter acetylcholine is produced and stored in intracellular vesicles. When a stimulus is applied to the motor nerve, vesicles are mobilized toward the cell membrane, where acetylcholine is released. Acetylcholine crosses the synaptic cleft and attaches to receptors on the motor end-plate of the muscle, causing depolarization of the muscle cell and muscle contraction. This period of receptor occupation is brief, because acetylcholine is quickly broken down by acetylcholinesterase located in the invaginations of the motor end-plate. The breakdown products are taken up at receptors on the nerve terminal, and are used for subsequent production and mobilization of acetylcholine.

Blockade of Neuromuscular Transmission

Neuromuscular blocking agents fall into two categories, depolarizing or nondepolarizing. The depolarizing relaxants behave very much like acetylcholine in that they attach to receptors on the motor end-plate and depolarize the muscle cell, causing contraction. The duration of attachment of the depolarizing relaxants to the end-plate receptors, however, is longer than for acetylcholine. Thus, paralysis occurs as a result of persis-

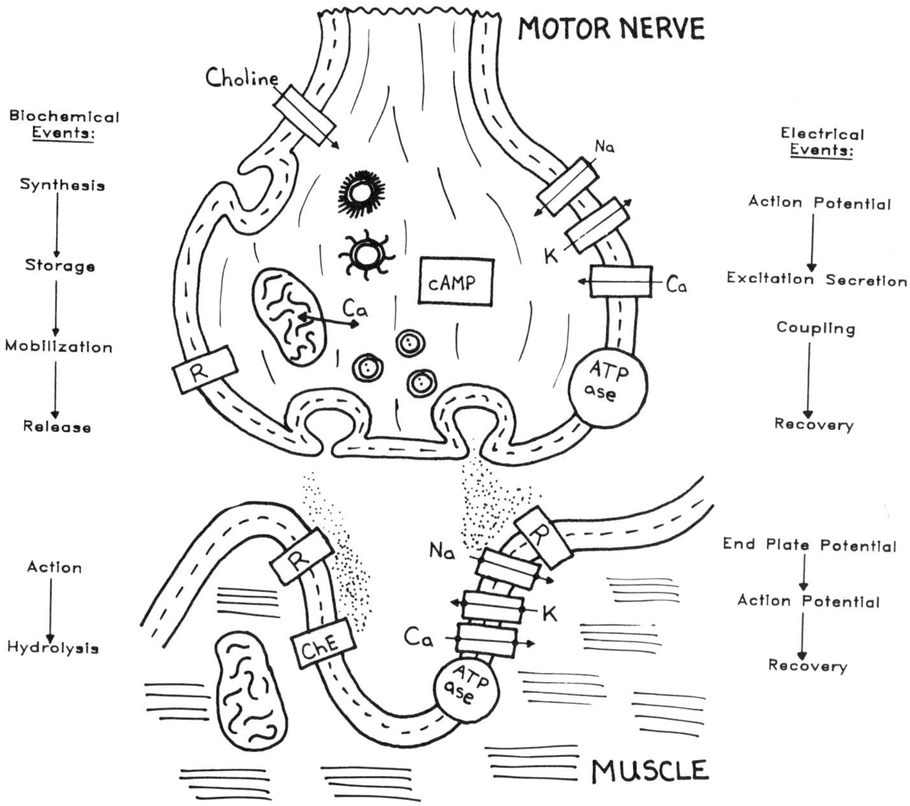

Figure 17–1. Diagrammatic representation of the motor nerve ending and the motor end-plate on the muscle, indicating the electrical and chemical events that occur when a motor neuron is stimulated. *R*, receptor; *ChE*, cholinesterase. *cAMP*, cyclic adenosine monophosphate; ◎, acetylcholine vesicle. (Courtesy of F. G. Standaert, MD.)

tent depolarization of the muscle. A familiar depolarizing relaxant is succinylcholine. It can be used to produce a rapid onset of muscle relaxation with a short duration of action. However, it can cause cardiac arrhythmias and a rise in serum potassium concentration, and may trigger a malignant hyperthermic response. Because of these complications and the advent of safer agents, succinylcholine is being replaced by other relaxants.

Rather than mimicking acetylcholine, the nondepolarizing relaxants compete with it for the motor endplate receptors. Once the receptor is occupied by the relaxant, the muscle cell is prevented from depolarizing. Spontaneous recovery of neuromuscular transmission occurs as the nondepolarizing relaxant diffuses away from the receptor site as plasma levels of relaxant decrease. With the exception of gallamine, nondepolarizing relaxants do not cross the placenta.

Nondepolarizing relaxants that have application to equine anesthesia fall into two categories based on their molecular structures. One includes the curariform relaxants such as atracurium. The other group are steroid-type molecules, examples of which are pancuronium and vecuronium.

Atracurium. Atracurium besylate (Tracrium) was recently developed as a result of continuing research to produce a nondepolarizing relaxant with a rapid onset and short duration of action, with no cardiovascular side effects. While onset and duration are dependent on the magnitude of the dose administered, recovery of neuromuscular transmission is very predictable because of the unique degradation of atracurium by Hofmann elimination. Because the molecule is unstable at body temperature and pH, it breaks down at a constant rate in the body. The breakdown products do not have neuromuscular blocking activity. Hepatic, renal, and cholinesterase functions are not necessary to terminate the action of atracurium. Because the molecule is also unstable at room temperature, atracurium must be refrigerated for storage. A second method of atracurium breakdown in the body is by ester hydrolysis. Despite this, anticholinesterases such as the anthelmintic trichlorfon do not alter the activity of atracurium in horses.

Atracurium is classed as a "mild" histamine-releasing agent. In humans, elevations in plasma histamine, with concurrent clinical signs including tachycardia, hypotension, and flushing, have been noted when large doses (approximately three times that which produces a 95% block) were given as a rapid intravenous (IV) bolus. When doses of that magnitude were given slowly over one minute, no signs of histamine release were noted, and no increases in plasma histamine were measured. No evidence of histamine release has been noted as a result of atracurium use in the equine species.

Pancuronium. Pancuronium bromide (Pavulon), like atracurium, has an onset time and duration of action that is dose dependent. Unlike atracurium, however, pancuronium depends to a large extent on hepatic breakdown to terminate its activity, and one of its metabolites has weak neuromuscular blocking capability. Cumulative effects are therefore possible with repeated doses, and recovery of neuromuscular blockade is less predictable than for atracurium. In addition, pancuronium has some vagolytic activity, and increased heart rate and blood pressure can occur with large doses or rapid bolus administration.

Vecuronium. Vecuronium bromide (Norcuron) is another recently developed relaxant. Vecuronium has the least effect on cardiovascular function of any of the neuromuscular blocking agents. Vecuronium is slightly more potent than its relative pancuronium. A large amount of both unchanged vecuronium and its metabolite can be found in the bile. A small amount is excreted unchanged in the urine.

Reversal of Neuromuscular Blockade

Rapid recovery of neuromuscular transmission after blockade by the nondepolarizing relaxants can be achieved by antagonizing their effects with anticholinesterases such as edrophonium (Enlon), neostigmine (Prostigmin), or pyridostigmine (Mestinon). Anticholinesterases inhibit cholinesterase activity and thus more acetylcholine is available to compete with the relaxant for receptor sites on the motor end-plate. For reversal to be effective, some spontaneous recovery of muscle contraction must be present.

CLINICAL USE OF NEUROMUSCULAR BLOCKING AGENTS

Selection of Cases

When is it appropriate to use neuromuscular blocking agents in equine anesthesia? In our recent review of 89 anesthetics in 88 horses given relaxants as an adjunct to anesthesia, equine patients ranged in age from 5 weeks to 25 years old, and weighed from 70 kg to 612 kg. Eighteen breeds were represented (Table 17–1).

In that clinical study, the decision to use relaxants was based on assignment of the patient to one of three selection categories. First, there were certain types of patients that benefited from, or surgical procedures that were facilitated by, improved muscle relaxation. In those instances, relaxants were planned as part of the preoperative anesthetic decision. For example, an elective decision to use relaxants would be made for horses known to have problems with hypotension and persistent movement under anesthesia. Surgical procedures that were facilitated by relaxant use included abdominal procedures such as removal of ovarian tumors and cesarean section. Ophthalmologic surgery, reduction of difficult fractures, and prevention of vigorous muscle movement induced by electrocautery were other examples of surgical procedures facilitated by relaxants.

A second category included anesthetics for which relaxant use was not planned, but intraoperative problems arose for which the best solution was the administration of relaxant. The most common problem encountered in this instance was severe hypotension

TABLE 17–1. BREEDS OF HORSES GIVEN CLINICAL GENERAL ANESTHESIA WITH ADJUNCT NEUROMUSCULAR BLOCKING AGENTS

Breed	Number
Thoroughbred	29
Arabian	17
Quarter Horse	12
Appaloosa	8
Mix	4
Saddlebred	3
Tennessee Walking Horse	2
Paint	2
Dutch Warmblood	1
Hanovarian	1
Morgan	1
Salle France	1
Pony of America	1
Palomino	1
Holsteiner	1
Shetland	1
American Miniature	1
Mustang	1

accompanied by persistent movement. Another common reason for intraoperative relaxant use was difficulty in obtaining adequate surgical exposure. One case cited was a Holsteiner presented for cryptorchid castration. This was a very large horse that became hypotensive during surgery, but was not relaxed sufficiently for the surgeons to exteriorize the retained testicle. Atracurium provided relaxation for the surgical exposure while sparing the horse the further cardiovascular depression that increased doses of anesthetic would have caused.

The third reason for selecting relaxant use was for teaching purposes. Types of surgical procedures that were performed under anesthesia with adjunct relaxants are noted in Table 17–2.

Monitoring Neuromuscular Blockade

Neuromuscular blocking agents should not be used without monitoring neuromuscular function. Fortunately, this is not difficult to do. There are, however, some limitations to monitoring neuromuscular blockade, since the neuromuscular junction, like many other organs, has a built-in "safety margin." That is, response to tests can appear normal when as many as 75% of the receptors on the neuromuscular junction are still occupied by relaxant. The most commonly used method of monitoring neuromuscular blockade is to place stimulating electrodes on either side of a nerve and observe muscle twitch response to nerve stimulus delivered by a hand-held peripheral nerve stimulator (Ministim; Professional Instruments). The stimulus mode has an important effect on muscle twitch response.

Single Twitch. The single twitch is given at a relatively slow frequency (Fig. 17–2). Stimulus frequency is measured in Hertz (Hz), or cycles per second. Single twitches are given at approximately 0.1 to 0.15 Hz, or a twitch every 6 to 10 seconds. To be most effective, the stimulus must be supramaximal voltage—in other words, increasing voltage will not increase the strength of muscle contraction. The single twitch has a duration of approximately 0.3 msec.

TABLE 17–2. TYPE OF SURGICAL PROCEDURES PERFORMED DURING CLINICAL GENERAL ANESTHESIA WITH ADJUNCT NEUROMUSCULAR BLOCKING AGENTS*

Abdominal	# of Animals	Orthopedic	# of Animals
Ovariectomy	19	Arthrotomy	6†
Exploratory laparotomy	12	Arthroscopy	2
Uterine torsion	2	Long bone fracture	5
Colopexy	2	Small bone fracture	2
Hysterectomy	1	Fracture jaw	2
Umbilical abscess	1	Joint flush	1
Dystocia	1	Arthrodesis	1
Remove twin	1	TOTAL	19
Hernia repair	1		
Uterine electrodes	1		
TOTAL	41		
Ophthalmologic	**# of Animals**	**Soft Tissue**	**# of Animals**
Keratectomy	4	Carotid relocation	5†
Corneal repair	4	Carotid catheterization	3
Corneal graft	3	Cholangiotomy	1
Cataract removal	2	Ethmoid hematoma removal	1
Eyelid mass	1	Cryptorchid castration	1
Ocular exploration	1	Penile retroversion	1
Strontium therapy	1	Penile retraction	1
Iridectomy	1	Melanoma removal	1
TOTAL	17	Esophagotomy	1
		TOTAL	15
Thoracotomy	**# of Animals**		
Persistent right aortic arch	1		

* From Hildebrand SV, Holland M, Copland VS, Daunt D, Brock N: Clinical use of the neuromuscular blocking agents atracurium and pancuronium for equine anesthesia. *J Am Vet Med Assoc* 1989;195:212–219.

† For four cases, carotid relocation and arthrotomy were performed on the same animal.

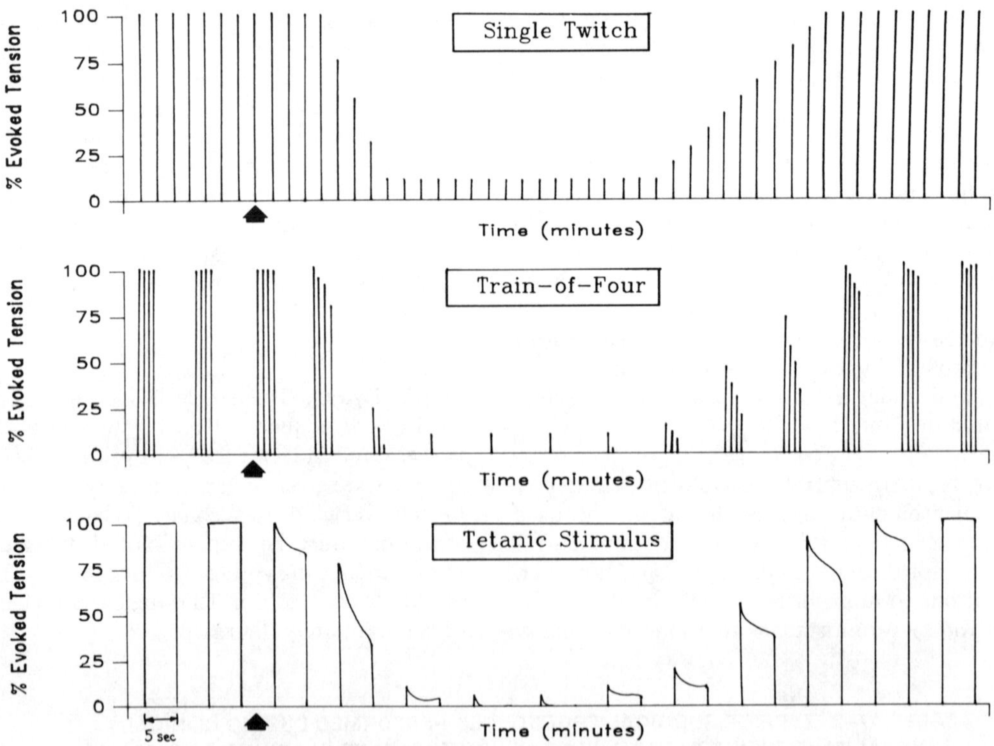

Figure 17–2. Drawing representing the evoked muscle tension (twitch) responses to single twitch, train-of-four, and tetanic nerve stimuli as they would appear on a polygraph trace if measured. In a clinical situation, the anesthesiologist observes or palpates these changes, and objectively assesses the reduction in twitch strength. Two features of muscle response are noted. First, a decrease in evoked tension is seen after administration of relaxant with all three stimulus modes. Second, with train-of-four and tetanic stimuli, fade is seen as an inability to sustain initial evoked strength. For train-of-four, fade progresses until only the first twitch in the train is seen. For tetanic response, the evoked tension rapidly decreases even though the stimulus is continuously administered for the same amount of time (usually 5 seconds) as it was before the relaxant was given. Large doses of relaxant can completely obliterate all twitch responses.

The single twitch generates a nerve action potential and subsequent neuromuscular transmission and muscle contraction that mimics the normal response. The drawback to this stimulus mode relates to the safety margin mentioned previously. The single twitch does not stress the neuromuscular junction very much, so twitch response can appear normal, even with as many as 75% of the receptors still occupied by relaxant. As an analogy, a very weak person walking slowly along a flat surface could appear perfectly normal at that slow, undemanding pace.

Train-of-Four. The train-of-four stimulus mode consists of four single twitches given in rapid succession at a rate of 2 Hz, or two twitches per second given for 2 seconds. The train is repeated no more frequently than every 12 seconds. This more rapid stimulus rate is more stressful to the neuromuscular junction than is the single twitch, but does not upset normal neuromuscular junction physiology. The train-of-four defines the influence of the relaxant on neuromuscular transmission better than does the single twitch. To use the same analogy as above, if people are asked to jog on a flat surface, it becomes clearer which individuals are weak now that demands on their muscle strength are increased. The train-of-four, then, gives the anesthesiologist better information about muscle strength than the single twitch.

The train-of-four also gives information that the single twitch cannot, that is, the ability of the muscle to sustain the strength it generates in response to nerve stimulus. There are receptors on both the motor endplate and the nerve terminal (Fig. 17–1). The former affect the strength of the twitch response and the latter affect the ability to sustain the response. The nondepolarizing muscle relaxants attach to both of those receptors. As a result, when a more demanding stimulus such as the train-of-four is applied during neuromuscular blockade with a nondepolarizing relaxant, a phenomenon known as fade will occur. Fade defines the inability of the neuromuscular junction to sustain muscle strength. An analogy to illustrate this is a weight lifter who can press 500 lb, but must quickly drop the weight because he is unable to continue suspending it in the air. Train-of-four fade is illustrated in Figure 17–2. Prejunctional receptor blockade may be very important for the horse recovering from anesthesia, because an animal with significant residual blockade of those receptors may be able to stand, but will quickly fall again because of its inability to sustain the strength needed to remain on its feet.

Train-of-four, then, is more informative than the single twitch, but it is not perfect. As many as 50% of receptors may still be blocked and the train-of-four can appear normal.

Tetanic Stimulus. Tetanic stimulus (Fig. 17–2) is the most rapid stimulus mode, and as such is very stressful to neuromuscular transmission. Tetanic stimulus is a series of single twitches given at 50 to 200 Hz over a 5-second period. At that rapid stimulus rate, the unparalyzed muscle cannot relax between stimuli and remains contracted for the duration of application. For clinical purposes, it is not necessary to exceed 50 Hz. Tetanic stimulus should not be repeated more often than every 12 seconds, or the enhanced mobilization and release of acetylcholine caused by this unphysiologic stimulus will make the next stimulus appear stronger than it really is. Tetanic stimulus is quite painful, and it is therefore important to make sure the horse is adequately anesthetized before giving a tetanic stimulus. Otherwise, the horse may respond quite vigorously. Indeed, peripheral nerve stimulators can be quite useful to assess an unparalyzed, anesthetized horse's response to stimulus before surgery to predict the reaction to an incision.

Tetanic stimulus is the strongest stimulus mode for stressing the neuromuscular junction, and as such provides even more information about residual blockade. To use the earlier analogy, tetanic stimulus would equate to asking the people jogging on the flat to run full tilt up a hill. This would reveal the weaker individuals during this more demanding exercise.

Like the train-of-four, tetanic stimulus also gives information about fade. With a relaxant such as atracurium, when the train-of-four is so reduced and faded that only the first twitch in the train is visible, the tetanic stimulus will look like a weak single stimulus since both its initial strength and its ability to sustain strength are affected.

Position of Stimulating Electrodes. The anatomic placement of the stimulating electrodes will also influence interpretation of the twitch response. The nerves most commonly used are the facial or the superficial peroneal nerve on the hind limb (Fig. 17–3). The response of the hind hoof extensor muscles to superficial peroneal nerve stimulus is much more sensitive to the effects of neuromuscular blocking agents than is the response of the facial muscles when the stimulus is applied to the facial nerve. This disparity in sensitivity is not unique to the horse, and has also been described in humans. It does have some practical significance since a relatively strong facial twitch will be present after a dose of relaxant that obliterates the hoof twitch. In addition, fade, which is an early response of the hind hoof response to train-of-four or tetanic stimulus, may not be seen at all with the facial muscles. This poses both advantages and disadvantages. For example, during colic surgery the hind limb is not available for monitoring twitch response. Because the response of the facial muscles will give less specific information about neuromuscular blockade, it is a little more difficult to determine the degree of block, to decide when additional doses are necessary, and to know the level of the block when it is time to recover the horse. During ophthalmologic surgery, the head is not available for monitoring, and the large doses of relaxant required to ensure a motionless eye will obliterate the hoof twitch. If the duration of ocular surgery dictates repeated doses

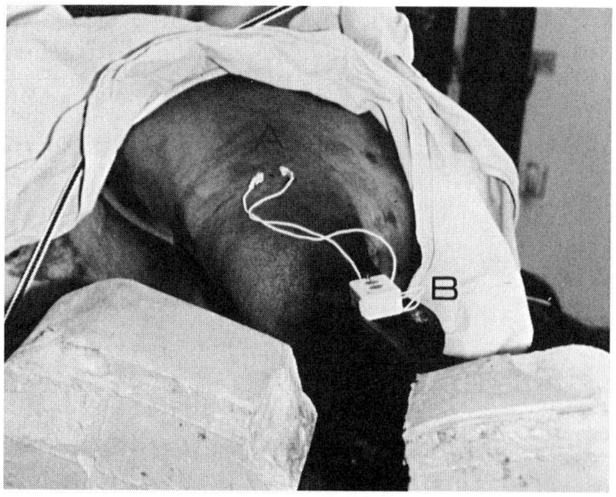

Figure 17–3. Placement of stimulating electrodes on the superficial peroneal nerve. For placement of the electrodes, palpate the tibial crest, then move in a caudal direction to a point about halfway across the lateral aspect of the leg. There the superficial peroneal nerve can be palpated as a mobile cordlike structure as it crosses the lateral head of the tibia. Stimulus causes extension of the hoof. *A*, the needle electrodes; *B*, a hand-held peripheral nerve stimulator.

of relaxant, these need to be given when hoof twitch becomes barely discernible again. When both face and hind limb are available for monitoring, the gradation in response is an advantage since one of those two sites will generally have a response to monitor at all times.

Selection of Relaxants

Positive pressure ventilation MUST be used when neuromuscular blocking agents are used. It is advisable to begin positive pressure ventilation before the relaxant is administered. This practice ensures that consistent ventilatory support is possible.

In our review of clinical cases, atracurium and pancuronium were used. However, atracurium was the relaxant of choice. In part that was related to the predictable action of atracurium, and its lack of effect on cardiovascular function. However, a major reason for selection of atracurium was cost. Atracurium proved to be as potent as pancuronium in horses, an unusual finding since atracurium is less potent than pancuronium in other species. Because of the potency relationship between the two relaxants, pancuronium was much more expensive than atracurium. Pancuronium was also inconvenient to use compared to atracurium. Pancuronium is provided in 2-mg/mL glass ampules, whereas atracurium is provided as 10-ml, 10-mg/mL, multiple-dose vials.

Atracurium was used in two dose ranges, depending on desired relaxation. An initial dose of 0.1 to 0.12 mg/kg (50 to 80 mg for an average adult horse) provided surgical relaxation, or 95% block of the hind hoof twitch. Onset of maximum relaxation occurred approximately 5 minutes after IV injection, with relaxation lasting 30 to 40 minutes. This dose proved adequate for most surgical procedures on the body and limbs. However, for ophthalmologic surgery or reduction of difficult fractures, larger doses of 0.15 to 0.2 mg/kg were used. Doses of that magnitude lasted approximately 60 minutes. Once recovery of hoof twitch began, recovery of muscle function proceeded at the same rate, regardless of magnitude of dose or how many times doses were repeated. Repeat doses were given as necessary, depending on the duration of surgery and the return of muscle strength (Table 17–3). It was considered desirable to have as long a time as possible elapse between the last dose of relaxant and the end of anesthesia, to allow spontaneous recovery of strength to proceed as much as possible before reversal and transportation to the recovery stall. Repeat doses ranged from 10 to 30 mg for average adult horses, for relaxation of up to 4 hours' duration. Pancuronium was used in a manner similar to atracurium.

Use of vecuronium has not been described in horses. Presumably, vecuronium would have many of the features of pancuronium and should be appropriate for use in equine anesthesia.

Monitoring Depth of Anesthesia

It is very important to ensure adequate depth of anesthesia when neuromuscular blocking agents are used. It is not unreasonable to assume that mistakes of "too light" or "too deep" will be made when the anesthesiologist is first learning to use relaxants as adjuncts to anesthesia. However, the same signs that are used to monitor depth of anesthesia in the unparalyzed horse are used when relaxants are given. For example, hyper-

TABLE 17–3. DOSES OF RELAXANT USED*,†

	Routine	High
1st dose (mg/kg)	0.01–0.15	0.2
Duration of 1st dose (min)	30–40	50–60
Repeat doses (mg/kg)	0.02–0.06	0.06–0.1
Duration of repeat dose (mg/kg)	15–20	30–50
	Pancuronium	**Atracurium**
Total dose (mg)		
$\bar{X} \pm$ SD	80 ± 27	87 ± 38
Range	40–114	50–240

* From Hildebrand SV, Holland M, Copland VS, Daunt D, Brock N: Clinical use of neuromuscular blocking agents atracurium and pancuronium for equine anesthesia. *J Am Vet Med Assoc* 1989;195:212–219.

† Dose magnitude is broken down into two categories, with the high dose representing the larger doses used for surgical procedures judged to require profound relaxation, for example, ophthalmic surgery or difficult fracture repair. Total dose given over the course of surgery for pancuronium and atracurium is also noted on the table.

tension, tachycardia, lacrimation, nystagmus, and pupillary dilation reliably indicate the need for deeper anesthesia, whether the horse is paralyzed or not. At the dose range cited for atracurium and pancuronium, muscle movement can also occur in the event that the horse is too lightly anesthetized, but the movement is slight. An advantage of relaxants in this case is that the error of inadequate anesthesia can be quickly corrected without the violent and devastating movement that can attend such errors. During surgery for colic, for example, horses are frequently very ill and have poor tolerance of the depressing effects of general anesthesia. Sudden movement can occur during surgery, when the anesthesiologist is trying to protect against further circulatory compromise by using light levels of anesthesia. If that movement is violent, bowel may be spilled onto the floor and contamination may occur.

It is probably possible to give anesthesia that is too light to be humane if larger doses of relaxant than are cited in this study are used, and the anesthesiologist is completely oblivious to the usual signs of depth of anesthesia. The signs of depth of anesthesia will also indicate that the horse is too deeply anesthetized. Both positive pressure ventilation and relaxant contribute to vaporizer dial settings that may be lower than those required for the unparalyzed, spontaneously breathing horse. Again, patient monitoring is the guide for determining the concentration of anesthetic to be administered. Augmentation of general anesthesia by relaxants can be seen during equine clinical anesthesia. Signs of anesthesia and vaporizer dial settings will be stable, but as spontaneous recovery from relaxant is noted, blood pressure may be seen to rise. When the relaxant dose is repeated, blood pressure returns to its previous stable level.

Reversal of Neuromuscular Blocking Agents

Because of the safety margin of neuromuscular transmission noted earlier, and the limitations of even the best monitoring guides, it is advisable to antagonize nondepolarizing blockade, regardless of how long it has been since the last dose of relaxant. Reversal drugs should be given at the end of anesthesia, when the horse is ready to be taken to the recovery stall. Even if it has been some time since the last dose of relaxant was given, administration of the reversal agent just before the horse is moved to the recovery stall will permit the reversal agent to have its maximal effect when it is needed most.

Edrophonium 0.5 to 1.0 mg/kg IV and neostigmine 0.04 mg/kg IV have been used to antagonize neuromuscular blockade in horses. Both drugs were effective reversal agents when the hoof twitch had recovered to 10% of its prerelaxant strength. Edrophonium had a slightly more rapid onset of action than did neostigmine, and the muscarinic side effects of edrophonium were much less than those for neostigmine. Because of those undesirable side effects, which included salivation, flatulence, and defecation, atropine 0.01 to 0.02 mg/kg IV should be used in conjunction with neostigmine. However, side effects were so minimal with edrophonium that atropine was not administered with it. This is a distinct advantage of edrophonium, since atropine can have prolonged undesirable side effects of its own.

In most species, additional muscarinic side effects of the anticholinesterase agents are bradycardia and hypotension. This does not appear to be the case in horses. Edrophonium, without atropine, consistently caused blood pressure to increase in horses (Fig. 17–4). In an experimental study, the decrease in heart rate, when it occurred, was after the rise in blood pressure. Neostigmine caused similar changes. In a clinical study, heart rate changes after edrophonium were quite variable, with no change or an increase in heart rate occurring in approximately half the horses (Table 17–4). When there was a reduction in heart rate, the decrease was generally slight, with no apparent deleterious effects on blood pressure. Rate of injection of edrophonium influenced cardiovascular changes, with a slow injection over 1 minute decreasing the changes. One horse in the clinical study developed total atrioventricular block after rapid injection of edrophonium. This block responded to treatment with atropine. It is therefore recommended that edrophonium be given slowly, and the electrocardiogram be monitored carefully during injection.

In most cases, additional edrophonium should not be required after the first 0.5 mg/kg dose. However, if there is any concern that the horse has residual weakness in the recovery stall, additional increments of 0.25 mg/kg edrophonium should be given slowly IV while palpating the pulse. It is difficult to differentiate residual weakness due to a muscle relaxant from the effects of general anesthesia. Signs to look for include shallow breathing pattern without a periodic large sigh and weak, minimal leg movement despite ocular responses that indicate the horse has regained consciousness. To help determine if residual weakness is present, one should consider the total dose of relaxant given during anesthesia and when the last dose of relaxant was given. Relaxant effects may be prolonged if the horse is acidemic or cold or has electrolyte abnormalities. In the clinical study cited above, only one animal clearly had a problem with inadequate reversal. A large dose of relaxant had been given in a relatively short period of time, and reversal attempted soon after the last dose of relaxant. The first additional dose of edrophonium in

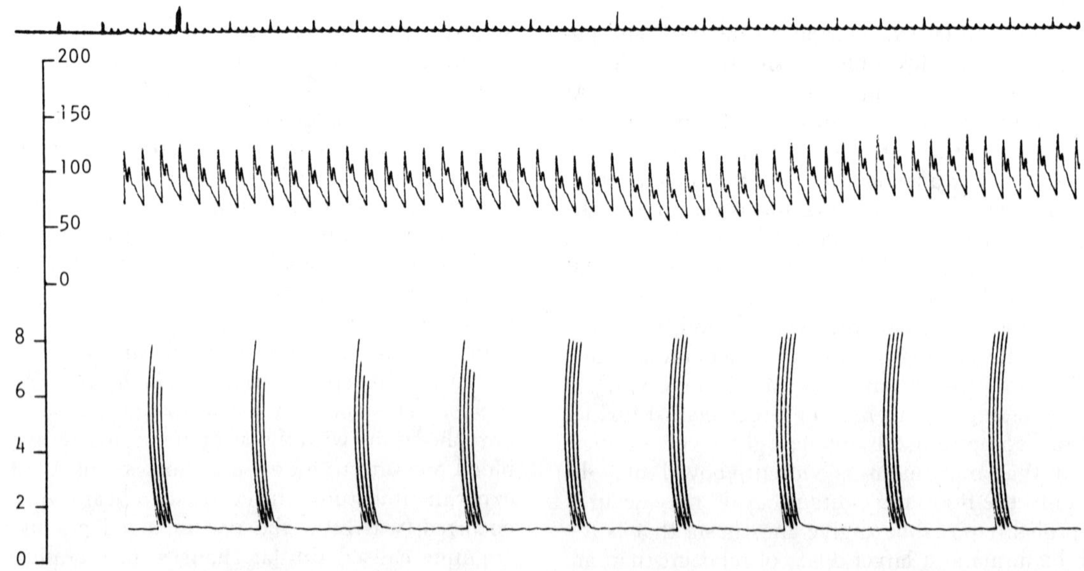

Figure 17–4. Actual polygraph trace to illustrate both cardiovascular and neuromuscular effects of edrophonium 0.5 mg/kg IV in a horse anesthetized with halothane. **Top.** Time elapsed, with each mark representing 1 second. Edrophonium is given at the heavy mark on the left of the time scale. **Middle.** Arterial blood pressure. Within 80 seconds of injection, blood pressure increased from 120/70 mm Hg to 130/75 mm Hg. Heart rate did not change. Scale on the far left indicates 0 to 200 mm Hg for the blood pressure trace. **Bottom.** Evoked twitch tension. Within 1 minute of injection, fade disappears and evoked tension of all four twitches in the train-of-four increases. Scale on the far left indicates 0 to 8 kg for evoked tension of hoof twitch. (From Hildebrand SV, Arpin D: Neuromuscular and cardiovascular effects of atracurium in healthy adult horses. *Am J Vet Res* 1988;49:1066–1071.)

recovery improved that animal's breathing pattern. The animal assumed sternal recumbency after the second additional dose, and stood well after the third dose of edrophonium.

Quality of Recovery to Standing after Muscle Relaxant Use

In both experimental and clinical studies, the majority of recoveries were rated excellent to good (Table 17–5). Some of the longest and most difficult cases recovered in an excellent manner. Examples of these included an apprehensive 7-year-old Arabian cross gelding that underwent a 4-hour pastern arthrodesis. Another was a 25-year-old Pony of America undergoing repair of a fractured tibia. Fracture repair took several hours and a blood transfusion was needed during surgery.

Two horses in the clinical study had recoveries that were rated as poor based on repeated, violent, unsuc-

TABLE 17–4. CARDIOVASCULAR EFFECTS OF EDROPHONIUM*

	Increase	No Change	Decrease
Blood pressure			
Number of animals	65	4	7
Magnitude (mm Hg)			
$\bar{X} \pm$ SD	16 ± 11	—	4 ± 2
Range	5–42	—	2–8
Heart rate			
Number of animals	30	13	36
Magnitude (beats/min)			
$\bar{X} \pm$ SD	10 ± 7	—	7 ± 4
Range	1–39	—	1–20

* From Hildebrand SV, Holland M, Copland VS, Daunt D, Brock N: Clinical use of neuromuscular blocking agents atracurium and pancuronium for equine anesthesia. *J Am Vet Med Assoc* 1989;195:212–219.

TABLE 17–5. RATINGS OF RECOVERY TO STANDING AFTER ANESTHESIA WITH ADJUNCT NEUROMUSCULAR BLOCKING AGENTS*,†

	Number of Animals			
	Excellent	Good	Fair	Poor
All animals	43	29	11	2
Pancuronium group‡	3	2	—	—
Isoflurane group	12	8	5	—
Halothane group	31	21	6	2

* From Hildebrand SV, Holland M, Copland VS, Daunt D, Brock N: Clinical use of neuromuscular blocking agents atracurium and pancuronium for equine anesthesia. *J Am Vet Med Assoc* 1989;195:212–219.

† To illustrate the quality of recovery associated with different agents, recovery ratings for the five animals that received pancuronium, and for the animals that received halothane or isoflurane for maintenance anesthesia, are separated from the total of all animals. Quality of recovery was not influenced by the different agents.

‡ All animals in the pancuronium group received halothane as the maintenance anesthetic.

cessful attempts to stand. It was difficult, however, to implicate any one factor as the cause of the poor recoveries in those two instances. Unknown history, temperament of the horses prior to anesthesia, pressure on muscles during anesthesia, and pain from surgery probably all contributed to those two poor recoveries.

Of all the horses in experimental and clinical studies, one horse developed a serious complication. That animal developed laminitis severe enough to necessitate euthanasia the day after anesthesia. Since that horse was a research animal with an unknown history, and anesthesia and surgery for subcutaneous carotid artery relocation were uneventful until the laminitis developed, it is difficult to determine what contribution atracurium may have had.

BIBLIOGRAPHY

Ali HH, Savarese JJ: Monitoring neuromuscular function. *Anesthesiology* 1976;45:216–243.

Hildebrand SV, Howitt GA: Antagonism of pancuronium neuromuscular blockade in halothane anesthetized ponies using neostigmine and edrophonium. *Am J Vet Res* 1984;45:2276–2280.

Hildebrand SV, Howitt GA, Arpin D: Neuromuscular and cardiovascular effects of atracurium in ponies anesthetized with halothane. *Am J Vet Res* 1986;47:1096–1100.

Hildebrand SV, Arpin D: Neuromuscular and cardiovascular effects of atracurium in healthy adult horses. *Am J Vet Res* 1988;49:1066–1071.

Hildebrand SV, Holland M, Hill T: Trichlorfon does not alter neuromuscular blocking activity of atracurium in halothane anesthetized horses. *Anesthesiology* 1987;67:A350.

Hughes R, Chapple DJ: The pharmacology of atracurium: a new competitive neuromuscular blocking agent. *Br J Anaesth* 1981;53:31–44.

Miller RD, Savarese JJ: Pharmacology of muscle relaxants and their antagonists, in Miller RD (ed): *Anesthesia*. New York, Churchill Livingstone, 1986, pp 889–943.

Scott RPF, Savarese JJ, Basta SF, Sunder N, Ali HH, Gargarian M, Gionfriddo M, Batson AG: Atracurium: Clinical strategies for preventing histamine release and attenuating the hemodynamic response. *Br J Anaesth* 1985;57:550–553.

Standaert FG: Basic physiology and pharmacology of neuromuscular junction, in Miller RD (ed): *Anesthesia*. New York, Churchill Livingstone, 1986, pp 835–870.

18 Management of Anesthetic Emergencies

Wayne N. McDonell
Doris H. Dyson

The best method of dealing with anesthetic emergencies is to anticipate and prevent them if at all possible. While temperament, size, preexisting disease, unavoidable equipment failure, and idiosyncratic drug reactions are responsible for some equine anesthetic emergencies, many clinical emergencies are a result of human error. This may take the form of inadequate preoperative evaluation and/or preparation of the animal, inattention to detail in drug selection, dosage, and administration, or inexperience or carelessness in the use of anesthetic and monitoring equipment.

BASIC DRUG AND EQUIPMENT REQUIREMENTS

Even when performing anesthesia in "field" conditions, the clinician who assumes the responsibility must also assume the responsibility of providing at least elementary emergency support if the animal responds adversely to the anesthetic. Recommended emergency equipment and drugs are shown in Tables 18–1 and 18–2. An E-sized oxygen tank with a reducing valve and flow control (Hudson 2 Stage Regulator, Model 2815; Hudson Oxygen Therapy Sales Co) provides a convenient portable source of oxygen; a full tank will provide 25 L/min oxygen flow for about 20 minutes. With the addition of a simple demand valve and appropriate regulator (Hudson Demand Valve, Model 5040, and Model 2830 demand valve regulator), it is possible to provide very effective short-term intermittent positive pressure ventilation (IPPV). Oxygen cylinders should be firmly secured in a reasonably central location (e.g., backseat area) when transported in a vehicle and the valve should be completely closed.

Emergency drugs and equipment should be readily available and organized in a consistent manner. Comparatively inexpensive multidrawer toolboxes work very well as emergency kits. An attached list of drug indications and recommended doses will save valuable time and minimize the chances of error in administration.

PERIANESTHETIC PROBLEMS

Intracarotid and Perivascular Injections

The carotid artery of the horse lies just under the jugular vein and it is surprisingly easy to go through the vein accidentally and enter the artery. Consequently, all injections should be given in the upper half of the jugular vein. To permit visual evidence of pulsatile blood flow if the needle tip is in the artery, no needle smaller than an 18-gauge bore should ever be used for equine jugular venipuncture. The needle should always be inserted before attachment to the syringe. Arterial blood will not spontaneously push back the plunger of a plastic syringe, and the color of blood drawn into a syringe is not a reliable indicator of needle (or catheter) placement.

Intracarotid injection of even small amounts (0.5 mL) of xylazine, acetylpromazine, lidocaine, or antibiotics will produce sudden collapse, in some cases with convulsions or apnea. Treatment is supportive (oxygen, IPPV, 10 to 20 mg diazepam intravenously [IV]), and directed toward maintaining oxygenation and preventing self-trauma.

The best way of protecting against accidental intracarotid and perivascular injections is by placement of an indwelling catheter. These are recommended even for field anesthetics because of the risk of serious tissue irritation caused by perivascular leakage of thiobarbiturates, guaifenesin, chloral hydrate, or sodium bicarbonate solutions. A secure indwelling catheter also provides a ready, reliable venous access if supplementary anesthetic or supportive drugs are required during the period of anesthesia. A 14-gauge over-the-needle

(*text continues on p. 109*)

TABLE 18–1. RECOMMENDED BASIC EQUINE EMERGENCY EQUIPMENT AND SUPPLIES

1. Oxygen source, regulator, and flow meter
2. Demand valve
3. Endotracheal tubes:
   25 mm (for orotracheal use)
   18–20 mm (for nasotracheal use and ponies)
   14–16 mm (for foals)
   10–12 mm (for pony foals)
4. Mouth gag (7.5–10-cm length of 7.5-cm plumbing pipe)
5. Foal stomach tube (for endotracheal oxygen administration)
6. Indwelling vascular catheters (14 gauge) and at least two fluid administration sets (for titration of catecholamine dose and fluid therapy)
7. Assorted needles and syringes
8. Needle for intracardiac injections (16–18 gauge, 15–20 cm long)
9. Sterile fluids:
   2 units 500 mL lactated Ringer's solution or 0.9% sodium chloride
   1 unit 500 mL 5% dextrose in water

TABLE 18–2. DRUGS USED FOR EQUINE ANESTHETIC EMERGENCIES

Classification and Generic Name	Preparation (Supplier)	Recommended Use	Dose		Remarks, Precautions
			Per kg	Total (450 kg)	
Respiratory stimulant					
Doxapram	Dopram-V 20 mg/mL (A. H. Robins Co)	To initiate or stimulate breathing (temporarily) when IPPV is not possible.	0.25–0.5 mg IV	5–10 mL	Best used with concurrent O_2 insufflation. Will not work in the presence of significant cerebral hypoxia. May lighten anesthesia to the point where movement occurs.
Cardiac stimulants					
Epinephrine	Adrenalin 1.0 mg/mL (Parke Davis)	For initiation of a heartbeat in an asystolic heart. Rapidly restores vascular tone unless phenothiazine tranquilizer used in premedication. Bronchodilator.	2–4 μg IV, IC, IT (repeat in 1–2 min if needed)	1.0–2.0 mL diluted in 10 mL saline	Most effective drug for use with asystole. May produce arrhythmias/fibrillation during halothane anesthesia; the risk of this may be lessened by giving 1–2 mg/kg lidocaine before epinephrine. Tachycardia and hypertension common if the heart starts, or if the drug is used when asystole not present.
Calcium chloride	100 mg salt/mL (1.36 mEq Ca/mL)	To increase myocardial contractility, stroke volume, and cardiac output. To reverse cardiodepressive effects of high K^+ levels in uremic animals. May be useful with electromechanical dissociation. Used with neostigmine to reverse neuromuscular blockade from aminoglycoside antibiotic.	0.05–0.1 mL IV	20–45 mL	Reflex bradycardia and atrioventricular block may be seen if infusion too rapid. Usually does not provide sustained effect.

Continued

TABLE 18–2. (*continued*)

Classification and Generic Name	Preparation (Supplier)	Recommended Use	Dose		Remarks, Precautions
			Per kg	Total (450 kg)	
Ephedrine	Ephedrine 50 mg/mL (Abbot)	To increase arterial blood pressure.	0.01–0.2 mg IV, IM	Usually given in 10-mg doses IV at 3–5-min intervals until desired response seen	Indirect and direct pressor effects. Slower onset and longer duration. May produce cardiac dysrhythmias. No reduction of uterine blood flow. Should not be used as a replacement for blood volume expansion.
Anticholinergics					
Atropine	0.6 mg/mL or 15 mg/mL	Treatment of sinus arrest, atrioventricular second- and third-degree block, severe bradycardia.	0.01–0.02 mg IV	4.5–9.0 mg (volume varies with preparation)	Always start with the lowest dose and see if it will work. High doses will produce prolonged tachycardia and gastrointestinal stasis.
Glycopyrrolate	Robinul-V 0.2 mg/mL (A. H. Robins Co)	Treatment of sinus arrest, atrioventricular second- and third-degree block, severe bradycardia.	1–5 μg IV	2.5–12.5 mL	Precautions as for atropine. Produces less tachycardia and may be associated with less gastrointestinal stasis than atropine.
Antiarrhythmics					
Lidocaine (without epinephrine)	20 mg/mL	Ventricular tachycardia and premature ventricular contractions.	0.5–1.0-mg IV bolus or 80 μg/min IV for continued effect	11–22 mL bolus or 90 mL in 500 mL 5% D/W at a drip rate of 10 mL/min	Convulsions may be seen with high doses in unanesthetized horses. Will produce mild myocardial depression but this should not preclude use.
Quinidine	80 mg/mL	Atrial fibrillation, supraventricular tachycardia.	1.0 mg IV every 10 min until a total of 4.0 mg/kg given	5–6-mL doses at each interval	May cause hypotension, or tachycardia. May worsen ventricular dysrhythmias.
Calcium borogluconate	230 mg salt/mL (0.96 mEq Ca/mL)	As for calcium chloride.	0.1–0.2 mL IV	45–90 mL	As for calcium chloride.

Continued

TABLE 18–2. (*continued*)

Classification and Generic Name	Preparation (Supplier)	Recommended Use	Dose: Per kg	Dose: Total (450 kg)	Remarks, Precautions
Dobutamine	Dobutrex 250 mg powder/ vial (Eli Lilly and Co)	To increase myocardial contractility, cardiac output, and blood pressure.	2.5–5.0 μg/ min IV	1 vial in 500 mL 5% dextrose (2–4 mL/ min for as long as needed)	Almost pure β_1 agonist. Improves myocardial contractility and blood pressure without tachycardia. Ventricular tachycardia and hypertension possible with overdose. Dose to effect.
Dopamine	Intropin 40 mg/ mL (Arnar-Stone Laboratories, Inc)	To increase myocardial contractility, cardiac output, and (at high doses) blood pressure.	2.5–5.0 μg/ min IV	1 vial (5 mL) in 500 mL 5% dextrose (2.5–5 mL/min for as long as needed)	Slightly more tendency to produce tachycardia than dobutamine at effective doses. Produces renal and splanchnic vasodilation with lower dose, and blood pressure may not rise. Dose to effect. Ventricular tachycardia is a sign of overdose.
Isoproterenol	Isuprel 0.2 mg/ mL (Winthrop Laboratories)	To correct atropine-resistant bradycardia. Bronchodilation.	0.5–0.1 μg/ min IV	1 vial (1 mL) in 500 mL NaCl and establish slow drip to effect	β_1 and β_2 agonist. Will produce severe tachycardia, dysrhythmias with overdose. Produces hypotension by vasodilation (β_2 effect).
Vasopressors					
Methoxamine	Vasoxyl 20 mg/ mL (Winthrop Laboratories)	For rapid increase of blood pressure when coronary perfusion threatened.	0.04 mg IV	1-mL bolus in emergency; otherwise dilute in 500 mL NaCl and give to effect	Almost pure α_1 agonist. Rapid effect IV—lasts for up to 1 h. May get reflex bradycardia. Will increase myocardial work and should only be used with life-threatening hypotension or when hypotension is due to peripheral vasodilation.

Continued

TABLE 18–2. (*continued*)

Classification and Generic Name	Preparation (Supplier)	Recommended Use	Dose		Remarks, Precautions
			Per kg	Total (450 kg)	
Phenylephrine	Neo-Synephrine 10 mg/mL (Winthrop Laboratories)	To increase arterial blood pressure.	0.01–0.02 mg IV, IM	0.5–1.0 mL, or add vial (1 mL) to 500 mL NaCl and give to effect	Rapid effect IV—lasts about 20 min. May get reflex bradycardia. Should not be used as a replacement for blood volume expansion.
Others					
Furosemide	Lasix 50 mg/mL (American Hoechst Corp)	To promote diuresis, reduce pulmonary edema.	0.5–1.0 mg IV	4.5–9.0 mL	Works well when the pulmonary edema is due to reduced oncotic pressure (fluid overload), not so well when edema has an inflammatory origin.
Prednisolone sodium succinate	Solu-Delta-Cortef 100 mg/mL (Upjohn Co)	Anaphylaxis, cerebral anoxia, electromechanical dissociation, pulseless idioventricular rhythm.	1–2 mg IV	1–2 vials (500 mg/vial)	Used as an initial dose, followed by dexamethasone for sustained effect.
Dexamethasone phosphate	Hexadrol 20 mg/mL (Organon)	As for prednisolone sodium succinate.	1–4 mg IV	22–100 mL	Should be administered slowly because may cause hypotension. Risk of inducing laminitis is suspected.
Flunixin meglumine	Banamine 500 mg/mL (Schering)	To modify circulatory response to endotoxin.	0.2–1.0 mg	2–10 mL	Should be given to all horses for treatment of endotoxemia or suspected endotoxemia.
Diazepam	Valium 5 mg/mL (Roche)	To stop convulsions.	0.02–0.1 mg IV	2-mL (1 vial) boluses to a total of 10 mL if needed	Mild antiarrhythmic effect. Produces little cardiopulmonary depression. Higher doses may leave the animal ataxic.
Sodium bicarbonate		To treat metabolic acidosis.	0.5 mEq IV at 10–15-min intervals as required (or as calculated by acid-base analysis)		May produce hypokalemia, paradoxical cerebrospinal fluid acidosis with higher doses given rapidly.

IV, intravenous; *IC*, intracardiac, *IM*, intramuscular; *IT*, intratracheal.

catheter is usually preferable, and it should be at least 2.5 in (7.5 cm) long; 5.5-in (15-cm) catheters are preferred because they stay in the vein better. These catheters may be left in place for up to 48 hours if they are inserted aseptically and are carefully secured in place.

The damage associated with accidental perivascular injections may be minimized by immediate dilution with large volumes of sterile saline, using at least ten times the estimated volume of the irritant solution. Hot compresses and massage will promote absorption and aid in resolution of the subsequent cellulitis.

Emergence Delirium

Emergence delirium is more likely if the induction was difficult or if problems were encountered keeping the horse asleep during anesthesia. In such instances, and whenever the duration of anesthesia is such that the preanesthetic sedative effect will have worn off, a small dose of xylazine (50 to 100 mg/450 kg IV) or acetylpromazine (10 to 15 mg/45O kg IV) should be given 3 to 5 minutes before the horse is disconnected from the anesthetic machine and moved to the recovery box. This seems to be a safe and efficacious procedure, even though these drugs have the potential to add to the degree of hypoxemia and circulatory depression characteristic of the recovery period. The objective should be to keep the horse quiet, sedated, and recumbent for about 30 minutes to provide time for clearance of the inhalant anesthetic. While halothane and isoflurane will wash out from the lungs and perhaps highly perfused visceral tissue sooner, clearance from the muscle and fat storage compartments is dependent upon circulation in these tissues. Accordingly, increasing ventilation for 5 or 10 minutes through the use of doxapram or a demand valve may not shorten the time to full recovery, especially if the circulation is poor. We believe doxapram administration is contraindicated as an equine recovery drug because of the generalized central nervous system stimulation that it produces, with the resultant tendency of early attempts of horses to stand.

Emergence delirium may be associated with airway obstruction and hypoxemia (see "Respiratory Insufficiency"), or with severe postorthopedic surgical pain. It is best to control this pain with reasonably heavy doses of opioid analgesics (meperidine, butorphanol, morphine) combined with small doses of xylazine, and to accept that the horse may remain recumbent for a longer time. Our clinical experience is that preoperative or prerecovery administration of anti-inflammatory drugs (phenylbutazone, flunixin) seems to reduce the chance of having a painful recovery after orthopedic surgery.

Prolonged postanesthetic recumbency (beyond 1 hour) occurs occasionally and may or may not be associated with unsuccessful attempts to rise. The possible causes include: (*a*) drug overdose (thiobarbiturate, guaifenesin); (*b*) unrecognized femoral or vertebral fracture; (*c*) myositis; (*d*) circulatory shock with secondary muscle weakness; and (*e*) generalized weakness or exhaustion. Successful treatment requires identification of the cause and institution of appropriate specific therapy; however, there is one important general principle. Repeated unsuccessful attempts at standing are always detrimental to a horse and will sooner or later lead to a long bone fracture or some other form of self-inflicted trauma. Occasionally a horse is able to stand on its front legs but cannot support itself on its hind legs. In these cases it is helpful to assist the animal using a rope on the tail. This can be passed through a ring or a hoist and used to aid and support the animal when it attempts to stand. When a horse is apparently unable to stand, it may be necessary to institute supportive therapy with intravenous crystalloid or colloid solutions as indicated, while keeping the horse quiet with heavy doses of opioid analgesics combined with small doses of xylazine, or by using chloral hydrate sedation to effect. Deep bedding, feed, and water should be provided if the horse is quiet enough to tolerate them. The horse should be cared for in the recumbent position and allowed to get up when it is strong enough to do so. A sling may be used to determine whether the horse can bear weight, but we have had little success with this technique for getting a horse to its feet. Many horses will not tolerate a sling, and other animals show submissive behavior (with no attempt to stand), indicating their dislike of being bodily suspended. Continued use of the sling in either case may be detrimental and may increase muscle damage.

RESPIRATORY INSUFFICIENCY

Apnea

A brief period of apnea (30 to 45 seconds) occurs commonly when a horse becomes recumbent upon induction of anesthesia. This postinduction apnea in the lightly anesthetized, nontympanitic animal is self-limiting and will correct itself when the arterial CO_2 levels rise. Twisting the ear or compression of the chest wall often provides enough stimulus to initiate a breath. Horses should not be positioned in dorsal recumbency until they are breathing regularly, preferably with oxygen supplementation. In the critically ill animal it is best to protect against the development of hypoxemia during the immediate postinduction period by preanesthetic oxygen administration through a nasotracheal catheter using flows of at least 15 L/min. A foal stomach tube works well as a catheter. Oxygen administration should be continued during the induction, if possible.

More threatening apnea episodes may be encountered on induction as a result of accidental drug overdose. This may occur when the animal's lean body weight is estimated incorrectly, if doses are based on total body weight in an obese animal, or if "cold"-blooded horses are given anesthetic doses developed for "warm"-blooded animals (see Chapter 13). Relative drug overdose may occur if unadjusted drug doses are used in heavily sedated, hypovolemic, or hypoproteinemic animals, or in the presence of other drugs that are highly protein bound (e.g., phenylbutazone). Animals with severe abdominal tympany (e.g., terminal pregnancy, colic) often show extreme hypoventilation and even apnea as soon as they become recumbent on induction. This eventuality should be anticipated, and the anesthetist needs to be prepared for immediate endotracheal intubation and IPPV.

Irrespective of the cause, apnea is best treated by rapid insertion of an endotracheal tube, followed by IPPV with oxygen. When inhalation anesthesia is being used, this is most easily accomplished by connecting the horse to the anesthetic machine and by manual or mechanical compression of the rebreathing bag at a rate of 4 to 6 compressions/min. During anesthesia away from the clinic, IPPV can be easily accomplished using an E-sized oxygen tank and a demand valve. A rate of 4 to 6 breaths per minute is adequate, and the lungs are inflated to produce visible chest expansion. If a demand valve is not available, an oro- or nasotracheal tube should be inserted quickly and oxygen insufflation should be started at a flow rate of at least 15 L/min. The resulting arterial oxygen tension (P_aO_2) levels are not normal, but life-sustaining hemoglobin saturation can be maintained for short periods of time. Usually the duration of apnea is short as a result of redistribution of the drugs. Doxapram (0.25 to 0.5 mg/kg IV) may help to establish spontaneous respiration in the drug-depressed animal if the animal is simultaneously oxygenated. External compression (4 to 6 times/min) of the chest wall provides little useful gas exchange between the lung and the exterior, but it may improve gas mixing when oxygen is being insufflated.

Airway Obstruction

Horses with preanesthetic evidence of upper airway obstruction (nasal or laryngeal edema or collapse, guttural pouch empyema, pharyngeal lymph node enlargement) will almost always develop far more severe obstruction once anesthetized. When possible, an 18- to 20-mm nasotracheal tube should be inserted with local anesthesia before induction. The nasal passage can be desensitized by spraying lidocaine into the nasal passage. A few minutes should be allowed before attempting to insert the nasotracheal tube. Alternatively, the anesthetist should have a range of endotracheal tubes available for rapid intubation shortly after induction. It is better to insert a relatively small tube (e.g., 20 mm) atraumatically and rapidly than to persist in trying to insert a larger (25- to 30-mm) tube that causes laryngeal trauma. The neck area should be clipped and prepared for an emergency tracheotomy before induction. If there is any real doubt about the ability to safely establish a secure airway following anesthetic induction, an endotracheal tube should be inserted via a tracheotomy under local anesthesia before induction.

A degree of airway obstruction is often observed when horses are extubated in the recovery period, particularly if the head has been positioned lower than the heart (dorsal recumbency) over 2 to 4 hours of anesthesia. This position leads to passive congestion and edema of the nasopharyngeal tissues. If significant airway obstruction occurs as the horse struggles to stand in the recovery period, the strong negative pressure on inspiration worsens the obstruction, with ensuing hypoxia and panic. In such instances it is very dangerous to even approach the horse in an effort to carry out an emergency tracheotomy. When the potential for partial or complete obstruction is present, it is best to recover the horse with an uncuffed orotracheal tube, or an 18- to 20-mm uncuffed nasotracheal tube taped in place. Horses tolerate this well.

Many horses that have undergone only short periods of anesthesia will demonstrate some respiratory stridor when the endotracheal tube is removed. This is related to the displacement of the soft palate above the epiglottis as a result of orotracheal intubation. If a foal stomach tube is inserted through the nostril and into the trachea, the stimulation usually causes a swallowing movement that realigns the epiglottis and soft palate, stopping the stridor. This same nasotracheal tube can be taped to the muzzle and will permit convenient oxygen insufflation (15 L/min) during the recovery period. While oxygen flows at these rates may not achieve normal P_aO_2 values, they improve P_aO_2 somewhat during the critical recovery period, lessening the chances of emergence delirium and sudden cardiovascular collapse.

Hypoventilation during Anesthesia

With short-duration (15- to 30-minute) field anesthetics, progressive hypoventilation (as distinct from apnea) is not likely to be a problem. If the horse is moving reasonable tidal volumes and the inspired oxygen concentration is enriched, arterial carbon dioxide tension

(P_aCO_2) and pH levels will not change enough to affect cardiovascular stability.

In contrast, progressive hypoventilation is always a distinct possibility with inhalation anesthesia, and many spontaneously breathing horses that are anesthetized longer than 60 minutes warrant the use of IPPV. The decision to use IPPV (controlled or assisted) is often made when P_aCO_2 levels reach 55 to 60 mm Hg or when pH is less than 7.20 (see Chapter 15).

Hypoxemia

The diagnosis of significant hypoxemia (P_aO_2 levels below 65 to 70 mm Hg) is not easy without the aid of arterial blood gas analysis. Advanced age, dorsal recumbency, obesity, size, abdominal tympany, endotoxemia, and low cardiac outputs all predispose to the development of arterial hypoxemia in horses, even when high levels of oxygen are administered and IPPV is used to keep P_aCO_2 levels in the eucapnic range. If nitrous oxide is being used as part of the anesthetic regimen, it should be discontinued. When possible, the horse should be repositioned into lateral recumbency or the abdomen should be rapidly decompressed by exteriorization of the distended bowel (e.g., abdominal surgery) to reduce the pressure on the diaphragm and the degree of lung collapse. If the circulation seems stable (mean blood pressure over 75 to 80 mm Hg, rapid capillary refill, and preexisting hypovolemia has been corrected), the duration of the IPPV inspiratory phase should be lengthened in an attempt to improve P_aO_2 levels. This often works, presumably through recruitment of ventilation to collapsed airspaces with a long time constant for inflation. With a Dräger AV-E Anesthesia Ventilator (North American Dräger) the inspiratory phase is lengthened by readjusting the inspiratory : expiratory ratio from the usual 1 : 2.5 to 1 : 3 setting to a 1 : 1 or 1 : 1.5 setting. With Bird ventilators (JD Medical Distributing Company) the inspiratory phase may be lengthened by reducing the inspiratory flow rate, or by switching off the air-mix setting (which serves to increase inspiratory flow when activated).

When the hypoxemia is not responsive to the measures listed above, or when the circulatory status will not permit prolongation of the inspiratory phase of the respiratory cycle, a dobutamine infusion at 2.5 to 5.0 μg/kg/min should be started. While healthy horses do not seem to improve their P_aO_2 levels as a result of dobutamine stimulation of cardiac output and blood pressure, a favorable response is often seen in the critically ill horse.

Pulmonary Edema

Pulmonary edema is rare during equine anesthesia, but it may be produced as an anaphylactic response to drugs (usually antibiotics), during endotoxemia, with pneumonia, or if excessive volumes of crystalloid solutions are administered, thereby reducing the plasma oncotic pressure by hemodilution. This latter situation is more likely to occur in hypoproteinemic animals, or when large amounts of protein are being lost intraoperatively into either the pleural or peritoneal cavity. Volume expansion should be carried out with plasma or dextran if the total protein level is below 4.0 g/dL. Pulmonary edema may occur as the left ventricle fails in terminal shock, and this edema is not necessarily due to overhydration.

Cyanosis, moist rales, and blood-tinged watery or frothy material in the trachea or endotracheal tube are all suggestive of pulmonary edema. If the animal is being ventilated, greater inflation pressures may be required to fully inflate the lungs (reduced compliance). High levels of oxygen should be administered and IPPV should be started if not already underway, using positive end-expiratory pressures of 5 to 10 cm H_2O if possible. Furosemide (0.5 to 1.0 mg/kg IV) should be administered. During anaphylactic reactions, epinephrine (2 to 4 μg/kg IV or intramuscularly [IM]) and a rapid-acting corticosteroid (prednisolone succinate 1 to 2 mg/kg IV) should also be administered.

CARDIOVASCULAR INSUFFICIENCY

Hypotension

During equine anesthesia sudden cardiopulmonary collapse is often preceded by serious arterial hypotension, and less severe prolonged arterial hypotension contributes to the development of postanesthetic myopathy. A primary goal during anesthesia is to maintain adequate blood pressure by influencing cardiac output and total peripheral resistance (Fig. 18–1). In most instances the hypotension is probably accompanied by a low cardiac output; however, cardiac output is seldom measured in routine clinical anesthesia.

It is not clear why the horse is so prone to the development of hypotension during general anesthesia, but the most likely culprits are the drugs used and the alterations in body position. Interestingly, adult cattle are not nearly as prone to the development of hypotension during inhalation anesthesia as the horse, despite the fact they should be subject to many of the same mechanical problems associated with recumbency and are often given similar drugs to induce general anesthesia. Cattle may actually become hypertensive during inhalation anesthesia.

In our clinical experience a degree of hypotension is very common early in the course of general anesthesia, especially during the period when transfer is being

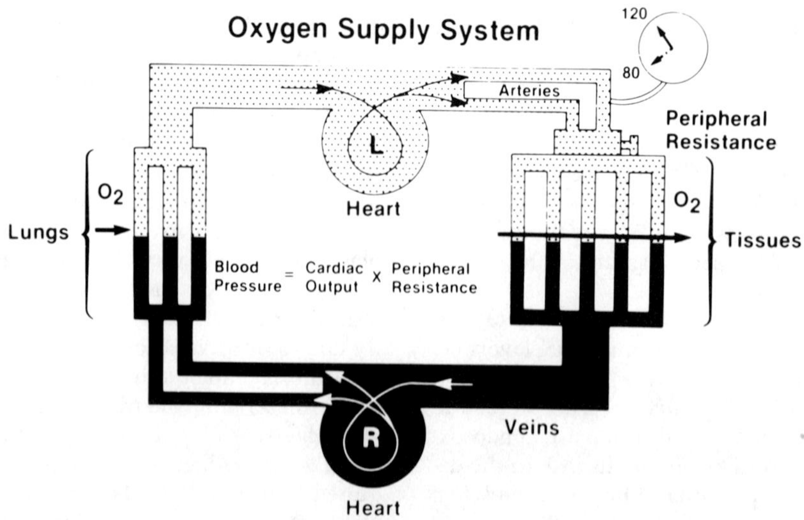

Figure 18–1. Schematic diagram of the circulation and oxygen supply system showing the interrelationship between arterial blood pressure, cardiac output (forward flow), and total peripheral resistance (made up of varying regional vascular resistances).

made from an intravenous agent to an inhalation agent. This hypotension seems to occur irrespective of the actual premedication and/or induction regimen chosen or the health of the horse, although inappropriate preanesthetic management certainly can worsen the situation in the critically ill animal. In individual animals the degree of hypotension can be life threatening and often it is the healthy, fit animal that is affected. It is important to recognize that large doses of anesthetic agents will almost always produce hypotension; there is a reasonably linear relationship between increases in the alveolar concentration of the inhalant anesthetics and the fall in cardiac output and blood pressure. Thus, the clinical message is clear: keep the horse in as light a plane of anesthesia as the surgery will permit.

Hypotension is best detected by the routine objective measurement of blood pressure during anesthesia using a direct or indirect system (see Chapter 16). Generally, severe hypotension will be detected by a reduction of pulse intensity on digital palpation and a prolongation of capillary refill time (>2.5 seconds), but earlier, less severe, and more easily treated degrees of hypotension will not be detectable by these clinical signs.

Whenever hypotension is detected a thorough examination should be made for potential contributing factors. Is the animal hypovolemic? Are there known or suspected arrhythmias or electrolyte, blood gas, or acid-base abnormalities? Is the disease state likely to be producing endotoxemia? When these factors are present, the priority should be to correct the primary problem if time allows and the blood pressure is stable. The therapy for a hypotensive episode will depend on its severity. With a mean pressure less than 50 mm Hg or a systolic pressure below 65 mm Hg there is a risk that coronary perfusion will be insufficient and cardiac arrest may occur. Electrocardiographic evidence of myocardial anoxia may show up as depression of the ST segment, T wave enlargement or reversal, bradycardia, or tachycardia. A weak corneal reflex and irregular respiratory pattern may also be seen. In this situation the inhalant is turned off, and the fluids (if already connected) are increased up to a flow of 1 mL/kg/min. In the spontaneously breathing animal it is important that IPPV *not* be suddenly instituted in an attempt to more readily clear the lungs of anesthetic, because this may further reduce venous return, leading to a further reduction of cardiac output and blood pressure that may precipitate cardiac arrest. Instead, the rebreathing bag should be emptied of anesthetic and refilled with oxygen using the flush valve at 90-second intervals, letting the horse continue to breathe spontaneously. If the horse is already on IPPV (or becomes apneic), the anesthetic concentration in the circuit and lungs is reduced with the use of the flush valve and the rate of ventilation is set at 4 to 6 breaths/min to provide a good interval for cardiac filling between breaths.

The next step is to prepare a vasopressor, which will be used to provide an immediate increase in arterial pressure. Doses are given for three vasopressors in Table 18–2. Ephedrine is probably the agent of choice because it has a greater effect in reducing venous capacitance than on arteriolar constriction. It also possesses some β_1 activity, so it will give an improvement in cardiac performance. Phenylephrine increases both arteriolar and venous constriction, whereas methoxamine has its predominant activity on the arteriolar side. This makes it the least desirable of the three vasopressors. Nevertheless, the authors have used methoxamine on many occasions and found it to be effective at increasing blood pressure. It must be appreciated that the use of an α adrenergic stimulant such as methoxamine or phenylephrine will actually increase the myocardial workload, and prolonged administration will lead to peripheral tissue anoxia. Therefore, usage of these drugs should be restricted to those life-threatening emergencies in which coronary perfusion seems at risk and that factor becomes the overriding concern. Other effective alternatives in severe hypotension are dobutamine or dopamine. Either should be started at an infusion rate of 5 μg/kg/min and adjusted to produce a sufficient rise in blood pressure while monitoring for tachycardia. Their use is described in more detail below as a treatment for moderate hypotension.

If the mean blood pressure is above 50 but less than 70 mm Hg (systolic 70 to 90 mm Hg), there is less immediate danger but therapy should still be instituted. As before, the inhalant is reduced so that the animal is in the lightest anesthetic plane possible. The rate of fluid administration is increased and time is allowed for these therapies to take effect. If the pressure is falling or there is little or no improvement within 10 minutes, a dopamine or dobutamine drip (1 to 5 μg/kg/min) is started to provide direct cardiac stimulation and improve cardiac output along with blood pressure. Clinical and experimental studies have demonstrated the efficacy and safety of these drugs. They are best administered by slow continuous infusion to effect using a minidrip administration set. An overdose is reflected by tachycardia or hypertension, and is easily treated by either reducing or discontinuing drug administration because the drugs have a short half-life. Our preference is to use dobutamine because we find it more reliably increases blood pressure with lower doses and has slightly less tendency to produce tachycardia. Since the drug is quite expensive and only a small portion of the total drug is needed for an individual animal, a sterile dilute solution (one vial in a 500 mL 5% dextrose solution with a minidrip set attached) is prepared at the start of a week and used as needed for the week. Nothing else should be added to the solution and the fluid is kept sterile and refrigerated between anesthetic cases over the week. At the end of the week any remaining solution is discarded. Loss of potency as a result of this system of utilization has not been apparent and is of no real consequence, since the drug is administered to effect anyway. With this method the resultant cost of having dobutamine readily available is less than $4.00 per animal. It is important that cardiac output and blood pressure not be sustained with dobutamine or dopamine while persisting with too deep a level of anesthesia, or while neglecting treatment of hypovolemia. In such cases, when the drug is subsequently discontinued at the termination of anesthesia, the full degree of cardiovascular depression will soon become evident and may lead to problems during the recovery period.

Bradycardia, Tachycardia, and Arrhythmias

When disturbances of heart rate and rhythm produce hypotension and poor peripheral perfusion in the anesthetized horse, treatment is necessary. Unless the arrhythmia is leading to circulatory insufficiency, the best approach is generally the conservative one of lightening the anesthesia as much as possible, ensuring that oxygenation and CO_2 removal are adequate, and correcting any underlying acid-base and electrolyte problems.

Heart rates of 25 to 30 beats/min, sinus arrhythmias, brief periods of sinus arrest, first- and second-degree atrioventricular block, and isorhythmic atrioventricular dissociation (regular PP and RR intervals but varying PR intervals) rarely produce hypotension. These arrhythmias often disappear spontaneously if the depth of anesthesia is lightened or as the anesthetic period progresses and the degree of surgical stimulation increases. Bradycardia (heart rates below 25 beats/min), prolonged periods of sinus arrest (especially in foals with ruptured bladders), and third-degree atrioventricular heart blocks will usually produce hypotension and prolonged capillary refill times. In such instances the first response should be to administer an anticholinergic agent (atropine, glycopyrrolate) (Table 18–2), remembering that the response to IV administration may be slow because of the prolonged circulation time. If this is not successful in reestablishing a normal heart rate and rhythm, consideration should be given to using dopamine at a drip rate that will increase heart rate to a satisfactory level. An isoproterenol drip can also be used successfully to reverse anticholinergic-resistant bursts of sinus arrest in foals with ruptured bladders.

The most common cause of ventricular tachycardia is persistent abdominal pain, hypovolemia, and endotoxemia in horses with colic. If the tachycardia persists throughout the operation despite aggressive shock treatment, the prognosis is often poor. Treatment must be directed toward improving myocardial perfusion and oxygenation. Rarely, severe ventricular tachycardia occurs as a transient arrhythmia leading to ventricular fibrillation.

Intraoperative atrial fibrillation occurs rarely in the

horse and may lead to circulatory insufficiency. The recommended treatment is to give quinidine in 1.0-mg/kg boluses at 10-minute intervals until a response occurs, or a total dose of 4 mg/kg is given. Ventricular premature beats are rare and generally need not be treated. If they occur in rapid succession or at frequent intervals (more than 10 beats/min), a bolus of 0.5 to 1.0 mg/kg lidocaine should be administered to reduce their frequency, followed by a continuous lidocaine infusion of 60 to 80 μg/kg/min.

Cardiovascular Collapse

Absence of heart sounds and a pulse on digital palpation, cessation of bleeding or cyanosis of blood at the surgical site, absent corneal and possibly anal reflexes, pupillary dilatation, and apnea or an irregular gasping respiratory pattern are all signs of acute cardiovascular collapse. In the anesthetized horse, this collapse is often associated with profound hypotension with at least temporary persistence of cardiac electrical activity. Occasionally, however, asystole or fibrillation may occur spontaneously before these signs develop. If blood pressure and electrocardiographic monitoring are being used, the nature of the cardiovascular collapse is immediately evident. When this monitoring is not available, there is no option other than to treat the situation as an asystolic cardiac arrest.

Cardiovascular collapse that is related to profound hypotension without cessation of electrical activity should be treated as outlined above for severe hypotension. Rapid fluid administration should be commenced, the horse should be positioned in lateral recumbency, and external cardiac massage should be commenced at a rate of 20 to 30 beats/min using forceful compression with both knees over the seventh to tenth intercostal space one third of the way up the thorax. In foals two-hand compression is used instead. Positive pressure ventilation with 100% oxygen at a rate of 4 to 6 breaths/min using *normal* tidal volumes should be carried out simultaneously. There is no need to discontinue the cardiac compression for IPPV, or to synchronize the breaths between the periods of chest wall compression. Improvement in circulation is most readily seen by restoration of the corneal-reflex and resumption of spontaneous respiratory efforts. If no improvement is seen within 2 to 3 minutes, epinephrine (2 to 4 μg/kg IV) should be administered through the venous access using external cardiac massage to move the drug toward the heart and through the coronary vasculature. Alternatively, the drug can be given by intracardiac injection using a 16- to 18-gauge needle that is 15 to 20 cm long inserted through the eighth intercostal space. This is only done as a last resort because it may produce fatal ventricular fibrillation in the anoxic heart.

Ventricular asystole is treated as described above for profound hypotension, only epinephrine is given as soon as possible. Although epinephrine may produce ventricular fibrillation in the halothane-anesthetized horse, particularly if the horse has not been premedicated with a phenothiazine tranquilizer, it is a risk that must be taken to achieve rapid reversal of the asystole. Sodium bicarbonate should be administered intravenously at a rate of 0.5 mEq/kg/10 min until the circulation is restored. If a cardiac beat is established but is weak, cardiac contractility can be improved with calcium chloride, a dobutamine drip, or both. Corticosteroids should be administered after resuscitation to minimize hypoxia-induced cerebral and pulmonary edema. Although internal cardiac massage has been reported, the results have not been good.

In foals with ventricular fibrillation it is possible to attempt electrical defibrillation using external placement of the paddles and a 300- to 450-joule discharge. We have not been able to achieve electrical or chemical defibrillation in adult full-sized horses, and at present we discontinue resuscitation attempts when ventricular fibrillation is confirmed.

BIBLIOGRAPHY

Blaze CA, Robinson NE: Apneic oxygenation in anesthetized ponies and horses. *Vet Res Comm* 1987;11:281–291.

Klein L: Equine anesthetic emergencies, in Mansmann RA, McAllister ES, Pratt PW (eds): *Equine Medicine and Surgery*, ed 3. Santa Barbara, CA, American Veterinary Publications, 1982, pp 282–300.

Muir WW, Bednarski RM: Equine cardiopulmonary resuscitation—Part I. *Compend Contin Educ Pract Vet* 1983;5:S228-S235.

Muir WW, Bednarski RM: Equine cardiopulmonary resuscitation—Part II. *Compend Contin Educ Pract Vet* 1983;5:S287–295.

Swanson CR, Muir WW: Dobutamine-induced augmentation of cardiac output does not enhance respiratory gas exchange in anesthetized recumbent healthy horses. *Am J Vet Res* 1986;47:1573–1576.

Swanson CR, Muir WW, Bednarski RM, Skarda RT, Hubbell JAE: Hemodynamic responses in halothane-anesthetized horses given infusions of dopamine or dobutamine. *Am J Vet Res* 1985;46:365–370.

19
Postanesthetic Lameness

Peter J. Pascoe

When a horse becomes lame following surgery or is showing signs of pain or limb swelling, the animal should be examined thoroughly. It is necessary to differentiate the myopathy/neuropathy syndromes from fractures or sprains occurring during the recovery or from conditions related to the surgery. The condition of the spinal cord must also be considered when ataxia or paralysis is present following surgery. Postoperative lameness may be manifested as a localized condition in which there are one or two affected limbs, or as a generalized condition in which lameness, stiffness, or weakness is apparent in all four legs.

LOCALIZED MYOPATHY/NEUROPATHY

Pathogenesis

Localized myopathy/neuropathy is thought to be due to an ischemic process. When this condition was first described it was termed "radial nerve paralysis," because the condition was seen in the forelimb and presumed to be related to direct pressure on the nerve. However, damage occurring at the point where the nerve is most vulnerable would not cause this type of lameness. It has become clear that the most common cause of this lameness is related to muscle damage. However, both types of injury can occur because nerve damage may be caused by direct pressure or it may occur indirectly as a result of the muscle swelling and ischemia.

Ischemia to the tissues during surgery arises as a result of combinations of reduction in arterial flow, increased venous back pressure, and increased muscle pressure due to the weight of the horse or the position of the muscle. In addition, horses are also prone to develop arterial hypoxemia even when breathing 100% oxygen. Although the exact contribution of each of these factors is unknown, there is good evidence to suggest that each is important.

The development of hypotension during anesthesia increases the risk of damage to the muscle. For example, mean arterial pressures maintained at 55 to 65 mm Hg for 3.5 hours under halothane anesthesia resulted in a 100% incidence of post anesthesia forelimb lameness. Because isoflurane produces a vasodilation in the muscles, it was hypothesized that this agent might protect the horse against the development of myositis. When systemic arterial pressures were maintained at 50 to 65 mm Hg for 3 hours of isoflurane anesthesia, three out of six horses developed severe lameness and one horse showed some minor signs. The other two horses recovered uneventfully. Although these findings lend some credence to the hypothesis, the study indicates that horses anesthetized with isoflurane can still develop myositis.

The arterial flow to the muscles may also be interrupted by the position in which the animal is placed. Radiographic studies indicate that if the foreleg is allowed to hang down without support there will be pressure on the brachial vessels, resulting in a decreased flow. Similarly, when the horse is placed in dorsal recumbency and the legs are flexed, the deep peroneal nerve and the cranial tibial vessels may be compressed against the inelastic connective tissue and the blood supply interrupted. Recently another "ischemic" syndrome has been described, an adductor myositis (involving the adductor, gracilis, and pectineus muscles) occurring when animals have been positioned in dorsal recumbency. Compression of the medial circumflex femoral artery, which supplies these muscles, is postulated as the cause of this myopathy. Although venous compression itself has not been proven to be part of this syndrome, the collapsibility of the vessels and the weight of the horse make it likely that venous compression contributes to the condition.

Many of the muscles in the limb are enclosed by fascial compartments that are inelastic and limit the expansion of the muscle. When pressure is applied, or if the tissue within the compartment swells, there will be a reduction in capillary blood flow. Compartmental syndrome is a well-known entity in humans and can result in muscle and nerve damage that becomes permanent unless a timely fasciotomy is performed. In this syndrome the ischemia leads to tissue damage and the injured tissue swells. Tissue swelling increases the compartment pressure, which reduces the capillary flow and may occlude venous drainage, initiating a vicious cycle that increases compartment pressure until the pressure is relieved or there is a sufficient restoration of blood flow to overcome the effects of ischemia. True compartmental syndrome is rare in the horse and swelling is either not present or subsides before the onset of muscle necrosis. The elevated pressures affect other structures passing through the compartment, including the nerves. In experimental studies it has been shown that nerves are more susceptible to ischemic damage than muscle and so the clinical manifestation of the condition may be due to nerve paralysis with or without muscle damage.

Capillary blood flow throughout the compartment is affected by the pressure within the compartment. The exact pressure at which the capillary closes has not been established in the horse, but in humans it is thought that a pressure within 30 mm Hg of the diastolic pressure will eventually lead to ischemia. Muscle pressure greater than 30 mm Hg may lead to muscle necrosis. The length of time for which a given pressure is applied is also important because poor circulation may be as detrimental as no circulation, if present long enough. With the compartmental syndrome in humans it is recommended that a fasciotomy be performed if the pressure exceeds 40 mm Hg for more than 20 to 30 minutes. The pressure is monitored continuously in any patient with compartmental syndrome until it falls below 30 mm Hg.

To minimize the muscle pressure while the horse is under anesthesia, the surface on which the horse is placed must provide uniform support. Various experiments have shown that a water bed, or a very thick foam pad (>10 cm), will reduce the intracompartmental pressures when the animal is in lateral recumbency. With the limbs positioned correctly and on a good surface, pressures in the lower triceps muscle have been about 30 mm Hg. With a hard surface and poor positioning, these pressures may exceed 60 mm Hg. Therefore, even under the best of conditions horses will often have a pressure in the lower triceps that would be regarded as critical in humans, and it is very easy to exceed these values. In most of these experiments it has been difficult to find any relationship between the weight of the animal and the pressures generated, but it has been shown very clearly that a person leaning on the animal will raise the pressures immediately. In certain surgeries, it is very difficult to avoid this (e.g., flank ovariectomies and midline cystotomies) and these procedures have been associated with a high incidence of postanesthesia myopathy.

Another risk factor that hypothetically relates to the intracompartmental pressure is the fitness of the animal. Horses that are anesthetized when they are in peak condition appear to have an increased risk of myositis. When one looks at a horse that is well trained there is an impression that the muscles are "hard." Although not proven, this "fitness" may produce higher intracompartmental pressures when compared with the untrained animal. If this is the case, then it would take less external pressure to generate a muscle pressure that could lead to ischemia. Also, in the horse that is trained for short bursts of high-speed activity, there is an increase in the number of type II fibers in the muscle. These are the cells that are affected first when the muscle is rendered ischemic. If there is an increased proportion of these fibers present in the trained muscle, the overall damage to the muscle could be more severe.

Occasionally a horse will recover normally from the surgery only to become lame shortly afterward. The muscle swells and hardens and the horse shows the characteristic signs of pain and lameness. This is likely to be the result of postischemic swelling. Cells that have been deprived of oxygen become energy depleted, and xanthine dehydrogenase, an enzyme involved in the breakdown of purine bases, is converted to xanthine oxidase. When the cell's oxygen supply is restored, the presence of oxygen and xanthine oxidase leads to the formation of hydroxyl radicals that will damage the cell. This is referred to as a reperfusion injury and may be the cause of these delayed-onset myopathies.

Prevention

With the attention that has been paid to this condition in recent years, it has been possible to reduce the incidence to some degree. The following factors should be considered.

History. When dealing with the fit animal I have routinely asked for a "let down" period of at least a week before an elective surgery is performed. No absolute recommendation can be made about the length of time required before an animal is to be anesthetized. Some "let down" period is desirable, but the fitness of the animal, the duration and nature of the surgery, and the type of surface on which the horse will be lying should all be factors in deciding how long this period will be. In any case it is wise to reduce the horse's grain intake in an effort to prevent rhabdomyolysis.

Preoperative Workup. During the preoperative period, the animal should be assessed for conditions that might predispose it to intraoperative hypotension (e.g., dehydration, blood loss). These conditions should be treated appropriately before the horse is anesthetized.

Intraoperative Care. The three main features include proper positioning, padding, and avoiding hypotension. If the horse is in lateral recumbency, it should be positioned with the lowermost front leg brought forward and the uppermost leg lifted so that the legs are parallel

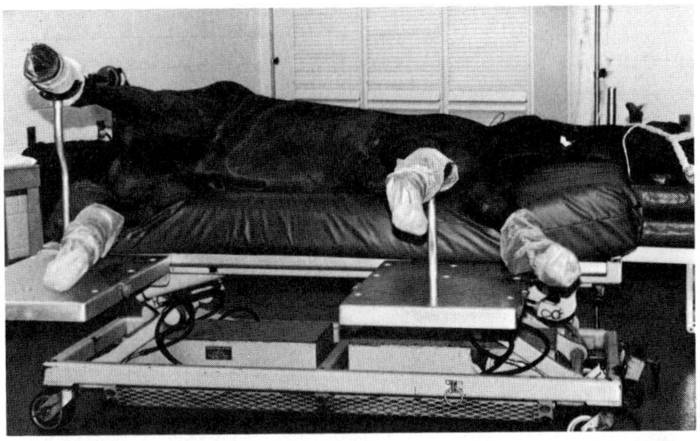

Figure 19–1. Horse in lateral recumbency showing the position of the legs. The lowermost front leg is pulled forward, with the upper legs being supported in their normal anatomic positions.

and at right angles to the body (Fig. 19–1). Some authors recommend hobbling the legs together and hoisting the legs up so that the triceps is not touching the surface of the table. If not done properly, however, this can increase muscle damage. If the horse is in dorsal recumbency, the shoulders must be supported with a soft pad and the hind legs must not be allowed to splay without some support to prevent total abduction. Occasionally a horse has to be placed in a dorsolateral position (e.g., cesarean, colostomy). This position can cause postanesthetic myopathy and so the time that the horse is in this position should be made as short as possible.

The padding used for the animal also appears to be critical. A water bed is probably the best contact surface for a horse, and some clinics have used this technique successfully. The disadvantage with this surface is that the animal tends to move once suspended on the bed. Alternatively, very thick foam pads (10 to 12 in) may be used. These are now being used in many clinics and, although there are no hard data to support this, their use appears to have reduced the incidence of postanesthetic myopathy.

Because prevention of hypotension depends on knowing the blood pressure, this should be monitored routinely during anesthesia. The methods for dealing with this are described in Chapter 16. In selected cases in which hypotension is expected (e.g., a fit hunter weighing 650 kg), it may be worth using a dopamine or dobutamine infusion starting immediately after induction of anesthesia.

It is also quite feasible to monitor the intracompartmental muscle pressure in the lower triceps or gluteal muscle using a standard 14-gauge catheter. The catheter is inserted into the muscle and connected to a pressure transducer with a constant low-flow infusion of saline. This keeps the catheter patent without increasing the compartmental pressure. In several cases in which compartmental pressure was monitored, pressure began to climb rapidly during the surgery. This finding has permitted the anesthesia personnel to treat the horse appropriately and thereby prevent further damage to the muscle.

Therapy

Once a postoperative lameness is detected that is thought to be related to the above conditions, the therapy will depend on the severity of the signs. An animal with some mild swelling and little lameness should be treated with an analgesic and intravenous fluid therapy and monitored for signs of exacerbation of the condition. Other therapies noted below may be used in the more severe cases.

Analgesics. Horses with signs of acute pain should be treated immediately. Since the lesion involves local tissue damage, there will be a local generation of prostaglandins. Nonsteroidal anti-inflammatory drugs are therefore indicated. Since the pain is acute, the drug should be given intravenously. If the condition is severe, the horse should be treated with an opioid as well. Examples include meperidine 2 mg/kg, butorphanol 0.05 to 0.1 mg/kg, or morphine 0.5 mg/kg, all given intramuscularly. Xylazine can be used once the horse is standing, and detomidine may prove to be an even more effective agent for more prolonged analgesia and sedation.

Sedation. Horses with a severe myopathy and pain struggle continuously even when it is obvious that they are not going to be able to stand. Some horses will tolerate the disability with equanimity but others will continue to struggle, causing injury or exhaustion, and may fracture a leg in the process. To control these horses sedation is often necessary. To date I have had the best results with chloral hydrate given to effect (0.03 to 0.06 g/kg). Sedation is administered carefully since heavily sedated horses may lie down and cause further to damage their muscles. If the horse is to remain recumbent, it must be on deep bedding or a thick (10- to 12-inch) foam pad. The horse may respond to being put in a sling and hoisted to a standing position periodically, unless this causes more struggling or appears to increase the pain.

Fluids. Horses affected with myositis may often sweat profusely and will become dehydrated. Furthermore, the damaged muscle cells will release myoglobin, which in high enough concentrations will cause renal tubular injury. Consequently, monitoring of hydration and acid-base balance is necessary. Intravenous fluids at a volume of 20 to 40 mL/kg should be given over 2 to 3 hours. The urine output should be monitored and diuretics used if the urine flow is not adequate. Mannitol is the diuretic of choice in an animal with overt muscular swelling because it is effective in reducing the intracompartmental muscle pressure and enhancing the ability to initiate urine flow. A dose of 0.5 to 1 g/kg is used as an initial bolus followed by an infusion of 0.25 to 0.5 g/kg/hour for 2 hours. Mannitol therapy must be accompanied by adequate volume expansion with crystalloid solution and continuous monitoring during its use.

Muscle Relaxants. These have been advocated to reduce the contraction and help to break the vicious cycle. Centrally acting muscle relaxants such as methocarbamol and guiafenesin have been advocated. They can be given intravenously and, if they work at all, it is probably by relieving some of the muscle stimulation and pain. Guaifenesin should be given at a dose of 20 to 30 mg/kg and will provide relaxation for 20 to 30 minutes; methocarbamol at a dose of 15 to 25 mg/kg will give relaxation for several hours.

Miscellaneous Therapies. Other treatments that have been recommended are primarily aimed at reducing any inflammatory responses. Dimethylsulfoxide (DMSO) has been used either by rubbing it over the affected area or by administering it intravenously. Dimethylsulfoxide also has been shown to be a free radical scavenger, and these radicals are thought to be part of the reperfusion injury to tissue following ischemia. It is not known whether DMSO has any beneficial effects in these conditions. Corticosteroids have also been suggested but are probably best avoided because of the risk of inducing laminitis.

GENERALIZED MYOSITIS

Pathogenesis

The other factors that predispose the horse to postoperative lameness include exertional rhabdomyolysis and malignant hyperthermia. Both are relatively rare in the horse but either can occur during or after anesthesia. In both of these conditions the final common pathway for the disease involves excess calcium entry into the sarcoplasm of the muscle cell. Calcium initiates the contractile process and, if it cannot be removed from the sarcoplasm, causes continuous contraction of the muscle. The energy used to maintain this process releases heat. It is this continued release of energy that leads to the hyperthermic response in the animal. The entry of calcium into the cytoplasm may also cause cell damage in ischemic myositis. Evidence to date suggests that malignant hyperthermia is related to a defect in the sarcoplasmic reticulum that allows excessive amounts of calcium to remain in the sarcoplasm. Equine susceptibility to malignant hyperthermia has a lower prevalence than in some other species (e.g., pigs) and, although, this syndrome is triggered by stress in humans and pigs, this has not been reported in the horse.

The manifestation of the condition can range from a mild stiffness following halothane exposure to a full-blown hyperthermic response. The inhalant agents and the depolarizing muscle relaxants (e.g., succinylcholine) are known to be potent triggers for malignant hyperthermia, and in most of the overt cases reported to date both halothane and succinylcholine were used during the anesthetic period. Other factors that appear to be associated with malignant hyperthermia include recent stress, a difficult induction, difficulty controlling blood pressure during the anesthetic period, a widening pulse pressure, increasing end-tidal carbon dioxide and arterial carbon dioxide tension (P_aCO_2) levels, metabolic acidosis, and an anesthetic period lasting more than 2 hours.

Some clinical cases of postanesthetic equine rhabdomyolysis and malignant hyperthermia have been reported to have abnormal sensitivity to halothane-caffeine contracture tests and have been treated successfully with dantrolene. These findings suggest that similarities exist between the two conditions. However, this evidence is not specific because there may be other defects in the cell that can be triggered by the halothane-caffeine contracture test. The dantrolene therapy only prevents the calcium entry into the cell, a pathway common to both these diseases.

Prevention

History. The owner should be asked about any history of "tying up" in the horse or in the horse's family. The owner should also be asked if any other members of this animal's family have had problems during anesthesia. It is worth taking the time to ask the question even though malignant hyperthermia is an extremely rare condition in the horse. If the answer is yes, then further details should be solicited to determine if there is a possibility of malignant hyperthermia.

Preoperative Workup. There is almost no way of predicting which animal will develop generalized rhabdomyolysis. Heavy horses should be handled with extra care and heavily muscled animals should also be watched carefully. If an elevated serum creatine kinase level exists preoperatively (which cannot be explained by the injury to the animal), this horse should be considered as a likely suspect for exertional rhabdomyolysis. I have recommended that these horses be treated with oral dantrolene before the surgery (see below).

Therapy

The therapy for a generalized myopathy would include the treatments used for the localized form as well as dantrolene.

Dantrolene Sodium. This benzothiazepine is the drug of choice for the treatment of malignant hyperthermia responses in the horse. The drug acts by reducing the release of calcium from the sarcoplasmic reticulum to the sarcoplasm and hence breaks the vicious cycle initiated during the onset of malignant hyperthermia. Dantrolene has much less affinity for other types of muscle, but it does have some minor effects on the heart, vascular smooth muscle, intestine, and bladder. In the horse the administration of dantrolene preoperatively may be associated with some hypotension during anesthesia.

The drug is available as an oral or an intravenous preparation. The oral form consists of capsules containing 100 mg of dantrolene mixed with starch, talc, magnesium, stearate, and lactose. The capsules are normally opened, the contents dissolved in warm water, and the fluid given by stomach tube. The commercial intravenous preparation is a lyophilized powder containing 20 mg dantrolene, 3 g mannitol, and sodium hydroxide in a vial that must be dissolved in 60 mL of water. Because this preparation is very expensive and has a relatively short shelf life, some people have made their own intravenous drug from the oral preparation. This can be done by dissolving thirty-two 100-mg capsules in 4 L of sterile water containing 16 mL of sterile 0.1 M sodium hydroxide and stirring for 30 minutes. This is then filtered through 201-grade filter paper and sterilized by passing it through a 0.45-μm Millipore filter. The resulting solution can be used after adjusting the pH to 7.4 using citric acid, or the dantrolene can be precipitated out using 80 mL of 10% citric acid and then collected using vacuum filtration. The crystals are then dried in a laminar flow hood overnight. When these crystals are redissolved, it may be necessary to readjust the pH with a few drops of sodium hydroxide. Obviously, this is not a procedure that can be done quickly or with the equipment available in a normal practice pharmacy. Furthermore, the use of homemade intravenous dantrolene preparations in humans has been associated with higher mortality rates. Therefore, in veterinary practice one has to be prepared either to accept the limitations associated with the use of the oral preparation or to expend a considerable amount of effort or money to have an intravenous preparation on the shelf.

Dantrolene has been used by some clinicians as a routine part of premedication for the horse. It is difficult to justify this approach since the incidence of generalized myositis is low and that of malignant hyperthermia even lower. Preoperative use could be justified under the following circumstances:

1. A horse with a known history of malignant hyperthermia or rhabdomyolysis, or with a strong family history of the condition.
2. A horse with an elevated serum creatine kinase activity that cannot be explained on the basis of the known history.
3. A fit racehorse that has had no "let down" period and is expected to be in surgery for more than 2 hours.
4. Any horse admitted for emergency orthopedic surgery where the animal has been stressed by the accident and subsequent transport.

Although postoperative use of dantrolene is even less well defined, it should receive consideration because of its action on the release of calcium. Entry of calcium into the cell will exacerbate an injury initially caused by ischemia. The use of dantrolene apparently has been beneficial in a number of clinical cases, but it is going to be difficult to prove this scientifically because of the low incidence of the condition.

A therapeutic dose of dantrolene has not been established in the horse but the pharmacokinetics and bioavailability have been reported. The therapeutic blood levels have been extrapolated from humans. A dose of 2 mg/kg given intravenously should provide adequate blood levels for about 20 minutes and a dose of 4 mg/kg should maintain blood levels in the therapeutic range for 2 hours. An oral dose of 10 mg/kg will reach its peak blood level after 1.5 hours and will maintain a therapeutic level for about 2 hours. If it is necessary to keep the blood levels in this range, a further oral dose of 2.5 mg/kg, given every hour, would be needed. Muscle weakness is possible with high doses of Dantrolene so it is recommended that the initial dose be 1 to 2 mg/kg intravenously, and 4 to 6 mg/kg orally. The half-life of the drug is much shorter in the horse than in humans (1 hour versus 6 to 9 hours) and the bioavailability is roughly half that reported for humans (38 versus 70%).

Intraoperative Management of Malignant Hyperthermia

It is impossible to confirm a diagnosis of malignant hyperthermia during surgery, but a high index of suspicion would be aroused when a horse demonstrates some or all of the features indicated above. The first step that should be taken is to remove the animal from the causative agent. This will usually be an inhalant anesthetic, so at the very least the vaporizer should be turned off and the system flushed with oxygen for several minutes. The horse should be connected to a new machine that has not been used with an inhalant for the last 24 hours, if one is available. If it is necessary to continue the surgery, then the anesthesia should be continued with nitrous oxide and a barbiturate. Ventilation should be controlled and it will be necessary to use an increased minute ventilation to cope with the rising production of carbon dioxide The horse may fight the ventilator and make it difficult to achieve a reduction in P_{CO_2}. One can cope with this by removing the ventilator and allowing the patient to breathe spontaneously, or alternatively, one can paralyze the horse using a nondepolarizing muscle relaxant such as pancuronium or atracurium and continue the ventilation.

Dantrolene sodium should be given intravenously as soon as possible. This will take some time if the commercial preparation is to be used since one will have to make up about 50 bottles for an average-sized horse. Metabolic acidosis is likely to be present and this can be partly compensated for by hyperventilating the horse, but it is usually necessary to administer sodium bicarbonate. The dose needed will depend on the degree of acidosis.

The body temperature will rise in a true malignant hyperthermia episode, and the most effective way of dealing with this is by evaporative cooling. This will mean turning a hose on the horse and having several fans blowing over the animal. Ideally the water coming out of the hose should be lukewarm because it will evaporate more rapidly and will not cause as much vasoconstriction as ice-cold water. The use of cold intravenous solutions will also help, and these should be given rapidly in order to diurese the horse to prevent myoglobin damage to the renal tubules. Since the animal is anesthetized at this stage, it is relatively easy to pass a urinary catheter, and it would be prudent to maintain this into the postoperative period to allow urine volume to be monitored. Ventricular arrhythmias should be treated with procainamide rather than lidocaine since some local anesthetics can trigger malignant hyperthermia.

If the horse survives to the recovery period it should be monitored very carefully to ensure that a further episode does not occur. In a recent report on equine rhabdomyolysis one animal showed evidence of another myolytic episode while standing in its stall. It is possible that a malignant hyperthermic reaction in a horse may be further triggered by the perioperative stress and the strange environment. The creatine kinase value should start to decline over the first 24 to 48 hours, and should be measured daily until it returns to near-normal.

BIBLIOGRAPHY

Court MH, Engelking LR, Dodman NH, Anwer MS, Seeler DC, Clark M: Pharmacokinetics of dantrolene sodium in horses. *J Vet Pharmacol Therap* 1987;10:218–226.

Dodman NH, Gray L, Williams R, Goldspink G: Intracompartmental muscle pressure, temperature and pH in the horse under general anesthesia. *Equine Vet Sci* 1985;5:11–15.

Grandy JL, Steffey EP, Hodgson DS, Woliner MJ: Arterial hypotension and the development of postanesthetic myopathy in halothane-anesthetized horses. *Am J Vet Res* 1987;48:192–197.

Hutton M, Rhodes RS, Chapman G: The lowering of postischemic compartment pressures with mannitol. *J Surg Res* 1982;32:239–242.

Lindsay WA, Pascoe PJ, McDonell WN, Burgess MLF: Effect of protective padding on forelimb intracompartmental muscle pressures in anesthetized horses. *Am J Vet Res* 1985;46:688–691.

Manley SV, Kelly AB, Hodgson D: Malignant hyperthermia-like reactions in three anesthetized horses. *J Am Vet Med Assoc* 1983;183:85–89.

Mubarak SJ, Hargens AR: Acute compartment syndromes. *Surg Clin North Am* 1983;63:539–565.

Serteyn D, Mottart E, Michaux C: Laser Doppler flowmetry: Muscular microcirculation in anesthetised horses. *Equine Vet J* 1986;18:391–395.

UNIT III

Wound Healing

20
Principles of Wound Healing

William A. Lindsay

The treatment of wounds of the equine integument is a common component of equine practice. The Veterinary Medical Data Program, located at Purdue University, has provided information concerning equine wounds. Of a total of 122,642 equines presented at nineteen participating veterinary teaching hospitals and clinics during the years 1982 to 1986 for treatment of any problem, 2,489 required wound treatment. Lacerations accounted for 84.8% of these wounds, contusions 11.0%, abrasions 3.4%, and purulent lacerations 0.7%. Of the horses receiving treatment for these wounds, 61% were débrided only. Suture repair was performed in 30.4%, débridement and suture in 3.4%, application of a lower leg cast in 3.0%, and application of a full leg cast in 1.8%. All of the breeds presented followed this pattern (Table 20–1).

The most frequent sites of injury are reported in Table 20–2 and depicted in Figure 20–1. In the front leg, the hoof was most often injured (72%) followed by the shoulder (9.7%), metacarpus (8.8%), and carpus (6.5%). In the hind limbs, the hoof was again most commonly injured (51%), then the metatarsus (34.1%) and tarsus (7.5%). When comparing the front and hind limbs, it was interesting that the hoof injuries of the front limb required treatment at an increased frequency ($P \leq 0.001$) and that the metatarsus was more often involved than the metacarpus ($P < 0.001$). The type of wound seen in any particular geographic area will depend upon local management practices. Lower limb lacerations are frequent in areas where horses are confined by barbed wire; facial lacerations occur when horses are confined in stalls.

In addition to classifying wounds by their location on the body, they may also be described as either open or closed. Closed wounds such as hematomas and seromas rarely require treatment. Open wounds frequently require treatment. Partial-thickness wounds such as abrasions with an intact, supporting dermis will heal by regeneration of the epithelial cells. Wound cleansing and protection from further trauma are required. Full-thickness wounds include incisions, lacerations, avulsions, and punctures. These wounds may be closed by suture or left to heal by second intention depending upon the severity and location of the injury. First-intention healing refers to that which occurs in wounds that have been created under aseptic conditions and apposed by sutures (Fig. 20–2). Second-intention healing occurs in wounds that are not sutured but are left to heal through the processes of epithelization and wound contraction (Fig. 20–3). The formation of a granulation bed is a prerequisite for healing by second intention. Third-intention healing (delayed closure) is defined as delayed suture of wounds after allowing for the initial formation of a granulation bed (Fig. 20–4).

Wound healing may be studied in a variety of ways. The most simple is the clinical observation of wounds for the cardinal signs of inflammation: heat, pain, swelling, and redness. Serosanguinous discharge from a wound may herald wound dehiscence, and the dehydration of surrounding skin may signal avascular necrosis. Wound fluids may be assayed for concentrations of various humoral agents and tissues examined microscopically for cellular infiltrates. Collagen is elaborated by fibroblasts and may be studied using electron microscopy and histochemical techniques.

Wound healing is traditionally considered to occur in three stages: the initial inflammatory phase, followed by the repair (glycosaminoglycan) phase, and finally the remodeling phase. Thus, the major biologic processes of tissue repair will involve inflammatory cells, humoral components, collagen metabolism, epithelization, wound contraction, and reduction and remodeling of the original scar.

The initial inflammation that follows injury is essential to the repair process, and it is important that neither the client nor the veterinarian do anything to disrupt this portion of the process. The inflammatory response is initiated immediately after the injury as thrombus formation occurs in damaged capillaries and humoral substances cause local vasodilation. Histamine, serotonin, kinins, and prostaglandins are the primary mediators implicated in this response.

Histamine is released from mast cells and effects an immediate, but short-lived (30-min), increase in vascular permeability. Serotonin (5-hydroxytryptamine) is also released from mast cells and platelets and has a similar action. This substance may be of little significance in species other than the rat. The kinins are released from the α_2-globulin fraction of plasma. They are also relatively short lived and increase the separa-

TABLE 20–1. AN ANALYSIS OF THE INCIDENCE AND TREATMENT OF EQUINE WOUNDS AT 19 VETERINARY COLLEGES FOR THE YEARS 1982 TO 1986 INCLUSIVE*

Breed	Total Accessions	Wounds Debrided	Wounds Sutured	Wounds Debrided and Sutured	Half Cast Applied	Full Cast Applied
Quarterhorse	49,071	682	383	41	32	22
Thoroughbred	21,947	250	99	15	14	6
Arabian	12,553	98	55	4	8	7
Standardbred	12,138	89	27	3	2	2
Mixed breed	10,629	193	80	12	8	4
Appaloosa	7,522	115	77	5	7	4
Paint	2,779	44	18	2	2	1
Ponies (American, Connemarra, Shetland, Welsh)	2,373	19	7	2	0	0
American Saddle Horse	1,930	15	8	0	0	0
Belgian	1,700	24	2	0	1	0

* Data from the Veterinary Medical Data Program, Purdue University, West Lafayette, IN.

tion between adjacent endothelial cells in the small venules. Prostaglandins (PGs) E_1 and E_2 are also potent vasodilators that are generated locally by the actions of the phospolipases on cell membranes of injured cells. The initial inflammatory response evoked by PGE_1 and PGE_2 may later be replaced by anti-inflammatory effects of other prostaglandins. Surrounding blood vessels dilate, capillary permeability increases, and polymorphonuclear leukocytes and monocytes migrate into the wound. These cells are phagocytic and remove bacteria and debris within the wound. In addition to their involvement in coagulation, platelets serve to attract macrophages and also activate fibroblasts, which surround the wound.

The repair process begins as fibroblasts migrate into the wound and secrete collagen. This stage in wound healing has been termed the "glycosaminoglycan phase." Fibroblasts secrete the mucopolysaccharides of the ground substance and also synthesize collagen from hydroxyproline and hydroxylysine. Fibronectin, a group of high-molecular-weight proteins that are present in high levels in immature granulation tissue 24 to 48 hours after wounding, is responsible for the adherence of different protein fractions and also of fibroblasts to fibrin. Thus, fibronectin is important as an "anchoring strand." Fibronectin disappears when type III collagen synthesis commences. Collagen molecules are crossed-linked into larger fibrillar complexes result-

TABLE 20–2. A SURVEY OF THE INCIDENCE OF WOUNDS BY LOCATION IN THE FRONT AND HIND LEGS OF THE HORSE*

	Total Accessions	Wounds of the Forelimbs						Wounds of the Hindlimbs					
		Foot	Fetlock	Metacarpus	Carpus	Elbow	Shoulder	Foot	Fetlock	Meta tarsus	Tarsus	Stifle	Thigh
Quarterhorse	51,204	407	15	59	46	7	73	185	17	135	22	7	4
Thoroughbred	22,436	98	1	8	10	0	1	31	1	14	8	0	0
Arabian	12,873	49	2	6	1	0	7	13	3	12	1	1	0
Standardbred	12,317	54	1	3	1	0	1	11	0	7	1	1	0
Mixed breed	11,041	80	3	7	5	0	12	27	4	17	7	0	1
Ponies	2,419	3	0	2	1	0	2	4	0	3	1	1	1
American Saddle Horse	1,990	16	0	1	0	0	0	6	0	0	1	0	0
Belgian	1,740	7	0	1	0	1	0	7	0	2	1	0	0

* Data provided by the Veterinary Medicine Data Program, Purdue University, based on case material presented to 19 veterinary schools during the years 1982 through 1986 inclusive.

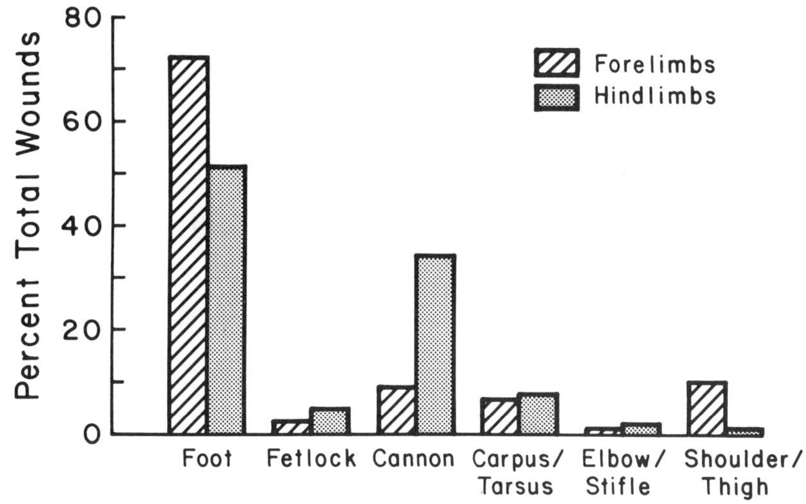

Figure 20–1. The incidence of wounds in various locations regardless of breed in a total of 2,489 equine wounds evaluated during the years 1982 through 1986. (The information was provided by the Veterinary Medical Data Program, Purdue University, West Lafayette, IN.)

ing in a mature, polymerized, collagen structure. Collagen content of the wound increases rapidly 4 to 5 days after injury and stabilizes after 3 weeks. At this stage, permanent adhesions may occur, particularly following tendon repair or abdominal surgery. These adhesions are the result of the polymerization of collagen.

Collagen synthesis and degradation should occur in equilibrium during this stage of wound healing, which lasts from 2 to 4 weeks. Epithelization also begins and involves the mitosis and migration of epithelial cells from the stratum basale. The epithelial cells are mobilized and migrate into and across the defect. In first-intention healing, active mitosis had been noted in epithelial cells at the wound edge as early as 8 to 12 hours after injury, and epithelium may cover the wound as early as 48 hours. Wounds that heal by second intention will require considerable time for epithelization to be complete. Epithelium that has no supporting dermal structure, but only a thin layer of epithelial cells, will provide little strength or integrity to the wound. Note that wound contraction is the most important phenomenon in the healing of wounds by second intention. Wound contraction is effected by the myofibroblast, a fibroblast with smooth muscle capabilities.

The final stage of scar remodeling goes on for many months after the initial wounding. Old collagen is lysed as the new collagen is synthesized. In general, the size of the original scar will be reduced. The final

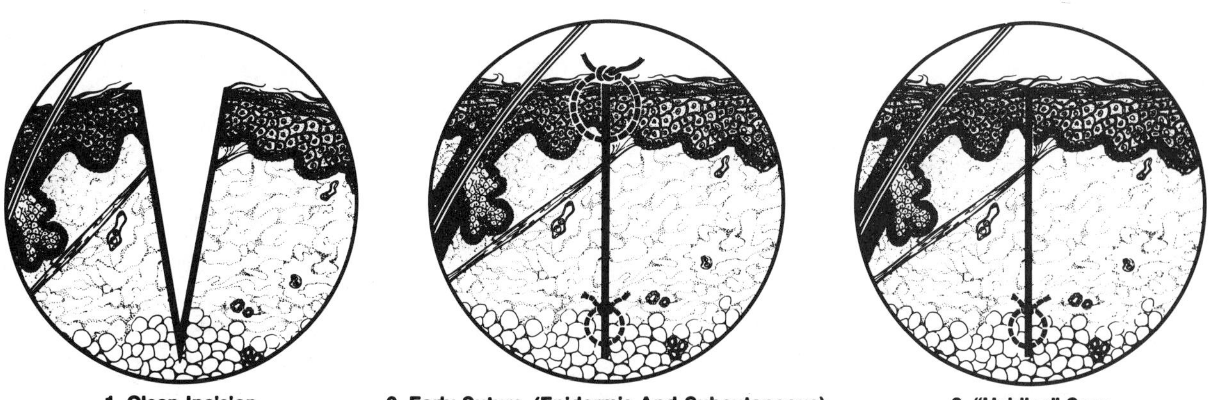

Figure 20–2. First-intention healing occurs in wounds in which aseptic conditions prevail and the tissues have been accurately reapposed by suture. (Reprinted with permission from Lindsay WA: Wound treatment in horses: Guidelines for classification. *Vet Med* 1988; 83(4):387–395.)

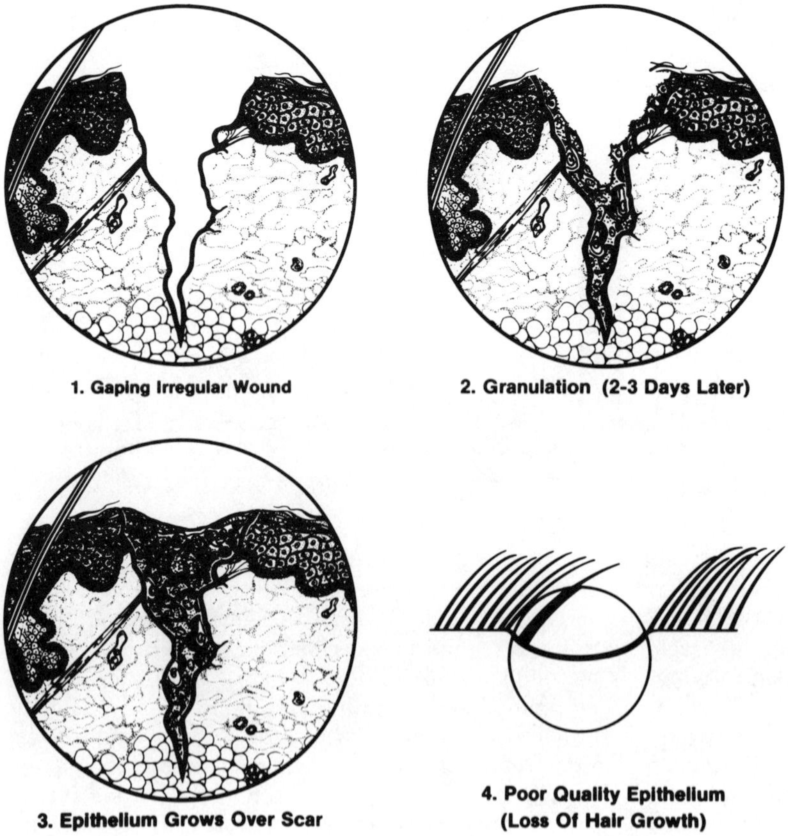

Figure 20–3. Second-intention healing progresses as granulation tissue fills the wound. Epithelial cells migrate over the defect; wound contraction causes a reduction in surface area. (Reprinted with permission from Lindsay WA: Wound treatment in horses: Guidelines for classification. *Vet Med* 1988; 83(4):387–395.)

amount of scar in the wound will depend upon the tension and pressure across the wound and the amount of oxygen delivered to the tissue.

Some authors do not use the terms "inflammatory phase," "glycosaminoglycan phase," and "remodeling phase." Synonyms for the same processes are lag phase, fibroblastic phase, and scar maturation phase. Following wounding, there is a *lag phase* of 4 to 6 days with no increase in tensile strength. However, the tensile strength increases rapidly and peaks between day 14

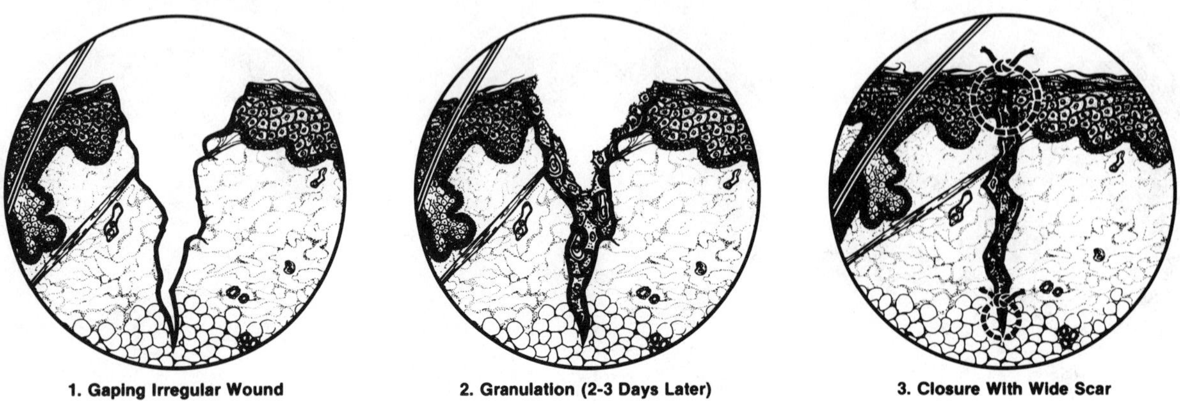

Figure 20–4. In third-intention healing, wound closure is delayed for several days, until the full extent of damage to skin and deeper structures has been assessed. (Reprinted with permission from Lindsay WA: Wound treatment in horses: Guidelines for classification. *Vet Med* 1988; 83(4):387–395.)

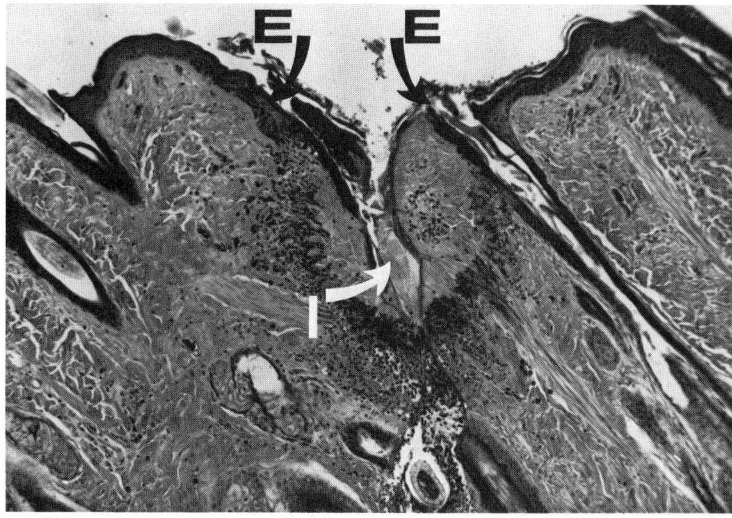

A

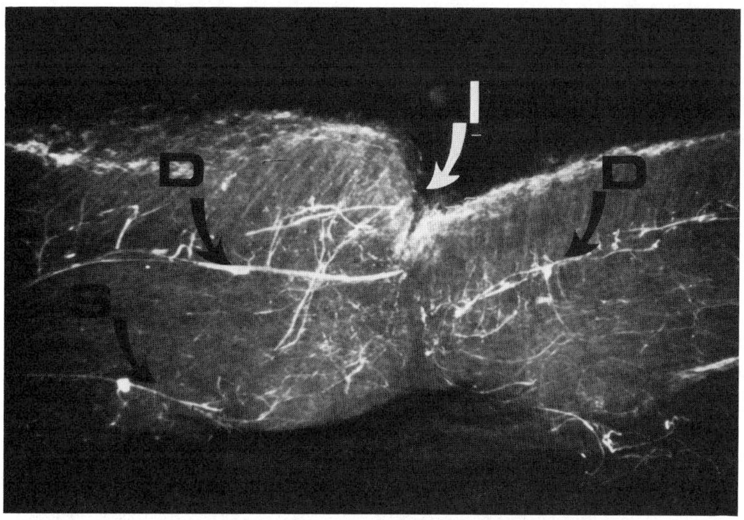

B

Figure 20–5. **A.** Twenty-four hours after skin incision and suture, note the inversion of the epithelial edges (*E*, epithelium) and the loss of epithelial margin on the right side of the incision (*I*) (Hematoxylin-eosin; original magnification × 36, actual magnification this print × 100). **B.** The dermal (*D*) and subdermal (*S*) plexuses are visualized on either side of the incision (*I*). The capillaries on either side of the incision no longer interlock. (Original magnification × 3.3; actual magnification this print × 9.)

and day 16; days 4 to 16 are termed the *fibroblastic phase*. Canine skin regains only 20 to 30% of normal strength by that time. There are differences between species and also marked differences between different tissues (skin, fascia, tendon, or bladder) of the same species. The final stage of wound healing, the *maturation phase*, allows for a constant, but less dramatic, increase in tensile strength. There is no further gain in collagen content but rather a cross-linking of collagen fibers and ongoing remodeling and replacement of collagen fibers. This process may be rather time consuming; tendon and fascia that have been divided and repaired under experimental situations will require 6 to 12 months for completion of this process. Even then, the resulting tensile strength will only be 70 to 80% of unwounded tissue.

Of importance to the surgeon is the rate of gain of tensile strength of the healing wound. Unfortunately, there is little information that relates directly to wound healing in the equine species. Consequently, we must extrapolate from studies performed primarily in laboratory animals. Also, close attention must be paid to the methods used for evaluating tensile strength or breaking strength testing in each particular study. The species and age of animal, method of wounding, and type of suture repair also vary from study to study. Biochemical studies may also be performed to quantitate collagen production. Hydroxypro-

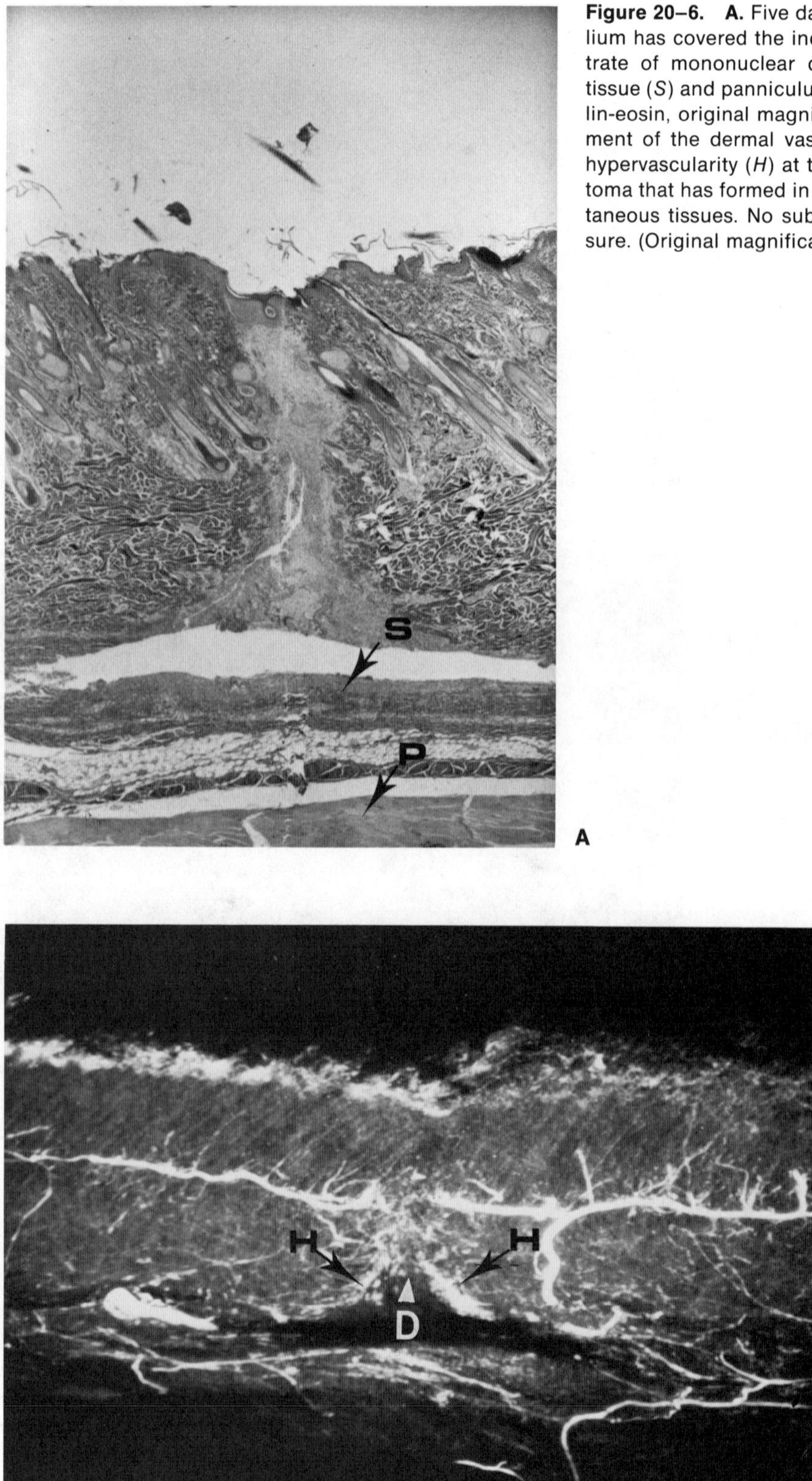

Figure 20–6. **A.** Five days after incision and suture, epithelium has covered the incisional defect. There is a mild infiltrate of mononuclear cells in the dermis. Subcutaneous tissue (*S*) and panniculus muscle (*P*) are visible. (Hematoxylin-eosin, original magnification × 5.5.) **B.** Note the realignment of the dermal vascular plexus. There is evidence of hypervascularity (*H*) at the dermal margins. Note the hematoma that has formed in the dead space (*D*) between subcutaneous tissues. No subcutaneous suture was used in closure. (Original magnification, × 20.)

Figure 20–7. **A.** Histologic examination of skin 8 days after suture. There is accurate reapposition of epidermis and dermis. Fibroblasts are plentiful. (Hematoxylin-eosin, original magnification × 5.5.) **B.** Dermal and subdermal plexuses are apparent. A hematoma is evident at the base of the dermis; hypervascularity is still observed at the dermal margins. (Original magnification × 5.5.)

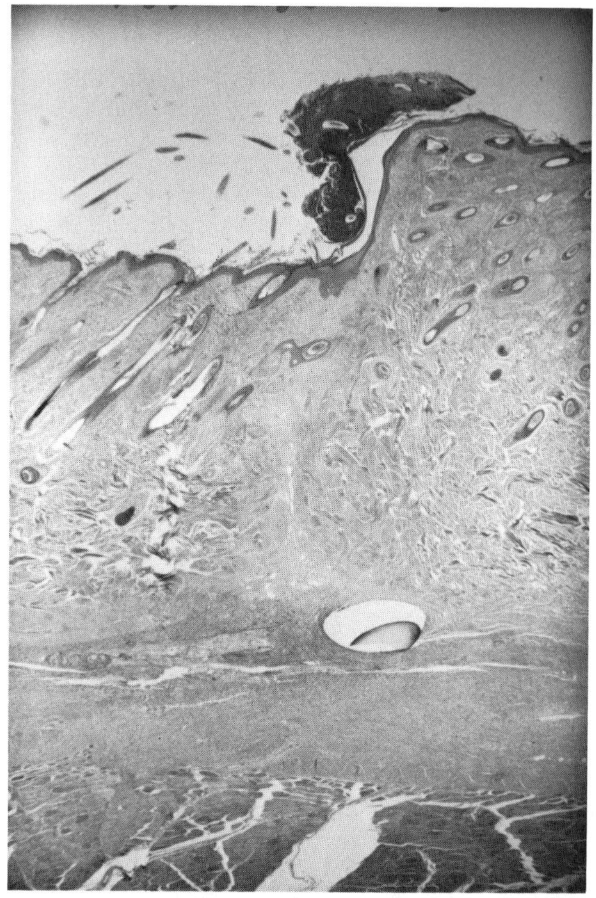

A

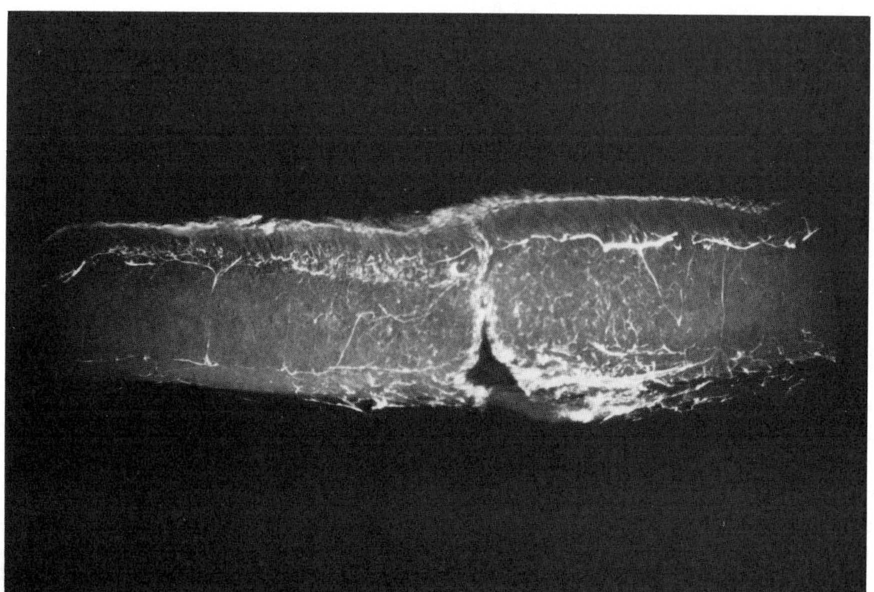

B

line, hexosamine, and uronic acid may be assayed to detect the rate of collagen synthesis.

Using correlated microangiography and histology, the healing of equine incisions has been studied in our laboratory. Full-thickness skin incisions 15 cm in length were made on the lateral body wall of ponies and sutured immediately with monofilament nylon under aseptic conditions. The ponies were euthanized and perfused centrally with a finely divided barium sulfate solution at physiologic pressures. The sutured wounds were examined sequentially during the various phases of wound healing. All tissues were excised and fixed in formalin. After embedding in paraffin, full-thickness skin sections 1 to 2 mm thick were cut and oriented at right angles to the incision. High-detail radiographs were obtained, and the sections then stained histochemically. Thus, both vascular phenomena and cellular detail were studied on the same tissue section.

The wound margins of all incisions were inverted 24 hours after the incision, despite the meticulous placement of sutures (Fig. 20–5). Although there was a disruption of the capillary continuity, no areas of avascularity were noted. As would be expected with first-intention healing, the inflammatory response was minimal and epithelialization was evident by day 5 (Fig. 20–6A). Because the capillaries crossed the healing incision, hypervascularity was noted (Fig. 20–6B). Fibroblasts were plentiful by day 8 (Fig. 20–7A). A consistent finding was the presence of a hematoma at the subcutaneous level (Fig. 20–7B). No subcutaneous sutures were used in wound closure, but obviously they would be appropriate in the clinical situation.

These studies substantiate the similarity between wound healing as described in previous studies in laboratory animals and that seen in the horse. Even so, further studies in the basic physiology of equine wound healing must be done to improve management of traumatic injuries.

BIBLIOGRAPHY

Baur PS, Parks DH: The myofibroblast anchoring strand—the fibronectin connection in wound healing and the possible loci of collagen fibril assembly. *J Trauma* 1983;23:853–862.

Boucek, RJ: Factors affecting wound healing. *Otolaryngol Clin North Am* 1984;17:243–264.

Chvapil M, Koopmann CF: Scar formation physiology and pathological states. *Otolaryngol Clin North Am* 1984; 17:265–272.

Jacobs KA, Leach DH, Fretz PB, Townsend HGG: Comparative aspects of the healing of excisional wounds on the leg and body of horses. *Vet Surg* 1984;13:83–90.

Peacock EE: *Wound Repair*, ed 3. Philadelphia, WB Saunders Co, 1984.

Silver IA: Basic physiology of wound healing in the horse. *Equine Vet J* 1982;14:7–15.

21 Second-Intention Healing and Delayed Closure

Lawrence C. Booth

There are many wounds that cannot and should not be sutured at the time they are first seen. Loss of skin, excessive swelling, gross contamination, and severely traumatized and devitalized tissues are all reasons to leave a wound open. Client expectations and economics may also dictate how the wound is handled. The wound may be allowed to heal by second intention or it may be sutured at a later date, which is called delayed closure.

Second-intention healing relies upon granulation tissue formation, wound contraction, and epithelialization. Delayed closure can be classified as delayed primary closure or secondary closure. Delayed primary wound closure is usually performed 3 to 5 days after injury. Secondary closure is performed later than 5 days after injury, when granulation tissue has formed.

SECOND-INTENTION HEALING

The goal of second-intention healing is a cosmetic and functional scar. One factor in predicting the cosmetic result is wound location. Wounds on the upper extremity, body, and neck almost always heal with better cosmetic results than wounds on the distal extremities and the head (Fig. 21–1 and 21–2). This is because wound contraction is usually successful in these relatively loose-skinned areas over abundant soft tissue and muscle. In contrast, wound contraction is often incomplete on the head and distal extremities because of a lack of redundant skin. This may leave a wide, epithelialized scar devoid of hair and other dermal appendages.

Another problem in allowing distal leg wounds to heal by second intention is the frequent development of exuberant granulation tissue, which will inhibit wound contraction and epithelialization. Dermal fibrosis and collagen deposition become excessive, elevating the wound bed above the surrounding skin. The reason for this deposition is not completely understood. Studies have shown that collagen formation occurs very early in horse wounds and tends to be excessive when compared to that in the rat. The fact that exuberant granulation tissue does not occur above the carpus or the tarsus suggests that continual disruption of the wound bed as a result of joint and tendon movement and the lack of underlying soft tissues are also important factors. Exuberant granulation tissue does not occur in wounds with underlying muscle tissue. The muscle probably serves to stabilize the wound bed and can contribute to the new vascular supply. Below the carpus and tarsus, there are only tendons, ligaments, and fascia. Movement of the joints produces movement of the deep tissues in relation to the skin. Abnormal collagen deposition may occur in an effort to stabilize the wound margins.

Because of the above limitations, second-intention healing is utilized mainly for upper body wounds or small superficial lacerations or abrasions on the distal legs. It is also used for wounds created by destructive methods such as electrodessication, cryosurgery, or chemical cautery.

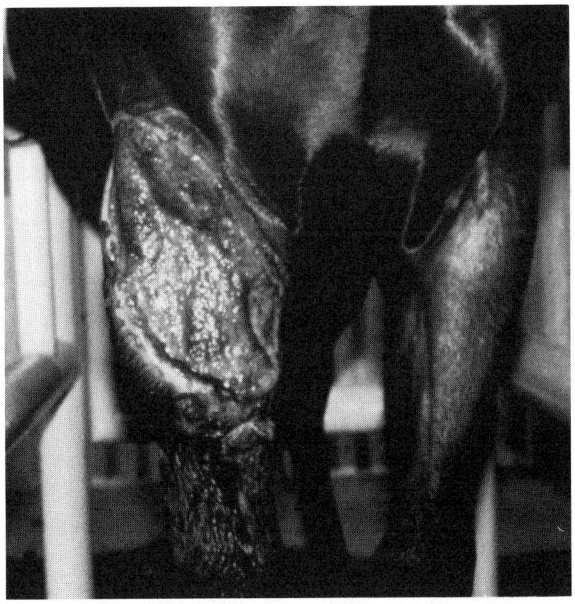

A

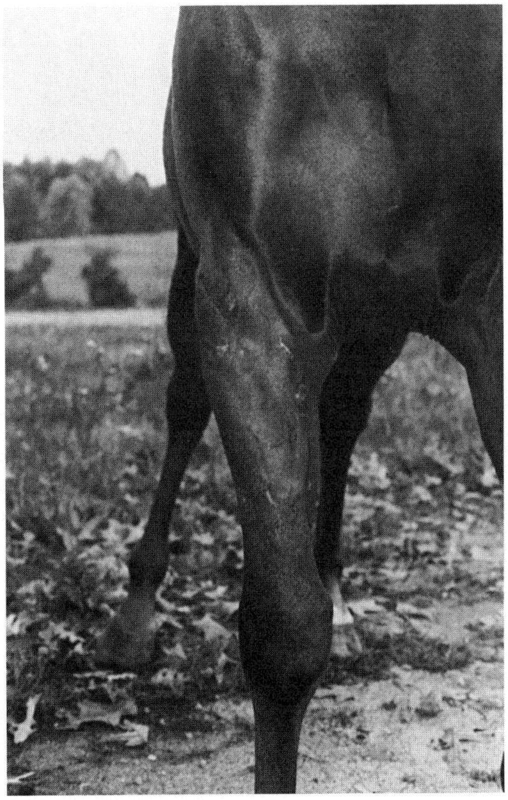

B

Figure 21–1. A. A 3-week-old wound of the forearm, demonstrating a healthy granulation tissue bed. **B.** The same horse approximately 9 months later. Note that wound contraction was sufficient to allow a cosmetic scar.

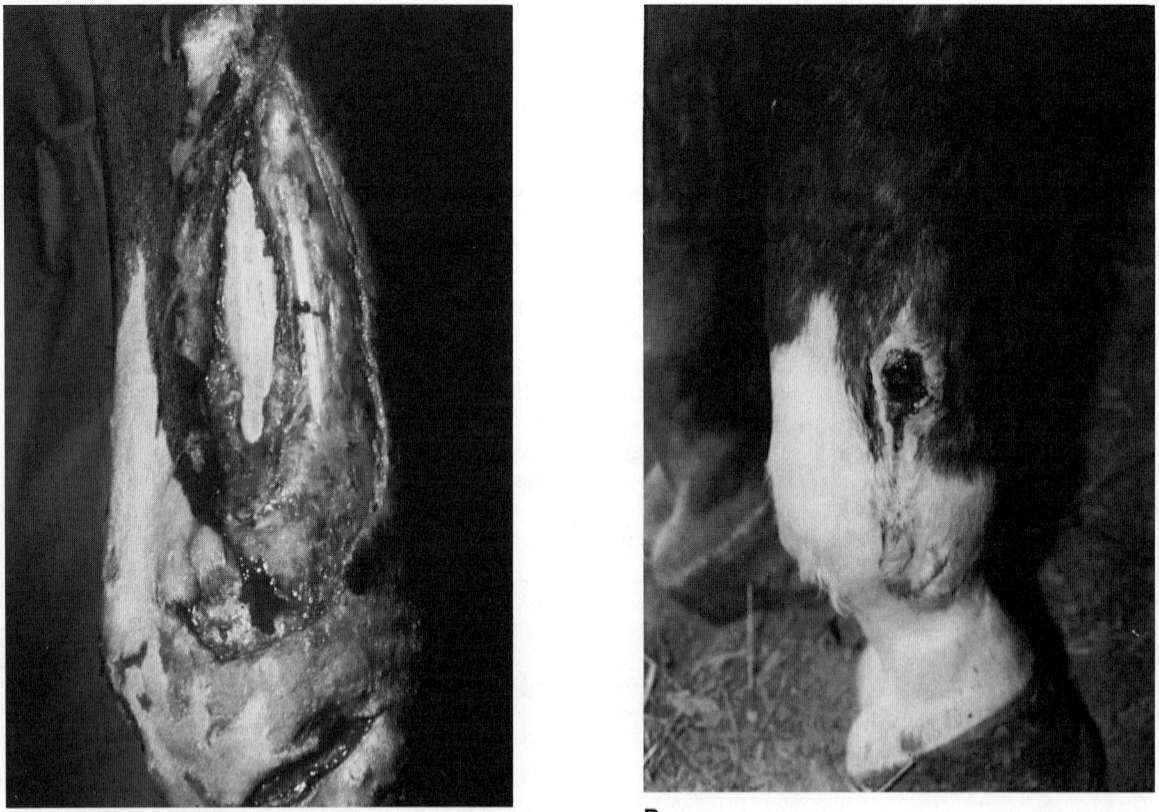

A

B

Figure 21–2. A. Appearance of an acute wound to the lateral aspect of the metacarpus following surgical débridement. Note the exposed tendon and bone. B. Appearance of the same wound approximately 6 months later, demonstrating incomplete healing and a wide epithelialized scar. A central area of granulation tissue persists and is surrounded by a wide epithelialized scar devoid of hair.

Wound Management

Wound management during second-intention healing is simple, requiring only periodic wound cleansing, topical medication, and dressing changes in most cases. Treatment can be performed by the owner at home, which saves the cost of hospitalization and reconstructive procedures.

Bandaging and Dressing. Whenever possible, wounds should be bandaged. Bandages serve to maintain a moist environment, control bacterial numbers by "wicking away" exudate, and provide protection to the wound. They also prevent dependent edema when the wound is on the extremity. The components of a bandage often include several layers. Ointments generally constitute the first layer, followed by a contact layer, an absorbent layer, a protective layer, and a securing layer. All wounds do not require all layers.

Ointments help maintain a moist environment, and they should have antibacterial properties. The type of topical medication used is often a matter of personal preference. Polymyxin B-bacitracin-neomycin (triple antibiotic) ointment (Neosporin) is a good choice because it is effective against a wide spectrum of bacteria. It has also been shown to stimulate epithelialization because of the presence of the bacitracin zinc. In contrast, nitrofurazone (Furacin dressing), which is a widely used topical antimicrobial, has been shown to delay epithelialization by 30%. Gentamicin ointment (Garamycin 0.1%) is a good choice for wounds infected with gram-negative bacteria, especially *Pseudomonas species*.

The contact layer of the bandage usually consists of a nonadherent material. The type of material depends upon the conditions of the wound. Initially a nonadherent fine-mesh gauze (Adaptic nonadhering dressing; Johnson & Johnson) should be used. This dressing allows wound exudate to escape into the overlying absorbent layer. When there is a complete healthy granulation tissue bed with minimal discharge, a rayon-polyethylene (Release nonadhering dressing; Johnson & Johnson) or cotton nonadherent film (Telfa adhesive pads; The Kendall Co) dressing should be used since they provide a moist, semiocclusive environment that enhances epithelialization and minimizes pain.

Synthetic gas-permeable dressings, (Op Site; Smith and Nephew Rolyan, Inc) will increase the rate of epithelialization, but they should be used with caution since they create an occlusive environment that allows bacteria to thrive and multiply. These dressings can be helpful over skin graft donor sites and minor skin abrasions. They can also be used in the final phases of wound healing when infection is not a concern.

Biologic dressings such as pigskin xenografts and equine cadaver allografts stimulate healing and control exuberant granulation tissue. They are discussed further in Chapter 22.

The absorbent layer of the bandage generally consists of dry gauze sponges or bulky stretch gauze (Kerlix roll; The Kendall Co). The function of this layer is to absorb exudate and "wick" it away from the wound surface. This aids in reducing bacterial numbers and the amount of proteolytic enzymes on the wound surface. The protective layer is composed of sheet cotton or roll cotton. This layer helps immobilize the wounded part and provides compression to prevent swelling. The final securing layer utilizes a variety of elastic bandages and tape.

Bandages should be changed as needed, depending upon the amount of wound discharge. When the absorbent layer becomes saturated, it should be changed. Bandages may need to be changed daily at first and then every 3 to 5 days as healing progresses. A bandage can be detrimental to the final stages of wound healing in instances in which the new epithelium is traumatized by continual movement of the bandage in relation to the skin. This may occur over movable joints. If the bandage cannot be adequately secured to the surrounding skin and the wound is small, then removing all bandages and allowing a scab to form on the wound is preferred.

Control of Granulation Tissue. Recent studies have shown that allowing the wound to heal under a scab without bandages is effective in preventing and controlling exuberant granulation tissue. However, this technique is only effective after a period of proper wound management and wound immobilization under a bandage or a cast that produces a complete granulation tissue bed and stable wound margins. One major advantage of leaving the wound open is the cost savings of bandage materials and reduced labor.

Exuberant granulation tissue formation in small wounds can also be readily controlled by the periodic application of 0.1% triamcinolone ointment (Panalog). This treatment works best on immature granulation tissue. The bed will usually flatten within 24 hours. If not, additional applications may be necessary. Continual use of steroids should be avoided since delayed epithelialization may occur. Granulation tissue can be removed surgically by taking the back of a scalpel handle or a tongue depressor and raking it across the wound bed with firm pressure. This will quickly avulse the granulation tissue down to its fibrous bed. Older, more mature granulation tissue requires scalpel excision. Bleeding is easily controlled with a compression bandage. Large wounds in which exuberant granulation tissue is a continual problem should be handled by delayed closure, skin grafting, or cast immobilization.

Exposed Bone or Tendon. Bone or tendon devoid of periosteum or paratenon presents special problems to healing. Exposed tendon is very slow to slough portions that become dessicated or infected and necrotic. In addition, unless the limb is immobilized sufficiently to prevent tendon movement, granulation tissue will not bridge the defect for an extended period. Treatment consists of meticulous débridement of all necrotic tissue and cast immobilization of the limb for 2 to 3 weeks.

Exposed bone very often develops superficial osteitis. The periosteum provides the blood supply to approximately the outer one third of the bone cortex. Loss of the periosteum allows bacteria within the wound to colonize the ischemic bone quickly. With the establishment of infection, the bone attempts to wall off the process by the proliferation of granulation tissue in the haversian canals and marrow spaces. Primitive mesenchymal cells in the haversian canals, in the periosteum, and along the trabeculae are stimulated to produce new reactive bone to further isolate the necrotic bone. The isolated bone is termed a "sequestrum." The new bony shell is termed the "involucrum."

The goals of therapy are to provide immediate coverage of the bone with bandages and to induce granulation tissue to cover the bone. If the area of exposure is small, systemic antibiotics combined with the liberal and frequent application of triple antibiotic ointment under a nonadherent pad, which allows escape of exudate, may prevent desiccation, necrosis, and infection. At the time of bandage changes, any adherent clot that was formed over the bone should not be disturbed since it will serve as a scaffold for new granulation tissue. All other debris and exudate should be removed. Scraping the edges of the granulation tissue in contact with the bone to encourage clot formation may also be helpful. Unfortunately, granulation tissue coverage proceeds very slowly, often taking 60 to 90 days to cover large defects.

Lameness, excessive exudate, purple granulation tissue, or necrotic tracts are all suggestive of superficial cortical osteitis. Characteristic radiographic changes are observed within 7 to 12 days. Bone resorption due to hyperemia of adjacent bone may be visible. Later, the central area of necrotic bone becomes surrounded by granulation tissue and separated from the rest of the bone by the osteoclastic resorption of bone. Radiographically, the granulation tissue appears as a zone of relative radiolucency surrounding the radiodense sequestrum. The granulation tissue is surrounded by an area of increased radiodensity, the involucrum (Fig. 21–3).

Small pieces of bone may be resorbed or extruded relatively quickly. Resorption of large pieces is slow because of the dense mass of cortical bone relative to its surface area. Wound healing is delayed until the infected bone is removed. Sequestrectomy is desirable in most all cases. At surgery, dead bone is easily identified as a free-floating or loosely attached fragment in the involucrum. All involved bone is curetted or chiseled away. Healthy granulation tissue will quickly fill in the defect.

DELAYED WOUND CLOSURE

Wound management by delayed closure is indicated for lower limb wounds in which the level of contamination and/or the amount of devitalized tissue prevent primary suture closure. The wound should not be sutured for at least 4 days. This allows the local body defenses to overcome any bacterial contamination and to remove any necrotic tissue. This does not mean that the wound can simply be packed with an antibiotic ointment and bandaged. Clipping and cleansing of the skin, followed by surgical débridement and lavage of the wound, must be performed with the same care taken as if the wound were to be sutured immediately.

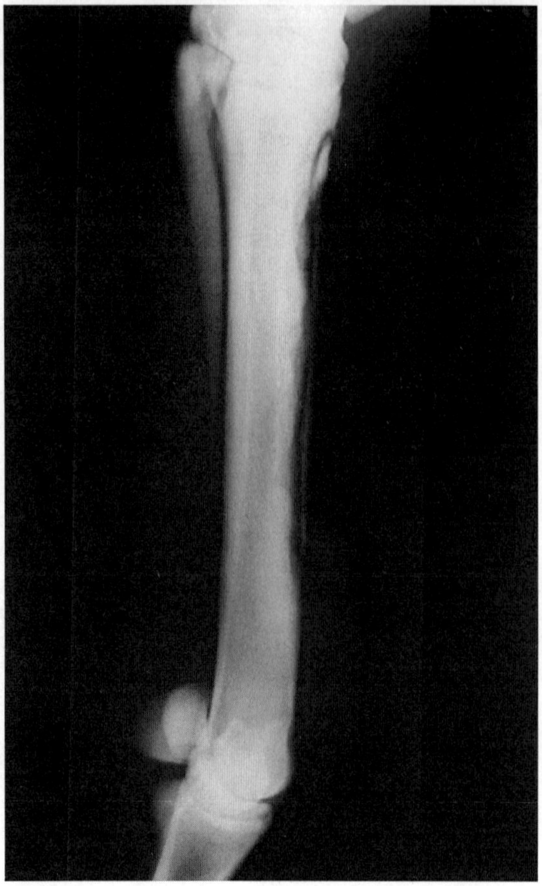

Figure 21–3. Radiographic appearance of a large avulsion wound to the metatarus that resulted in superficial osteitis and sequestrum formation of the dorsal cortex.

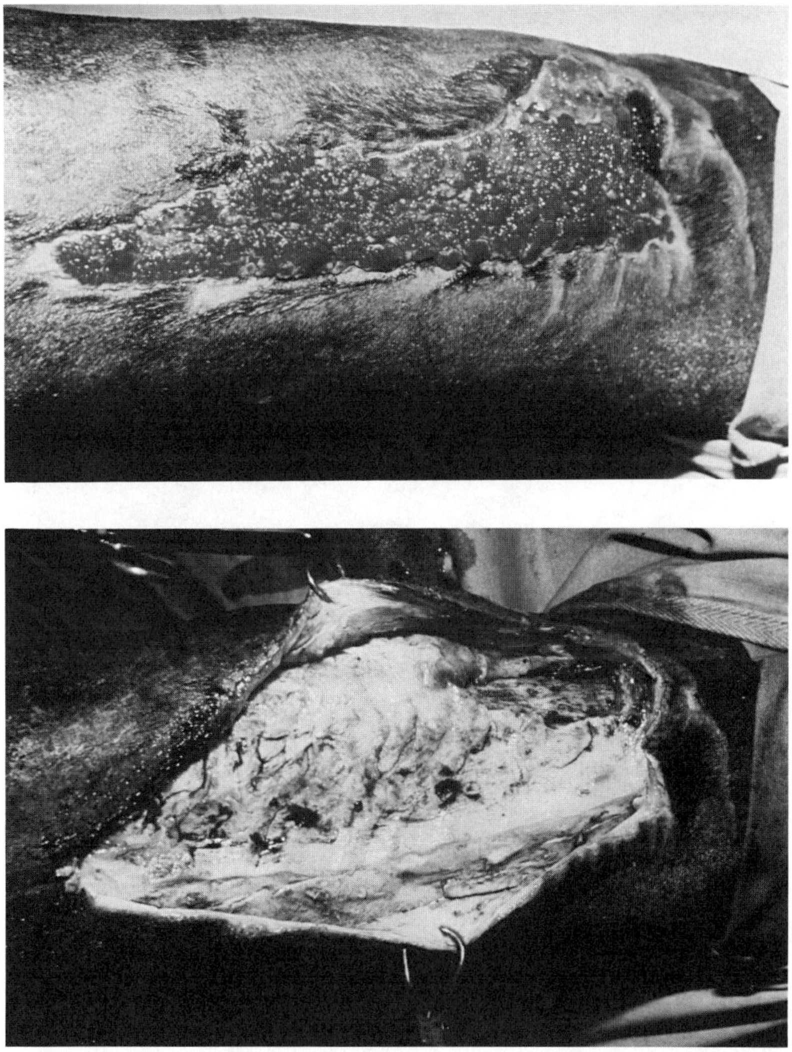

A

B

Figure 21–4. A. A large metatarsal wound of several weeks' duration, demonstrating incomplete wound contraction. **B.** The granulation tissue has been removed and the skin edges have been undermined. The skin is fibrotic and inelastic. (*Figure continues.*)

The wound must be maintained in a sterile bandage. The bandage should be changed at 24- to 48-hour intervals. Any additional nonviable tissue that is identified during bandage changes should be removed surgically. Saline-soaked sponges are used to gently clean the wound. A dilute antiseptic solution such as 0.05% chlorhexidine (Nolvasan solution; Fort Dodge Laboratories, Inc) in water or a 1% povidone-iodine (Betadine solution; Purdue Frederick Co) in saline may be used to lavage the wound under pressure using a spray bottle. Lavage with sterile saline is also acceptable. Triple antibiotic ointment is applied topically. Prophylactic systemic antibiotics are of little value in preventing infection unless they are given prior to initial wound débridement. Even then, their importance is often overestimated.

On, or anytime after, the fourth day following injury, the wound may be closed with less risk of infection providing the tissues appear healthy. At this time, the horse will have developed granulation tissue. The skin edges will be fibrotic and inelastic. The granulation tissue should be removed because it contains numerous clefts and crevices that make aseptic preparation difficult. The skin edges should be dissected free from the underlying tissues and undermined sufficiently to mobilize the skin for closure. Undermining should be done deep to the subcutaneous fascia to preserve the blood supply to the skin (Fig. 21–4).

If undermining does not allow skin closure without undue tension, mesh expansion of the skin can be used. This technique is simple to perform, is cosmetically acceptable, and provides drainage of the dead space cre-

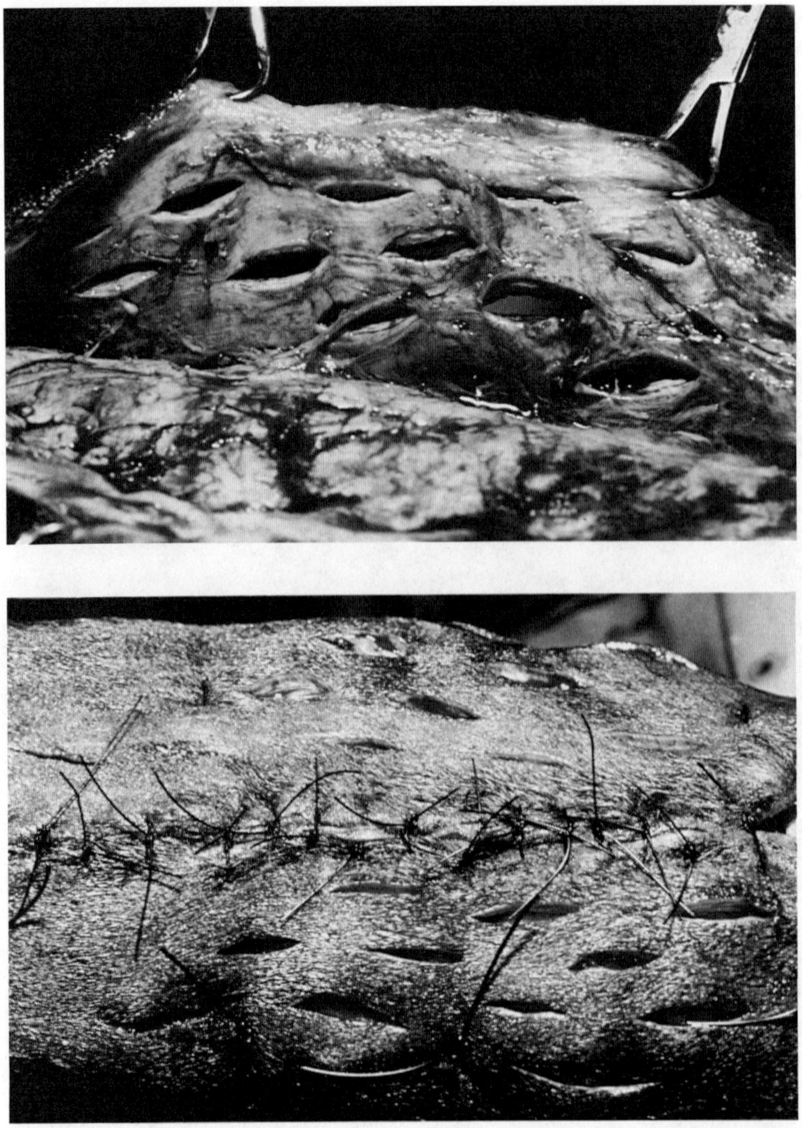

C

D

Figure 21–4. *(Continued).* **C.** Full-thickness staggered release incisions have been performed in the undermined skin edges. **D.** Completed closure accomplished by using mesh expansion and vertical mattress sutures to reduce skin tension.

ated by undermining. Meshing the skin consists of making several full-thickness release incisions in a staggered pattern on either side of the wound. The incisions should be at least 1.5 to 2.5 cm in length and at least 1 cm apart, and must be made parallel to the wound margins (Fig. 21–4C). Fewer, larger incisions will provide more expansion than multiple small incisions in fibrotic skin.

Tension sutures may be required, with or without skin expansion. Size 2 monofilament nylon in a vertical mattress pattern works well (Fig. 21–4D). A vertical mattress pattern is preferred to a horizontal mattress pattern because it is less likely to interfere with the blood supply to the wound margins. These sutures should be preplaced at least several centimeters from the skin edges and then tied when the skin edges have been apposed by sutures or by towel clamps. This method prevents the tension sutures from being tied too tightly. Tension sutures can be removed in 5 to 7 days unless the limb is immobilized in a cast.

If the skin has been undermined extensively, the drainage of any hematoma or seroma that forms will be necessary to minimize scar formation and decrease the risk of infection. If the skin is not meshed, a drain may be used. It should exit the skin away from the suture line and at the ventral aspect of the wound cavity. The drain should not be placed directly beneath the suture line or it will prevent healing. Closed suction units (TLS Surgical drainage system; Porex Medical) are also available that utilize vacutainer tubes for collection of wound fluids. These drains are small, compact, and easy to maintain and can be tucked into bandages or taped to the outside of casts. Drains should be removed when fluid collections decrease significantly, usually within 24 to 72 hours.

The decision to use a bandage, a bandage and splint, or a cast will depend upon the location of the wound and the degree of tension on the closure. A cast used for laceration immobilization is generally left in place for 2 to 3 weeks. Bandages are continued for at least 4 to 6 weeks following the repair to limit thickening of the limb and improve the scar.

Delayed closure can also be used when hypertrophic scar elevates the skin and limits wound contraction and epithelialization. As exuberant granulation tissue and scar build up underneath the skin, the skin is stretched by a process called intussusceptive growth. Debulking of all the scar tissue from the wound bed and undermining and mobilizing the skin edges will often allow suture closure. Tension sutures, drainage, or meshing are utilized as necessary. A cast or a splint is usually necessary to immobilize the repair.

BIBLIOGRAPHY

Bailey JV, Jacobs KA: The mesh expansion method of suturing wounds on the legs of horses. *Vet Surg* 1983;12:78–82.

Bertone AL, Sullins KE, Stashak TS, Norrdin RW: Effect of wound location and the use of topical collagen gel on exuberant granulation tissue formation and wound healing in the horse and pony. *Am J Vet Res* 1985;46:1438–1444.

Fretz PB, Martin GS, Jacobs KA, McIlwraith CW: Treatment of exuberant granulation tissue in the horse, evaluation of four methods. *Vet Surg* 1983;12:137–140.

Hacket RP: Delayed wound closure, a review and report of use of the technique on three equine limb wounds. *Vet Surg* 1983;12:48–53.

Jacobs KA, Leach DH, Fretz PB, Townsend HGG: Comparative aspects of the healing of excisional wounds on the leg and body of horses. *Vet Surg* 1984;13:83–90.

Lee AH, Swaim SF, McGuire JA, Huges KS: Effects of nonadherent dressing materials on the healing of open wounds in dogs. *J Am Vet Med Assoc* 1987;190:416–422.

Stashak TS: Reconstructive surgery in the horse. *J Am Vet Med Assoc* 1977;170:143–149.

Swaim SF, Lee AH: Topical wound medications: A review. *J Am Vet Med Assoc* 1987;190:1588–1593.

22 Skin Grafting

Lawrence C. Booth

Skin grafting is an established practice in equine surgery. It utilizes various techniques, including pinch grafts, punch grafts, postage stamp grafts, strip grafts, tunnel grafts, and sheet grafts. The indications for each type of graft depend upon the size and location of the wound, the expertise of the surgeon, and the economic considerations and cosmetic expectations of the client. Sheet grafting will be discussed here.

CLASSIFICATION OF GRAFTS

Grafts are classified according to their thickness and also according to their source. A split-thickness graft includes the epidermis and a varying amount of the dermis. The thickness may vary from approximately 0.008 to 0.030 in. A full-thickness graft includes the epidermis and all of the dermis.

A graft taken from the same individual and transplanted to a different area is called an autograft. If a graft is taken from a different individual of the same species, it is termed an allograft or homograft. A xenograft or heterograft is a graft taken from another species. Pigskin is the most notable example of a xenograft. The most common indication for the use of autografts in companion animals is reconstruction of traumatic injuries to the extremities in which there is excessive skin loss. Skin grafting can also be used to cover large defects created by excision of skin tumors or scars. Traumatically avulsed skin may also be replaced with a graft.

Full-thickness sheet grafts give the most functional

protection to underlying structures and the most acceptable cosmetic appearance in horses. Unfortunately, their acceptance rate is low. Both clinical and experimental investigations have shown that split-thickness, mesh expansion skin grafting has a high acceptance rate and an acceptable cosmetic appearance in horses.

PREPARATION OF THE WOUND BED

Most of the initial effort in grafting is directed at obtaining an acceptable recipient bed of young, healthy granulation tissue. Grafting success is largely determined by the level of bacterial growth on the wound bed. A bacterial level of 10^5 or greater organisms/g of tissue will interfere with graft acceptance. Techniques for quantifying bacteria in a contaminated wound have been described; however, their use in veterinary medicine to date has been limited. Bacterial counts can be reduced in an acute wound by surgical debridement since most bacteria are concentrated in necrotic tissue and around foreign bodies on the wound surface. Irrigation can also be helpful if the fluid is delivered with enough pressure to mechanically dislodge bacteria from the wound surface. Seven pounds of pressure per square inch is effective. This level of pressure can be generated using a 35-mL syringe and an 18-gauge needle or a simple plastic spray bottle.

Once the wound has developed a granulation tissue bed, systemic antibiotics are not effective in reducing the bacterial count. At least one study has shown that an aerosol containing neomycin, polymyxin B, and bacitracin was effective in eliminating bacterial infections of granulating wounds. Avulsion of the granulation tissue bed is the most effective way of dealing with an established infection. The back of a scalpel handle is pressed into the granulation tissue and scraped along the base, removing the tissue in total. Bleeding is then controlled by a compression dressing.

Exuberant granulation tissue should be trimmed 24 to 48 hours prior to grafting. This delay results in a proliferation of capillaries and allows a fresh, fine granular surface to reform. Since granulation tissue has no nerve supply, excision can be accomplished in the standing horse with minimal restraint. This eliminates unnecessary anesthesia time during grafting, because hemorrhage from the wound bed in the horse can be profuse and difficult to control in a short time.

BIOLOGIC DRESSINGS

Biologic dressings such as allografts or xenografts act as temporary physiologic bandages. They can be helpful in preparing the wound bed for the eventual application of an autograft. An allograft will "take" or become vascularized initially and may survive for a short time, but rejection will occur because it is immunologically different from the host. Freeze-dried pigskin never becomes vascularized. Although it is not known how these grafts mediate their beneficial effects, to some extent it depends upon their capacity to become vascularized, suggesting that fresh-stored allografts are preferable to reconstituted freeze-dried skin. However, stored porcine xenografts (Porcine skin dressing; Genetic Laboratories, Inc) have been used successfully in horses.

The reported advantages of allografts and xenografts include reduction of the bacterial count of the wound bed to which they are applied; reduction of wound pain; reduction of protein, electrolyte, and fluid loss; prevention of exuberant granulation tissue; and stimulation of epithelialization.

As allograft skin is changed every 48 hours, it will eventually become adherent to the wound bed, suggesting early vascularization. The application of an autograft at that time should be successful because the proper wound bed conditions for graft "take" have already been established. Equine cadaver allografts can be easily collected aseptically with a dermatome and stored for later use in a nutrient medium that supplies a physiologic concentration of electrolytes, nutrients, and buffers to ensure continued metabolic survival of the graft. McCoy's 5A Medium (Flow Laboratories, Inc) plus 10% horse serum (GG-Free Horse Serum; Gibco Lab) is recommended. Gentamicin sulfate (Gentocin) (80 mg) is added to each liter of storage medium. Damage to the graft from antigenic reactions can be prevented by using commercially prepared antibody-free equine serum.

Individual strips of collected skin are placed on separate layers of gauze. Then they are rolled up like a jelly roll and placed in a sterile container. Medium is added at a ratio of 1 to 1.5 mL of medium/cm^2 of skin. Skin should be stored at 4 °C to reduce tissue metabolism to a basal level. Air must be present in the storage container to provide oxygen for cellular metabolism. Skin can be stored in this manner for up to 3 weeks. Meshing the graft as described later is optional.

PHYSIOLOGY OF GRAFT TAKE

Initial adherence of a graft to its recipient bed is by fibrin adhesion, and this fibrin is later converted to fibrous tissue. During the first 24 to 48 hours following placement of a graft, there is absorption into the graft of a plasma-like fluid from the recipient bed by capillary action. This has been termed "plasmatic imbibition." This fluid carries enough nourishment to permit the graft to survive during this critical period. By 48 hours, a fine network of vascular channels is established in the fibrin layer binding the graft. This occurs by capillary budding from the blood vessels of the recipient granulation bed. These vascular channels connect with the blood vessels existing in the graft and blood flow in the graft is restored. This process has been termed "inosculation." At the same time that inosculation is taking place, capillary ingrowth from the bed directly into the graft occurs. Circulation may be completely reestablished anywhere from 4 to 12 days following grafting.

GRAFTING TECHNIQUE

Prior to collecting the graft, the recipient wound bed is gently scraped with a scalpel blade to remove the fibrin coagulum that has formed. This ensures direct contact of the graft with the capillary bed.

Split-thickness skin can be obtained from anywhere on the body, but the ventral pectoral region caudal to the elbow seems most satisfactory. This area hides any resulting scar. If possible, the area where the girth strap will cross should be avoided to prevent possible irritation. As in other species, skin thickness and hair density in the horse are greater over the dorsal body and neck and thinner over the ventral body regions. Graft thickness will depend upon where it is taken. Grafts 0.025 to 0.030 in thick from the pectoral area are most satisfactory. Grafts can be harvested with a razor blade or free-hand knife, but because of the amount of skin generally needed, an electric (Electric Dermatome; Stryker Electro-Surgical Unit, Orthopedic Fram Co) or pneumatic dermatome works best (Fig. 22–1).

Meshing the graft has been criticized because it still leaves a large area of the wound to heal by epithelialization. However, hematomas, seromas, and wound exudate account for the majority of skin graft loss. Making a few cuts in a large graft, called "pie crusting," is not very effective in allowing fluid accumulations to escape because the edges of the cuts in the graft stick to the graft bed, forming a seal. The expansile mesher (Mesh Graft Expander, No. P-160; Padgett Instruments), on the other hand, is a very effective method of "pie crusting" and will allow survival of the majority of a graft even if other portions are lost. The expansile mesher consists of a bed of staggered razor blades on which the skin is cut with a Teflon roller, producing a 3:1 expansion ratio (Fig. 22–2). The grafts are applied to the wound partially expanded and fixed to the wound margins with sutures, stainless steel skin staples (Elite Disposable Skin Stapler; United States Surgical Corp), or cyanoacrylate glue (Nexaband Liquid; CRX Medical, Inc) (Fig. 22–3).

DRESSING TECHNIQUE

A nonadherent petrolatum dressing (Adaptic nonadhering dressing; Johnson & Johnson) is applied over the graft and secured to the surrounding skin with additional sutures, staples, or glue. This allows early inspection and dressing changes without fear of graft disruption. An absorbent layer of 4 × 4–in gauze sponges

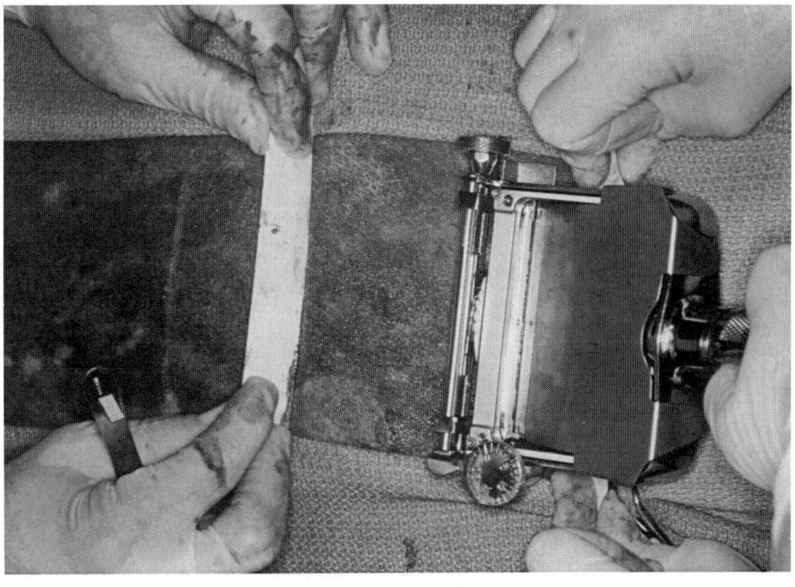

Figure 22–1. Collection of a split-thickness sheet graft using an electric dermatome.

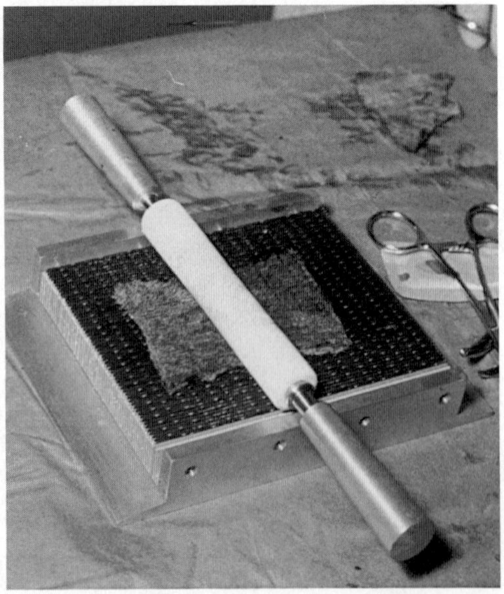

Figure 22–2. Split-thickness skin meshed on a bed of staggered razor blades.

is used, followed by an elastic adhesive bandage (ExpAndover elastic tape; ExpAndover, Inc) applied circumferentially around the limb to produce gentle, even pressure. The dressings are changed daily (except the nonadherent layer) until graft take is assured, usually about 5 days. The bandages are then changed every 3 to 5 days. Wounds over joints should be immobilized in a splinted bandage if possible. Frequent dressing changes are not an absolute prerequisite to success if the wound bed is healthy. Consequently, if a cast is deemed necessary, it should be left in place at least 2 weeks.

When wound drainage ceases, the petrolatum dressing is changed to a semiocclusive rayon-polyethylene (Release nonadhering dressing; Johnson & Johnson) dressing that enhances epithelialization. Polymyxin B–bacitracin-neomycin antibiotic ointment (Neosporin) is applied topically. When epithelialization is complete, the new graft is kept under a light cotton bandage for protection for an additional 2 to 3 weeks.

One important note is that any leftover donor skin from a grafting procedure should be saved for possible future use in case the original graft does not take completely. The storage procedure is as described for allograft skin (Fig. 22–4).

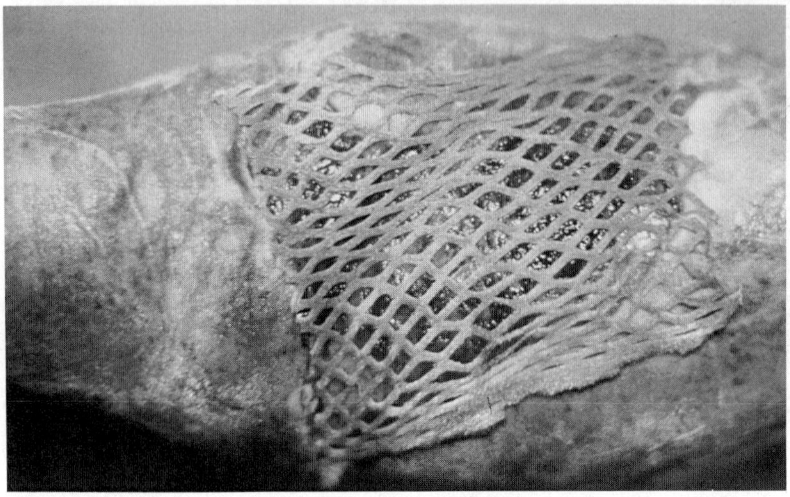

Figure 22–3. Split-thickness mesh graft being applied to a wound in a partially expanded manner to allow drainage.

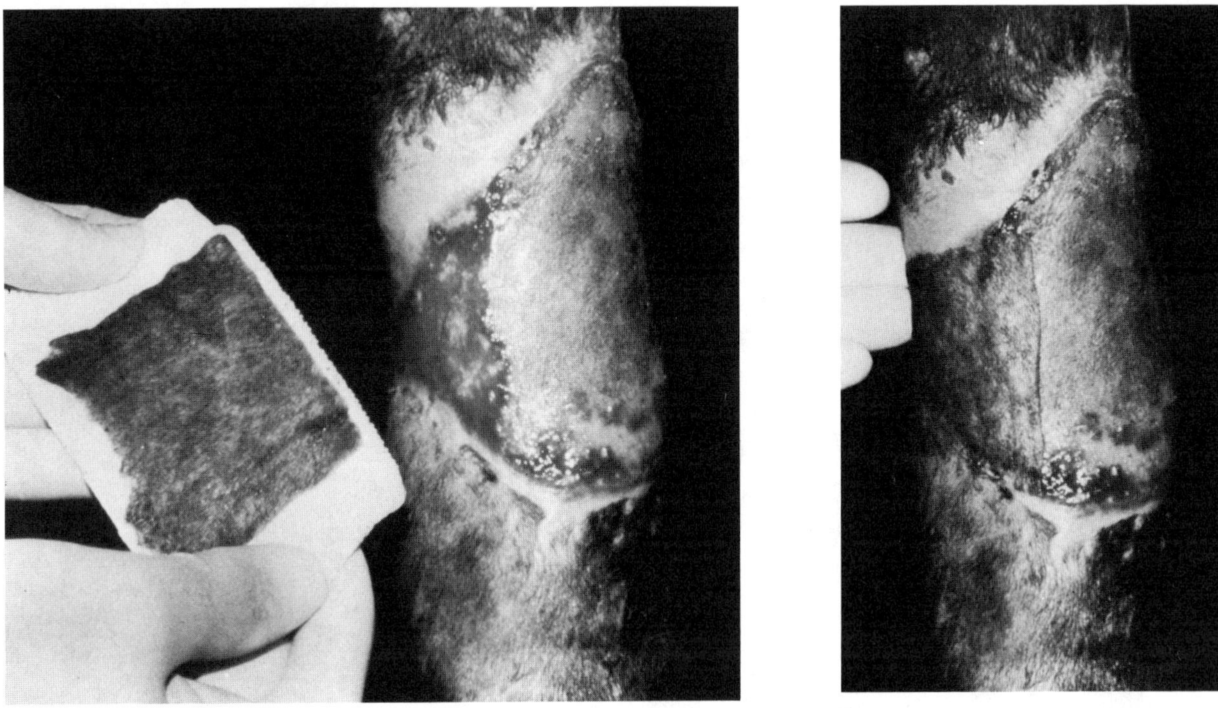

A B

Figure 22–4. A. Stored autograft skin is about to be applied to a wound in a standing horse where graft take was incomplete initially. **B.** The stored sheet graft is fixed to the recipient bed by gluing it to the surrounding skin.

HEALING OF THE DONOR SITE

Protection to the donor site is best accomplished with a spray cyanoacrylate bandage (New Skin; Medtech Laboratories, Inc). It not only keeps the wound clean and dry, but also seems to reduce the pain and swelling. Alternatively, a semiocclusive dressing can be secured to the site with elastic tape around the horse's trunk. In the case of a split-thickness graft, the donor site heals by epithelialization from hair follicles and sebaceous glands. Hair regrowth may be sparse with thick split-thickness grafts, but still remains functionally and cosmetically acceptable.

DELAYED GRAFTING USING STORED SKIN

Delayed grafting of stored skin can also be used in selected cases to provide late coverage of wounds not suitable for grafting at the time of initial surgical débridement. The advantage of this technique is that it eliminates the need for an additional anesthetic and surgical procedure. At the time of initial wound therapy, when the horse is under anesthesia, autogenous skin grafts are collected, meshed, stored in McCoy's medium, and banked in a refrigerator. Such autogenous equine grafts have been successfully stored for up to 3 weeks. Then, when the recipient bed is ready, the stored graft can be applied to the wound with the horse standing and sedated. The graft should be secured to the wound margins with cyanoacrylate glue and bandages as previously described. Another advantage of this procedure is that a 2-day delay in grafting a newly created or newly freshened wound along with simultaneous graft storage reduces plasmatic imbibition time by production of anaerobic metabolites that stimulate vascularization.

GRAFTING PROBLEM WOUNDS

Problem wounds with exposed bone or tendon or with an open tendon sheath or joint may still be grafted, but persistent bacterial contamination or excessive drainage make the task more difficult. Typically, large areas of the wound are ready for grafting while other areas undergo delayed healing. Meshing the graft in these cases is essential to allow the escape of collections of fluids, exudate, or blood that might separate the graft from its underlying vascular supply (Fig. 22–5).

Thin skin grafts (approximately 0.020 in) are harvested and mechanically meshed on a 3:1 expansion ratio meshing device. The grafts are applied, partially expanded, and fixed to the wound margins with stainless steel skin staples. Sterile petroleum-impregnated gauze is applied and stapled to the skin at a distance from the wound margins. This allows both good wound drainage and frequent bandage changes without graft disruption. A thick dressing of absorbent cotton (Combine Roll; Johnson & Johnson), wet with antibiotic solution, is applied to immobilize the graft and to remove wound fluids by a wicking action. This absorbent layer is changed daily to remove exudate and to inspect the graft. Elastic wraps are used to secure the dressings. If

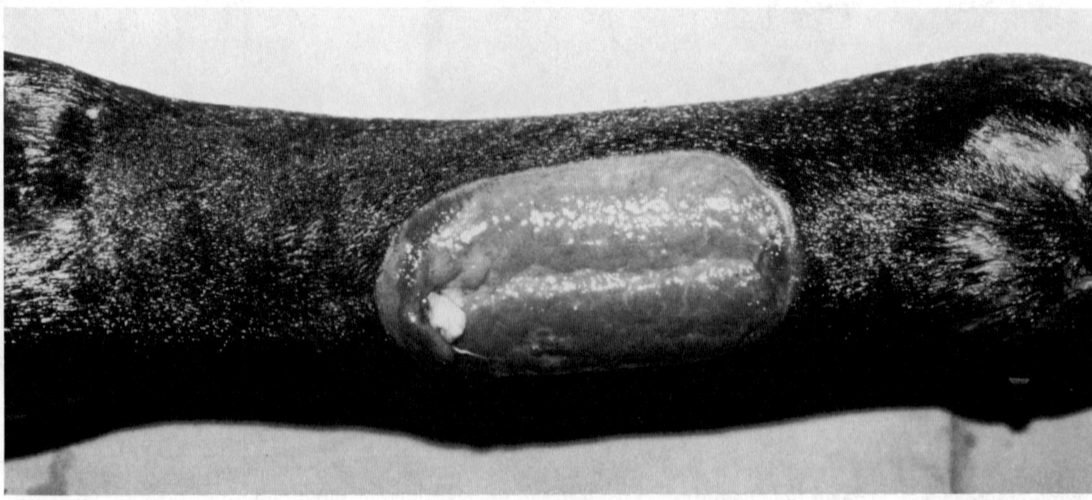

A

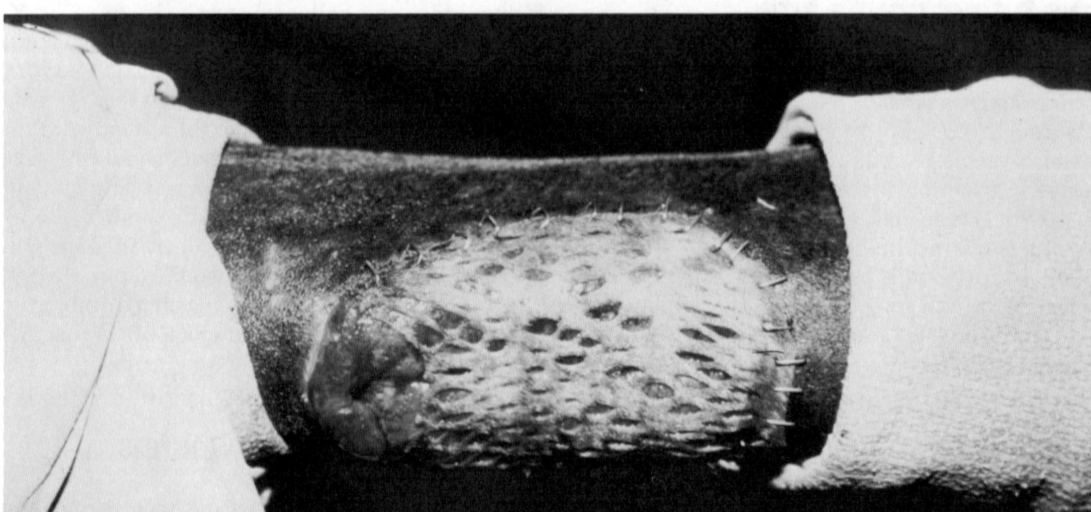

B

Figure 22–5. A. This wound on the palmar aspect of the metacarpus has a healthy granulation tissue bed except for a section of necrotic superficial flexor tendon visible at one end. Wound drainage from the tendon was excessive. **B.** The necrotic portion of tendon has been débrided and a mesh graft has been applied to the majority of the wound. Note the area left open where further wound drainage is anticipated.

necessary, joint immobilization is accomplished with fiberglass (Delta Lite "S" fiberglass casting tape; Johnson & Johnson) or Orthoplast splints (Johnson & Johnson).

Topical antibiotic solutions are applied at least every 4 hours to maintain a wet environment. This can be accomplished by incorporating perforated polyethylene tubing within the bandage or pouring the solution into the bandage from the top and allowing gravity to spread it over the wound. Topical treatment is discontinued following graft take, which is usually evident by the fifth day. The appropriate antibiotic solution is best determined by culture and sensitivity. Prophylactic antibiotics should be directed at preventing β-hemolytic streptococcus infections, since they occur commonly in the horse. These organisms produce proteolytic enzymes that can dissolve the fibrin scaffold that fixes the graft to the wound bed.

One final indication for grafting is treating extensive traumatic avulsion flaps on the distal extremity. In those cases in which significant flap death is expected, salvaging the avulsed skin as a graft should be considered. The flap can be removed, converted to a full-thickness or split-thickness skin graft, meshed, and reapplied. A fresh wound is an acceptable recipient bed *only* if complete débridement can be accomplished. If not, the skin can be banked in the refrigerator until the wound bed is ready for grafting.

BIBLIOGRAPHY

Diehl M, Ersek RA: Porcine xenografts for treatment of skin defects in horses. *J Am Vet Med Assoc* 1980;177:625–628.

Hurst LN, Brown DH, Murray KA: Prolonged life and improved quality for stored skin grafts. *Plast Reconstr Surg* 1984;73:105–109.

Peyton LC, Connelly MB: Evaluation of quantitative bacterial counts as an aid in the treatment of wounds in the horse. *Equine Vet J* 1983;15:251–252.

Schumacher J, Chambers M, Hanselka DV, Morton LD: Preservation of skin by refrigeration for autogenous grafting in the horse. *Vet Surg*, 1987;16:358–361.

Spence RJ, Ruas EF: The banking and clinical use of human skin allograft in trauma patients: Clinical use of allograft skin. *Md Med J* 1986;35:205–212.

Swaim SF: Principles of mesh skin grafting. *Compd Contin Educ* 1982;4:194–200.

Tobin GR: The comprised bed technique, an improved method for skin grafting problem wounds. *Surg Clin North Am* 1984;64:653–658.

23
Distal Limb Lacerations

Eric L. Reinertson

Lacerations of the distal limbs occur frequently in the horse. Wire fencing, protruding objects in stalls, and discarded metal or glass objects, in addition to kicks, may cause these injuries. It is important that the veterinarian determine the depths of these wounds and the involvement of deeper structures. The potential for disfigurement and the possibility of diminished athletic ability from leg lacerations are often a concern to horse owners. Clients should be instructed in proper first aid procedures. In most instances, the best care is a sterile, or at least clean, compression bandage. Hemorrhage and swelling will be controlled, and the wound will be protected from further trauma and contamination, and will be partially immobilized. Clients should be cautioned against applying medications to a wound. Many of the medications available to laymen are oily preparations or contain irritants that may interfere with wound healing.

In some instances, injuries may go unnoticed for extended periods of time. Wounds that are very swollen and necrotic and are producing exudate or are starting to show evidence of granulation tissue are probably at least 2 to 5 days old. Surgical closure of these wounds should be delayed; alternatively, they may best be left to heal by second intention.

WOUND HISTORY AND INSPECTION

A history pertaining to the wound should always be obtained. If possible, an accurate estimation of the duration of the wound should be determined. It may be necessary to determine when the horse was last seen in order to estimate the possible duration of the injury if the wounding was not witnessed. Determining what made the wound may give some indication about the type of wound. Glass or sheet metal cuts tend to be sharper and less traumatic to tissues than blunt trauma or a rope burn. The depth of the wound and degree of contamination can also be estimated if the source of the wound is known. Although owners tend to overestimate the amount of hemorrhage, the possibility of severe blood loss should not be ignored.

An episode of colic or a neurologic disease may be the underlying cause of wounds to the extremities. Oftentimes the most obvious wound is not the most serious one. A gaping, bleeding leg wound should not allow a puncture wound to the chest, abdomen, or a joint to go unnoticed. Examination of the wound should follow with examination of the entire horse. Uneasiness, tachycardia, and pale mucous membranes may indicate significant blood loss.

Sedation may be necessary to allow a thorough examination if the horse is untrained, excited, or in pain. However, most tranquilizers cause hypotension and should not be used if the horse is showing any signs of hypovolemia (blood loss) or neurogenic (pain) shock. Local or regional anesthesia should not be used until the integrity of supporting bones and tendons is assured, because attempts at weight bearing may result in further tissue damage and contamination.

A sterile gloved hand is used to explore the wound, being cautious to avoid introducing further contamination. Careful exploration and examination of the wound allows the clinician to assess the degree of injury to the skin, joints, ligaments, tendons, bones and coronary band. An attempt should be made to evaluate the blood supply to the wound area and the distal limb. It is important to recognize that wounds caused by blunt trauma, such as a pastern caught in a wooden gate, commonly develop areas of devitalized tissue much larger than the original wound. These wounds may enlarge as the necrotic skin sloughs over the following days.

When a wound is in close proximity to a joint, it is vitally important to determine if the joint has been penetrated. A small wound that would otherwise be inconsequential is potentially disastrous if it enters a joint and results in septic arthritis. Thus, early recognition and vigorous therapy are necessary to prevent a contaminated joint from becoming infected. If careful manual exploration of the wound is not conclusive for joint penetration, further examination is indicated. A needle aseptically placed into the joint at a site distant to the wound may be used to inject sterile Ringer's solution into the joint. If fluid runs out of the wound, it confirms an open joint capsule. If the entire periarticular area is swollen and potentially septic, this technique should not be used because it might introduce contamination into the joint with the needle. In this instance, radiographs may reveal the presence of air within the joint spaces, confirming joint involvement. Injecting contrast media through the wound should be avoided because it may force more contamination into the joint. If any doubt remains concerning the integrity of the joint, it is best to proceed with surgical exploration as if the joint were open.

DEVELOPING A TREATMENT PLAN

After the wound has been carefully explored and the extent of injuries determined, a treatment plan can be formulated. The extent of injury, the intended use of the horse, the prognosis for recovery, the wishes of the owner, and the projected cost of treatment must be taken into account when selecting a treatment regimen. A partially severed superficial flexor tendon may not be a serious wound to a child's pony, yet it might be an impossible injury to resolve for the intended use of a race gelding. Likewise, a disfiguring scar may be acceptable on a brood mare, yet may be the end of a career for a horse shown at halter.

Most wounds heal faster and with a better cosmetic appearance if they can be sutured and heal by first intention. Fresh, clean, incised wounds are ideal candidates for primary wound closure. Older, more contaminated wounds containing damaged tissue require meticulous preparation before they can safely be closed under suture. Some wounds are best handled as open wounds. Any extremity wound that is severely swollen, contains draining exudate, or is over 8 to 10 hours old should not be sutured closed in hopes of first intention healing. Wounds associated with injury to deeper structures (i.e., joints and tendon sheaths) may benefit from the extra effort to prepare them for primary closure.

Fresh, clean, small skin wounds on the extremities can often be closed in the standing horse. Local anesthesia in conjunction with chemical restraint (tranquilization) and/or physical restraint (twitch) may be all that is necessary in many instances. Selective nerve blocks or "ring blocks" are preferable to the infiltration of local anesthesia because local infiltration risks spreading contamination and adds to the local inflammatory response. Local anesthetics with epinephrine should be used sparingly because the vasoconstrictor effect may further compromise the blood supply in some wounds.

Wounds requiring extensive débridement, tissue mobilization, or repair of deeper structures (tendons, bones, joints) are best repaired under general anesthesia. The horse is positioned to provide the best access to the wound and the bandage and sterile compress is removed. The area is then prepared for aseptic surgery.

MANAGEMENT OF SIMPLE LACERATIONS

Cleansing and Débridement

Prior to cleansing the wound, the skin around it should be aseptically prepared. The wound cavity is packed with sterile gauze sponges moistened with sterile isotonic fluid. Sterile, water-soluble lubricating jelly can also be used to help protect the wound from dirt and hair while the surrounding area is being clipped. The area should be liberally clipped to allow the wound to be enlarged, to explore fascial planes, or to allow placement of drains distant from the wound. The skin is then scrubbed with a suitable surgical soap. Soap or disinfectants should be kept from entering the wound. The gauze packing is then removed and the wound lavaged with sterile isotonic fluids. The use of a sterile plastic spray bottle similar to those used for household cleaners has proved to be a very simple, effective wound lavage system.

Wound débridement involves the surgical removal of contaminated and devitalized tissue from a wound in an effort to transform an accidental wound into a surgically clean wound. In some wounds, this may be a relatively easy process. In other wounds, débridement may actually entail removing an entire layer of tissue, creating a new surgically clean wound a few millimeters larger than the original wound. This is referred to as wound excision. In severely contaminated wounds, débridement may be done in two stages. The majority of the contaminated and devitalized tissue is removed in the first stage, and new gloves, drapes, and instruments are used for the final débridement. Wound débridement should be done in an orderly fashion, working from one end of the wound to the other. Care should be taken to avoid recontamination of an area that has been débrided. The careful use of wound lavage with sterile Ringer's solution using a spray bottle is helpful in flushing particles away from the clean area. A large volume of lavage solution should be used because dilution is a very effective means of reducing contamination.

The temptation to trim off an avulsed flap of skin should be resisted unless is it of no value for wound coverage. In nearly all instances, if skin can be preserved, it can be utilized to provide coverage for the healing wound. Débridement should be done by sharp dissection whenever possible. Although scraping a wound surface may make it look cleaner, this is very traumatic to tissues. Tendons, ligaments, blood vessels, and nerves should be preserved if they appear viable. Bone that has been stripped of periosteum and appears contaminated should be cautiously débrided with a sharp currette. Débridement of the skin edges should be conservative, especially if there has been skin loss with the original wound. Along with débridement, a thorough exploration of the wound is conducted. The external skin wound should be enlarged if necessary to adequately explore the wound, searching for foreign bodies, contaminated pockets of tissue, or previously unrecognized damage to deeper structures. During débridement, culturing the wound is advised, particularly if deep structures are involved or if pockets are discovered. Bacterial identification and antibiotic sensitivity detected early in the course of treatment will help selection of antibiotic therapy.

Primary Wound Closure

Deep fascial planes should be sutured with carefully spaced, fine, synthetic absorbable sutures. Unnecessary sutures within the wound act as foreign material and should be avoided. Various drain systems and/or compression bandaging are alternatives to suture closing of dead space. No tissue plane should be closed with excessive tension on the suture line. This is especially true of the skin. Excess tension may lead to tissue ischemia and result in suture "pull out." Ischemic, necrotic tissue also predisposes to wound infection. Tension sutures may be used to alleviate tension on the primary suture line, but they too can cause ischemic tissue. If the wound cannot be closed without excessive tension on the sutures, then it should be left at least partially open. Likewise, if the surgeon is not satisfied that débridement and lavage have left the wound clean enough to close, it should also be left at least partially open. Carefully placed large tension sutures may be utilized to hold large avulsed skin flaps in position even when a primary closure is not attempted. The sutured wound must be monitored very closely and at least partially reopened if signs of infection become evident.

Bandaging and Casting

Bandaging of distal limb wounds is a very important part of any treatment regime. A properly applied padded compression bandage is not only an excellent first-aid tool but also a very important postoperative aid. Bandages help prevent further trauma and contamination of the wound. They help reduce swelling and hematoma formation within the wound. Bandaging also protects the suture line by providing external support and minimizing motion at the wound site.

Some exterior wounds occur in areas that are subject to excessive motion in the wound bed. These wounds may benefit from more rigid immobilization than may be provided by a heavy bandage. Alternatively, a cast may be necessary to provide the immobility needed for the wound to heal. Wounds on the palmar or plantar aspect of the pastern, whether sutured or not, often benefit from immobilization within a cast. Injuries to the hoof and bulbs of the heels are very difficult to stabilize and immobilize without the use of casts.

Drug Therapy

The use of systemic antibiotics is indicated in the treatment of extensive wounds or those involving deeper structures. Combinations of antibiotics are often utilized to achieve broad-spectrum coverage in wound therapy. Gentamicin and penicillin provide such coverage in most cases. Simple skin wounds or wounds left open to heal by second intention may not need treatment with systemic antibiotics. To be effective, systemic antibiotics should be started as early as possible in the course of therapy, prior to wound débridement.

Tetanus prophylaxis in the form of tetanus toxoid is indicated in any equine wound. The concurrent use of tetanus antitoxin may be indicated if there is no history of previous tetanus toxoid immunization. The use of nonsteroidal anti-inflammatory agents is often helpful to control the inflammatory response and the pain of injury without interfering with wound healing.

MANAGEMENT OF COMPLEX WOUNDS

Joint or Tendon Sheath Lacerations

Lacerations involving joints or tendon sheaths generally benefit from surgical débridement and closure. Initial first aid therapy should include clipping, preparing, and bandaging the wound as previously described. Splinting may also be utilized if concurrent tendon or ligament injury requires more stability than a bandage can provide. Systemic antibiotic therapy should be instituted early in the treatment regimen. The surgical treatment of an open joint should be undertaken without unnecessary delay. The horse should be placed under general anesthesia and positioned to provide maximum exposure of the wound and affected joint. The wound is surgically prepared and draped for débridement as described. When possible, a 14-gauge needle or catheter is placed into the affected joint at an area distant to the wound and a continuous flush of sterile Ringer's solution is maintained throughout the surgical procedure. This maintains an egress flow of fluid that helps prevent the inadvertent introduction of further contamination into the joint. The wound is then systematically explored and débrided, working from the joint to the skin surface. A visual assessment of damage to the joint surfaces should be made if possible. This may help establish a prognosis for future soundness.

Careful curettage of contaminated or nonviable cartilage and bone is performed. After thorough débridement and lavage of the joint has rendered it as clean as possible, the joint capsule should be closed by suture if possible. A closed-system continuous suction drain (TLS Surgical Drainage System; Porex Medical) (Fig. 23–1) placed within the joint is helpful in preventing the accumulation of exudate and abnormal joint fluid. The drain system is usually left in place for 2 to 4 days. Closure of the remainder of the wound is then performed. As with any sutured wound, if evidence of infection within the joint is noted, it should be opened and adequate drainage established. This may include leaving the joint open for drainage in rare instances. Postoperative immobilization of joint wounds has been very helpful in protecting the suture line and relieving pain. This immobilization can be accomplished by incorporating splints or casting materials within the pressure bandage.

Lacerations that involve tendon sheaths deserve the same rigorous therapy as joint wounds. Thorough exploration of the wound in conjunction with débridement and lavage may result in a wound that would benefit from primary closure. Closed-suction drainage has been utilized to advantage in the carpal canal and deep digital flexor tendon sheaths. The wound should be monitored closely for signs of infection and the initial closure reopened if necessary.

Puncture Wounds and Rope Burns

Small puncture wounds or rope burns of the digit may go unnoticed or seem inconsequential to the owner until sepsis is established. These wounds then present as a warm, swollen tendon sheath. A grade 5/5 lameness (non—weight bearing) is common and may be difficult to differentiate from fractures or joint sepsis. Careful palpation of the area, radiography, and laboratory examination of centesis fluid from the tendon sheath and joints may be helpful in establishing a definitive diagnosis.

Surgical placement of a through-and-through Penrose drain ensures adequate drainage and allows daily flushing of the sheath. Heavy bandages, with or without splints, have been useful to control motion initially, which seems to provide some relief of pain. Nonsteroidal anti-inflammatory agents and appropriate

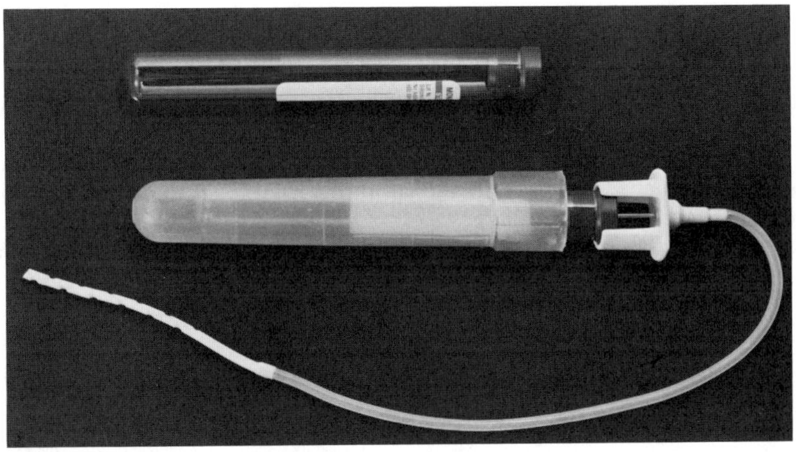

Figure 23–1. An example of a closed-system continuous suction drain that utilizes evacuated tubes to maintain negative pressure within the system.

antibiotic therapy are also indicated. Improvement is often dramatic initially, but some degree of lameness may persist for months following resolution of the sepsis.

Flexor Tendon Lacerations and Fractures

Lacerations of the flexor tendons or fractures may occur with an accidental wound. These injuries may require definitive surgical repair. Aggressive early wound therapy will ensure that these horses reach the surgery room in the best possible condition. The wound should be prepared as previously described and placed in a sterile bandage. Splinting or casting is indicated to provide additional support prior to transportation or induction of anesthesia. Systemic broad-spectrum antibiotics should be initiated as soon as possible.

Coronary Band Wounds

Wounds to the coronary band present a unique situation. Because the coronary band produces the hoof wall, injuries to the coronary band are manifested as changes in the hoof wall. A full-thickness coronary band wound results in a permanent defect in the hoof wall. Wounds that disrupt the coronary band must be carefully repaired in order to minimize the hoof wall defect. Stabilization of the hoof wall with wire sutures or incorporation of the entire foot in a cast to immobilize the wound for 3 to 4 weeks is often beneficial. The

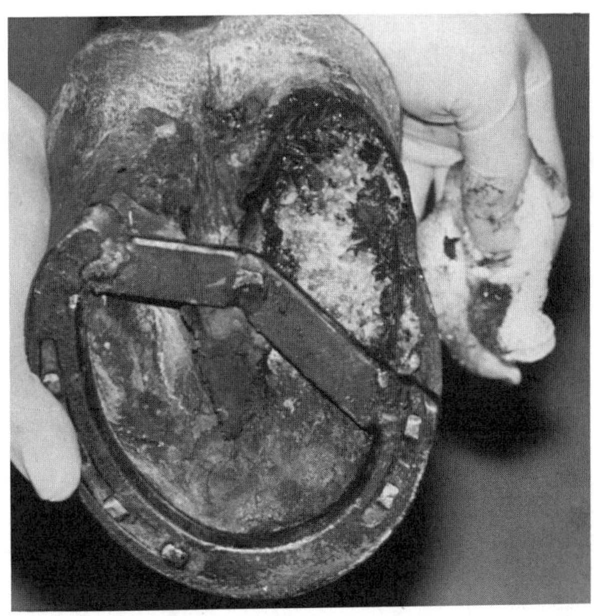

Figure 23–2. A corrective shoe with clip is placed to reduce movement and weight bearing at the site of injury.

hoof will grow out with a permanent defect associated with the coronary band scar. However, with proper shoeing, the hoof can still be sound and functional. If the wound involves only a small portion of the coronary band (15% or less), amputation of the involved segment of coronary band is an alternative technique. This will produce a void in the hoof wall rather than a defect. A bar shoe or some other form of corrective shoe may be necessary to span the defect (Fig. 23–2) and prevent weight bearing at this site of injury. Corrective shoeing will be required for the life of the horse because the coronary band can not regenerate.

SUMMARY

Because of extreme variations in types and severity of distal limb lacerations, it is impossible to present a "best" way to handle them. However, a few premises hold true in nearly all instances. A thorough examination of both the entire horse and the wound to determine the full extent of the injury is always indicated. Careful lavage, débridement, and exploration of the wound is indicated no matter how the wound will be managed. Do not hesitate to leave a wound at least partially open if there is any doubt about the cleanliness of the wound. There is no suitable substitute, cosmetically or functionally, for full-thickness skin covering a wound. Therefore, skin should be preserved whenever possible. A properly applied, padded compression bandage is always beneficial in at least the initial stages of therapy for any distal leg wound. Many wounds involving the distal aspect of the limb benefit from more complete immobilization within a cast.

24 Equine Sarcoid

Eric L. Reinertson

Equine sarcoid is a benign, yet locally invasive, fibroblastic neoplasm of the equine species. It is the most commonly occurring equine neoplasm. Sarcoids affect horses, donkeys, and mules with no known age, sex, or color predisposition. Sarcoids are thought to have no breed predisposition, though one study suggested that Standardbreds may be more resistant to sarcoid formation. Sarcoids occur singly or at multiple sites. Sarcoids may occur at any site, although the head, neck, and legs are the most common. Healing wounds and areas that are often traumatized seem to be common sites for sarcoid formation. There is growing evidence that a transforming retrovirus may be associated with sarcoid formation. Individual horses seem to be predisposed to sarcoid formation, suggesting a possible immunologic predisposition.

MORPHOLOGY

Morphologically equine sarcoids occur in verrucous, fibroblastic, or combined forms. Individuals may have more than one type present at different sites. Verrucous sarcoids appear as dry, scaly areas that are partially or totally hairless. Although they may be quite large, these sarcoids are usually 6 cm or less in diameter. Because of their tendency to be circular, verrucous sarcoids are often mistaken for "ringworm" by laymen. Verrucous sarcoids may remain quiescent for long periods of time yet tend to transform into the fibroblastic type when disturbed by trauma or biopsy.

Fibroblastic sarcoids present as a hard, fibrous, nodular mass within the dermis (Fig. 24–1). The surface epithelium is often ulcerated, although in some instances it remains intact. Fibroblastic sarcoids may be broad based or pedunculated. They are commonly rapid growing. Clinically, fibroblastic sarcoids are most often confused with exuberant granulation tissue, although cutaneous habronemiasis, phycomycosis, and squamous cell carcinoma all have a similar ulcerated appearance. Nonulcerated fibroblastic sarcoids are very difficult to distinguish clinically from fibromas.

In the combined form nodular fibroblastic masses are present in or adjacent to the verrucous plaque.

The definitive diagnosis of sarcoid must be made by histopathologic examination. Care should be taken to submit specimens to a qualified veterinary pathologist because equine sarcoids can be quite confusing to inexperienced histopathologists.

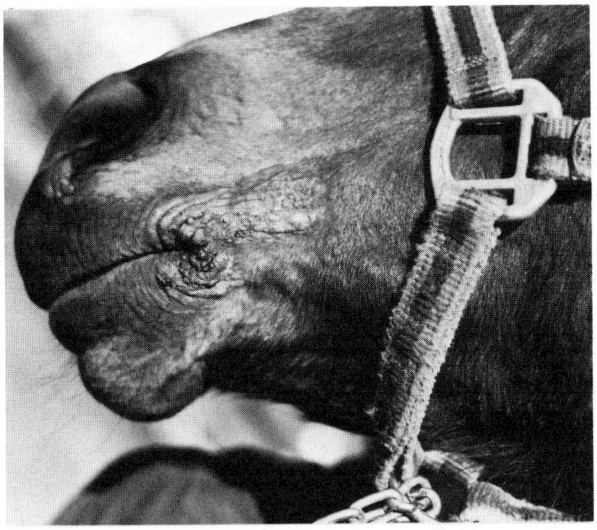

Figure 24–1. A fibroblastic sarcoid located at the lateral commissure of the lips.

THERAPY

There are many modes of therapy commonly used to treat equine sarcoids. Surgical excision, cryotherapy, hyperthermia, and immunotherapy are all currently used for therapy. No one mode of therapy has been determined to be best for the treatment of equine sarcoid. Selection of treatment, variations in technique, frequent reexaminations, early retreatment, and the individual patient's resistance all play a part in determining the outcome of a particular case. Some horses may lack the ability to resist sarcoid formation and be very difficult or impossible to maintain in remission.

Surgical Excision

Surgical excision of sarcoids has been associated with inconsistent results and no greater than 60% remission. It is often difficult to define the margins of these lesions. Another contributing factor may be the surgeon's tendency to be conservative when creating a wound that must subsequently be sutured. Careless handling of instruments may also result in contamination of the wound bed with cells from the tumor mass, resulting in recurrence by implantation. Surgical excision can be successful when small tumors are located in areas where adequate redundant skin in the surrounding area allows excision of at least a 1-cm margin around the tumor mass and primary closure of the wound. Surgical debulking is often utilized in conjunction with other forms of therapy.

Cryotherapy

The utilization of cryonecrosis to treat sarcoids has produced very good results and has become a popular mode of therapy. The tumor mass and approximately 0.5 cm of normal tissue surrounding it are frozen to −25 °C in a series of two or three rapid-freeze/slow-thaw cycles. Within a few hours after treatment, the area undergoes an intense inflammatory response to the cellular destruction. Pretreatment with nonsteroidal anti-inflammatory agents may be helpful in controlling this response in patients with large or multiple areas requiring treatment.

Within a few days following treatment, a line of demarcation will be evident as dead tissue is sloughed. Varying amounts of exudate and necrotic tissue odor accompany this phase. It is important to inform owners of this.

In approximately 10 to 14 days the necrotic tissue will slough off, leaving behind a healthy bed of granulation tissue. This step may be delayed somewhat if the freeze involves deep tissues. The granulating wound that remains undergoes contraction and epithelialization. Bandaging to control swelling and motion in the wound bed is helpful in aiding the contraction process. Skin grafting or surgical scar revision may be necessary if the sarcoid was large, resulting in a large granulating wound. This is especially true of sarcoids involving the distal aspects of the limbs. Careful monitoring of the healing wound is also necessary to detect recurrence of the tumor.

The most commonly used cryogen in the treatment of equine sarcoid is liquid nitrogen. Nitrous oxide can be used, but it is not as cold, which limits its use to very small lesions. Application of the cryogen commonly involves the use of a contact probe or direct contact with either a spray tip or area flooding.

The contact probe freezes tissue by transferring cold from the cryogen to a metallic probe and then to the tissue. It requires intimate tissue contact for most efficient freezing. The area of cryonecrosis is fairly easy to estimate and control because a visible "iceball" forms in the tissue that closely approximates the area of cryonecrosis (Fig. 24–2). Temperature monitoring with thermocouple probes is not as critical with this technique. Inadvertent freezing of adjacent tissues by "run-off" is not a problem with the contact probes. The size of the probe, however, severely limits the area of cryonecrosis that can be achieved with this technique, so that tedious multiple applications may be necessary to adequately treat a large area.

Direct application with a spray tip or flooding of the area are more efficient ways to rapidly freeze large tumor masses. The necessity to monitor the tissue temperature with thermocouple probes (C2–76; Frigi-

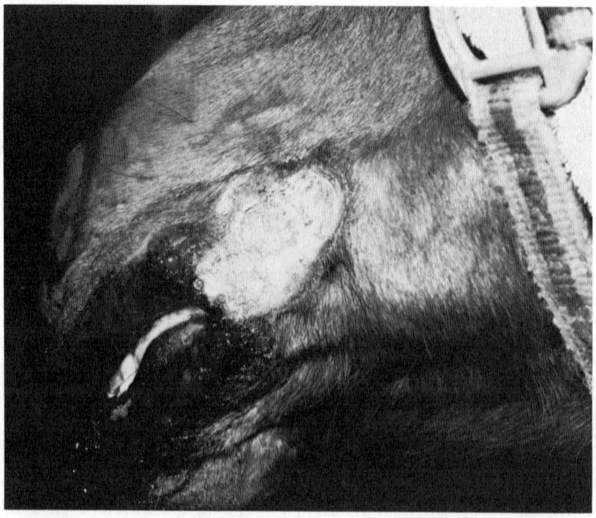

A

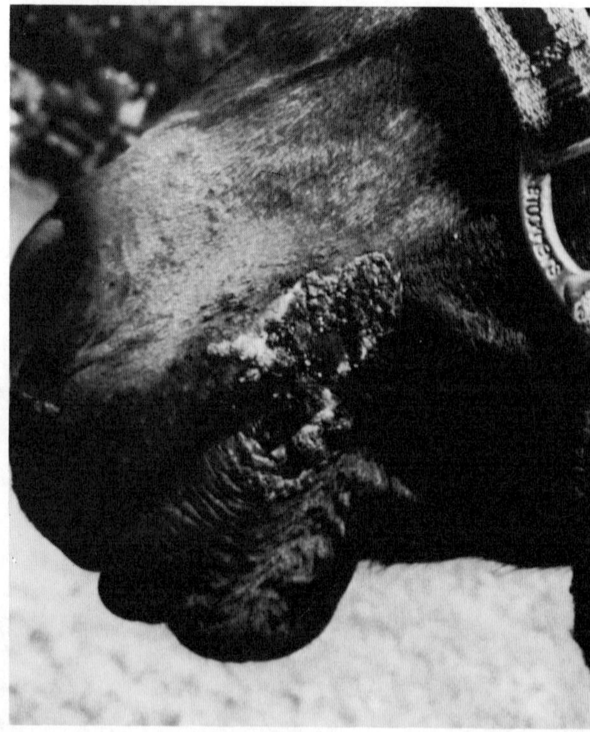

B

Figure 24–2. A. The area that has been treated with liquid nitrogen is well demarcated by iceball formation. **B.** The appearance of the wound 6 weeks after a double freeze-thaw application of liquid nitrogen. There is evidence of tumor recurrence at the margins of the granulating wound.

tronics of Connecticut, Inc) cannot be overemphasized when direct application methods are used. It is necessary to monitor the temperatures both deep to the lesion and at the periphery. This will prevent inadvertent damage to deep structures or creation of an excessively large wound. Monitoring tissue temperature also ensures an adequate freeze to achieve cryonecrosis of the tumor mass. Extreme care must also be taken to adequately protect adjacent tissues from "runoff" of the cryogen. Careful application of insulators such as

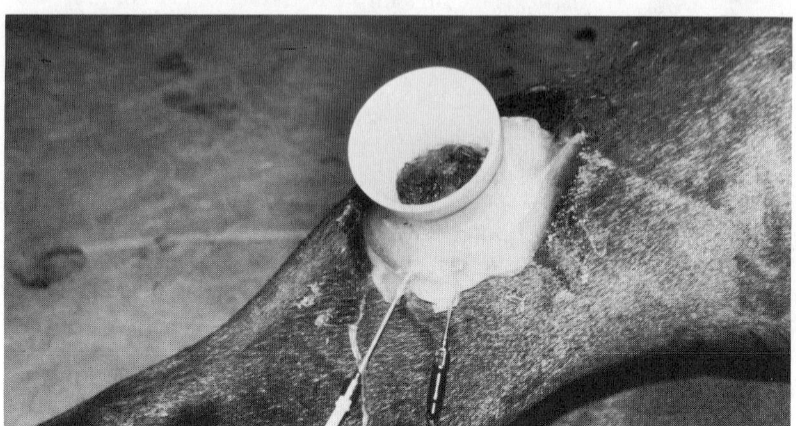

Figure 24–3. A disposable polystyrene beverage cup is trimmed to fit the lesion and sealed with petroleum jelly. Liquid nitrogen is then applied directly to the area. Thermocouple needles are placed at the periphery of and deep to the lesion to monitor tissue temperature.

sheets of polystyrene sealed in place with petroleum jelly have proven effective in containing the cryogen in the desired area (Fig. 24–3).

Surgical debulking is often employed prior to cryotherapy to decrease the amount of tissue that must be frozen. When possible, the use of tourniquets to control hemorrhage following debulking is advantageous. It is very difficult to adequately freeze actively bleeding tissues. Alternatively, cryotherapy can be postponed for 6 to 24 hours following debulking to allow for hemostasis.

Hyperthermia

Tumor destruction from radiofrequency current-induced hyperthermia has been used to effectively treat equine sarcoid. A localized current field (LCF) device (Thermoprobe LCF Device; Ideal Instruments) is used with either piercing probes or surface probes to heat tissue to approximately 50 °C. This temperature is maintained for 30 seconds, resulting in tumor cell death. The surface probes treat an area 1 cm^2 and 3 to 4 mm deep, whereas the piercing probes treat approximately 1 cm^3 per application. The small area treated with each application makes it very easy to precisely control the amount of tissue destruction with this technique. This is particularly advantageous when treating periocular sarcoids. However, it limits the application of this technique to relatively small sarcoids. Multiple treatments at 2- to 3-week intervals may be necessary to achieve tumor clearance.

Immunotherapy

Intralesional injection of potent immune stimulants has proven to be an effective means of treating equine sarcoid. Either Bacille Calmette-Guérin (BCG vaccine), which is an attenuated *Mycobacterium bovis*, or mycobacterial cell wall preparations (Nomagen; Fort Dodge Laboratories, Inc) have been used (see Chapter 6). Tumor masses are injected with BCG preparation utilizing approximately 2 mL/cm^3 of area. Multiple injection sites utilizing a 25-gauge needle are used to infiltrate the tumor mass. Care should be taken to adequately infiltrate the interface between the sarcoid and normal tissue. Surgical debulking may be helpful in minimizing the tumor mass to be injected. The BCG stimulates an intense immune response manifested as a local rejection reaction. The injected area becomes swollen and painful. The intensity of the reaction usually increases with successive treatments. The tumor mass may become ulcerated or necrotic. Repeated injections at 2 to 4-week intervals are usually necessary to achieve regression. Successive injections are made after the reaction to the previous injection has subsided and the clinician has been able to evaluate the status of the tumor.

Regression usually requires three to four injections, although more injections may be required to achieve total remission. Because of the necessity to completely infiltrate the tumor mass, immunotherapy is best reserved for the treatment of small tumor masses. The clinician also has relatively precise control over the area treated, making immunotherapy a desirable therapeutic technique when preservation of surrounding tissues is important, as in cases of periorbital sarcoids.

Although an anaphylactic reaction is not commonly reported with BCG products, it can occur and patients should be observed for 30 minutes following treatment. This reaction has not been reported with mycobacterial cell wall extracts.

BIBLIOGRAPHY

Cheevers WP, Fatemi-Nainine S, Anderson LW: Spontaneous expression of an endogenous retrovirus by the equine sarcoid-derived MC-1 cell line. *Am J Vet Res* 1986;47:50–52.

Hofman KD, Kainer RA, Shideler RK: Radio-frequency current-induced hyperthermia for the treatment of equine sarcoid. *Equine Pract* 1983;5:24–31.

Lavach JD, Severin GA, Leuker D: Immunotherapy of periocular sarcoids in horses. *Vet Clin North Am Large Anim Pract* 1984;6:513–518.

25 Casting Materials and Techniques

William A. Lindsay

Certain injuries to the limb of the horse may require protection or immobilization beyond that provided by bandages or splints. Casting may be combined with methods of internal fixation such as plate fixation and intramedullary pin placement or with external fixation devices such as the Kirschner apparatus or modified Thomas splints. External coaptation may be provided by casting the foot, lower leg, or entire limb.

Plaster of Paris bandages have been in use for over a century. Calcium sulfate crystals (gypsum or plaster of Paris) are incorporated into cotton gauze. When immersed in warm water, the gypsum rehydrates and recrystallizes, resulting in an exothermic reaction:

$$(2CaSO_4) \cdot H_2O + 3H_2O \rightarrow 2(CaSO_4 \cdot 2H_2O) + \text{heat}$$

The cast is applied, and as it dries the calcium sulfate crystals interlock. Plaster is easy to apply and mold to different shapes. It is relatively strong and dries with a smooth surface. Unfortunately, plaster is untidy to work with, bulky, and heavy, and weakens when it becomes wet. Plaster is not considered "cured" to full strength until at least 24 hours after application. A plaster bandage reinforced with a melamine-formaldehyde polymer and catalyst (Zoroc) was the standard material used in equine casts for many years. It cured more quickly and was more moisture resistant than plaster of Paris.

New cast materials have replaced the plaster of Paris compounds and offer many distinct advantages, such as lightness and rapid curing. These synthetic compounds include fiberglass tapes impregnated with a water-activated polyurethane or polyester polymer or resin. Because these tapes do not conform well, it is advisable to apply an initial two layers of plaster when using tapes constructed solely of fiberglass. Also available are blended tapes of fiberglass and polyester that permit limb contouring. Several companies also offer polymers that are "low tack." These tapes are easier to unroll and apply and have the added benefit of not sticking to the gloved hand. These casts are smoother to touch when finished than fiberglass and are also less radiodense. A list of some of the materials currently available is included in Table 25–1, but the reader must be aware that new developments are constantly being made in this area. An example is the cast-reinforcing resin that can be applied to synthetic casting tapes to provide extra strength (Delta-Form cast reinforcing resin; Johnson & Johnson Orthopedic).

GENERAL RECOMMENDATIONS

The newer, synthetic materials offer many advantages over plaster in regard to weight, strength, durability, and cure time. The "low tack" synthetic products have markedly improved handling characteristics. The fiberglass-polyester tapes conform easily to limb contours, are more radiolucent and have a smoother finish. It is advisable to become familiar with one product and the recommendations of the manufacturer. Observe expiration dates and do not use rolls with damaged wrappers or with polymer unevenly dispersed throughout the weave of the tape.

Indications for casts in the horse include avulsion injuries of the hoof wall, coronary band lacerations, heel bulb lacerations, tendon lacerations, joint luxations, wounds over joints and tendons, angular limb deformities, and fractures that are not amenable to other methods of internal or external fixation. Many veterinary orthopedic surgeons will apply a cast to protect an operative site or implants during recovery of the horse from general anesthesia.

CAST APPLICATION

Most casts are applied to anesthetized horses. Preparation and selection of cast materials prior to anesthesia minimizes anesthesia time. All necessary equipment for cast application should be readily at hand. The veterinarian must be thoroughly familiar with the product and tolerate no distractions because cure time may be as short as 3 minutes. Basic principles of large animal cast application dictate that the cast should extend at least one joint above the fracture, that the cast should *not* terminate in the middle of a long bone and that the entire hoof should be contained within the cast. Table 25–2 lists items required for cast application in the horse.

The patient is positioned in lateral recumbency with the affected limb uppermost. The hoof is trimmed level, pared out, and scrubbed until clean and dry. Particular attention is paid to the sulci of the frog. After cleansing, this area may be packed with an antiseptic cream. The limb to be cast must be clean and dry and any surgical wounds must be covered with a sterile, nonadherent dressing. This dressing should be secured with a light wrap of conforming gauze and elastic tape to avoid slippage as the cast is applied. This elastic tape should contact the hair above and below the wound dressing. Cotton stockinette is used under plaster of Paris, whereas polyester or polypropylene stockinette is recommended for use under synthetic casting tapes. The stockinette is measured and rolled; the contact layer is rolled to the outside; the outer layer to the inside. The inner roll is applied and secured proximally to the limb. The stockinette is then twisted over the hoof and the second layer applied over the first. In general, a 3-in stockinette will fit the front leg of an average-sized adult horse, whereas 4-in stockinette may be needed for a hind limb. A piece of orthopedic felt 2-in wide and 1/4 in thick is placed at the proximal extent

TABLE 25–1. CASTING MATERIALS

Casting Material	Manufacturer	Composition	Roll Size	Directions	Set Time (min)	Time to Weight Bearing
Caraglas	Carapace	100% fiberglass substrate	2, 3, 4, 5 in × 4 yd	Immerse in 70–75 °F water; squeeze 3–4 times	4	20 min
Delta-Lite Conformable Casting Tape	Johnson & Johnson	Fiberglass substrate, polyurethane resin (low tack)	2, 3, 4, 5 in × 4 yd	Immerse in 21–27 ° F water; squeeze 4–5 times	7	20 min
Flex-Plus	Orthopedic Casting Laboratories	100% fiberglass	2, 3, 4, 5 in × 5 yd	Immerse in room-temperature water; squeeze 3–4 times	3–5	20–30 min
Hexcelite	Hexcel Medical	Thermoplastic polyester polymer cotton base	2, 3, 4, 6 in × 2 yd	Heat in water to 80 °F for 4–5 min	3–4	When cool
K-Cast	Kirschner	100% fiberglass	2, 3, 4, 5 in × 4 yd	Immerse in water at 20 °C for 5–6 s; squeeze 2 times	6–7	20 min
Lightcast II	Orthopedic Products (Surgical Products Division, 3-M)	Fiberglass tape, photosensitive resin	1, 2, 3 in × 2 yd; 6 in × 3 yd	Expose to near-ultraviolet lamp	3	20 min
Orthoflex	Johnson & Johnson	Plaster of Paris	2, 3, 4 in × 5 yd	Immerse in 80–85 °F water for 5 s	5–8	24–72 h (completely dry)
Readi-Cast	AOA/CHICK	Plaster of Paris	2, 3 in × 3 yd, 4, 5, 6, 8 in × 5 yd	Immerse in 80 °F water for 5 s	2–4	24–72 h
Scotch Cast II	Animal Care Products/3m	Fiberglass bandage, polyurethane resin	2, 3, 4, 5 in × 4 yd	Immerse in 20 °C water for 15 s	5–6	30 min
Specialist	Johnson & Johnson	Plaster of Paris	2, 3, 4, 5, 6, 8 in × 5 yd	Immerse in 70–75 °F water for 5 s	5–8 (blue label) 2–4 (green label)	24–72 h (completely dry)
Tack-Free	Orthopedic Casting Laboratory	90% fiberglass, 10% polyester, water-activated polyurethane resin (low tack)	2, 3, 4, 5 in × 4 yd	Immerse in room-temperature water; squeeze 3–4 times	3–5	20–30 min
Vet Cast	Animal Care Products/3M	Fiberglass tape, polyurethane resin	2, 3, 4, 5 in × 5 yd	Immerse in warm water	5–7	20–30 min
Zim-Flex Casting Tape	Zimmer	Fiberglass tape, polyurethane resin	2, 3, 4, 5 in × 4 yd	Immerse in warm water	5–7	20 min

TABLE 25–2. EQUIPMENT AND SUPPLIES USED IN CAST APPLICATION

Hoof Preparation	Limb Restraint	Cast Padding
Hoof pick Hoof knife Hoof nippers Rasp Bristle brush	Electric drill Electric drill bit Flexible wire or nylon suture Wood: 1 × 1 × 12 in	3-in stockinette, double thickness Adhesive tape Orthopedic felt Wound dressings
Casting Materials	**Walking Bars**	**Sole Reinforcement**
Protective drapes Plastic pail with liner Water of specified temperature Rubber gloves with hand cream Casting materials	1 × ¼-in aluminum bar, 6–8 ft in length	Acrylic resin (Technovit)

of the cast and secured in place with tape (Fig. 25–1). No other padding is required. Excessive padding will be compressed and slip, thus predisposing to movement of the limb within the cast as the horse bears weight. Movement will result in cast sores. Padding may be required over the accessory carpal bone and the point of the hock (Fig. 25–2) with full leg casts, particularly if the limb is not in a relaxed position when the cast is applied.

Stabilizing wires may now be applied to the hoof. Small openings are made in the stockinette and holes are drilled in the hoof using an electric drill and 1/8-in bit; wire or nylon suture (#8 Vetafil) is threaded through the holes in a horizontal mattress pattern (Fig. 25–3). A piece of wood may then be applied to the sole of the foot, secured with the suture and used to support the leg (Fig. 25–4). Alternatively, the wires or sutures may be attached to a rope used to exert tension and stretch the leg into a straight position. In certain instances, it may be desirable to cast the limb in a flexed

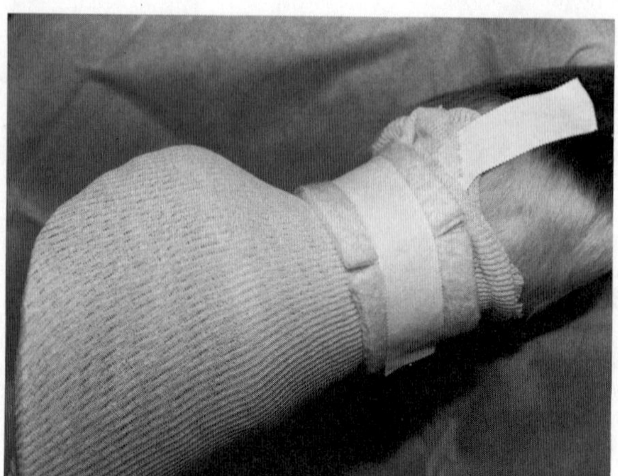

Figure 25–1. Orthopedic felt is secured at the top of the cast site. This may be at the pastern, just below the carpus or hock, or just below the elbow or stifle.

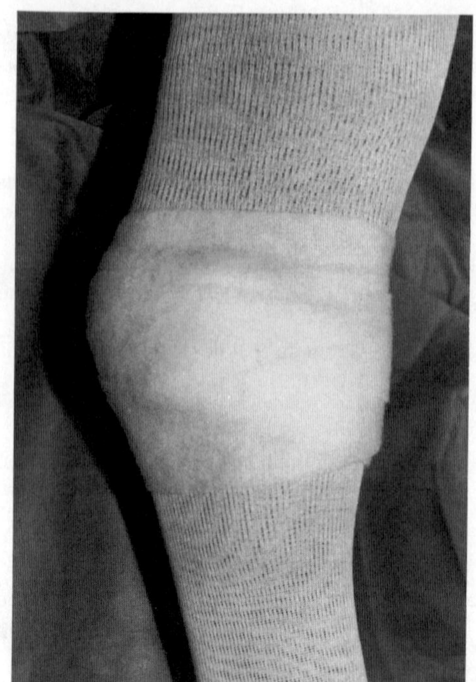

Figure 25–2. Cast padding is placed on either side of the calcaneal bone. The padding serves to make the hock joint of more uniform diameter.

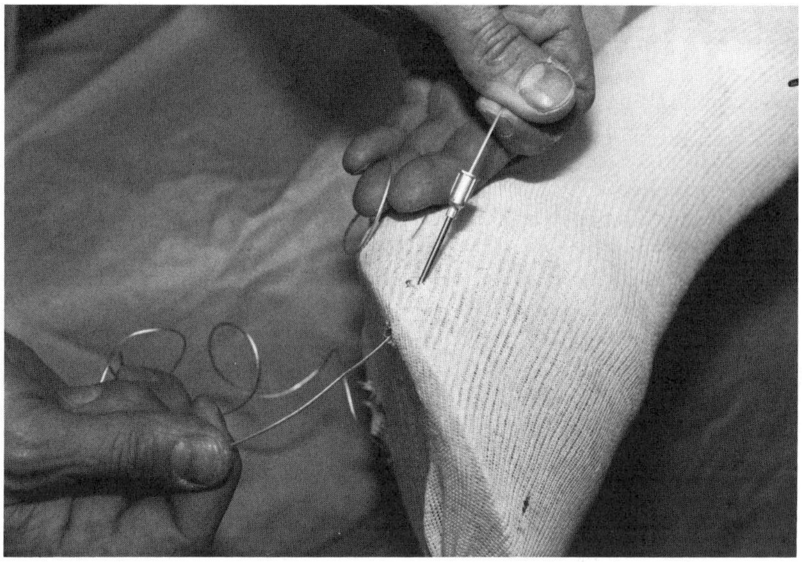

Figure 25–3. The hoof and pastern are covered with a double thickness of stockinette. An electric drill is used to drill holes in the insensitive laminae. A disposable 14-gauge hypodermic needle is inserted and used as a cannula to permit placement of wires or sutures that can be used to apply tension to the leg or to apply a board to the foot for leverage.

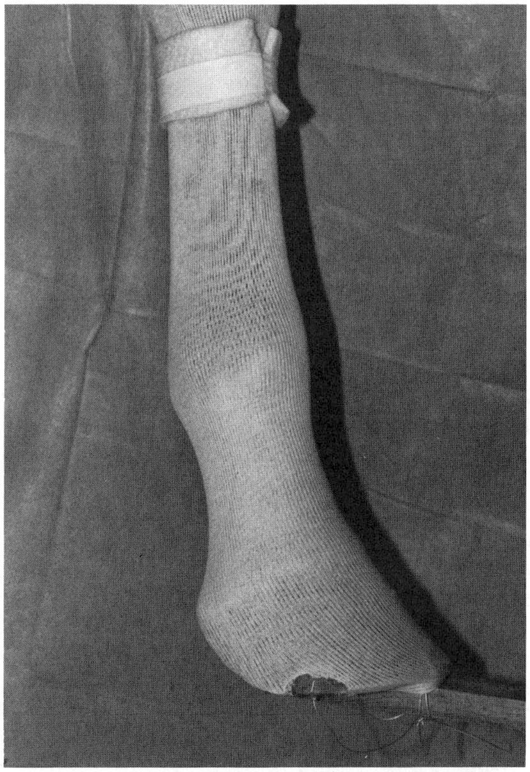

Figure 25–4. The forelimb has been prepared for application of a lower leg cast. A double thickness of stockinette and orthopedic felt are in place. The limb is maintained in the desired position using the board secured to the foot.

position, such as following repair of traumatic flexor tendon lacerations.

Positioning of the limb is crucial during cast application. The leg must be maintained in one position throughout the entire period. The limb should not be allowed to "bow" downward as it is supported. Individuals assisting with support of the limb should not indent the cast material with their fingers or thumbs, but rather keep their digits extended. This is especially true when applying full-leg hind limb casts.

Fiberglass casting tapes do not readily conform to the contours of the limb, and two to three rolls of plaster material must first be applied to achieve a snug fit. Orthoflex is very useful for this purpose because it is constructed of conforming elastic gauze impregnated with plaster. These initial rolls of plaster must be allowed to dry thoroughly (10 to 20 minutes) before the fiberglass materials are applied. If this cast material does not dry, the heat produced during curing of the fiberglass may leave the plaster moist. The opposite leg and the surrounding work area must be protected. Two assistants are very useful during cast application: one to hold the leg in a fixed position, and the other to prepare rolls for application and continually moisten and "work" the curing cast. Each packet of fiberglass casting tape should be squeezed prior to opening to ensure that the roll is compressible and has not hardened during storage. After the leg is placed in the desired position, usually that achieved during normal weight bearing, the roll of tape is dipped in water of the correct temperature. It is preferable to err on the side of too cool rather than too warm, because hot water accelerates the curing process. The assistant must secure the free end of the roll during the dipping process. When applying multiple rolls of fiberglass cast material to large animal patients considerable heat is produced, making the final rolls difficult to apply. It may be advisable to apply the first roll dry and the second damp, and gradually increase the amount of moisture by squeezing less water from each successive roll.

The first roll is applied starting at the middle of a long bone and is snugly wrapped in successive layers up the leg to the top of the cast. Approximately 1 in of the orthopedic felt is left exposed and cast application proceeds down the limb toward the hoof. Each spiral wrap should overlap the previous wrap by approximately one-half the width of the casting tape (Fig. 25–5). The person applying the casting tape must select that width of tape that will result in easy contouring of the tape around the limb, usually 3- or 4-in rolls. As the fetlock joint is covered, a "figure-of-eight" may be required to cover limb contours with a smooth layer. All casts (with the exception of the sleeve cast for angular limb deformities) should incorporate the hoof. It is difficult to wrap the awkward contours of the hoof with the nonconforming fiberglass tapes, and a "figure-of-eight" application and judicious folding over of loose ends on the sole are required (Fig. 25–6). These tucks should not contact the skin directly.

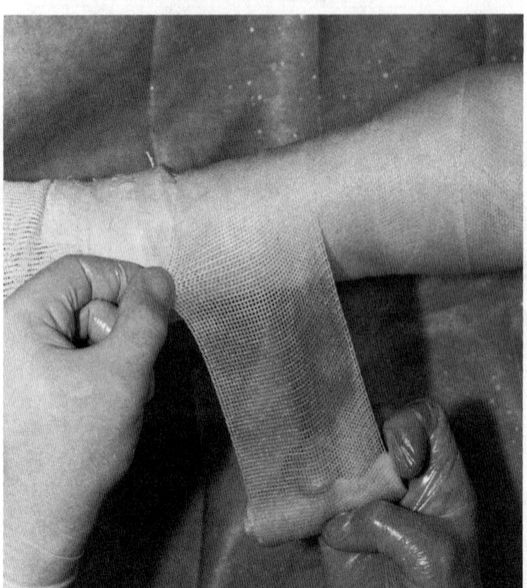

Figure 25–5. After the plaster is allowed to dry, the fiberglass casting tape is applied. The casting tape is stretched to its full width. Each successive wrap is overlaid by one half of the tape's width.

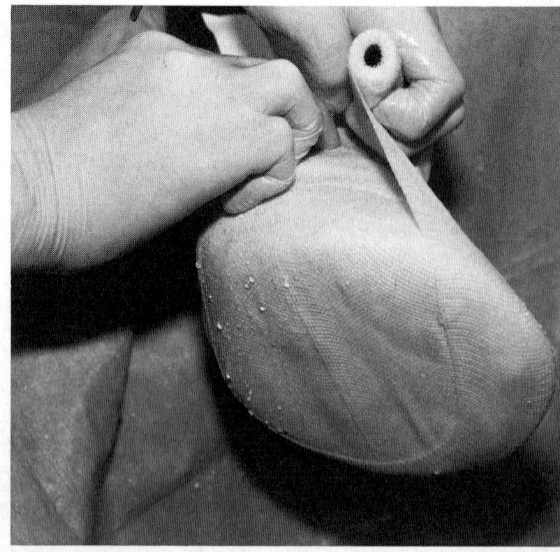

Figure 25–6. The casting tape is wrapped snugly: each roll must bond securely to the previous layer. Note that the tape has been stretched to its full width. The cast must include the entire hoof but also conform to the bulbs of the heel. A fiberglass polyester tape (Tack-Free) has been selected to permit accurate contouring of the hoof and pastern.

The first layer of cast material is applied snugly—successive layers are then applied more tightly to achieve bonding. Each successive layer must become bonded to the previous layers (Fig. 25–7). This can be facilitated by keeping the cast moist and by rubbing or working each successive layer of tape as it is applied. Air bubbles between layers must be avoided. After three or four layers of tape have been applied, wider tape (of the same brand) may be used to complete the cast. The casting tape is applied up and down the leg until four to six rolls have been applied for a lower leg cast, ten to 12 rolls for a full front leg cast, and 12 to 14 rolls for a full hind leg cast, the total number depending on the horse's size. Ideally, the cast should be a cylinder conforming exactly to limb contours and should be constructed of an equal thickness of cast material throughout. Compression during application is the most effective way to laminate successive layers. If additional contouring of the cast is required—for example, at the bulbs of the heels or at the bony prominences of the accessory carpal or fibular tarsal bones—gentle palm pressure may be applied for 5 to 10 seconds to further mold the cast.

The tape may be folded, twisted, spread, or tucked. Twists or tucks, however, should *not* contact the patient's skin (Fig. 25–8). Casts are frequently weak just below the tarsus and the fetlock because a uniform

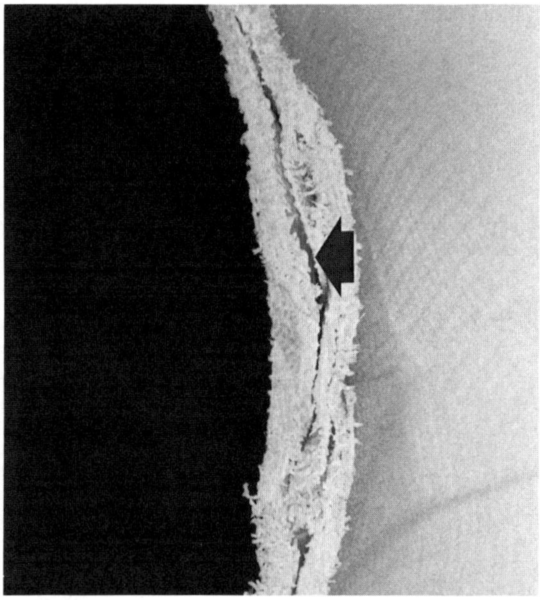

Figure 25–7. This is the cut edge of a cast in which the cast material was not properly laminated. Each layer must be moist and snugly wrapped; likewise it should be lightly rubbed while moist.

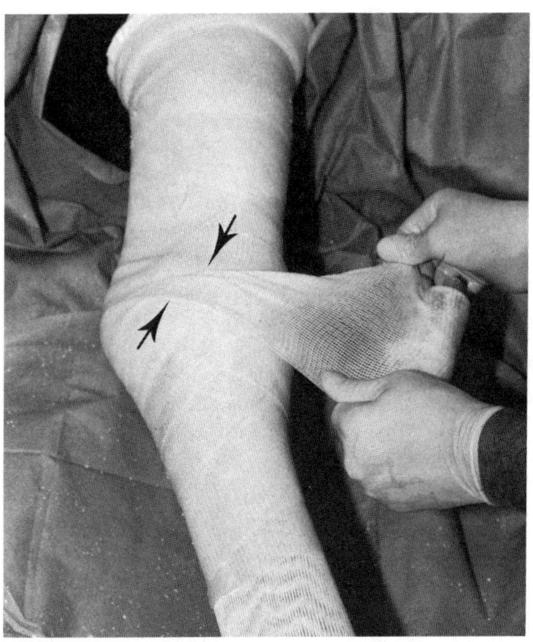

Figure 25–8. Casting tape constructed of a fiberglass-polyester blend (Tack-Free) is applied directly over stockinette. The tape must be contoured to the hock. Note that a "tuck" (arrows) should *not* contact the patient's skin.

thickness of material has not been applied. Likewise, the top of the cast is frequently neglected. In the early stage of cast application, the most proximal part of the cast should be reinforced. At cast completion, the number of rolls applied and the date may be inscribed on the cast. It has been traditional to incorporate longitudinal splints in plaster casts to provide additional stability; however, this particular technique has not been evaluated objectively. Such splints are not required when constructing a fiberglass cast.

Immediately after the final roll has been applied, the cast is wrapped snugly with moistened conforming gauze to aid in the curing process and to prevent the free end of the last roll from curling. This gauze is removed in 2 to 3 minutes. We recommend that the sole be reinforced with an acrylic compound such as Technovit because this area of the cast wears quickly (Fig. 25–9). Alternatively, a piece of rubber tubing may be secured with duct tape. We also recommend that the top of the cast and the exposed orthopedic felt be covered with conforming elastic tape to prevent bedding and feces from entering the top of the cast. This tape should be changed at 2- to 3-day intervals.

Walking bars are occasionally incorporated in plaster casts and may be used in conjunction with fiberglass materials (Fig. 25–10). These bars are useful in protecting the sole of the foot from excessive wear, and may reinforce the cast. A 1-inch aluminum bar should be available and preformed to the leg prior to anesthetizing the horse. This is applied to the cast after six rolls of casting tape have been applied. An additional roll of

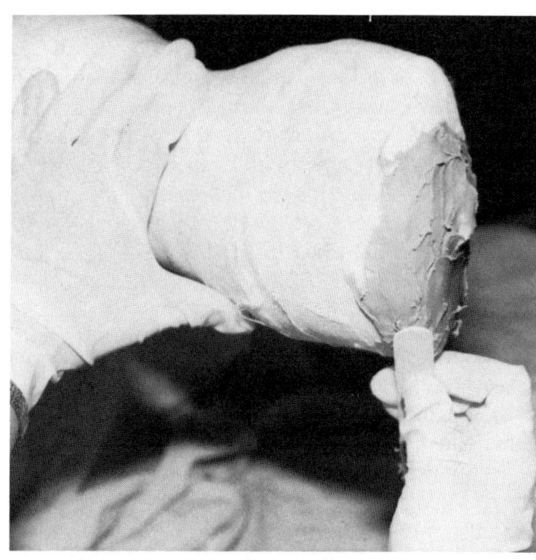

Figure 25–9. The sole should be protected with an acrylic compound to prevent excessive wearing of the cast.

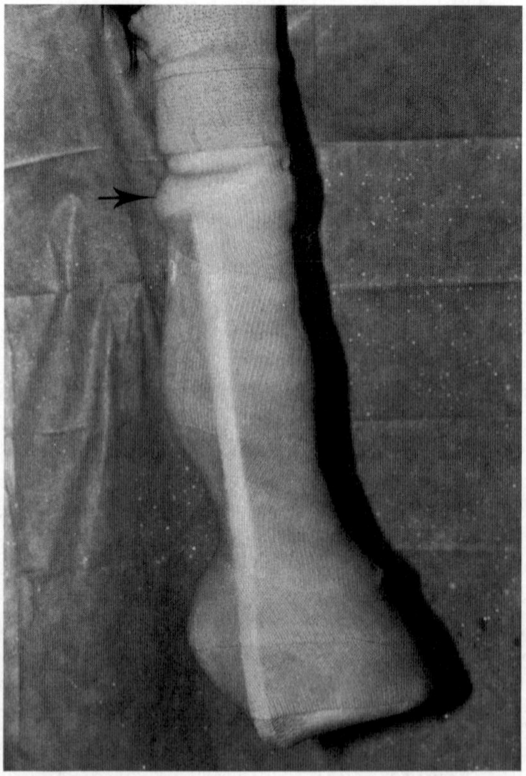

Figure 25–10. A walking bar of 1-in aluminum stock rests against a collar of casting material (*arrow*). The collar is constructed by twisting a roll of cast tape as it is applied. The walking bar is incorporated into the cast with additional cast tapes.

cast tape is twisted and wrapped at the top of the cast to make a narrow collar against which the walking bar may rest. The walking bar should contact the sole of the foot and also the collar at the top of the cast. The walking bar is then secured and incorporated into the cast with several additional rolls of casting tape applied in spiral fashion. Excessive length of this bar below the foot will make weight bearing awkward.

CAST CARE

A 20- to 30-minute wait is recommended after application of the last roll of cast material before weight bearing is permitted. The sole of the cast may be reinforced during this time. If using acrylic resins, one must be sure to observe instructions and wear gloves.

Recovery from general anesthesia requires close supervision, especially if a full leg cast has been applied to the hind limb. The horse is always positioned with the cast limb uppermost. The patient is encouraged to remain recumbent as long as possible. Premedication with acetylpromazine may help recovery; judicious administration of small increments of xylazine (100 mg intravenously) may also assist recovery, especially if the patient is recovering on a tilt-type table. If a recovery stall is available, tail and head ropes may be passed through overhead eye bolts to help stabilize the horse after standing. An occasional horse will not tolerate a full leg hind limb cast but will kick out incessantly after recovery. These patients require constant supervision, distraction, or sedation.

Casts that are damaged, even if only partially creased or wrinkled, must be removed and replaced. Patching the cast after recovery is not sufficient and never eliminates movement within the cast. This usually necessitates a second anesthetic. The patient must be carefully evaluated before induction, and closely observed during recovery.

The patient and cast must be monitored at least twice daily by an experienced observer. It may be advisable to keep the horse in a clinic environment. To ensure client compliance, the guidelines in Table 25–3 are recommended. Temperature, pulse, and respiratory rates must be recorded and the cast evaluated. A slight increase in temperature may herald a full-thickness skin erosion. Slight increases in pulse and respiration rate often precede obvious lameness as cast sores de-

TABLE 25–3. GUIDELINES FOR TWICE-DAILY OBSERVATIONS OF CASTS IN HORSES

1. Stall rest is *MANDATORY.*
2. Walk the horse a *few* steps twice a day to see if it is bearing full weight on the cast—a change in weight bearing usually indicates a problem.
3. Palpate the entire cast for local areas of heat (heat over a wounded area may be acceptable).
4. Check the top of the cast for any rubbed areas, discharge, or foul odor.
5. Keep the top of the cast wrapped to prevent hay and debris from falling inside the cast. The wrap should be reset regularly.
6. Check the leg above the cast for swelling.
7. Check the toe of the cast for excessive wear.
8. If the opposite leg has a support bandage on, it should be reset every other day.
9. Casts should *not* be left on longer than the specified time.
10. If there are any problems with the cast or the horse appears uncomfortable, act immediately. *IT MAY BE AN EMERGENCY* and immediate removal of the cast may be necessary.

velop or excessive movement occurs at an unstable fracture site. The administration of anti-inflammatory agents may mask complications associated with the original injury or the cast.

Casts are applied for varying periods of time. Repair by internal fixation of phalangeal or third metacarpal or metatarsal fractures may be protected during recovery from anesthesia by a lower leg cast. Heel bulb lacerations, wounds over joints, and flexor tendon lacerations benefit from an immobilization period of 2 to 3 weeks. If used as a primary method of fracture immobilization, the cast may be removed initially at 3 to 4 weeks and replaced at similar time intervals until the fracture no longer requires immobilization. Do not hesitate to change a cast earlier than planned. A reluctance to bear weight, or the persistence of areas of warmth or defects in the cast, are reasons for removal. Casts applied to rapidly growing foals should be changed at 10- to 14-day intervals.

COMPLICATIONS

Most complications result from a failure to observe the manufacturer's recommendations in regard to storage and handling of casting materials, from using excessive padding or inadequate contouring, or from applying insufficient amounts of casting tape (Fig. 25–11). Frequent examination of the cast and twice-daily patient assessment may allow early identification of fracture instability or cast sores.

Some erosion of skin may be anticipated in virtually any cast worn for more than 3 weeks because some movement within the cast is inevitable during weight bearing. Abrasions are frequently located at the heel bulbs, the palmar or plantar surfaces of the proximal sesamoid bones, the accessory carpal bone, the fibular tarsal bone, and the dorsal aspect of the top of the cast. If the abrasion is superficial, clipping of hair and gentle cleansing is indicated. If the abrasion is full thickness, the wound should be bandaged and medicated daily until filled with granulation tissue. If necessary, a second cast may be applied over such wounds, taking care that the top of the cast extends beyond the wound. Cutting wedges from cast tops only delays their inevitable removal. The client should be informed that hair regrowth may be without pigment.

Other complications less frequently observed include rupture of the peroneus tertius, fractures of the radius and tibia, and unpleasant odors. Laminitis and angular limb deformity may develop in the contralateral limb if the patient does not bear weight on the cast limb. The peroneus tertius may be ruptured if a horse struggles against a full leg cast. The top of the cast, if poorly fitted and unpadded, may abrade skin, muscle, and then tendon. Treatment consists of stall confinement for 2 to 3 months until the clinical signs are no longer present. Resulting wounds are usually left to heal by second intention.

Long bone fractures have been observed when full-limb casts terminate just above the carpus or tarsus. In these cases, the top of the cast acts as a fulcrum and, if sufficient forces are applied, a fracture may occur, usually during recovery from anesthesia. It is important that the cast extend as high on the radius and tibia as possible. The top of the cast must conform snugly to the muscles of the fore or hind limb.

CAST REMOVAL

The equipment required for cast removal includes an oscillating cast cutter and cast spreaders. Many horses will tolerate cast removal in the standing position, but

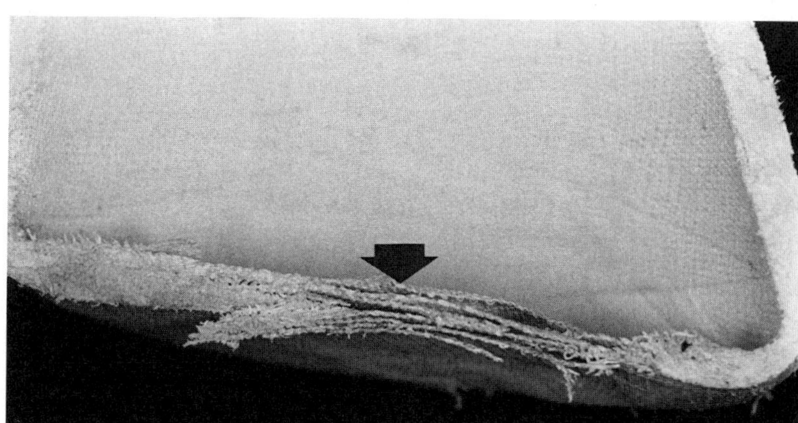

Figure 25–11. Inadequate cast material has been applied to the sole of this foot cast. Also note a failure of bonding between layers (*arrow*), which diminishes the strength of the cast.

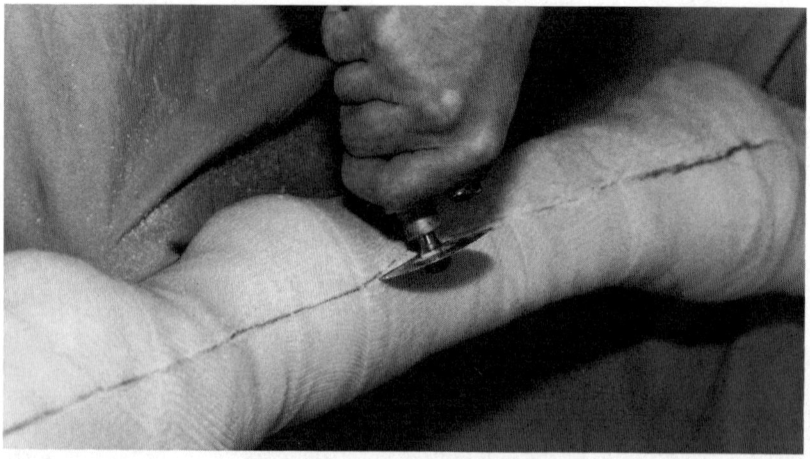

Figure 25–12. The cast must be "scored" initially with a partial thickness saw cut for the entire length of both sides of the cast. The complete thickness of the cast is penetrated for the width of one saw blade. This process is repeated methodically over both the entire medial and lateral aspects. Particular attention must be paid to depth of penetration when the cast cutter is used over the fetlock and coronary band regions.

it is a false economy to jeopardize the surgical repair or risk injury to horse or handler. A cast may also be removed following administration of an intravenous anesthesia. It is advisable to wear safety glasses and a surgical mask when removing cast material. The cast must be removed in two complete halves. It should be scored completely from one side to the other, including the hoof surface, so as to permit an even, regular cut (Fig. 25–12). The full-thickness cut is then begun at the top of the cast. The blade is pressed inward with a controlled motion using the thumb as a depth gauge. At this point, one may gauge whether the horse will tolerate standing cast removal. In addition to the noise of the saw, the horse will become apprehensive of the heat and vibrations of the saw close to the skin. Twitching and sedation will aid patient restraint, but may also reduce the ability of the horse to forewarn the operator that the cast has been completely penetrated.

As the full thickness of the cast is penetrated, the blade should not be advanced, but rather pressed inward until it is felt to drop through the cast material. After one blade width of the blade has been completely cut, the saw is removed and replaced on the area immediately adjacent. The entire cast is sequentially perforated. It is important to avoid excess pressure when penetrating the cast, especially over the fetlock joints and coronary band. Although the oscillating blade is designed to reduce the risk of cutting skin beneath the cast, it can easily lacerate skin held tightly against the cast. Even under general anesthesia, one must proceed methodically as the cast is removed. The full length of the cast must be scored and then penetrated with the cast cutter before any attempts at removal are made. Cast spreaders may then be placed to separate the two halves of the cast (Fig. 25–13). The stockinette must also be cut. If the cast has been removed under general

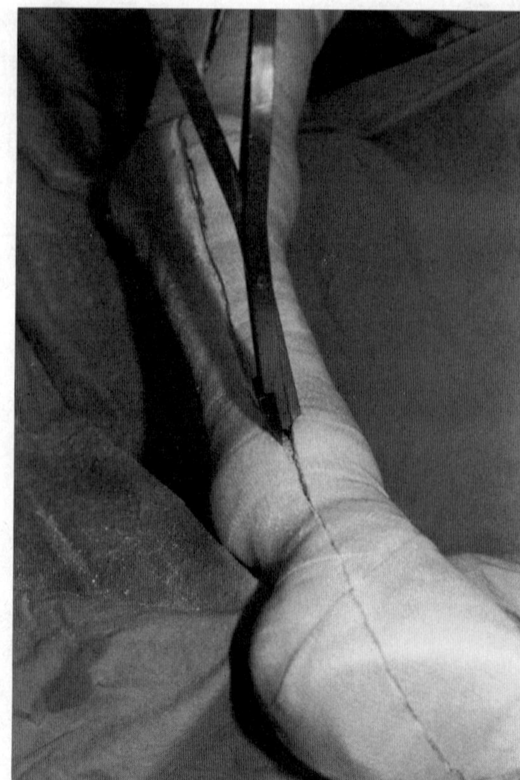

Figure 25–13. The cast spreaders are inserted in the separation of the full-thickness cut in the cast. The entire length of the cast must be cut before the cast will separate by spreading.

anesthesia, a well-padded bandage is usually applied to the injured area and the palmar or plantar half of the cast used as a splint to prevent limb trauma during recovery. Alternatively, the cast is bivalved during short-acting intravenous anesthesia and secured with duct tape. The tape is cut and the two halves removed after recovery from anesthesia and a bandage applied.

Although the cast cutter is an oscillating instrument, the blade is quite capable of lacerating skin. This is especially true of thin-skinned foals. Skin over the fetlock, carpus, and tarsus and the coronary band are also prone to injury. Movement of the horse during standing cast removal may result in laceration. Because the awake horse is able to move to avoid the saw blade, these wounds are usually small and only of partial skin thickness. Full-thickness lacerations are more likely to be inflicted when a cast is removed during general anesthesia. It may be difficult to assess the amount of tissue damaged by thermal necrosis or the amount of fiberglass dust remaining in the wound. Lacerations that involve a joint frequently have an unfavorable outcome. If sutured, these wounds frequently dehisce and then must be allowed to heal by second intention. Despite vigorous systemic and intraarticular therapy, septic arthritis and osteomyelitis may ensue.

BIBLIOGRAPHY

Bartels KE, Denwick RC, Freeman LJ, Lowery RL, Alexander T, Appleman K, Bount C: Mechanical testing and evaluation of eight synthetic casting materials. *Vet Surg* 1985;14:310–318.

Bramlage LR: Long bone fractures. *Vet Clin North Am Large Anim Pract* 1983;5:285–310.

Dingwall JS, Horney FD, McDonell W, Duncan DB, Fretz PW: A comparison of breaking strengths of various casting materials. *Can Vet J* 1973;14:62–65.

Houlton JEF, Brearley MJ: A comparison of some casting materials. *Vet Rec* 1985;117:55–58.

Moll HD, Slone DE, Humburg JM, Jagar JE: Traumatic tarsal luxation repaired without internal fixation in three horses and three ponies. *J Am Vet Med Assoc* 1987;190:297–300.

Multiclinic Evaluation Group, Leach RE, et al: New fiber glass casting system. *Clin Orthop Rel Res* 1974;103:109–117.

Pope MH, Callahan G, Lavalette R: Setting temperature of synthetic casts. *J Bone Joint Surg Am* 1985;67:262–263.

Schneider RK, Milne DW, Gabel AA, Groom JJ, Bramlage LR: Multidirectional in vivo strain analysis of the equine radius and tibia during dynamic loading with and without a cast. *Am J Vet Res* 1982;43:1541–1550.

Stashak TS: Methods of therapy, in Stashak TS (ed): *Adams' Lameness in Horses*, ed 4. Philadelphia, Lea & Febiger, 1987, pp 847–855.

UNIT IV

Neurology and Ophthalmology

26 Palmar Digital Neurectomy

John V. Yovich

Palmar digital neurectomy is used as a palliative treatment for painful diseases of the palmar one third to one half of the distal portion of the digit and the sole. The most common indication for palmar digital neurectomy is navicular disease. Pain from some fractures of the palmar process of the distal phalanx and navicular bone fractures can be alleviated by palmar digital neurectomy. This surgery is contraindicated in diseases that involve the dorsal one half of the distal digit since this area will not be desensitized. Surgery should not be done to provide relief for infectious disease, which can then progress without a pain response being detected.

In horses in which palmar digital neurectomy is considered, the lameness should be relievable by local anesthesia of the palmar digital nerves. Horses with a concomitant source of lameness should not undergo the surgery. After localizing the lameness to the area supplied by the palmar digital nerve, a definitive diagnosis should be made from clinical findings and radiographic examination. Since there are complications associated with palmar digital neurectomy, conservative methods of treatment are recommended before resorting to surgery.

Palmar digital neurectomy is not universally legal in competition horses. However, since the procedure does not involve the dorsal branch of the digital nerve, horses retain afferent sensations from the dorsal half of the distal digit and may perform safely.

Several modifications of palmar digital neurectomy have been described. Each modification involves a different method of handling or treating the proximal nerve stump, after nerve transection, in an attempt to decrease the incidence of painful neuroma formation or reinnervation. Some of the techniques that have been employed in palmar digital neurectomy include simple neurectomy or the guillotine method, neurectomy with nerve ligation, nerve crushing, epineural capping, capping the nerve with silicone rubber tubing, electrocoagulation and ligation of the nerve, and cryotherapy of the nerve. Ligation of the nerve with a radioactive chromic phosphate—impregnated ligature resulted in inhibition of neuroma formation but persistent pain in horses. Stainless steel caps placed over the nerve stump have been evaluated, but these cause pain during exercise, probably from bending of the nerve over the sharp edge of the cap. Insertion of the proximal nerve stump into a hole drilled in the proximal phalanx has been described but not pursued.

At the present time it is not known which technique of palmar digital neurectomy results in the least complications and longest pain-free interval. The choice of technique is largely based on personal preference, and three methods will be described in this chapter.

SURGICAL PREPARATION

Palmar digital neurectomy can be done with the horse sedated and using regional anesthesia of the digital nerve at the level of the proximal sesamoid bones or with the horse under general anesthesia. General anesthesia is recommended because it facilitates aseptic technique, atraumatic surgery, and good visualization for identification of accessory nerve branches. When the more involved techniques of epineural capping or cryotherapy are used, general anesthesia is indicated.

The area between the fetlock joint and coronary band should be clipped and prepared for aseptic surgery. Plastic adhesive drapes are convenient for draping the hoof.

SURGICAL ANATOMY AND TECHNIQUE

The palmar digital nerve lies immediately palmar to the digital artery and vein and is about 1 cm deep to the skin, below the ligament of the ergot at the point where the ligament crosses the digital artery. Slight variation in the relationship of the digital vein, artery, nerve, and ligament of the ergot occurs and the nerve should be carefully identified. Approximately 50% of horses have a small accessory branch of the palmar digital nerve near the ligament of the ergot. In 5% of horses there are two nerves of nearly equal size.

The surgical incision is made midway between the fetlock and the coronary band. A 2- to 3-cm skin incision is made parallel and just dorsal to the superficial digital flexor tendon. The jaws of a hemostat can be used to separate the tissues. The ligament of the ergot lies subcutaneously. It is preferable to preserve the ligament, rather than transect it, in order to minimize scar tissue formation. Accessory branches of the palmar digital nerve often lie near the ligament of the ergot and these should be transected. With continued dissection through the subcutaneous tissue, the palmar digital nerve is identified. The nerve is freed from the subcutaneous tissues and the adjacent palmar digital artery by spreading the jaws of a hemostat in the tissue adjacent to the nerve in a motion parallel to the nerve. With the nerve supported by the hemostat the longitudinally arranged nerve fascicles should be visible. When stretched by traction with an instrument placed under the nerve and then released, the nerve should pucker and undulate. This is in contrast to the artery, which retracts back into the incision in its original shape after being stretched out of the incision. The nerve is transected distally and handled according to the specific technique selected.

Guillotine Technique

The palmar digital nerve is transected distally. A hemostat is placed on the proximal end of the nerve. Traction is applied to the nerve, which is then transected at the most proximal portion exposed. The nerve should retract proximally into the previously undisturbed tissue. A sterile tongue depressor can be used to stretch the nerve and act as a firm cutting surface for transection. This is probably the least traumatic technique.

Epineural Capping Technique

A 3- to 4-cm long incision is required for this technique. A 3-cm portion of the nerve is isolated and freed from surrounding tissue. The nerve is transected as distally as possible. The proximal nerve end is manipulated with a rolling motion between thumb and forefinger, exposing the nerve fascicles. The nerve fascicles are secured with mosquito forceps. Using another mosquito forceps with the jaws partially closed against the nerve, the epineurium is stripped in a proximal direction. The most proximal portion of the nerve fiber stripped of epineurium is incised halfway through from one side and then a few millimeters distal to this it is incised halfway through from the opposite side. The nerve is then transected 5 mm distal to these partial transections. The epineurium is then pulled distally over the transected nerve end and ligated with 4–0 nonabsorbable monofilament suture material.

Epineural capping should prevent reinnervation by sprouting, regenerating axons, but this is not always the case. Minute tears in the epineurium or reflection of axons with the epineurium when it is stripped are possible ways for axons to exit the epineural cap.

Cryotherapy Technique

In the cryotherapy technique the palmar digital nerve is transected distally and the epineurium reflected proximally as in the epineural capping method. A sterile wooden tongue depressor is placed under the proximal nerve stump, isolating the nerve from surrounding tissues. A sterile cryoprobe is used to freeze the nerve stump to −30 °C using a double rapid-freeze/slow-thaw method. Adequate freezing takes approximately 25 seconds and slow thawing takes 3 minutes. The proximal nerve stump is transected so that 5 mm of nerve that was frozen can be covered by epineurium. The epineurium is pulled distally over the nerve stump and ligated with a single suture of nonabsorbable monofilament material.

Cryotherapy of the proximal nerve stump is presumed to delay axon sprouting. The connective tissue elements of the perineurium can survive freezing so that axons must regenerate a longer distance in the nerve structure before becoming randomly oriented in extraneuronal tissue. During this period of regeneration within the perineurium, a fibrous scar covers the transected nerve end, limiting the penetration of regenerating axons into extraneuronal tissue, and perhaps decreasing the formation of painful neuromas.

Closure and Bandaging after Neurectomy

After any of the neurectomy techniques is complete, the subcutaneous tissue is apposed with a continuous absorbable suture and the skin is closed with interrupted sutures of nonabsorbable material. The surgical site should be covered with a sterile dressing and wrapped with an elastic bandage pressure wrap. The lower limb is wrapped with a firm support bandage.

POSTOPERATIVE CARE

Phenylbutazone is administered preoperatively and for 4 days postoperatively to minimize the inflammatory response to the surgical procedure. Skin sutures are removed at 10 days after surgery. The limb should be kept bandaged for 2 to 3 weeks with bandage changes every few days. Stall rest for 2 to 3 weeks and controlled walking only for another 3 weeks is recommended.

The hoof must be cleaned and examined daily after palmar digital neurectomy. This is to identify and treat penetrating wounds, or bruising that will not be evidenced by lameness. Unidentified septic processes within the denervated foot can cause severe complications or even loss of the foot.

If navicular disease is being treated, continued corrective hoof care, including pads, is recommended for protection of the foot.

PROGNOSIS AND POSTOPERATIVE COMPLICATIONS

The prognosis for soundness after palmar digital neurectomy is excellent in the short term given that the source of lameness is in the region innervated by this nerve. Although exact figures based on large studies are unavailable, it is estimated that 60 to 70% of horses will still be sound at 1 year after surgery. With time, this percentage decreases. Lameness returns because of painful neuroma formation or reinnervation in most cases.

Painful neuroma formation is the most common complication of neurectomy. Neuromas develop in all transected nerves. It is thought that in painful neuromas, it is the nerve fibers that extend from the fibrous swelling at the nerve end and into the surrounding healing connective tissue that are the source of pain. No method consistently prevents neuroma formation. In humans, sharp nerve transection and allowing the nerve stump to retract into an environment of soft tissue away from an area exposed to trauma, weight bearing, or scarring is considered to result in the lowest frequency of painful neuroma formation. Unfortunately, these conditions are not always met when a palmar digital neurectomy is performed in the horse. It is likely that careful tissue handling, minimal dissection, and careful postoperative protection of the surgical site are important in minimizing the incidence of painful neuroma formation. A painful neuroma may be identified by return of lameness, sensitivity to palpation of the transected nerve end or palpable neuroma, and relief of lameness by local anesthesia of the palmar digital nerve proximal to the neuroma. These signs usually are observed 3 to 6 months after surgery. The definitive treatment for a painful neuroma is another neurectomy proximal to the neuroma, which is left undisturbed.

Incomplete desensitization of the palmar third of the distal digit occurs when all nerve fibers supplying this area are not transected. Accessory branches located more superficially near the ligament of the ergot must also be transected. Occasionally there is a palmar branch originating from the dorsal digital nerve and providing collateral innervation to the palmar aspect of the hoof. This branch is not within the usual surgical field. A check for sensation in the palmar distal digit should be made before discharging the horse. If sensation is present and the clinical response to neurectomy is poor, selective local anesthesia can be used after healing of the initial surgery, to identify the site of persistent innervation. Another surgery can be performed to transect the accessory branches.

Regeneration of the palmar digital nerves with reinnervation of the heel and return of sensation in the palmar hoof can occur after about 4 to 6 months postoperatively. This complication can occur following application of any of the special procedures described herein. A return of lameness and a response to local anesthesia is indicative of reinnervation if a painful neuroma is absent. Another neurectomy is indicated.

Other reported postoperative complications are less common. Rupture of the deep digital flexor tendon can occur if the tendon is weakened by degeneration and is attached by fibrous adhesions to the navicular bone. With normal use of the limb after pain relief by neurectomy, the adhesions can be torn and the degenerate tendon can rupture. Rupture of the tendon may occur months after surgery and is diagnosed by the observation of the toe of the hoof tipping up. There is no specific treatment.

BIBLIOGRAPHY

Bramlage LR, Gabel AA, Kuhn WE: Evaluation of stainless steel nerve caps for palmar digital neurectomy. *Vet Surg* 1982;11:23–29.

Fackelman GE, Clodius L: New technique for posterior digital neurectomy in the horse. *Vet Med* 1972;67:1339–1346.

Schneider RK, Mayhew IG, Clarke GL: Effects of cyrotherapy on the palmar and plantar digital nerves in the horse. *Am J Vet Res* 1985;46:7–12.

Stashak TS: Navicular disease (podotrochleosis), in Stashak TS (ed): *Adams' Lameness in Horses*, Philadelphia, Lea & Febiger, 1987; pp 499–513.

Tate LP, Evans LH: Cryoneurectomy in the horse. *J Am Vet Med Assoc* 1980;177:423–426.

27 Aerophagia

Alan J. Nixon

Crib biting in the horse is an acquired vice in which the animal places its upper incisors on a ledge or other firm surface, arches its neck, retracts its larynx, resulting in elevation of the soft palate, and engulfs a bolus of air. When air is swallowed, the vice is known as aerophagia or windsucking. The sequelae to crib biting can be debilitating to the animal as well as damaging to the objects on which the horse cribs. The upper incisors become worn, occasionally almost down to the gum line. The horse ingests sufficient air that appetite is depressed and occasionally flatulence and colic develop. Weight loss and poor performance can occur. The sternocephalicus muscles hypertrophy and can become disfiguring. Moreover, the vice and associated noise is often objectionable and irritating.

This repetitive and apparently pointless habit usually occurs in stabled horses. While it is probably the result of boredom or frustration, aerophagia can occur in pastured horses as well. Some horses can swallow air without the need for a fixed object to brace against, simply by arching the neck and retracting the larynx. These horses are quite difficult to treat.

The usual methods to discourage aerophagia include various plain and spiked collars or straps, electric collars, and a change in the animal's environment. Many horses stop cribbing when turned out to open pasture. The presence of other horses or a companion such as a goat frequently reduces the boredom of the stall environment and hence the frequency of aerophagia. Recent studies also indicate that systemically administered narcotic antagonists such as nalmefene and naloxone eliminate crib biting for variable periods. Sustained-release preparations of nalmefene are under investigation and may result in prolonged suppression of crib biting.

SURGERY

There are five recognized surgical procedures to control aerophagia in the horse. Forssell's procedure was probably the most widely used and involves removal of extensive portions of the sternocephalicus, omohyoideus, and sternothyrohyoideus muscles. The Peterson modification of Forssell's procedure involves removal of only a 10-cm portion of each muscle and is less disfiguring. Neurectomy of the ventral branches of the spinal accessory nerve (cranial nerve XI), either in the anesthetized or standing horse, has also been described. This nerve partially innervates the sternocephalicus muscle on either side of the neck. Unfortunately, published results were poor and the technique has been largely abandoned. The fourth technique, bilateral buccostomy, was used in horses that swallow air without grasping a solid object. The disadvantages of this procedure are the tendency for spontaneous closure of the buccal fistula, poor aesthetic appearance, and the daily care needed for the plastic or brass tube placed in the buccostomy. This procedure is now largely obsolete.

The poor results after the neurectomy procedure and the disfiguring nature of Forssell's operation led to the development of a combined neurectomy of the accessory nerves and myectomy of the cranial portions of the omohyoideus and sternothyrohyoideus muscles. This procedure, first described in Germany, combines the cosmetic advantage of neurectomy of the sternocephalicus muscles with myectomy of the smaller but still important omohyoideus and sternothyrohyoideus muscles. Furthermore, all procedures are accomplished through one incision. Three reports of the procedure appear in the literature, and this is currently the most acceptable technique for surgical control of aerophagia.

The horse is anesthetized and positioned in dorsal recumbency. The ventral neck and throatlatch region from the midcervical to the intermandibular region are shaved and prepared for aseptic surgery. A 25-cm midline skin incision is made extending caudally from the level of the cricoid cartilage of the larynx (Fig. 27–1A). The skin is dissected from the omohyoideus muscles and retracted laterally. Care is taken to identify and preserve the linguofacial vein on either side. A plane of dissection is developed on the medial surface of the sternocephalicus musculotendinous junction. This plane is extended 8 cm caudally to expose the cranial limits of the sternocephalicus muscle belly (Fig. 27–1B). By exposing the medial surface of the muscle belly, the arterial supply to the cranial portions of the sternocephalicus, is evident. Within the white fascia accompanying the artery lies the ventral branch of the spinal accessory nerve (Fig. 27–1C). The nerve can be

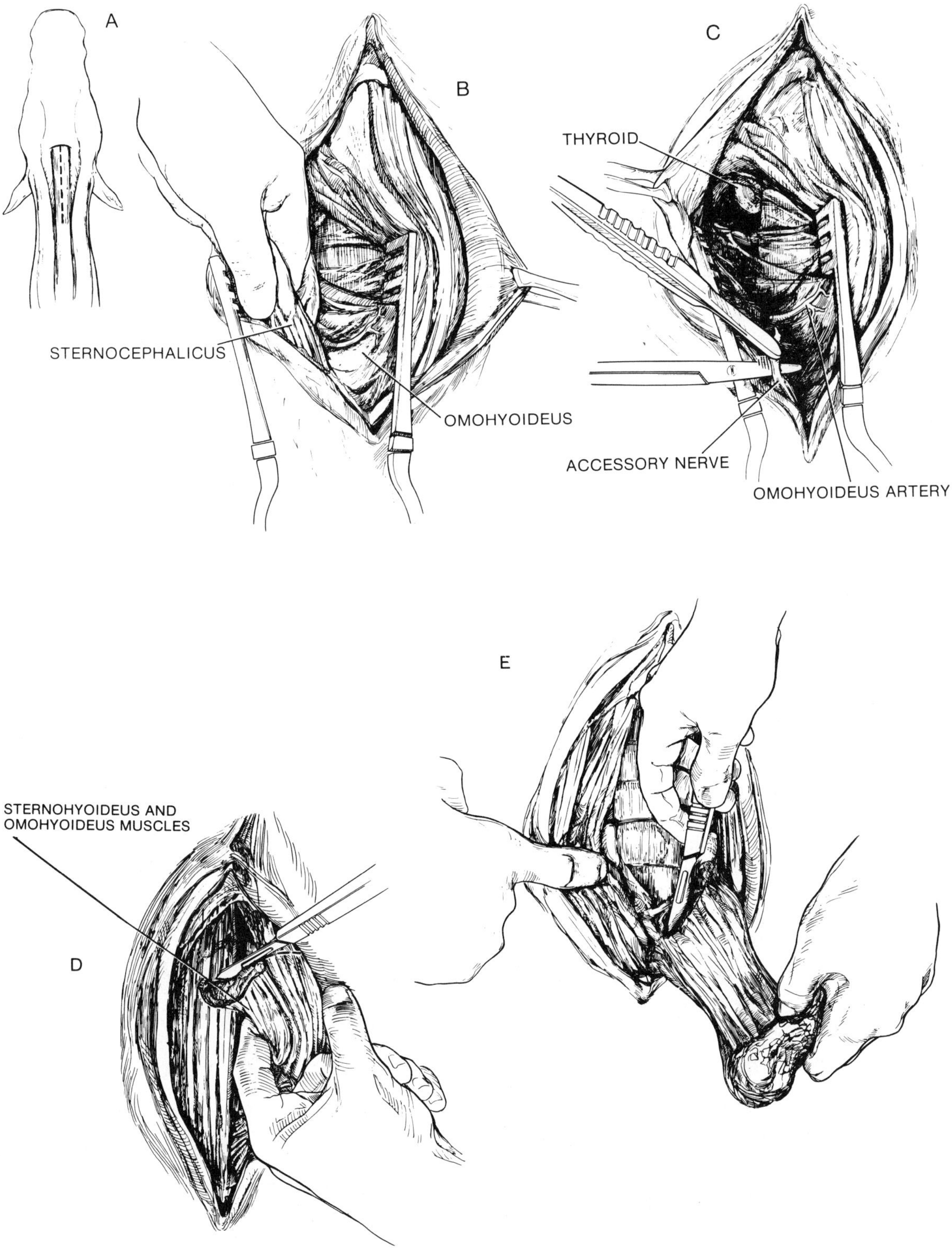

Figure 27–1. A. A 25-cm skin incision is made on midline extending caudally from the cricoid cartilage. **B.** The medial surface of the muscle belly of the sternocephalicus muscle is exposed. **C.** The ventral branch of the spinal accessory nerve is identified. **D.** The combined bellies of the omohyoideus and sternohyoideus muscles are severed cranially. **E.** The muscle bellies of the omohyoideus and sternohyoideus are severed caudally to permit removal of 15 cm of muscle. (Drawings by Jane Teichner.) (Courtesy of Dr. N. A. White.)

clamped momentarily, resulting in contraction of the muscle and verification that the correct nerve has been dissected. Curved hemostats are used to isolate this nerve, allowing both forefingers to be inserted under the nerve and spread, withdrawing and exposing as much as 10 cm of nerve. The isolated nerve is transected proximally and distally, removing as much nerve as possible. The procedure is performed bilaterally.

The myectomy then commences by isolating the cranially combined bellies of the omohyoideus and sternohyoideus muscles. These muscles are carefully dissected laterally where they form a close attachment to the linguofacial vein. A plane of dissection is developed between the muscles and the trachea and larynx. After elevating these muscles they are severed 2 cm from their insertions using a scalpel or Mayo scissors (Fig. 27–1D). The muscle bellies are then retracted caudally, severing attachments to the trachea, linguofacial veins, jugular veins, and sternocephalicus muscles as the dissection continues caudally. The omohyoideus and sternohyoideus muscle bellies are then severed obliquely, removing about 15 cm of muscle (Fig. 27–1E). The thin, straplike sternothyroideus muscles are then exposed, still loosely attached to the trachea. These muscles are elevated and severed at their insertions to the larynx, and 15 cm of each is removed.

A 1-in diameter Penrose drain is placed longitudinally in the wound and exteriorized through separate 3-cm stab incisions cranially and caudally to the skin wound. The subcutaneous tissue is closed with 2–0 synthetic absorbable suture placed in a continuous horizontal mattress pattern and the skin is closed with single interrupted sutures of 2–0 monofilament nylon or with stainless steel staples. To reduce the extensive dead space, a stent bandage can be secured over the incision using a continuous horizontal mattress suture of 0 monofilament nylon.

POSTOPERATIVE CARE

Box stall confinement is recommended for 3 weeks after surgery. Antibiotics are administered for 5 to 7 days after surgery to reduce the development of infection associated with the drain exit sites. The drain is removed 5 to 7 days after surgery depending on the quantity of discharge. The stent bandage is maintained for 8 to 10 days if the bandage is dry. If the bandage is soiled, it is removed and replaced by another sterile hand towel secured in place with adhesive tape. The drain exit sites are cleaned daily and the skin sutures or staples are removed 12 days after surgery. Horses are stall rested for the first 3 weeks of convalescence and then turned out to pasture.

Some horses develop an incisional seroma even as late as 2 weeks postoperatively. This can be prevented by making generous skin incisions at the site of the drain exit and maintenance of a bandage on the wound for a week after the drain is removed.

PROGNOSIS

The success rate of the combined neurectomy and myectomy procedure for total elimination of aerophagia is between 50 and 60%. A marked reduction in the frequency of crib biting was noted in a further 30% of horses, and 10 to 20% continue to crib unabated. These figures compare favorably with success rates ranging from 53 to 80% for the original Forssell procedure. Late return of the habit has been noted in several horses 5 and 6 months after combined neurectomy and myectomy, and a minimum of 12 months' postoperative absence of cribbing is recommended before the surgery can be classified as a success.

The combined surgery is superior to neurectomy alone. The poor results of neurectomy probably reflect the interplay of other muscles, such as the sternothyrohyoideus and omohyoideus, in the act of crib biting. Some authors have considered collateral innervation to the sternocephalicus muscle as being potentially important, but others claim these additional nerve branches are not motor branches.

The cosmetic nature of the neurectomy and myectomy procedure is clearly an advantage compared to the original Forssell procedure. Forssell's procedure produces a thin neck and a steplike defect where the sternocephalicus muscle bellies were transected. The Peterson modification of Forssell's procedure is less cosmetically disfiguring but the three separate skin incisions are time consuming and the proximity of vital structures and the risk of multiple seromas and wound management problems are clearly drawbacks.

Meticulous attention to hemostasis has been cited in the literature as an important consideration in reducing seroma formation. The sequence of performing the neurectomy before the myectomy is important to facilitate the identification and removal of the spinal accessory nerves. Hemorrhage from the severed muscle bellies can be profuse, and spot electrocautery is difficult in the fasciculating muscle. Pressure and occasionally ligation are needed.

Although aerophagia is not normally life-threatening, chronic weight loss, poor reproductive performance, and the possibility of more severe colic secondary to flatulent colic are potentially important factors when considering the use of this surgery.

BIBLIOGRAPHY

Dodman NH, Shuster L, Court MH, Dixon R: Investigation into the use of narcotic antagonists in the treatment of a stereotypic behavior pattern (crib-biting) in the horse. *Am J Vet Res* 1987;48:311–319.

Forssell G: The new surgical treatment against crib-biting. *Vet J* 1926;82:538–548.

Greet TRC: Windsucking treated by myectomy and neurectomy. *Equine Vet J* 1982;14:299–301.

Hamm D: A new surgical procedure to control crib biting, in *Proceedings of the American Association of Equine Practitioners.* 1977, pp 301–302.

Turner AS, White N, Ismay J: Modified Forssell's operation for crib biting in the horse. *J Am Vet Med Assoc* 1984; 184:309–312.

28 Scapular Wedge Resection for Management of Suprascapular Nerve Injury

Michael F. Clem
Richard M. DeBowes

The suprascapular nerve originates from the sixth and seventh cervical spinal cord segments to innervate the supraspinatus and infraspinatus muscles overlying the scapula. The nerve reflects around the cranial edge of the scapula at the scapular notch, passing beneath a small tendinous band. In this position the nerve is susceptible to direct trauma and resultant compression of the nerve against the underlying bone. There is histologic evidence of chronic demyelination and remyelination at the point where the nerve reflects over the edge of the scapula in "normal" suprascapular nerves in horses without clinical evidence of lameness or muscle atrophy. These findings suggest that recurrent trauma with subclinical neuronal damage is commonly present, a situation that is similar to suprascapular entrapment neuropathy in humans. The presence of underlying, chronic neuronal injury may render the nerve more susceptible to an acute traumatic insult and the development of clinical disease.

CLINICAL FINDINGS

Suprascapular neuropathy may occur at any age, with previous reviews reporting cases in patients from 1 month to 20 years. The disease was originally reported as most commonly occurring in draft breeds and was believed to be associated with repeated trauma from poorly fitted harness collars. With the decline in draft horse use, the condition is now more commonly associated with acute trauma and no breed predilection is shown. Although most cases are associated with a known history of trauma, the condition may develop spontaneously.

Suprascapular nerve paralysis is associated with varying degrees of lameness in the acute case. The lameness is characterized by lateral instability of the scapulohumeral joint during weight bearing. This instability is the result of a loss of the stabilizing function of the supraspinatus and infraspinatus muscles, which serve as lateral collateral support for the scapulohumeral joint. The acute lameness may be followed by complete recovery over a 2- to 3-month period, or denervation atrophy of the suprascapular musculature may become permanent. Following an injury to the nerve, atrophy may become apparent as early as 7 to 10 days after trauma. Subsequent chronic lateral instability and subluxation of the scapulohumeral joint may predispose to the development of degenerative joint disease.

A presumptive diagnosis of suprascapular nerve paralysis may be made from the clinical signs and a history of trauma to the area of the distal scapula. Radiographs of the scapulohumeral area should be obtained to rule out the possibility of fracture or degenerative joint disease in chronic cases. Confirmation of the diagnosis is made by an electromyographic evaluation, which demonstrates selective denervation of the suprascapular musculature. The presence of electromyographic findings of denervation of muscles supplied by other branches of the brachial plexus should prompt further neurolgic evaluation to rule out injuries to the brachial plexus or focal central neurologic involvement, such as occurs with protozoal myelitis.

TREATMENT

Initial therapy is directed toward reducing inflammation in the area of the nerve. Stall rest and the systemic administration of nonsteroidal anti-inflammatory agents or corticosteroids may produce a resolution of the clinical signs. In patients that continue to have clinical signs of suprascapular nerve dysfunction for 10 to 12 weeks, surgical decompression of the nerve is indicated.

The horse is positioned in lateral recumbency, with the affected limb uppermost. Following aseptic preparation, an 18- to 20-cm skin incision is made just cranial to the spine of the scapula and ending 5 cm beyond the distal end of the spine. This incision is carried through the subcutaneous tissues and deep fascia to expose the supraspinatus muscle. The supraspinatus muscle is bluntly elevated from the spine of the scapula and retracted cranially. The suprascapular nerve is identified as it reflects over the cranial edge of the scapula at the scapular notch, just distal to the distal end of the scapular spine (Fig. 28–1). The nerve is freed from the overlying fibrous tissue along the cranial border of the scapula or underlying bony proliferation by careful dissection. The nerve is then gently retracted dorsally. The periosteum underlying the normal path of the nerve is incised and removed along the cranial border of the scapula. A subtotal ostectomy is performed at the cranial edge of the scapular notch to remove an approximately 2 × 4 cm portion of the bone underlying the normal position of the nerve. The ostectomy may be performed utilizing an air drill, an osteotome, a wire saw, or a combination of these instruments. When using an osteotome or chisel, it has been recommended that care be taken to orient the longitudinal cut away from the scapulohumeral joint to avoid inadvertently creating a fracture into the joint. Following ostectomy, the nerve is replaced such that its course traverses the deficit in the scapula (Fig. 28–2). Some authors have described insertion of a Teflon sheet beneath the nerve to prevent incorporation of the nerve in any new bone growth that may occur at the ostectomy site.

Closure is achieved by apposition of the supraspinatus muscle to the scapular spine using synthetic ab-

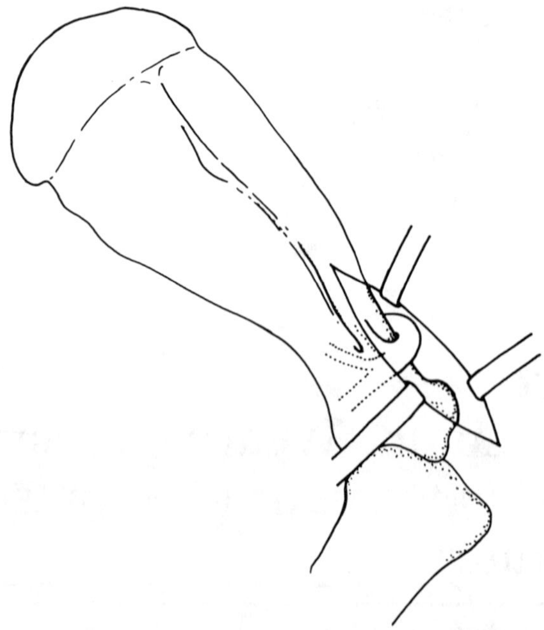

Figure 28–1. The suprascapular nerve is accessed through a longitudinal incision along the cranial edge of the scapula and beneath the supraspinatus muscle.

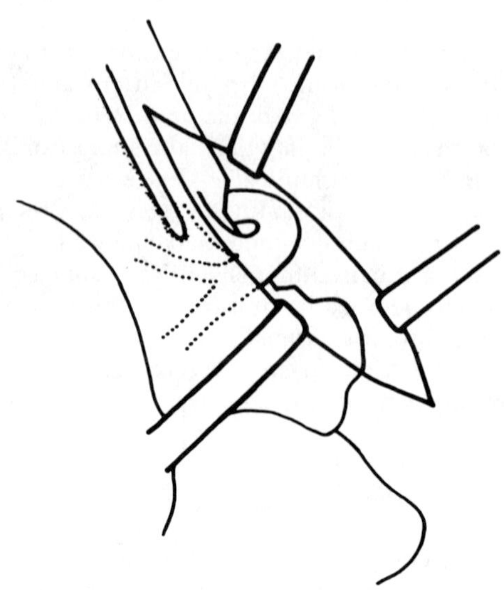

Figure 28–2. A section of the cranial edge of the scapula has been removed to minimize entrapment and compression of the suprascapular nerve.

sorbable suture material in a simple continuous pattern, followed by similar closure of the deep and subcutaneous fascia. The skin is apposed with nonabsorbable suture or skin staples in an interrupted fashion. A stent bandage is recommended for the recovery period and is left in place for the first 3 to 5 postoperative days.

Postoperative therapy consists of phenylbutazone administration for 1 week and stall rest. Sutures are removed 14 days postoperatively. Exercise should be restricted for 1 to 2 months postoperatively to reduce the development of degenerative changes within the scapulohumeral joint as a result of continued instability prior to return of suprascapular muscle function.

PROGNOSIS

Previous reports of the technique have indicated encouraging results, with approximately 80% of the surgical patients having return of normal muscle function. Resolution of muscle atrophy is also reported to be good, although results will certainly vary with duration of denervation and magnitude of the original injury to the nerve. Prolonged entrapment of the nerve may produce irreversible damage, and it has been recommended that surgery is best performed within 12 weeks of injury in any patient that has failed to respond to conservative therapy. In view of the fact that no other surgical therapies have been identified for use in suprascapular nerve paralysis patients that fail to respond to medical management, this technique should be considered as one that may provide a clinical resolution in otherwise intractable cases.

BIBLIOGRAPHY

Adams OR, Schneider RK, Bramlage LR, et al: A surgical approach to treatment of suprascapular nerve injury in the horse. *J Am Vet Med Assoc* 1985;187:1016–1018.

Duncan ID, Schneider RK: Equine suprascapular neuropathy (Sweeney): Clinical and pathologic observations, in *Proceedings of the American Association of Equine Practitioners.* 1985, pp 415–428.

Duncan ID, Schneider RK, Hammang JP: Subclinical entrapment neuropathy of the equine suprascapular nerve. *Acta Neuropathol* 1987;74:53–61.

Schneider JE, Adams OR, Easley KJ, et al: Scapular notch resection for suprascapular nerve decompression in 12 horses. *J Am Vet Med Assoc* 1985;187:1019–1020.

29 Static Compressive Spinal Cord Lesions

Alan J. Nixon

Cervical vertebral malformation has been broadly divided into two categories, cervical vertebral instability and cervical static stenosis. Although overlap occurs between the categories, bony malformations that result in static, nonvarying compression of the spinal cord are known as cervical static stenosis.

The cause of these bony malformations is largely conjectural; however, the majority are the direct or indirect result of degenerative joint disease (DJD) of the diarthrodial (synovial) articulations of the caudal cervical vertebrae. Initiation of DJD in these joints can be due to congenital malformations of the size and shape of the vertebral facets, osteochondritis dissecans of the facets, or trauma with fracture or simple cartilage injury to a portion of the facet. The thickened and osteosclerotic dorsal laminae of affected vertebrae are a secondary phenomenon due to DJD of the adjacent facet and a change in stress applied to this vertebral junction.

Because of the time delay in the development of DJD, most horses with cervical static stenosis are older than those in the cervical vertebral instability group. Cervical static stenosis is rarely diagnosed in horses less than 18 months old; the usual age of onset of clinical signs is 2 to 4 years. Many horses present with a history of neurologic symptoms beginning with a fall or training incident. Although occasionally subtle, the progression of symptoms can be rapid and many horses have grade 2 or grade 3 ataxia (on a scale of 4) at the time of presentation. The early phases of neurologic symptoms are frequently mistaken for unilateral or bilateral hind limb lameness, often with stifle disease as the tentative diagnosis.

Some horses become neurologically stable, and others occasionally progress to recumbency. Incoordination, weakness, spasticity, and dysmetria are typical symptoms of this condition. Generally the symptoms are mildly asymmetric and the hind limbs are more obviously affected than the forelimbs. Extraordinarily severe forelimb symptoms are usually associated with direct pressure on the cervical intumescence and associated nerve roots. These horses often show considerable difficulty in backing up, manifested as a reluctance or inability to step backward with the forelimbs. Localized, unilateral pectoral and forelimb muscle atrophy, an atypical sign of cervical static stenosis, can occasionally result from lateral foraminal stenosis.

DIAGNOSIS

The diagnosis of cervical vertebral malformation is made by radiography and the type of lesion and treatment is categorized by myelography. Cervical static stenosis occurs almost exclusively at C5–6, C6–7, or C7–T1. The C6–7 articulation is the most common site. Radiographic changes include signs of DJD such as osteophytosis, osteosclerosis, and obliteration of the joint space. Sclerosis and thickening of the dorsal lamina is frequently seen, resulting in narrowing of the vertebral canal diameter (Fig. 29–1). Angular fixation or ankylosis with reduced range of motion is also occasionally seen. Measurements of the sagittal diameter of the vertebral canal are not used routinely, but reference minimum values have been published. Myelography is preferred for confirmation of a static compressive lesion. Both normal horses and horses with symptoms due to intramedullary lesions may present with radiographic evidence of cervical static stenosis at C5–6 or C6–7. It is critical that myelography be performed to differentiate these incidental findings from true lesions. Even so, myelography is not always definitive and questionable myelographic features can be difficult to interpret.

Myelography techniques using either metrizamide, iopamidol or iohexol by cisternal injection are safe and result in few side effects. The technique of standing myelography does not appear to be as safe and precludes assessment of flexed, extended and ventrodorsal

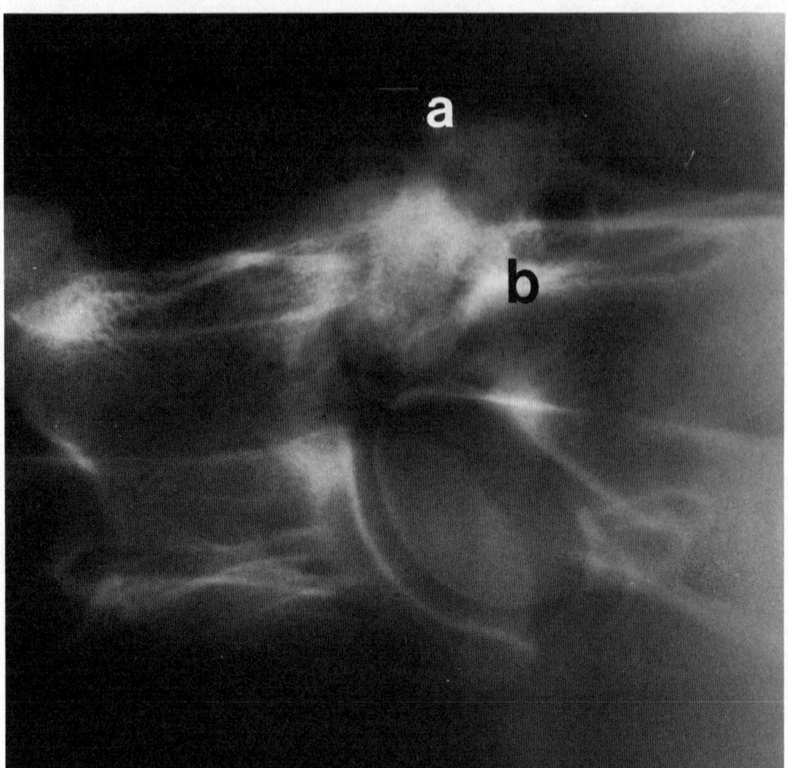

Figure 29–1. A plain radiograph showing characteristic changes of cervical static stenosis at C6-7. Osteophytes and subchondral sclerosis (*a*) indicate degenerative joint disease. Sclerosis of the dorsal lamina is also present (*b*).

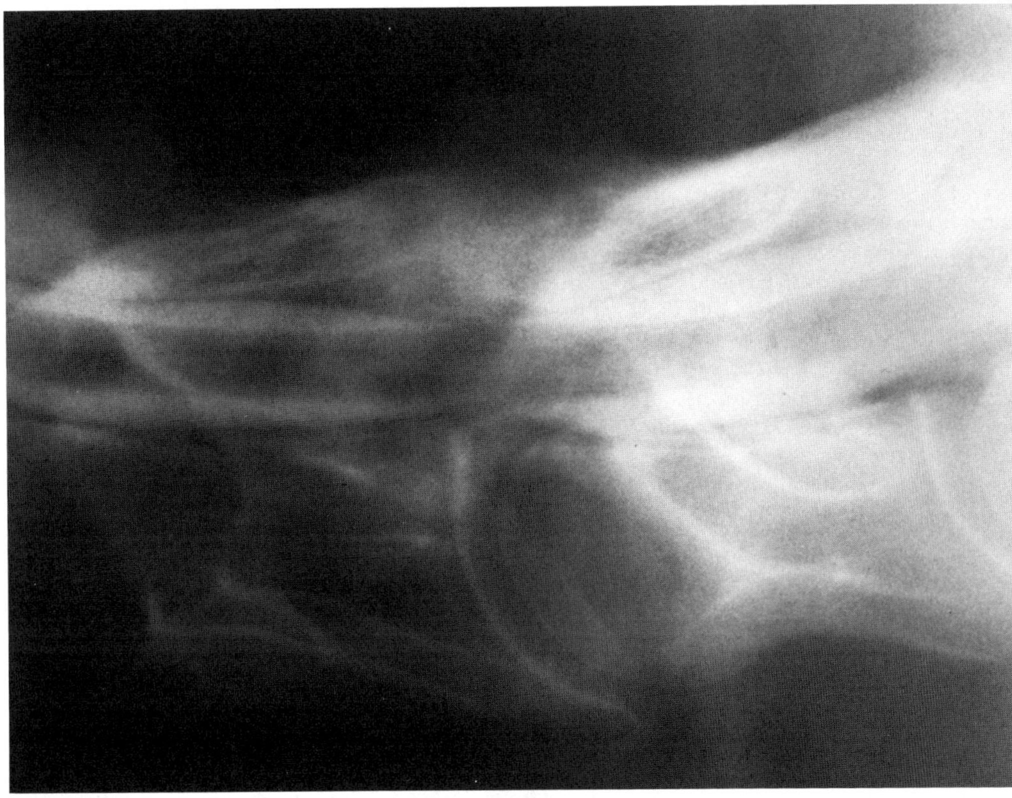

Figure 29–2. A neutral-position myelogram showing cervical static stenosis at C6-7 in a horse. Considerable narrowing of both dorsal and ventral contrast columns is evident.

views. Myelography is particularly useful to demonstrate compressive soft tissue components of cervical static stenosis such as hypertrophied ligamentum flava and joint capsules. These structures enlarge secondary to DJD of the articular facets. The hypertrophy of the joint capsule occasionally results in lateral spinal cord compression, which is difficult to appreciate on a lateral myelographic view. Ventrodorsal views of the caudal cervical vertebrae are rarely of diagnostic quality because of the thickness of the neck and associated radiation scatter. Spinal cord compression in horses with cervical static stenosis is generally directed to the dorsal and dorsolateral areas of the spinal cord. For a focal compressive lesion to exist, both dorsal and ventral contrast columns must be narrowed at the same level (Fig. 29–2). A 50% narrowing of the contrast columns has been considered sufficient to indicate spinal cord compression. However, this general rule has not always correlated histologically with a focal spinal cord lesion. Fortunately, most cases of cervical static stenosis result in considerable thinning of both contrast columns compared to cervical vertebral instability cases in the midcervical area, where equivocal lesions are more frequent. In early cases of cervical static stenosis, particularly those with significant soft tissue compression from the joint capsules and ligamentun flavum, the lesion is best demonstrated on neutral and extended views and is partially relieved by flexion. Chronic lesions often develop varying degrees of ankylosis of the vertebral junction, and compression is not relieved by flexion. A complete dynamic study is important.

Multiple-level lesions can occur, including stenosis at both C5–6 and C6–7, and the literature cites cases in which stenosis at C6–7 was coexistent with cervical vertebral instability in the midcervical area.

Other diagnostic tests that are useful aids include cerebrospinal fluid analysis, serology, and electromyography. Cerebrospinal fluid is frequently normal, although an elevated protein level is occasionally seen. Serology and electromyography are useful to eliminate other diseases in the differential diagnosis.

SURGICAL TREATMENT

Few horses affected with cervical static stenosis permanently respond to conservative therapy. Surgical decompression is recommended to relieve the impinging bone and soft tissue structures. Dorsal laminectomy is the procedure of choice for immediate decompression. Slower decompression can be achieved to a variable extent by ventral fusion of the affected junction, which decompresses the spinal cord as the bone remodels and hypertrophied soft tissues atrophy. Immediate ventral decompression by ventral slotting provides poor spinal cord exposure, severely weakens the vertebral bodies, and is not currently recommended for use in horses.

Several descriptions of dorsal laminectomy appear in the literature. Lateral or ventral recumbency can be used depending on available facilities. After induction of anesthesia, the horse is placed in left lateral recumbency with the neck flexed and the dorsal surface of the neck extended beyond the edge of the surgery table. Following sterile skin preparation and draping, a 25- to 30-cm skin incision is made on the dorsal midline commencing at the withers and extending cranially. The exposed nuchal fat is incised down to the funicular portion of the ligamentum nuchae. The ligamentum is separated on the midline, beginning near the caudal limits. The lamellar portions of the ligamentum nuchae separate readily, exposing the spinalis, semispinalis, and multifidus muscles (Fig. 29–3). Exposure is maintained by large self-retaining retractors (Finochietto Rib Retractors; Scanlan Instruments). The dorsal spinous processes of C7 and T1 are used as landmarks to identify the level of dissection. The insertions of the multifidus muscles on the dorsal spinous processes of the vertebrae are severed and these muscles are dissected from the affected dorsal laminae by large periosteal elevators (Cobb Periosteal Elevator; Orthopedic Equipment Co). The synovial capsule of the facet joints is also opened axially to expose the medial limits of the facets. Hinged self-retaining retractors (Beckman-Eaton Laminectomy Retractors; Codman & Shurtleff) are essential to maintain adequate exposure (Fig. 29–4). The ligamentum flavum is excised with scissors and removed to prevent entanglement in the air drill. The dorsal laminae are removed using an air drill to form a full-thickness channel around the bone fragment to be removed. The free segment of bone is then grasped in a bone-holding forceps, freed of its soft tissue attachments, and removed (Fig. 29–5). Curved cartilage scissors are useful to sever these tissues. Remnants of bone and soft tissue are removed with Kerrison rongeurs. If lateral compression is evident, the dura mater is gently retracted with a thin retractor and the encroaching tissue removed with a diamond burr. The dura should bulge evenly into the bone defect in the lamina.

After liberal lavage to remove bone debris and blood clots, a free autogenous fat graft is harvested from the nuchal fat and placed snugly into the laminectomy defect (Fig. 29–6). The multifidus muscles are reapposed over the laminae and fat graft using #1 synthetic absorbable suture. A 5-mm fenestrated suction drain is placed over the sutured multifidus muscles and exteriorized from the lateral aspect of the neck immedi-

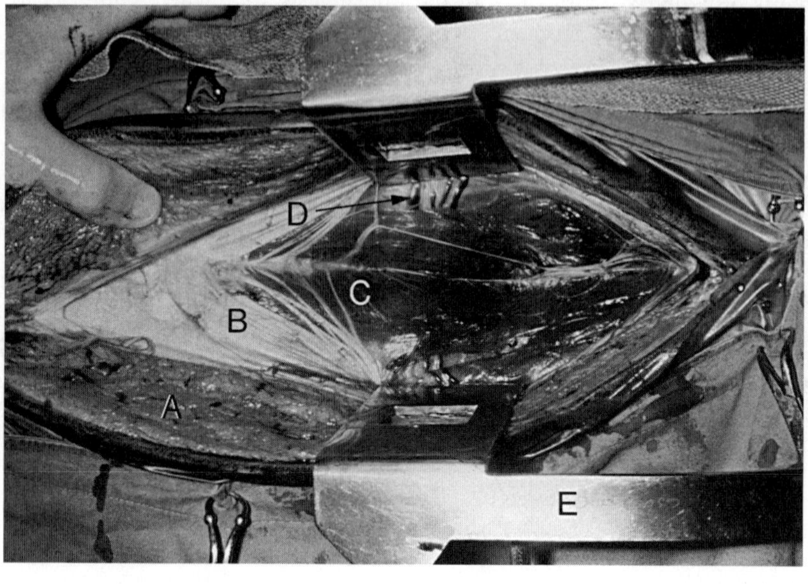

Figure 29–3. Dorsal approach to expose the caudal cervical vertebrae. *A*, subcutaneous nuchal fat; *B*, lamellar ligamentum nuchae; *C*, spinalis muscles; *D*, deep cervical blood vessels; *E*, Finochietto self-retaining retractors. (From Dorsal laminectomy in the horse. I. Review of the literature and description of a new procedure. *Veterinary Medicine* reproduced with permission of JB Lippincott Co.)

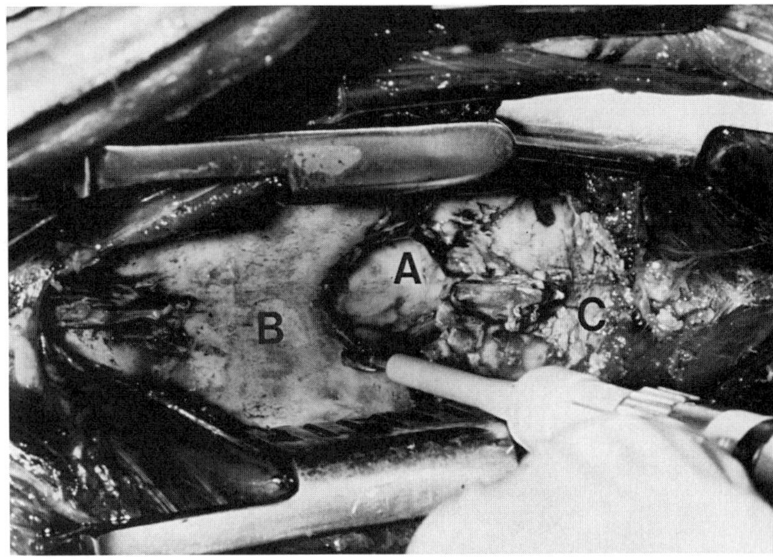

Figure 29–4. Exposed dorsal laminae ready for laminectomy with a high-speed burr. The ligamentum flavum has been removed, exposing the dura mater (*A*), between the cranial vertebra (*B*) and the caudal vertebra (*C*). The multifidus muscles are retracted with Beckman-Eaton laminectomy retractors.

ately deep to the funicular portion of the ligamentum nuchae. The funicular ligamentum nuchae, nuchal fat, and subcutaneous tissues are sutured sequentially with #2 synthetic absorbable suture placed in simple continuous patterns. The skin is apposed with a simple continuous layer of #0 monofilament nylon. A stent bandage is secured over the wound.

Recovery from anesthesia is usually slow and tranquilization with 125 mg xylazine is used to discourage premature attempts to rise. Supervision and occasional assistance is important in recovery. A sling is unnecessary.

Recently, intervertebral fusion for treatment of cervical static stenosis has been described. The surgical procedure is similar to the ventral cervical interbody fusion technique described for the treatment of cervical vertebral instability (see Chapter 30). The anesthetized horse is positioned in dorsal recumbency with the neck extended and stabilized (Fig. 29–7). The forelimbs are retracted caudally to increase access to the caudal cervical vertebrae and the rear of the horse is lowered to level the surgical field. After exposing the ventral surface of the vertebrae, the appropriate vertebral junction is identified by the broad parallel transverse pro-

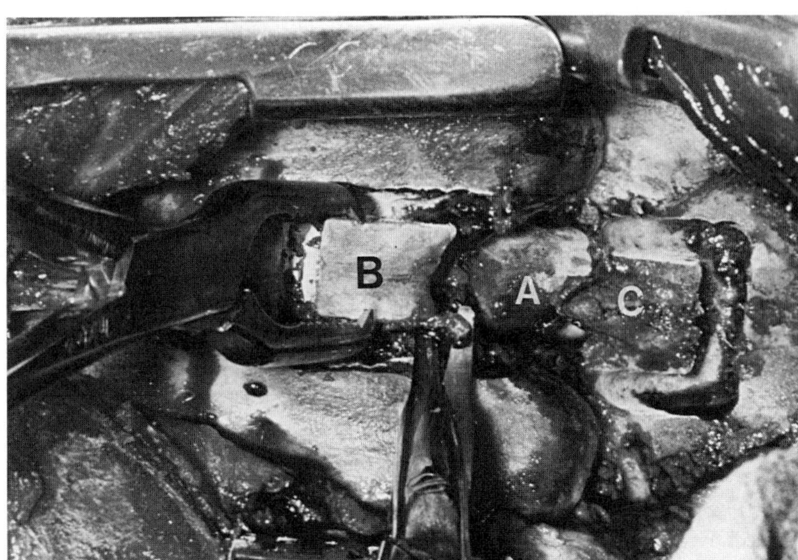

Figure 29–5. Completed burring results in a free fragment of bony lamina (*B*), which is gripped in a bone-holding forceps and its soft tissue attachments severed using curved scissors. The fragment of lamina from the caudal vertebra (*C*) is then removed in a similar manner. The dura mater (*A*) appears in the intervertebral space.

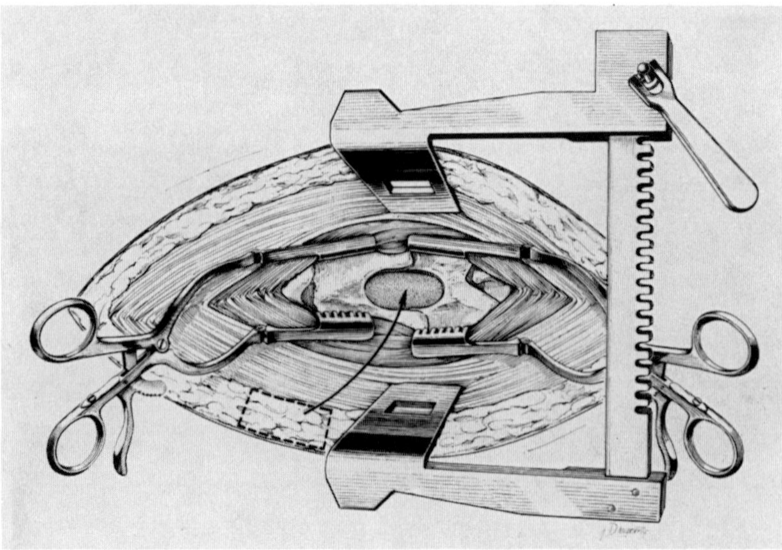

Figure 29–6. A free fat graft is harvested from the nuchal fat and transplanted to cover the dura mater in the laminectomy defect.

cesses of C6, the prominent ventral spinous process of C5, and the short seventh cervical vertebra. If C5-6 is to be fused the ventral crest of C5 is removed with a curved osteotome and mallet. A small portion of the caudoventral aspect of C6 is removed when C6-7 is operated. After drilling a 25-mm diameter hole to the predetermined depth a perforated stainless steel cylinder 22 mm in length is impacted into the site and seated below the level of the vertebral bone. The cylinder is packed with autogenous cancellous bone from the drillings and the previously removed ventral crest. When C6-7 is being fused a plastic spinal plate (Lubra plate; Lubra Co) is placed over the stainless steel cylinder and secured to the vertebrae with cancellous bone screws (Fig. 29–8). The C5-6 junction has a greater tendency to flex and a spinal plate is generally unnecessary to prevent the cylinder from migrating. Surgery times are longer than those for midcervical interbody fusions because of the depth of soft tissues ventral to the vertebral column and the need for more elaborate retraction and dissection. Long-term effectiveness of fusion for cervical static stenosis is not yet known.

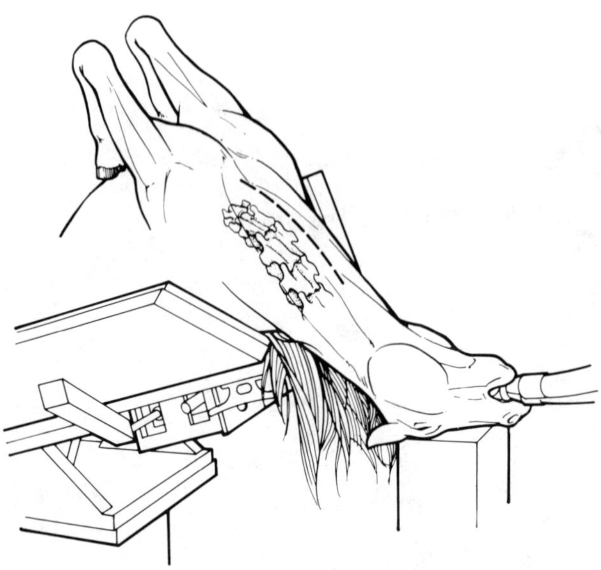

Figure 29–7. Positioning of a horse for ventral fusion of the caudal cervical vertebrae. The table is lowered caudally to extend and level the cervical spine.

POSTOPERATIVE CARE

Risk of acute postoperative exacerbation of clinical signs is greater following dorsal laminectomy than after interbody fusion. The exposed spinal cord is at risk of pressure from hematoma, seroma, or edema and the inflammation directly surrounding the spinal cord can occasionally lead to increased neurologic deficits. Nevertheless, the majority of laminectomy cases are unchanged in their neurologic status in the immediate postoperative period. Preoperative antibiotics and phenylbutazone are continued after surgery for 5 days. Accumulated fluid is usually removed from the drain at approximately 60 mL/h during the initial 24-hour

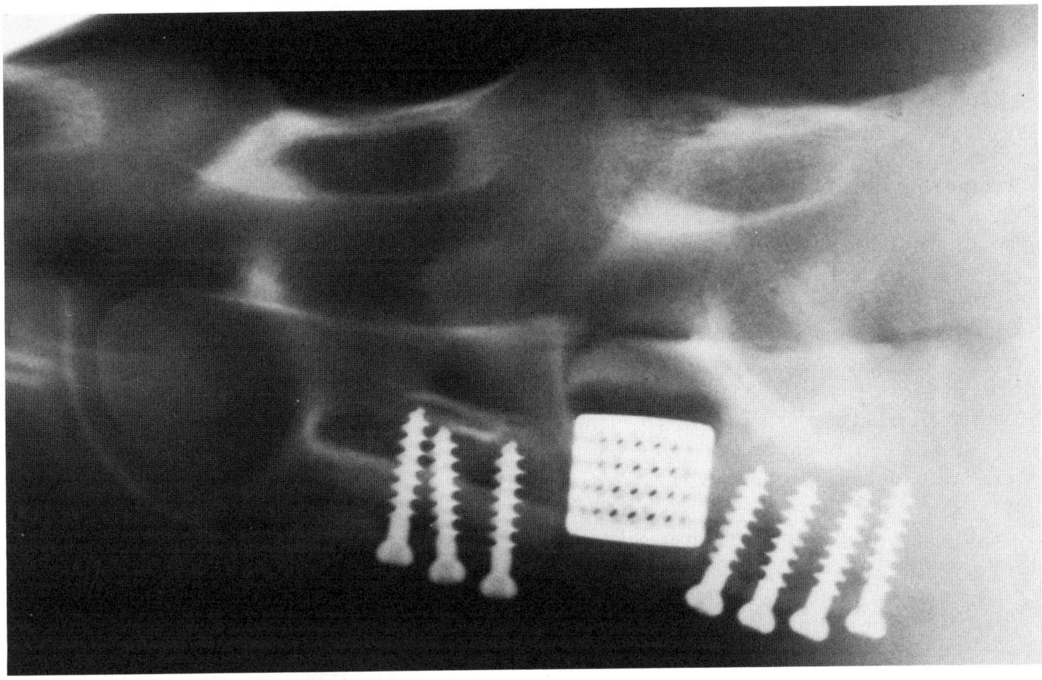

Figure 29–8. Postoperative radiograph 3 weeks following ventral fusion for cervical spinal stenosis at C6-7. A plastic spinal plate (Lubra) has been secured over the stainless steel cylinder to prevent migration.

period. The drainage diminishes over the first 4 days and the drain is removed when production is less than 10 mL/h. A radiograph is taken to ensure that the correct vertebral junction was decompressed and the vertebrae are intact. The horse is confined to a stall for 2 weeks. The stent bandage is removed after 10 days and the skin sutures at 12 to 14 days. Increasing periods of controlled walking exercise commence after 14 days, and many horses begin to show improved neurologic capabilities at that time. Depending on the neurologic status and travel distances, horses are discharged to the care of their owners 2 to 3 weeks after surgery.

Postoperative care following caudal vertebral fusion is similar to that following dorsal laminectomy. Because the spinal canal is not broached during a fusion procedure, there is less risk of acute exacerbation of clinical signs. Radiographic examination of the surgery site is important after a fusion procedure to ensure that the implant is located at the correct interspace and has not migrated from the drill hole. Most implants migrate a few millimeters for up to 2 weeks after surgery, and repeat radiographs during this time are important. Feeding hay from a feedrack level with the neck and head is recommended to avoid overextension of the cervical vertebrae, which can lead to reduced force on the perimeter of the implant and an increased tendency for the cylinder to drift ventrally. Neck cradles or casts are not used.

RESULTS

Results of dorsal laminectomy in 30 horses evaluated from 2 to 6 years after surgery indicated 17 horses had recovered full neurologic function. Eight were left with residual deficit (grade 1) and five deteriorated after surgery as a result of concurrent instability, fracture of a vertebral pedicle, or inflammation at the surgery site. Three horses had a double laminectomy at C5-6 and C6-7. Two of these became completely normal. However, of the racebred animals only two out of eight entered and maintained a race career. The only other published results of dorsal laminectomy revealed 8 of 16 horses died as a result of failure of the surgery or anesthesia and none of the 16 had raced at the time of evaluation. Long-term results of a large series of laminectomy cases have not been published.

Poor results can occur if concurrent instability exists, and these horses are better treated by vertebral fusion rather than laminectomy. While myelography is important in detecting these cases, excessive flexion of C6–7 can occasionally be seen on a standing lateral cervical radiograph and is the first indication of vertebral instability there.

The major complications associated with laminectomy have been laceration of aberrant branches of the vertebral venous sinuses, fracture of articular facets, and continued cord trauma due to concurrent instability. The aberrant venous branches were contained within proliferative scar tissue at the junction of the enlarged ligamentum flavum and thickened fibrous layer of the joint capsule. Hemorrhage is profuse but it can be effectively controlled using bipolar cautery and gelatin sponge. Fracture of the articular facets 2 to 4 days after surgery occurred in three of 30 cases described in one report. The change in shape of the laminectomy from rectangular to oval prevented further fractures in the subsequent 14 cases.

After laminectomy, recovery from neurologic disability is quite slow, and may take as long as 15 months. Some degree of improvement can usually be observed at the time the patient is discharged from the clinic. The final neurologic status is frequently dependent upon the duration of symptoms prior to surgery and the severity of signs. The chances of success are fair provided all levels of compression are detected and treated appropriately.

Little neurologic change is evident by 3 months after spinal fusion, since spinal cord decompression comes only as the compressing bone and soft tissues remodel and atrophy. Of eight horses described in the literature, seven had shown improved neurologic status 5 months after surgery. Ten months after surgery none of the eight animals were normal but most had only slight residual deficits. By 18 months four of the animals were lost to follow-up but were apparently being ridden, and another four had residual deficits but these were sufficiently mild that three were in performance work.

PROGNOSIS

No technique yields excellent return to function following caudal cervical static stenosis. Frequently, the long duration of compression and severity of symptoms at the time of presentation make the chances of a complete return to function poor. Worse still, the 12- to 18-month convalescent period makes many racing animals unlikely to be ready to perform until they are 4 years old, and this is often an unacceptable delay.

Although the literature contains only eight cases of caudal cervical static stenosis treated by interbody fusion, the early results revealed improved neurologic status and some of the animals went on to become riding horses, including racing. Ventral fusion is safer than dorsal laminectomy and may return some horses to a neurologic status suitable for athletic activity.

BIBLIOGRAPHY

Grant BD, Hoskinson JJ, Barbee DD, Gavin PR, Sande RD, Bayly WM: Ventral stabilization for decompression of caudal cervical spinal cord compression in the horse, in *Proceedings of the American Association of Equine Practitioners*, 1985, pp 75–90.

Mayhew IG, deLahunta A, Whitlock RH, Krook L, Tasker JB: Spinal cord disease in the horse. *Cornell Vet* 1978;68:1–207.

Nixon AJ, Stashak TS: Dorsal laminectomy in the horse. I. Review of the literature and description of a new procedure. *Vet Surg* 1983;12:172–176.

Nixon AJ, Stashak TS: Surgical therapy for spinal cord disease in the horse, in *Proceedings of the American Association of Equine Practitioners*, 1985, pp 61–74.

Nixon AJ, Stashak TS, Ingram JT: Dorsal laminectomy in the horse. III. Results in horses with cervical vertebral malformation. *Vet Surg* 1983;12:184–188.

Wagner PC, Bagby GW, Grant BD, Gallina AM, Ratzlaff M, Sande RD: Surgical stabilization of the equine cervical spine. *Vet Surg* 1979;8:7–12.

30
Cervical Vertebral Interbody Fusion for Management of Instability and Malformations

Richard M. DeBowes

Cervical vertebral malformation has been considered to involve at least three primary types of spinal cord lesions. The type I lesion is a true stenotic lesion, which places continuous pressure on the spinal cord regardless of whether the cervical spinal column is flexed or extended. Type II lesions are an intermittent type of spinal cord compression associated only with flexion or extension of the cervical spinal column. The type III lesions are multifocal lesions comprised of a mixture of both types I and II lesions.

DIAGNOSIS

Cervical vertebral malformation most commonly affects male horses. Although the condition has been observed throughout a wide range of age groups, most horses affected with type I lesions are 6 months to 4 years of age. Horses with type II lesions tend to be older than horses with type I involvement and range in age from 2 to 10 years. Although many breeds have been affected, the Thoroughbred and Quarter Horse breeds are most commonly represented in the veterinary literature.

The diagnosis is made based on a history of spinal ataxia, incoordination, or spasticity of acute onset. Occasionally, owners may be aware of a progressive deterioration in the clinical signs. Often, the acuity of the lesions or the observation of an incident of stumbling and falling leads the owner to suspect that the horse has suffered a traumatic injury. Some horses are presented for evaluation of a possible hind limb lameness and are subsequently demonstrated to have a cervical vertebral malformation.

CLINICAL FINDINGS

The typical patient affected with a midcervical compressive cord lesion will demonstrate clinical signs of truncal ataxia, weakness, spasticity, and proprioceptive deficits that are most evident in the hind limbs. The difference in severity of clinical signs from the forelimbs to the hind limbs is generally 1 to 2 grades on a scale of 1 to 4, in which 1) constitutes minimal proprioceptive deficits; 2) enhanced proprioceptive deficits and weakness, which are evident at the trot; 3) moderate proprioceptive deficits and weakness evident at the walk; and 4) extreme proprioceptive deficits and weakness, barely able to stand. The clinical signs on the left and right sides of the patient's body usually appear to be symmetric. Horses with caudal cervical lesions may demonstrate forelimb signs equal in severity to those of the hind limbs. This is assumed to be associated with the involvement of the cervical intumescence. Patients with type I lesions will generally not demonstrate a worsening in their clinical signs with flexion, extension, or turning of the cervical vertebral spine. Conversely, manipulation of the head and neck may result in a significant worsening of clinical signs for those patients with types II or III lesions.

DIAGNOSIS

The diagnosis of cervical vertebral malformation is confirmed with positive contrast myelography. A plain-film radiographic examination is helpful in ruling out vertebral fractures or severe vertebral luxations and should be performed prior to a myelographic examination. Plain-film radiography may also be used to detect evidence of osteochondrosis, degenerative joint disease, or remodeling of the articular facets. However, considering the difficulties associated with the analysis of minimum flexed spinal canal diameters as measured on plain-film radiographs, myelographic studies are required for accurate diagnosis of compressive spinal cord lesions.

The specific technique of equine cisternal myelography using either iohexol or metrizamide has been previously described. The demonstration of a focal area in which the dorsal column of myelographic agent is

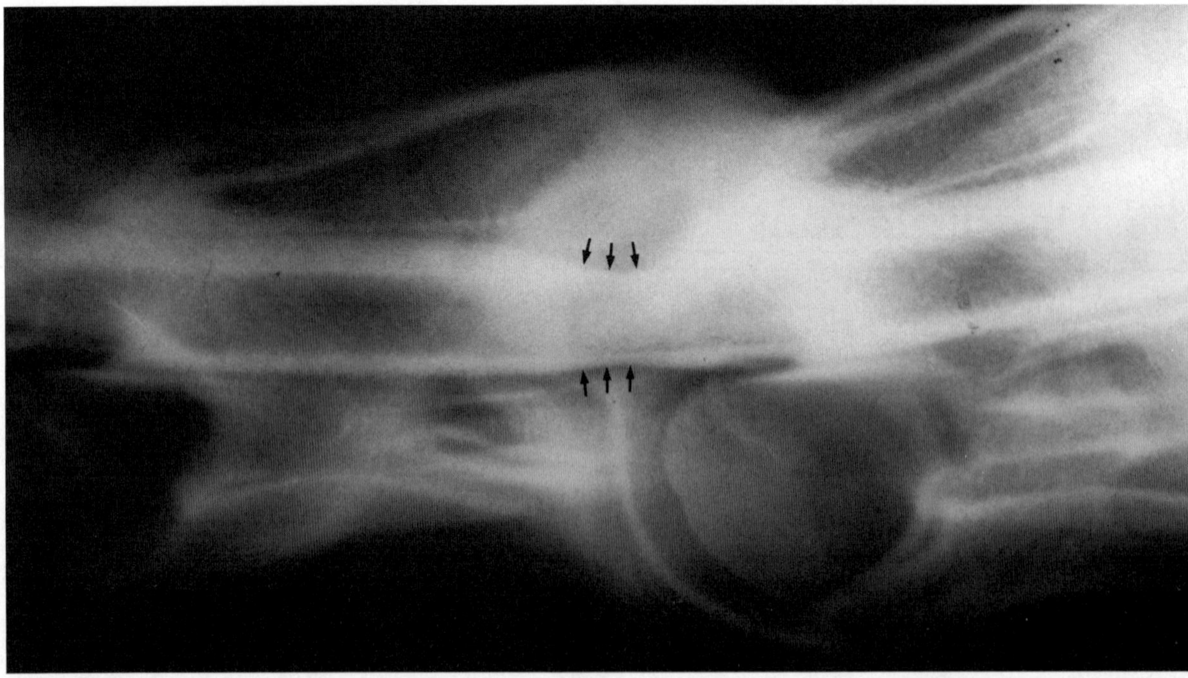

Figure 30–1. A type I lesion is demonstrated with significant compression of the dorsal dye column (*arrows*).

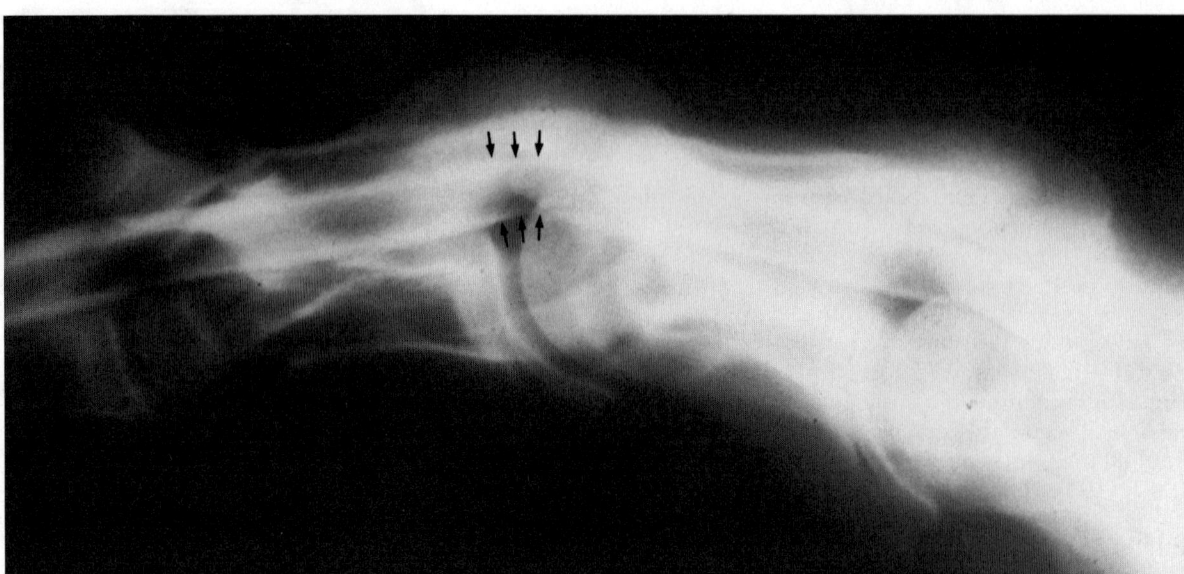

Figure 30–2. A type II lesion is demonstrated with compression of the dorsal dye column on flexion of the neck (*arrows*).

compressed by at least 50% is considered to be diagnostic. Horses that demonstrate myelographic evidence of cervical spinal cord compression in neutral, flexed, and extended lateral radiographs are suspected of having a type I lesion (Fig. 30–1). Horses with evidence of spinal cord compression of the dorsal dye column with the cervical spine held in flexion that is alleviated by repositioning the spine in a neutral position are considered to have type II lesions (Fig. 30–2).

Clarification of the specific type of lesion is important to permit selection of the correct surgical treatment. Osseous type I or static compressive cord lesions are treated by dorsal decompressive laminectomy (see Chapter 29). Type I lesions associated with soft tissue hypertrophy may be treated by either laminectomy or ventral interbody fusion. Type II lesions are best treated with cervical interbody fusion using an adaptation of the Cloward technique.

VERTEBRAL INTERBODY FUSION: SURGICAL TECHNIQUE

Following anesthetic induction, the horse is positioned in dorsal recumbency and secured with its neck in extension. The neck is supported ventrally to cause extension and straightening. The horse is prepared for aseptic surgery and draped to permit adequate access to the ventral cervical midline. A 30-cm skin incision is made on the ventral midline centered over the affected intervertebral junctions. Correct patient positioning and accurate identification of the affected level may be confirmed by preoperative lateral cervical radiographs with hypodermic needles placed in the skin as reference markers. With careful dissection and adequate hemostasis, the sternothyrohyoideus muscles are divided and retracted. Similarly, the sternocephalicus muscles are dissected free from the trachea. The trachea is mobilized and retracted to the horse's left side with the right carotid sheath, taking care to preserve the integrity of the vagosympathetic trunk, the right recurrent laryngeal nerve, and the right common carotid artery (Fig. 30–3). The ventral spinous processes of the vertebrae are identified by palpation using the preplaced skin markers and the large transverse processes of the sixth cervical vertebrae as reference points.

The paired longus coli muscles are divided on the midline and elevated from the ventral surface of the vertebral body and spinous process using a Cobb periosteal elevator. Beckman hinged self-retaining retractors or Inge self-retaining laminar retractors are adequate to maintain exposure.

The ventral spinous process is removed with either double-action bone rongeurs or an osteotome and mallet to provide a flat surface on which to locate the drill guide (Fig. 30–4). An 18-mm drill guide is positioned over the affected interbody space with the caudal surface of the guide aligned with the caudal physeal scar of the vertebra cranial to the interbody space. An 18-mm twist drill, driven either by hand using a Hudson cranial brace or by a high-torque air drill (Air Driver II; 3M Corp) is used to drill a pilot hole over the affected disk space to a premeasured depth 6 mm short of the spinal canal (Fig. 30–5). The pilot hole is then overdrilled with a 25-mm core saw or twist drill, making adjustments as needed to center the hole directly over the intervertebral disk space (Fig. 30–6). The 25-mm hole is then contoured using a rotary osteotome to level and smooth the implant hole (Fig. 30–7). Bone fragments removed from these drilling processes are cleared of disk material and saved for subsequent utilization in the stainless steel basket implant (Bagby Basket; Dr. George Bagby, Spokane, WA).

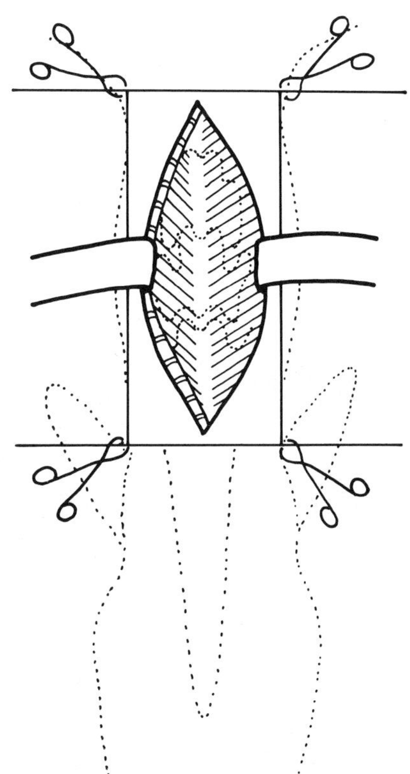

Figure 30–3. The surgical approach to the ventral midline of the neck is facilitated by the retraction of the trachea to the left side.

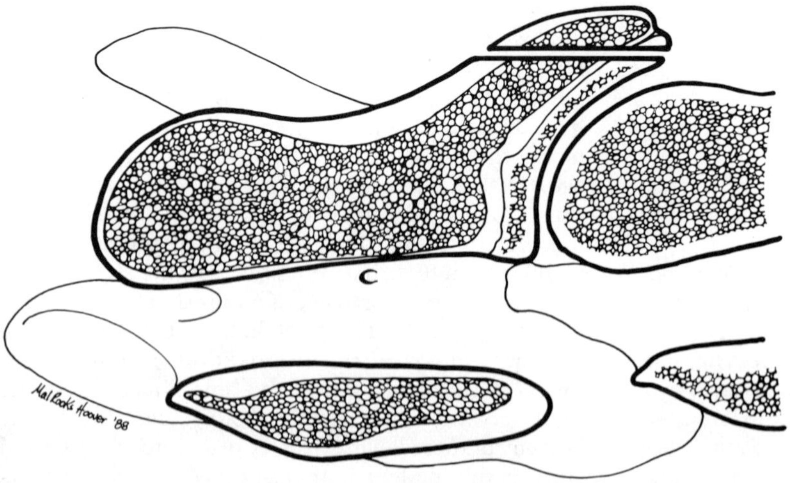

Figure 30–4. The ventral spinous process is removed to create a flat surface from which to drill the 16-mm diameter pilot hole.

The implant is packed with the autogenous mixed corticocancellous bone graft, which is harvested during the drilling procedure. The basket is then attached to an impacting instrument and driven into the intervertebral space with a mallet (Fig. 30–8). The basket remains in position by virtue of the principle of distraction-compression. The basket is the same shape as and slightly larger than the hole. When the basket is driven into the hole, the vertebrae are forced apart against the elastic constraints of the surrounding soft tissues, which normally hold the vertebrae in close apposition. These soft tissues tend to pull the vertebrae together,

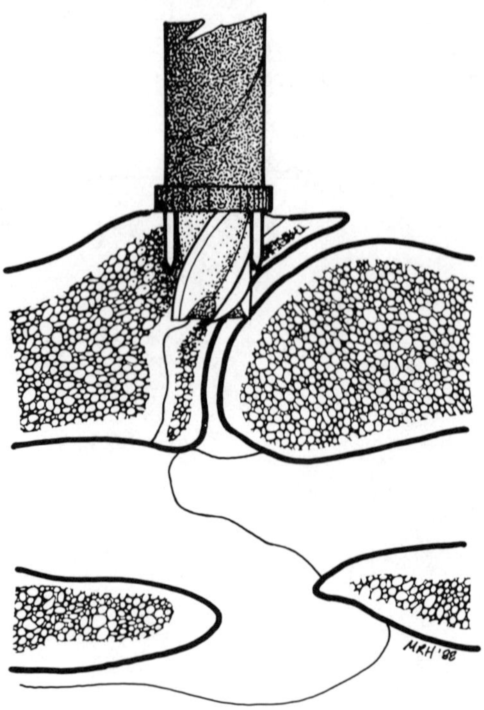

Figure 30–5. A pilot hole is drilled with the 16-mm twist drill bit centered cranial to the physeal scar.

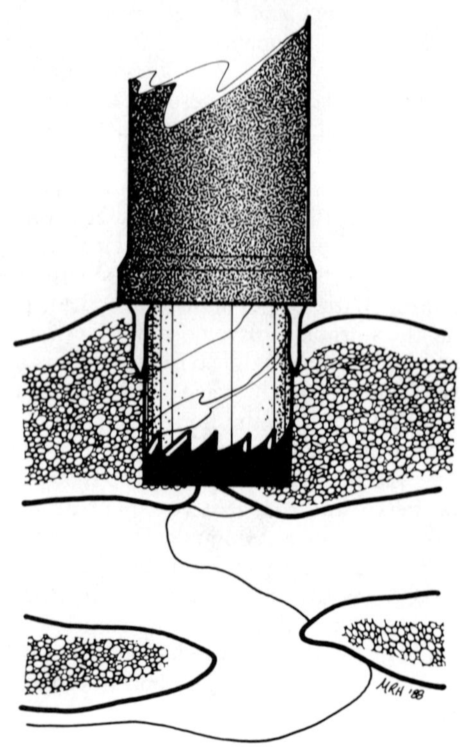

Figure 30–6. The 16-mm pilot hole is overdrilled with a 25-mm core saw.

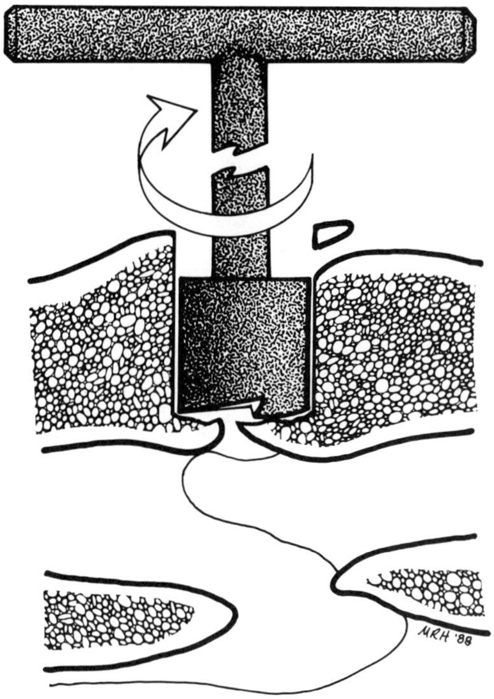

Figure 30–7. The 25-mm diameter hole is smoothed with a circular osteotome.

securing the stainless steel basket in position. The remaining corticocancellous graft material may be placed over the ventral aspect of the implant and the longus coli muscles apposed with 2–0 synthetic absorbable suture in a simple continuous pattern.

The technique of cervical interbody fusion may be modified when applied to the sixth and seventh cervical vertebrae. Implants placed in this location appear to be more likely to drift or migrate ventrally, possibly because of the naturally hyperextended position of the caudal cervical spine. To prevent ventral displacement of the stainless steel basket, a plastic spinal plate; (Lubra plate; Lubra Co) may be applied across the ventral surface of the operated interbody space and secured with cancellous bone screws to the juxtaposing vertebrae (see Chapter 29).

The incision is lavaged and then closed by apposing the sternothyrohyoideus muscles with 0 synthetic absorbable suture in simple interrupted fashion. The subcutaneous tissues are apposed with 2–0 synthetic absorbable suture in a simple continuous pattern and the skin is closed with either simple interrupted sutures of nylon or stainless steel staples. Surgical drains are not required. The incision may be covered with a stent bandage or a self adhesive elastic wrap.

POSTOPERATIVE CARE

Aftercare for postoperative patients begins in the recovery stall, where a controlled and smooth transition to a standing position is important. Affected individuals may have a difficult time standing because of the destabilizing effect of the general anesthesia superimposed on their preexisting neurologic problem. The degree of assistance may range from simply helping the horse to its feet with cautious applications of halter pressure and a tail lift to more extreme forms of assistance such as the use of a recovery sling.

Postoperative medical treatment includes the administration of broad-spectrum antibiotics and phenylbutazone (4.4 mg/kg by mouth twice daily) for 5 to 7 days following surgery. Feed and water should be elevated to the level of the patient's shoulder to minimize the need for movement of the neck. A radiographic examination is indicated to evaluate the position of the implant following recovery from anesthesia. Hyperextension of the neck may cause the implant to drift 1 to 4 mm out of its hole. Minimal amounts of drift are of no consequence. Nevertheless, a horse could theoretically displace its implant completely during a violent recovery from anesthesia.

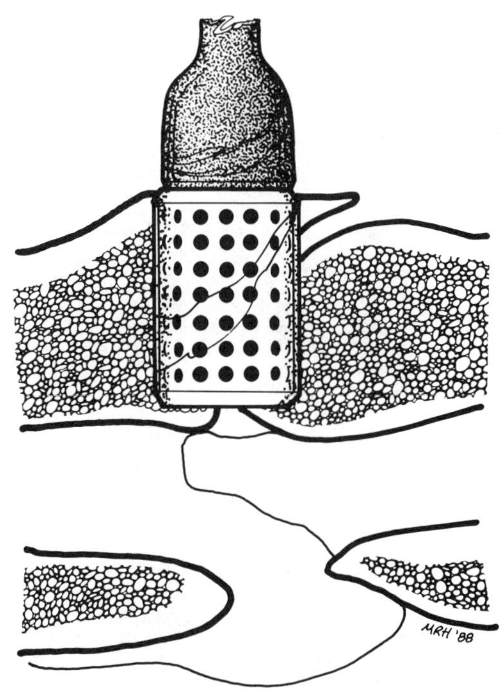

Figure 30–8. The stainless steel bone cage is packed with a mixed corticocancellous autogenous bone graft and positioned in the hole with an impacting device.

Recently, the author has encouraged the use of walking on a lead over low obstacles as a form of physical therapy. As yet, there is no objective evidence to support the suspicion that physical therapy is beneficial in the recovery of equine patients with neurologic diseases. However, it is the author's impression that controlled physical exercise and coordination exercises may be of benefit to horses affected with grades 1 and 2 neurologic deficits.

The patient should be rechecked at 3, 6, and 12 months following surgery. The operative site should be radiographed on three occasions at 2-week intervals following surgery and on the 3-month postoperative evaluation to assess the position of the implant. If there is radiographic evidence of an osseous fusion of the operated vertebrae (Fig. 30–9), the horse may be turned out for pasture exercise. Under no circumstances should the horse be tied by its halter until the vertebrae are fused, 6 to 12 months following surgery.

PROGNOSIS

The treatment of type II lesions by cervical interbody fusion is associated with a guarded to good prognosis (>50%) for returning a patient to riding soundness if the lesion is less than grade 2 in severity and operated early in the course of the disease (<3 months). The prognosis for recovery to a level of competitive athletic soundness appears to decrease with increasing severity of clinical signs and increasing duration of the condition. Although exceptions have been noted, severely affected animals (grade 4 ataxia) are often improved only to the extent that they may serve as breeding stock. Generally, the optimal response to the timely application of interbody fusion techniques is a clinical improvement of 1 to 2 grades of ataxia.

The prognosis for treatment of Type I lessions involving the fifth and sixth or sixth and seventh cervical vertebrae by interbody fusion is guarded. The degree of clinical success depends to some extent on the amount of osseous compression of the spinal cord that has developed. Although immediate decompression of the spinal cord is not an early benefit of the interbody fusion technique, cervical fusion is believed to result in size reduction of the hypertrophied dorsal longitudinal ligament and ligamentum flavum. Remodeling of the vertebral bone to effectively decompress the spinal cord may also be observed over time. Although this decompression requires time to occur, the technique of interbody fusion is generally safer than dorsal decompressive laminectomy and has been shown with chronic postoperative myelograms to effectively decompress the spinal cord.

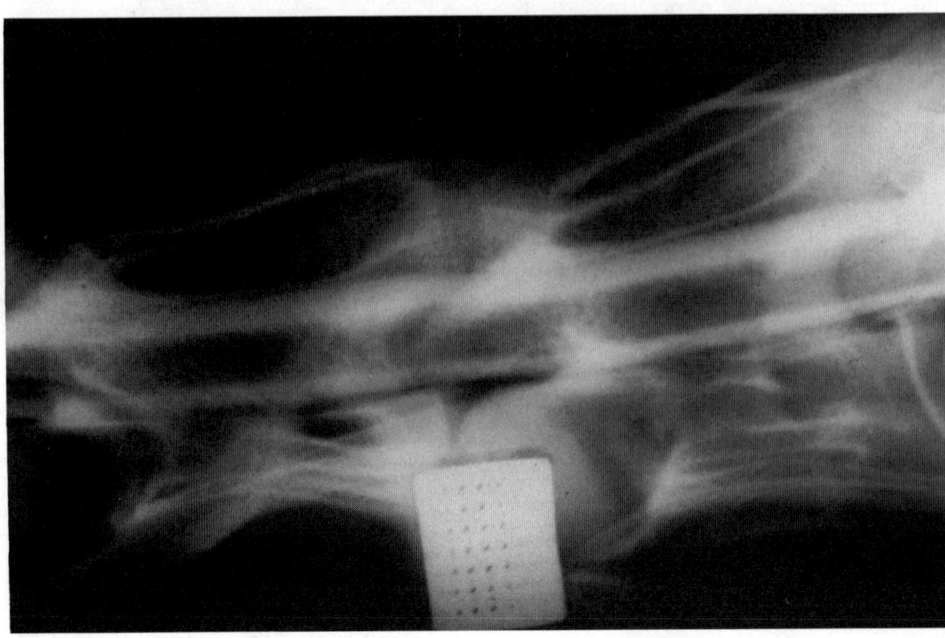

Figure 30–9. A postoperative myelogram of an affected interbody space reveals the restoration of an uncompromised dorsal dye column.

BIBLIOGRAPHY

DeBowes RM, Grant BD, Bagby GW, et al: Cervical vertebral interbody fusion in the horse: A comparative study of bovine xenografts and autographs supported by stainless steel baskets. *Am J Vet Res* 1984;45:191–199.

Grant BD, Barbee DD, Wagner PC, et al: Long term results of surgery for equine cervical vertebral malformation. *Proc Am Assoc Equine Practit* 196; pp 91–96.

Grant BD, Hoskinson JJ, Barbee DD, et al: Ventral stabilization for decompression of the caudal cervical spinal cord compression in the horse. *Proc Am Assoc Equine Practit* 1986; pp 79–90.

Mayhew IG, deLahunta A, Whitlock RH, et al: Spinal cord diseases in the horse. *Cornell Vet* 1978;68(suppl 6).

Nixon, AJ, Stashak TS: Surgical therapy for spinal cord disease in the horse. *Proc Am Assoc Equine Practit* 1986; pp 61–74.

Wagner PC, Bagby GW, Grant BD, et al: Surgical stabilization of the equine cervical spine. *J Vet Surg* 1979;8:7–12.

31
Management of Vertebral Fractures

Richard M. DeBowes

Although vertebral injuries may affect horses of any age, young horses are more commonly injured as a result of training or competitive activities. While vertebral fractures may occur at any level of the spine, clinical experience and reports in the literature suggest that the cervical spine is most commonly injured. Foals are more likely to injure the cranial cervical spine, in particular fracturing the dens (Fig. 31–1). Older horses are more likely to injure the caudal cervical spine (Fig. 31–2) and the thoracolumbar region. Hyperextension, hyperflexion, and torsional and compressive forces that are applied to the spine have been associated with the creation of these injuries. Collisions with immovable objects, failure to negotiate jumps, and serious falls are commonly reported by owners and trainers when presenting affected horses.

CLINICAL SIGNS

There are a wide variety of neurologic signs that may be evident on physical examination (Table 31–1). Some horses with severe vertebral fractures may be recumbent and tetraplegic, whereas, other individuals with seemingly similar injuries are relatively unaffected. This variation in symptomatology may be explained in at least two possible ways. It is important to recognize that the radiographic appearance of any vertebral fracture may not truly represent the degree of fragmentary displacement and resultant cord compression that occurred at the time of the injury. Second, the relatively smaller size of the spinal cord compared to the greater diameter of the vertebral canal permits some displacement of the spinal cord within the vertebral canal in response to spinal trauma. Usually, the clinical signs are related to the location of the injury. However, if the patient has been recumbent for an extended period of time, the extensive loss of condition or recumbency myopathy may make this association less distinct.

Cervical injuries are commonly accompanied by some degree of ataxia, paresis, or paralysis. When a severe injury involves the most cranial cervical vertebrae, the affected individual may be reluctant or unable to raise its head and neck. Occasionally, cranial cervical fractures with marked displacement result in acute death. More caudal cervical lesions may permit some mobility of the head but prevent the patient from rising to a standing position. Fractures involving the vertebral bodies, transverse processes, or articular processes may be associated with minimal symptomatology except some lameness or reluctance to move. Fractures of the thoracolumbar spine tend to affect the cranial thoracic (T1–3), midthoracic (T9–16), and lumbar (L1–6), regions. Fractures of the dorsal spinous processes are the most innocuous and may be accompanied only by localized swelling and pain. Fractures of the vertebral bodies that produce lesions in the spinal cord may be associated with hind limb ataxia or paraplegia. Diffuse

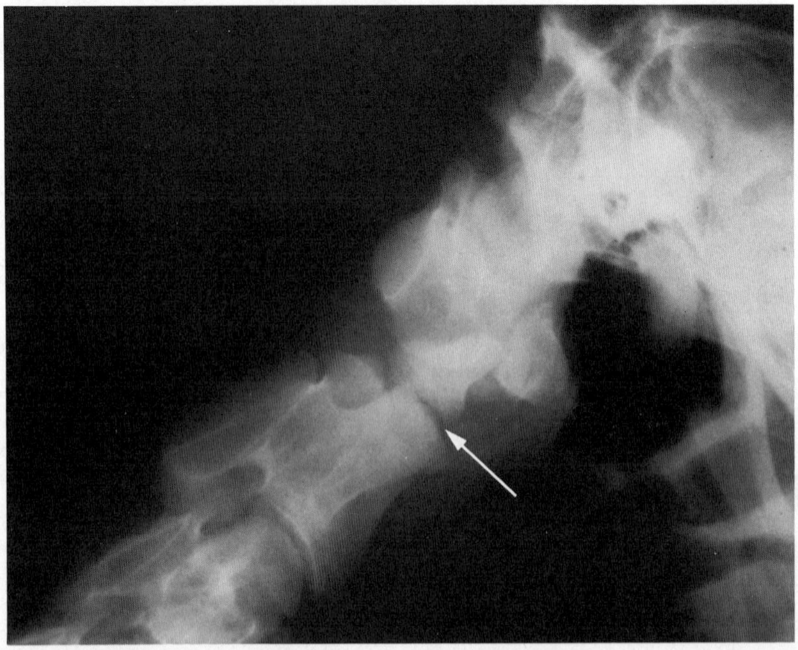

Figure 31–1. Fractured odontoid process (*arrow*) in a young foal.

sweating may be noted if the descending sympathetic tracts are affected. The Schiff-Sherrington sign is not commonly observed in horses but may be seen if anatomic or functional transection of the spinal cord occurs caudal to T2. Fractures affecting the caudal spinal segments are generally associated with injury of the cauda equina. Depending on the severity of the injury, the clinical signs may be present acutely or develop slowly over time with concomitant hemorrhage or edema. Clinical signs may include fecal and urinary incontinence, paresis/paralysis of the tail, and altered perineal sensation.

DIAGNOSIS

The diagnosis of suspected vertebral fracture or subluxation injuries should include a thorough physical ex-

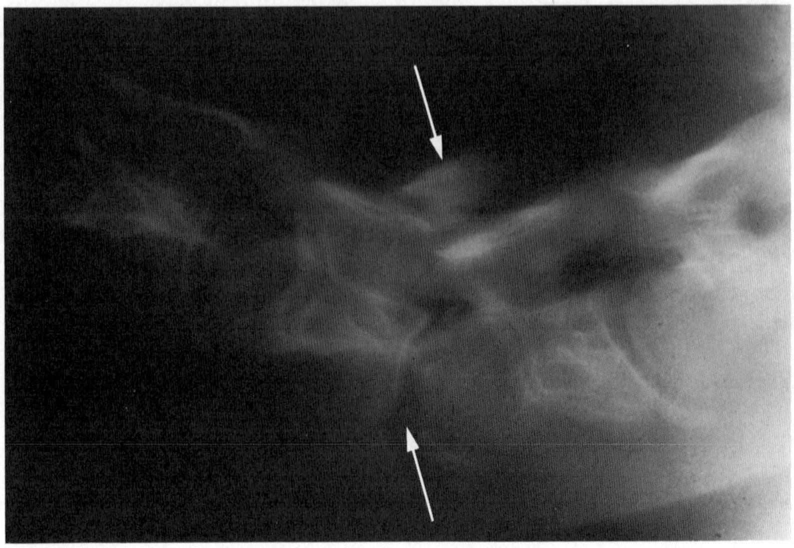

Figure 31–2. Fracture-luxation of the fifth and sixth cervical vertebrae (*arrows*).

TABLE 31–1. SIGNS, TREATMENT, AND PROGNOSIS OF VERTEBRAL FRACTURES

Location	Signs	Management	Prognosis
C1	Respiratory distress, reluctance to move, tetraparesis, tetraplegia	Conservative, lag screw, IM pins, decompression	Guarded to poor for pasture soundness (poor with severe cord compression)
C2 (dens)	Respiratory distress, tetraparesis to tetraplegia	IM pins, orthopedic wire, decompression	Guarded to poor (poor with severe cord compression)
C3-C4	Ataxia (forelimbs > hind limbs)	Modified Bagby basket, D-C plates (foal)	Guarded dependent on degree of cord compression
C5-T1	Ataxia (forelimbs = hind limbs)	Modified Bagby basket	Guarded to poor
Dorsal spinous processes	Swelling and pain ± drainage	Excision of fragments if nonresponsive to conservative therapy	Guarded to good
T2-L3	Paraparesis to paraplegia, ± Schiff-Scherrington	Wire or lag screw in dorsal facets, laminectomy for compression fractures	Guarded for facet fractures, poor for vertebral body fractures
L4-S3	Paraparesis to paraplegia, hind limb areflexia	Laminectomy for compression fractures	Guarded to poor for vertebral body fractures
Sacral-coccygeal	Urinary & fecal incontinence, ± posterior paresis	Laminectomy for decompression of acute injuries	Guarded for acute, poor for chronic

amination, a neurologic examination, and a complete historic account of the injury when available. Occasionally, a complete description of the causative trauma may direct the clinician's attention to a particular spinal segment. The physical examination should be utilized to evaluate the patient completely and attend to life-threatening medical conditions. The neurologic examination should be used to specifically localize the lesion to a particular level or segment of the spine. Detection of crepitation or palpable instability is possible in the cervical spine but considerably more difficult in other locations. Occasionally, a rectal examination may be of some benefit in examining the lumbosacral spine.

Diagnosis of vertebral fractures is facilitated by radiographic examination and occasionally myelography. Electromyographic studies may not be contributory to a diagnosis until 7 to 10 days after the injury and are not routinely performed. The collection of cerebrospinal fluid (CSF) is commonly performed in neurologic cases. Evaluation of CSF from individuals suffering from vertebral fractures may be normal. However, when abnormalities are noted, xanthochromia is the most commonly observed finding. Elevation of the protein concentration and evidence of hemorrhage in the CSF may also be observed, the latter being difficult to evaluate as being a true finding or a collection artifact. A myelogram is often necessary in cases of vertebral fracture or luxation to determine the degree of spinal cord involvement. Certainly in the cervical cord this can aid in determining which type of therapy will be instituted. The decision to decompress the cord either by treating bony or soft tissue swelling or by treating hematoma will be based on this diagnostic technique.

TREATMENT

The demonstration of a vertebral fracture with clinically detectable neurologic deficits usually indicates the need for therapeutic intervention. In those cases in which minimal displacement of vertebral fragments is evident and the neurologic signs are minimal, the horse should be treated conservatively with stall rest and medical therapy. The potential complication of fracture callus formation with resultant spinal cord compression may be dealt with by laminectomy techniques after the fracture has healed.

Surgical options available for management of equine vertebral fractures are generally limited to stabilization or decompression techniques (Table 31–1). Pins and lag screws are used to stabilize vertebral fractures in foals. Given the general size and level of activity of the horse, the author recommends the use of the dynamic self-compression bone plate whenever possible. Unfortunately, many efforts to stabilize fractured vertebrae have resulted in clinical failures because of the inability of the implants or the vertebral bone to tolerate the stresses to which they are subjected. The use of intrafragmentary compression techniques for repair of vertebral fractures applied in conjunction with vertebral interbody fusion techniques may permit the surgeon to achieve some degree of spinal stabilization. A modification of the Bagby stainless steel bone cage (Fig. 31–3) presently used for vertebral interbody fusion (see Chapter 30) may be applied across unstable interbody spaces following hyperextension trauma. Depending on the degree of neurologic compromise, concurrent application of dorsal decompression techniques may be indicated (see Chapter 29).

Most horses with neurologic compromise that have been subjected to surgical therapy will also be treated with medical therapy. Usually, the administration of anti-inflammatory agents with or without diuretics or analgesics is indicated. Therapy is directed at the control of spinal cord swelling and inflammation. Glucocorticoid therapy may be initiated with intravenous dexamethasone (0.1 to 0.2 mg/kg) every 8 hours for a series of three treatments. If improvement is noted, corticosteroid therapy may be continued with oral prednisolone (10 mg/kg). The administration of glucocorticoids has been associated with the development of laminitis, and appropriate caution and clinical monitoring should be initiated. Phenylbutazone (4.4 mg/kg) or flunixin meglumine (1.1 mg/kg) may be administered intravenously for their analgesic and anti-inflammatory effects.

If neurologic signs fail to stabilize within 4 to 6 hours of treatment, additional therapy may be warranted. The intravenous administration of osmotic diuretics such as mannitol (2 g/kg) is no longer recommended. Rather, the systemic administration of 90% medical-grade dimethyl sulfoxide has been recommended for management of spinal cord swelling and inflammation. Although controversial with respect to its true efficacy, this agent is commonly administered as a 10% solution in lactated Ringer's solution at doses not to exceed 1 g/kg. This dose is used by the author in the treatment of spinal cord injuries twice daily for a period of 3 days. The dose is subsequently reduced to once daily for an additional 3 days.

PROGNOSIS

The likelihood of successful resolution of neurologic injury attendant on vertebral fractures or subluxations is generally difficult to predict (Table 31–1). Past experience with these injuries suggests that the cases most likely to resolve are those involving the cranial cervical spine that were accompanied by minimal displacement and neurologic dysfunction. Similarly, vertebral fractures that do not involve the spinal canal or impinge on the spinal cord are likely to resolve without significant complication. In general, it has been the author's experience that the prognosis for recovery depends on the severity of the neurologic signs and the patient's response to treatment during the first 24 to 48 hours following the trauma.

BIBLIOGRAPHY

DeBowes RM, Wagner PC, Gavin PR: Vertebral compression fracture in a foal following electric shock. *J Vet Orthop* 1981;2:14–19.

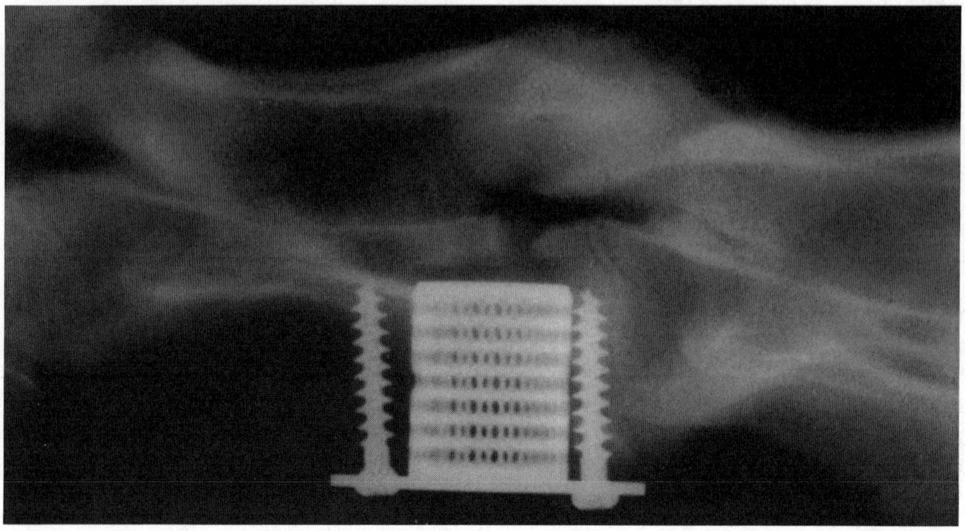

Figure 31–3. Cervical interbody fusion using a modified Bagby basket with cortical bone screws.

Jeffcott LB: Disorders of the thoracolumbar spine of the horse—a survey of 443 cases. *Equine Vet J* 1980;12:197–210.

McCoy DJ, Shires PK, Beadle R: Ventral approach for stabilization of atlantoaxial subluxation secondary to odontoid fracture in a foal. *J Am Vet Med Assoc* 1984;185:545–549.

Nixon AJ: Vertebral fractures, in Stashak TS (ed): *Adams' Lameness in the Horse*. Philadelphia, Lea & Febiger, 1987; pp 779–782.

Reed SR: Spinal trauma, in Robinson NE (ed): *Current Therapy in Equine Medicine*, ed 2. Philadelphia, WB Saunders Co, 1987; pp 374–376.

32 Corneal Lacerations

Claire A. Latimer

Corneal laceration must be considered as a potential diagnosis in any horse with a history of acute onset of ocular pain. Blunt trauma may occur through closed lids or directly to the cornea following contact with gates, trailers, whips, ropes, or airborne objects. Sharp trauma can result from contact with nails, wire, tree limbs, thorns, grooming implements, or other barn equipment.

CLINICAL FINDINGS

Clinical signs of corneal laceration vary with the depth, duration, size, and degree of contamination. All lacerations cause ocular pain manifested by blepharospasm, lacrimation, and photophobia. Partial-thickness lacerations may be accompanied by perilesional edema, secondary uveitis, and hyphema. Full-thickness lacerations are usually accompanied by iris prolapse, a shallow anterior chamber, and pupil distortion toward the wound. Aqueous humor may be leaking through full-thickness wounds if the laceration has not been temporarily sealed by uvea and/or fibrin. Hyphema and/or fibrin may partially or completely fill the anterior chamber. Severe trauma can result in expulsion of intraocular contents and partial collapse of the globe.

Complete examination of the wound is best performed with the animal under heavy sedation and regional anesthesia or under general anesthesia. Any pressure exerted on the globe by the examiner or by the patient's resistance to examination can cause further prolapse of intraocular contents and dramatically lessen the chance of a successful surgical repair.

TREATMENT

The decision to surgically repair, enucleate, or medically manage a lacerated globe depends on the intended use of the patient, prognosis for vision, estimated cost, and potential complications and their management. Clean partial-thickness lacerations have the best prognosis, whereas large full-thickness lacerations extending past the limbus with marked prolapse of intraocular contents have the worst prognosis.

Preparation for surgery includes the administration of tetanus antitoxin and a systemic nonsteroidal anti-inflammatory drug (e.g., flunixin meglumine). If the wound is full thickness, systemic antibiotics are also indicated. Samples for culture and sensitivity testing are obtained from the wound. Care must be taken not to incur further ocular damage while preparing the patient and the globe for surgery. Eyelashes and tactile hairs are cut with wet scissors and the eyelids are hand shaved to prevent contamination of the ocular surface with hair. The periocular skin is prepared routinely, and the ocular surface is irrigated with sterile saline that may contain aqueous potassium penicillin (2,000 U/mL) or dilute povidone-iodine solution (1:50). Adequate exposure is achieved using a speculum, manual eyelid retractor, or sutures placed in the eyelids. If necessary, a lateral canthotomy may be performed.

Superficial Lacerations

A superficial laceration is one that penetrates through less than one half the thickness of the cornea. If the wound is deep enough and of sufficient length, it can be sutured with a synthetic absorbable suture in a simple interrupted pattern. Wound margins are not débrided in order to maintain adequate tissue for complete closure. Wounds that involve a flap of cornea may be sutured if acute, but are débrided and treated as an ulcer if the flap is devitalized. Wounds that are superficial, chronic, or infected are best treated as ulcers. Culture and cytology should be used to direct medical management. Healing may involve vascularization and fibrosis if the wound is deep and/or infected.

Deep Lacerations

Lacerations that extend through one half or more of the corneal thickness should be sutured as soon as possible. Accurate reapposition of the wound edges will decrease both healing time and resultant scar formation.

Wound closure is achieved with 6–0 or 7–0 synthetic absorbable suture (e.g., polyglactin 910; Ethicon Inc) swaged on a micropoint spatula needle in a simple interrupted and/or horizontal mattress pattern. Sutures are placed approximately 2 mm apart and 2 to 4 mm from the wound margin depending on the degree of edema. If tissue has been avulsed or the wound margins are necrotic, a combination of direct closure with a conjunctival flap may be necessary. Some degree of vascularization and scarring can be expected during healing, but this will subside following suture removal and subsequent corneal remodeling.

Full-Thickness Lacerations

In most instances, the full extent of a penetrating injury can only be appreciated during surgical exploration. The fibrin clot is teased off the wound with forceps and a cyclodialysis spatula until prolapsed uvea and the wound margins can be identified. If the uvea has been prolapsed for any length of time or is traumatized, necrotic, or not easily reduced, it is excised at the level of the cornea using scissors or electrocautery. The wound margins are freed of fibrin, adherent uvea, and clotted blood. Blood and fibrin clots may be gently irrigated from the anterior chamber or engaged with a blunt iris hook and removed. If the lens is displaced or its capsule ruptured, it is removed at this time. The wound margins are accurately reapposed using preplaced simple interrupted or horizontal mattress sutures of 6–0 or 7–0 synthetic absorbable material. An iris repositor or cyclodialysis spatula may be used to prevent incarceration of uvea in the wound as the sutures are tied. Additional simple interrupted sutures may be necessary for optimum reapposition of the wound margins. The anterior chamber is reformed with balanced salt solution or lactated Ringer's solution plus an air bubble to inhibit iridocorneal contact. These are introduced via the wound or through the limbus using a 25- or 26-gauge needle or cannula.

If the amount of prolapsed uvea is small and the wound is acute and uncontaminated, the uvea may be repositioned in the anterior chamber. In this instance, sutures may be preplaced before collapsing the anterior chamber.

When the laceration extends to the limbus, the adjacent conjunctiva is elevated and the sclera inspected. Chemosis and subconjunctival hemorrhage can obscure a scleral laceration. If the laceration crosses the limbus, the first suture is placed in the limbus to ensure accurate realignment.

If the anterior chamber cannot be reformed after suturing the wound margins because of loss of corneal tissue, a conjunctival flap may be placed over the sutured wound to facilitate closure and healing.

Healing will generally involve vascularization of the wound and scarring. The final outcome will be known only after suture removal, and several months of corneal remodeling. Sutures are removed at 10 to 21 days depending on the degree of healing and adverse response to the suture material.

POSTOPERATIVE CARE

The goals of medical management are to prevent or control infection and to control the secondary uveitis that always accompanies a full-thickness laceration. Systemic antibiotics are continued for at least 5 days after surgery. Topical antibiotics are selected on the basis of culture results or to cover the spectrum of known pathogens in the horse. Most gram-positive isolates are sensitive to cephalothin, chloramphenicol, erythromycin, and carbenicillin. Gram-negative isolates are usually sensitive to polymyxin B, tobramycin, and gentamicin.

Systemic nonsteroidal anti-inflammatory drugs are used to improve patient comfort and to control uveitis. Flunixin meglumine appears to be the most effective of the nonsteroidal drugs in relieving acute ocular discomfort and inflammation. After administration of flunixin meglumine at 1.1 mg/kg for 3 to 5 days, the dosage may be tapered to alternate days or the patient switched to phenylbutazone or aspirin. Anti-inflammatory drugs may be necessary over a prolonged period to control uveal inflammation. Aspirin has been advocated for this long-term management at a dose of 25 mg/kg for 30 to 60 days, then 30 mg/kg daily for as long as necessary.

Atropine (1% atropine ophthalmic solution or ointment) is used topically to achieve and maintain mydriasis and to improve patient comfort by relieving ciliary spasm. Atropine also decreases the outpouring of protein and inflammatory cells into the aqueous humor by restoring the permeability of uveal vessels toward normal.

PROGNOSIS

The major determinant of prognosis is the severity of the injury. Severity is evaluated on the basis of wound size, location, and configuration as well as amount of uveal and lens involvement and presence of sepsis, gross contamination, or necrosis. Lacerations involving only the cornea have a better prognosis than those involving cornea and sclera. Wounds caused by sharp trauma are usually more isolated and manageable than those caused by blunt trauma. Blunt trauma is typically associated with greater damage to intraocular structures.

Duration of the wound is of less importance than the severity of the injury, but delayed treatment increases the chance of intraocular infection. Intraocular inflammatory processes also become established, and after 36 hours progressive intraocular organization and fibrosis may lead to irreversible damage. While there are eyes that have been successfully repaired 5 to 7 days after injury, there are also many that present in this time frame with complicating factors that preclude successful repair.

Clinical signs that imply severe ocular damage and thus a grave prognosis are severe or continuous hemorrhage; lens rupture, dislocation, or expulsion; vitreous humor prolapse; or massive prolapse of intraocular contents with partial collapse of the globe. Surgical alternatives for these patients include enucleation and intraocular prosthesis. An intraocular prosthesis placed through a wound in the cornea has a higher risk of dehiscence as a result of corneal compromise than when placed through a planned scleral incision. Primary wound repair may also be performed with the knowledge that phthisis bulbi will likely result. This retains the option of a shell prosthesis fit to the phthisical globe for improved cosmesis.

A number of complications can occur following primary repair of corneal lacerations. *Corneal scarring* with vascularization and fibrosis is expected, but may compromise vision more than anticipated. Persistent *corneal edema* can result from endothelial damage or ongoing inflammation. Supportive treatment with saline ointment and a topical corticosteroid may be beneficial. *Synechia* formation is also a common sequela to surgery. When posterior synechia are present, *cataract* formation may result. Cataracts may also result from alterations of the aqueous humor as a result of inflammatory products, toxins, and infection. Unidentified laceration of the lens capsule can also result in cataract formation and *lens-induced uveitis. Retinal detachment* can result from rapid decompression of the globe at the time of injury or subsequent organization of inflammatory debris in the vitreous cavity. *Retinal atrophy* may occur over time, particularly following blunt trauma. *Phthisis bulbi* will result if uveal damage is severe or subsequent uveitis is uncontrolled. *Wound dehiscence* and infectious *endophthalmitis* or keratitis are more immediate but equally devastating complications.

BIBLIOGRAPHY

Lavach JD: *The Handbook of Equine Ophthalmology.* Fort Collins, Co, Giddings Studio Publishing, 1987.

Lavach JD, Severin GA, Roberts SM: Lacerations of the equine eye: A review of 48 cases. *J Am Vet Med Assoc* 1984;184:1243–1248.

McLaughlin SA, Brightman AH, Helper LC, Manning JP, Tomes JE: Pathogenic bacteria and fungi associated with extraocular disease in the horse. *J Am Vet Med Assoc* 1983;182:241–242.

Moore CP, Heller N, Majors LJ, Whitley RD, Burgess EC, Weber J: Prevalence of ocular microorganisms in hospitalized and stabled horses. *Am J Vet Res* 1988;49:773–777.

33 Deep Stromal and Perforating Corneal Ulcers

Claire A. Latimer

A deep stromal corneal ulcer is one in which epithelium and more than one half of the stroma are lost. A deep stromal ulcer can rapidly progress to a descemetocele in which only one cell layer (corneal endothelium) and its basement membrane (Descemet's membrane) retain ocular integrity. Deep stromal ulcers and descemetoceles may perforate, producing a corneal defect that is plugged by fibrin (plasmoid aqueous humor), uvea, or, less commonly, lens or vitreous humor.

A number of factors can promote rapid progression of corneal ulceration after an initial traumatic incident. Loss of epithelial integrity allows infection by opportunistic microorganisms. These microorganisms may cause liquefactive necrosis of the cornea through release of proteolytic enzymes. Further destruction of corneal ground substance and collagen lamellae may be caused by proteases and collagenases produced by corneal epithelial cells, keratocytes, and polymorphonuclear leukocytes. Thus, corneal liquefaction can continue after the elimination of viable bacteria. Keratomalacia and sloughing of necrotic cornea may occur more rapidly than corneal healing, resulting in corneal rupture. Corticosteroids potentiate both infection and enzymatic activity, thus further compromising healing. Corneal exposure due to inadequate spreading or production of the precorneal tearfilm will also impair healing.

CLINICAL FINDINGS

Deep stromal ulcers present with an obvious defect in the corneal surface. The remaining stroma will stain positive with fluorescein and the perilesional cornea is usually edematous and infiltrated with cells. Keratomalacia may develop and is recognized by the gelatinous appearance of the involved cornea. The affected cornea may actually slide ventrally and overhang the peripheral cornea and lid margins. Corneal vascularization may be noted at the limbus within 1 to 5 days of injury. Rapidly progressive keratomalatic corneal ulcers are often accompanied by a secondary anterior uveitis. Hypopyon and fibrin may be present in the ventral anterior chamber, but these are a response to local chemotactic and inflammatory factors and do not usually represent intraocular infection. Pain is variable and dependent on the degree of secondary anterior uveitis and depth of the ulcer. The more superficial the ulcer, the more pain is typically manifest.

Descemetoceles have similar clinical signs but the deepest aspect of the ulcer has a clear, glassy appearance and does not retain fluorescein. The corneal defect in perforated ulcers is typically filled with fibrin and incarcerated uvea, which may protrude above the surface of the cornea. The protruding uvea is usually covered by a layer of fibrin that imparts a glistening grey or yellow-green cast to the uvea. The anterior chamber may be collapsed, with apposition of the intraocular iris to the corneal endothelium, or formed, with anterior displacement of iris adjacent to the perforation. Hyphema, hypopyon, and plasmoid aqueous humor may obscure all intraocular structures.

Surgery is indicated when deep stromal ulcers progress despite aggressive medical management, particularly when keratomalacia is present. Descemetoceles of any size and corneal perforations also require surgery in almost every instance. Because it is always preferable to operate on an intact globe, surgical intervention must be prompt.

MANAGEMENT

The goals of combined medical and surgical management are to: (*a*) identify, remove, and treat the inciting etiology and or complicating factors; (*b*) create an ideal environment for healing; and (*c*) prevent progression of the lesion. This latter goal includes surgical intervention to prevent or repair corneal rupture. In assessing the degree of ocular damage, pressure on the globe must be avoided to prevent iatrogenic rupture or further expulsion of intraocular contents. In most patients, the preoperative examination must be performed under sedation or general anesthesia. Systemic antibiotics, flunixin meglumine, and tetanus antitoxin are often administered preoperatively.

Specimens for culture and sensitivity and cytologic evaluations should be obtained before the surgical preparation begins. Débridement of necrotic cornea may provide additional specimens for histopathology. Information obtained from these evaluations will guide postoperative medical management.

Preparations for aseptic surgery are routine. Special care must be taken not to introduce hair or other foreign material onto the ocular surface. The lids may be hand shaved with a scalpel blade, surgical razor, or straight-edged razor blade and the vibrissae clipped with wet scissors. Sterile atropine and broad-spectrum antibiotic solutions may be instilled at the end of the surgical prep if the cornea has not been ruptured.

Direct Suturing

Direct suturing of descemetoceles and perforated ulcers is possible provided that the lesion is no greater than 5 mm in diameter and the surrounding cornea is healthy enough to retain sutures. If the viability of the surrounding cornea is questionable, a conjunctival flap may be placed over the sutured lesion to lessen the risks associated with dehiscence.

Débridement of the ulcer margins is usually minimal because this procedure is reserved for relatively "clean" lesions. Sutures are preplaced at three-quarters corneal depth in a simple interrupted horizontal mattress pattern using 6–0 or 7–0 absorbable suture (e.g., polyglactin 910; Ethicon Inc). If the globe is intact, closure of sutures should be done over 3 to 5 minutes to allow aqueous humor to exit from the anterior chamber. Additional simple interrupted sutures may be necessary for accurate closure. Postoperatively the cornea will be flattened but the distorted curvature will normalize over time.

When the ulcer has perforated, prolapsed devitalized uvea is excised using electrocautery or scissors. It is preferable to preplace sutures before excising incarcerated uvea and fibrin because the anterior chamber will collapse and more uvea will usually present in the perforation site. An iris repositor may be used to keep iris away from ulcer margins as each suture is tied. The anterior chamber is reformed using sterile balanced salt solution, or lactated Ringer's solution plus an air bubble to inhibit iridocorneal contact. These are introduced via the wound or limbus using a 25- or 26-gauge needle or air-injection cannula.

Conjunctival Flap

The conjunctival flap has many advantages as a graft of healthy fibrovascular tissue directly to the ulcer. The flap provides structural support and a source of fibroblasts to help fill the stromal defect. Flaps provide a blood supply to the healing ulcer and, with it, direct access to systemic antibiotics and serum that has anticollagenase, antiprotease, and antimicrobial activity. Conjunctival flaps are indicated for deep stromal ulcers that deteriorate despite appropriate medical management. They are also appropriate for descemetoceles that are unsuitable for direct suturing or corneal grafting because of ulcer size or keratomalacia of the surrounding cornea (Fig. 33–1). Conjunctival flaps can also be used for corneal perforations, either in addition to direct suturing or as the sole reparative procedure.

A sliding fornix-based conjunctival flap can usually be mobilized adequately to cover even large ulcers (Fig. 33–2). The ulcer bed should be débrided of necrotic tissue before flap placement. If the flap is to be placed over a perforation, it is best not to amputate prolapsed uvea and deflate the anterior chamber, because a tight seal of conjunctiva to cornea may then be difficult to obtain.

The conjunctival incision is made parallel to the closest limbus. The conjunctiva is elevated 2 to 3 mm from the limbus and incised with blunt tenotomy scissors. Blunt dissection is continued toward the fornix and to either side, carefully freeing conjunctiva from Tenon's capsule. The incision is extended along the limbus and the procedure repeated until adequate conjunctiva has been mobilized to cover the lesion without undue tension. Conjunctiva is then sutured to the cornea such that even tension is applied over the lesion. Sutures of 6–0 or 7–0 absorbable suture material are placed through conjunctiva and one-half thickness through the cornea. Sutures may be placed at the limbus to minimize tension on the graft.

If the conjunctiva cannot be mobilized sufficiently using the above technique, a 360-degree flap may be done. The same dissection technique is employed around the entire limbus. The conjunctiva is then closed using a continuous or simple interrupted mattress pattern of 6–0 absorbable suture material.

Conjunctival grafts adhere to the ulcer site but not to epithelialized cornea. Sutures are removed in 7 to 14 days. Those in 360-degree flaps are best left for 14 days. The flap should be left in place for 2 to 3 months. At that time the cosmetic appearance of the healed ulcer may be improved by cutting the conjunctiva free peripheral to the area of corneal adherence. This can usually be achieved with tranquilization and/or an auriculopalpebral nerve block plus topical anesthesia. The island of adhered conjunctiva will remodel into a smooth corneal leukoma and the released conjunctiva will retract and reattach at the limbus. There is no advantage to cutting the flap free early, and in cases in which the initial lesion was very deep and/or large it may be safer to leave the pedicle attached.

Complications are usually due to inadequate dissection (resulting in incorporation of Tenon's capsule or excessive tension) or improper suture placement. Either may result in premature contracture of the flap.

CORNEAL SCLERAL CONJUNCTIVAL TRANSPOSITION

A lamellar graft of cornea, limbal sclera, and adjacent conjunctiva can be used to repair a partial- or full-thickness corneal defect provided there is adequate healthy cornea peripheral to the lesion. The thickness of the grafted cornea is desirable to restore corneal integrity, and the visual impairment associated with scarring and vascularization of deep lesions may be lessened by this technique. The lack of blood supply makes the transposed cornea vulnerable to the enzymatic and infectious processes of degradation present in the ulcerated cornea. A vascular graft (i.e., conjunctival flap) may be preferable when keratomalacia and rapid deterioration are features of the ulcer.

Two moderately divergent midstromal incisions are made with a blade encompassing the lesion and extending to the limbus. A third incision joins these at their origin. The perilesional and healthy cornea are then dissected toward the limbus in the midstromal plane (half the thickness of the cornea) using a blade or corneal dissector. Dissection is continued through the limbal sclera and beneath the conjunctiva. The conjunctiva is mobilized adequately to allow the attached cornea to be advanced into the prepared ulcer bed. The perilesional cornea is cut from the end of the graft and may be submitted for culture and histopathology. Healthy transposed cornea is then sutured into the ulcer bed with 6–0 or 7–0 absorbable material in a simple interrupted or simple continuous pattern. Additional sutures secure the graft along its course to the limbus.

The complications of dehiscence and erosion of the graft by enzymatic and infectious processes can be minimized by careful patient selection and appropriate postoperative care. Eventual scarring and pigmentation of the transposed cornea may occur.

Corneal Transplant

Lamellar and full-thickness free grafts may be considered when adequate donor tissue and a skilled surgeon are available. Partial-thickness donor cornea may be obtained from the affected or normal eye of the patient. Because the majority of ulcers requiring surgical management in the horse are malatic and infected, free transplants are rarely the procedure of choice.

Tissue Adhesive

Cyanoacrylate tissue adhesive has been used successfully to manage corneal ulcers, perforations, and lacerations in small animals. Among the potential benefits of tissue adhesives is their apparent ability to arrest stro-

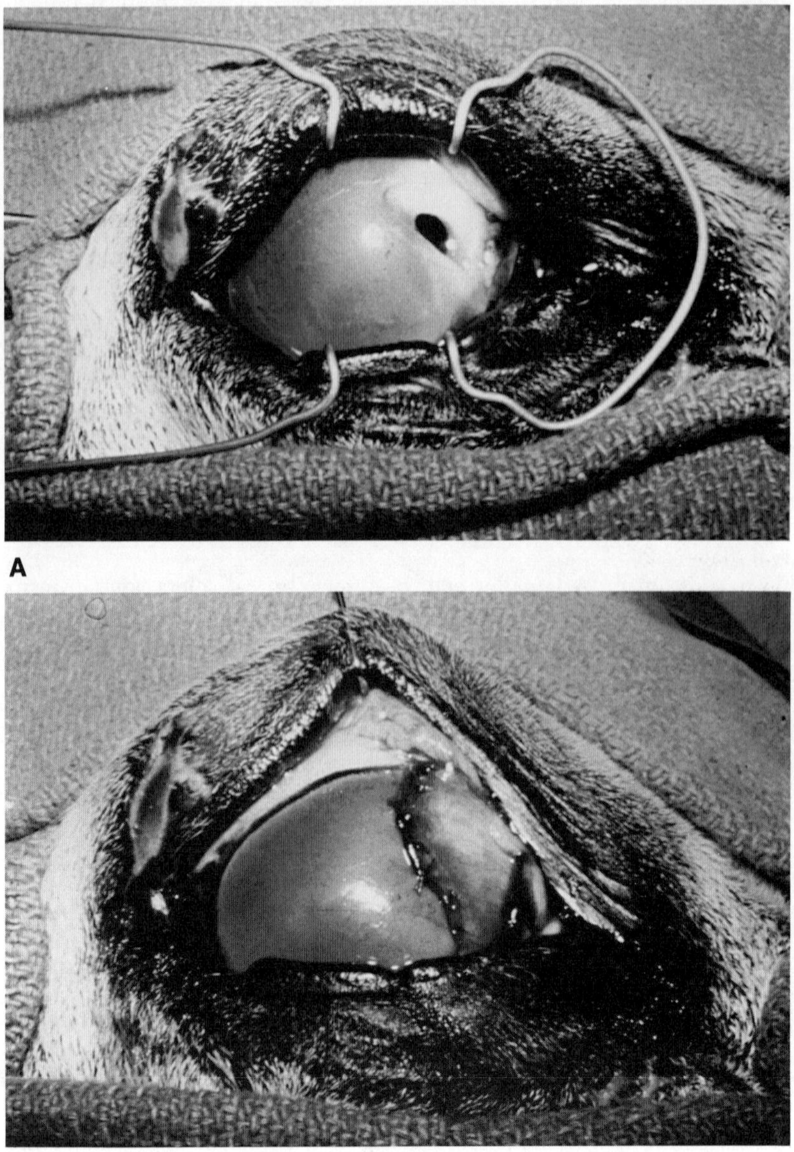

A

B

Figure 33–1. Immediate preoperative (**A**) and postoperative (**B**) appearance of a conjunctival flap used to repair a large descemetocele with significant infiltration and edema of the perilesional stroma. Vision was maintained after healing of the defect.

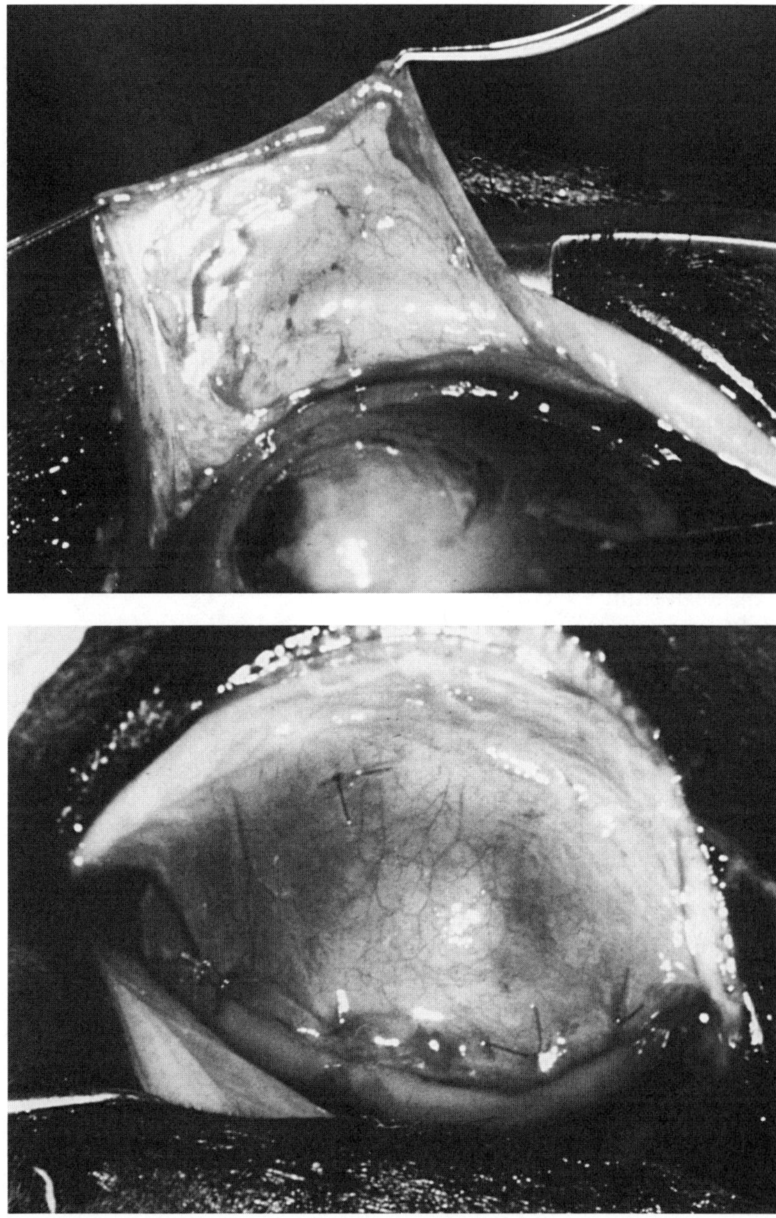

A

B

Figure 33–2. Intraoperative (**A**) and postoperative (**B**) appearance of a fornix-based conjunctival flap used to manage a large, axial, mycotic corneal ulcer. The flap was ultimately adherent only to the ulcer bed and vision was preserved.

mal melting. The adhesive excludes polymorphonuclear cells in tears, thus protecting stroma from their collagenolytic and proteolytic activity. To date, successful use of tissue adhesives for deep stromal or perforating corneal lesions in the horse has not been reported.

POSTOPERATIVE CARE

Postoperative patient management strives to create an ideal environment for healing. Therapy is guided by cytology, culture, and histopathologic results augmented by repeated clinical observations and knowledge of common complicating factors.

Systemic nonsteroidal anti-inflammatory drugs are used to relieve patient discomfort, thus minimizing blepharospasm and facilitating administration of topical medications. Anti-inflammatory agents also help control secondary anterior uveitis. Clinical observations suggest that these anti-inflammatory agents may enhance keratomalacia; thus they must be used with caution and supervision in patients with infection and/or enzymatic degradation of the cornea.

Topical antibiotics are selected on the basis of culture and sensitivity results. When preoperative cultures are uninformative, selection is based on the clinician's knowledge of the most commonly observed pathogens. Although pathogens may vary by region, *Streptoccus*, *Staphylococcus*, *Pseudomonas*, and *Aspergillus* species should always be considered. Most gram-positive isolates are sensitive to cephalothin, chloramphenicol, erythromycin, and carbenicillin. Gram-negative isolates are usually sensitive to polymyxin B, tobramycin, and gentamicin. Systemic antibiotics may be helpful in the initial postoperative period for infectious ulcers covered with a conjunctival flap.

Inhibition of proteolytic enzymes can be achieved by topical administration of 5 to 10% acetylcysteine diluted with an artificial tear compound. This preparation should be kept refrigerated. Serum may also be used to inhibit proteolytic enzymes. The antiproteolytic enzyme activity of serum has been attributed to an α_2 macroglobulin. Experimental inhibition of the proteoglycanases of lysosomal lysates has been achieved with serum but not with cysteine. This may indicate that serum is necessary to inhibit the proteases released by polymorphonuclear cells. Patients with conjunctival flaps do not need these medications. Patients with nonvascular grafts or ulcers closed by direct suturing may benefit from the use of antiproteolytic medication.

Atropine is used to help preserve the pupillary aperture and to improve patient comfort by reversing ciliary spasm and miosis. It also tends to restore the permeability of inflamed uveal vessels toward normal, thus decreasing the outpouring of protein and inflammatory cells into the aqueous humor.

PROGNOSIS

Prognosis depends on the severity of the original lesion, efficacy of the surgical repair, and control of postoperative complications. Perforating lesions always carry a guarded prognosis for vision, and in some patients maintenance of a cosmetic globe is the best result that can be achieved. Small perforations sealed by fibrin and uvea with a formed anterior chamber carry the best prognosis, whereas large lesions, extensive keratomalacia, and active hemorrhage all lessen the chance of a successful outcome. Severe secondary iridocyclitis or uveal damage may result in synechia, cataract, or phthisis bulbi.

Nonperforating lesions carry a better prognosis for maintenance of a cosmetic globe. Vision will depend on the extent and location of the lesion and the degree of secondary uveitis. All deep stromal ulcers will heal with some degree of vascularization and fibrosis. The resulting scar will fade with time. Secondary uveitis can result in synechia and cataract formation, but these changes do not usually become significant in adequately managed nonperforating lesions.

BIBLIOGRAPHY

Lavach JD: *The Handbook of Equine Ophthalmology.* Fort Collins, CO, Giddings Studio Publishing, 1987.

McLaughlin SA, Brightman AH, Helper LC, Manning JP, Tomes JE: Pathogenic bacteria and fungi associated with extraocular disease in the horse. *J Am Vet Med Assoc* 1983;182:241–242.

Moore CP, Fales WH, Whittington P, Bauer L: Bacterial and fungal isolates for Equidae with ulcerative keratitis. *J Am Vet Med Assoc* 1983;182:600–603.

Peruccio C, Bosio P, Cornaglia E: Indications and limits of the cyanoacrylate tissue adhesive in corneal ulcers and perforations, in *Proceedings of the Fourteenth Annual Scientific Program of the American College of Veterinary Ophthalmologists,* 1983, pp 135–153.

Wyman M: Ophthalmic surgery for the practitioner. *Vet Clin North Am Small Anim Pract* 1979;9:311–348.

34 Glaucoma

Claire A. Latimer

Glaucoma is either rare or infrequently recognized in the horse. It is most often seen in association with or as a sequel to iridocyclitis, or in association with multiple congenital ocular anomalies. Despite the relative frequency of extensive anterior and posterior synechiae and deposition of inflammatory debris in the iridocorneal angle of horses with recurrent uveitis, secondary pressure elevations appear to be rare. Significant aqueous humor outflow via unconventional routes (uveosclera and uveovortex) may account for this apparent species resistance to secondary glaucoma.

CLINICAL FINDINGS

The most consistent clinical signs associated with glaucoma are mild buphthalmia, corneal edema, and corneal scarring and/or vascularization. Other clinical signs include corneal striae, lens luxation or subluxation, cataract, dilated or fixed midrange pupil, retinal and/or optic atrophy, retinal detachment, and uveitis. Pain is variable and may be manifest as lacrimation, blepharospasm, photophobia, or personality change.

DIAGNOSIS

Definitive diagnosis of glaucoma is made by tonometry. Mean intraocular pressure obtained following topical anesthesia has been reported as 28.6 mm Hg using a Mackay-Marg applanation tonometer. The use of acetylpromazine or xylazine to facilitate examination has been demonstrated to lower recorded values by an average of 6.2 mm Hg (20%) and 7.9 mm Hg (27%), respectively.

MANAGEMENT

The response to medical management of glaucoma is variable, unpredictable, and generally poor. When active uveitis is present, the inclusion of a systemic nonsteroidal anti-inflammatory drug and a topical corticosteroid in the treatment plan is generally beneficial. Parasympathomimetic, sympathomimetic, and β-antagonist drugs have all been utilized in an attempt to lower intraocular pressure.

Surgical procedures used to manage glaucoma in the horse are dictated by clinical signs, vision, intended use of the horse, and economic concerns. A sighted, glaucomatous eye in a performance horse presents a different treatment goal from that of a blind, painful glaucomatous eye in an aged broodmare.

Cyclocryotherapy

Cyclocryotherapy is the application of intense cold through the sclera and bulbar conjunctiva to the ciliary body with the intent of lowering aqueous humor production. The desired effect is thought to result from selective destruction of the secretory epithelial layer of the ciliary processes or alterations in capillary blood flow within these processes.

This technique is indicated when intraocular pressure cannot be controlled medically in a sighted eye. It may be preferable to other forms of surgical management when cosmesis is a major goal of therapy. It is also preferable to other forms of surgical management in that it is noninvasive, less expensive, repeatable, and technically easier.

The technique used in the horse has followed after that used in the dog. Liquid nitrogen and nitrous oxide are the cryogens of choice. Nitrous oxide is preferred by many surgeons because of its ease of storage and handling, its availability, and the wide variety of cryoprobe tips available for use with nitrous oxide units. A cryoprobe with an incorporated thermocouple to monitor tip temperature is ideal. A ciliary body temperature of −10 to −13 °C is adequate to produce hypotony in dogs. Nitrous oxide systems achieve this ciliary body temperature after 2 minutes at a cryoprobe tip temperature of −70 to −80 °C using a 2.5- to 3-mm probe tip. Liquid nitrogen systems with a 2.5 × 6.5 × 58–mm brass probe tip at −185 °C achieve this ciliary body temperature after 15 to 25 seconds, or when the edge of the resultant iceball extends 1 mm into clear cornea.

Following the induction of general anesthesia, the cryoprobe is positioned over the ciliary body, approximately 5 to 6 mm posterior to the limbus (Fig. 34–1). A rapid-freeze/slow-thaw cycle is carried out at each of three to eight sites depending on the size of the cryoprobe tip and the degree of pressure elevation. The long posterior ciliary arteries at 3:00 and 9:00 are avoided, and the freeze sites are preferably confined to the inferotemporal quadrant to avoid inadvertent damage to the peripheral retina with subsequent detachment.

Immediate postoperative therapy is directed at control of the resultant chemosis, conjunctivitis, and uveitis. Flunixin meglumine (1.1 mg/kg) should be administered preoperatively and for 3 to 7 days postoperatively as dictated by clinical signs. A topical ophthalmic corticosteroid should be administered four times daily postoperatively until clinical signs of inflammation abate. A transient rise in intraocular pressure occurs in a significant percentage of dogs postoperatively, and a similar rise has been noted in a few of the horses observed by the author. In these patients, postoperative medical management should include any drugs previously shown to lower intraocular pressure in that individual. If no drugs have been effective, a β-antagonist might be the best choice because it will not aggravate the uveitis as will some of the miotics.

The long-term prognosis for horses following cyclocryotherapy is unknown because of limited experience with the technique. The opportunity to maintain vi-

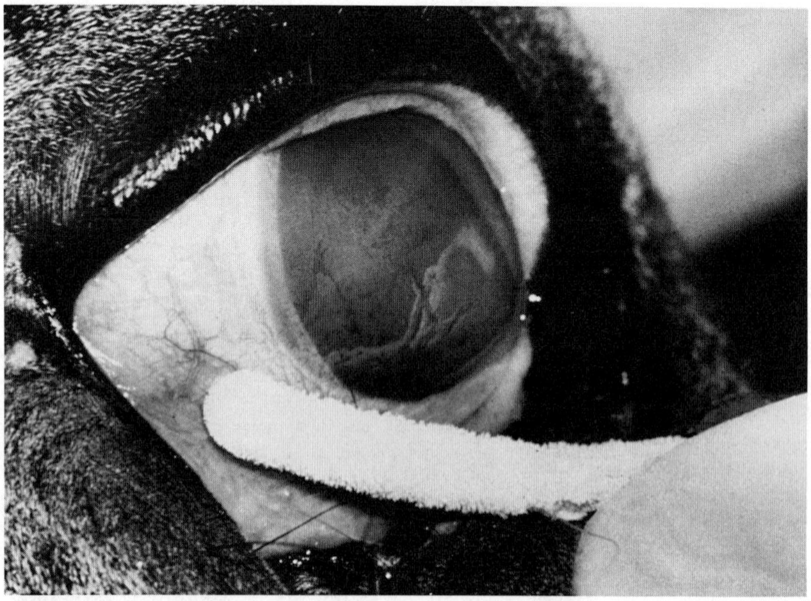

Figure 34–1. A cryoprobe in position over the ciliary body at the 8:00 position on a glaucomatous eye.

sion and cosmesis makes this technique attractive as compared to other surgical procedures. The most frequent complication observed to date has been a lack of therapeutic effect. Phthisis bulbi and retinal and choroidal detachments have been reported in the dog as major postoperative complications but have not been observed to date in the horse.

Intraocular Prosthesis

An intraocular prosthesis is a cosmetic alternative to enucleation in patients unresponsive to previous medical and surgical therapy. A silicone sphere (Jardon Plastics Research Corp) is placed within the corneoscleral shell following evisceration of intraocular contents through a scleral incision. The procedure provides definitive relief of patient discomfort, and following a somewhat prolonged postoperative course, the resultant globe is maintenance free.

An intraocular prosthesis is contraindicated in the presence of intraocular neoplasia, septic endophthalmitis, or panophthalmitis. When neoplasia cannot be ruled out by ophthalmic examination because of cloudy ocular media, ultrasonography may be helpful. Corneal damage, including endothelial cell loss and damage due to chronic pressure elevation, is also cause for increased concern about implant extrusion. The cosmetic result will be less satisfactory over time in globes that have not achieved adult size.

The periocular skin and ocular surface are prepared routinely for aseptic surgery following induction of general anesthesia. The head should be positioned to provide access to the dorsal limbus. Small tenotomy scissors are used to incise and elevate a 160-degree dorsal limbal-based conjunctival flap. Tenon's capsule is reflected to expose the sclera 3 to 4 mm posterior to the limbus. The sclera is grooved parallel to the limbus over 160 degrees using a blade or electrocautery. A 4- to 5-mm scleral incision is made and a cyclodialysis spatula introduced and rotated 360 degrees to separate uvea from sclera. The scleral incision is extended and cyclodialysis repeated before delivering the entire intraocular contents (i.e., iris, lens, and retina) using forceps with traction. Low-vacuum suction and irrigation can facilitate visualization of the corneoscleral shell and removal of blood clots. A sterile black silicone sphere is rinsed in saline and introduced into the corneoscleral shell. Sphere size should be the maximum comfortably accommodated by the globe. This will vary from 33 to 45 mm depending on the age of the horse. Since the anterior-to-posterior axis of the globe is the smallest, fit will be loose in the vertical and horizontal dimensions. The sclera, Tenon's capsule, and conjunctiva are each closed as a separate layer using a 6-0 absorbable suture material in a continuous pattern.

Postoperative care includes systemic antibiotics for 5 days and flunixin meglumine (1.1 mg/kg) or phenylbutazone (4.4 mg/kg) for analgesia, if necessary. Immediately after surgery, blood will usually be observed between the cornea and prosthesis. Corneal edema will occur followed by vascularization, varied pigmentation, and scarring. The corneal response with subsequent scarring takes about 2 to 3 months. During this time the globe contracts around the implant with a resultant shape that is notably spherical compared to a normal eye (Fig. 34–2).

Potential complications include unsatisfactory corneal appearance, extrusion, infection, and dehiscence of sutures. Corneal ulcers that occur during healing can be very serious in an already compromised cornea. They require careful management. In the long run, these globes may also be more susceptible to trauma as a result of blindness and a possible decrease in corneal sensitivity.

Enucleation

Enucleation is an acceptable alternative to an intraocular prosthesis for treatment of a blind, painful, glaucomatous eye. It is also indicated when a loss of corneal or scleral integrity occurs as a result of chronic glaucoma. Transconjunctival and transpalpebral techniques have been previously described for the horse.

If a more cosmetic result is required following enucleation, two options may be considered. A silicone sphere may be placed in the orbit inside the extraocular muscle cone and orbital fascia. The sphere may be sutured to the apex of the muscle cone to help prevent migration. After closure of muscle and fascia, the conjunctiva and skin are closed. The result is a more normal contour to the enucleated orbit.

Alternatively, the bulbar conjunctiva may be closed as a separate layer and the nictitans and eyelids retained in preparation for fitting with a shell-like conjunctival prosthesis. Impression molds of the enucleated and normal eyes and photographs of the normal eye assist an ocularist in preparing a cosmetic shell prosthesis. A duplicate conformer shell may have to be worn with some regularity to prevent contracture of the eyelids. Because of problems with achieving proper fit and the necessity for regular removal of the prosthesis for cleaning, this procedure is only recommended for the highly motivated client and tractable patient.

Intravitreal Gentamicin Injection

Intravitreal injection of gentamicin is an inexpensive alternative to surgery for blind, painful, glaucomatous eyes. Advantages of the technique are short anesthesia time, minimal expense, technical ease, and retention of the globe. The procedure should not be performed in the presence of intraocular neoplasia, and it will cause blindness as a result of retinal degeneration and opacification of the ocular media. The therapeutic effect of intravitreal gentamicin is due to its toxic effects on the ciliary epithelium, with resultant decrease in aqueous humor production and hypotony.

A 20- to 22-gauge needle is inserted through the sclera 8 to 10 mm posterior to the limbus in the dorsolateral quadrant. The needle is directed into the vitreous humor and 0.5 to 1.0 mL is aspirated. Twenty-five milligrams of gentamicin for injection is injected. One milligram of dexamethasone may also be injected to help control resultant intraocular inflammation.

Postoperative response may include chemosis, hyphema, corneal edema, uveitis, and retinal detachment. More chronic changes include corneal scarring with pigmentation, vascularization, degeneration, synechia, cataract, and phthisis bulbi. Postoperative

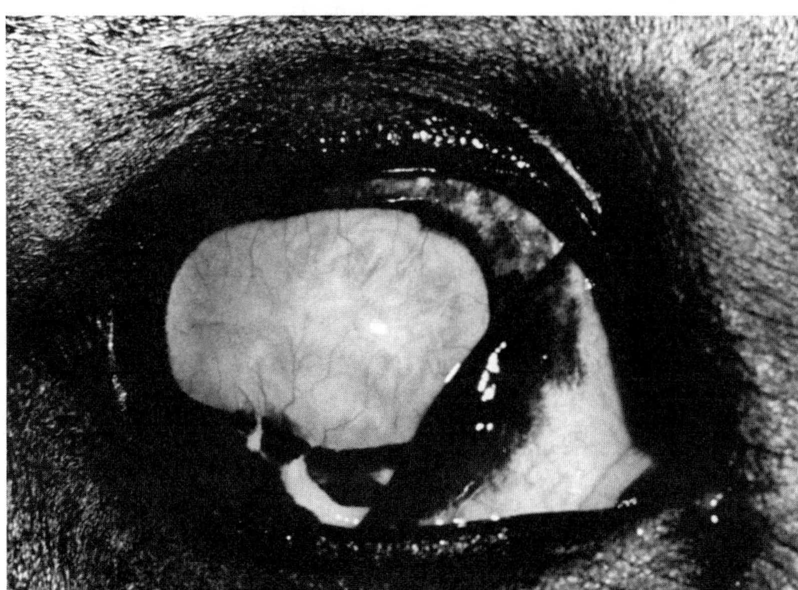

Figure 34–2. The cornea is opaque and has conformed to the shape of the intraocular prosthesis 3 months after surgery.

treatment with flunixin meglumine and a topical corticosteroid for control of pain and uveitis is symptomatic.

This technique has been successful in dogs with intractable glaucoma, but limited use in the horse precludes a meaningful discussion of prognosis following injection. At best, the result will be a hypotonic, cosmetic, comfortable eye. At worst the eye may become phthisical or develop secondary changes (e.g., uveitis or corneal degeneation) that require further management.

BIBLIOGRAPHY

Lavach JD: *The Handbook of Equine Ophthalmology.* Fort Collins, CO, Giddings Studio Publishing, 1987.

McClure JR, Gelatt KN, Gum SG, Manning JP: The effect of parenteral acepromazine and xylazine on intraocular pressure in the horse. *Vet Med/Small Anim Clinician* 1976;1727–1730.

Roberts SM, Severin GA, Lavach JD: Cyclocryotherapy—Part II. Clinical comparison of liquid nitrogen and nitrous oxide cryotherapy on glaucomatous eyes. *J Am Anim Hosp Assoc* 1984;20:828–833.

Smith PJ, Samuelson DA, Brooks DE, Whitley RD: Unconventional aqueous humor outflow of microspheres perfused into the equine eye. *Am J Vet Res* 1986;47:2445–2453.

Vestre WA: Cryosurgical techniques in veterinary ophthalmology. *Compend Contin Educ Pract Vet* 1984; 6:481–490.

Whitley RD, Shaffer KW, Albert RA: Implantation of intraocular silicone prostheses in dogs. *Compend Contin Educ Pract Vet* 1985;7:802–811.

35 Cataracts

Milton Wyman

A cataract may be defined as any opacity of the lens or its capsule. There are many methods of classifying cataracts: chronologically, geographically, or by location, appearance, cause, and degree of progression. Discussion of classification is not within the scope of this chapter; however, certain degrees of progression do affect the postoperative result of cataract extraction. For example, an incipient cataract will cause less postoperative irritation than a hypermature cataract. I believe this is due to the nature of the proteins released into the anterior chamber when an extracapsular procedure is performed. If this theory is correct, it adds credence to the requisite of classifying the cataract according to stage of progression.

The success of cataract extraction is determined in part by patient selection. Patients with secondary cataracts or concomitant uveitis, regardless of its cause, are poor candidates for cataract extraction. Secondary cataracts are those due to antecedent disease, such as anterior uveitis, trauma, or toxins. Older animals with mature or hypermature cataracts are also poor candidates. These patients respond to the mechanical trauma of the surgery and the release of the abnormal cataractous lens protein with excessive postoperative inflammation. Recurrent iridocyclitis is often the result and is the most devastating ocular disease to affect horses. The best candidates are, therefore, young foals with congenital, bilateral, blinding cataracts.

Cataract extractions require surgical skill, appropriate instruments, and knowledge of ocular anatomy and response of ocular tissue to surgical manipulation. I do not recommend attempting this surgery without proper preparation of the surgeon and adequate patient selection.

CLINICAL FINDINGS

Congenital cataracts are usually bilateral, but they vary in location and degree of lens fiber involvement. They can be restricted to the central core of the lens (embryonal or fetal nuclei) (Fig. 35–1) or can be generalized and involve the cortex and lens capsule. Nuclear opacities often become smaller as the animal grows, matures, and lays down new normal cortical lens fibers. Thus, there may be a significant decrease in functional difficulties with age. Opacities that affect both lens cortices and compromise the animal's function are those selected for surgery.

The younger the patient, the more probable the success. This is due to the less inflammatory nature of lens proteins and the softer lens material in young patients.

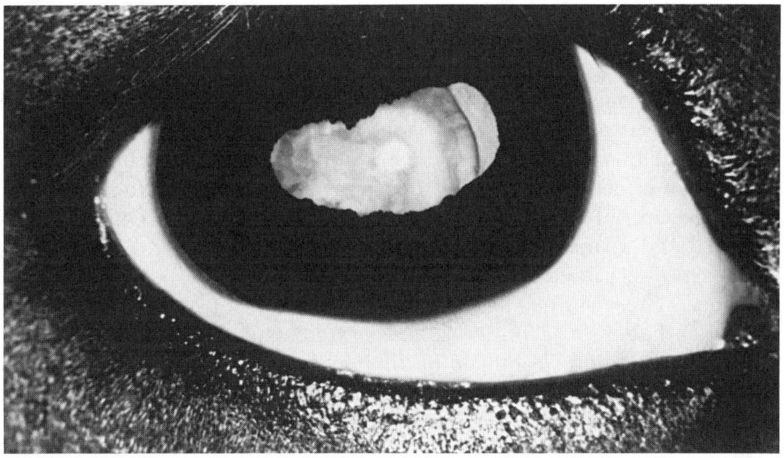

Figure 35–1. Left eye of standardbred foal with congenital cataract involving the embryonal and fetal nuclei.

The younger animal also has less chance of previous anterior uveitis. The more normal the lens protein, the less inflammation it causes when it comes in contact with the anterior uveal tissue. A horse's eye previously sensitized by an inflammatory insult will respond more severely to additional insult. Furthermore, ocular function may be more reliably salvaged if the animal's sight is restored as soon as possible. This is hypothetically true based on extrapolated information from humans and kittens deprived of sight as neonates. These animals may remain blind if visual stimuli are restored after a critical age. A foal that presents with a unilateral cataract is not a good candidate for surgery unless corrective lenses are used. The disparity in projected image size in the operated and unoperated eye causes the animal a greater problem than if the foal remains clinically blind in the cataractous eye.

SURGICAL TREATMENT

Preoperative therapy includes producing adequate and effective mydriasis. I have found that 1% atropine sulfate ophthalmic ointment administered four to six times during the 24 hours prior to surgery produces adequate mydriasis. In addition, a combination of 10% phenylephrine hydrochloride and 0.3% scopolamine hydrobromide (Murocoll-2 Solution) is administered two to three times starting 1 to 2 hours before surgery. Because of the release of potent prostaglandins within the eye that directly affect the pupillary sphincter, I premedicate the animal with a nonsteroidal anti-inflammatory drug (flunixin meglumine, 1 mg/kg intravenously) one-half hour prior to scheduled surgery. In addition, 2 mg/kg of prednisolone is administered systemically one-half hour prior to scheduled surgery.

The lens can be delivered by extracapsular extraction, phacoemulsification (ultrasonic fragmentation and aspiration of lens material), or decission-aspiration. Phacoemulsification requires an expensive unit to fragment the lens material and aspirate it. The lens material must be soft for successful aspiration. This technique is fast, clean, and very successful when performed correctly, and other than cost and the technical skill necessary for the surgeon and technicians, there are no disadvantages.

Decission-Aspiration

The decission-aspiration technique works on the same principle as phacoemulsification but can be performed with balanced salt solution, a three-way valve, a 30-mL syringe, a decission blade, two (14- and 16-gauge) Sovereign indwelling catheters, plastic administration tubing, fixation forceps, lid speculum, and other appropriate hand instruments. The technique is reserved for soft lenses, particularly those seen in very young foals. An extracapsular extraction is necessary if the lens material is hard and cannot be fragmented (see below).

A small stab incision is made so that the catheter may be inserted watertight in its outside diameter to prevent escape of aqueous humor. The smaller gauge catheter is inserted and used to deliver balanced salt solution to the anterior chamber. The descission knife enters the eye through a second perilimbal corneal stab incision and is directed toward the anterior capsule to make a jagged incision in the capsule. This is known as a "Christmas tree" capsulotomy. The lens materials is fragmented and delivered into the anterior chamber.

The knife is withdrawn, and the 14-gauge catheter with a three-way valve attached is inserted. A 30-mL syringe is used to gently remove the lens material by aspiration through the 14-gauge catheter. During this procedure, warmed balanced salt solution is placed in the anterior chamber by gravity flow to maintain the anterior chamber depth during the aspiration process. All lens material must be removed. The catheters are removed and a small 6–0 absorbable suture in a mattress pattern is placed to close each of the corneal stab incisions. These sutures can be placed prior to inserting the catheters to accommodate accurate closure.

Additional fluid or a bubble of air may be injected with a tuberculin syringe and 27-gauge needle inserted at the limbus to reform the anterior chamber, if necessary.

Postoperative therapy is for anterior uveitis, using nonsteroidal anti-inflammatory drugs, cycloplegic/mydriatics, topical antibiotics/steroids, and systemic antibiotics. The duration of therapy is dependent on the degree of inflammation and rate of healing. Reevaluation at 3- to 5-day intervals is indicated to regulate duration and frequency of medication. Corneal sutures should be removed in 10 to 14 days.

The prognosis for cataract surgery is dependent on the selection process as described above. Success is defined as an animal that can be used safely for its intended purpose with functional and cosmetically acceptable vision. The younger the animal the better the postoperative results. Our success rate is about 85%. The owners should be informed that cataracts may be inherited and be cautioned against using the patient for breeding.

Extracapsular Extraction

Patient selection is similar to that previously described. In some instances the lenses in these young animals resist fragmentation and cannot be aspirated. Consequently, it becomes necessary to do an extracapsular extraction. The patient is routinely prepped and anesthesized. Using a #64 Beaver blade or a razor blade and blade breaker, a corneal incision extending 150 to 180 degrees is made as close to the dorsal limbus as possible. The incision should penetrate two thirds the thickness of the cornea, especially at the 12:00 position. A preplaced 7–0 absorbable double-armed suture is positioned in the bottom of the incision trough. A large loop is made in order to remove the suture from the surgical site. This suture provides accurate realignment when the wound is closed.

A stab incision is made with a #11 Bard Parker Blade through the cornea into the anterior chamber adequate to insert one blade of a corneal scissor. The incision is continued in both directions. A pair of forceps are used to grasp the preplaced sutures and carefully elevate the cornea, exposing the anterior lens capsule. The capsule is grasped with an Arruga capsule forceps and gentle but firm pressure is applied to tear the capsule at the equator. Counterpressure is sometimes necessary with a Colibri forceps to accomplish the tear. When the capsule is removed, a cyclodialysis cannula attached to a 15-ml squeeze bottle of sterile balanced salt solution is inserted between the posterior capsule and the lens. Irrigation is used to elevate the lens. Counterpressure exerted externally on the corneal surface with a blunt strabismus hook will accomplish lens extraction. The preplaced suture is central, and suturing continues in both directions from it to accomplish closure and accurate realignment of the cornea. Sutures must be placed accurately and carefully to accomplish perfect watertight closure. The anterior chamber is reformed by forcing sterile balanced salt solution through the incision line.

Postoperative therapy includes topical mydriatics, cycloplegics, antibiotics/steroid solutions, and systemic administration of a nonsteroidal anti-inflammatory agent (flunixin meglumine) intravenously once daily, starting the first postoperative day at a dose of 1 mg/kg. Administration of systemic antibiotics for 7 days is also indicated. Reevaluation of the patient should be done according to problems that are identified during the postoperative period. Sutures are removed in 14 days.

BIBLIOGRAPHY

Gelatt KN, Myers VS, McClure JR: Aspiration of congenital and soft cataracts in foals and young horses. *J Am Vet Med Assoc* 1974;5:611–616.

Van Kruninger HJ: Intracapsular cataract extraction in the horse. *J Am Vet Med Assoc* 1964;145:773–777.

Whitely RD, Moore RP, Slone DE: Cataract surgery in the horse: A review. *Equine Vet J* 1983;(suppl 2):127–134.

36 Ocular and Periorbital Squamous Cell Carcinoma

Milton Wyman

Squamous cell carcinoma is reported in the literature as the most frequent neoplasm of the horse's globe and adnexa. Mean age of onset is reported as 9.8 years. The neoplasm involves the conjunctiva and third eyelid most frequently, but can also invade the eyelids, cornea, sclera, and orbit and is malignant and locally invasive. The reported incidence of metastasis to the thorax, parotid salivary glands, and regional lymph nodes is 10 to 15%. The possibility of metastasis and rapid local growth necessitates early recognition and appropriate therapy for the best possible outcome.

CLINICAL FINDINGS

Clinically, squamous cell carcinoma is characterized as a proliferative, pink enlargement of the third eyelid, conjunctiva, or eyelids. The involved tissue is often quite friable and may bleed when handled, particularly if involving the conjunctiva. Squamous cell carcinoma involving the conjunctiva can invade the cornea or sclera by extension. Deviation of the globe as a result of orbital invasion or erosion of the eyelid margins occurs infrequently.

Periocular soiling with mucopurulent to purulent discharges is often observed in the more advanced conditions. Ocular discharge warrants a complete and thorough evaluation of the eye and adnexa prior to initiating treatment. An accurate diagnosis of the condition is necessary. Often the lesion can be successfully managed at this stage, but topical medication is ineffective and can cause a delay in use of appropriate treatment until such treatment is no longer effective.

TREATMENT

Conjunctival Squamous Cell Carcinoma

Squamous cell carcinoma may be found anywhere on the conjunctiva, but the third eyelid, particularly the free margin, appears to be the site for which there is the greatest predilection. Limbal conjunctival squamous cell carcinoma, when allowed to progress, has a tendency to invade the cornea (Fig. 36–1). These cases require a more involved surgical procedure, which is another reason for early recognition and therapy. Conjunctival squamous cell carcinomas are easily excised with regional or general anesthesia. The animal or the ocular region is appropriately anesthetized depending on the extent of the lesion. The surgeon may elect either general or regional anesthesia. (i.e., retrobulbar or local, such as topical proparacaine hydrochloride in conjunction with an auriculopalpebral block). The conjunctival cul-de-sacs should be thoroughly irrigated with sterile saline. A lid speculum is used to provide adequate exposure, and scleral fixation forceps are used to immobilize the globe and provide exposure of the involved region. A #64 Beaver blade and handle or #15 Bard Parker blade and handle can be used to excise the mass, ensuring that normal adjacent conjunctiva is included in the excision.

An alternative for small lesions is to grasp the lesion with forceps and "tent" it so as to expose normal conjunctiva at the base of the elevated tissue. The normal tissue at the base of the tent is engaged between the blades of blunt-tipped, moderately curved scissors and the lesion is excised, incorporating a margin of normal tissue 360 degrees around the lesion. Small lesions do not usually invade the subconjunctival tissue so that conjunctivectomy is adequate. Closure of the resultant conjunctival defect is dependent on its size. Large gaping conjunctival wounds are closed with buried 7–0 absorbable sutures. Precaution should be taken to prevent knot exposure, which may irritate the adjacent cornea and conjunctiva. Topical administration of ophthalmic antibiotic ointments is indicated for 5 to 7 days.

Lesions involving the conjunctiva and extending into the fibrous tunic (cornea or sclera) may not be amenable to simple excision alone. When the neoplasm involves the cornea or sclera, the mass should be excised by superficial keratectomy or sclerectomy. Excised tissue must be submitted for histopathologic diagnosis. In many instances it is possible to completely excise the neoplastic tissue; however, when it extends too deep to permit excision, ancillary therapy is advised. Radiation therapy using a strontium 90 β-ray applicator has been used successfully following partial excision when the remaining involved tissue is less than 2 mm thick. The dosage ranges from 25,000 to 45,000 reps and the treated area should extend at least 2 mm beyond the visible edges of the lesion. This method has resulted in an 89% regression rate for at least 1 year.

Treatment after surgery and radiation therapy should include topical antibiotic and steroid therapy for 5 to 7 days. Follow-up in 5 to 6 weeks is prudent and, if regrowth is apparent, the lesion should be retreated.

Squamous Cell Carcinoma Involving the Third Eyelid

The third eyelid is the ocular structure most frequently involved with squamous cell carcinoma. It often presents with a fleshy enlargement or indurated, crusted appearance in the medial canthus. It is frequently accompanied by a mucopurulent exudate and periocular soiling.

Well-circumscribed lesions may be easily excised, whereas those that extend toward the base of the third eyelid may require ancillary modalities of therapy. Simple excision is preceeded by anesthesia. This can include general, regional (retrobulbar), or local anesthesia. The horse should be sedated, and local anesthesia can be accomplished by topical administration of proparacaine hydrochloride until the surface conjunctiva and cornea are desensitized. The third eyelid can be elevated with thumb forceps, and a 22-gauge needle affixed to a 10-mL syringe is used to infiltrate 10 mL of local anesthetic into the base of the third eyelid. An auriculopalpebral block will enhance exposure by relaxing the upper eyelid. The third eyelid is elevated as far as possible to visualize the entire mass. Two large curved hemostats are placed beneath the lesion from either side of the third eyelid so that their tips touch one another. The involved tissue is excised by running a #15 Bard Parker blade along the dorsal edge of the curved hemostats. The excised tissue should include the lesion and a grossly normal margin of tissue. This should be histopathologically examined for possible local tumor invasion, which could require more extensive removal of the third eyelid. The hemostats should remain in place for a few minutes to control hemorrhage. Closure is unnecessary. Ophthalmic antibiotic-steroid solutions are used topically for 5 to 7 days at the discretion of the surgeon dependent on the postoperative reaction.

Lesions that extend further than the base of the third eyelid require adjunctive modalities of therapy. These include cryotherapy, radiation therapy, or radiofrequency hyperthermia. There are benefits and limitations to each modality. Cryosurgery is my choice for these lesions. Ideally, microthermocouple needles should be inserted 0.5 cm outside the margin of the neoplasm in normal tissue. When the margin is impossible to identify, the success rate drops significantly. The objective is to freeze the involved tissue rapidly and thaw it slowly. This results in direct cellular destruction and infarction as a result of vascular injury. Neoplastic tissue apparently is more cryosensitive than normal tissue. These injuries result in postfreeze swelling and discoloration, and within 24 hours the tissue appears swollen and dark. Necrosis results in shrinking and drying of the involved tissue and is manifest within a week of surgery. Pain is not apparent, presumably because of the analgesia associated with

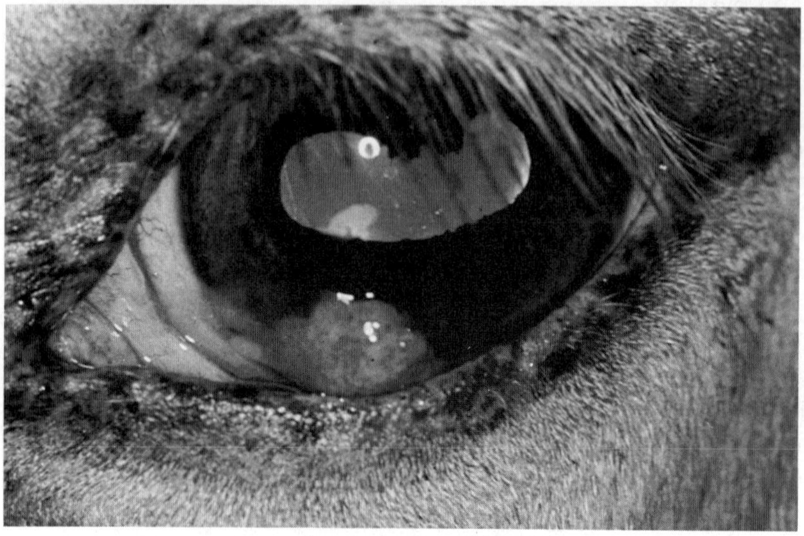

Figure 36–1. A 9-year-old Quarter horse with a limbal conjunctival squamous cell carcinoma invading the cornea.

sensory nerve cryoinjury. The cryogen can be applied as a spray or via solid cryoprobes. The efficacy of either is good when applied correctly. Liquid nitrogen is readily available, inexpensive, noncombustible, and nontoxic and it boils at −195.6 °C. It should be applied to the center of the mass from a stationary position 1 or 2 cm away for best results. The perilesional temperature should reach −20 to −25 °C before the tissue is allowed to slowly thaw. A double freeze-thaw cycle is optional. The disadvantage of liquid nitrogen spray is the lack of defined control. The surgeon must take every precaution to protect the perilesional normal tissue with Styrofoam barriers and petrolatum jelly. Solid, variable-sized probes have the advantage of better control to the involved tissue. There are many units available using nitrous oxide as the cryogen, but they are more expensive than liquid nitrogen units. Cryosurgery is also a very effective way of removing neoplastic tissue that remains after debulking.

Squamous Cell Carcinoma of the Lids

Small lesions involving the eyelid may be excised by simple V-plasty. More extensive lesions require bold excision and often complicated blepharoplastic techniques to repair. Alternatives to this include surgical debulking combined with cryosurgery, radiofrequency hyperthermia, or radiation therapy. My choice is cryosurgery. Available cryogens are liquid nitrogen and nitrous oxide as previously described for conjunctival tumors. The tissue temperature must be dropped rapidly to −20 °C, and then the tissue allowed to slowly thaw. This procedure is repeated once.

The cornea and adjacent normal tissue must be protected from the cryoprobe/cryogen to prevent unnecessary tissue injury. This is achieved using petrolatum-coated Styrofoam placed around the lesion as a "dam." The tissue swelling that will occur following cryosurgery can be minimized with systemic nonsteroidal anti-inflammatory agents. A marked reduction in neoplastic tissue occurs within 2 to 3 weeks. The procedure may be repeated if necessary.

Extension of Squamous Cell Carcinoma into the Orbit

Surgical debulking, in conjunction with various forms of ionizing radiation, may be used for squamous cell carcinomas that extend into the orbit. Gamma and x-rays can be applied by implanting the neoplasm with cesium or radioactive cobalt needles. These are removed when approximately 5,000 rads have been delivered. The radiation hazard is an obvious and important consideration in selecting this method of therapy. Radioactive gold (Au) seeds have the advantages of a short half-life (2.7 days) and they do not produce tissue reaction, so they may be left in situ. The disadvantages are cost and the need to be close to a source for activating the isotope. The same dosage is required as for cesium or cobalt needles, and calibration is necessary to obtain the proper dosage. This depends on the size of the neoplasm, and a reasonably accurate measurement is pivotal to satisfactory treatment.

POSTOPERATIVE CARE

Postoperative care is directed at control of swelling and pain and prevention of secondary bacterial infection. Systemic nonsteroidal anti-inflammatory drugs effectively control swelling and pain. Systemic antibiotics are also indicated prophylactically following blepharoplastic techniques, cryosurgery, or radiation therapy. Ulcerative lesions of the lids, conjunctiva, or cornea may require topical medication. However, the eyelids can be effectively medicated by systemic antibiotics, either prophylactically or therapeutically. When surgical reconstruction is necessary, sutures are removed in 10 to 14 days.

PROGNOSIS

Prognosis depends on the size and extent of involvement, in addition to evidence of metastasis. In general, when the lesion is not extensive, the prognosis is good for survival, cosmesis, and function.

BIBLIOGRAPHY

Fraunfelder HC, Blevins WE, Page EH: Sr for treatment of periocular squamous cell carcinoma in the horse. *J Am Vet Med Assoc* 1982;180:307–309.

Fraunfelder FT, Wingfield D: Management of intraepithelial conjunctival tumors and squamous cell carcinomas. *Am J Ophthalmol* 1983;95:359–363.

Gelatt KN, Myers VS, Perman V, Jessen C: Conjunctival squamous cell carcinoma in the horse. *J Am Vet Med Assoc* 1974;165:617.

Grier RL, Brewer WG Jr, Paul SR, Theilen GH: Treatment of bovine and equine ocular squamous cell carcinoma by radiofrequency hyperthermia. *J Am Vet Med Assoc* 1980;177:55–61.

Hilbert BJ, Farrell RK, Grant BD: Cryotherapy of periocular squamous cell carcinoma in the horse. *J Am Vet Med Assoc* 1977;170:1305–1308.

37 Blepharoplastic Techniques

Milton Wyman

Some general concepts should be considered when eyelid surgery is undertaken in horses. The tissue must be handled as gently as possible. This requires proper instrumentation with no substitutions because of the relatively delicate tissues involved. Tissues must be identified and repaired in layers; for example, conjunctiva must be reapposed to conjunctiva as well as muscle to muscle and skin to skin.

Sutures placed in the conjunctiva must not protrude and irritate the cornea or adjacent conjunctiva. This concept is also applicable to sutures placed in the free lid margin. The surgeon should use the very smallest suture possible to accomplish successful closure. One third of the length of the lid in dogs and young cats can be removed without concern for effective closure; however, this is not possible in the horse. The rigid medial and lateral canthal attachments in the horse restrict the amount of tissue that can be removed from the free lid margins without impairing functional closure of the defect.

Preparation of the surgical site must also be meticulously performed. Overzealous clipping, scrubbing, and mechanical irritation will compromise postoperative healing. Povidone-iodine surgical soaps and sterile saline are the preferred detergent and irrigant to minimize irritation of the lid skin, cornea, and conjunctiva. I recommend thorough wetting with saline followed by gentle periocular scrub with a sterile sponge saturated with povidone-iodine surgical soap. The site is irrigated carefully to minimize corneal irritation by beginning at the lid margins and enlarging circumferentially. This can be repeated twice before shaving is performed. I prefer to shave the immediate surgical site with a bare Schick injector blade. The site is lathered and the skin tensed by digital pressure. The blade is positioned almost parallel to the skin surface and moved in the direction of the hair growth. The long tactile hairs can be removed with the blade or with wet surgical scissors. One or more scrubs should be done after appropriate shaving.

The horse often has potential pathogenic fungi on the facial hair and I prefer to moisten and lather the entire face, including the ear and muzzle, to minimize possible contamination of the surgical site. While the surgeon is preparing the involved eye, it is equally important to protect the uninvolved eye from soap and unnecessary irritation. Although an inflated inner tube can be used to elevate the head and keep the eye off the table, irrigating the eye will eliminate any unnecessary injury.

V-PLASTY

The V-plasty procedure can be effectively used to excise small lid masses; repair trauma-induced, small, notchlike defects; and shorten the lid margins in response to a shrinking globe.

The area is properly scrubbed and prepared and the tissue to be removed is determined. A common mistake is to be too conservative in the depth of excision. Depth is defined as the distance between the free lid margin and the fornix conjunctiva. The surgeon can excise the entire depth and into the fornix conjunctiva everywhere but in the dorsal lateral lid. Care must be exercised in this region to avoid invading the ducts of the primary lacrimal gland. Therefore, the surgeon can excise to but not into the fornix without risking severing these important structures.

The tissue can be removed by dissection with a scalpel blade or by using mosquito forceps and scissors. A forceps is placed on either side of the tissue to be removed in the form of a "V" with the apex toward the fornix. The forceps are removed and scissors are used to cut along the resultant indentations. When excising a neoplasm, the surgeon should include all abnormal tissue plus a small margin of normal tissue to assure complete excision. The excised tissue should be submitted for histopathologic examination for diagnostic and prognostic purposes.

Closure is accomplished by closing the tissues in two planes, the conjunctiva and skin. The conjunctiva is closed first, beginning at the apex and continuing to the free lid margin. The conjunctiva is identified and grasped with small forceps; my preference is a Colibri forceps. An intraconjunctival 6-0 or 7-0 absorbable suture is placed in the apex and tied. The closure is continued by placing a "running" horizontal mattress suture to the free lid margin. The free lid margin is then meticulously reapposed so that the two edges are as accurately realigned as possible. I prefer an intratarsal mattress suture; however, a figure-of-eight pattern can also be used. The remaining wound can be closed with simple interrupted sutures. Suture material used in the skin should be no larger than 5-0 nonabsorbable material using a swaged-on needle.

Postoperative care should include systemic prophylactic antibiotic therapy for at least 5 days. Skin sutures should be removed in 10 to 14 days.

The prognosis for repair of a laceration or notch defect using this technique is excellent and unless the neoplastic tissue has invaded to the margin of excised tissue, it is excellent for excisional biopsies as well.

MODIFIED HOTZ-CELSUS TECHNIQUES FOR ENTROPION

Congenital entropion has been reported in foals. I am convinced that the condition as diagnosed in neonates is acquired and secondary to either keratoconjunctivitis or enophthalmos due to dehydration. Painful superficial ocular inflammatory disease may result in the patient squinting, with subsequent inturning of the lid margins further irritation and discomfort, which initiates a vicious circle. Enophthalmos due to ocular pain or dehydration results in the lids falling over the orbital rim and turning into the cornea, initiating additional keratoconjunctivitis, discomfort, and further inversion of the lid.

Some patients respond to temporary eversion of the lids using vertical mattress sutures to effect turning of the free lid margins. Size 3-0 or 4-0 nonabsorbable sutures are placed in the tarsal plate but not through it, approximately 2 mm from the free lid margin. The second bite is taken about 1 cm below or above the free lid margin of the lower or upper lid, respectively. A surgeon's throw is placed and tension applied until adequate eversion is accomplished, at which time the knot is completed. These are left in place for 2 to 3 weeks or at the discretion of the surgeon.

When this technique is inadequate, the Hotz-Celsus technique has proven effective. Proper instrumentation and patient preparation are similar to those for the V-plasty. Anesthesia can be regional or general.

The amount of tissue to be removed is determined prior to chemical restraint or nerve blocks. Digital pressure is applied to the lid skin adjacent to the entropic region to evert the lid until the free lid margin is in an acceptable position. The distance necessary to accomplish this is the width of the widest part of the elliptical piece of skin to be excised from the involved lid. The ends of the incisions should extend 1 mm medial and lateral to the entropic region. The first incision, made with a #15 Bard Parker blade and handle, is parallel to the free lid margin as close to the tarsus as possible without invading it. This provides rigidity, which enhances eversion. The second incision is made in an elliptical fashion so that the center of the ellipse is the width predetermined by the digital technique described above. Both incisions must be perpendicular to the surface and just through the skin. It is not necessary to excise orbicularis muscle to successfully correct uncomplicated entropion. A suture is placed at an angle on either side of an imaginary line bisecting the wound so that the sutures form an arrow pointing toward the free lid margin (Fig. 37–1). The arrow pattern accentuates eversion and minimizes the amount of skin that must be removed. Additional sutures are placed parallel to the first two sutures, 1.5 to 2 mm apart, working medially and laterally until the wound is closed. Suture material should be the smallest possible for effective closure (no larger than 5-0) and nonabsorbable.

Postoperative care should include topical therapy for keratoconjunctivitis, if present. Topical medication is not necessary for the skin incision. Systemic prophylatic antibiotics can be used for 5 days or more but are usually unnecessary. Sutures are removed in 10 to 14 days.

The prognosis for uncomplicated entropion is excellent provided the primary cause is identified and eliminated.

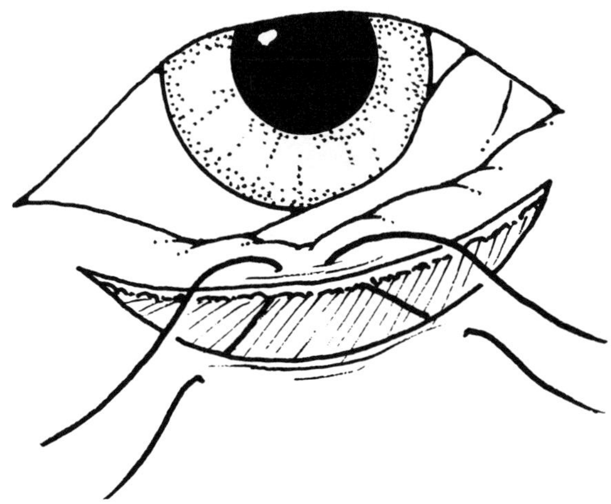

Figure 37–1. "Arrow suture" placement for closure of modified Hotz-Celsus entropion repair techniques.

SURGICAL MANAGEMENT OF EYELID LACERATIONS

Traumatic eyelid lacerations are common in horses. These lacerations can occur as a result of blunt trauma because of the relatively sharp orbital rim and large, thin upper eyelid. Contact with objects such as nails, wires, low-topped trailers, whips, and ropes, and kicks and bites from other horses, have been incriminated.

Clinical signs provide an easy diagnosis. Characteristically, there are tears anywhere in the free lid margin, severe hemorrhage and facial soiling, patient discomfort of variable degree, and, depending on the duration of injury, discoloration and swelling of the pedicle and adjacent tissues.

Examination should include evaluation of the cornea and anterior segment to eliminate corneal lacerations and traumatic anterior uveitis. The next important consideration is the integrity of the nasolacrimal drainage apparatus. This is rarely involved in my experience; however, both the upper and lower canaliculi should be examined to determine their integrity. The upper canaliculus need not be repaired; however, if the lower one is involved it should be identified, canulated, and repaired appropriately.

Lid lacerations should be repaired regardless of the duration of the wound. Healing without repair may result in deformity, predisposing to exposure keratopathy. Under ordinary circumstances the problem is quickly recognized, and, because of the nature of the wound, client concern stimulates early veterinary consultation. The following medications are administered after the cornea and anterior segment have been evaluated: tetanus antitoxin, a systemic nonsteroidal anti-inflammatory/analgesic agent, and systemic antibiotics.

The procedure can be performed under regional anesthesia with tranquilization or under general anesthesia. Because local infiltration with an anesthetic agent will distort the tissue and cause further insult to the injury, I recommend regional blocks or general anesthesia. The extent of the wound, temperament of the horse, agility of the surgeon, and health status of the patient are determining factors.

The wound must be cleaned adequately with warmed sterile saline to which may be added 2,000 U of aqueous penicillin/mL. The irrigation is best accomplished with a Water-Pic or bulb syringe. Although necrotic tissue must be removed, it is imperative that minimal débridement be done to preserve as much lid tissue as possible. As a rule, if the wound edge bleeds, the tissue is viable and will heal if appropriate repositioning is accomplished. The defect is repaired in two layers, the conjunctiva and skin. The conjunctiva is identified and an intraconjunctival suture is placed at the apex of the wound by driving the swaged-on needle into the dense fibrous connective tissue layers of the conjunctiva and continuing with a continuous horizontal mattress to the free lid margin. This is done with 7-0 absorbable ophthalmic suture. Care should be taken to bury the knots so that corneal irritation does not occur. The lid margin is repaired by meticulously placing a 5-0 nonabsorbable ophthalmic suture in a mattress pattern intratarsally to bring the free lid margin into accurate apposition. This is followed by simple interrupted sutures to complete the closure.

Swelling and possible posttraumatic infection may be controlled by systemic administration of nonsteroidal anti-inflammatory analgesics and antibiotics. These drugs should be administered for at least 5 days. No topical medication is indicated unless corneal involvement is manifest.

Because of the excellent blood supply and healing ability of the eyelids, the prognosis is excellent. The surgeon should not excise the pedicle because this can result in a significant lid defect requiring more extensive blepharoplastic repair.

BIBLIOGRAPHY

Gelatt, KV: "Blepharoplastic procedures in horses. *J Am Vet Med Assoc* 1967;151:27–44.

UNIT V

Respiratory Tract Disorders

38 Pathophysiology of Upper Airway Obstruction

John R. Pascoe

A major function of the upper airway is to provide a conduit for the movement of air between the environment and the lung. Other upper airway functions include phonation, respiratory defense, and air modification. The biomechanics of the upper airway depend to a large extent on the airflow and the shape and size of the airway. Unlike humans, horses are obligate nasal breathers and do not switch to mouth breathing with strenuous exercise. However, since many of the commonly encountered equine upper airway obstructions occur in the laryngeal region, mouth breathing would offer no advantage.

NORMAL UPPER AIRWAY ANATOMY AND PHYSIOLOGY

The extrathoracic airway is composed of valve-like structures (nostrils, soft palate, larynx) and both elastic (naso- and laryngopharynx) and relatively rigid (nasal cavity) components. Both static and dynamic changes in airway geometry can influence the resistance to airflow. Static changes in airway geometry occur when the aperture of the valves changes (e.g., laryngeal hemiplegia) or the contour of the elastic or rigid components is altered (e.g., retropharyngeal masses, nasal bone fractures). The vascular network of the nasal submucosa has characteristics similar to erectile tissue, so changes in vascular capacitance can also influence nasal airway caliber.

Because the respiratory tissues are compliant, dynamic changes in airway caliber occur with breathing. Inspiration is accompanied by decreases in intraluminal pressure and expiration by increases in intraluminal pressure. The magnitude of these intraluminal pressure changes is determined by the distribution of resistance along the airway, the compliance of the airway walls, and the magnitude of the forces that determine airflow. For airflow to occur there must be a pressure gradient between the environment and the alveoli of the lung. This gradient is established by changing the pleural pressure, a function of the elastic recoil of the lungs and chest wall and the degree of respiratory muscle activation.

With the onset of inspiration, the abdominal muscles relax and the thoracic muscles contract, changing thoracic shape and decreasing pleural pressure, which decreases alveolar pressure. As the alveolar pressure falls below the environmental pressure (barometric pressure), a flow gradient is established between the nostrils and the alveoli and air flows through the upper airway into the lungs. Air flows out of the lung when alveolar pressure rises above environmental pressure. Because the upper airway is composed of compliant structures, the driving pressure for airflow across the upper airway is not solely dependent on thoracic events. It is also influenced by regional changes in airway geometry and by the velocity of the airflow.

Figure 38–1 illustrates the pressures acting in the upper airway during respiration. For a given region, the upper airway pressure (P_{ua}) is a function of the lateral pressure (P_{lat}), measured perpendicular to the airflow, and the velocity-dependent convective acceleration of the air. The pressure acting on the airway wall, the transmural pressure (P_{tm}), is the difference between the pressure of the tissues surrounding the airway (P_{tis}) and the lateral pressure of the airflow. For a given airflow, narrowing a section of the airway decreases the bulk flow of air at this site but increases the particle velocity. Since the convective acceleration of the air is a function of the square of the particle velocity, narrowing of the airway segment has a profound effect on the lateral pressure, making it more negative and consequently increasing the transmural pressure ($P_{tis} - P_{lat}$). If the airway wall distal to the narrowing is at all compliant, the net effect of this increased transmural pressure is to cause further narrowing of the airway.

Thus, flow through a compliant airway is affected by the airway cross-sectional area and the transmural

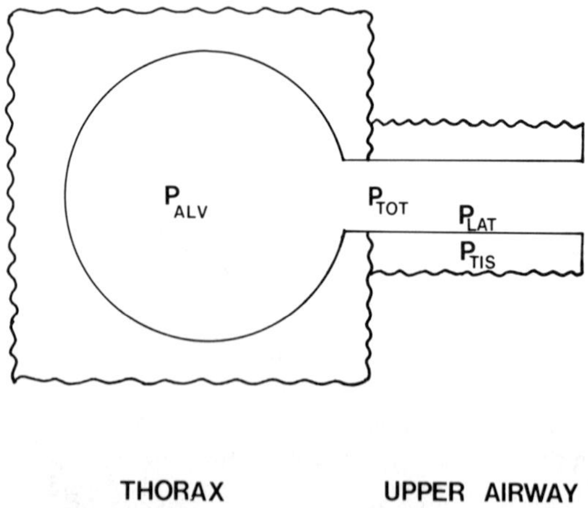

Figure 38–1. Pressures in the upper airway during respiration. The pressure acting on the airway wall (the transmural pressure) is the difference between the tissue pressure (P_{TIS}) and the lateral pressure (P_{LAT}). P_B = barometric pressure, P_{TOT} = total upper airway pressure, P_{ALV} = alveolar pressure.

pressure. For the upper airway this means that flow is dependent on the relative magnitude of the driving pressures and the extent to which the airway walls can be deformed. Muscular tone and activation therefore play an important role in maintaining airway geometry and efficient breathing. Since dynamic collapse is more likely to be of concern during inspiration, when intraluminal pressures become increasingly negative, muscular activity to prevent airway collapse assumes paramount importance. For example, failure of the dilator muscles of the "valves" of the upper airway is likely to have the greatest dynamic impact on impedance to airflow. This, of course, is the situation that exists in horses with laryngeal hemiplegia.

PHYSIOLOGY OF IMPAIRED AIRWAY FUNCTION

Recent experimental studies have demonstrated the significant physiologic consequences of impaired laryngeal function during exercise. In normal horses, increasing exercise intensity from rest to a gallop (7.2 m/s on a 6.38-degree incline) results in large increases in respiratory frequency (sixfold), trans—upper airway pressure (tenfold), and flow (15-fold) but no change in inspiratory impedance and a decrease in expiratory impedance. To achieve flow increases of this magnitude without increasing the impedance to flow, there must be progressive dilation of the upper airway. This is achieved by dilation of the nostrils, vasoconstriction of the nasal mucosa, tensing of the muscular walls of the pharynx and abduction of the vocal cords and arytenoid cartilages of the larynx. The decrease in expiratory impedance probably largely reflects maintenance of laryngeal abduction since the larynx acts to brake expiratory flow during resting breathing.

Transection of the left recurrent laryngeal nerve mimics the "worst case" clinical scenario for laryngeal hemiplegia and has been the method of choice for studying the naturally occurring disease. Endoscopic observation of the hemiplegic larynx at rest, reveals a stationary left arytenoid cartilage and vocal fold that occupy a median position in the airway. It was widely believed that during exercise the left arytenoid and vocal fold continued to maintain this median position because of the loss of both abductor and adductor muscle function. However, videoendoscopic observation has shown that this loss of muscular control allows progressive deformation of the larynx and narrowing of the laryngeal aperture with increasing exercise intensity. Although the right arytenoid and vocal fold abduct maximally during inspiration at higher flow rates, the paralyzed left arytenoid and vocal fold are drawn across the midline toward the right side, effectively narrowing the laryngeal aperture. With increasing effort this dynamic inspiratory collapse is accentuated until the left side touches the abducted right side. During expiration the left side returns to its median position and the right side remains abducted.

These observations suggest that dynamic collapse of the larynx could be expected to have a marked effect on upper airway pressure-flow characteristics. When horses performed the same submaximal exercise test after left recurrent neurectomy, inspiratory impedance increased threefold. Despite a twofold increase in trans—upper airway pressure, these horses were unable to attain the inspiratory flows generated before neurectomy. In fact it would appear that, even during submaximal exercise, flow limitation occurs. This means that despite increasing muscular effort and thus increased driving pressure, no further increases in flow can be achieved.

To meet the metabolic demand of increased muscular activity, alveolar ventilation ([tidal volume − dead space volume] × respiratory frequency) must increase. Since dead space volume changes little during exercise, increases in alveolar ventilation must be achieved through increases in tidal volume and respiratory frequency. With flow limitation, increases in respiratory frequency will result in smaller tidal volumes and thus decrease alveolar ventilation. So, with flow limitation, an increase in alveolar ventilation requires an increase in tidal volume, which is achieved by decreasing respiratory frequency. Because respiratory and locomotor events are coupled in horses during the canter and gallop, changes in respiratory frequency will likely result in changes in speed and consequently impaired performance.

Respiratory frequency is coupled with stride frequency in a 1:1 ratio at the canter and the gallop, a relationship that is believed to be energetically efficient. Different coupling ratios occur in pacers and trotters. If respiratory frequency decreases, then either stride frequency must decrease or locomotor-respiratory uncoupling must occur. Studies in maximally exercised ponies have shown that laryngeal hemiplegia results in decreased respiratory frequency without alteration of stride frequency. However, despite this locomotor-respiratory uncoupling and the respiratory adjustments (decreased respiratory frequency and increased driving pressure), alveolar hypoventilation (elevated arterial carbon dioxide tension) and hypoxemia occur and strenuous exercise cannot be maintained. Before recurrent neurectomy, these ponies were capable of sustained maximal exercise for 4 minutes, whereas after neurectomy the same exercise intensity could only be sustained for 45 to 90 seconds. With training, this interval could be extended to 120 seconds. Thus, it is apparent that dynamic collapse of the upper airway and, in particular, flow limitation significantly impair exercise potential.

INFLUENCE OF SURGERY

It is clear from the preceding discussion that reversal of these changes in airway function requires stabilization of the collapsing airway segments. Although a variety of surgical techniques have been used to correct laryngeal hemiplegia, only three—ventriculectomy, laryngoplasty, and arytenoidectomy—are currently practiced. Recent airway function studies have provided some objective evaluation of the efficacy of these techniques.

Removal of the laryngeal ventricle is believed to promote scarring between the vocal fold and the thyroid cartilage and thus enlarge glottic dimensions and stabilize the vocal fold. Such changes are not readily apparent on endoscopy. Furthermore, since this technique does not stabilize the arytenoid cartilage, little improvement in airway function would be expected. Experimental studies have shown that 30 days after ventriculectomy, there is no improvement in inspiratory impedance or trans—upper airway pressures.

In *laryngoplasty* techniques, the left arytenoid cartilage is maintained in abduction by sutures placed between the cricoid cartilage and the muscular process of the arytenoid cartilage, the site of insertion of the principal abductor muscle of the larynx. The intent of this procedure is to lateralize and stabilize the arytenoid cartilage and vocal fold. Some surgeons also perform a ventriculectomy during the same operative period. There has been considerable controversy about the efficacy of laryngoplasty. Most of this controversy has focused on the difficulty in obtaining a degree of abduction that increases glottic dimension without compromising airway protection, especially during swallowing. Experimental treadmill studies have shown that laryngoplasty effectively restores airway function by reversing the increase in inspiratory impedance and trans-upper airway pressure and improving arterial blood gases. These findings have also been verified under racetrack conditions with horses galloping at 16 m/s (mean heart rate, 230 beats/min; mean respiratory frequency, 145 breaths/min). Thus, although it is not possible to obtain maximum static abduction of the left arytenoid cartilage without compromising airway protection, the partial abduction achieved with laryngoplasty not only increases glottic dimension but either prevents or minimizes the tendency for dynamic collapse of the laryngeal aperture. Unfortunately, there is no objective means for determining the ideal position for abduction, and some surgeons use intraoperative endoscopy to determine what each believes to be adequate abduction. Although detractors would argue that this is sufficient reason to abandon the technique, clinical experience and airway function studies have demonstrated that it is the only technique currently available that results in adequate restoration of function.

Subtotal arytenoidectomy involves the removal of most of the arytenoid cartilage. Depending on the method utilized, the muscular process and the corniculate process are not removed. The aim of the surgical procedure is to increase glottic dimension by cartilage removal and to attempt to stabilize the laryngeal wall by mucosal scarring to the underlying musculature and the thyroid lamina. A ventriculectomy and cordectomy are often combined with this procedure. Recent racetrack studies with horses galloping at 16 m/s have shown that while this technique is capable of reversing the increase in translaryngeal pressure that occurs with hemiplegia, it does not return pressures to control values. The reason for this is unknown but it is probable that even though glottic dimension is improved, dynamic collapse of the vocal fold and corniculate process still occurs. These results support clinical experience and suggest that subtotal arytenoidectomy is not a satisfactory technique for palliation of laryngeal hemiplegia. While its use is advocated for treatment of arytenoid chondropathy, it should be recognized that dynamic airway collapse probably still occurs and only limited improvements in performance should be anticipated.

Recently there has been renewed interest in reinnervation techniques either through direct nerve transplant or nerve-muscle pedicle grafts in an attempt restore neuromuscular function. To date these techniques have not been objectively evaluated. In light of the previous comments it should be apparent that the success of these techniques will depend on their ability to increase and maintain glottic dimensions during maximal exercise.

BIBLIOGRAPHY

Derksen FJ, Stick JA, Scott EA, et al: Effect of laryngeal hemiplegia and laryngoplasty on airway flow mechanics in exercising horses. *Am J Vet Res* 1986;47:16–20.

Manohar M: Blood flow in respiratory muscles during maximal exertion in ponies with laryngeal hemiplegia. *J Appl Physiol* 1987;62:229–237.

Manohar M: Right heart pressures and blood gas tensions in ponies during exercise and laryngeal hemiplegia. *Am J Physiol (Heart Circ Physiol)* 1986;251:H121-H126.

Manohar M, Goetz TE, Nganwa D: Costal diaphragmatic O_2 and lactate extraction in laryngeal hemiplegic ponies during exercise. *J Appl Physiol* 1988;65:1723–1728.

Shappell KK, Derksen FJ, Stick JA, et al: Effect of ventriculectomy, prosthetic laryngoplasty and exercise on upper airway function in horses with left laryngeal hemiplegia. *Am J Vet Res* 1988;49:1760–1765.

Williams JW. *Evaluation of Upper Airway Function in the Maximally Exercising Horse,* MS thesis. University of California, Davis, 1989.

39 Nasal Turbinates and Septum

Eric P. Tulleners

TURBINATES

Disease involving the turbinates is unusual. Differential diagnosis includes congenital deviation (wry nose foals), thickening from inflammation, granulation tissue secondary to trauma or surgery, polyps, tumors, granulomas, and fungal infections.

Clinical signs include decreased exercise tolerance with variable continuous respiratory noise. Horses with tumors or infection may present with a chronic scant, usually malodorous unilateral nasal discharge that may be intermixed with blood. Exercise intolerance will range from slight to incapacitating depending on the amount of airway reduction and whether there is unilateral or bilateral nasal passage involvement.

The head should be examined and palpated for alterations in contour, facial deformity, tearing, nerve deficits, or pain. The airflow from each nostril should be compared by holding the palms or a pledget of cotton a few inches from the nares. In horses with a unilateral problem, temporary occlusion of the affected nares should eliminate the respiratory noise. Auscultation and percussion of the nasal passages may reveal dullness or changes in resonance. More rostrally located lesions may be palpated, or observed with a strong light source by elevating the nostril and alar cartilage.

Lesions further in the nasal cavity can usually be observed by endoscopy. Alterations in turbinate contour such as deviation or thickening caused by polyps may be seen, but the surface will still be smooth and covered by normal-appearing mucous membrane. Granulation tissue, granulomas, fungal plaques, and tumors are irregular and slightly to severely raised, and may be erosive. There may be a mucopurulent or hemorrhagic exudate. It may be difficult or impossible to bypass the deformity and enter the pharynx and larynx. Both nasal passages should be examined to rule out bilateral involvement and also to allow for comparison of normal and abnormal structures. It is important to examine the contour of the ethmoturbinates and the septum. If a standard 11.0-mm outer diameter gastroscope cannot be passed into the pharynx, a pediatric endoscope with a 9.0-mm outside diameter should be tried, if available.

Radiography, including a dorsoventral, a lateral, and two oblique views, is useful in evaluating the extent and site of the disease. Sinus and tooth root involvement may also be diagnosed with the aid of radiographs.

Biopsy instruments passed through the biopsy channel of the endoscope may not be of sufficient size to obtain representative, diagnostic tissue samples. Often biopsies obtained superficial to the depths of the lesion will show nonspecific inflammatory changes. An accurate histologic diagnosis or tissue cultures may require an endoscope-guided biopsy with a Ferris-Smith rongeur or uterine biopsy forceps. In the fractious horse or for examination and biopsy of lesions between the dorsal and ventral turbinates, general anesthesia may be necessary.

Endoscopic Anatomy of the Nasal Passages

The paired nasal passages are separated at the midline by the vertically oriented nasal septum and contain dorsal and ventral turbinates (conchae) that emanate laterally. The dorsal turbinate is slightly smaller than the ventral. The turbinates divide each nasal passage into three meati. The narrow dorsal meatus is situated between the nasal bones and the dorsal turbinate and ends blindly. The middle meatus is between the two turbinates. It contains the slitlike nasomaxillary opening, which on endoscopic examination in adult horses is situated approximately 30 cm from the external nares. The ventral meatus is fairly large, allowing for passage of the endoscope into the pharynx. The mucous membrane appears thick, pink, and highly vascular.

Passing the endoscope into the right ventral meatus, the septum appears as a pink, smooth, vertical wall on the viewer's right. The turbinates should be smooth, glistening, pink, and slightly rectangular-appearing structures on the viewer's left. At a distance of 15 to 20 cm, the middle meatus becomes apparent as a gradually widening, horizontally aligned space between the dorsal and ventral turbinates on the observer's left. At approximately 30 to 35 cm, the shelf is fairly deep, and in most horses the slit nasal maxillary opening is not visible. At a distance of 30 to 35 cm, the smooth bulbous outpouching of the ethmoturbinates is seen dorsally within the confines of a distinct recess or alcove in the roof of the nasal passage. At this level the caudal extent of the nasal septum is seen angling obliquely from ventral to caudodorsal at the viewer's right. The caudal edge of the septum is smooth, whitish-pink, and rounded. Continuing into the pharynx beyond the nasal septum is the soft palate and lateral pharyngeal walls containing the obliquely oriented pharyngeal openings of the auditory tube diverticula (guttural pouches).

Congenital Septal Deviations

Congenital lateral deviations (wry nose) are often complicated by a strong spiraling component to the nasal and incisive bones, hard palate, turbinates, and nasal septum. Flattening and twisting of the nostrils can affect both nasal passages, causing stertorous and stridulous breathing. Dysphagia and aspiration pneumonia are serious, common sequela necessitating humane destruction of most affected neonates.

Surgical repair is expensive and yields only a guarded to poor prognosis for future athletic ability if the foal survives. Owner commitment to the expense of a staged repair in the face of this guarded prognosis is essential. Reconstruction is done with the foal positioned in ventral recumbency under general anesthesia. A vertical intraoral incision is made through the mucous membrane over the hard palate in the interdental space at the most convex aspect of the deformity. The hard palate is cut transversely with an oscillating bone saw. The cut is completed at the most concave aspect of the deformity. The initial deformity in most foals causes some degree of brachygnathism. Consequently, manually realigning the incisive bone after the osteotomy results in an open-angle wedge defect on the concave side of the hard palate. The septum and turbinates are flexible enough to straighten considerably without incision or fracturing. Stability is achieved by inserting Steinmann pins passed from rostral to caudal just above the roots of the incisors into the marrow cavity of the incisive bones and maxilla. The pins are cut flush with the gum line. If stability is tenuous, an approximately 1-cm gap between the cheek teeth can be created by fashioning bilateral polymethylmethacrylate or acrylic bite blocks positioned between the cheek teeth and wired to the mandible. This allows protrusion of the tongue for nursing while still restricting chewing movement. Pins may usually be removed in approximately 6 to 8 weeks if the fracture site is stable. Pin tract infection is treated with gentle daily cleansing and flushing with 0.5% chlorhexidine in physiologic saline solution.

Broad-spectrum antibiotics begun prior to surgery may be necessary to treat concomitant aspiration pneumonia. If pneumonia is present, transtracheal aspiration is recommended for cytologic examination and definitive bacteriologic culture and susceptibility determination.

The prognosis for strenuous athletic activity is guarded to poor because of the severe decrease in airway area and pronounced alteration in airway geometry. Residual thickening and deformity of the nasal turbinates and/or nasal septum may require total or subtotal resection when the animal is a yearling. Physical examination, endoscopy, and radiology will determine the extent and location of any obstruction.

Thickening of the Turbinates

Nasal turbinectomy may be necessary to remove a thickened turbinate, which is usually due to trauma or chronic infection. Fractures through the nasal cavity will commonly result in turbinate thickening.

The horse is typed for a possible blood transfusion and placed in lateral recumbency under inhalation anesthesia with the affected side up. Aggressive pre- and intraoperative intravenous fluid therapy (25 to 50 mL/kg body weight) using one or more 14-gauge intravenous catheters is strongly recommended because of the possible extent of blood loss.

The skin incision is made just off and parallel to the midline over the length of the involved turbinate. Each end of the incision is curved laterally approximately 2.5 to 5 cm. Sharp dissection is continued through the periosteum. A three-sided nasal bone osteotomy flap is created just lateral to the nasal septum with an oscillating saw. The bone flap and overlying skin and periosteum are elevated, fracturing the fourth (lateral) side of the rectangle. Removal of the turbinates is achieved with blunt and sharp dissection and double-action rongeurs. Hemorrhage is profuse, necessitating a quick, well-executed procedure. Affected portions of the septum can be sharply excised, if necessary. If the turbinate deformity is bilateral, it may be preferable to perform two separate surgeries spaced approximately 6 to 8 weeks apart, depending on the amount of hemorrhage encountered.

The nasal passage is packed tightly with sterile, dry gauze packing or gauze packing that has been soaked in 1:10,000 epinephrine in saline solution. About 10 to 20 feet of packing material is usually necessary. One end of the packing is positioned to exit through the nares. The flap is replaced and small-diameter holes are made 5 mm from the cut edge with a Kirschner wire and a Jacobs chuck at the corners of the flap, and the midportion if it is fairly long. Holes are made through the parent nasal bone at corresponding sites, and the flap is secured with synthetic monofilament nonabsorbable suture material. Subcutaneous tissue is closed with synthetic absorbable sutures and the skin with synthetic nonabsorbable sutures, both in a simple interrupted pattern. The exiting end of the packing is secured to the nares with a nonabsorbable suture in a horizontal mattress pattern, closing the nares over the packing to prevent dislodgment during recovery. If there is concern about difficult respiration from partial obstruction of the other nasal cavity or if bilateral turbinectomy has been done, a midcervical tracheotomy is performed and the horse is recovered from general anesthesia with a cuffed endotracheal tube in place.

Procaine penicillin G (22,000 IU/kg given intramuscularly twice daily) is given perioperatively until the packing is removed in 48 to 72 hours. The packing is removed with the horse lightly sedated with xylazine, preferably in a quiet, well-bedded stall. Light bleeding is common but usually stops in minutes. Heavier bleeding may respond to elevation of the horse's head. Packing can also be introduced through the nares, but it is difficult to impossible to repack the nasal civity in a standing horse when there is profuse bleeding. If severe hemorrhage is encountered, intravenous fluids should be started, the horse anesthetized, and the nasal cavity repacked. An additional 48 hours should be allowed before attempting pack removal again.

Incisional healing proceeds remarkably unimpeded in spite of contamination with organisms from the nasal passage. This is probably due to an excellent blood supply and local defense mechanisms. Low-grade infection can be treated with hot packing, removing adjacent sutures, and gentle cleansing. Parenteral antibiotics based on culture and susceptibility results may be necessary if infection is serious or persistent. Serosanguinous nasal exudate is common for several days to weeks because of sloughing of necrotic nasal tissue. Stall confinement should be recommended for 45 to 60 days to allow for the early phases of bony and mucous membrane healing.

Nasal Polyps

It may be possible to excise solitary polyps during endoscopic observation with the horse under general anesthesia. Custom-designed snares made with obstetric wire passed through a mare urinary catheter, Ferris-Smith rongeurs, or uterine biopsy forceps may be useful depending on the polyp's location and how pedunculated the stalk is. Transendoscopic excision or vaporization with a Nd-YAG laser should be possible. Cryotherapy may be possible using liquid nitrogen and a custom-designed insulated delivery system.

Neoplasia

The most common tumors of the nasal passage are squamous cell carcinomas and fibromas. Although slow to metastasize, gradual enlargement of the tumor in this confined area causes progressive respiratory embarrassment. Total excision through a flap procedure may be attempted, followed by cryotherapy of the base if it can be observed. Retrospective studies are lacking; however, the prognosis for recovery appears to be guarded to poor.

Fungal Infection

Fungal granulomas are reported to be most commonly caused by *Entomophtera coronata,* and in North America are seen primarily in the Southwest and the Southeastern United States. Several other organisms, including *Aspergillus, Coccidioides,* and *Rhinosporidium,* have been reported, hence definitive diagnosis requires biopsy and fungal cultures. A scant, fetid unilateral nasal discharge that may be bloody is characteristic. The presumptive diagnosis is made by direct or endoscopic observation of lesions.

Surgical excision is recommended for solitary or well-defined lesions; however, total excision is usually impossible because of location and size. If partial excision can be achieved, Haynes recommends that the remaining area or base be injected with amphotericin B (40 to 50 mg/10 to 15 mL of fungal volume). This treatment should be followed with daily topical therapy with a 0.05% solution of amphotericin B in dimethyl sulfoxide (DMSO) for 14 to 21 days.

Nasal aspergillosis has been treated successfully with excision followed by topical application of natamycin solution (25 mg in 100 mL sterile water) for 3 to 5 days and intranasal insufflation of nystatin for 7 to 11 days.

NASAL SEPTUM

Nasal septal abnormalities are rare. Thickening and/or deviation of the nasal septum causes decreased exercise tolerance and a lowpitched, continuous respiratory noise. Even a slight thickening of the septum can cause markedly reduced airflow. Horses less than 4 years of age are most commonly affected. Trauma, congenital cystic dilatation and inflammation secondary to severe respiratory infections are the most common causes of thickening. Rarely, neoplasia, including carcinomas, lymphosarcoma, and chondrosarcoma, causing thickening has been diagnosed. Septal deviation may result from congenital deviation of the face or trauma or may be secondary to expansile sinus disease, such as congenital dental cysts, chronic maxillary sinus empyema, or neoplasms of the maxillary or frontal sinuses.

In most horses septal abnormalities extend far enough rostrally to be palpable through the nares. Elevation of the nares and visual inspection with a strong light source may reveal thickening or deviation. Endoscopic examination may be useful in delineating the extent of the problem; however, severe involvement may cause sufficient obstruction of the nasal passage to preclude endoscopic inspection. Radiographs, particu-

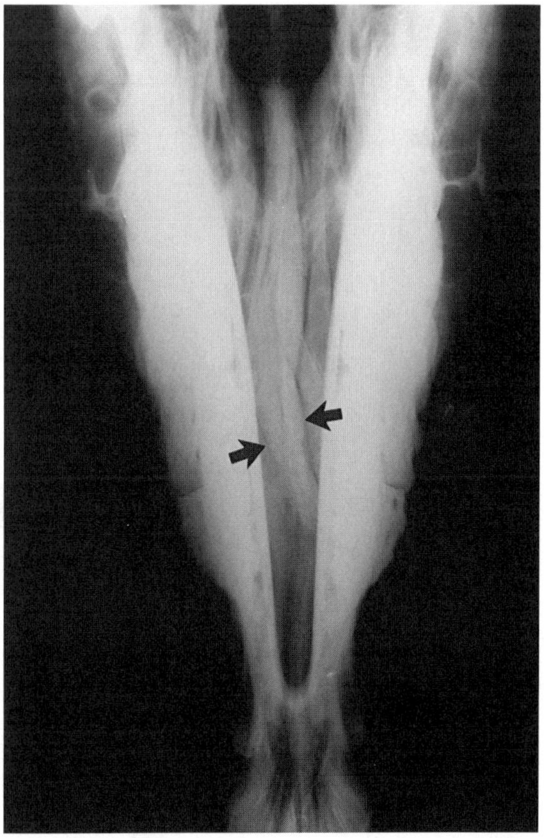

Figure 39–1. Dorsal ventral radiograph demonstrating extreme deviation and thickening of the nasal septum (between the *arrows*).

larly the dorsal ventral view, are very useful because the cartilaginous nasal septum and its mucosa contribute substantially to midline radiodensities and the cartilaginous nasal septum is not totally obscured by the bones dorsal and ventral to the nasal cavity (Fig. 39–1). In horses with discrete lesions located very rostrally, intraoral occlusal films are useful (Fig. 39–2).

Anatomy

The vertically positioned septum separates the two nasal cavities. The septum is composed of hyaline cartilage except caudoventrally, where it becomes osseous as it blends with the perpendicular plate of the ethmoid and vomer bones. The dorsal border of the cartilage is expanded on either side to form the narrow dorsolateral cartilages. The ventral border is thick and rounded and rests for most of its length in a groove in the vomer bone. The surfaces of the cartilage are covered with a highly vascular mucous membrane marked by faint grooves for the vessels and nerves that course over it. On each side lateral and parallel to the septum are dorsal and ventral nasal conchae (turbinate bones) that occupy most of the space in each nasal cavity. Rostrally, the nasal septum is attached to the alar carti-

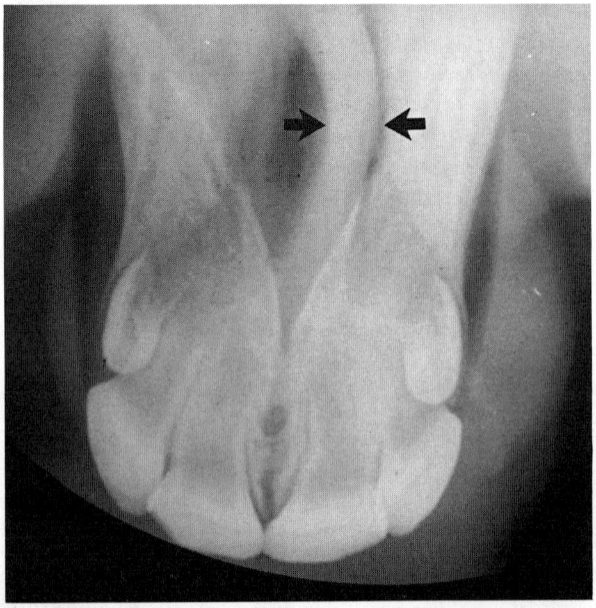

Figure 39–2. Dorsal ventral occlusal (intraoral) radiograph of the upper jaw demonstrating deviation of the rostral aspect of the nasal septum (between *arrows*). The septal deviation and fractured incisive bones resulted from a kick and produced stertorous respiration and severe dyspnea at rest.

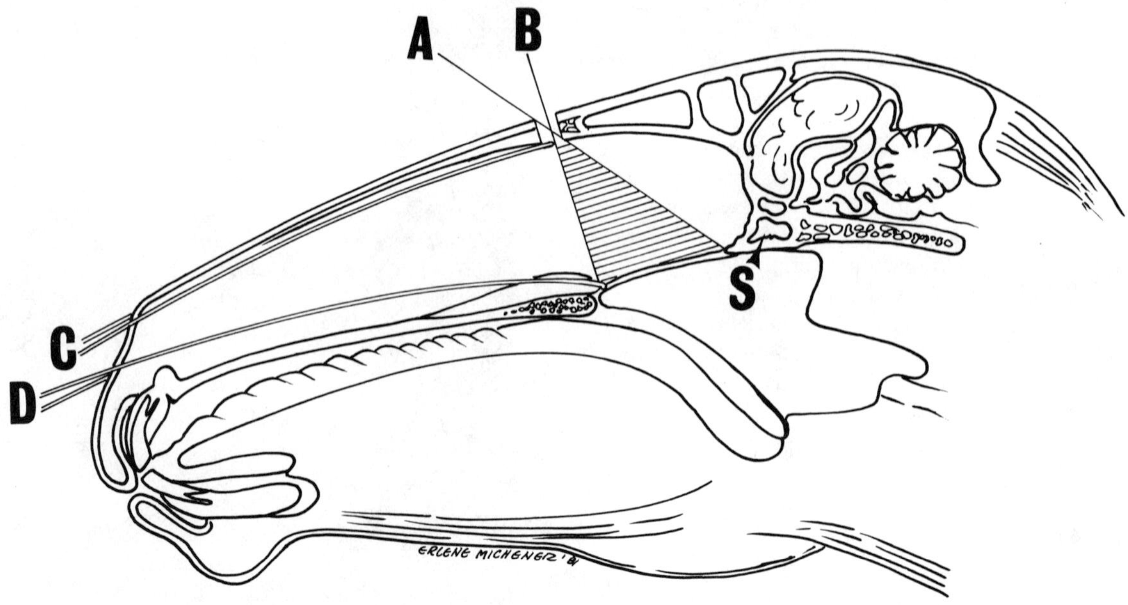

Figure 39–3. Sagittal section of an equine head, several millimeters left of the median plane, showing the additional area of septum (*shaded area*) that could be removed following an incision at a 60-degree angle to the nasal bones (*A*) compared with a vertical incision (*B*). The position of the dorsal (*C*) and ventral (*D*) obstetric wires are shown prior to removal of the nasal septum. This 60-degree angle incision ends rostral to the sphenopalatine sinus (*S*).

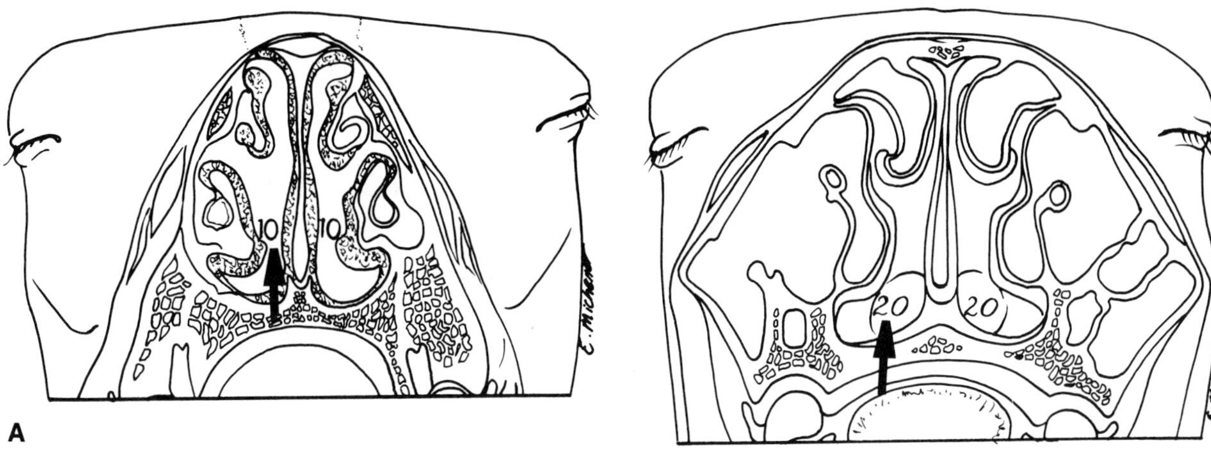

A

B

Figure 39–4. A. Frontal section through the dorsal half of the equine head at the rostral end of the facial crest. This is the level at which the septum would be removed when using a vertical caudal incision. Note the narrow space (*arrow*) approximately 10 mm between the turbinates and the septum. **B.** Frontal section through the dorsal half of the equine head at the level of the last molar teeth. Using an incision at a 60-degree angle to the nasal bones, the granulating septal stump will be in a wider area, approximately 20 mm from the ventral turbinates (*arrow*) near the nasopharynx.

lages by strong fibrous tissue that allows movement, and in some horses an actual joint may exist.

Surgery

Prior to surgery, a complete physical examination, complete blood count, and typing for a blood transfusion are necessary. Hemorrhage can be profuse, necessitating a carefully planned and executed general anesthetic and surgical procedure. Large volumes (25 to 50 mL/kg of body weight) of a balanced polyionic electrolyte solution should be administered pre- and intraoperatively through one or more 14-gauge intravenous catheters. While blood transfusions are rarely necessary, previously determined compatible donors should be immediately available.

Surgical excision is completed with the horse positioned in lateral recumbency and using inhalation anesthesia. An 18-mm circular trephine hole is made on the midline of the face at a point just rostral to the frontal sinuses, where the nasal bones begin to diverge. Dorsal and ventral longitudinal incisions are made in the septum using obstetric wire. One end of the wire is inserted into a #10 French catheter to achieve rigidity and then passed through the nostril along the ventral meatus into the pharynx. Following extubation, the end of the wire is retrieved through the mouth. A second wire is passed up the opposite nostril in similar fashion. After removing the catheters, the two wire ends protruding from the mouth are twisted together and the connected piece is pulled through the nasal cavity. After disconnecting one wire, handles are attached to the remaining wire protruding from each nostril. The wire is snugly seated dorsal to the junction of the hard and soft palate and along the ventral attachment of the septum to the vomer bone (Fig. 39–3).

In a similar fashion a wire is passed up each dorsal meatus, exiting through the trephine hole (Fig. 39–3). These wires are connected and one wire is pulled through and seated along the dorsal attachment. The rostral incision in the septum is made with a hard-backed scalpel just caudal to the alar cartilages from dorsal to ventral through the rostral aspect of the septum; the incision is curvilinear with the convexity facing rostrally. The dorsal and ventral attachments are severed using the obstetric wire. The caudal incision is made at approximately a 60-degree angle to the nasal bones using either a 12-mm osteotome or a standard wide screwdriver, each modified by grinding a sharp concave tip at the end. The septum is removed through the nostril by heavy Vulsellum forceps (Fig. 39–3).

Hemorrhage is usually reduced by the use of the obstetric wire; however, the nasal cavity can be packed with sterile cotton gauze (up to 24 feet may be needed) either dry or soaked in a 1:10,000 solution of epinephrine in saline. The nostrils are sutured closed with nonabsorbable suture material to retain the packing and prevent dislodgment during recovery from general anesthesia. Prior to extubation, a tracheotomy tube is placed.

This technique is recommended based on a consideration of the regional anatomy and the nature of the septal abnormalities being treated (Fig. 39–4). The technique, first reported in 1916, has largely been abandoned because of problems with granulation tissue formation at the caudal cut edge and in some horses incomplete removal of the affected septum.

A second technique is effective in removing very discrete and rostrally located lesions. Exposure of the affected portion of the septum is made by a longitudinal incision through the dorsal aspect of the nasal diverticulum. Using a hard-backed scalpel all attachments of the abnormal septum are severed and the rostral one third of the septum is removed. Packing is placed as described and the incised tissues of the nasal diverticulum are apposed with synthetic absorbable suture placed in a continuous pattern.

Phenylbutazone (4.4 mg/kg intravenously) is administered after surgery. Parenteral procaine penicillin G (22,000 IU/kg given intramuscularly twice daily), begun preoperatively, is continued for 3 to 5 days. Packing is removed either 48 or 72 hours after surgery. The following day twice-daily flushing of the nasal cavity is begun through the trephined opening using water at an ambient temperature from a hose or physiologic saline administered through a large syringe. Xylazine may be needed for restraint. Flushing facilitates removal of dried blood, debris, and tissue fragments. Larger fragments of tissue may need to be removed through the nostrils with forceps.

The trephine hole and tracheotomy are cleaned twice daily with gauze sponges soaked in povidone-iodine or chlorhexidine solution. Most horses heal without complications; however, occasionally mild to moderate cellulitis around the tracheotomy site or intranasal inflammation will result in transient fever. This short-term complication responds to hot packing of the tracheotomy site or flushing the necrotic debris from the nasal passages, and parenteral antibiotic administration. Most adult horses are rested for approximately 2 months before being returned to work.

Ninety percent of operated horses will still produce respiratory noise during exercise, although most owners believe that it is less than prior to surgery. The prognosis for successful return to strenuous exercise is estimated to be about 50%. Continued decreased exercise tolerance and noise may result from excessive granulation tissue on the caudal cut edge and/or alterations in airway geometry.

The cosmetic results are excellent in approximately 75% of cases. Occasionally some flattening of the bridge of the nose appears near the nasal diverticulum in spite of an effort to leave sufficient cartilage support. The alar fold and floor of the nasal diverticulum may need to be removed in a second procedure either unilaterally or bilaterally in an attempt to further increase airway size. The need for this surgery is determined by observation, palpation, and response to elevation of the alar fold.

In foals the cartilaginous nasal septum appears to be important in providing support for the developing nasal bones and nostrils. Septal removal may result in flattening of the bridge of the nose, especially when surgery is performed on foals less than 6 months of age. The result is partial upper airway obstruction caused by the tissues of the alar folds and floor of the nasal diverticulum occluding the nasal passages. Based on these observations, it is recommended that the nasal septum not be removed if possible before the horse is approximately 18 months old. Conservative treatment of traumatic septal injuries suffered as a foal may include temporary repositioning.

BIBLIOGRAPHY

French DD, Haynes PF, Miller RI: Surgical and medical management of rhinophycomycosis (conidiobolomycosis) in a horse. *J Am Vet Med Assoc* 1985;186:1105–1106.

Greet TRC: Nasal aspergillosis in three horses. *Vet Rec* 1981;109:487–489.

Hare WCD: Equine respiratory system, in Getty R (ed): *The Anatomy of the Domestic Animals.* Philadelphia, WB Saunders Co, 1975, pp 498–504.

Haynes PF: The respiratory system, in Jennings PB (ed): *The Practice of Large Animal Surgery*, vol 1. Philadelphia, WB Saunders, 1984; pp 398–405.

Stillson AE, Herring DS, Robertson JT: Contribution of the nasal septum to the radiographic anatomy of the equine nasal cavity. *J Am Vet Med Assoc* 1985;186:590–592.

Tulleners BP, Raker CW: Nasal septum resection in the horse. *Vet Surg* 1983;12:41–47.

40
Paranasal Sinuses

Dennis M. Meagher

The paranasal sinuses of the horse are composed of the maxillary, conchofrontal, ethmoid, and sphenopalatine sinuses. The frontal and maxillary are most often of concern from a surgical standpoint. The anatomic outline and the surgical landmarks of the frontal and maxillary sinuses are shown in Figures 40–1 and 40–2. Of particular importance are the bony canals, through which the nasal lacrimal duct and infraorbital nerve pass, and the position of the infraorbital foramen.

The large frontomaxillary aperture allows for drainage from the frontal to the maxillary sinus. The nasomaxillary aperture, which opens into the middle meatus, allows for drainage from the maxillary sinus to the nasal cavity. The frontal sinus is divided into caudal and rostral compartments that are separated by a thin, incomplete, irregular plate of trabecular bone. The rostral compartment is also called the dorsal conchal or turbinate portion of the frontal sinus. The maxillary sinus is also divided into rostral and caudal compartments, which are partially divided by a plate of bone. The rostral compartment has both medial and lateral sections, which are partially divided by the bony infraorbital canal. Since the drainage of the medial portion of the rostral compartment is via the lateral compartment, fluid or exudate may become trapped in this area as the bony infraorbital canal acts as a natural dam. The roots of the upper last premolar and three upper molars are in close contact with the floor of the maxillary sinus, which is formed by a thin plate of alveolar bone. In young horses the maxillary sinus is comparatively small, but as the horse ages and the teeth grow, the size of the maxillary sinus increases. The age of the horse needs to be kept in mind when planning any surgery involving the maxillary sinus.

COMMON SURGICAL PROCEDURES

The most common surgical procedures involving the frontal and maxillary sinuses include: drilling a small hole in the sinus for centesis, lavage, or biopsy; trephination for drainage, lavage, or repulsion of teeth; bone flap incisions for sinus exploration and removal of space-occupying lesions; and reduction and stabilization of compression fractures.

Sinus Centesis

Centesis of the frontal or maxillary sinus can be performed in the standing sedated horse. This procedure is of value primarily from a diagnostic standpoint but is also used for the placement of catheters for sinus lavage. After outlining the borders of the sinus and selecting a site, a small area is shaved, prepared for aseptic surgery, and infiltrated subcutaneously with local anesthetic. A stab incision is made down to the bone and a small hole is drilled with the trocar point of a Steinmann pin held in a Jacobs chuck. About 2 to 3 cm of the trocar point is left protruding from the chuck so that deeper structures will not be injured. The size of pin selected depends on the purpose of the procedure. Fluid can be collected with a needle or fine catheter. If an indwelling catheter is to be placed or a biopsy taken, a larger hole will be needed. If an infectious process is present, the stab incision should be left open to heal by granulation; otherwise it can be closed with a single suture.

Trephination

Careful attention to the topographic landmarks outlining the sinuses is important when selecting sites for trephination. The commonly used sites for trephination of the frontal and maxillary sinuses are shown in Figure 40–3. For tooth repulsion, the site needs to be selected so that the dental punch can be placed squarely over the tooth roots. This ensures that the repelling force will be directed through the long axis of the tooth. A hypodermic needle may be placed through the cheek, and directed over the center of the occlusal surface of the involved tooth. This provides an external marker for the selection of the trephine site. During tooth repulsion it is beneficial to have an assistant hold a finger on the occlusal surface of the involved tooth to ensure that the force is being directed through the correct tooth. Since the teeth are much longer and tend to curve caudally in young horses, the age of the horse needs to be considered.

Once the site has been selected, and following preparation for aseptic surgery, a round plug of skin, subcutaneous tissue, and periosteum is excised. The soft tissue plug needs to be slightly larger than the diameter of the trephine. When the rostral compartment of the

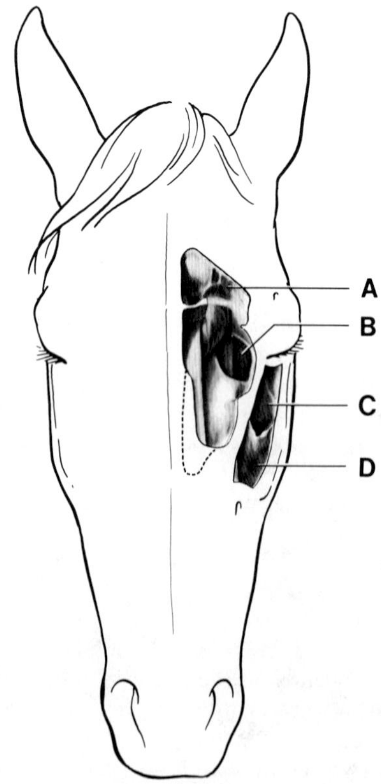

Figure 40–1. A line drawing showing the frontal and maxillary sinuses outlined: *A*, frontal sinus; *B*, frontomaxillary opening; *C*, caudal maxillary sinus; *D*, rostral maxillary sinus.

maxillary sinus is to be trephined, the levator labii maxillaris and levator nasolabialis muscles need to be retracted after the skin is removed to gain exposure to the periosteum. The trephine is then used to cut out the round plug of bone. Both the excised soft tissue and bone plug are discarded and the trephine opening is left to heal by second intention.

Sinus Bone Flap Incisions

Bone flap incisions were first described as a means of gaining wide exposure to the maxillary sinus. Since that time this technique has been applied to the frontal sinus and the nasal cavity (Fig. 40–4). Recently, a triangulated flap that exposes both the rostral compartment of the frontal sinus and the caudal aspect of the nasal cavity with a single bone flap has been described. A double bone flap technique that provides very wide exposure to both the frontal and maxillary sinus simultaneously has also been described.

The basic principle of sinusotomy via bone flap is that the soft tissues and bone are cut on three sides and the bone flap with its soft tissue, including the skin, is opened similarly to opening a door (Fig. 40–5). It is important to leave the soft tissues attached to the bone flap to ensure bone viability. The soft tissue also acts as a hinge along the fourth side. The bone flap is planned to gain the greatest amount of exposure to the lesion in question and may be hinged medially or laterally depending on the location of the lesion being explored.

The site for the bone flap is planned and an incision is made through the skin and soft tissues, including the periosteum. Following hemostasis, the periosteum is elevated for a width of 0.5 cm along the incision, exposing the bone, which is then cut on a 45-degree angle along three sides using an oscillating saw or a cutting burr attached to an air drill. The soft tissues are elevated and the bone on the fourth side is cut 0.5 cm in from each corner. Two wide-bladed elevators or osteotomes are used to elevate the bone flap until it fractures the bone along the remainder of the fourth side. The bone flap is then secured in the open position with a towel clamp and protected with a moistened towel or sponge. It is important not to traumatize the bone flap or separate it from the soft tissues during surgical manipulation.

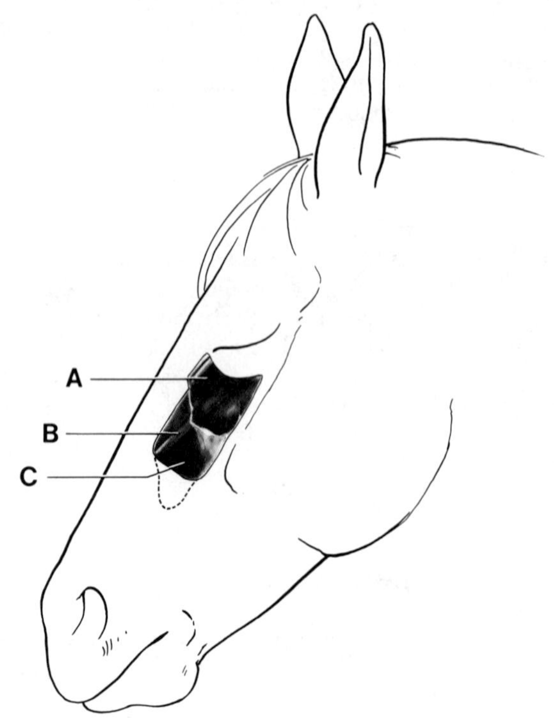

Figure 40–2. A line drawing of a lateral view of the maxillary sinus: *A*, caudal maxillary sinus; *B*, infraorbital canal; *C*, rostral maxillary sinus.

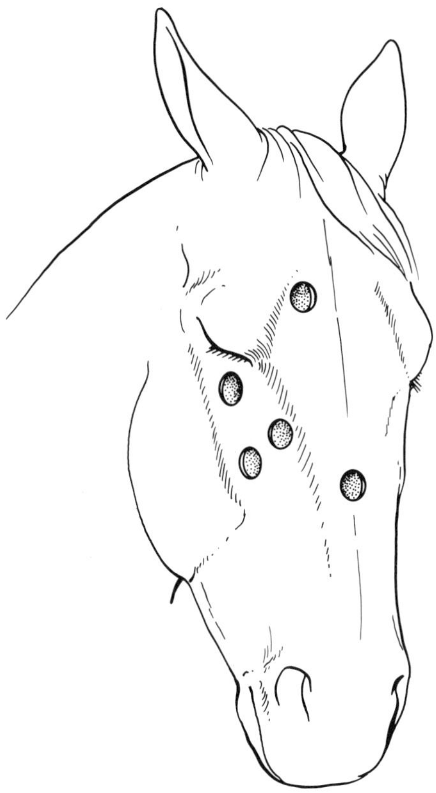

Figure 40–3. Line drawing showing common sites of trephination into the frontal and maxillary sinuses and the nasal cavity.

Surgery of the sinuses and nasal cavity frequently results in marked hemorrhage, which is best controlled by packing. Gauze soaked in povidone-iodine diluted 1:1 with either water or saline is partly pulled from the sinus through the nasal passage and out the external nares. The sinus is then packed through the sinusotomy and the nasal passage is packed via the external nares. The end of the pack is sutured to the external nares to secure it in place and prevent the horse from swallowing it should it become dislodged. The pack is removed from 48 to 96 hours following surgery and may be removed in stages if epistaxis occurs.

Once the surgical procedure is complete, the bone flap is replaced and the soft tissues are closed in layers. It is usually not necessary to secure the bone itself, since it will be held in place by the soft tissue, the irregular fracture line on one side, and the dovetail effect of cutting the bone flap on a 45-degree angle.

In most instances it is beneficial to lavage the sinuses for several days after pack removal to remove blood clots and exudate. It is preferable to place the lavage tube into the sinus at a site other than through the bone flap. This may be done at surgery or later utilizing the sinus centesis technique. The latter is preferable if the sinuses had to be tightly packed to control hemorrhage at the time of surgery. A #32 French mushroom catheter can be installed through a hole made with a #7 Steinman pin. This size catheter allows a stomach pump to be used to flush the sinus, which is more effective than a gravity flow system through a small sinus catheter. Sinus lavage is carried out once or twice daily for 5 to 10 days until the nasal discharge is markedly reduced. The hole is allowed to heal by granulation after catheter removal.

COMPRESSION FRACTURES OF THE FACIAL BONES

Compression fractures of the head occur relatively frequently in the horse and are usually the result of direct

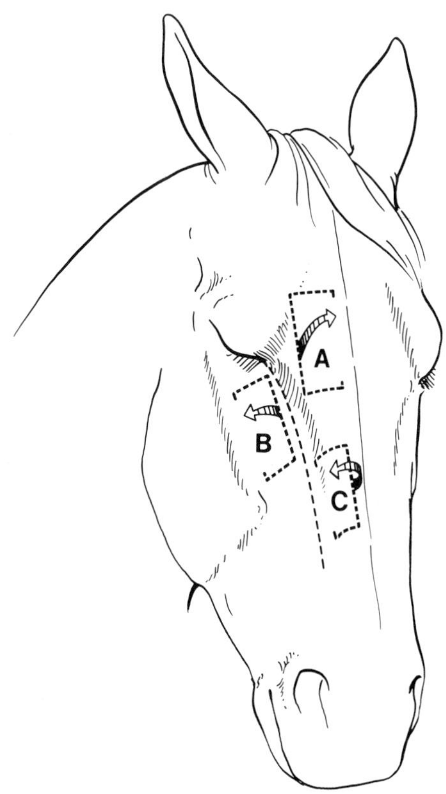

Figure 40–4. Line drawing of the common sites for bone flap incisions (heavy broken lines and arrows) to expose: *A*, the frontal sinus; *B*, the maxillary sinus, and *C*, the nasal cavity. The *lighter broken line* indicates the location of the nasolacrimal canal.

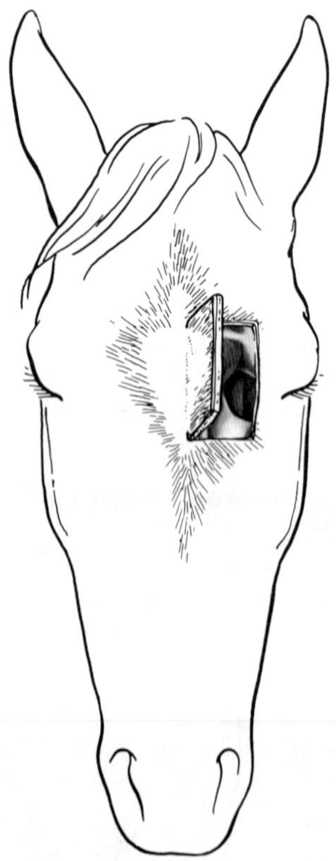

Figure 40–5. Line drawing of a sinus flap incision into the frontal sinus showing the bone flap and attached soft tissues in a partially open position.

trauma. The relatively thin bone over the frontal and maxillary sinuses is often involved, as well as the bony orbit and nasal bones; frequently more than one bone is involved. Aside from the cosmetic defects caused by such fractures, there may also be damage to the eye, contamination of the sinuses, reduction of the size of the nasal passage, and damage to the nasolacrimal duct and other structures. A very careful physical examination is the most important feature of the diagnostic workup. By standing directly in front of the horse and carefully viewing the entire head, comparing the affected and nonaffected sides, often the difference in symmetry can be identified. With careful palpation, the major features of the fracture can often be felt. A complete set of good-quality radiographs should then be taken, remembering that the multitude of overlapping lines present in radiographs of the skull may obscure some fractures. Total reliance on radiographic examination for fractures of the equine skull will result in a significant number of misdiagnosed fractures. In some instances, in spite of careful physical examination and good-quality radiographs, the full extent of the fracture is not appreciated until the area is exposed surgically.

Since these fractures may present in such a wide variety of configurations, it is not practical to attempt to describe an individual approach to their repair; therefore, the principles of repair will be presented. Unlike long bones in the horse, facial fractures heal readily with a minimum of fixation. The aim is to reduce the fracture so all fragments are in normal anatomic alignment, or as near to that as possible, and secured with the least amount of internal fixation that will maintain their normal position. There is no direct weight taken by these bones, they are under comparatively little tension, and the fracture lines are usually very irregular. For these reasons, elevation of the compressed fragments into their normal position is often all that is needed.

The fracture lines and compressed area are best exposed with a curved incision and elevation of the soft tissue flap. The location, size, and direction of the flap will depend on the size of the fracture as well as the location of vital structures such as the infraorbital foramen. Once the fractured area is exposed, bone hooks and elevators are used to pry the fragments into normal positions. In some instances, it may be necessary to drill small holes in the bone to position the bone hooks in such a way that the compressed fragments can be elevated. Some compressed fractures may be best managed by drilling holes a short distance from the edges of the compressed area so that the tip of an elevator can be inserted under the compressed bone to pry it into place and restore the facial contour. If the fragments cannot be reduced or they fail to stay reduced, it is often because there are additional fractures present that have not been identified. Following existing fracture lines will often help to identify these. Fragments that are stable after reduction usually do not require fixation. Unstable fragments may be fixed with fine stainless steel wire placed in a simple interrupted pattern through predrilled holes on either side of the fracture line.

The bony orbit will often fracture in two places. Usually one involves the subraorbital or zygomatic arch, but frequently a second fracture involves the sides or ventral rim of the orbit and is much less obvious. Both fractures must be reduced simultaneously in order to return the bony orbit to its normal shape and position. The supraorbital and zygomatic arch fractures may require only reduction, but they may need to be secured with stainless steel wire or a small bone screw. Curved incisions above and/or below the eye allow for exposure of the bony orbit and digital manipulation inside the orbit by carrying blunt dissections inside the orbital rim. Fractures that involve the orbit are best repaired soon after they occur to reduce the chance of permanent eye damage.

Fractures that are severely comminuted or have sustained significant bone loss may require the use of reconstruction bone plates in place of, or in combination with, stainless steel wire sutures.

Open fractures need to be carefully débrided and lavaged. When these involve a sinus, a large mushroom catheter should be placed into the sinus through a separate opening made with a #7 Steinmann pin or a small trephine, and the sinus flushed for several days after surgery to avoid the development of chronic sinusitis.

Some comminuted and open fractures will contain bone fragments that are severely contaminated and completely separated from soft tissues. In these cases, the detached and contaminated fragments are best discarded. When a bone defect results, it is sometimes possible to close, or at least partially close, the soft tissues. The bony defect will fill in with new bone over a period of several weeks.

Reduction of nasal bone fractures may be facilitated by manipulation of the nose and finger pressure inside the nasal passage or the use of a gauze pack, which forces the nasal bone into its normal position. Severe nasal fractures may result in a crushing injury to the nasal septum. However, it is best to reduce the fractures and allow time for healing, accepting the fact that there may be significant thickening of the nasal septum that requires resection at a later date. (see Chapter 39).

Closed compression fractures over the sinuses that do not involve other structures may be of only cosmetic significance, and therefore will not necessarily need to be repaired depending on the use of the horse and the interest of the owner. Facial fractures that are nondisplaced or minimally displaced will usually heal uneventfully without surgical intervention.

BIBLIOGRAPHY

Blackford JT, Goble DO, Henry RW, Geiser DR, Held JP: Triangulated flap technique for nasofrontal surgery. *Vet Surg* 1985;14:287–294.

Haynes PF: Surgery of the equine respiratory tract, in Jenning PB, (ed): *The Practice of Large Animal Surgery*. Philadelphia, WB Saunders Co, 1984, pp 388–486.

Koch DB, Leitch M, Beech J: Orbital surgery in two horses. *Vet Surg* 1980;9:61.

Levine SB: Depression fractures of the nasal and frontal bones of the horse. *J Eq Med Surg* 1979;3:186.

Little CB, Hilbert BJ, McGill CA: A retrospective study of head fractures in 21 horses. *Aust Vet J* 1985;14:62–89.

McIlwraith CW, Turner AS: *Equine Surgery Advanced Techniques*. Philadelphia, Lea & Febiger, 1987, pp 244–253.

Turner AS: Conditions of facial bones, in Jennings PB (ed): *The Practice of Large Animal Surgery*. Philadelphia, WB Saunders Co, 1984, pp 897–899.

41 Ethmoid Hematoma

Dennis M. Meagher

Ethmoid hematomas are slowly expanding angiomatous masses that originate from the mucosal lining of the ethmoidal conchae in the caudal nasal cavity. They occur in middle-aged to older horses and appear to be more common in Thoroughbreds. Intact and gelded males are more frequently affected than females. The most common presenting sign is an intermittent bloody nasal discharge that is usually unilateral, but may be bilateral, and ranges in character from serosanguinous to a slow drip of blood. The frequency and amount of hemorrhage is usually not affected by exercise or the position of the horse's head. As the hematoma enlarges, it may partially or completely occlude the nasal cavity, usually the ventral meatus, causing respiratory stridor and in some instances exercise intolerance. With progressive expansion, the hematoma may extend into the maxillary and frontal sinuses, and occasionally result in distortion of the facial bones.

DIAGNOSIS

The diagnosis is confirmed by endoscopic observation of a dark redish to purple colored mass protruding from the ethmoidal conchae. In some cases, there will be a yellow-brown to dark green hue on the surface or areas of ulceration and recent hemorrhage. As the hematoma enlarges, it may take on a bulblike form as it protrudes rostrally into the nasal cavity. It may be necessary to pass the endoscope beyond the rostral portion of the mass to identify its origin from the ethmoturbinate. Since this condition may occur bilaterally, it is important to examine both left and right ethmoidal conchae. It is also important to use an endoscope that is small and maneuverable enough to inspect the caudal recesses of the ethmoidal conchae. Occasionally, a very small hematoma not apparent on inspection of the rostral surface of the ethmoidal conchae can be identified. This is particularly important when a large mass has been identified on one side and the contralateral side is being examined.

In some long-standing cases, the hematoma may expand into the nasopharynx as well as into the frontal, dorsal conchal, and maxillary sinuses. Expansion into the nasopharynx may progress to the point where the hematoma expands into the opposite nasal passage, giving the endoscopic appearance of a bilateral ethmoid hematoma when, in fact, all of the abnormal tissue is originating from a single site. Careful observation of both ethmoidal conchae will aid in resolving this confusing appearance. Diagnostic-quality radiographs (lateral, dorsoventral, and oblique) are necessary to identify the extent of the hematoma, especially to assess the involvement of the paranasal sinuses. In chronic cases there may have been sufficient blood loss to cause anemia, and this needs to be considered when a treatment plan is being developed.

The original description of this condition referred to it as a progressive ethmoid hematoma. This appears to be an accurate description because the tissue mass continues to enlarge if untreated and, in some instances, continues to enlarge in spite of treatment. The etiology is unknown.

Histologically, these masses appear as expanding, poorly organized hematomas filled with blood in various stages of breakdown. There is a thin capsule that consists of normal nasal mucosa and thin sheets of connective tissue loosely distributed throughout the mass.

Surgery

Treatment has been directed toward surgical removal and/or procedures aimed at destroying the mass, including its origin in the ethmoid labyrinth. The ethmoidal conchae can be approached surgically, using a bone flap technique into the frontal sinus or the caudal nasal cavity. A triangulated flap technique has been described that provides exposure to both the rostral compartment of the frontal sinus and the caudal nasal cavity utilizing a single flap. The frontal sinus normally is separated from the nasal ethmoid labyrinth by a thin plate of bone (the internal lamina of the frontal bone), which forms the floor of the frontal sinus. Unless the hematoma has expanded into the frontal sinus through this bony plate, it will be necessary to remove the plate to gain access to the ethmoid labyrinth from the frontal sinus. This approach provides the most direct access to the ethmoidal conchae. When an ethmoid hematoma has expanded to fill the frontal or the frontal and maxillary sinuses, a rostral frontal or triangulated nasofrontal flap combined with a maxillary sinus flap may be needed to gain access to the entire mass.

The proximity of the nasal turbinates to the ethmoturbinate and the richly vascular lining mucosa results in significant hemorrhage during this surgical procedure. Therefore, it is necessary to be prepared to support the cardiovascular system during surgery with intravenous isotonic fluids as well as having cross-matched blood available for transfusion. Blood loss can be reduced markedly by temporary bilateral carotid artery occlusion during the time the ethmoid mass is being ablated. This requires a separate surgical approach to the carotid arteries in the rostral third of the neck and thus additional preoperative planning. On average, the arteries have been occluded for 11 to 13 minutes without untoward sequelae.

Once the hematoma has been exposed via sinusotomy, it should be quickly removed and the sinus cavity packed with gauze to minimize blood loss. The mass can be removed manually, but it tends to be friable, and a large currette facilitates removal by detaching the mass from its base. A large gauze pack soaked in 1:1 sterile saline and povidone-iodine can be packed into the sinuses and nasal cavity via the sinusotomy to temporarily control hemorrhage while any remaining hematoma is removed. By holding the pack firmly in place for a few moments and then progressively exposing small areas, additional dissection can be achieved with minimal hemorrhage. The origin of the hematoma is then frozen utilizing a large cryosurgical probe. This may be difficult because of hemorrhage, and care should be taken not to freeze this area too liberally because of the close proximity of the cribriform plate, which separates the ethmoidal conchae from the brain. An alternate method for removal is to apply the cryosurgical probe to the intact hematoma and then piecemeal remove the frozen sections, until the entire hematoma has been removed and the origin frozen. While this technique can result in significantly less hemorrhage, it requires a large cryosurgical unit, good surgical exposure, and a relatively hemorrhage-free surgical field.

Whether the hematoma is removed surgically, by combined surgical ablation and cryosurgery, or by cryosurgery alone, there usually is sufficient hemorrhage to require packing of the sinuses and the nasal cavity. A long forceps (Knowles forceps) is passed up the ventral meatus of the nasal cavity by an assistant until the jaws can be felt through the sinusotomy. The end of a 1- to 2-m sterile cotton gauze pack is passed into the jaws of the forceps and pulled through the sinus and out the nostrils. Sufficient material is pulled through the nostrils to allow packing of the nasal cavity. The frontal sinus and caudal nasal cavity are packed through the surgical incision by folding the pack firmly into place in an accordion-like manner until the cavity is filled sufficiently to control hemorrhage. The nasal cavity is then packed via the external nares using long forceps and the end of the gauze pack is sutured to the external nares to prevent the horse from swallowing the pack should it become dislodged. The flap incision(s) are closed in a routine manner and a large mushroom catheter is placed in the caudal compartment of the frontal sinus to facilitate lavage of the sinuses after pack removal.

Preparations should be made for a tracheostomy in case the horse experiences respiratory distress after removal of the endotracheal tube. Close observation for signs of respiratory distress is necessary until the pack and tracheostomy tube have been removed. The pack is left in place for 48 to 72 hours and then removed over a 48-hour period by pulling one third to one half of the pack out of the nose once daily. If epistaxis occurs, further removal of the pack is discontinued until the following day. Antibiotics are started preoperatively and continued for 24 hours after pack removal. Nonsteroidal anti-inflammatory drugs are used as needed to control pain, swelling, and edema.

Since there is a tendency for recurrence, some surgeons have taken a less aggressive approach to the management of ethmoid hematoma, particularly in older breeding horses. J. H. Johnson (Lexington, KY; personal communication) reports satisfactory results using cryosurgery applied directly to the hematoma via transnasal endoscopy. This treatment is directed at reducing the size of the hematoma, allowing the horse to be more comfortable and to maintain an adequate airway. Cryosurgical treatment is repeated once or twice a year as needed. I have also used this approach in two horses, with Freon delivered via a small plastic tube passed through the biopsy portal of an endoscope. One horse had a unilateral 3-cm diameter hematoma that was frozen four times in 8 days. There was no recurrence during 8 months of follow-up. The other horse had bilateral hematomas, with a 5-cm hematoma protruding into the left nasal cavity and a 2-cm mass on the right side. These were frozen with freon numerous times over a 4-month period, and although they were reduced in size by approximately one half, they failed to respond beyond that point, and if left untreated for 3 weeks would begin to increase in size.

Recently, several groups have used the Nd:YAG laser as a method of treating ethmoid hematomas. This may be done via transnasal endoscopy (see Chapter 7). Because of the precision and hemostasis afforded by photovaporization, it would seem to be an ideal way of removing these troublesome lesions. Although this has to some extent been true, the problem of recurrence persists. Vaporization of large lesions like ethmoid hematomas produces a large amount of smoke, and efficient evacuation of the smoke is critical to prevent smoke injury to the lung and also to maintain vision in the operative field. This method of treatment has only been used in a comparatively small number of cases, and with increased experience and modification of the technique, it may prove to be very useful.

PROGNOSIS

Long term, the most common complication is recurrence, which occurs with all the forms of therapy reported to date. In a series of 24 cases I have reviewed, the use of cryosurgery combined with surgical ablation resulted in a lower recurrence rate than did surgical ablation alone. Transnasal cryosurgical treatment and laser photovaporization and ablation have been used on too few cases to draw any conclusions on relative recurrence rates. Both of these techniques have the advantage of being performed in the standing sedated horse with topical anesthesia, thus avoiding the risks attendant with general anesthesia. Also, these techniques are not usually associated with serious blood loss, in contrast to surgical removal, wherein hemorrhage may be severe enough to warrant blood transfusion and, at least, is of concern from the standpoint of anesthetic management. The direct application of the cryosurgical probe to the origin of the hematoma may be beneficial in reducing recurrence, but does pose the potential risk of brain damage if it is not applied carefully or if the cribriform plate has been thinned by pressure from the expanding hematoma.

Transnasal cryosurgery may be palliative, but may be insufficient in most cases for the performing horse. The use of the Nd:YAG laser, although in its developmental stages, currently has the disadvantage of requiring specialized and expensive equipment as well as special knowledge and skill in its use.

The development of a management plan for progressive ethmoid hematomas requires consideration of the intended use of the horse, the equipment, facilities, and personnel available, and the wishes of the owner. Currently, a guarded prognosis needs to be given relating to a complete cure without recurrence. However, with the currently available surgical and treatment methods, the condition is not immediately life threatening and a number of horses have continued to function at their previous level.

BIBLIOGRAPHY

Blackford JT, Goble DO, Henry RW, Geiser DR, Held JP: Triangulated flap technique for nasofrontal surgery. *Vet Surg* 1985;14:287–294.

Boles CL: Abnormalities of the upper respiratory tract. *Vet Clin North Am Large Anim Pract* 1979;1:89–111.

Boles CL: Treatment of upper airway abnormalities. *Vet Clin North Am Large Anim Pract* 1979;1:127–147.

Cook WR, Littlewort MC: Progressive haematoma of the ethmoid region in the horse. *Equine Vet J* 1974;6:101–108.

Haynes PF: Surgery of the equine respiratory tract, in Jennings PB (ed): *The Practice of Large Animal Surgery*, vol. 1. Philadelphia, WB Saunders Co, 1984, p 404.

Leyland A, Baker JR: Lesions of the nasal and paranasal sinuses of the horse causing dyspnoea. *Br Vet J* 1975, 131:339–346.

Platt H: Haemorrhagic nasal polyps of the horse. *J Pathol* 1975;115:51–55.

Sullivan M, Burrell MH, McCandish IAP: Progressive haematoma of the maxillary sinus in a horse. *Vet Rec* 1984;114:191.

Wheat JD: Sinus surgery in the horse. *Arch Am Coll Vet Surg* 1973;2:25.

Wheat JD: Sinus drainage and tooth repulsion in the horse. *Proc Am Assoc Equine Pract* 1973;19:171.

42
Dorsal Displacement of the Soft Palate

David E. Freeman

Dorsal displacement of the soft palate is a common cause of upper airway obstruction in racehorses. The cause of the condition is unknown, and earlier explanations, such as overlong soft palate or soft palate paresis, are no longer tenable. Although soft palate paresis occurs in horses with pharyngeal paresis, it is manifested clinically as dysphagia and not as transient upper airway obstruction during fast work. If nerve damage was responsible for dorsal displacement of the soft palate during fast work, the tensor veli palatini muscle should be affected because its primary action is to depress the soft palate. The site of nerve damage would have to be specific in horses with dorsal displacement of the soft palate to explain the normal appearance and function of other muscles that have the same innervation as the tensor veli palatini. In addition, neither nerve damage nor muscle atrophy can be demonstrated in sections of soft palate from horses with the condition.

Cook proposed that idiopathic dorsal displacement of the soft palate in racehorses is probably caused by a functional defect that disrupts stability of the normal relationship between the soft palate and larynx rather than an abnormality in the soft palate alone. The caudal free border of the soft palate is continued on both sides of the pharynx by folds of mucous membrane that unite to form the palatopharyngeal arch (Fig. 42–1A). The opening bordered by these parts of the soft palate is called the ostium intrapharyngeum and, under normal conditions, this is completely sealed against the lingual surface of the epiglottis and the corniculate cartilages of the arytenoids (Fig. 42–1B). During strenuous activity, maintenance of this seal ensures that air inhaled through the nasal passages can flow through the nasopharynx at its maximum diameter. During full abduction of the arytenoid cartilages, the corniculate cartilages rotate laterally and rostrally, thereby enlarging the ostium intrapharyngeum and converting the pharynx and larynx into a continuous, smooth-walled tube. The relationship between the laryngeal cartilages and soft palate is analogous to the fingers and thumb of one hand stretching a rubber band, with the index and middle fingers as one corniculate cartilage, the ring and little finger as the other, the thumb as the epiglottis, and the rubber band as the borders of the ostium (Fig. 42–1B). Dorsal displacement of the soft palate is analogous to withdrawal of the thumb from within the rubber band, allowing it to collapse (Fig. 42–1C). When the epiglottis assumes a position beneath the soft palate, the caudal free border of the soft palate prolapses dorsally into the nasopharynx and reduces its diameter

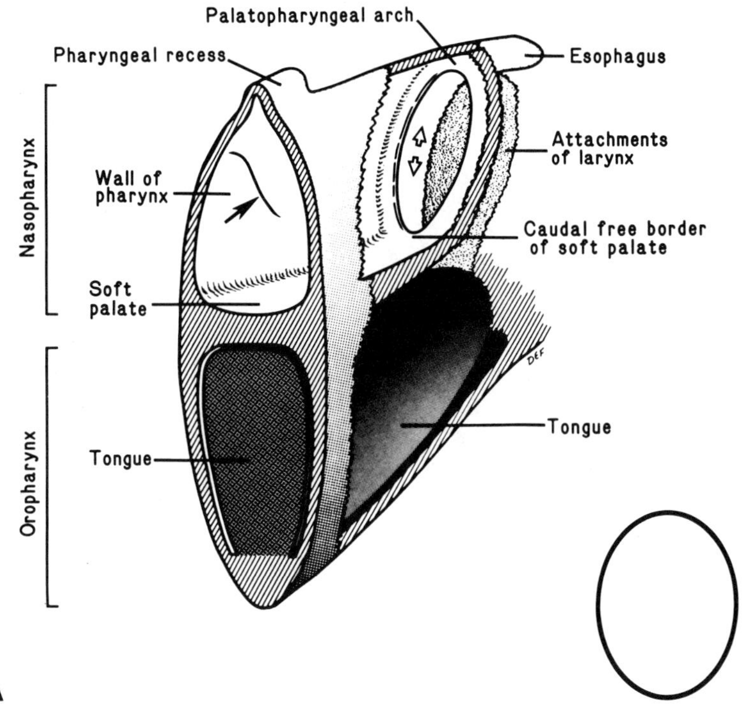

A

Figure 42–1A. Nasopharynx and oropharynx of the horse represented as two parallel tubes, cut transversely. The lateral walls of both structures and the entire larynx have been removed to show the anatomy of the soft palate. The soft palate is continued from the caudal free border by mucosal folds that follow the lateral walls of the pharynx to form the palatopharyngeal arch. The oval opening created by these structures is the ostium intrapharyngeum. Between the soft palate and the larynx is a narrow space, the piriform recess (*double* open arrows). The *single arrow* points to the pharyngeal orifice of the guttural pouch. In the lower right-hand corner, the ostium intrapharyngeum is shown as an ellipse. (*Figure continues*)

(Fig. 42–1C). Consequently, airflow through the pharynx is diminished.

Heffron and Baker conducted cine-endoscopic studies on horses prone to this condition and observed that displacement induced by manual occlusion of the nostrils was associated with caudal retraction of the larynx. Cook proposed that the muscles responsible for this movement of the larynx, the sternothyroideus, sternohyoideus, and omohyoideus muscles, can be regarded as accessory muscles of respiration and that they normally draw the larynx caudally during strenuous activity. The purpose of this caudal retraction is to indirectly tense and flatten the walls of the pharynx, which is coupled to the larynx through the ostium intrapharyngeum (Fig. 42–1A). Cook postulated that these muscles may be hyperactive in excitable or nervous horses and that they then retract the larynx sufficiently to disrupt the airtight seal between the pharynx and larynx. Consequently, the soft palate becomes displaced above the epiglottis. The problem may be compounded in horses that have a lower respiratory tract disease because the increased negative pressure created on inspiration can draw the larynx and trachea further caudally. The problem is favored also in horses that carry their heads in marked flexion and in horses that retract the tongue behind the bit. The latter maneuver forces the dorsum of the tongue against the oral surface of the soft palate and also displaces the larynx caudally.

Although soft palate displacement is most frequently seen in the absence of predisposing causes, it may occur secondary to any abnormality that can disrupt the normal relationship between the larynx and the ostium intrapharyngeum. Such abnormalities include any form of pharyngeal inflammation, laryngeal hemiplegia, loss of normal corniculate cartilage contour, hypoplastic epiglottis, subepiglottic fibrosis after surgery to correct entrapped epiglottis, or congenital malformation of the laryngeal cartilages. In the latter, rostral displacement of the palatopharyngeal arch is the more likely abnormality, but complete dislocation of the ostium intrapharyngeum can be seen in rare cases (Fig. 42–2).

Although largely speculative, the preceding mechanism of luxation of laryngopalatal dislocation provides a working hypothesis that is consistent with known mechanisms of normal pharyngeal function and that is compatible with the clinical manifestations of the disease. In addition, it has led to the development of a treatment for soft palate displacement that appears to have a more sound basis than other forms of treatment.

DIAGNOSIS

The most typical history of soft palate displacement is a report of the horse slowing down, apparently as a

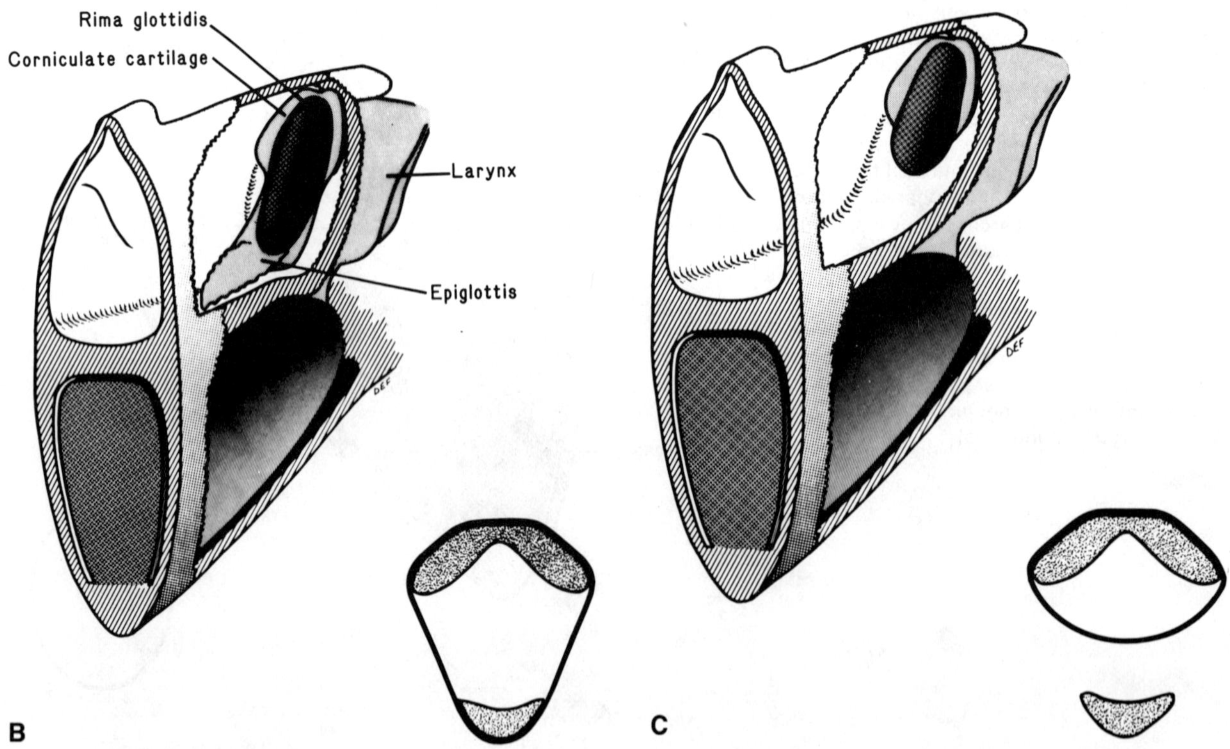

Figure 42–1B and C. **B.** As Figure 42–1A, but with the entire larynx in place to show its normal relationship with the ostium intrapharyngeum and the soft palate. In the lower right-hand corner, the borders of the ostium intrapharyngeum are stretched open by the corniculate cartilages and epiglottis. **C.** As **B** but with a dorsal displacement of the soft palate. The caudal free border is dorsal to and obscuring the epiglottis and the ostium intrapharyngeum is reduced in size (compare with **B**). In the lower right-hand corner, the epiglottis has slipped out of the ostium so that the ostium intrapharyngeum is no longer stretched open.

result of acute breathing difficulty, when it is asked to produce maximum effort. Concurrently, the horse makes a gurgling noise that is loudest on expiration and can be attributed to vibration of the caudal free border of the soft palate as air passes over it. In lay terms, these signs are usually described as "gurgling," "choking up," or "swallowing the tongue." Although the problem can be temporarily resolved by swallowing, apparently it is difficult for a horse to accomplish a swallowing maneuver under racing conditions. However, an important diagnostic feature of this condition is its sudden onset and its intermittent nature during work. In many cases, the history is unclear and the problem can only be described in vague terms that are weakly suggestive of the condition.

Because dorsal displacement of the soft palate rarely occurs in horses at rest, it cannot be seen consistently on endoscopic examination. Manual occlusion of the nostrils for a sufficient period to induce deep breathing may cause a displacement and the associated abnormal respiratory noise. When viewed through the endoscope, the caudal free border of the soft palate completely obscures the epiglottis and the lateral mucosal folds appear more prominent than normal. The displacement is usually accompanied by bulging of the cheeks as exhaled air is forced into the oropharynx. In some horses, the soft palate may maintain its normal position beneath the epiglottis but its rostral portion may billow into the pharyngeal airway. This change may or may not be accompanied by an abnormal respiratory noise. The impression may be gained in some of these horses that the epiglottis is flaccid and narrow and therefore unable to maintain its normal position above the soft palate.

If swallowing is induced by spraying the caudal pharynx and the larynx with a stream of saline through the endoscope, a transient displacement can be seen occasionally in normal horses; however, if the displacement occurs frequently or persists for a large part of the examination period, it may be considered abnormal. This assessment is purely subjective and can be influenced by potential effects of endoscopic examination and the amount of restraint required in some horses. Tranquilizers can alter pharyngeal muscle activity and therefore should not be administered. If an endoscopic examination can be performed after a training session of sufficient intensity to induce soft palate displacement, a definitive diagnosis can be made more readily than under resting conditions. Radiographs are of value in some cases, especially those in which some abnormality of the epiglottis or other laryngeal cartilages is suspected.

Frequently, the diagnosis is made when all other potential causes of an abnormal upper respiratory tract noise are eliminated by endoscopic examination. In such cases, a detailed history should be sought and a thorough examination of the lower respiratory and the cardiovascular systems should be conducted to rule out other possible causes of poor performance. Consideration should be given to racing these horses with a tongue tie (tongue tied to the lower jaw) because a favorable response would be strongly suggestive of soft palate displacement and would eliminate the need for more radical forms of treatment. The tongue is connected indirectly to the larynx through its attachments to the hyoid apparatus. Tying the tongue therefore prevents caudal retraction of the tongue and it also resists excessive caudal retraction of the larynx. Some horses may benefit from rest, especially those that have concomitant respiratory tract problems that resolve spontaneously with time.

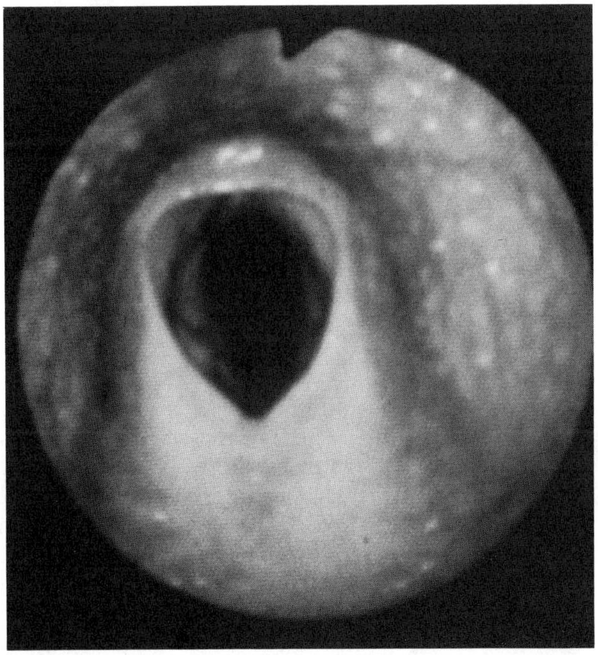

Figure 42–2. Endoscopic view of the pharynx in a horse with complete laryngopalatal dislocation. The entire ostium intrapharyngeum and its borders can be clearly seen rostral to the cartilages of the larynx, which are obscured behind the caudal free border of the soft palate and the palatopharyngeal arch. This horse had a congenital malformation of the laryngeal cartilages that produced instability of the relationship between the larynx and soft palate. (Courtesy of Dr. Ian Harrison.)

SURGERY

Soft Palate Resection

Soft palate resection is performed with the horse in dorsal recumbency, under general anesthesia, and a standard laryngotomy is used. If a gas anesthetic agent is used, the endotracheal tube should be removed and the soft palate will be seen in the caudal part of the pharynx, above the epiglottis. If the horse has been anesthetized with an intravenous anesthetic agent, the soft palate may be in its normal position beneath the epiglottis and will have to be displaced into the nasopharynx by passing a finger between its lateral mucosal folds and the epiglottis. Although visual inspection of the soft palate during surgery has been used as a means of assessing its length and degree of flaccidity, this is highly unreliable. Both will be influenced by the depth of anesthesia and by the degree of flexion of the head and neck. Ulceration of the caudal border of the soft palate has been described but is rare.

The soft palate is grasped on its midline by straight sponge forceps, placed so that the distal edge of the instrument can serve as an approximate guide for the most rostral edge of the incision (Fig. 42–3). The limit for this is 2.5 cm from the caudal edge with the free border under tension. The soft palate is then grasped approximately 2 to 2.5 cm lateral to the sponge forceps by means of an Allis tissue forceps (Fig. 42–3). The caudal free border is brought up close to the laryngotomy and it is incised immediately rostral to the tips of both forceps (Fig. 42–3). A double-curved Satinsky thoracic scissors or long-handled Mayo dissecting scissors is used. Another Allis tissue forceps is placed on the free border on the other side of the sponge forceps and the soft palate is trimmed in similar fashion from that point until it joins the other incision (Fig. 42–3). In this way, a crescent-shaped segment of the soft palate is resected, approximately 4 to 5 cm long and 2.0 cm wide at its midpoint. Alternatively, a V-shaped notch may be cut in the caudal border of the soft palate. In horses with a deeply concave or notched caudal border, most of the resection is lateral to the midline and the width

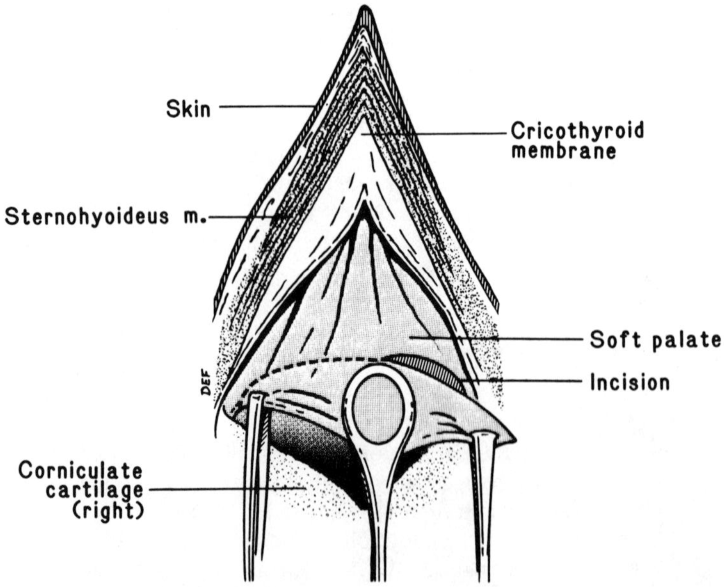

Figure 42–3. Illustration of a method of resecting the caudal free border of the soft palate through a laryngotomy. The soft palate has been grasped on its midline by the sponge forceps, which are then used to draw it caudally toward the laryngotomy. The left side of the soft palate has been incised from the point where it was grasped with Allis tissue forceps (note that the left side of the palate is toward the reader's right because the horse is in dorsal recumbency). An Allis tissue forceps has been placed on the other side of the soft palate to mark the most lateral extent of the remaining incision, represented by a *broken line*. The soft palate can be incised in either direction along the broken line to complete the line of resection. The most rostral part of the laryngotomy is uppermost.

of the resected strip at its midpoint is reduced in proportion to the degree of concavity. Any mucosal tags on the soft palate are trimmed and the incisions are left open to heal by second intention. Hemorrhage is usually mild and cautery is rarely required.

Postoperative Care. The horse should be given phenylbutazone intravenously (4.4 mg/kg body weight) immediately before or after surgery to reduce postoperative laryngeal edema. After the horse is fully recovered from anesthesia, it can be returned to its stall and fed; however, all food should be placed on the ground to encourage ventral drainage from the incision and from the pharynx. The horse should be checked at hourly intervals during the first 8 to 14 hours after surgery for breathing difficulties. Although some water may escape from the laryngotomy while the horse drinks over the next 4 to 5 days, this problem is usually of little consequence and resolves spontaneously.

Postoperative care includes daily cleaning of the laryngotomy wound with gauze sponges soaked in warm water. Some petrolatum is applied to the surrounding skin edges and the intermandibular space to reduce excoriation from draining serum. The horse should be confined to a stall at least during the first 3 to 4 weeks after surgery. The open incision usually seals with granulation tissue within 14 days after surgery and healing is complete 7 to 14 days later. The horse can be returned to work 4 to 6 weeks after surgery.

An endoscopic examination should be conducted periodically during the postoperative period. Edges of the soft palate incision are usually edematous and congested for the first 2 to 4 days after surgery, but this resolves rapidly. Ideally, the soft palate should assume a normal position beneath the epiglottis throughout the period of endoscopic examination. In some horses, the epiglottis can be seen clearly through the notch that remains in the soft palate after resection, and it cannot assume a normal position above the pharyngeal surface of the soft palate. This is most likely to occur if the epiglottis is severely hypoplastic and indicates a poor prognosis for recovery of normal athletic potential.

Special Precautions. If too much soft palate is resected, the remaining defect in the caudal free border may allow the contents of the oropharynx to enter the nasopharynx during swallowing. This will cause coughing, sneezing, and, in severe cases, aspiration pneumonia. This complication is rare (1 to 4%), but the owner should be advised of this risk beforehand. If there is any evidence of muscle necrosis, severe postoperative swelling, or infection in the laryngotomy site or if the horse develops a fever, antibiotic therapy should be initiated; however, antibiotics are not administered routinely.

Success Rate. A successful response to soft palate resection would appear to defy current concepts about the anatomic and physiologic relationship between the pharynx and larynx. However, the estimated rate of improvement after resection is 40 to 50%. A successful outcome following this procedure can be attributed to reduction of the amount of tissue that obstructs the nasopharynx if displacement persists during work or racing. Alternatively, if soft palate displacement tends to recur, repositioning of the soft palate beneath the epiglottis may be facilitated when the caudal free border is shortened. According to Raker, approximately 50 to 60% of horses with a diagnosis of soft palate "elongation" may respond favorably to this procedure; however, there is no convincing evidence that this specific defect exists. Soft palate resection is used successfully as a prophylactic measure in horses that undergo resection of the aryepiglottic fold to correct an entrapped epiglottis, because dorsal displacement of the soft palate is a frequent complication following this procedure.

Myectomy

Heffron and Baker proposed that caudal retraction of the larynx is responsible for soft palate displacement. On this basis, they proposed that resection of the muscles responsible for caudal retraction of the larynx should be an effective method of treatment. If segments of the omohyoideus, sternohyoideus, and sternothyroideus muscles are resected, general anesthesia is required because dissection is quite extensive. The procedure has been modified currently so that only segments of the sternothyroideus and sternohyoideus muscles are removed, and this can be done on the standing horse. It is possible that the action of the omohyoideus may be diminished when the other muscles are removed and therefore its resection is not essential.

The horse is sedated, the proposed surgical site is infiltrated with local anesthetic, and the skin is prepared for sterile surgery. The horse's head is raised and a 10-cm long incision is made on the ventral midline of the neck, usually in the upper half, above the level of divergence of the paired sternocephalicus muscles. The incision is extended by sharp dissection through the underlying cutaneous colli muscle to expose the underlying sternothyroideus and sternohyoideus muscles. Exposure of these muscles can be improved by blunt dissection, either with curved scissors or by digital disruption of their fascial attachments. The muscles are then elevated from the trachea and clamped at each end of the incision by means of Rochester-Pean forceps, applied approximately 6 to 8 cm apart. The intervening segment of muscle is then removed by transecting it with a scalpel along the inner edges of both forceps. Although the paired sternothyroideus and sternohyoideus muscles are closely grouped, care should be taken to avoid separating individual muscle bellies from the remainder of the group. The segment removed from each side should therefore be inspected to ensure that two pairs of muscles can be identified within it. The sternothyroideus is the more lateral of the two muscle pairs and also is smaller and more tendinous, especially in the rostral part of the neck. Some surgeons attempt to include a portion of the omohyoideus muscles in their resection, but there is little critical evidence that this is necessary.

After the myectomy has been completed, the Rochester-Pean forceps are kept in place for approximately 1 to 2 minutes to minimize hemorrhage from the severed muscle ends. A half-inch Penrose drain is placed in the space between the severed muscle ends, which retract considerably, and tunneled subcutaneously to exit through a stab wound caudal to the skin incision. It can be secured to the skin close to the exit point by a simple interrupted suture. The cut edges of the cutaneous colli muscle are apposed with interrupted sutures of absorbable suture material and the skin is closed in routine fashion.

Postoperative Care. The horse should be confined to a stall and exercised by walking in hand for 5 to 10 days after surgery. After that, it can return to work. The Penrose drain should be removed after 3 to 5 days and skin sutures should be removed 10 to 14 days after surgery. In rare cases postoperative swelling is severe, but this usually responds to local hydrotherapy or to the application of hot compresses. If infection develops, antibiotics should be administered, and consideration given to opening the incision for drainage. In most cases, the incision heals by first intention with minimal postoperative problems.

Special Precautions. In the rostral third of the neck, the sternothyroideus muscles diverge from the midline caudal to the larynx and are directed dorsally to insert on the thyroid cartilage. If the approach is rostral to this point, these branches can be missed and the surgery may fail to achieve its objectives.

Success Rate. According to Cook, a favorable response was achieved in 71% of the first 21 horses subjected to this surgery, whereas Harrison and Raker obtained a 58% success rate. A major advantage of the procedure is that horses can be returned to work within a short period after surgery so that their training routine suffers minimal interruption. In addition, the risk of complications is low compared with soft palate resection. As with any method of treating the condition, a poorer prognosis must be issued in cases with concomitant abnormalities of the epiglottis and other laryngeal cartilages. Because of its apparently higher success rate, freedom from serious complications, and simplicity, myectomy is the treatment of choice in horses with dorsal displacement of the soft palate. If it fails, soft palate resection may then be considered as further treatment. Evidence that the condition can be treated successfully by two procedures that appear to have opposite effects on the normal relationship between the pharynx and larynx provides a strong measure of our failure to understand the pathophysiology of this disease.

BIBLIOGRAPHY

Blythe LL, Cardinet GH, Meagher DM, et al: Palatal myositis in horses with dorsal displacement of the soft palate. *J Am Vet Med Assoc* 1983;183:781–785.

Cook WR: Some observations on form and function of the equine upper airway in health and disease: I. The pharynx. *Proc Am Assoc Equine Pract* 1981;27:355–391.

Cook WR: The diagnosis of respiratory unsoundness in the horse. *Vet Rec* 1965;77:516–528.

Harrison IW, Raker CW: Sternothyrohyoideus myectomy in horses: 17 cases (1984–1985). *J Am Vet Med Assoc* 1988;193:1299–1302.

Haynes PF: Surgery of the equine respiratory tract, in Jennings PB (ed): *The Practice of Large Animal Surgery*. Philadelphia, WB Saunders Co, 1984, pp 423–431.

Haynes PF: Surgical failures in upper respiratory surgery. *Proc Am Assoc Equine Pract* 1978;24:223–250.

Heffron CJ, Baker GJ: Endoscopic observations on the deglutition reflex in the horse. *Equine Vet J* 1979;11:137–141.

Heffron CJ, Baker GJ: Observations on the mechanism of functional obstruction of the nasopharyngeal airway in the horse. *Equine Vet J* 1979;11:142–147.

Raker CW: Soft palate defects, in Mansmann HA, McAllister ES, Pratt PW (eds): *Equine Medicine and Surgery*, ed 3. Santa Barbara, CA, American Veterinary Publications, 1982, pp 752–756.

43
Epiglottic Entrapment

Gregory L. Ferraro

Epiglottic entrapment occurs when the ventral mucosal folds of the epiglottis become dorsally displaced, trapping the epiglottic cartilage in a pouchlike fold of tissue. This freely moveable tissue is attached to the ventral border of the epiglottis, is continuous with its mucosal covering, and forms a series of overlapping layers that alternately stretch to allow deglutition and then fold up upon themselves in an accordion-like fashion when the epiglottic cartilage returns to its horizontal position. The fold of this tissue is not normally seen during endoscopy, althouqh its caudal attachments can usually be observed at the base of the epiglottis during endoscopic examination (Fig. 43–1).

When entrapment occurs, this tissue can be readily observed as a saclike mucous membrane surrounding the epiglottis dorsally and laterally, (Fig. 43–2), giving an appearance similar to a hand in a pants pocket. The shape of the epiglottis is distinguishable, but its edges appear thickened and rounded because of the overlying tissue. Closer inspection reveals that the normal reticulated vascular pattern on the dorsal surface of the epiglottis and the slightly irregular serrations of the left and right edges of the epiglottis are not visible. These findings differentiate the condition from dorsal displacement of the soft palate, in which the tip and the borders of the epiglottic cartilage cannot be delineated. Entrapment of the epiglottis by this arytenoepiglottic fold can be caused either by abnormalities of the fold itself or by abnormalities of the epiglottic cartilage.

CLINICAL FINDINGS

Horses with aryepiglottic entrapment may or may not present with a clinical complaint. It is possible for horses to have an apparently benign entrapment that causes no clinical signs. Other horses will have intermittent entrapment of the epiglottis, and are also usually asymptomatic. The presenting complaint for affected horses is usually exercise intolerance. Rarely is there an associated noise during respiration, especially in the racehorse. Normally the presenting complaint is that the horse seems to tire suddenly, and that this sudden onset of fatigue is associated with an apparent choking-like behavior that is followed by coughing, especially when the horse is being eased after a race. Some gurgling or expiratory noise may be heard subsequently. This noise is probably associated with secondary dorsal displacement of the soft palate. Horses will

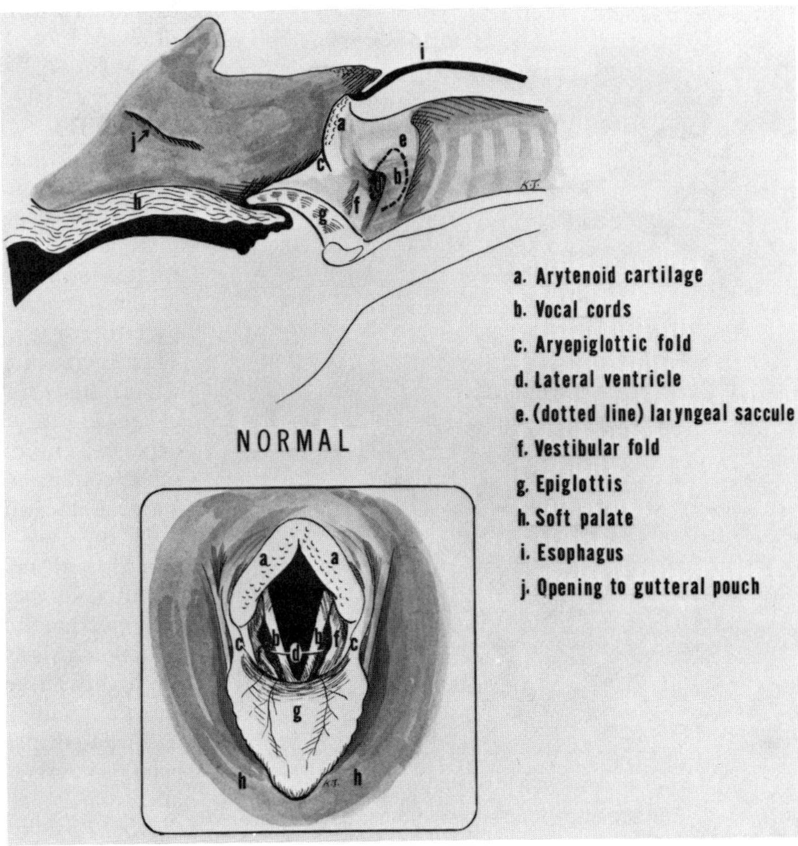

Figure 43–1. Normal pharyngeal anatomy: sagittal section and endoscopic view. (From Honnas CM, Wheat JD: Epiglottic entrapment: A transnasal surgical approach to divide the aryepiglottic fold axially in the standing horse. *Vet Surg* 1988;17:246–251.)

sometimes cough while eating because of the entrapment.

In trying to analyze these presenting complaints, it is important to understand the mechanical factors that cause the animal to become distressed. Entrapment of the epiglottis has two primary effects—it alters respiratory airflow and limits deglutition. Its effect on airflow is primarily obstructive, in that the entrapping tissue balloons into the airway, especially during expiration, increasing resistance to airflow. If the tissue is severely inflamed and swollen, the obstruction can be quite severe. However, the effects of entrapment on swallowing may be the more important factor associated with poor performance. A normal horse will swallow approximately six times during a brisk 1-mile gallop. Deglutition is necessary to clear accumulated respiratory secretions, and each swallow must be completed within the rhythm of locomotion and always interrupts respiration during the single stride in which it occurs. In horses with an entrapped epiglottis, normal swallowing and therefore clearing of secretions cannot occur within a single stride because of restricted epiglottic movement. Presumably this results in a gradual increase in fluid within the pharynx and contributes to the tiring and sudden stopping associated with choking and coughing.

PHYSIOLOGIC EVALUATION

In preparation for successful correction of epiglottic entrapment, the clinician must make a careful evaluation of its underlying cause and of the various sequelae that may be associated with it. The first and most important determination is whether or not the epiglottis is of normal size. Congenital epiglottic hypoplasia has been reported and is frequently associated with entrapment. In addition, normal-sized epiglottic cartilages that have been entrapped for a prolonged period or those entrapments associated with infected, inflamed, or severely ulcerated entrapping mucous membrane may have undergone degenerative changes, contributing to a hypoplastic configuration. Abnormalities in epiglottic size or shape are the single most important factors affecting prognosis.

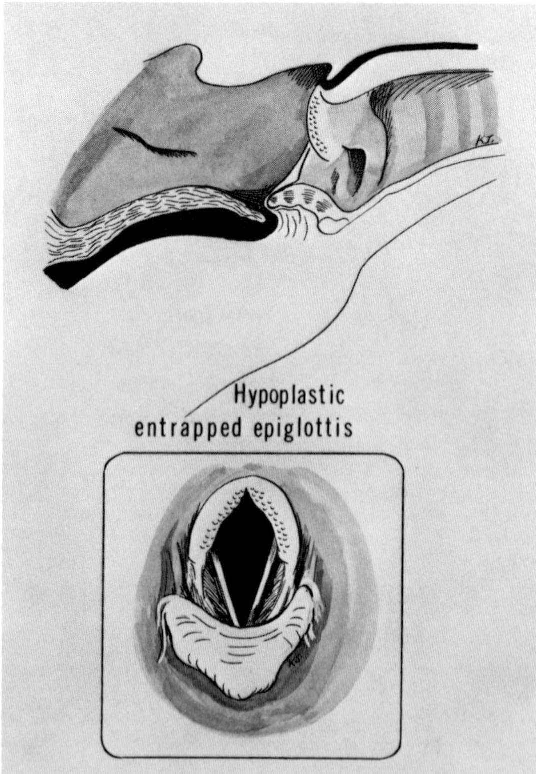

Figure 43–2. Entrapped hypoplastic epiglottis: sagittal section and endoscopic view. (From Honnas CM, Wheat JD: Epiglottic entrapment: A transnasal surgical approach to divide the aryepiglottic fold axially in the standing horse. *Vet Surg* 1988;17:246–251.)

Horses with an abnormal epiglottis cannot be expected to function well as athletes regardless of whether or not the entrapment is corrected. Estimation of epiglottic size can prove difficult endoscopically, especially when inflamed tissue is present. Radiography of the pharynx and measurement of the thyroepiglottic length is useful to determine abnormalities in configuration. Thyroepiglottic length in the normal Thoroughbred, corrected for radiographic magnification, is considered to be 8.76 ± 0.44 cm. Horses having a shorter thyroepiglottic length should automatically be given a poor prognosis for athletic competition because even when the entrapment is corrected, these horses often have continued clinical signs.

When the epiglottic size is normal, several other important factors need to be considered before correction is undertaken. These include the severity and duration of the inflammation associated with the entrapping tissue. The effect of these other factors on prognosis is explained within the context of the method of correction.

SURGERY

Surgery is required for correction of epiglottic entrapment, and success is variable and dependent upon the method used, the presurgical health of the involved tissue, and the postsurgical care. One surgical method involves general anesthesia and access to the epiglottis by either a ventral laryngotomy or a pharyngotomy. This approach is best employed in chronic cases in which there is evidence of adhesion between the epiglottis and the entrapping tissue and in which there is excessive chronic granulation tissue or the presence of other conditions of the larynx or pharynx that need surgical attention.

Of the two methods, the ventral pharyngeal approach is advantageous because it provides better visualization of the entrapment and avoids the necessity for reflecting the epiglottis caudally when resecting the entrapping tissue. The epiglottis and ventral pharynx are highly susceptible to inflammation. Furthermore, surgical trauma followed by excessive inflammation can lead to many unwanted sequelae, including soft palate paresis, aberrant deglutition, and aspiration pneumonia. The retraction of the epiglottis needed in the laryngotomy approach adds significantly to this inciting trauma and is therefore undesirable. Additionally, the visualization possible using the ventral pharyngotomy allows a more careful and discerning excision of the entrapping tissue. It is important that no more of the arytenoepiglottic fold than necessary be excised to avoid nerve damage. Regardless of the approach employed, however, careful atraumatic excision is imperative, and careful attention to postsurgical control of inflammation is essential, because this type of repair is often fraught with postsurgical problems and eventual failure of the animal's ability to return to athletic activity.

A method of surgical repair that has a much lower incidence of postsurgical complications and a much higher percentage of individuals able to compete athletically postsurgery is the nasal approach using a hook-bladed resection knife (Scanlon Instruments). With the horse standing and sedated, the pharynx is anesthetized topically using 4% lidocaine or 2% butacaine solution administered in a pharyngeal spray. The horse is twitched, the fiberoptic endoscope is placed up one nostril for visualization, and the guarded epiglottic resection knife is placed up the other nostril (Fig. 43–3). The entrapping tissue is hooked by the blade and incised along its midline, thereby freeing the

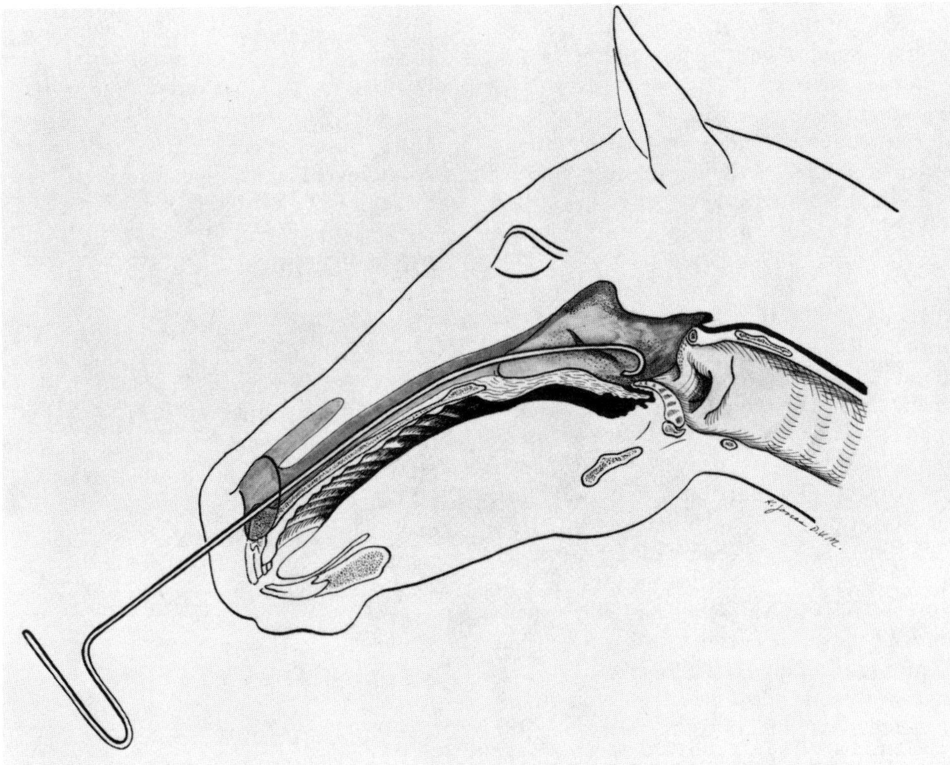

Figure 43–3. Sagittal section of the head showing the transnasal position of a hooked bistuory immediately rostral to a normal epiglottis. (From Honnas CM, Wheat JD: Epiglottic entrapment: A transnasal surgical approach to divide the aryepiglottic fold axially in the standing horse. *Vet Surg* 1988;17:246–251.)

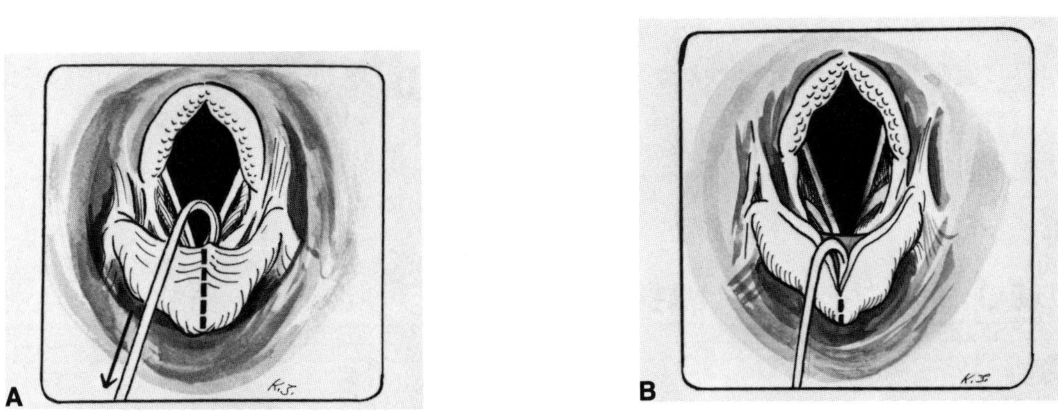

Figure 43–4. Endoscopic view of transnasal axial division of aryepiglottic entrapment using a curved bistoury. **A.** Hooked bistoury positioned at caudal edge of the entrapment. *Dotted line*, line of axial division; *arrow*, the direction of pull of the bistoury. **B.** The appearance of the entrapment during axial division. (From Honnas CM, Wheat JD: Epiglottic entrapment: A transnasal surgical approach to divide the aryepiglottic fold axially in the standing horse. *Vet Surg* 1988;17:246–251.)

epiglottis (Fig. 43–4). It is important that the blade be extremely sharp and of the proper configuration so that it cuts easily on demand. A gentle, slow pull is used on the knife so that as long a cut as possible is made in the fold. Tugging or hard pulling with a dull or improperly shaped knife can reduce the entrapment without adequate resection. If inadvertent deentrapment occurs during the procedure, stimulating the horse to swallow several times will usually result in reentrapment, allowing the resection to be completed.

This is a safe and efficient procedure that can be completed in under 10 minutes provided that the proper instrument is used and the operator has sufficient skill. It should not be attempted with inadequate equipment or by those with insufficient manipulative skills. Adequate restraint is also critical because incorrect placement of the blade or inadvertent movement of the horse may result in accidental transection of the soft palate or laceration of the turbinates, with attendant complications. This procedure does, however, result in correction of the epiglottic entrapment with minimal trauma. This allows for a rapid and usually successful return to athletic competition if the proper pre- and postsurgical therapy is employed.

All evidence of infection and inflammation should be corrected medically before any surgery is done. Initially, entrapments often appear inflamed and swollen. Many have ulcerative lesions, especially rostrally, and there may even be a fistula in the entrapping tissue that allows protrusion of the epiglottic apex. Topical application of a mixture of hydrocortisone powder, dimethyl sulfoxide, and polyethylene glycol can be administered via a pharyngeal spray for several days and is effective in eliminating most of the inflammation. This anti-inflammatory therapy should be continued until the entrapping tissue looks benign in nature and there are no other secondary lesions present. Attempted surgical correction before this usually results in ineffective resection, severe postsurgical inflammation, and reentrapment. Following resection, the local pharyngeal spray is administered several times daily until all evidence of inflammatory tissue and swelling has subsided. This generally takes from 5 to 10 days. Once the laryngeal region appears normal on endoscopic exam, training can resume.

PROGNOSIS

The prognosis for this type of surgical correction can be extremely good if the horse has a normal epiglottis, adequate resection is achieved, and inflammation is carefully controlled both before and after surgery. Entrapment of the epiglottis is one of the few upper respiratory conditions in which one can expect a return to athletic competition with no impairment of performance following surgical correction, provided the entrapment is fully corrected and the case properly managed postsurgically.

BIBLIOGRAPHY

Boles CL: Epiglottic entrapment and follicular pharyngitis: Diagnosis and treatment. *Proc Am Assoc Equine Pract* 1975; pp 29–34.

Boles CL, Raker CW, Wheat JD: Epiglottic entrapment by arytenoepiglottic folds in the horse. *J Am Vet Med Assoc* 1978;172:338–342.

Speirs VC: Entrapment of the epiglottis in horses. *J Equine Med Surg* 1977;1:267.

Linford RL, O'Brien TR, Wheat JD, et al: Radiographic assessment of epiglottic length, pharyngeal and laryngeal dimensions in the Thoroughbred. *Am J Vet Res* 1983;44:1660.

Fretz PB: Endoscopic differentiation of epiglottic entrapment and elongation of the soft palate: Including surgical correction of epiglottic entrapment. *Can Vet J* 1977;18:352.

44
Guttural Pouch Empyema

David E. Freeman

Guttural pouch empyema is an uncommon disease in horses. It usually develops following rupture of retropharyngeal lymph node abscesses into the guttural pouch cavity or as a sequela to streptococcal infections. It can be associated also with guttural pouch tympany and may occur as an iatrogenic complication of guttural pouch infusion with irritating solutions. The condition is usually unilateral but bilateral involvement has been reported.

DIAGNOSIS

The major signs of guttural pouch empyema are intermittent nasal discharge, swelling of adjacent lymph nodes, parotid swelling and pain, fever, extended head carriage, and, in severe cases, dyspnea. In some horses, the nasal discharge is only evident when the horse eats off the ground. On endoscopic examination of the pharynx, the dorsal roof of the nasopharynx may be collapsed and some purulent material can be seen draining from the pharyngeal orifice on the affected side. If a catheter or the endoscope is inserted into the involved guttural pouch, purulent material may flow freely from the opening. Endoscopic examination of the guttural pouch should reveal an accumulation of purulent exudate, and the lining is usually inflamed and thickened. A fluid line should be evident on standing lateral radiographs of the head. Fluid aspirates and saline washes of this material should be submitted for bacterial culture and sensitivity testing. A history of a recent outbreak of strangles on the farm can help in making the diagnosis.

SURGERY

The majority of horses with guttural pouch empyema respond to medical therapy. Such therapy is usually directed at removing the purulent contents of the guttural pouch by repeated saline lavage and systemic antibiotics. Anti-inflammatory agents may be indicated in some cases, especially if the inflammation is sufficient to cause neuritis and neurologic signs.

Drainage Techniques

Normally, the pharyngeal orifice of the guttural pouch allows ventral drainage from the cavity while the horse's head is lowered; however, in severe cases of guttural pouch empyema, the lining of the orifice may be so inflamed that it becomes obstructed and thick exudate is retained. In rare cases, the purulent contents are dehydrated, forming ovoid masses called chondroids. If medical treatment is not sufficient to remove inspissated exudate or chondroids, then the guttural pouch should be drained by one of the following approaches.

Hyovertebrotomy. An incision is made 2 cm cranial to and parallel with the wing of the atlas for a length of 10 cm. Sharp dissection is continued through the dense fascia that invests the caudal edge of the parotid gland, and this and the overlying parotidoauricularis muscle are reflected cranially. The second cervical (caudal auricular) nerve is reflected caudally and the areolar tissue is broken down by blunt dissection medial to the mandibular and parotid salivary glands. The lining of the guttural pouch is carefully punctured by the closed tips of a scissors or by a hemostat, taking care not to damage the underlying nerves and arteries. The incision should be enlarged carefully by spreading it with the fingers or by spreading the jaws of a scissors or hemostat within its edges. The inspissated pus and chondroids are removed by a combination of lavage and swabbing the mucosal surface with saline-soaked sponges. In many cases, the inspissated pus forms dense, tightly adherent plaques on the mucosal surface and frequently these are impossible to remove without damaging the guttural pouch. The hyovertebrotomy incision can be closed by suturing the fascia of the parotid gland to the fascia beneath the wing of the atlas with an absorbable suture material, followed by simple interrupted sutures in the skin. Because the hyovertebrotomy approach is dorsal to the floor of the guttural pouch, it should be combined with an incision in Viborg's triangle to provide ventral drainage.

Viborg's Approach. Viborg's triangle is bordered by the tendon of the sternocephalicus muscle, the linguofacial vein, and the vertical ramus of the mandible. A vertical or horizontal approach can be made in this area. When used as the primary approach the fascia is separated by dissection, and a finger, directed rostrally and slightly dorsally medial to the mandible, is used to palpate the stylohyoid bone. If the pouch is distended with exudate, it is easily palpated and can be opened for drainage. When this approach is used in combination with a hyovertebrotomy, a metal probe or the index finger is passed through the incision and directed ventrally until it can be palpated at Viborg's triangle. An incision is then made in Viborg's triangle, taking care to avoid the parotid duct and the branches of the vagus nerve along the floor of the guttural pouch. Once the overlying tissues have been incised, a hemostat or curved scissors is inserted through the hyovertebrotomy incision and the tip is used to puncture the mucosa within the edges of the skin incision. This incision is usually left open to heal by second intention, and it can be packed with antiseptic-soaked gauze or a soft rubber drain can be inserted through it to provide an ingress for irrigating solutions.

Whitehouse Approach. The classic Whitehouse approach is made on the ventral midline over the larynx with the horse in dorsal recumbency. Dissection is continued through the septum joining the paired sternohyoideus and omohyoideus muscles and is then directed along the lateral aspect of the larynx. The direction of dissection can be guided by palpating the ventral edge of the stylohyoid bone deep in the incision. The guttural pouch is opened medial to the stylohyoid bone and the external carotid artery. The incision is left open to heal by second intention, and a soft rubber tube or similar catheter system can be placed through the incision to allow irrigation of the guttural pouch cavity.

Modified Whitehouse Approach. The Whitehouse approach can be modified by placing the skin incision along the ventral edge of the linguofacial vein and extending it rostrally for 12 cm from the jugular vein. The fascia attaching the vein to the surrounding structures is incised and the lateral aspect of the larynx is exposed. The incision is then continued as described for the preceding approach until the guttural pouch cavity has been entered. The major advantage of this approach is that the incision through the sternohyoideus and omohyoideus muscles is avoided and dissection is through a natural fascial plane.

Postoperative Care

The open incisions in the guttural pouch are cleaned daily with gauze sponges soaked with warm water and dilute antiseptic solutions. A small amount of petrolatum can be applied to the surrounding skin edges to reduce excoriation from draining serum and pus. The guttural pouch cavity should be flushed through the open incision daily with a nonirritating solution, such as a 0.5% povidone-iodine—saline solution, to remove any accumulated purulent material. The incision will close spontaneously within 14 days, by which time the infection should have resolved. Until the infection has resolved, the horse should be fed from the ground to facilitate ventral drainage. The horse can have antibiotics administered postoperatively if desired. Antibiotics may be especially indicated in those cases in which a deep incision was made, such as for a Whitehouse or modified Whitehouse approach, or when healing by first intention is needed, as in a sutured hyovertebrotomy approach.

Special Precautions

Surgery of the guttural pouch should be regarded as a last resort because it is fraught with the risk of iatrogenic nerve damage, regardless of the approach used. Although the above-described incisions start at different points externally, they are all directed internally toward the floor and caudal aspect of the medial compartment of the guttural pouch (Fig. 44–1). The mucosal incision is restricted to this small area of the guttural pouch by the ventral straight muscles of the head medially and by the stylohyoid bone, the stylohyoid and occipitohyoideus muscles, and the jugular process of the occipital bone laterally. The internal carotid artery, sympathetic trunk, the cranial cervical ganglion, the vagus nerve, the hypoglossal nerve, and glossopharyngeal nerve, are all contained in a fold of the guttural

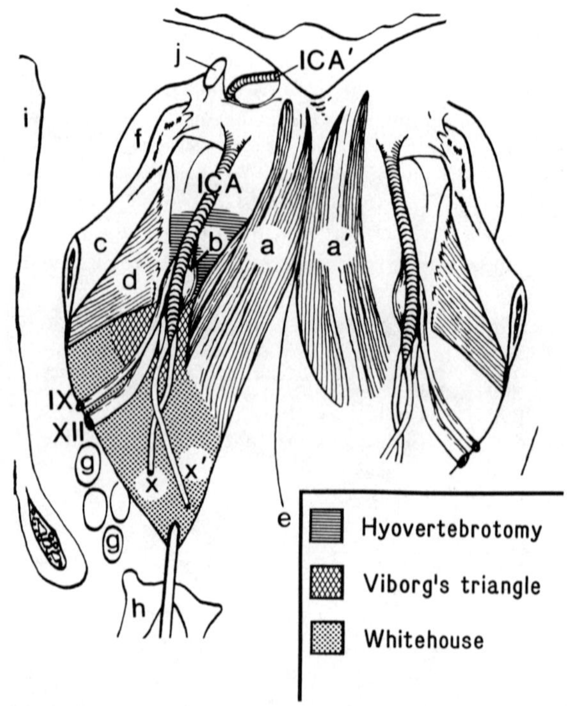

Figure 44–1. Transverse section of head viewed from front to back in a slightly oblique direction. *Shaded segments* along the floor and caudal part of the right guttural pouch are points of entry through the incisions identified in the lower right-hand inset. The hyovertebrotomy and Whitehouse incisions usually overlap the incision through Viborg's triangle.

ICA = internal carotid artery; *ICA'*, internal carotid artery within the venous sinuses; *a* and *a'*, ventral straight muscles of the head; *b*, cranial cervical ganglion; *c*, stylohyoid bone; *d*, occipitohyoideus muscle, *e*, median septum dividing right and left guttural pouches; *f*, lateral compartment of the right guttural pouch; *g*, retropharyngeal lymph nodes; *h*, arytenoid cartilage of the larynx; *i*, vertical ramus of the mandible; *j*, cut edge of the medial lamina of the eustachian tube; *IX*, glossopharyngeal nerve, *XII*, hypoglossal nerve; *x*, cranial laryngeal nerve; *x'*, pharyngeal branch of the vagus nerve. (From Freeman DE: Diagnosis and treatment of diseases of the guttural pouch (Part I). Compend Contin Educ Pract Vet 1980;2:S3-S11.)

pouch mucosa in the caudal wall of the medial compartment. The pharyngeal and laryngeal branches of the vagus nerve, the glossopharyngeal and the hypoglossal nerve, and the external carotid artery and its linguofacial trunk lie beneath the mucosa on the floor of the guttural pouch.

Identification of the guttural pouch lining is extremely difficult and may be facilitated by prior insertion of a lighted endoscope into the medial compartment. Because the mucosa tends to collapse away from the plane of dissection, a fixed structure within the guttural pouch should be identified by palpation and used as a guide for the Whitehouse approach; the stylohyoid bone can be used. Because the external carotid artery and the glossopharyngeal and hypoglossal nerves pass along the ventral edge of the stylohyoid bone, their course is fixed, and this makes it easier to identify and avoid them from this approach. If the guttural pouch lining is thickened and inflamed, identification of fine nerve branches may be facilitated by illuminating the mucosa with the endoscope. Once exposed, the mucosa should not be incised with a scalpel or scissors because of the risk of severing important nerves. Because all approaches to the guttural pouch are deep and restricted by the surrounding structures, considerable retraction may be necessary to gain adequate exposure but this must be done carefully so as not to damage nerves in the approach.

The four methods used to approach the guttural pouch each have distinct features that render them superior to the other approaches under different conditions. For example, the hyovertebrotomy approach is direct and it allows easy access to the caudal aspect of the medial compartment and roof of the guttural pouch. However, it does not allow ventral drainage. The approach through Viborg's triangle is restricted by the structures that surround this area so that only a small external incision can be made, and this prevents access to deeper structures within the guttural pouch. It is useful in foals with tympany because then it is enlarged by the underlying swelling.

The Whitehouse approach allows direct access to the roof of the guttural pouch and allows digital exploration of the lateral compartment. However, unless the guttural pouch is markedly distended, access by this approach involves careful dissection through structures associated with the pharynx, larynx, and parts of the hyoid apparatus. It has the advantages of allowing access to both guttural pouches through a common skin incision and it is the most ventral approach to the guttural pouch, thus allowing excellent drainage.

PROGNOSIS

Surgical treatment of guttural pouch empyema has a good prognosis, provided that the empyema is not part of a more generalized infection. Seven to 10 days are usually required for complete resolution of the infection. Neurologic signs are rarely seen as complications of bacterial infections in the guttural pouch but can be caused by surgical damage to the nerves. In such cases the prognosis is poor, because intractable dysphagia is the most common surgical complication, and can eventually lead to aspiration pneumonia and death.

45 Guttural Pouch Mycosis

David E. Freeman

Guttural pouch mycosis is a localized or diffuse fungal infection on the roof and walls of the medial and lateral compartments of the guttural pouch. There is no age, sex, or breed predisposition to this disease. The true cause of the infection is unknown, although fungi can be isolated from the lesion in most cases and an *Aspergillus* species is identified most frequently.

DIAGNOSIS

The diagnosis of guttural pouch mycosis is usually based on the clinical signs and on endoscopic examination. The wide variety of clinical signs produced by this disease can be explained by the close proximity of the predilection site for the infection to a number of important structures in the mucosal lining of the guttural pouch. In order of decreasing frequency of occurrence, the clinical signs of this disease are profuse and spontaneous hemorrhage (epistaxis), dysphagia, Horner's syndrome, nasal discharge, corneal ulceration, parotid pain, abnormal respiratory noise, abnormal head posture, facial nerve paralysis, and head shyness.

Hemorrhage is usually severe and intermittent, occurs without warning signs, and, if untreated, is fatal in most cases. It is caused by a fungal erosion of either the wall the internal carotid artery in the medial compartment of the guttural pouch or the wall of the external carotid artery in the lateral compartment. The neurologic signs of guttural pouch mycosis can be attributed to neuritis of the cranial nerves within the guttural pouch, such as the vagus nerve and its pharyngeal and cranial laryngeal branches, and the glossopharyngeal nerve. Neurologic abnormalities that can be detected on endoscopic examination include collapse of the pharynx, dorsal displacement of the soft palate, and laryngeal hemiplegia. Atrophy of the brachiocephalicus and trapezius muscles is seen when the accessory spinal nerve (cranial nerve XI) is involved, and Horner's syndrome occurs when there is damage to the sympathetic trunk and the cranial cervical ganglion. Many horses may not show evidence of sympathetic nerve damage until xylazine is administered; then the horse will sweat profusely on the affected half of the face. Of all the neurologic signs caused by this disease, Horner's syndrome is the most likely to resolve.

The diagnosis of guttural pouch mycosis is confirmed by inserting the fiberoptic endoscope into the affected guttural pouch and observing the characteristic lesion on the roof and walls of the affected compartments. The severity of the clinical signs cannot be correlated with the size of the lesion. Lesions involving the lateral compartment only rarely cause neurologic signs but may cause signs of facial nerve paralysis because this nerve courses along the roof of this portion of the guttural pouch. In addition, hemorrhage from a lesion in the lateral compartment can be attributed to an ulceration in the wall of the external carotid artery and its branches, whereas the internal carotid artery is the most likely source of hemorrhage when the lesion is confined to the medial compartment.

SURGERY

The success rate following medical treatment of guttural pouch mycosis is low. Therefore, treatment should be directed at nutritional support of horses with neuritis and dysphagia, combined with the administration of anti-inflammatory agents, and prevention of hemorrhage in horses in which this clinical sign is evident. The lesion resolves spontaneously in most cases, so that medical treatment is not advocated unless an effective and safe method becomes available.

Removal of the Diphtheritic Membrane

Removal of the diphtheritic membrane should not be attempted until after the involved arteries have been satisfactorily occluded (see below). The diphtheritic membrane can be removed from the lining of the guttural pouch via a modified Whitehouse approach. A combination of gentle swabbing with saline-soaked gauze sponges and peeling with sponge forceps can be used to detach the plaques. The guttural pouch cavity is then irrigated with copious amounts of sterile saline. Topical antifungal agents can be applied to the roof of the guttural pouch and allowed to bathe the tissues for several minutes before the horse is allowed to recover from anesthesia. The incision can be left open and rubber tubing or similar infusion apparatus can be sutured in place between the incision edges to allow daily irrigation of the guttural pouch.

Surgical removal of the lesion in this way is the only assured method of eliminating the infection from the affected guttural pouch; however, it does not ensure against the risk of subsequent hemorrhage from an eroded artery and it also fails to retard progression of neurologic signs. This procedure may be of benefit in those rare cases that have a protracted history of nasal discharge arising from a mycotic infection in the guttural pouch. In general, surgical débridement offers few advantages in the treatment of guttural pouch mycosis and carries the risk of iatrogenic nerve damage.

Arterial Occlusion

Arterial Ligation. Arteriography should not be used as a means of determining which vessels are involved; rather, this is determined by endoscopic examination of the guttural pouch. If the lesion is discrete and is situated on only one artery, attempts are made to occlude only that vessel. If the lesion is extensive and overlies both the internal and the external carotid arteries, then both vessels are occluded. The most frequently involved artery is the internal carotid artery as it courses in a fold of mucosa along the caudal wall of the medial compartment. This artery can be ligated close to its origin outside the guttural pouch (Fig. 45–1). Failure of this procedure to prevent subsequent bouts of hemorrhage has been attributed to backflow from the cerebral arterial circle. To obviate this problem, an additional ligature has been placed distal to the mycotic infection on the roof of the guttural pouch. However, this is difficult because the artery must be

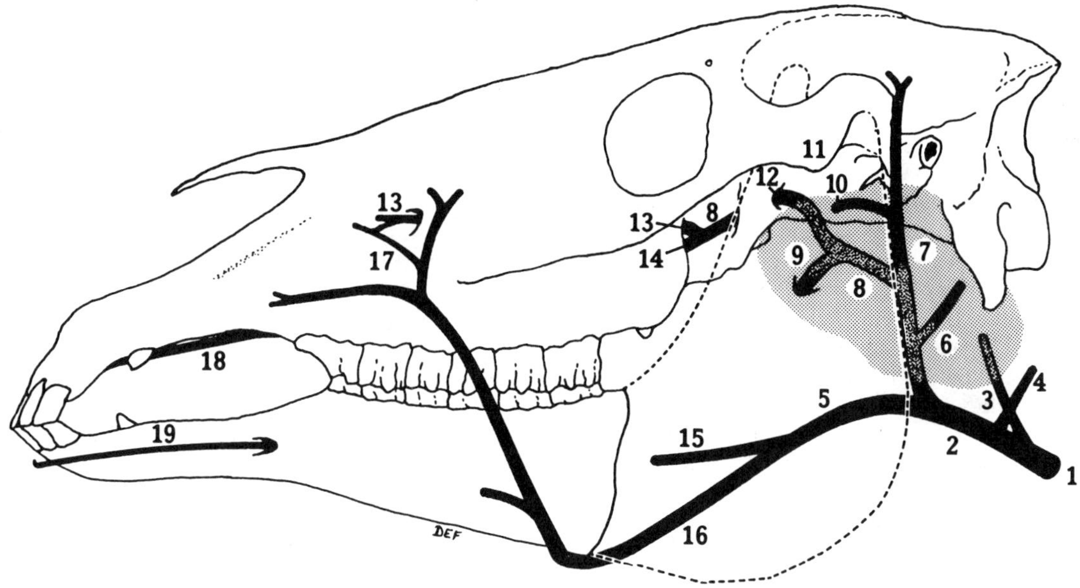

Figure 45–1. Anatomy of the major arteries of the head and their relationship to the left guttural pouch (*shaded area* beneath the skull). The vertical ramus of the mandible is represented by a *broken line* to allow more complete demonstration of the arteries medial to it. Those segments of arteries that are covered by the mucosal lining of the guttural pouch are stippled.

1, left common carotid artery; *2*, external carotid artery; *3*, internal carotid artery; *4*, occipital artery; *5*, linguofacial trunk; *6*, caudal auricular artery; *7*, superficial temporal artery; *8*, maxillary artery; *9*, inferior alveolar artery (which enters the mandibular foramen); *10*, transverse facial artery; *11*, articular tubercle of the temporal bone; *12*, caudal alar foramen (which marks the most caudal extent of the alar canal); *13*, infraorbital artery; *14*, descending palatine artery; *15*, lingual artery; *16*, facial artery; *17*, lateral nasal artery; *18*, major palatine artery; *19*, mental artery (this artery is a continuation of the inferior alveolar artery after it emerges through the mental foramen).

ligated close to the point where it enters the venous sinuses, and the involved segment may be obscured by the diphtheritic membrane. In this case the ligature has to be placed blindly, and may fail to include the vessel or may incorporate the sympathetic trunk and cause Horner's syndrome.

In recent reports, it has been shown that a single ligature on the internal carotid artery, close to its origin, is sufficient to prevent fatal epistaxis in most horses. The high success rate achieved with single ligation in this series was attributed to a reduction of blood pressure in the artery distal to the ligature and subsequent thrombosis of the vessel over the following days. Thrombosis is favored because there are no collateral channels to allow circulation through the infected segment, so that the column of blood distal to the ligature becomes stagnant. However, the author has measured blood pressure in the internal-carotid artery distal to a single ligature and did not observe a change in pressure over the next 3 days. Therefore, a single ligature would be unlikely to prevent severe hemorrhage within a short period after surgery. Hemorrhage at a later time after ligation can be attributed to occlusion of the wrong vessel. Both internal carotid arteries can be ligated simultaneously without any adverse effects.

The internal carotid artery is approached for ligation immediately distal to its origin from the common carotid artery. An approach similar to a hyovertebrotomy is used, but the ligature is positioned further ventrally in the neck, beneath the parotid gland. The internal carotid originates immediately before the occipital artery and travels deep to that vessel and in a more rostral direction (Fig. 45–1). Special care must be taken to distinguish between these vessels. Occasionally both arteries arise as a single trunk and bifurcate at a variable distance from the common carotid artery.

If the external carotid artery is the source of hemorrhage, it can be approached through a similar incision. However, exposure of this vessel at the desired point of ligation, distal to the origin of the linguofacial trunk (Fig. 45–1), is difficult and requires deep dissection to a point rostral to the caudal edge of the parotid gland.

The application of a single ligature to the external carotid artery is generally unsuccessful because this vessel has numerous collateral channels that allow retrograde flow to the infected segment (Fig. 45–1).

After the external carotid artery gives off the linguofacial trunk, it travels dorsally beneath the mucosa of the lateral compartment of the guttural pouch and gives off the caudal auricular and superficial temporal arteries (Fig. 45–1). After the latter, it is continued as the maxillary artery (Fig. 45–1). This vessel continues along the roof of the lateral compartment, passes above the tensor veli palatini muscle, and enters the alar canal (Fig. 45–1). Before it reaches this level, it gives off several branches within the guttural pouch, but the one most likely to provide retrograde flow is the inferior alveolar artery (Fig. 45–1). This artery travels through the mandible and joins its fellow artery on the opposite side to form a complete arterial loop around the lower jaw (Fig. 45–1). After the maxillary artery enters the caudal alar foramen it gives off the external ophthalmic and external ethmoidal arteries, which unite with the cerebral arterial circle through their corresponding internal branches and the common (median) artery of the corpus callosum. After it leaves the alar canal, the maxillary artery gives off the infraorbital artery, and this anastomoses with the facial artery on the same side through several arterial connections (Fig. 45–1). The maxillary artery is then continued as a large vessel, the major palatine artery, and this joins the contralateral major palatine artery behind the upper row of incisor teeth to form a large arterial loop around the upper jaw (Fig. 45–1). Although all the preceding arterial connections can provide retrograde flow to the lesion, the most likely source, based on size alone, is the major palatine artery (Fig. 45–1). No attempts have been made to ligate the maxillary artery distal to the site of infection, largely because access to this area would be extremely difficult.

Balloon Catheter Occlusion of the Internal Carotid Artery. To prevent retrograde flow from the cerebral arterial circle to the infected segment of internal carotid artery, a surgical procedure was devised to allow intravascular occlusion of the full length of the artery beneath the mucosa of the guttural pouch. The internal carotid artery is isolated close to its origin from the common carotid artery and freed from surrounding fascia. It is then ligated and a small arteriotomy is made in its wall distal to the ligature. A #4 to #8 French (1.32- to 2.64-mm) balloon-tipped catheter is then inserted through the arteriotomy for a distance of 13 cm (Fig. 45–2). Fluoroscopy is not required. This distance usually places the balloon tip of the catheter at the second flexure of the sigmoid, within the venous sinuses on the roof of the guttural pouch and therefore distant to the site of infection (Fig. 45–3). The catheter is inflated with sterile saline and secured in position by a ligature applied distal to the site of insertion. The redundant portion of the catheter is buried in the deeper tissues and the incision is closed in routine fashion. Different types of catheters have been used for this purpose, and the most suitable are a silicone rubber catheter constructed especially for this purpose, an embolectomy/thrombectomy catheter (Bard Parker), or a venous thrombectomy catheter (Fogarty; Edwards Laboratories). The last two catheters are quite stiff and therefore carry the risk of inadvertent penetration of the arterial wall at the site of infection.

Special Precautions. If the catheter penetrates the defect in the artery, it can be withdrawn and attempts made to redirect the tip distally. Alternatively, the

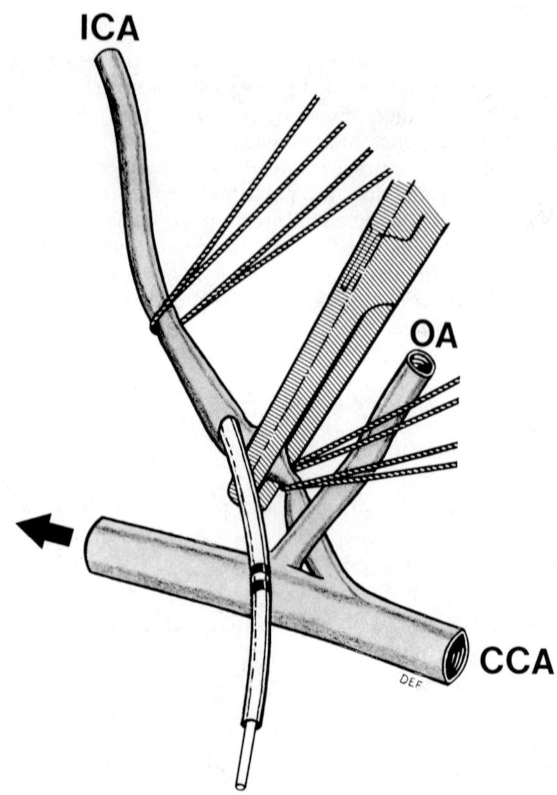

Figure 45–2. Method of inserting a balloon-tipped catheter into the left internal carotid artery (*ICA*). The artery has been exposed between two double loops of 0 silk suture material and a small arteriotomy made distal to the forceps, which is applied to obstruct normograde flow. The tip of the catheter is directed distally and marks on the catheter body are used to measure the distance of insertion before the balloon is inflated. *OA*, occipital artery; *CCA*, common carotid artery. The *arrow* points cranially.

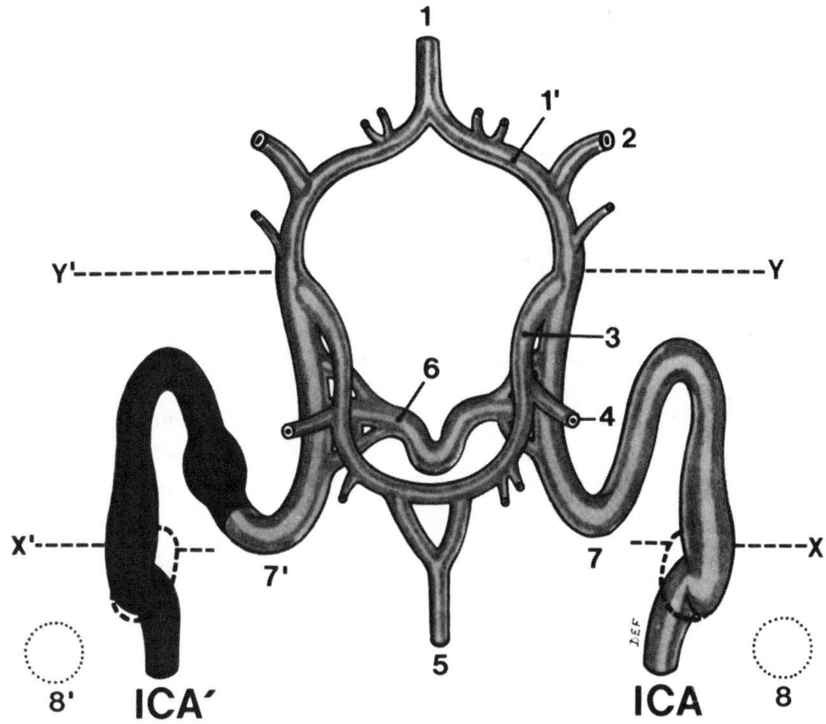

Figure 45–3. Diagram of the dorsal aspect of the cerebral arterial circle and distal parts of the internal carotid arteries of the horse. The *dark shading* on the left internal carotid artery (*ICA'*) represents the segment occupied by the catheter and balloon tip, with the balloon inflated midway between the first and second flexures of the sigmoid. The internal carotid artery terminates by dividing into the rostral (*1*) and middle (*2*) cerebral arteries. *X* and *X'* indicate the roof of the guttural pouch, and this is the typical location of the mycotic infection. Between this point and *Y* or *Y'*, the artery is contained in the ventral petrosal and venous cavernous sinuses, where it is surgically inaccessible and beyond the view of an endoscope placed in the guttural pouch. *ICA*, right internal carotid artery; *3*, caudal communicating artery; *4*, caudal cerebral artery; *5*, basilar artery; *6*, intercarotid artery; *7* and *7'*, second flexures of the sigmoid; *8* and *8'*, right and left styloid processes of the petrous part of the temporal bone. (From Freeman DE, Donawick WJ: Occlusion of internal carotid artery in the horse by means of a balloon-tipped catheter: Clinical use of a method to prevent epistaxis caused by guttural pouch mycosis. *J Am Vet Med Assoc* 1980;176:236.)

catheter can be left in place and another catheter directed alongside it. While the tip of the first catheter is positioned in the defect, it will divert the second catheter into the distal segment of artery. It is recommended that an endoscope be placed in the guttural pouch before surgery and the internal carotid artery be observed during catheter placement to ensure that the correct vessel is catheterized and that the catheter does not penetrate a defect in the infected segment of artery.

Complications associated with this procedure are few and mild and the most common is infection in the surgical site. This can be easily resolved by removal of the catheter and establishing drainage. Fortunately, this complication is rare and can be prevented by inflating the balloon to sufficient diameter (6 to 8 mm) to ensure that arterial pressure distal to it does not force it in retrograde fashion into the infected segment. It is unnecessary to remove the catheter after surgery unless infection tracks along it and invades the surgical incision. Alternatively, the catheter can be removed after 14 to 21 days, once a thrombus has formed distal to the catheter occlusion.

Success Rate. The balloon catheter technique has been used on several horses in several clinics and found to be successful in preventing hemorrhage from guttural pouch mycosis. The technique is not difficult to perform and only requires one additional step beyond the application of a single ligature to the internal carotid artery. In addition, it immediately occludes the entire length of the internal carotid artery within the guttural pouch, so that the risk of hemorrhage after surgery is completely abolished.

Balloon Catheter Occlusion of the External Carotid Artery and Its Branches. Attempts have been made to occlude the external carotid artery by means of a balloon-tipped catheter. This approach has proven to be unsatisfactory because it is impossible to control the direction of the catheter tip in the distal branches of the artery and it can readily enter the superficial temporal artery rather than the maxillary artery (Fig. 45–1). In this event, the catheter accomplishes little more than the single ligation procedure because the most common site of infection is on the maxillary artery, distal to the superficial temporal artery. This problem can be resolved by inserting a catheter into the external carotid artery via the transverse facial artery and by withdrawing the partially inflated balloon until it impacts at the origin of the superficial temporal artery (Fig. 45–1). A catheter inserted into the external carotid artery is then directed into the maxillary artery and inflated at the level of the caudal alar foramen (Fig. 45–1). The distance to this point from the origin of the linguofacial trunk was measured in a number of horses and was found to be 10.6 cm (range 9.5 to 13.3 cm, n = 14). The catheter in the transverse facial artery is removed, and the arteriotomy used for its insertion is closed by double ligation. The purpose of this procedure is to occlude the external carotid artery at the beginning and end of its course under the guttural pouch mucosa (Fig. 45–1) so that blood flow to the lesion from both directions is reduced or eliminated.

An alternative approach of occluding the external carotid artery involves ligation of the external carotid artery at its origin and insertion of a #6 French Fogarty venous thrombectomy catheter into the major palatine artery. (Fig. 45–1). This catheter is directed in retrograde fashion so that the distended balloon will occlude the maxillary artery, caudal to the caudal alar foramen (Fig. 45–1). The artery is isolated through a cutdown procedure 3 cm caudal to the corner incisor tooth, approximately 1 to 2 cm medial to the edge of the interalveolar space. The distal tip of the catheter is advanced into the artery a distance approximately 2 to 3 cm longer than the shortest distance from the arteriotomy site to the articular tubercle of the temporal bone (Fig. 45–1). The balloon is then partly filled with sterile saline until it is felt to make contact with the wall of the vessel. It is then gently withdrawn until some resistance is encountered. At this point, the partly inflated balloon has become impacted at the level of the caudal alar foramen (Fig. 45–1). It is then fully inflated with sterile saline.

The external carotid artery can be occluded by ligation immediately distal to the origin of the linguofacial trunk. In large horses, exposure at this point is difficult so that the artery can be ligated further proximally and the linguofacial trunk is also ligated to eliminate backflow from it. The external carotid artery also can be occluded by inserting a catheter through the transverse facial artery beneath the articular tubercle of the temporal bone (Fig. 45–1). This catheter is advanced so that its tip is approximately 12 cm from the arteriotomy and then it is partly inflated with saline. When the partly inflated balloon makes contact with the wall of the artery, it is gently withdrawn until resistance is encountered. It is then assumed that the tip of the catheter is in the external carotid artery (Fig. 45–1). The catheter is then advanced approximately 2 to 3 cm more into the external carotid artery and the balloon is fully inflated until it is impacted at this level. The redundant ends of the catheters in the transverse facial and major palatine arteries are folded upon themselves and secured with tape. They are then incorporated into a stockinette hood and secured to the halter. This method is most valuable in horses with involvement of the external carotid artery alone because, without the need to occlude the internal carotid, a difficult and deep dissection is obviated.

Precaution. The major complication of external carotid occlusion is blindness. However, this has not been observed in the small number of cases treated regardless of whether the external carotid artery was occluded alone or in combination with occlusion of the internal carotid artery. However, the owner of the horse should be advised of this potential risk and the effects of unilateral blindness in the horse's future use should be considered before proceeding with the surgery.

This surgery appears to be completely effective in preventing hemorrhage in cases in which the external carotid artery is involved. However, there are several branches given off from the maxillary artery in the segment intervening between the points of balloon inflation, and it is possible that these may still provide some retrograde flow to the infected segment. Another potential risk is inadvertent withdrawal of the catheters if they become hooked on stall fittings. To minimize this risk and the potential spread of infection from the oral cavity along the major palatine catheter, these catheters are removed after 7 to 10 days. Removal is easy and does not require sedation or local anesthesia.

Postoperative Care. All methods of occluding the internal carotid and external carotid arteries require minimal postoperative care. Antibiotics should be given, especially when balloon catheters are used. However, vigorous forms of treatment are ineffective and the lesion resolves spontaneously, usually without creating further problems. When catheters are placed in superficial vessels, such as the major palatine or the superficial temporal artery, they must be covered to prevent accidental removal on stall fittings.

Success Rate. Based on our experiences to date, it is clear that hemorrhage from the external carotid or the maxillary artery can only be prevented by occluding these vessels at both ends of their course through the guttural pouch mucosa. Their collateral channels are numerous and they can maintain a constant circulation of blood through the infected segment (Fig. 45–1). Both methods used to accomplish these goals need further evaluation before definite conclusions can be drawn about which is preferable. The single catheter technique diverted into the maxillary artery by a temporary balloon catheter in the superficial temporal artery carries the slight risk of providing an avenue for infection to spread to the surgery site. The second technique, with catheterization of the major palatine artery, carries the risk of accidental catheter displacement after surgery. However, the procedure has the advantage that the catheters can be inserted through superficial vessels so that deep dissection beneath the parotid gland is obviated.

BIBLIOGRAPHY

Caron JF, Fretz FB, Bailey JV, et al: Balloon-tipped catheter arterial occlusion for prevention of hemorrhage caused by guttural pouch mycosis: 13 cases (1982–1985). *J Am Vet Med Assoc* 1987;191:345–349.

Church S, Wyn-Jones G, Parks AH, et al: Treatment of guttural pouch mycosis. *Equine Vet J* 1986;18:362–365.

Colles CM, Cook WR: Carotid and cerebral angiography in the horse. *Vet Rec* 1983;113:483–489.

Cook WR: Clinical observations on the anatomy and physiology of the equine upper respiratory tract. *Vet Rec* 1966;79:440–446.

Freeman DE: Diagnosis and treatment of diseases of the guttural pouch (Part I). *Compend Cont Educ Pract Vet* 1980;2:S3-S11.

Freeman DE: Diagnosis and treatment of diseases of the guttural pouch (Part II). *Compend Cont Educ Pract Vet* 1980:2:S25-S31.

Freeman DE, Donawick WJ: Occlusion of internal carotid artery in the horse by means of a balloon-tipped catheter: Clinical use of a method to prevent epistaxis caused by guttural pouch mycosis. *J Am Vet Med Assoc* 1980;176:236–240.

Freeman DE, Donawick WJ: Occlusion of internal carotid artery in the horse by means of a balloon-tipped catheter: Evaluation of a method designed to prevent epistaxis caused by guttural pouch mycosis. *J Am Vet Med Assoc* 1980;176:232–235.

Greet TRC: Outcome of treatment in 35 cases of guttural pouch mycosis. *Equine Vet J* 1987;19:483–487.

Smith DM, Barber SM: Guttural pouch hemorrhage associated with lesions of the maxillary artery in two horses. *Can Vet J* 1984;25:239–242.

46 Guttural Pouch Tympany

David E. Freeman

Tympany of the guttural pouch generally occurs in foals shortly after birth but may not be noticed in some horses for up to 1 year. The condition occurs predominantly in fillies. The affected guttural pouch becomes distended with air and the resultant swelling in the parotid region is nonpainful and tympanic. In severe cases, the foal may develop stertorous breathing and may have mild dysphagia. The cause of the condition is unknown but it is probably a functional problem rather than a structural defect. It has been postulated that the pharyngeal orifice of the affected guttural pouch allows the ingress of air during expiration but that it acts as a one-way valve to prevent its egress. Consequently, the pouch becomes progressively larger and displaces the trachea, larynx, and pharynx ventrally and to the contralateral side. Most cases are unilateral, although the swelling is so extensive that it appears that both pouches are involved. Bilateral cases have been reported.

DIAGNOSIS

Diagnosis is made on the basis of the foal's age, the history, and the physical appearance of the swelling. The foal may appear in good health and be thriving. On radiographs, the air-filled guttural pouch outline will appear larger than normal and will extend as far caudally as the caudal edge of the axis. Surrounding soft tissue structures and cavities will be markedly displaced. A fluid line may be evident within the guttural pouch, and this can be attributed to a secondary empyema. In severe, long-standing cases and in those foals with dysphagia, aspiration pneumonia may occur.

In severe cases, when the swelling on the affected side bulges under the parotid gland on the opposite side, it can be difficult to determine if involvement is unilateral or bilateral. If a needle inserted in one side decompresses most of the swelling, it can be concluded that the condition is unilateral.

SURGERY

Surgery is the treatment of choice for guttural pouch tympany. The purpose of surgery is to establish a communication between the affected guttural pouch and the normal pouch by creating a fenestration in the median septum between them. Air can then pass from the affected side through the normal pharyngeal orifice on the opposite side. The median septum can be approached through Viborg's triangle with the foal in lateral recumbency or through a modified Whitehouse approach with the foal in dorsal recumbency. The advantage of the latter is that it allows direct access to the median septum close to the point of entry into the guttural pouch. Viborg's triangle is usually enlarged in foals with tympany because the swelling has forced the guttural pouch lining to assume a subcutaneous position in this area. A long, shallow incision can then be made in Viborg's triangle to gain direct access to the guttural pouch. The septum is usually collapsed away from the incision and can be difficult to locate. A fiberoptic endoscope is therefore inserted in the contralateral guttural pouch and used to elevate the median septum into a more accessible position, (Fig. 46–1). The septum is then grasped and a 3-cm diameter segment is resected with scissors. Care is taken to remove the mucosa from both pouches so that the resection is complete. If bilateral guttural pouch tympany is suspected, a small segment of the cartilage on the medial lamina of the eustachian tube can be trimmed along the inner guttural pouch orifice, thereby enlarging the opening.

If the interior of the guttural pouch is healthy and contains only a small volume of mucopurulent fluid, the incision can be closed in routine fashion. If a large amount of purulent material has accumulated, an indwelling rubber tube or Penrose drain can be inserted through the incision and sutured in place to allow daily irrigation of the guttural pouch cavity. In these cases, the incision is left open to provide ventral drainage.

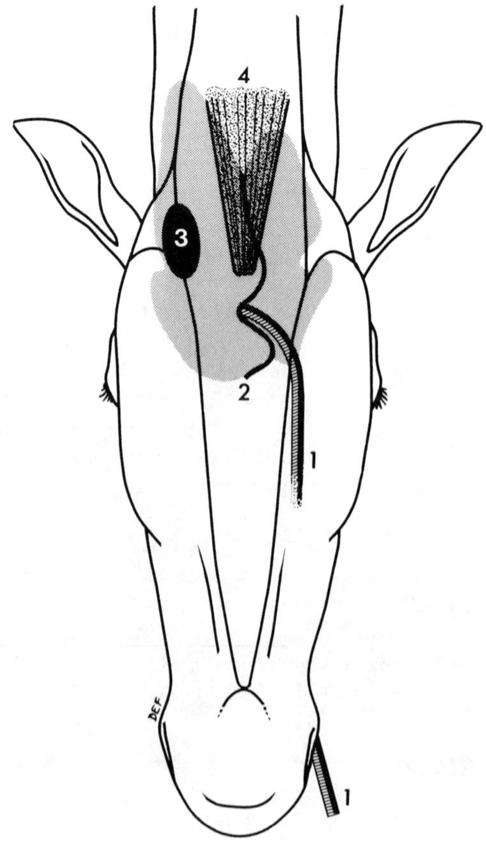

Figure 46–1. Method of using the fiberoptic endoscope to help identify the median septum in a foal with tympany of the left guttural pouch. In this diagram, the foal is in dorsal recumbency and the shaded segments represent the outlines of both guttural pouches. The endoscope (*1*) has been inserted through the right nasal passage and into the right guttural pouch and its tip has been directed medially to push the median septum (*2*) toward the modified Whitehouse incision (*3*). A Chamber's catheter or similar rigid instrument with an angled tip can be used instead of the endoscope. *4*, ventral straight muscles of the head, which divide the left and right guttural pouches caudally and dorsally.

A successful fenestration has also been performed by diathermy through a fiberoptic endoscope. The condition has also been treated by creation of a fistula between the guttural pouch and pharynx, close to the dorsal pharyngeal recess, again using diathermy. Fenestration of the median septum by Nd:YAG laser appears to be particularly promising and has the advantage that it can be performed on the conscious, tranquilized foal.

This procedure thus avoids the risks of nerve damage associated with incisions into the guttural pouch.

POSTOPERATIVE CARE

After surgery, the foal can be returned to the mare and no special aftercare is required. Antibiotics can be administered if indicated, as in those cases in which concurrent guttural pouch empyema is considered severe. Aggressive antibiotic therapy is warranted in foals that have developed secondary aspiration pneumonia or that had signs of dysphagia before surgery.

PROGNOSIS

The prognosis is excellent in uncomplicated cases, but a small number of foals develop fatal aspiration pneumonia. When the tympany resolves, all displaced structures regain their normal positions. In some cases the fenestration may seal after surgery, and a second procedure may be required. If the condition recurs and a patent fenestration is found during the second surgery, both guttural pouches are probably involved. Then the pharyngeal orifice should be enlarged by trimming a portion of the medial lamina of the guttural pouch opening on one side.

47 Laryngeal Hemiplegia

Gregory L. Ferraro

Of the currently diagnosed maladies of the equine upper airway, laryngeal hemiplegia is probably the best known and most often discussed. This condition usually affects the left arytenoid cartilage as a result of denervation of the ipsilateral intrinsic laryngeal musculature, primarily the left dorsal cricoarytenoid muscle. In spite of its long historic recognition, there are still many misconceptions regarding the diagnosis of laryngeal hemiplegia, the method of treatment, and the prognosis following surgical correction. The old horsemen's term, "roarer," is still the best and most encompassing term to describe the condition because it projects the concept of laryngeal dysfunction rather than merely the presence of an abnormal appearance. It is, of course, the horse's inability to perform a given level of exercise that is the underlying complaint with all upper respiratory tract conditions. The veterinarian must be cognizant of this during the examination and realize that the mere presence of anatomic or physiologic abnormalities of the larynx does not necessarily constitute grounds for treatment.

DIAGNOSIS

One must remember when evaluating the equine patient for suspected laryngeal hemiplegia or other upper respiratory maladies that the veterinarian is trying to make a functional diagnosis; that is, the animal's athletic performance in relationship to the function of its larynx should be consistent with reasonable expectations. Such an evaluation is made more difficult by the fact that it is being done in a relatively static situation by integration of physical findings with observation, and evaluation of rather circumstantial information. Laryngeal function per se cannot currently be measured or directly evaluated during field performance, although treadmill tests for upper airway function have been reported. Therefore, it is imperative that the clinician carefully follow all procedures used in a thorough diagnostic workup.

The first of these procedures is careful evaluation of the horse's past performance as it relates to the presenting complaint. Important questions include: Is the horse showing evidence of abnormal tiring during exercise, and is this exercise intolerance consistent with what one would expect from laryngeal dysfunction? Does the horse tire suddenly after a period of normal performance, or does poor performance commence at the onset of exercise? Is this early fatigue the result of some possible loss of respiratory function that corresponds with other signs, such as noise production, or does the fatigue result from lack of fitness? Is it possible that a sudden onset of poor performance during exercise could be the result of pain due to locomotor abnormalities? Is the character of the respiratory noise consistent or variable? What has been the duration of the problem, and was its onset sudden or gradual? These questions, as well as any others relating to performance, must be thoroughly explored before the diagnostic procedures take place. For racehorses, one should also look at the horse's recorded past performances, or "form." Following this investigatory procedure a clinical examination can be performed.

Since the introduction of the flexible fiberoptic endoscope, the equine veterinarian has too often been guilty of relying on its use as the sole basis for the diagnosis of an upper respiratory disorder. This is an unconscionable error that often leads to erroneous diagnoses. If the diagnosis of laryngeal hemiplegia is to be based on function, then several diagnostic procedures must be included in the examination. These should include the visual assessment of the horse's performance on the track or in the show ring, listening to and evaluating respiratory noise characteristics, endoscopic examination at rest and after exercise, digital palpation of the larynx for evidence of muscular atrophy, and use of the arytenoid depression test.

Observation should be made at a time when the horse is performing at maximal exercise. In the case of racehorses this is best done during a workout or speed drill. Work over a distance of five eighths of a mile or more is best, provided the horse is sufficiently fit, because this distance taxes the horse enough that he will tire if respiratory function is abnormal. Distances less than five eighths of a mile can often be successfully completed by superior athletes in spite of laryngeal dysfunction. The examiner should be looking for the horse to tire excessively during the last one eighth to one quarter of a mile during this exercise. Such fatigue is evident by a longer elapsed time for each succeeding one eighth of a mile, with perhaps a sudden slowing during the last eighth of a mile.

With the onset of fatigue, one should also hear an increased intensity of respiratory noise. While horses may exhibit noise throughout exercise, the intensity of the noise tends to increase with fatigue. This is particularly true during the early stages of laryngeal dysfunction before paralysis occurs. The noise heard should be the characteristic high-pitched, shrill sound or whistle that is made only on inspiration. If the roaring sound is produced on expiration as well, then arytenoid chondritis or some other physical obstruction in the upper airway, rather than laryngeal hemiplegia, should be suspected.

Upon returning to the stall, one should be able to palpate a definite lack of musculature over the dorsal aspect of the affected side of the larynx. A pit will often be palpable over the dorsal larynx on the affected side, and the muscular process of the arytenoid cartilage should be easily palpable. A sound similar to the one heard during exercise can be elicited by applying pressure over the affected arytenoid cartilage and turning the horse's head toward the same side (arytenoid depression test). Once these diagnostic tests have been performed, the information derived from the endoscopic examination can be more accurately evaluated. It must be stressed again that to avoid an erroneous diagnosis of laryngeal hemiplegia, one must remember that a functional evaluation is being made in a relatively static state.

The mere presence of apparently abnormal laryngeal anatomy or function does not necessarily constitute a definitive diagnosis of malfunction. Thus, recognition during endoscopic examination of asymmetry of the arytenoid cartilages or asynchronous movement does not constitute a diagnosis of laryngeal hemiplegia. Moreover, the existence of laryngeal hemiplegia does not necessarily indicate unsatisfactory performance. In evaluating the larynx, one must determine if the suspected dysfunctional arytenoid cartilage is capable of any voluntary movement; that is, can the horse abduct or adduct the arytenoid cartilages, and open or close the glottis at will? This can be determined by watching normal respiration and looking for laryngeal movements consistent with respiratory function. The larynx should dilate and the arytenoids should abduct during inspiration and adduct slightly during expiration. A lack of movement of one arytenoid cartilage or movement inconsistent with normal respiration may indicate dysfunction.

It has been stated that the paralyzed arytenoid loses adductor function before abductor function. This should be evaluated by observing the larynx during swallowing or using the slap or grunt test. One should also look for evidence of a relaxed vocal fold on the affected side; this occasionally results in the laryngeal saccule on the affected side appearing larger than the opposite saccule.

A misdiagnosis often made during examination for exercise intolerance is that of laryngeal hemiplegia when, in fact, arytenoid chondritis is the problem. One must remember that laryngeal hemiplegia is characterized by a complete lack of movement. Chondritis of the arytenoid, on the other hand, while giving the appearance of an asymmetric or stenotic larynx, will usually show some consistent but ineffectual movement. Also, chondritis often causes a visible thickening of the arytenoid cartilage. It is also widely known that about 95% of affected horses have left-sided laryngeal hemiplegia. While arytenoid chondritis can affect both left and right arytenoid cartilages, it should always be strongly considered in apparent right-sided laryngeal hemiplegia.

TREATMENT

Currently, there are four basic management options to consider for left laryngeal hemiplegia. The first three involve various surgical procedures that have been well documented. These are ventriculectomy, prosthetic laryngoplasty, and total or subtotal arytenoidectomy. The fourth method of treatment, however, and the one most frequently overlooked in the veterinary literature, is a change in athletic management.

Surgical Procedures

Ventriculectomy for the correction of laryngeal hemiplegia is the oldest known surgical method currently practiced in the United States, since the creation of a permanent tracheal fistula (tubing) is no longer considered a viable method of treatment. The chief advantage of ventriculectomy is that it can be performed upon the standing horse. For horses that present a high risk for general anesthesia (e.g., draft horses), this is a major consideration. It is fairly well accepted, however, that at best the procedure provides only marginal relief from laryngeal hemiplegia, and a marked improvement in athletic performance in horses engaged in speed-oriented events cannot be expected. It was this fact that prompted the development of the prosthetic laryngoplasty technique.

Laryngoplasty for the correction of left laryngeal hemiplegia was first described by Marks and colleagues in 1970. Since then, the procedure has become the standard method of correction employed in most horses. The technique has been modified and improved upon since its original description, and a good example of the basic technique has been described by Haynes. Most equine veterinarians are familiar with this technique, so a complete description of it will not be given. There are some aspects of the technique, however, that I believe are important enough to be discussed here.

Laryngoplasty is a procedure whose success rate is definitely related to the skill of the surgeon. Therefore, those attempting it should be familiar with both the regional anatomy and the surgical technique. Careful and atraumatic dissection is a must if undesirable sequelae are to be avoided. The surgical area is moderately supplied with nerves and vascular structures, and these should be compromised as little as possible. Nerves cut or damaged by rough handling can lead to aspiration, the presence of ingested feed at the nostrils, or chronic coughing. Disruption of vessels and inadequate hemostasis leads to excessive bleeding, making completion of the procedure difficult.

Careful and correct placement of the laryngoplasty sutures is essential for success. The technique of using towel clamps to retract the cartilage for easier placement of the sutures is considered to be excessively traumatic and therefore is not favored. A loop or blunt hook is preferable to place gentle traction on the muscular process of the arytenoid cartilage and make suture placement easier. The loop can be fashioned by redesigning a spay hook. Improper suture placement and the suture cutting through the cartilage after placement are the two most common causes for surgical failure.

Many types of suture can be used in this procedure. I prefer either #5 Ethibond (green braided cardiovascular suture MD-66, MS/4 taper cut V-37 needle; Ethicon, Inc) with a swaged-on needle or a 5-mm Mersilene tape suture (orthopedic white woven tape, polyester fiber suture 522 G, Ethicon 05-8 cutting needle). The second type is considered more advantageous because its ribbon-like configuration makes it less likely to cut through the cartilage than the round, braided configuration. The ribbon suture has a triangular-shaped swaged-on needle that cuts through the cartilage so that the flat side of the ribbon lies across the tension side of the tunnel created through the cartilage. Both types of suture material are placed directly through the cricoid and arytenoid cartilages using their swaged-on needles. No predrilling of the suture path is necessary with the needles supplied with these suture materials.

It is also believed that the horse should be extubated and the larynx observed endoscopically before the suture is tied. This ensures that proper retraction of the arytenoid cartilage occurs. Inadequate abduction may result in continued exercise intolerance, whereas excessive abduction can lead to aspiration of food material postsurgically. It has been demonstrated that the abducted position of the arytenoid cartilage following laryngoplasty is not as significant a factor as the need for rigid fixation of the cartilage.

Once the suture has been placed and tied, the operative site should be thoroughly lavaged with saline and carefully closed. This surgical wound has a propensity for seroma formation. Approximately 15 to 20% of operated horses show some degree of seroma formation postsurgically. This can be minimized by gentle surgical manipulation, attention to hemostasis, adequate flushing of the wound before closure, and careful closure technique. The cavity created during the procedure cannot be completely reduced no matter how thoroughly one attempts to do this. Therefore, it is best to avoid implanting an unnecessary amount of suture material in the wound during closure. Simply closing the muscles overlying the prosthetic implant with two or three simple interrupted sutures followed by a simple interrupted closure of the subcutaneous tissues and skin in separate rows is sufficient. I prefer synthetic absorbable suture material rather than more reactive suture material such as catgut.

After laryngoplasty, the laryngeal saccule on the affected side is traditionally removed. This is accomplished by using the standard ventriculectomy approach. This is recommended to prevent the vocal cord or the saccule from interfering with airflow during exercise. However, recent treadmill testing after only laryngoplasty indicates that, if proper abduction is obtained, the airflow returns to normal without a ventriculectomy.

Total or subtotal arytenoidectomy, while being successful in horses with chondroma formation, is not a preferred treatment for laryngeal hemiplegia. Removal of the arytenoid cartilage in the absence of a normally functioning dorsal cricoarytenoid muscle can result in laryngeal failure because of the lack of formation of a rigid laryngeal tube during exercise. This flaccid tissue becomes drawn into the airway during exercise, causing obstruction to airflow. While it may sometimes be tried as a last resort after failure of a laryngoplasty, it is not generally recommended for laryngeal hemiplegia.

Postoperative Care

The postsurgical care is similar for each of these procedures. The horse should be fed hay placed in a hay net or feeder in an elevated position immediately upon return to the stall. Mastication and swallowing for the first few hours after surgery helps to reduce swelling and pain. It is important that the feed be presented off the ground so that the horse's head remains elevated. The laryngotomy incision must be cleansed daily until closure (approximately 2 weeks). If seroma formation occurs within the laryngoplasty incision, drainage is achieved by removing one or two sutures and flushing the wound once daily for 2 or 3 days with either sterile saline or a dilute povidone-iodine solution. If the incision is opened, probing or rigorous flushing should be avoided to prevent the prosthesis from becoming contaminated.

The horse should be hand walked starting the day after surgery, and this should continue until the laryngotomy incision is closed. Then, the horse can be ridden under tack for an additional 4 to 6 weeks. At that time, an endoscopic examination should show healing and no postsurgical swelling. The horse can then be returned to its chosen athletic endeavor. In the case of racehorses, it has been found preferable to keep the convalescence as short as possible and to try to maintain some fitness so as to make the return to training less stressful.

PROGNOSIS

As has been previously mentioned, the success rate of each of these procedures in terms of athletic performance is very low. It is estimated that the laryngoplasty technique is only 30 to 50% successful for racing horses depending on the surgeon and the type of athletic endeavor in which the horse is engaged. Horses used in athletic endeavors less strenuous than racing are more likely to return to performance. In these cases simple stabilization of the arytenoid is often (80 to 90%) successful in improving performance and can lessen or stop the associated respiratory noise.

The most common cause of failure of laryngoplasty is the suture cutting through the cartilage, resulting in relaxation of the abducted arytenoid cartilage. This may not occur immediately, and, indeed, horses that look well abducted at 6 to 8 weeks may appear poorly abducted at 3 to 4 months. Complete exit of the suture from the cartilage is also not necessary because only slight relaxation of the affected cartilage can be enough to alter airflow dynamics so that maximal performance is not achieved. It is the low level of success achieved by surgery that makes its use desirable only as a last resort.

A more desirable course of action in most cases is a change in athletic management. Horses with laryngeal hemiplegia can often be made useful by changing the athletic event for which they are trained. Some racehorses with laryngeal hemiplegia can be quite successful if they compete in shorter races or drop in class. For this reason, management changes should always be the first course of action in afflicted horses, and I believe that surgical correction should be chosen as a last resort. In general I believe that horses with laryngeal hemiplegia should be considered as permanently debilitated given the current state of the veterinary art. These horses almost never become top-class racehorses regardless of the treatment applied, and young horses afflicted with the condition rarely even make it to their first race. Veterinarians, therefore, must guard against giving an overly optimistic prognosis to the owner of a horse afflicted with laryngeal hemiplegia.

BIBLIOGRAPHY

Cook WR: The diagnosis of respiratory unsoundness in the horse. *Vet Rec* 1965;77:516–528.

Derksen FJ, Stick JA, Scott EA, et al: Effect of laryngeal hemiplegia and laryngoplasty on airway flow mechanics in exercising horses. *Am J Vet Res* 1986;47:16–20.

Greet TRC, Baker GH, Lee R: The effect of laryngoplasty on pharyngeal function in the horse. *Equine Vet J* 1979;11:153–158.

Haynes PF: Surgery of the equine respiratory tract, in Jennings PB (ed): *The Practice of Large Animal Surgery*, vol 1. Philadelphia, WB Saunders Co, 1984, pp 388–487.

Marks D, Mackay-Smith MP, Cushing LS, et al: Use of a prosthetic device for surgical correction of laryngeal hemiplegia in horses. *J Am Vet Med Assoc* 1970;157:157–163.

Raker CW: Complications related to the insertion of a suture to retract the arytenoid cartilage to correct laryngeal hemiplegia in the horse. *Arch Am Coll Vet Surg* 1975;4:64–66.

48 Arytenoidectomy

Eric P. Tulleners

The rima glottidis is the narrowest portion of the upper respiratory tract in horses at rest. The normal resting diamond-shaped appearance of the larynx seen endoscopically is created by the dorsolaterally situated arytenoid cartilages and the ventrolaterally positioned vocal cords. The normal glottic opening becomes kite-shaped during maximal abduction of the arytenoid cartilages. Arytenoid abduction tenses and elongates the vocal cords, pulling them laterally and flat against the laryngeal wall, obliterating the saccule openings.

Compared with the other dilatable components of the upper respiratory tract, the greatest enlargement of the rima glottidis in proportion to its resting cross-sectional area occurs during sustained exercise. Diseases that reduce this ability to enlarge the rima glottidis increase airway resistance. Changes in airway geometry and vibration of unsupported soft tissue structures may also change aerodynamics, causing an increase in airway resistance.

ETIOLOGY OF GLOTTIC APERTURE NARROWING

Narrowing of the glottic aperture is most commonly caused by idiopathic left laryngeal hemiplegia, resulting in reduced cross-sectional airway area due to loss of abductor function of the dorsal cricoid arytenoid muscle. Endoscopically, the arytenoid cartilage and vocal cords appear structurally normal. Horses with laryngeal hemiplegia are best treated with a prosthetic laryngoplasty and sacculectomy.

Structural abnormalities, which are less common, are most commonly termed chondrosis or chondritis, and cause thickening and/or distortion of the arytenoid cartilage, resulting in a decreased cross-sectional area. Arytenoid cartilage thickening results in a decreased range of motion, and, because of its anatomic position, lateral movement (abduction) is restricted by the adjacent thyroid cartilage. Gradual and increasing impingement on the laryngeal lumen reduces the cross-sectional area of the airway, resulting in a decreased ability of the horse to tolerate high-speed exercise and progressive development of increasing respiratory noise during exercise. Except in horses with primarily a loss of abductor muscle function and only minor concomitant structural cartilaginous changes, prosthetic laryngoplasty and sacculectomy techniques are ineffective in abducting the affected cartilage out of the airway, making arytenoidectomy necessary.

Laryngoplasty Failure

Horses with primary laryngoplasty failure not due to infection and without endoscopic evidence of cartilage changes may be treated with a partial arytenoidectomy or an attempt can be made to replace the prosthesis. If the latter procedure is chosen, a standard approach is made to the lateral aspect of the affected side of the larynx. If fairly normal anatomic landmarks are present, the failed prosthesis can be removed and an attempt made to replace it with a new one. If proper suture placement is achieved in a desirable location, the prosthesis should be tightened and tied and the results examined endoscopically intraoperatively. If a desirable degree of abduction has been achieved, closure is routine. If abduction is inadequate, the prosthesis is removed, the incision is closed, and a partial arytenoidectomy is performed through a laryngotomy incision made with the horse in dorsal recumbency. Intralaryngeal observation and palpation of the arytenoid cartilages and vocal cords after removal of the endotracheal tube will often afford the surgeon an estimation of the degree of abduction or a sense of whether the cartilage is abnormal compared to the normal side. A partial arytenoidectomy can then be done, if necessary, depending on the results of this intraoperative evaluation.

Partial arytenoidectomy is recommended for horses with failed left laryngoplasty in which there are endoscopically visible cartilage changes in addition to loss of abductor function. It is also recommended for horses in which laryngoplasty has failed because of infection at the prosthesis site. Infection usually causes irreversible damage to the cartilage, loss of normal anatomic landmarks from excessive scar tissue infiltration, and a loss of normal range of motion at the diarthrodial cricoarytenoid joint.

Arytenoid Chondropathy

Arytenoid chondropathy is primarily a disease of young racehorses 2 to 4 years old. Thoroughbred racehorses are overrepresented and Standardbred racehorses are underrepresented. The male-to-female ratio is approximately 2 : 1. The disease has been reported in most other breeds and ponies, in older horses, and in horses not used as racehorses.

In most affected horses, arytenoid chondropathy results in a slowly progressive enlargement of one or both arytenoid cartilages over several months to 2 years. Horses usually present with variable degrees of reduced exercise tolerance and a low-pitched whistling or roaring noise similar to that associated with laryngeal hemiplegia. Occasionally affected horses will be presented in acute respiratory embarrassment, needing an emergency tracheotomy, with no previous history of stridor or decreased exercise tolerance.

The cause of arytenoid chondropathy is unknown but is probably multifactorial. Some horses have a history of previous laryngeal surgery, such as laryngoplasty for left laryngeal hemiplegia. Others have had serious respiratory infections such as *Streptococcus equi*, bacterial pneumonia, or retropharyngeal abscesses. However, the majority or horses present with no specific known inciting cause.

PHYSICAL EXAMINATION, RADIOGRAPHY, AND ENDOSCOPY

External examination and palpation of the head and neck often reveals increased firmness and loss of resiliency to the laryngeal cartilages. Firm compression of the laryngeal cartilage may induce dyspnea and an audible noise at rest. Lateral laryngeal radiography should be performed in horses suspected to have mineralization of their laryngeal cartilages. Racehorses with increased mineralization of the laryngeal cartilages have a poor prognosis for returning to racing following arytenoidectomy compared to those horses without mineralization. Increased mineralization of the laryngeal cartilages may also develop after routine laryngeal surgery in approximately 5% of horses, causing severe narrowing of the glottis with endoscopically normal-appearing arytenoids.

Structural abnormalities of the arytenoid cartilages are diagnosed by endoscopic examination. The arytenoid cartilage may have a limited range of motion with medial projection of the affected cartilage, suggestive of laryngeal hemiplegia. In early cases the corniculate portion of the affected cartilage appears only slightly thickened or may have a peculiar wrinkled or *S*-shaped appearance with no alteration in the typical cobblestone texture of the overlying mucous membrane. The presence of partial-thickness erosions to full-thickness ulcerated defects in the mucous membrane is common, particularly on the medial surface of the corniculate cartilage. The perimeters of these defects usually are slightly raised and reddened, with the central portion being depressed and somewhat whitish in appearance. Because of the thickness of this cartilage, the slightly raised areas often contact the opposing arytenoid cartilage, causing defects in the mucous membrane. In some horses intraluminal projections of granulation tissue emanate from these ulcerated areas. These projections, which often cause defects on the medial surface of the mucous membrane of the contralateral cartilage during adduction, vary in size from a few to 20 mm in diameter. Occasionally, purulent exudate can be seen exuding from ulcerated areas.

In rare cases, the arytenoid cartilage may be just mildly thickened and have an apparently normal range of motion. Alterations may be restricted to a large, circular, granular-appearing growth protruding from the medial surface of the corniculate portion of the arytenoid cartilage just above the vocal cord attachment. These lesions can range in size from 5 to 10 up to 30 mm in diameter (Fig. 48–1).

As the lesions become more advanced, the arytenoid cartilage appears more vertical than normal and projects into the airway. The vocal cord appears shortened and often there is distortion with loss of definition of the laryngeal saccule because of obliteration by abnormal tissue. With more advanced unilateral or bilateral involvement the rima glottidis becomes a mere slit, with the opening becoming more rectangular than normal because of the vertical position of the vocal cords and grossly thickened arytenoid cartilages. In these horses the palatopharyngeal arch also may appear more prominent or displace rostrally (Fig. 48–2).

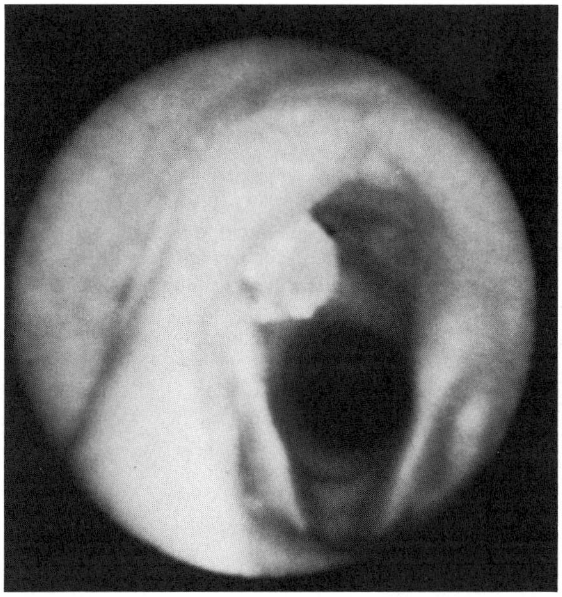

Figure 48–1. Endoscopic view of granulation tissue mass protruding from the medial aspect of the corniculate process of the right arytenoid.

Other concurrent endoscopic abnormalities are uncommon; however, retropharyngeal abscesses, entrapment of the epiglottis by the aryepiglottic folds, epiglottic hypoplasia, and dorsal displacement of the soft palate have also been seen concomitantly.

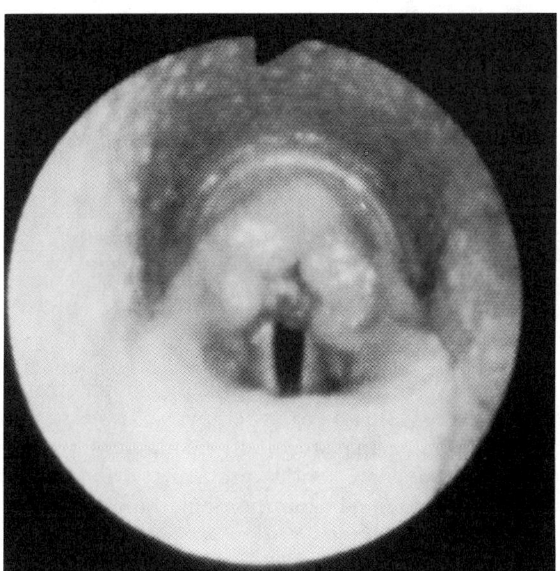

Figure 48–2. Bilateral arytenoid chondropathy seen by endoscopy. Note the extremely narrow rectangular-shaped glottic opening and the prominent palatopharyngeal arch.

SURGICAL PROCEDURE

Surgery is performed with the horse in dorsal recumbency using inhalation anesthesia administered through a midcervical tracheotomy. A laryngotomy is performed, with incision of the cricoid or thyroid cartilages rarely necessary.

A vertical incision is made with a #15 Bard Parker scalpel around the rostral aspect of the vocal fold and around the perimeter of the laryngeal saccule, which is then dissected free and removed. The vertical incision is extended dorsally on the medial surface of the arytenoid cartilage from the saccule to the dorsal midline, elliptically excising any mucosal defects. The mucous membrane is then carefully elevated circumferentially from the corniculate cartilage and vocal process with Freer elevators and straight or curved Beaver blades (Arista Surgical Supply Co). Partial arytenoidectomy is recommended since this preserves the muscular process. Defects in the mucous membrane are excised, and the mucous membrane is trimmed and apposed with synthetic absorbable suture material in a simple interrupted or continuous pattern. The ventral portion of the mucous membrane need not be sutured if drainage is needed. Particular attention should be paid to reconstructing the dorsal one-half of the mucosal incision since this is commonly the site of wound dehiscence.

Submucosal cartilage removal with mucosal closure as described is recommended and most likely to be achieved in horses with primary laryngeal hemiplegia or following failed laryngoplasty and in those horses with early to moderate degrees of unilateral or bilateral arytenoid chondropathy. In horses with advanced unilateral or bilateral chondropathy with extensive damage to the mucous membrane, only partial mucosal closure can be achieved.

In some horses with advanced unilateral or bilateral disease, it may be preferable or necessary to perform a partial arytenoidectomy without mucosal closure. The procedure begins with removal of the vocal fold and laryngeal saccule as previously described. With scalpel or scissors the vertical incision is continued dorsally to the midline, leaving a 3-mm wide rostral, vertical strip of corniculate cartilage. The incision is continued around the dorsal, caudal, and ventral perimeter of the arytenoid cartilage (Fig. 48–3). Lateral attachments are incised and the body of the cartilage is removed en bloc, leaving a portion of the muscular process. Experimentally, in normal horses even large defects created in the laryngeal mucous membrane healed in 12 to 16 weeks without excessive granulation tissue. Healing was by granulation tissue to the luminal surface with a gradual, time-related transition to mature dense con-

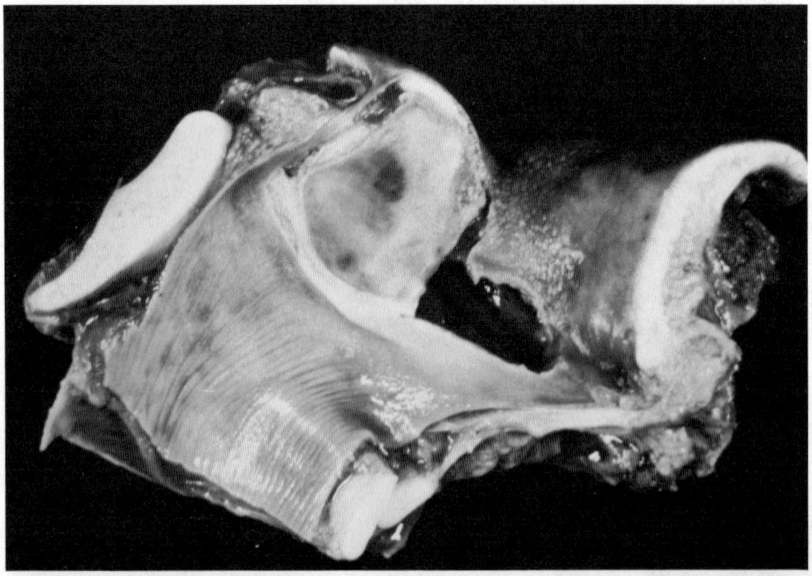

A

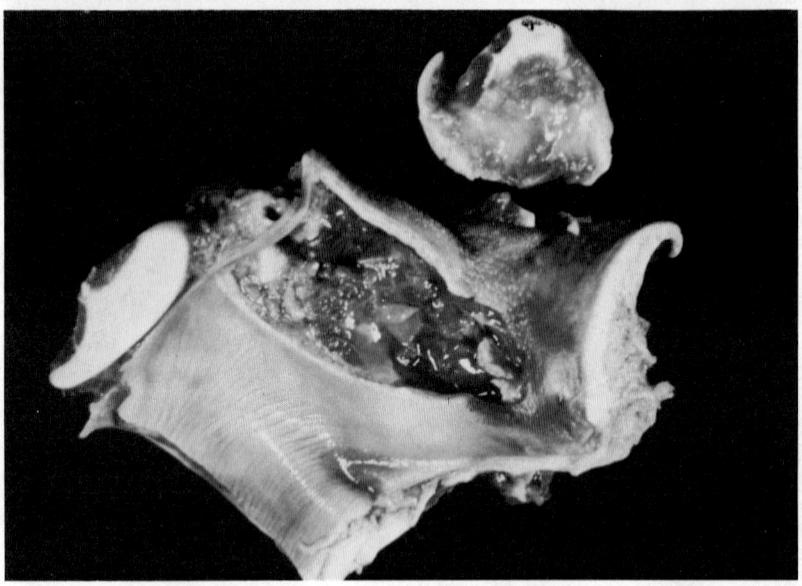

B

Figure 48–3. A. Sagittal section of the left hemilarynx with the lumen visible. The epiglottis is to the right; the cricoid cartilage is on the left. An open left arytenoidectomy is seen in which the laryngeal ventricle has been removed (ventrally) and an incision has been made around the perimeter of the left arytenoid cartilage (dorsally). **B.** Sagittal section of the left hemilarynx with the lumen visible. Muscular attachments of the lateral (abaxial) surface of the left arytenoid have been severed and the cartilage has been removed en bloc. An estimated 3-mm wide rostral vertical strip of corniculate cartilage and mucosa remains, as does the muscular process.

nective tissue. Epithelialization from the periphery gradually covered this connective tissue.

Based on these observations, it is probably preferable to leave even large defects in the mucous membrane rather than attempting mucosal closure of a poor-quality tissue under tension. All remaining mucous membranes should have vertical margins and should be firmly anchored to underlying cartilage to avoid medially directed flaps.

In both techniques special attention must be paid to preserving the rostral and laterally located mucous membrane of the corniculate process, which forms the piriform recess. Inadvertent removal of excessive mucous membrane may result in insufficient tissue remaining to prevent serious problems with dysphagia and/or coughing and aspiration pneumonia, rendering the horse useless (Fig. 48–4).

Routine postoperative care includes cleansing of the laryngotomy and tracheotomy sites twice daily, administration of phenylbutazone (4 mg/kg twice daily by mouth, usually for 3 to 7 days), and procaine penicillin G (22,000 IU/kg, twice daily intramuscularly, usually for 3 to 5 days). Tracheotomy tubes are changed daily and usually removed in 3 to 5 days when endoscopic examination confirms that the horse has sufficient airway to breathe comfortably. Most horses are confined to a box stall for 1 to 2 months and given an additional 1 to 2 months of paddock or pasture turnout prior to returning to active exercise.

COMPLICATIONS

Problems encountered during surgery include difficult access and visualization, large defects in the mucous membranes, and hemorrhage. Affected arytenoid(s) are often so thickened and dense that surgical access and visualization is often difficult. Meticulous submucosal dissection and elevation may be difficult or impossible because of large granulation tissue projections, draining tracts, and extremely dense, often mineralized cartilage with tightly adherent mucous membranes. Excessive hemorrhage usually results from dissection into soft tissue structures (the vestibularis, vocalis, and lateral cricoid arytenoid muscles and the lateral ventricle) on the lateral aspect of the cartilage. Mucous membrane defects, abnormal-appearing mucous membrane, and partially avascular mucous membrane resulting from the density of the cartilage and the distance to be undermined often require extensive trimming, which makes careful apposition with fine absorbable sutures difficult to impossible.

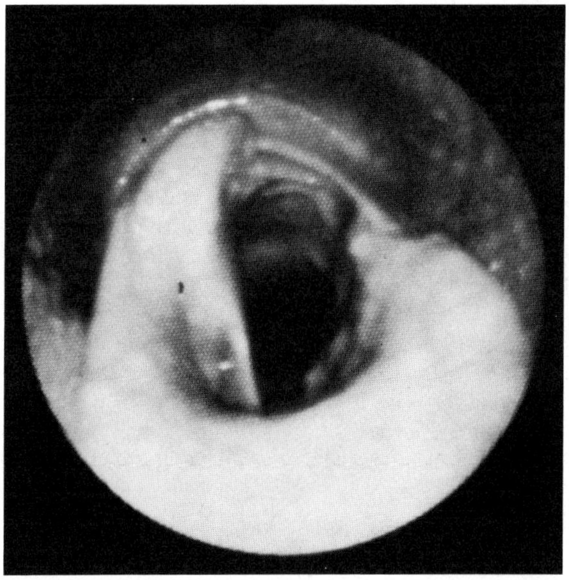

Figure 48–4. Endoscopic view of partial arytenoidectomy resulting in insufficient rostral corniculate mucous membrane remaining. This horse had excessive coughing, dysphagia, and aspiration pneumonia.

Postoperative complications include partial to complete suture line dehiscence, either traumatically during difficult recoveries from general anesthesia or structurally from sutures tearing through poor-quality mucous membrane. Dehiscence may result in medially directed mucosal flaps with defects adjacent to the flap that must heal by second intention. In some horses hemorrhage during surgery leads to postoperative submucosal hematoma formation that either resolves or undergoes fibroplasia, resulting in medial thickening where the cartilage has been removed.

Partial wound dehiscence usually occurs dorsally and is difficult to detect endoscopically during the early phases of wound healing, when swelling obscures the view; hence the surgeon may not be aware of its existence when the horse is discharged from the hospital. Partial dehiscence appears to be fairly common and may be due to movement of the opposing arytenoid, inaccurate mucosal apposition, excessive tension, or poor blood supply to the remaining mucous membrane. This area is most ventral during the surgery and hence most difficult to visualize and suture. Dorsally positioned granulation tissue buds seen endoscopically 60 to 90 days postoperatively are probably caused by this dehiscence.

Many horses that perform successfully after partial arytenoidectomy continue to make a respiratory noise. Long-term athletic failure, especially in horses undergoing maximal exercise, is usually caused by continued upper airway obstruction. There may be medial thickening in the area where the arytenoid cartilage(s) have been removed. Dorsal cicatricial formation decreasing the normal dorsal-to-ventral height of the larynx has been seen after bilateral partial arytenoidectomy, particularly using the technique without mucosal closure. Some horses will have exercise-induced dorsal displacement of the soft palate or an increased prominence or rostral displacement of the palatopharyngeal arch as a result of loss of the support provided by the corniculate process of the arytenoid cartilage.

Most laryngotomy and tracheotomy incisions heal without complications; however, approximately 5% of horses will develop extensive mineralization of the laryngeal cartilage secondary to arytenoidectomy, rendering the horse useless for performance. This complication is not unique to arytenoidectomy, but has also been documented following most types of laryngeal surgery. There is no way to predict the occurrence of this complication, so owners should be appraised of this possibility preoperatively.

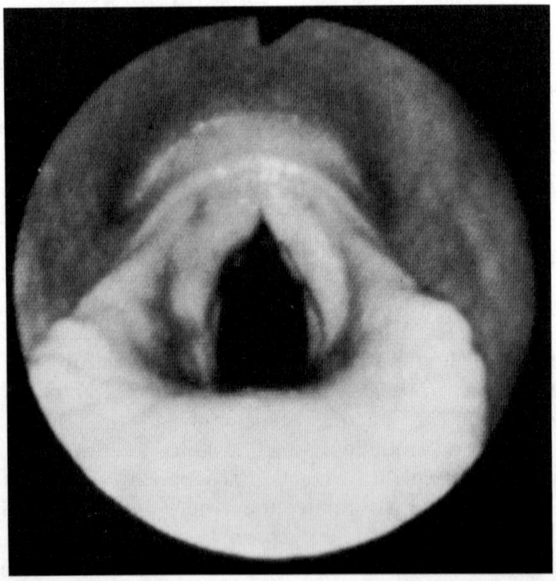

Figure 48–5. Endoscopic appearance of a bilateral partial arytenoidectomy 80 days postoperatively. This Thoroughbred racehorse was able to compete successfully but continued to make a respiratory noise.

Occasionally, horses will have bouts of coughing while eating, probably as a result of being unable to completely protect the glottis during swallowing. Rarely, a horse may have serious problems with coughing during exercise, rendering it useless or, as a result of aspiration with pneumonia, occasionally necessitating euthanasia.

PROGNOSIS

Progressive arytenoid cartilage enlargement usually renders the horse useless for maximal exercise, and may be life endangering in many horses. However, some horses make only a slight respiratory noise and have minimal exercise intolerance and apparently early minor cartilage changes, such as slight thickening, asymmetry, wrinkling, alterations in contour, erosions, ulcerations, or minor projections, in which there is fairly normal abductor muscle function; these horses may be able to train and race successfully for approximately 1 to 2 years after the diagnosis. Palliative treatment with rest, nonsteroidal anti-inflammatory drugs, antibiotics, or local sprays containing anti-inflammatory medications and antibacterial agents may be beneficial if the arytenoid cartilage is inflamed or if there are obvious draining tracts. Alternatively, or in addition, a laryngotomy might be considered to facilitate excising any projections of granulation tissue and cauterizing any defects and for performing a ventriculectomy. A ventriculectomy may improve the stability of the arytenoid cartilage, thereby reducing airway resistance.

In the rare horse with only a protruding soft tissue mass, transendoscopic excision with a Nd:YAG laser is recommended. The mass is usually granulation tissue, and excision generally allows for healing of the mucous membrane over the concave defect.

Horses with only minor cartilage changes that inadvertently undergo laryngoplasty rather than an arytenoidectomy are sometimes able to train and race successfully for up to 2 years. This is particularly true for Thoroughbreds raced at shorter distances.

Horses with respiratory noise, exercise intolerance, reduced abductor function, and obvious cartilage changes decreasing the cross-sectional area of the airway are generally unable to train and race competitively without surgery. The overall success rate in returning a horse to a competitive level of racing following partial arytenoidectomy is approximately 50% for horses with unilateral involvement and 20 to 25% for horses with bilateral involvement (Fig. 48–5). Horses with right-sided involvement appear to have a slightly better prognosis, approximately 70%, than horses in which there is left-sided involvement. Presumably this difference is because of greater right-sided residual abductor function after surgery allowing for greater airway dilatation. Horses with left-sided chondropathy or left laryngeal hemiplegia undergoing arytenoidectomy generally have a much higher prevalence of previous laryngeal surgery and may also have reduced abductor function compared to horses with right-sided involvement.

It may be possible to use horses with obvious unilateral abnormalities in which the progression appears to be slow as broodmares or breeding stallions for a period of time without having surgery. Close observation by owners and periodic endoscopic examinations are recommended to monitor changes in the airway. Horses with rapidly progressive bilateral lesions will require surgery to save their lives; however, almost all of these horses can be salvaged as comfortable breeding stock.

BIBLIOGRAPHY

Derksen FJ, Stick JA, Scott EA, et al: The effect of laryngeal hemiplegia and the laryngoplasty on airway flow mechanics in exercising horses. *Am J Vet Res* 1986;47:16–20.

Haynes PF: Subtotal arytenoidectomy in the horse: An update. *Proc Am Assoc Equine Pract* 1984; pp 21–33.

Haynes PF, Snyder TG, McClure JR, et al: Chronic chondritis of the equine arytenoid cartilage. *J Am Vet Med Assoc* 1980;177:1135–1142.

Martin GS, Beadle RE, Haynes PF, et al: Cross-sectional area of the attidus laryngis and rima glottidis before and after transection of the left recurrent laryngeal nerve in the horse. *Am J Vet Res* 1986;47:422–426.

Speirs VC: Partial arytenoidectomy in horses. *Vet Surg* 1986;15:316–320.

49
Tracheotomy and Tracheostomy

John R. Pascoe

Relief from acute, life-threatening obstructive upper airway disease requires provision of a secure patent airway. While this can sometimes be rapidly achieved by passage of a length of tubing (e.g., nasogastric tube) through a nostril into the trachea, thus bypassing the site of obstruction, the nature of the airway obstruction may preclude safe or unobstructed passage of the tube. Caution must be exercised to avoid undue stimulation of airway irritant receptors and exacerbation of the respiratory distress by further excitement. Exaggerated breathing efforts against an obstructed airway may cause pulmonary edema and cardiorespiratory arrest and result in significant patient morbidity or death.

With knowledge of the regional anatomy, a temporary midcervical tracheotomy can be performed efficiently without eliciting any additional stress. Prior experience with the technique will facilitate its completion, especially if the foal or horse is markedly distressed or displaying agonal signs. Care is needed in such situations to avoid injury to the surgeon and personnel involved in restraint. Fortunately, in most situations where tracheotomy is indicated for palliation of airway obstruction, noticeable abnormal respiratory noise often forewarns the owner to seek veterinary attention before an emergency tracheotomy is needed. Exceptions include airway obstruction secondary to acute laryngitis associated with arytenoid chondropathy, inhaled foreign bodies, tracheal compression by retropharyngeal masses, tracheal crush injuries, and acute laryngeal edema, in which situation progression of signs may occur rapidly.

Elective tracheotomy is necessary for tracheal intubation in some surgical procedures of the upper airway, so that access to the lumen of the naso- or oropharynx, larynx, or rostral trachea is not impeded by the endotracheal tube. This tracheotomy may be maintained during the early postoperative period if temporary airway obstruction from inflammation is anticipated or if hemorrhage has been controlled by gauze packing of the nasal cavity. Permanent tracheostomy is indicated when economics or the extent of the airway lesion preclude successful surgical correction. Permanent tracheostomas are also used in chronic, experimental studies of lung function when it is desirable to bypass the upper airway.

DIAGNOSIS

Recognition of upper airway obstruction that warrants tracheotomy is based on clinical signs, palpation of the cervical trachea, endoscopy, and radiography. Clinical signs include abnormal respiratory noise at rest, reduced airflow at the nostrils, palpable fremitus over the larynx or trachea, distortion of the normal outline of the throatlatch or peritracheal tissues, and exaggerated or inappropriate respiratory effort. Endoscopy and radiography provide useful adjunctive information and will usually guide decisions as to the need for interim relief via tracheotomy or palliation with medical treatment until surgical correction is possible.

In true emergency situations, endoscopy and radiography are initially impractical and the course of action must be guided by clinical signs and the degree of distress the horse or foal is showing. Initially, respiratory noise will become progressively more audible and be accompanied by exaggerated flaring of the nares and vigorous respiratory movements of both the thorax and abdomen. With progression of the signs, the horse will become agitated, distressed, and finally frantic. The concurrent appearance of foam, blood-tinged foam, or blood at the nostrils is strongly suggestive of the development of marked pulmonary edema. Recumbency, agonal struggling, and death can occur rapidly after the onset of pulmonary edema if the airway obstruction is not relieved. Considerable care is needed in such situations to avoid personal injury. Sedation or anesthesia is generally impractical because of the lack of a secure patent airway and the risk of drug-related cardiorespiratory depression and death.

TRACHEOTOMY

Surgical Technique

Although temporary tracheotomy can be performed anywhere along the length of the cervical trachea, easiest access is usually at the junction of the proximal and middle thirds of the neck. However, it is important that the tracheostomy be distal to the airway obstruction. The tracheal rings can usually be palpated beneath the skin and strap muscles. An 8 × 15–cm area is shaved and aseptically prepared before line infiltration of the skin and underlying cutaneous muscle with local anesthetic.

With the horse's head stabilized and the skin tensed proximally, a 6 to 8-cm longitudinal incision is made through the skin and cutaneous muscle (cutaneous colli muscle) to expose the paired bellies of the sternothyrohyoid muscles. Hemorrhage is usually limited to vessels within the skin edges. The thin raphe joining the left and right sternothyrohyoid muscles is separated longitudinally with a scalpel or scissors to expose the trachea. The tracheotomy is performed by transverse incision of the annular ligament between two centrally located cartilaginous rings. This incision is best accomplished by stabilizing the trachea and carefully stabbing the blade through the annular ligament and tracheal mucosa. The incision is then extended for about 1 cm to the left and right of midline and should be slightly wider than the tracheotomy tube for ease of placement. It is preferable not to incise more than one third of the circumference to maintain tracheal stability and to minimize complications associated with local tracheal collapse and stricture formation.

Special Concerns

If the horse is sedated, it is often helpful to have an assistant elevate the horse's nose by supporting the rostral portion of the mandible. This tenses the skin and strap muscles and facilitates the skin incision and muscle separation. In a stocks, the same effect can also be achieved by use of a rope from a ring on the nose band of the halter over the top beam of the stocks.

Self-retaining tracheotomy tubes (Dyson, Papes) should be positioned so that the front plates are external to the muscles and skin rather than lying against the trachea. This reduces the extent of the postoperative cleaning, minimizes subcutaneous emphysema, and can be readily achieved by avoiding unnecessary separation of the strap muscles. It is also helpful to have greatest exposure in the skin and subcutaneous tissue to minimize pocketing of serum draining from the incision.

Care must be taken during tube insertion to ensure that the tube is actually placed in the tracheal lumen and not tunneled peritracheally beneath the sternothyrohyoid muscles. Incorrect tube placement occurs more easily with those tubes having two interlocking parts (e.g., Dyson and Papes tracheotomy tubes).

Adequate restraint is especially important in foals and American Miniature horses. The smaller tracheal size requires considerable care to prevent perforation of the dorsal surface of the trachea when making the stab incision and also to avoid unnecessary transection of the annular ligament. In noncritical cases, sedation with xylazine or diazepam and passage of a nasogastric tube into the trachea beyond the obstruction to secure a patent airway should be considered before attempting tracheotomy. Besides providing an airway, this improves identification and stabilization of the trachea and reduces the likelihood of inadvertent perforation of the dorsal tracheal surface or esophagus.

Postoperative Care

Initially the tracheotomy tube may need replacement more than twice daily depending on the accumulation of respiratory mucus and the configuration of the tube. After removal of the tube, the tracheotomy site should be cleaned with saline or diluted povidone-iodine moistened sponges. The surrounding skin, especially that ventral to the stoma, is protected with petroleum jelly. Because the inspissated mucus is normally tightly adherent to the tube lumen and requires soaking for removal, a new tube is replaced in the stoma at each cleaning. Once the tube is no longer needed, the tracheotomy site is cleaned twice daily until healed. Depending on the size of the stoma and the length of time the tube was maintained, healing occurs in 10 to 21 days.

Complications

Hemorrhage, granuloma formation, chondritis and stenosis can occur. It is uncommon to encounter significant hemorrhage, and any skin or muscular bleeders can be adequately controlled by clamping. Occasionally excessive bleeding may be encountered in the tracheal submucosa. Blood streaking of the trachea is often seen during endoscopy immediately after tracheotomy and is usually of no consequence.

Granulomas will occasionally form at the margins of the healing mucosa and can cause luminal obstruction. Removal can be accomplished with a wire snare passed through the biopsy channel of an endoscope. If the granuloma recurs or if the base is not pedunculated, it may be necessary to remove the granuloma under general anesthesia by recreating the tracheotomy, excising the granuloma, and, if possible, suturing the tracheal mucosa. Further closure of the surgical site will depend on whether the original tracheotomy had healed. If healing was incomplete, it is probably preferable to leave the muscle and skin to heal by granulation or at least only partially close the wound after débridement to allow for drainage.

Chondritis, chondroma formation, and tracheal ring deformities are more difficult management problems and may require tracheal ring resection and anastomosis. These complications are often associated with inadvertent incision of a cartilage ring during tracheotomy, prolonged maintenance of a tracheotomy tube, and either use of a tube that is larger than the stoma or incision of greater than two thirds of the tracheal circumference to accommodate a larger tube. Both the latter situations often result in inversion of the tracheal rings on either side of the tube and subsequent ring deformities or stenosis of the trachea. Excessive circumferential incision of the annular ligament can also result in stenosis by mucosal cicatrix during healing.

These complications can be minimized by removal of a semicircular portion of cartilage from the tracheal rings on each side of the stoma, to fashion a stoma that will accommodate the tube without causing ring inversion, deformity, or excessive retraction of the rings. This technique is also advocated if a tube is to be maintained for an extended period. However, chondroma formation may be a sequel to excision of the tracheal cartilage. Axial (longitudinal) division of the tracheal rings is not advocated. Although this may be the only choice in life or death situations, inversion or overlapping of the tracheal rings during healing often leads to tracheal stenosis.

Inadvertent perforation of the dorsal tracheal surface can occur with an overzealous stab incision through the annular ligament, especially in foals and miniature horses. Granuloma or chondroma formation may occur. With complete penetration of the dorsal tracheal surface there is also risk of esophageal perforation and subsequent suppurative cellulitis of the periesophageal and peritracheal tissues. Laceration or perforation of the esophagus can also occur if the incision in the annular ligament is extended too far lateral and caudal. It can be difficult to visualize such esophageal perforations endoscopically, but this complication should certainly be considered if inappropriate inflammation and soft tissue swelling develop in the region of the tracheotomy.

TRACHEOSTOMY

Surgical Technique

With the aid of general anesthesia, the horse is positioned in dorsal recumbency with the head and neck slightly extended to tense the skin and trachea. If the obstructive lesion is rostral to the cricotracheal junction, the tracheostoma is made in the rostral third of the trachea; otherwise it is sited distal to the obstruction. After adequate skin preparation, a 10-cm longitudinal median incision is made through the skin and cutaneous colli muscle. The paired bellies of the sternothyrohyoid muscles are separated by incision of the median raphe and are then retracted laterally to expose the trachea.

Three or four centrally located tracheal rings are selected. After removal of loose connective tissue, the selected rings are incised through the full thickness of the cartilage with a sharp scalpel, taking care not to incise the underlying submucosa and mucosa. Paramedian incisions are then made through the same tracheal rings lateral to the initial incision. Spacing of the paramedian incisions will depend on the diameter of the trachea, since removal of greater than one third of the tracheal circumference may predispose to tracheal collapse. In adult horses these paramedian incisions are made about 1 cm lateral to the median incision without penetrating the submucosa. The cartilaginous rectangles formed on each side of midline are then dissected from the underlying submucosa. This dissection can be tedious because of blood oozing from the exposed submucosal tissues.

Before incising the tracheal mucosa, longitudinal portions of the adjacent sternothyrohyoid muscles are removed to facilitate mucoepidermal closure. Removal of this muscular tissue is also important to prevent aspiration of the muscular edges into the stoma during forced inspiration. A double *Y* pattern is used to incise the mucosa and stay sutures are used to minimize mucosal retraction during closure. The triangular flaps created at each end of the incision are reflected and sutured with nonabsorbable suture to the corresponding edges of the skin incision. The lateral flaps are reflected similarly and sutured to the adjacent skin edges.

Postoperative Care

Perioperative antibiotics and tetanus prophylaxis are given. Nonsteroidal antiinflammatory drugs may be indicated to limit incisional swelling. Petrolatum jelly is applied to the skin ventral to the tracheostoma to prevent scalding from respiratory secretions and incisional drainage. The tracheostoma should be gently cleansed each day with saline-moistened sponges. Sutures can be removed in 10 to 14 days. An adequate opening can be maintained by making a flexible tracheostomy tube from silicone, which can be easily inserted and removed. This may be used long term, but must be cleaned daily.

Long-term care consists of daily cleaning of respiratory mucus from the edges of the stoma. Although this is desirable from an aesthetic viewpoint, functional obstruction from accumulated mucus is unlikely, and horses maintained at pasture experience little problem if the stoma is not cleaned regularly.

Complications

Incisional dehiscence can occur if the mucoepidermal closure is under excessive tension. This can be avoided if an adequate amount of the edges of the adjacent sternothyrohyoid muscles are removed. If partial dehiscence occurs, additional muscle should be removed and the wound resutured or the wound should be allowed to granulate.

Airway obstruction may occur from tracheal collapse at the stoma or obstruction from the edges of the sternothyrohyoid muscles. Tracheal collapse usually occurs because too many ring segments have been removed, the stoma has been eccentrically placed, or the ring segments removed were too wide relative to the diameter of the trachea. Sternothyrohyoid muscle obstruction of the stoma may occur during forced inspiration if insufficient muscle edge was removed during creation of the stoma. Stomal obstruction has also occurred from regrowth and apposition of the surrounding skin.

Breathing through a tracheostoma bypasses the defense mechanisms of the upper airway and potentially exposes the horse to increased risk of respiratory infection. Recent experience with a group of research ponies that had chronic tracheostomas suggested, however, that this occurs uncommonly. Visual inspection of the mucosal surface opposite the stoma reveals that this exposed mucosal area is often relatively dry, erythematous, and covered with inhaled material when compared with the remainder of the trachea.

BIBLIOGRAPHY

Haynes PF: Surgery of the equine respiratory tract, in Jennings PB (ed): *The Practice of Large Animal Surgery.* Philadelphia, WB Saunders Co, 1984, pp 388–487.

Shappel KK, Stick JA, Derksen FJ, Scott EA: Permanent tracheostomy in Equidae: 47 cases (1981–1986). *J Am Vet Med Assoc* 1988;192:939–942.

Turner AS, McIlwraith CW: *Techniques in Large Animal Surgery*, ed 2. Philadelphia, Lea & Febiger, 1988, pp 219–221.

50
Laser Surgery of the Upper Respiratory Tract

K. C. Kent Lloyd

Innovations in laser technology have recently been introduced as an alternative strategy in surgery of the equine upper respiratory tract. In some instances, the laser has sparked new ideas for solving old difficulties related to tissue inaccessibility and hemorrhage, problems inherent in conventional methods of nose and throat surgery. Understanding the principles, indications, and potential complications of laser use in surgery is essential to a rational application of this new technique to common problems of the upper airway in horses.

PRINCIPLES OF LASER USE

The details of laser physics are described elsewhere (see Chapter 7). Two types of lasers are currently used in surgery of the equine upper respiratory tract: the Carbon Dioxide (CO_2) laser and the Neodymium—yttrium-aluminum-garnet (Nd:YAG) laser. Differences in their physical characteristics make predictions about the biophysical interactions between laser energy and living tissue possible. The shallow depth of penetration of the CO_2 laser enables precise cutting and vaporization. However, since the CO_2 laser is absorbed primarily by intracellular water, the control of hemorrhage is minimal. In contrast, the deeper tissue penetration and coagulation effect of the Nd:YAG laser results in less hemorrhage, but also more diffuse thermal damage.

Because laryngeal and pharyngeal structures have irregular shapes and thicknesses, and contain varying amounts of pigment and water (e.g., cartilage and mucosa), they possess nonuniform absorption characteristics. Care must be exercised during lasing to control the depth of penetration of thermal energy by altering the power output (watts), lasing time (continuous or intermittent mode), or distance from the target tissue. Low power output, short duration, and long distance produce a low thermal effect over a large tissue area, depending on the type of laser used. High power output, long duration, and short distance produce the most energetic effects. Practical experience is essential to become comfortable with determining the appropriate power settings, time, and distance factors.

Minimal laryngeal and pharyngeal edema, less pain, improved outcome, and reduced healing time have also been attributed to laser ablation therapy when compared to other methods. Therefore, selection of the appropriate surgical laser depends on the properties of the beam, the absorptive characteristics of the target tissue, and the desired effect.

ADVANTAGES AND DISADVANTAGES OF THE SURGICAL LASER

Of the surgical lasers currently in use, the Nd:YAG laser has a special advantage in that it can be used through the biopsy channel of a flexible fiberoptic endoscope. Directing the laser beam endoscopically allows certain procedures to be performed in the standing horse that would otherwise require general anesthesia. In addition, the cost and risk of general anesthesia and recovery may be avoided by an endoscopic approach. The combination of xylazine (0.5 to 1.0 mg/kg IV) and butorphanol tartrate (0.01 to 0.2 mg/kg IV) provides adequate sedation and minimizes anxiety during endoscopic lasing. Butacaine sulfate (2%, 50 to 100 mL) sprayed liberally onto the target tissue through the biopsy channel of the endoscope produces adequate topical anesthesia for 1 to 2 hours. After lasing, eschar and coagulated tissue can be gently débrided through the nose using long-handled instruments.

The major disadvantages of lasers are related to their expense and potential for unwittingly injuring the patient. Depending on the number and kinds of accessories purchased, the cost of a Nd:YAG laser begins at approximately $65,000 to $90,000. Although a CO_2 laser is generally cheaper, it lacks the benefit and convenience of use through a flexible endoscope.

Adherence to special precautions when using a surgical laser will help avoid inadvertent injury to the patient or the operator. For general anesthesia, the endotracheal tube should be made of a nontransparent rubber material or wrapped with metal tape to prevent the ignition of anesthetic gases. Dull-surfaced instruments lessen the chance for thermal damage from reflection of the primary beam. A strong suction system should be used to scavenge smoke and aerosolized particulate debris produced during high-power lasing. During laser endoscopy, evacuation of the smoke plume can be efficiently performed through a narrow-diameter flexible catheter secured to the outer surface of the endoscope or through a nasopharyngeal catheter advanced up the opposite nasal cavity. Aiming the laser is more precise, with less risk of thermal damage to nontargeted tissue, when visualization is not hampered by the smoke plume.

APPLICATIONS

Lasers are indicated as a supplement to conventional surgical methods if their use would (*a*) promote hemostasis, (*b*) improve visualization of and accessibility, to target tissue, (*c*) shorten operating time, and (*d*) enhance the overall effect and outcome of the surgical procedure. During an arytenoidectomy, the mucosa can be elevated from the underlying cartilage of the corniculate and articular processes of the arytenoid cartilage using the CO_2 laser. More cartilage can be excised with less risk of perforating the overlying mucosa this way when compared to other techniques. Alternatively, the Nd:YAG laser may be used through a laryngotomy during general anesthesia or transnasally via endoscope in the sedated horse to ablate the nonfuctional cartilage. Early clinical trials have indicated adequate second-intention healing and reepithelialization after laser ablation. Exuberant granulation tissue causing partial upper airway obstruction or laryngeal disfigurement may require additional lasings. Photoablation via endoscopy has reportedly been performed considerably faster than the time required for a conventional arytenoidectomy. Further, a temporary tracheostomy may not be necessary after laser surgery because minimal laryngeal edema occurs.

The Nd:YAG laser may be advantageous for controlling hemorrhage, thus eliminating the need for blood transfusions during ethmoid hematoma removal via frontal sinusotomy. If accessible endoscopically, the base or stalk of the ethmoid hematoma may be lased, preferentially by first coagulating to a depth of 5 to 7 mm and then ablating the thermally treated tissue. In this way, removal of the ethmoid hematoma is faster and hemorrhage is comparatively less than if high-power lasing was used in a single step to ablate the entire tissue. The base of the ethmoid hematoma on the floor of the ethmoturbinate may be difficult to visualize and treat without first laser ablating the ventral lip of the entrance to the turbinate. Additional lasings through the endoscope are necessary several days or weeks after the necrotic tissue and eschar are gone and the remaining ethmoid hematoma becomes visible.

Redundant aryepiglottic tissue, dorsally displaced soft palate, and nasal polyps may all be more amenable to endoscopic laser therapy since they are difficult to clearly visualize and access through a laryngotomy or pharyngotomy. The sapphire point attachment of the Nd:YAG laser allows direct contact of the laser with the target tissue and enables deep and diffuse thermal treatment. An entrapped epiglottis can be effectively released by thorough ablation of the excess rostral tissue, which can sometimes result in reentrapment if it is not completely removed. The risk of damaging the soft palate is also reduced using the laser. Thermal injury to the underlying epiglottis may occur if the free beam of the Nd:YAG laser is used instead of the contact tip. Direct tissue contact may also facilitate shortening of the soft palate either endoscopically or through a pharyngotomy, if indicated. A nasal polyp can be excised quickly, easily, and almost hemorrhage free using a transnasal Nd:YAG laser via the endoscope.

A subepiglottic or laryngeal cyst clearly evident endoscopically may be ablated using the Nd:YAG laser. Occasionally, these structures can be visualized better through a pharyngotomy or laryngotomy, and endoscopically directed lasing may not have any advantage over electrocauterization. Similarly, laser treatment of chronic pharyngeal lymphoid hyperplasia may provide more effective results than that from freezing or electrocautery. Reconstruction or enlargement of the nasomaxillary opening, widening of a partially obstructed nasal meatus, turbinate excision, transnasal sinusotomy, and removal of the nasal septum may be amenable to laser therapy principally because of hemorrhage control and accessibility.

COMPLICATIONS

The benefits of laser technology in upper airway surgery in the horse are accompanied by several potential complications. Ignition of anesthetic gases with the laser beam through an unprotected endotracheal tube can cause an explosion and fire in the airway. Therapy directed at shock and pulmonary edema, airway lavage, and oxygenation should be instituted immediately. If adequate scavenging is unavailable, aerosolized particulate debris generated during prolonged high-power lasing may cause problems related to smoke inhalation, including airway irritation and burns, pneumonia, pulmonary edema, and allergic lung disease.

Although pain and edema are reportedly less after laser therapy than for other surgical methods, difficulty in breathing may result from laryngeal irritation. Flunixin meglumine (1.1 mg/kg intravenously) administered preoperatively will provide relief. The horse should be observed during the first 24 hours and an emergency tracheostomy set should be available if needed. Feeding coarse hay is not advisable for several days after lasing.

Estimating the distance between the laser tip and target tissue endoscopically is especially difficult because of a lack of depth perception and the necessity for wearing safety goggles. The quartz fiber can be burned if flecks of blood or debris accumulate on the fiber tip by accidentally touching the tissue or neglecting to clean the fiber during use.

Although the laser is a powerful and potentially dangerous instrument, practical knowledge and training in the basics of laser use can lead to a clear and reasonable approach to laser safety protocol. Several guidelines for laser use provided by the federal government and safety features incorporated into the laser by manufacturers have already been described (see Chapter 7). However, avoiding complications of laser use in upper airway surgery is the sole responsibility of the surgeon.

FUTURE APPLICATIONS OF THE LASER IN UPPER AIRWAY SURGERY

The number of technologic advances in surgical laser therapy are increasing rapidly in human medicine. With carefully controlled and critically evaluated clinical trials in horses, the application of the laser to many conditions of the upper respiratory tract will become evident. In the next few years, long-term results from prospective studies currently underway will provide suggestions for improving established laser procedures and new indications for using a specific laser for a particular problem. Because precision, hemostasis, and accessibility are enhanced by the laser, it may eventually become the preferred mode of therapy for cysts and neoplasms of the nasal sinuses and oral cavity, guttural pouch empyema and mycosis, and tracheal stenosis. Lasers may become useful in surgery of the lung and pulmonary vasculature with advances in thoracotomy techniques in the horse.

BIBLIOGRAPHY

Carrell BL: Laser treatment of laryngeal polyps. *J Assoc Operat Room Nurses*. 1983;38:232–236.

Dixon JA: Surgical applications of lasers. *J Assoc Operat Room Nurses* 1983;38:223–230.

Lipow M: Laser physics made simple. *Curr Probl Obstet Gynecol Fertil* 1986;9:445–493.

Tate LP, Newman HC, Cullen JN, Sweeney C: Neodymium (Nd):YAG laser surgery in the equine larynx: A pilot study. *Lasers Surg Med* 1986;6:473–476.

51 Diaphragmatic Hernia

Clifford M. Honnas

Diaphragmatic hernias are an infrequent cause of abdominal crisis in the horse. Respiratory compromise may accompany abdominal pain as a result of herniation of abdominal viscera into the thoracic cavity. The size and location of the diaphragmatic defect determines which abdominal organs herniate into the thorax. With small hernial rings, segments of small intestine generally herniate, whereas with larger defects the large intestine may be involved. Abdominal organs observed in the thorax at surgery and necropsy have included small intestine, cecum, large and small colon, stomach, liver, omentum, and spleen. Partial or complete intestinal obstruction may occur, necessitating surgical intervention.

In horses, the diaphragm consists of a peripheral muscle (pars costalis), which is pliable and provides for attachment to the ribs, and a central, rigid, tendinous portion (centrum tendineum). The tendinous portion is perforated by three foramina, from dorsal to ventral: the aortic hiatus, the esophageal hiatus, and the foramen for the caudal vena cava. Most diaphragmatic hernias occur in the centrum tendineum at the junction of the tendinous and muscular portions of the diaphragm (Fig. 51–1). This is a logical point of weakness between the pliable muscle and the rigid tendinous portion of the diaphragm.

ETIOLOGY

Defects in the diaphragm may be either congenital or acquired. Congenital defects usually result from incomplete fusion of the pleuroperitoneal folds, causing an enlarged esophageal hiatus, whereas acquired defects are thought to result from sudden increases in intrathoracic or intraabdominal pressure. Rupture of the diaphragm may be associated with external trauma, such as blows to the abdomen or thoracic injuries resulting in rib fractures. Internal factors such as gastrointestinal distention and pregnancy have also been implicated. The occurrence of diaphragmatic hernias in pregnant and postparturient mares suggests that the gravid uterus may increase the risk of hernia formation in these animals. Strenuous exercise has also been reported to precede diaphragmatic hernia. In some horses there is no history of injury and no other apparent predisposing cause can be identified. Postmortem rupture of the diaphragm occasionally occurs on the midline, dorsal to the xiphoid cartilage, and is of no clinical significance. Hemorrhage, inflammation, or fibrosis along the edges of the hernial ring suggests that the hernia is antemortem and acquired. Diaphragmatic hernias with smooth edges and an absence of hemorrhage and fibrosis are believed to be of congenital origin.

CLINICAL FINDINGS

Diaphragmatic hernia may occur in any age, breed, or sex of horse but has been observed most frequently in adults. Once a diaphragmatic defect exists, it is possible for abdominal organs to pass through the hole and become incarcerated. Such hernias result in clinical signs if the function of the herniated abdominal viscera or thoracic organs is compromised. Clinical signs of diaphragmatic hernia in the horse are variable because of the variety of organs that can be incarcerated and are also influenced by the size of the diaphragmatic defect. Presumably the potential for herniation increases with larger defects, whereas the risk of visceral strangulation probably decreases.

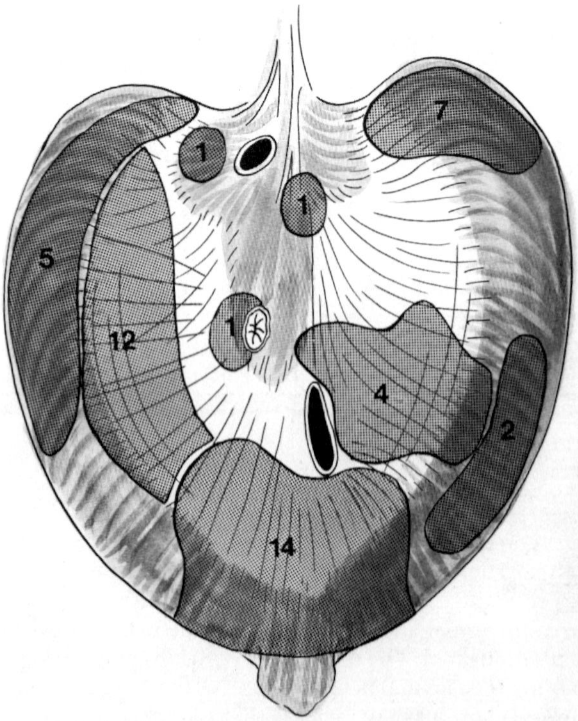

Figure 51–1. Abdominal view of the diaphragm showing the location of diaphragmatic hernias in 47 horses. These cases were compiled from a review of the literature (25 horses) and from horses admitted to the Veterinary Medical Teaching Hospital, University of California, Davis (22 horses). Numbers indicate number of cases of herniation in each location.

The predominant sign associated with diaphragmatic hernia is generally abdominal distress, which may vary from mild, recurrent episodes of colic to severe, unrelenting pain necessitating surgical exploration. Abdominal pain occurs as a consequence of interference with intestinal blood flow, intestinal obstruction, or mesenteric strain. After passage of the intestine into the thoracic cavity, incarceration may occur as a result of ingesta or gas accumulation in the herniated intestinal segment, adhesion formation within the thoracic cavity, or stricture of the hernial ring around the intestine. Although rapid, shallow breathing is often observed with other more common causes of abdominal distress, these alterations in respiration may occur with diaphragmatic hernia as a result of a decrease in lung volume after intestinal displacement into the thorax. Herniation of the large intestine into the thorax has been reported to result more often in respiratory distress than in abdominal pain, because the large size of the colon limits full lung excursion. Occasionally, signs of respiratory compromise occur without evidence of abdominal pain when there is a nonstrangulating diaphragmatic hernia. Generally, however, the majority of horses exhibit both respiratory and abdominal signs. Two foals were found to have only respiratory signs associated with large diaphragmatic defects that allowed large portions of the gastrointestinal tract to occupy the thoracic cavity. Some cases of diaphragmatic hernia are chronic, with acute abdominal signs occurring intermittently and for some time after the initial diaphragmatic tear and visceral herniation.

DIAGNOSIS

A definitive antemortem diagnosis of diaphragmatic hernia can be difficult to make and, in some cases, may be confirmed only during exploratory celiotomy. None of the diagnostic methods routinely used to evaluate abdominal crisis in the horse will consistently help to identify a diaphragmatic hernia. Diaphragmatic hernia should certainly be considered in the differential diagnosis in all horses presented for colic, and especially in those having suffered from trauma and in periparturient mares exhibiting abdominal distress. Abdominal palpation per rectum may reveal an empty caudal abdomen if a large portion of intestine occupies the thorax. Often abnormal rectal findings are not noted. Abnormal rectal findings in other cases of diaphragmatic hernia have included dilated small intestine, taut mesenteric bands, and displaced large intestine. Peritoneal fluid obtained by abdominal paracentesis generally has normal characteristics because the devitalized intestine lies within the thorax. In these horses, thoracentesis may yield fluid of diagnostic value.

While auscultation of the thorax may reveal borborygmi in the caudoventral thorax, referred gastrointestinal sounds are frequently heard over the thorax in normal horses, and thus should be regarded only as suggestive of diaphragmatic hernia. Increased regions of thoracic dullness or reduced cardiac sounds on the involved side of the thorax may increase suspicion of a diaphragmatic hernia.

Thoracic radiography and ultrasonography are used to definitively diagnose diaphragmatic hernia. Radiographic signs include gas-filled loops of intestine in the thoracic cavity, increased ventral thoracic density as a result of the presence of abdominal viscera or pleural fluid, absence of the cardiac shadow, and discontinuity of the ventral diaphragmatic shadow. Contrast radiography may confirm the diagnosis provided the hernia is nonstrangulating and there is progressive gastrointestinal motility.

SURGERY

Careful presurgical consideration should be given to acid-base status, electrolyte balance, and ventilatory capability when a definitive presurgical diagnosis of diaphragmatic hernia has been made. Severe hypercapnia and hypoxemia may occur as a result of decreased ventilatory capacity due to ventilation-perfusion mismatch in a lung compressed by abdominal viscera. The horse may survive by making maximal conscious efforts to inspire, with those efforts being diminished or abolished by anesthesia. Successful surgical correction of diaphragmatic hernia requires positive pressure ventilation to ensure adequate ventilation to overcome both visceral compression and loss of negative thoracic pressure when the abdomen is opened. The caudal mediastinum is usually fenestrated in the horse, thus bilateral pneumothorax can develop once the abdomen is opened or the hernia is reduced. This necessitates the need for positive pressure ventilation to prevent atelectasis and further pulmonary collapse.

The surgical approach to a diaphragmatic hernia is via ventral median celiotomy. If diagnosed preoperatively, the incision begins immediately caudal to the xiphoid cartilage and extends caudally. Otherwise, if diagnosed during exploratory celiotomy, the incision is extended cranially to the xiphoid cartilage. Surgical correction involves reduction of herniated viscera, resection and anastomosis of devitalized intestine, and repair of the diaphragmatic defect. Successful surgical repair of diaphragmatic hernia has been reported in two 3-month-old foals and two adult horses. The chief complaint in both foals was difficult breathing and neither foal exhibited abdominal pain. Both adults exhibited abdominal pain as the primary presenting sign. The defects were closed with sutures in both foals and one adult, and synthetic mesh was used to cover the defect in the other adult. Both foals grew normally, and showed no evidence of abdominal or respiratory distress 5 and 18 months after surgery.

Surgical success is often determined by the size of the diaphragmatic defect as well as its accessibility via ventral median celiotomy. Complicating factors include the friability of the diaphragmatic tissue, the surgeon's ability to reduce the incarcerated viscera, and the viability of the herniated organ. Just prior to final suture tightening and knot placement, the lungs should be inflated maximally to evacuate free air from the thoracic cavity.

POSTOPERATIVE CARE

Immediate postsurgical care requires close monitoring, especially for pneumothorax. Thoracic auscultation and radiography are useful to monitor the degree of pneumothorax. Residual free thoracic air can be evacuated via percutaneous centesis or by placement of a chest tube. If normal, unlabored respiratory rates resume following surgery, it may not be necessary to evacuate residual intrapleural air because this will be gradually absorbed and the lungs fully inflated within 2 weeks. Other postsurgical considerations include antibiotic therapy, especially if there has been resection and anastomosis of devitalized intestine. Exercise should be restricted for 60 to 90 days until the abdominal incision has healed. Following this, graded exercise can resume until the horse is performing as required.

PROGNOSIS

In most adult horses, the prognosis for surgical repair of diaphragmatic hernias has been poor, because of the mechanical difficulties associated with inadequate exposure, inability to adequately retract the abdominal viscera, and the friability of the injured diaphragmatic tissue. The size of the diaphragmatic defect may also preclude surgical repair. Alternate access to diaphragmatic hernias may be possible via lateral thoracotomy, if the correct side of the hernia can be determined. Conversely, surgical repair of diaphragmatic hernias in foals is somewhat easier because of improved surgical exposure associated with smaller body size. Overall, the prognosis for survival of horses with diaphragmatic hernia is poor, usually because of delay in diagnosis and the relative surgical inaccessibility of the defect.

BIBLIOGRAPHY

Firth EC: Diaphragmatic hernia in horses. *Cornell Vet* 1976;66:353–361.

Haynes PF: Surgery of the equine respiratory tract, in Jennings PB (ed). *The Practice of Large Animal Surgery*. Philadelphia, WB Saunders Co, 1984, pp 480–481.

Levine SB, Myhre GD: Surgical repair of a traumatic diaphragmatic hernia in a horse. *Equine Pract* 1983;5:31–34.

Orsini JA, Koch C, Stewart B: Peritoneopericardial hernia in a horse. *J Am Vet Med Assoc* 1981;179:907–910.

Pearson N, Pinsent PJN, Polley LR, Waterman A: Rupture of the diaphragm in the horse. *Equine Vet J* 1977;9:32–36.

Scott EA, Fishback WA: Surgical repair of diaphragmatic hernia in a horse. *J Am Vet Med Assoc* 1976;168:45–47.

Speirs VC, Reynolds WT: Succeesful repair of a diaphragmatic hernia in a foal. *Equine Vet J* 1976;8:170–172.

Wimberly HC, Andrews EJ, Haschek WN: Diaphragmatic hernias in the horse: A review of the literature and an analysis of six additional cases. *J Am Vet Med Assoc* 1977;170:1404–1407.

52
Postoperative Pleuropneumonia

John R. Pascoe

Parapneumonic pleural effusion occurs as a postoperative complication in 0.4% of the major surgical procedures performed in our practice. Postoperative pleuropneumonia is associated with significant morbidity, including prolonged hospitalization and increased client cost, and mortality. Survivors often have limited exercise endurance, and since most affected horses are young racehorses, exercise intolerance is an important sequela to consider when discussing therapy and prognosis.

RISK FACTORS

In humans, pneumonia is the third most common complication of general surgery after wound infection and urinary tract infection. Postoperative pneumonia accounts for 50% of hospital-acquired pneumonias and is associated with higher mortality than infection at any other site. Recognized risk factors include low serum albumin concentrations, high preanesthetic physical status classification, duration of preoperative hospitalization, length of operative procedure, thoracic and upper abdominal procedures, smoking history, and preexisting pulmonary disease.

Similar risk factors have not yet been identified in equine cases. Most horses (>90%) are apparently healthy young (<5 years) racehorses, primarily Thoroughbreds, Standardbreds, and Quarter Horses. Preoperative hospitalization is usually less than 2 days, mean preanesthetic physical status classification is 1 (a patient having no systemic disease who is undergoing a surgical procedure), and mean anesthetic time less than 2.25 hours. Although one study reported that 5 of 7 postoperative pleuropneumonias were associated with upper respiratory tract surgery, our cases have included a variety of elective operative procedures, with over 80% being elective orthopedic procedures and less than 2% occurring after respiratory tract procedures. Although aspiration pneumonia has occurred as a complication in some emergency abdominal procedures, pleuropneumonia has not been recognized in this group.

In most horses, abnormalities of the respiratory system are not detected during the preoperative physical examination, nor are abnormalities detected in the preoperative complete blood count, including serum fibrinogen concentration. Although thoracic radiographs were not routinely taken, our prospective study of surgical patients considered to be at risk for developing postoperative respiratory complications (young racehorses scheduled for elective surgery) failed to reveal any distinguishing preoperative radiographic features. Most horses developed bilateral pleural effusions and in those cases in which the effusion was unilateral there was no apparent correlation between the recumbent side and the involved lung.

The incidence of postoperative pneumonia without pleural effusion in horses is unknown. In our experience young racehorses scheduled for elective surgery appear to be the group at greatest risk for developing postoperative pleuropneumonia. If the frequency of postoperative pleuropneumonia is considered in terms of this group only, then the risk increases from 0.4% to 1%. Probable contributing factors include a relatively high incidence of subclinical respiratory disease in racehorses and stresses associated with racing, injury, and transport to a surgical facility. This situation is then compounded by the effect of anesthesia on respiratory defense mechanisms. General anesthesia, particularly inhalant anesthesia and tracheal intubation, are known to result in depression of the cough reflex, decreased mucociliary clearance, and suppression of alveolar macrophage activity for up to 96 hours after anesthetic recovery. Damaged cilia of respiratory epithelial cells can take 2 to 7 days to repair after injury.

Minimizing the Risk

Because of the potentially devastating consequences of postoperative pleuropneumonia, thorough preoperative evaluation is important. This includes obtaining an accurate history of the vaccination status for viral respiratory disease, and of recent respiratory infection in the patient, in the stable, or at the racetrack. Knowledge of whether the horse has had prior episodes of pneumonia, is a "bleeder" (exercise-induced pulmonary hemorrhage), or has functional upper respiratory disorders (particularly laryngeal dysfunction) should be elicited. Impaired upper airway function, particularly impaired laryngeal function, may predispose to aspiration during recovery from anesthesia. Careful auscultation of the thorax with and without a rebreathing bag is indicated to improve detection of abnormal respiratory sounds. If abnormal sounds are detected or if there is reason to believe the horse may have "subclinical" respiratory disease, preoperative thoracic radiographs are warranted. Identification of abnormal radiographic findings is, I believe, justification for performing a preoperative transtracheal aspirate for cytology, Gram stain, and culture.

Abnormalities in the preoperative complete blood count require additional investigation. Slight increases in serum fibrinogen (>400 mg/dl) especially if combined with abnormal lung sounds and/or equivocal thoracic radiographic changes, also warrant transtracheal aspiration and endoscopy. Abnormal cytology or positive culture mandate further workup and postponement of elective surgery if the risk of postoperative respiratory complications is to be minimized. All preoperative physical findings should be evaluated in the context that the horse may be receiving nonsteroidal anti-inflammatory therapy, especially if this information is not available, because these drugs may mask subtle elevations in body temperature and obtund changes in other physical signs that might alert the surgeon to existing or impending respiratory disease.

After surgery, careful postoperative monitoring and awareness of subtle changes in the patient's status, especially if postoperative antibiotics and nonsteroidal anti-inflammatory drugs are being administered, is important if early changes are to be detected. Early recognition and appropriate adjustments in postoperative treatment may limit the inflammatory process before pleural infection becomes established.

CLINICAL SIGNS

Early signs include diminished appetite, listless demeanor, fever, elevated respiratory rate, and an alteration in the pattern of breathing. Affected horses will often stand with their elbows slightly abducted and have decreased excursion of the chest wall with a variable degree of compensatory abdominal effort. Excursion of the chest wall may be asymmetric, and this can be best appreciated by viewing the horse from above and behind. A painful response to thoracic percussion is an early and sensitive indicator of pleural pain and can often be elicited before pleural effusion accumulates. A positive response may be limited to grunting or attempts to bite the clinician or may elicit escape maneuvers where the horse deliberately tries to avoid further attempts at percussion. With accumulation of fluid the painful response may lessen, but percussion is also useful to delineate the level of fluid within the thorax.

Auscultable changes in lung sounds consistent with pneumonia may be detected before fluid accumulation occurs. These sounds range from increased harshness, moist sounds, and inspiratory crackles and pops, to complete loss of sound. With fluid accumulation, there is likely to be loss of sound in the ventral lung fields and, depending on the degree of chest excursion, increased sounds dorsally. Provided the horse is not in respiratory distress, auscultation during rebreathing is strongly recommended to improve sound detection. Rubbing and musical sounds are indicative of pleural inflammation, adhesion, and loculation of pleural fluid. With progressive fluid accumulation, heart sounds can be detected over an increased area radiating dorsocaudally from the normal area of auscultation. Slight elevations in heart rate occur initially in association with chest pain and may increase as the inflammation and effusion progress.

The temporal sequence of hematologic changes in acute pleuropneumonia has not been well documented. In our experience, the most sensitive early changes are a slight decrease in total erythrocyte count, increased fibrinogen concentration, and variable leukocytosis. In fact less than 25% of our affected horses had leukocytosis (>10,000 cells/μL) at the time of initial signs, yet over 80% had elevated fibrinogen concentrations (>400 mg/dL). About 50% of the cases with normal total leukocyte counts had a relative neutrophilia. With progression of the infection and inflammation, fibrinogen concentration continues to rise and the leukocyte differential usually reflects neutrophilia with variable cell toxicity.

DIAGNOSIS

Early diagnosis requires careful observation and a high index of suspicion. This is particularly important in those horses being given nonsteroidal anti-inflammatory agents in the immediate postoperative period. A retrospective review of the temporal changes in perioperative rectal temperature revealed that horses not receiving nonsteroidal anti-inflammatory drugs had a 4 to 5 °F increase in temperature within 12 hours of the onset of signs, whereas the response was 2 °F or less in horses receiving these drugs. This spike in rectal temperature occurred within 1 to 6 days of surgery, with most horses becoming febrile before the third postoperative day.

Since the homeostatic response to surgical stress and inflammation includes fever, variable depression, some degree of inappetence, and minor hematologic changes, delineation of this response from the onset of postoperative respiratory complications requires careful observation and physical examination. In our practice another consideration is apparent nosocomial infection with a virus that can elicit similar premonitory signs. Confirmation of pleuropneumonia requires presence of the previously mentioned clinical signs and isolation of pathogenic microbes from pleural fluid, tracheobronchial secretions, bronchoalveolar lavage fluid, or lung tissue. Since the pleural effusion may be sterile (about 30% of cases), simultaneous collection of tracheobronchial secretions is recommended to improve the probability of bacterial isolation. Unless the specific location of the pneumonic lung is known, transtracheal aspiration is more likely to yield representative cells and microorganisms than bronchoalveolar lavage. If pleural fluid is detected in both pleural cavities, samples for cytology, Gram stain, and culture should be obtained from both cavities, because the fluid character and infectious agents may differ.

Ultrasonography, thoracic radiographs, and lung ventilation-perfusion scans are additional useful diagnostic methods. Thoracic radiography is of limited value until pleural effusion has been drained, and even then may only serve to confirm the presence of pulmonary consolidation. Ultrasonography generally provides more information about the nature of the pleural fluid, its relative volume and degree of loculation, the involvement of adjacent lung, and the presence of pleural adhesions. It is also a very effective noninvasive method of monitoring the response to therapy. Ventilation-perfusion scans are useful during convalescence to monitor the return of air and blood flow to affected lung regions, especially when resolution appears to be slow as judged from radiographic interpretation.

TREATMENT

Therapeutic goals include administration of appropriate systemic antibiotics, pain relief, drainage of the pleural space, maintenance of caloric intake, and good nursing care.

Selection of antimicrobial therapy should be based on susceptibility patterns of the microorganisms isolated from pleural fluid and tracheobronchial secretions. Since most are mixed infections, it is usually prudent to begin with intravenous broad-spectrum antibiotics. In our practice, procaine penicillin G (20,000 to 40,000 IU/kg four times daily) and gentamicin sulfate (2.2 mg/kg three times daily) are given initially and, unless susceptibility patterns or clinical response indicate otherwise, will be continued. Anaerobes (commonly *Bacteroides* and *Clostridium* species) are isolated in about half of the reported pleuropneumonia cases, and if they are β-lactamase producers, metronidazole (15 mg/kg intravenously or orally four times daily) should also be given. If *Mycoplasma* species are isolated, treatment with tetracycline (10 mg/kg intravenously twice daily) is recommended. Because prolonged antimicrobial therapy is often necessary, intravenous administration via catheter is preferred to intramuscular injections. Provided the microorganisms have appropriate susceptibility, oral antibiotics (trimethoprim-sulfamethoxazole, 3–5 mg/kg trimethoprim fraction, two or three times daily) are then used for another 2 to 4 weeks when the clinical response indicates the infection has been controlled.

Relief from thoracic pain is important for patient comfort and to help stimulate appetite. Phenylbutazone (4.4 mg/kg twice daily) or flunixin meglumine (0.5 mg/kg twice daily) is used. Careful monitoring of hydration and renal function is critical to minimize renal complications when aminoglycoside and nonsteroidal anti-inflammatory therapies are used, concurrently. Loss of fluid from pleural space drainage and reduced water intake because of inappetence can predispose to drug-associated nephrotoxicity. Supplementation with either oral or intravenous fluids (and electrolytes, if indicated) and periodic monitoring of serum aminoglycoside concentrations with appropriate adjustment of dosing interval can minimize renal damage.

Inappetence and anorexia in conjunction with the catabolic effects of an active inflammatory and infectious process often lead to rapid and marked weight loss. Stimulation of appetite with grazing and exposure to diets different from those normally offered can help to encourage renewed interest in eating. Generally, improved appetite occurs with increased patient comfort, normal temperature, and remission of the pleuropneumonia. In refractory cases, tube feeding or intravenous hyperalimentation may be necessary to offset weight loss. Supplementation with B vitamins and hematinics during treatment and convalescence should be considered when anemia of chronic disease is anticipated or recognized. Good nursing care, including grooming, leg bandages, and controlled exercise, is also very important for patient attitude and response.

Drainage of the Pleural Space

Guidelines for drainage of the pleural space and for surgical intervention are still not firmly established. Generally, drainage is indicated if any of the following conditions exists: (*a*) purulent exudate, (*b*) pleural exudate with a positive Gram stain or positive culture, (*c*) pleural fluid with more than 5,000 leukocytes/μL (*d*) more than 2 L of effusion, and (*e*) respiratory distress associated with fluid accumulation. The method of drainage depends on the character of the fluid, its rate of accumulation, and the degree of loculation within the pleural cavities. Loculated fluid may require thoracentesis in several locations to achieve complete removal. Ultrasonography is particularly useful in these instances to localize fluid pockets and to assess the effectiveness of fluid removal.

In acute postoperative pleuropneumonia, the volume of pleural fluid initially present can vary considerably from several hundred milliliters to several liters. Rapid removal of fluid from the pleural space can result in reexpansion pulmonary edema and a worsening hypoxemia. Although arterial blood gas analysis is not routinely performed in such cases, careful observation of respiratory effort, heart rate, mucous membrane color and refill time before and during pleural drainage is advised to avoid additional complications.

Intermittent Drainage. The choice of intermittent versus continuous drainage also depends on the characteristics of the effusion and the degree of loculation of the pleural space. Intermittent drainage can be satisfactorily achieved by thoracentesis with a cannula inserted percutaneously, after infiltration with local anesthetic, in the sixth to ninth intercostal spaces at the level of the costochondral junctions. It is usually advisable to insert a three-way stopcock in the hub of the cannula to minimize aspiration of air into the pleural space, although this is not usually a problem when larger volumes of fluid are present. Drainage can be achieved by aspiration or free flow, and measurement of the fluid volume is recommended so that the response to therapy can be assessed. If the effusion is too viscous to flow freely through a metal urinary or peritoneal cannula, a larger diameter plastic cannula (Argyle trochar catheter, Sherwood Medical) should be used or thoracostomy should be considered. In fibrinous pleural effusion, drainage is often hindered by occlusion of the cannula with fibrin tags.

Continuous Drainage. Closed drainage can be achieved by tube thoracostomy, using a large-diameter plastic cannula (#28 to #32 French Argyle trochar catheter, Sherwood Medical) attached to a one-way valve (Heimlich chest drain valve, Becton-Dickinson) or an underwater seal (Argyle Sentinel seal chest drainage unit, Sherwood Medical). This technique is advantageous in large-volume pleural effusion with rapid reaccumulation of fluid after drainage. It avoids the need for multiple thoracic entries and, provided the insertion site is managed carefully, can minimize problems with local cellulitis. Use of the one-way valve minimizes the need for patient restraint but does not allow quantitation of the fluid production and does result in environmental contamination. The underwater seal method allows quantitation of fluid production and this can be used as a guide for tube removal.

Open Drainage. Thoracostomy is indicated when the fluid is too viscous to drain through a large-bore cannula or if the infected space is well demarcated. After delineating the abscess with ultrasound, a site that allows ventral drainage is selected and a 5- to 10-cm thoracotomy is performed in the appropriate intercostal space. If the horse is tractable, this procedure is performed in the standing position. The abscess cavity is lavaged with sterile physiologic saline and gently débrided using gauze sponges and a sponge or other suitable forceps. Lavage is continued twice daily as needed until the cavity is obliterated. Local wound care is similar to that for any draining abscess cavity, with application of petrolatum to surrounding skin to prevent scalding. Dilute povidone-iodine solutions (0.1% iodine) or other antiseptics in solution can be used to débride the cavity. With resolution of the infection in the cavity lining, the thoracostomy incision heals by granulation.

Bronchopleural fistula and hemorrhage are two complications that can be encountered during this method of treatment and usually result from continued necrosis of the adjacent lung. If bronchopleural fistula occurs within the open abscess cavity and there is no associated lung collapse in the remainder of the thorax, resolution will usually occur with healing of the cavity. Caution must be exercised during lavage to minimize flooding of adjacent lung through the patent airway.

Lobectomy and Pleural Decortication

Although resection of the cranial lung lobes has been described in healthy horses, most pleuropneumonia cases have consolidation or abscessation of the ventral regions of the caudal lobes. To date attempts at resection of these affected regions have been unsuccessful. Several factors have contributed to this experience. The limited and incomplete lobation of the equine lung combined with the thickness of the caudal lobe results in a lung that does not readily lend itself to partial resection. Equally importantly, the decision to intervene surgically has usually been reserved until euthanasia was imminent, and thus the advanced state of the lung and pleural disease combined with the poor metabolic status of the patient have largely precluded success.

Attempts to decorticate the affected pleural surfaces have likewise been unsuccessful. This technique is intended to denude the thorax of infected pleural tissue and promote reexpansion of collapsed lung and obliteration of the pleural space. The advanced state of necrosis of the pleura and underlying tissues has precluded successful decortication. Improved success with these techniques will require earlier acceptance of either the failure of medical therapy or recognition that pleural empyema, loculation, excessive fibrin deposition, or formation of pleural rind are indications for surgical treatment, so that tissues are less devitalized at the time of intervention. Improved instrumentation and development of techniques for partial resection of consolidated caudal lung lobes are also needed.

PROGNOSIS

With early recognition and appropriate treatment, recovery can be expected in at least 50% of these horses. Return to a comparable level of previous activity occurs in about 50% of the survivors. The importance of early recognition, fastidious efforts to isolate and identify the infectious agent (including anaerobes and *Mycoplasma* species), systemic administration of appropriate antibiotics, and good nursing care cannot be overemphasized if improvements in survival and reduction of postoperative morbidity are to be accomplished.

In my experience the mean increase in postoperative hospitalization for horses with pleuropneumonia was 58 days, with survivors being hospitalized for an average of 43 days after surgery. This represents a significant increase in cost of hospitalization and must be considered when discussing therapeutic approaches and expectations if the horse recovers from the pleuropneumonia.

BIBLIOGRAPHY

Garibaldi RA, Britt MR, Coleman ML, et al: Risk factors for postoperative pneumonia. *Am J Med* 1981;70:677–680.

McIlwraith CW, Turner AS: Infections of the respiratory tract, in *Equine Surgery Advanced Techniques*. Philadelphia, Lea & Febiger, 1987 pp 46–52.

Raphel CF, Beech J: Pleuritis secondary to pneumonia or lung abscessation in 90 horses *J Am Vet Med Assoc* 1982;181:808–810.

Sweeney CR, Divers TJ, Benson CE: Anaerobic bacteria in 21 horses with pleuropneumonia. *J Am Vet Med Assoc* 1985;187:721–724.

UNIT VI

Gastrointestinal Tract Disorders

53
Cleft Palate

Karl Frederick Bowman
Lloyd P. Tate, Jr.
James T. Robertson

Developmental defects of the primary palate result in clefts of the lip and maxilla. These may be accompanied by cleft hard and soft palate as secondary anomalies. Failure of fusion of the secondary palate results in isolated cleft of the hard or soft palate. All repairs described in clinical reports of the condition in horses have involved clefts of the hard or soft palate.

DIAGNOSIS

Cleft palate results in bilateral nasal discharge during eating, dysphagia, and possibly aspiration pneumonia. In most cases, nasal regurgitation of milk becomes obvious soon after suckling. Confirmation of cleft palate is by observation of a cleft in the palate by endoscopic examination. Cleft soft palate can be difficult to detect by oral examination; therefore, endoscopy should be performed. Endoscopic findings include lack of palatal tissue in contact with the ventral border of the epiglottis, visualizing the epiglottis in the oral cavity, and seeing the tongue in front of the epiglottis. Submucous clefting, a dehiscence of the soft palatal muscles with intact overlying mucosa, may also be present. Auscultation of the lungs and thoracic radiography should be used to detect pneumonia due to aspiration. Microbiologic culture and antibiotic susceptibility testing of transtracheal aspirates are indicated to guide selection of appropriate antibiotic therapy for treatment of aspiration pneumonia. Our experience indicates that many animals will have mixed bacterial infection of the pulmonary system that may limit the success of treatment with broad-spectrum antibiotics. Dysphagia often contributes to failure of passive transfer of maternal immunoglobulin via colostrum and chronic malnutrition, which may require specific therapy. Although all affected foals should be examined for other congenital defects, these are not discovered frequently.

Adult horses that have exhibited postprandial nasal discharge since birth have been reported to have cleft soft palate. Individual horses were reported to be serviceable for intended use; however, one affected Thoroughbred racehorse died soon after exercise of fatal pulmonary hemorrhage that was attributed to subclinical aspiration pneumonia. Excessive partial soft palate resection used to treat dorsal displacement of the soft palate may result in clinical signs similar to cleft palate.

SURGERY

Currently, there are few reports of successful cleft palate repair in horses, and the surgical procedures that have been described reflected the surgeon's preference. This is particularly true in regard to the choice of suture material and patterns. At the outset of cleft palate repair, we advise owners of the possible heritability of the condition, the modest surgical success rate, the potential for complications, the period of intensive nursing care required, and the expenses associated with these cases. We do not believe that nonoperative treatment of foals with cleft palate will be associated with resolution of aspiration pneumonia and normal growth. Therefore, euthanasia, as an alternate to cleft palate repair, should be discussed.

Foals affected by cleft palate unaccompanied by aspiration pneumonia should be operated upon as soon as possible. Complicated cases benefit from therapy to prevent and/or treat aspiration pneumonia, including muzzling, feeding through either a nasogastric tube or esophagostomy, and antimicrobial therapy, prior to cleft palate repair. We prefer to operate upon foals younger than 6 weeks, because the depth of the surgical field is less than that in older patients, and the foal is still nursing, which allows coarse food to be withheld.

The surgical approaches for cleft palate repair include the intraoral route, bilateral buccotomy, pharyngotomy, and mandibular symphysiotomy, or various combinations of these techniques. Intraoral repair of cleft palate is limited by inadequate exposure of the defect; however, in at least one case ventral retraction of the tongue with a suture allowed successful repair. Mandibular symphysiotomy provides adequate exposure of the hard and soft palates, enabling repair with standard surgical instruments. Exposure of the caudal aspect of the soft palate has been accomplished via pharyngotomy.

The foal is anesthetized and placed in dorsal recumbency, and the ventral head and neck regions are prepared for aseptic surgery. An endotracheal tube is passed through a tracheostomy performed after induction of anesthesia, that allows unrestricted access to the oral cavity. The oral cavity is lavaged liberally with dilute povidone-iodine solution and the surgical site is draped routinely.

A mandibular symphysiotomy is performed according to the description by Nelson et al. Briefly, an intermandibular skin incision, extending rostrally from the hyoid apparatus to the lower lip, is made and deepened to the level of the mandibular lymph nodes caudally. Rostrally, the incision is deepened to divide the musculature of the chin, exposing the mandibular symphysis, labial mucosa, and gingiva. The labial mucosa is incised on the midline and that incision is extended to the space between the central incisors. The mandibular lymph nodes are separated by dissection, allowing the mylohyoideus muscle to be incised along its insertion from the lingual process of the hyoid bone to the mandibular symphysis. The mandibular symphysis is then separated, using an oscillating bone saw. The lingual gingiva, oral mucosa, and submucosal fascia are incised on the midline to the level of the frenulum. At this point, the mandibles may be separated approximately 2 cm, improving the exposure of the geniohyoideus and genioglossus muscles. Approximately 1 to 2 cm from their mandibular origins, the geniohyoideus and genioglossus muscles are severed and reflected. The polystomatic portions of the sublingual salivary gland and duct of the mandibular salivary gland, which are interposed between the muscular origins and the oral mucosa, must be avoided.

The incision is deepened along the natural plane of dissection, which is bordered laterally by the salivary structures and vertical portion of the mylohyoideus muscle and medially by the geniohyoideus and styloglossus muscles and the hypoglossal and lingual nerves. By spreading the mandibles, the oral mucosa can be visualized. The oral mucosa is opened with scissors caudally to the level of the rostral pillar of the soft palate. The exposed intermandibular tissue is draped with moistened towels or laparotomy drapes, and the tongue is retracted laterally. A self-retaining retractor, such as a Gelpi retractor or Finochietto rib spreader, is positioned to aid lateral retraction of the mandibles, and a hand retractor may be used to elevate the base of the tongue.

The cleft soft palate is injected along its oral margins with lidocaine with epinephrine (1:100,000 or more dilute) to tense the tissue and provide hemostasis. The margins of the cleft soft palate are incised in preparation for three-layer closure. Lateral relief incisions are made that extend rostrally from the caudal extent of the cleft to the level of the hard palate (Fig. 53–1). Occasionally, a stay suture is used to join and stabilize the caudal-most extent of the repair by passing the suture caudally through a separate laryngotomy incision. In addition to the lateral relief incisions, osteotomy and medial reflection of the hamulus of the pterygoid bone lessens (presumably) the pull of the tensor veli palatini muscle and relaxes the soft palate. Reconstruction of the levator veli palatini muscle "sling," which is performed in affected children to help restore pharyngeal function, has not been successful in the horse.

Once adequate tissue is free, the nasal mucosa is apposed with synthetic absorbable suture in a simple interrupted pattern. The palatal musculature is united with interrupted, horizontal mattress sutures. The knots should not be placed between the apposed muscle; rather they should be located within the lateral relief incisions. The oral mucosa is closed with similar suture in a simple interrupted or continuous pattern.

Caudal defects of the hard palate (up to 7 × 2 cm) are repaired by mucoperiosteal sliding-flap technique combined with cleft soft palate repair as described above. The margin of the cleft hard palate is incised and extended deeply to the bony palate. Incisions, paralleling the lingual margin of the teeth and located approximately 1 cm medially, are made through the oral mucosa and underlying periosteum for the length of the hard palate defect. The mucoperiosteum is elevated from rostral to caudal, avoiding damage to the greater palatine arteries. Using careful dissection and gentle traction, additional mobility of the greater palatine artery within its foramen can be achieved facilitating sliding of the mucoperiosteal flaps medially, and closure of the hard palate defect. Following its elevation, the medial margin of the mucoperiosteal flap is separated from its bony attachment with delicate scissors. The apposed mucoperiosteum is closed with synthetic absorbable suture in an interrupted horizontal mattress pattern. The oral mucosa is oversewn with similar suture in a simple continuous or interrupted pattern. Larger clefts of the hard palate repaired by this method should be protected postoperatively by use of an acrylic bridge between the molars to prevent trauma from lingual movement and pressure.

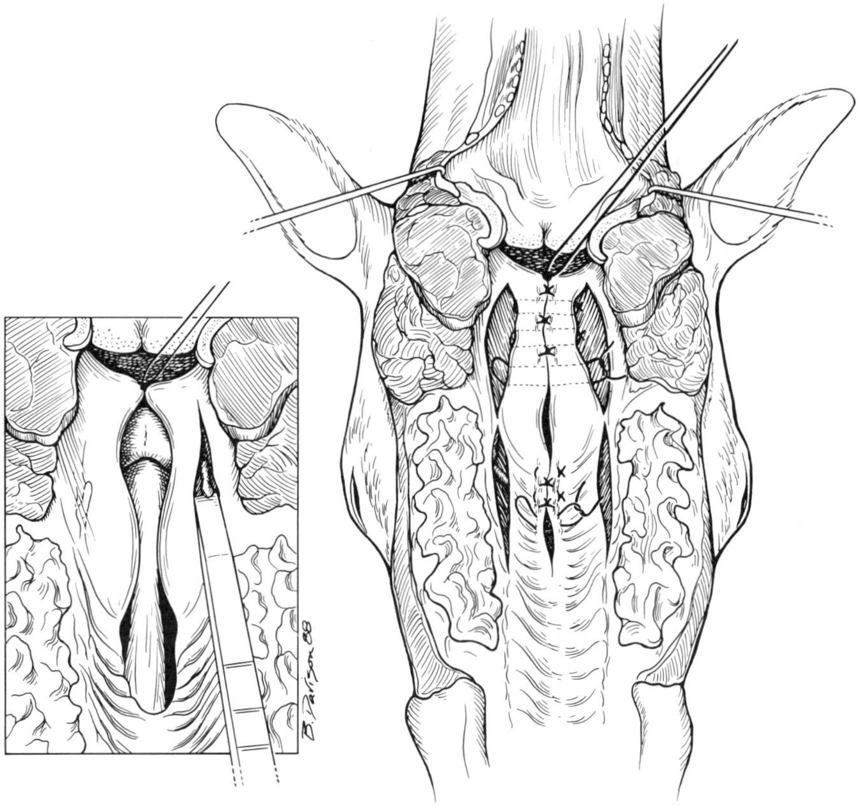

Figure 53–1. Hard palate repair by mucoperiosteal sliding-flap technique combined with cleft soft palate repair. A stay suture has been used to join and stabilize the caudal soft palate; it has been exited via separate laryngostomy incision. An osteotomy and medial reflection of the hamulus of the pterygoid bone may be completed to lessen tension on the sutured soft palate. The musculature is united with large horizontal mattress sutures and the oral mucosa is sutured with a simple interrupted or continuous suture.

POSTOPERATIVE CARE

Broad-spectrum antibiotic therapy and tetanus prophylaxis should be administered. A nonsteroidal anti-inflammatory drug should be used to help reduce postoperative swelling. Suckling foals having repair of a cleft soft palate should be allowed to nurse as soon as possible after surgery. Older foals or foals with defects in the hard palate should be fed through a feeding tube placed through the nasal passage or by esophagostomy, or alternatively by parenteral nutrition. Either of these feeding techniques should be continued for about 10 days to give the oral mucosa adequate time to heal. The oral cavity should be examined daily and trapped food particles removed gently by lavage. Although additional surgical procedures may be necessary to close defects in the palate, these are usually best done after 3 to 4 weeks once the wound has been assessed for healing. Secondary repairs after this period become more difficult because of a lack of sufficient tissue to close the defects without a second major dissection of the palate.

PROGNOSIS

Cleft soft palate repair is considered to have a better prognosis than reconstructions involving the hard and soft palates; however, variable tissue thickness and muscle in the cleft soft palate or presence of asymmetric defects may complicate its repair and diminish the prognosis. Dehiscence of the palatoplasty, especially in the caudal portions of the soft palate, occurs in up to 90% of cases. Large clefts of the hard palate, especially those extending rostrally to the incisors, are usually quite wide, and this prevents successful repair. Foals with these extensive defects usually have advanced aspiration pneumonia, which reduces the prognosis to the point where euthanasia is recommended.

Osteomyelitis, nonunion of the mandible, and lower lip dehiscence are also complications of mandibular symphysiotomy. These can be major complications that reduce the overall success of the surgery and are best prevented by careful attention to symphysiotomy fixation and the lip-sparing technique as described by Grossman et al.

Since the heritability of cleft palate in the horse is not known, horses that have had correction of the cleft palate should not be used for reproduction or should be neutered.

BIBLIOGRAPHY

Bertone JJ, Traub-Dargatz JL, Trotter GW: Bilateral hypoplasia of the soft palate and aryepiglottic entrapment in a horse. *J Am Vet Med Assoc* 1986;188:727–728.

Bowman KF, Tate LP, Evans LH, Donawick WJ: Complications of cleft palate repair in large animals. *J Am Vet Med Assoc* 1982;180:652–657.

Cooper HK, Harding RL, Krogman WM, Mazaheri M, Millard RT (eds): *Cleft Palate and Cleft Lip: A Team Approach to Clinical Management and Rehabilitation of the Patient.* Philadelphia, WB Saunders Co, 1979, pp 109–143, 200–262.

Grossman BS, Brinkman JF, Grant B: A new approach for intra-oral surgery in the horse: A lip-sparing modification of mandibular symphysiotomy. *Equine Vet Sci* 1981;1:107–109.

Haynes PF, Qualls CW: Cleft soft palate, nasal septal deviation, and epiglottic entrapment in a Thoroughbred filly. *J Am Vet Med Assoc* 1981;179:910–913.

Jones RS, Maisels DO, DeGeus JJ, Lovius BBJ: Surgical repair of cleft palate in the horse. *Equine Vet J* 1975;7:86–90.

Mason TA, Speirs VC, MacLean AA, Smyth GB: Surgical repair of cleft soft palate in the horse. *Vet Rec* 1977;100: 6–8.

Nelson AW, Curley BM, Kainer RA: Mandibular symphysiotomy to provide adequate exposure for intraoral surgery in the horse. *J Am Vet Med Assoc* 1971;159:1025–1031.

54 Esophageal Obstruction

John A. Stick

Esophageal diseases in the horse include obstruction, stricture, rupture, diverticulum, fistula, cyst, megaesophagus, and neoplasia. Of these, obstruction or "choke" is the most common disorder. Stricture formation is a possible sequela to obstruction. This chapter discusses the diagnosis and medical and surgical management of esophageal obstruction caused by feed impaction or foreign body.

DIAGNOSIS

Presenting Signs

Horses with obstructive esophageal disease present with regurgitation of food, water, and saliva through the mouth and nostrils, coughing, dysphagia, and excessive salivation. Attempts to eat are often followed by painful swallowing, indicated by repeated extension of the head and neck, distress, and agitation. These signs may mimic those of abdominal pain. The time interval from swallowing until these signs are shown by the horse depends on the location of the obstruction within the esophagus. Retching and discomfort may occur 10 to 12 seconds after swallowing when the obstruction is in the lower esophagus, whereas signs may occur immediately when a cervical obstruction is present. Intermittent signs of choke followed by periods of relief may indicate a disease other than simple feed impaction, and further diagnostic procedures are warranted. Anorexia, electrolyte imbalances, and dehydration accompany cases of long duration. Aspiration pneumonia frequently follows esophageal obstruction, and signs may be present as early as 1 day after the onset of choke.

Confirmatory Tests

Clinical evaluation of the horse with esophageal disease may be completed with physical and radiographic examinations. Occasionally esophagoscopy may be necessary to recognize some disorders or to clarify the extent of some injuries of the esophagus. Most often clinical features and physical and radiographic techniques will permit identification of common disorders so that medical management may be instituted.

Physical Examination. A thorough oral examination should be performed to rule out oral foreign body, dental disease, cleft palate, and oropharyngeal neoplasia from the differential diagnosis. Observation and palpation of the neck in the area of the jugular furrows may reveal an enlargement in the cervical esophagus. Simple food impaction of the cervical esophagus may be localized in this manner. Crepitation or a diffuse, firm enlargement may indicate a loss of integrity of the esophagus. Nasogastric tube passage often confirms luminal obstruction and localizes the site of involvement. Gentle lavage of warm water through the tube may permit material to be flushed free of the obstruction if feed or consumed bedding is the cause of the problem. Sedation of the animal with xylazine (Rompun; 1.1 mg/kg intravenously) will lower the head and prevent further aspiration. Lavage may be continued until the obstruction is relieved; if this occurs further diagnostic studies may be unnecessary. However, if reobstruction occurs, this is considered an indication that another esophageal disease may be present and a diagnosis should be pursued further.

When esophageal disease has been present, auscultation and radiography of the thorax are indicated to monitor the development of aspiration pneumonia. This complication is common and should be treated when the primary problem is encountered.

Radiography of the Esophagus. Esophagography in the adult horse is diagnostic in most instances and should be considered a part of the complete esophageal examination if reobstruction occurs. A survey film may establish the presence of a feed impaction or foreign body (Fig. 54–1). Frequently an area of dilatation will extend from the distal point of the obstruction to the upper esophageal sphincter after impaction of the esophagus has been relieved. Dilatation will present as air contrast in the esophagus, occasionally with a fluid line in the dilatation, and will serve to localize the lesion.

Barium paste (Solo-O-Pake, 120 ml, 85% w/v with water; E-Z-EM Co, Inc) given by mouth will outline the longitudinal mucosal folds of the esophagus with the lumen undistended and will permit identification of the location of the obstruction or any disruption of the

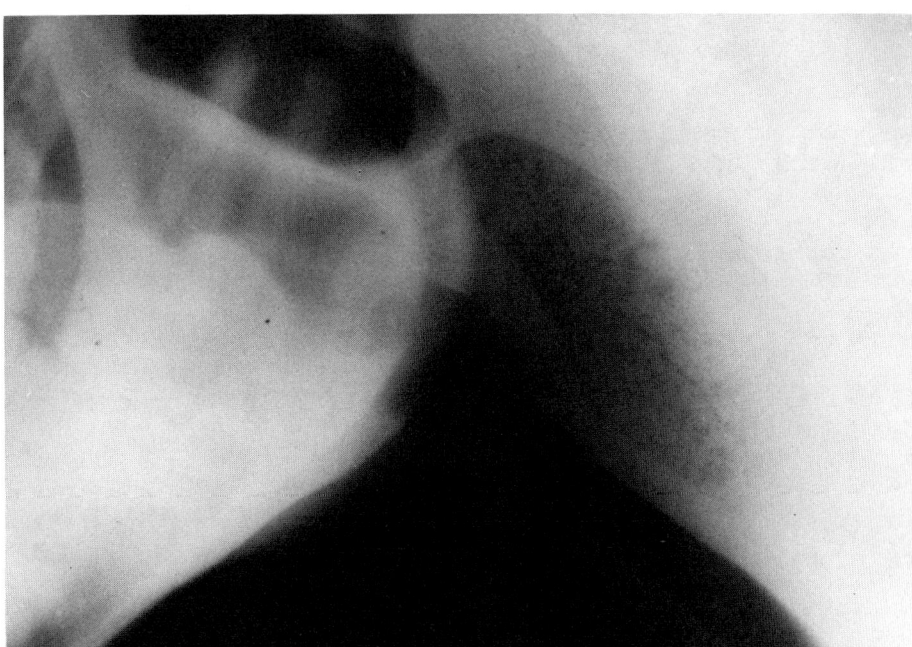

Figure 54–1. Survey radiograph of the proximal cervical region illustrates the typical appearance of a feed impaction of the esophagus.

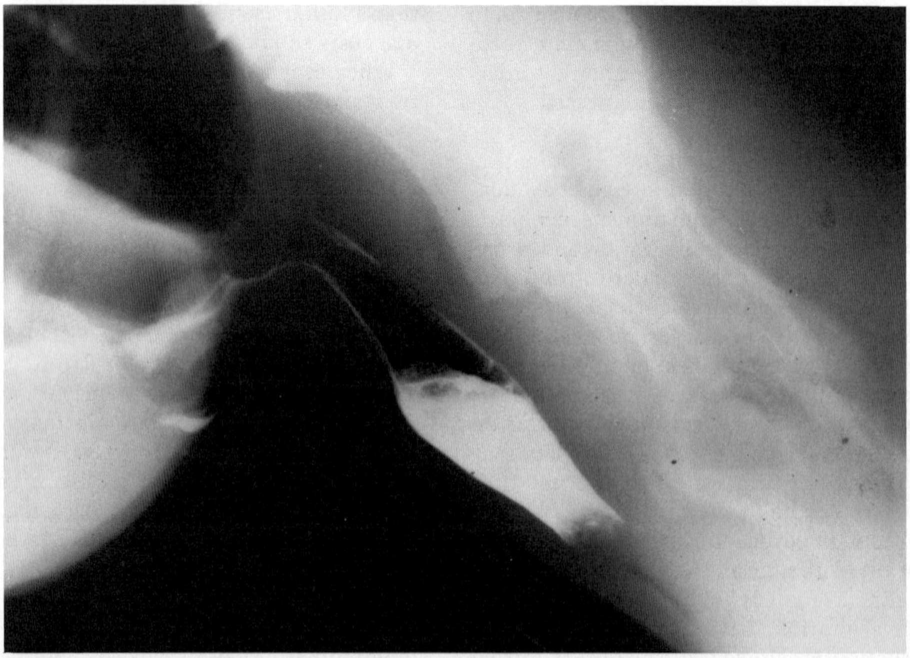

Figure 54–2. Barium swallow esophagogram shows a complete esophageal obstruction in the proximal cervical esophagus. Note the dilatation proximal to the obstruction.

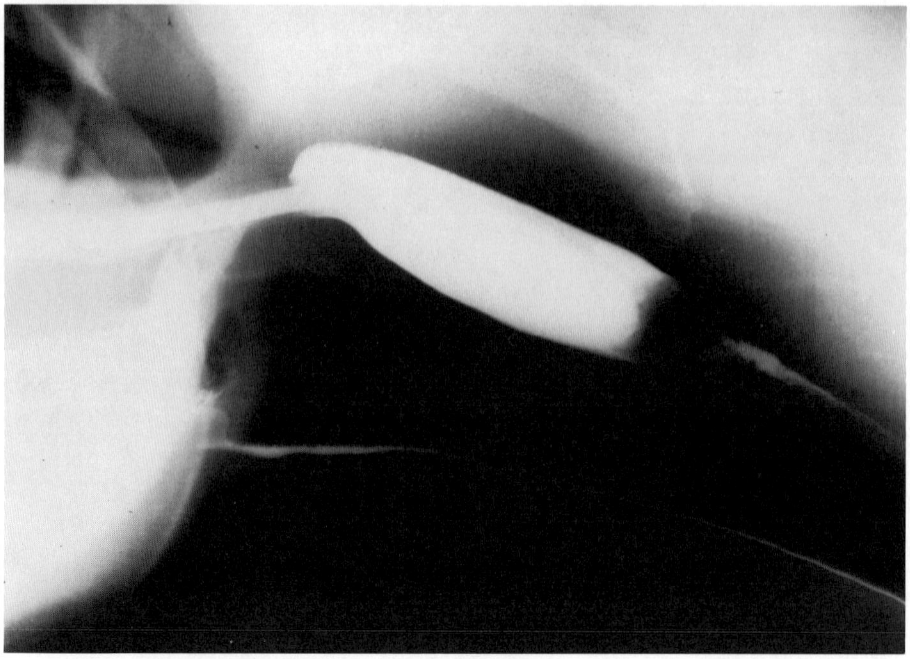

Figure 54–3. Barium liquid administered under pressure through a nasogastric tube clearly demarcates a stenotic lesion in the cervical esophagus.

lumen. Feed in the esophagus will become coated with the barium, a complete obstruction will stop the barium at the site of the lesion (Fig. 54–2), and rupture of the esophagus will permit barium to escape into the surrounding soft tissues. Sedation of the patient should be avoided if possible during this procedure, because it suppresses the swallowing reflex and barium will be held in the mouth, reducing the amount available to coat the esophagus.

Liquid barium (Solo-O-Pake, 480 ml, 72% w/v with water; E-Z-EM Co, Inc) administered under pressure by a dose syringe through a nasogastric tube will demonstrate strictures and associated prestenotic dilatation of the esophagus (Fig. 54–3). Liquid barium (480 ml) followed by air (480 ml) delivered by dose syringe under pressure provides a double-contrast study, permitting examination of mucosal folds with the esophagus distended. This latter technique gives the best definition of mucosal lesions, such as circumferential mucosal ulcers following feed impaction (Fig. 54–4). Although a diagnosis can often be made without using all three techniques, each technique will demonstrate lesions not seen with the other two.

Swallowing during contrast studies when the lumen is being distended will produce false signs of esophageal stricture. Xylazine (1.1 mg/kg intravenously) given 5 minutes prior to the barium-under-pressure or double-contrast esophagogram will help eliminate a swallow artifact by decreasing the reflex "secondary swallows" that follow luminal distention.

Endoscopy of the Esophagus. Esophagoscopy may better define the severity and extent of esophageal lesions diagnosed by radiography and can be used as an ancillary diagnostic aid. Endoscopic examinations always should be performed when radiographic findings are not diagnostic. If the endoscope is 150 cm or longer the entire esophagus may be examined, and esophageal lesions in the thorax of the adult horse undetected on radiographic examination may be identified. A flexible endoscope that allows irrigation and insufflation is necessary to provide good observation of mucosal disease and changes in luminal size.

Endoscopic examination may be safely performed on the restrained standing animal in most instances. Diagnostic observations are best made by starting with the endoscope fully inserted and the esophageal lumen insufflated. The endoscope is then slowly withdrawn craniad. After each swallow, the endoscope should be cleared by irrigation and the esophagus again dilated before the endoscope is withdrawn further. Several

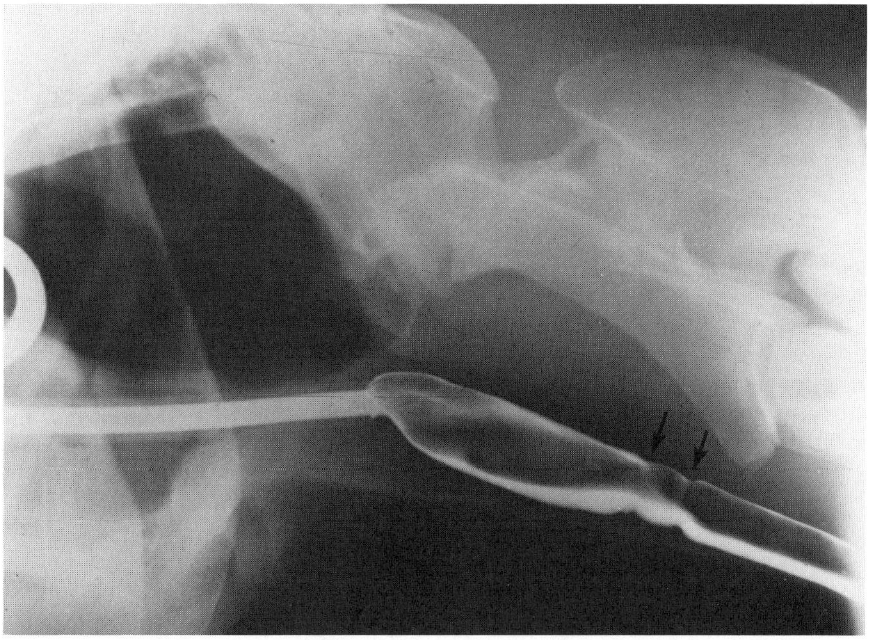

Figure 54–4. Barium liquid followed by air under pressure provides a double-contrast study that outlines a circumferential ulcer of the esophagus (*arrows*).

passes should be made over any area of suspected disease.

Normal longitudinal mucosal folds of the esophagus are seen when the endoscope tip is moved craniad and the esophagus is in the relaxed position. Insufflation flattens these folds and permits observation of luminal size. Transverse folds can be iatrogenically produced by moving the endoscope tip aborally. When the cervical esophagus is properly insufflated, the outline of the trachea can often be seen through the esophageal wall. Swallowing produces changes in the lumen that give the appearance of diverticula and strictures to the untrained observer. The mucosa should appear white to light pink in color. Reddened colorations are signs of mucosal injury.

The cranial aspect of the cervical esophageal sphincter is difficult to examine because of repeated stimulation of the swallowing reflex and because the larynx directs the endoscope tip dorsally. Radiographic assessment of this area may be more diagnostic. Additionally, the longitudinal mucosal folds found along the rest of the esophagus are absent in this area.

Frequently, the endoscopic appearance of an esophageal obstruction is obscured by saliva mixed with ingesta that collects cranial to the obstruction. This fluid should be removed by suction through a nasogastric tube and the endoscope should be immediately reinserted to observe the obstruction.

An inability to insufflate the esophagus and flatten the longitudinal mucosal folds usually indicates a disease process. This will be noted cranial and caudal to a stricture. Additionally, transverse mucosal folds, when not iatrogenic from endoscope manipulation, should be considered pathognomonic for mural lesions.

MEDICAL MANAGEMENT

The most common type of obstructive esophageal disease is impaction with ingesta. Nasogastric tube passage and gentle warm water lavage under xylazine sedation is usually successful in relieving the obstruction. Several alternative techniques may be necessary if gentle lavage fails. A cuffed nasogastric tube (Bivona, Inc) may be placed, the animal sedated, and water lavaged under pressure with a dose syringe or stomach pump. The tube helps prevent reflux of ingesta into the pharynx while permitting pressure of the water to push the obstruction distally. External massage and to-and-fro movement of the water will resolve most impactions. If this technique is not successful, the animal should be muzzled to prevent food and water intake and left alone for 8 to 12 hours, and the treatment should be repeated. Frequently, the initial treatment softens the impaction and it will become dislodged by swallowing or is easily relieved by a second treatment.

Refractory cases or intractable horses may benefit from general anesthesia and water lavage under pressure. This method has the advantages of providing some esophageal muscular relaxation, lessening the chances of aspiration because the horse's head may be inclined downward, and decreasing the risk of esophageal perforation with the tube in an intractable horse. Gentle manipulation is mandatory with this technique to avoid rupture of the esophagus.

One aftermath of simple impaction is fusiform dilatation of the esophagus that predisposes to reobstruction (Fig. 54–5). This condition will resolve in 24 to 48 hours provided the dilatation is kept free of ingesta. Food should be withheld or only small quantities of a soft diet fed for 2 days after an episode of choke to permit the lumen to return to a normal diameter. An electrolyte solution for drinking should be provided in addition to fresh water so that electrolyte abnormalities secondary to salivary losses may be corrected.

Broad-spectrum antimicrobial therapy is indicated for 5 to 7 days because the risk of aspiration pneumonia is increased after choke. I prefer procaine penicillin G (22,000 IU/kg twice a day) and gentamicin sulfate (Gentocin; 2.2 mg/kg three times a day). If pneumonia is not the major limiting factor in this disease, simple obstruction has a favorable prognosis.

When an obstruction has been present for several days or is refractory to the initial treatment, a postobstruction examination using radiography, endoscopy, or both is warranted. Circumferential mucosal ulceration is common in these cases and often results in esophageal stricture.

Impactions that do not respond to conservative therapy should be definitively identified, and if amenable should be relieved by longitudinal esophagotomy. Surgery is preferable to repeated trauma of the esophagus with a nasogastric tube.

SURGERY

Anatomy

The esophagus of the horse is 125 to 150 cm long, depending on the size of the animal, and can be classified into cervical, thoracic, and abdominal parts. As it courses caudally, it deviates from a position dorsal to the trachea in the cranial third of the neck to the left side of the median plane in the middle third of the neck and comes to lie ventral to the trachea at the thoracic inlet. The cervical part of the equine esophagus is most accessible to surgery and comprises over 50% of the total length of the esophagus.

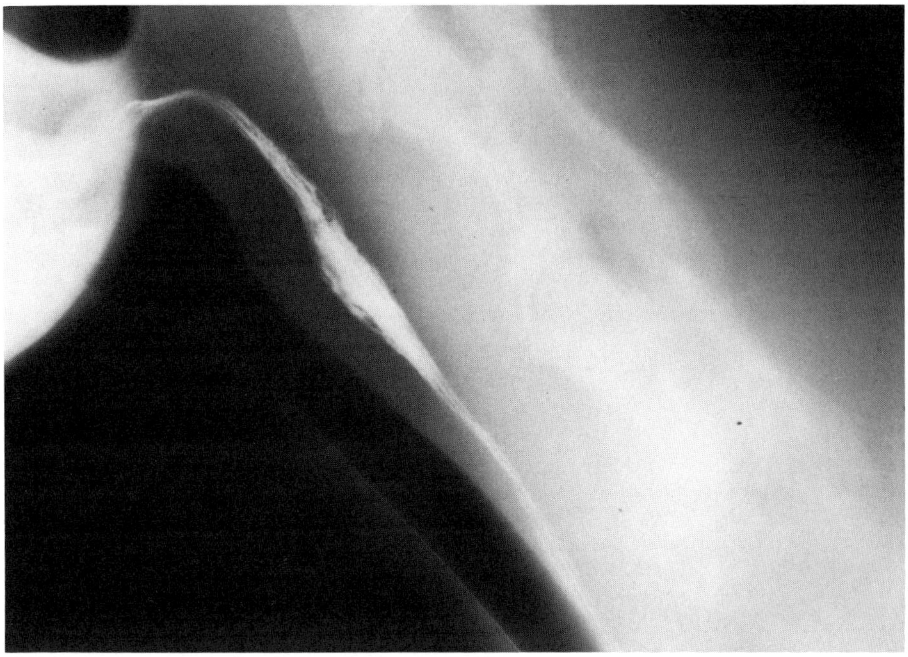

Figure 54–5. Barium swallow of a horse 24 hours after relief of a feed impaction shows a fusiform dilatation at the site of the previous obstruction.

The wall of the esophagus comprises four layers: a fibrous layer (tunica adventitia), muscular layers (tunica muscularis), a submucosal layer (tela submucosa), and mucous membrane (tunica mucosa). The muscular layers are striated from the pharynx to the base of the heart, where they gradually blend into smooth muscle. As the esophagus courses caudally, its muscular layers increase in thickness while the lumen diminishes. Except at the upper esophageal sphincter, the two muscular layers are spirally and elliptically arranged. On surgical incision, the esophageal wall separates easily into two distinct layers. The elastic inner layer, composed of mucosa and submucosa, is freely movable within the relatively inelastic outer muscular layer and adventitia (Fig. 54–6). The mucosa, which provides the greatest tensile strength upon closure of an esophageal incision, is covered with stratified squamous epithelium and lies in longitudinal folds that obliterate the lumen except during deglutition.

The arterial supply to the cervical part of the esophagus originates from the carotid arteries. The thoracic and relatively short (2- to 3-cm) abdominal esophagus are supplied by the bronchoesophageal and gastric arteries. The vascular pattern is arcuate but segmental, without generous collateral circulation, necessitating careful preservation of vessels during surgery.

Esophagotomy

Passage of a nasogastric tube as far as the foreign body (or beyond if possible) will facilitate identification of the esophagus during surgery. General anesthesia is preferred if closure is to be attempted.

The patient is placed in dorsal recumbency and the skin of the ventral surface of the neck is prepared and draped for aseptic surgery. An 8-cm incision made on the ventral midline of the neck over the area of the obstruction will provide exposure necessary to make a 5-cm longitudinal esophageal incision. The paired sternothyroid, sternohyoid, and omohyoid muscles are separated along the midline to expose the trachea. Blunt separation of fascia along the left side of the trachea permits identification of the esophagus containing the nasogastric tube. Retraction of the trachea to the right of the median plane and gentle sharp dissection of overlying loose adventitia exposes the ventral wall of the esophagus. Care should be taken to preserve the small vessels that supply the esophagus. Elevation of the esophagus from its bed of adventitia should be avoided. The left carotid sheath, containing the carotid artery and the vagus and recurrent laryngeal nerves, should be retracted laterally. Pediatric-size Balfour abdominal retractors will aid exposure to the esophagus, which then can be sharply incised through the muscle,

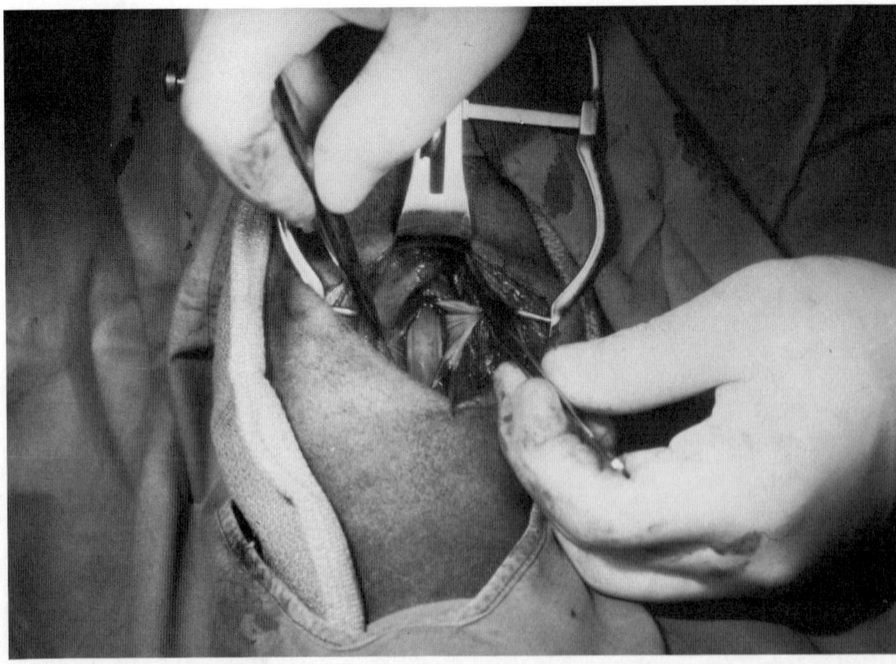

Figure 54–6. Photograph of an esophagotomy demonstrates the elasticity of the mucosal-submucosal layer of the equine esophagus. Note the preplaced nasogastric tube in the esophageal lumen.

submucosa, and mucosa craniad, caudad, or directly over the foreign body (Fig. 54–7). The location of the incision in the esophagus depends on the mobility of the foreign body within the lumen and the amount of swelling in the esophageal wall.

After removal of the foreign body, if the esophagus has a normal appearance in the area of the incision, closure should be completed using a simple continuous suture of 3–0 polypropylene suture material (Prolene; Ethicon Inc), with the knots tied in the lumen. Esophageal musculature may be apposed with simple interrupted sutures of 3–0 monofilament nonabsorbable suture material or polydioxanone according to the surgeon's preference. Muscular layers and subcutaneous tissues are apposed with 2–0 monofilament absorbable or nonabsorbable suture material in a simple interrupted pattern.

If the surgeon expects to invade the esophageal lumen, broad-spectrum antibiotics are indicated preoperatively, based on sound surgical principles, expected complications, and recognized bacterial colonization of this organ, as well as the probable existence of aspiration pneumonia. Before anesthetic induction, a nasogastric tube should be passed as far into the esophagus as the surgical site (or beyond if possible) to facilitate identification of the esophagus at surgery. A polyethylene drain (Hemovac, 0.25-in outer diameter; Snyder Laboratories) placed beside the esophagus, brought out ventral to the skin incision through a small stab wound, and maintained under constant suction for 48 hours removes serum and blood from the surgical site and will provide early detection of salivary leakage should dehiscence occur.

If removal of the foreign body is necessary through an obviously diseased segment of the esophagus, the incision may be made closer to the stomach or an esophagostomy tube may be placed directly into the esophagotomy incision. Feeding of a complete pelleted diet (Complete Horse Feed No. 705; 7 g/kg in 5 L of water twice daily; The Andersons) can be started immediately after surgery through the esophagostomy tube. Particular attention to the water and electrolyte balance of the patient is necessary when closure of the esophagus is not possible (see "Prognosis and Special Considerations" below).

POSTOPERATIVE CARE

If longitudinal esophagotomy has been performed with primary closure, feed should be withheld for 48 hours.

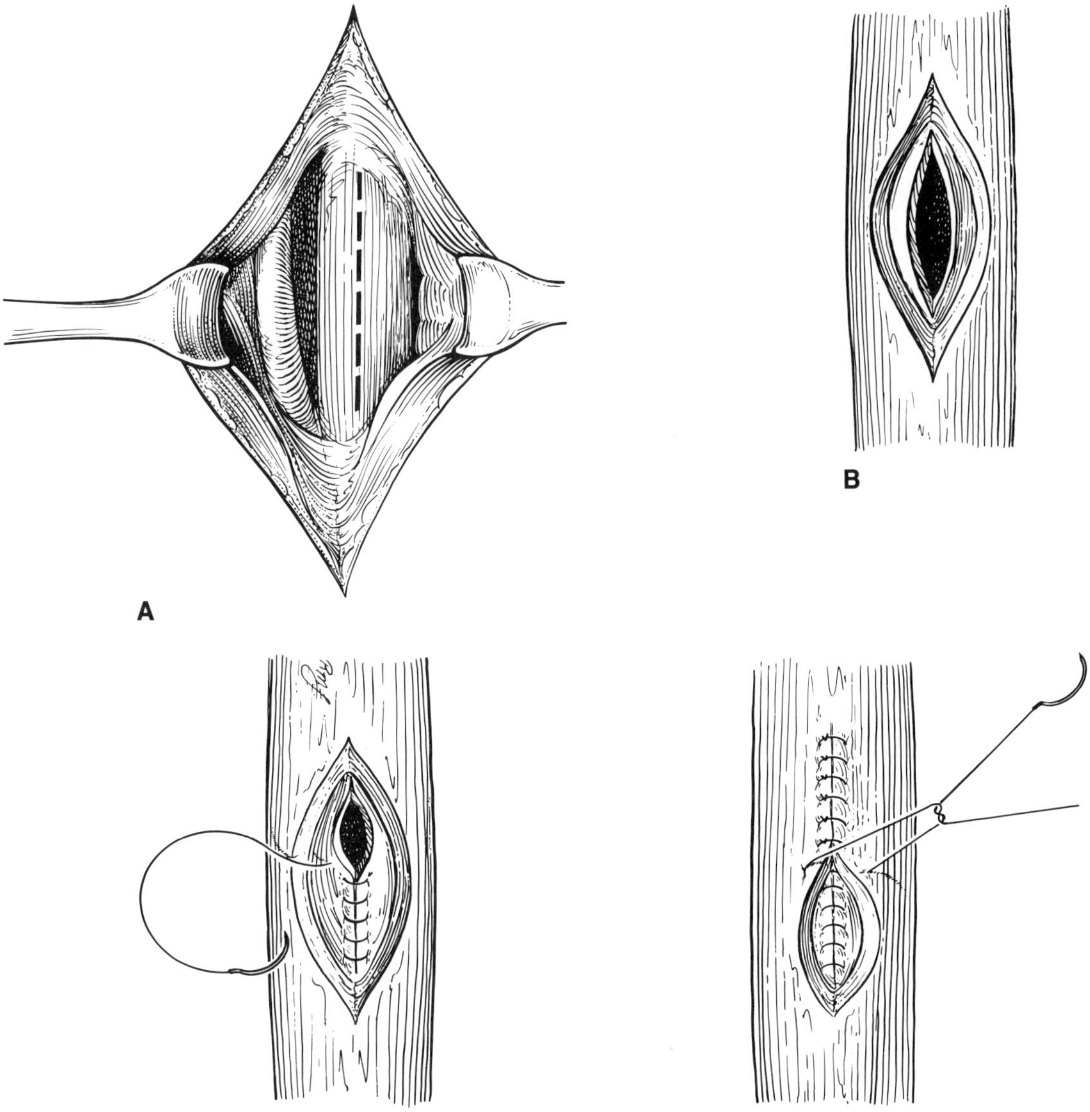

Figure 54–7. Esophagotomy. **A.** The ventral wall of the esophagus is exposed after abaxial retraction of the trachea (right). Note the left carotid sheath adjacent to the esophagus. The *dashed line* represents the direction of incision. **B.** Longitudinal incisure of the esophageal wall shows separation into two distinct layers, the muscularis and mucose-submucosa. **C.** Closure of the mucosal-submucosal layer is accomplished with a simple continuous suture of 3–0 polypropylene (Prolene), with the knots tied in the lumen. **D**. The esophageal musculature is apposed with simple interrupted sutures of 3–0 monofilament nonabsorbable suture material or polydioxanone according to the surgeon's preference.

Parenteral administration of electrolyte solutions may be used to maintain hydration. Small quantities of pelleted feed in a slurry should be fed between days 2 and 10 after surgery before normal feeding can be resumed. The drain is removed in 24 hours unless salivary leakage is observed. Reexamination of the esophageal lumen with the endoscope should be avoided for 10 days. A complete radiographic and endoscopic examination should be made every 14 days until mucosal healing has occurred.

PROGNOSIS AND SPECIAL CONSIDERATIONS

Longitudinal esophagotomy with primary closure of the incision results in minimal complications when performed in a region of normal esophagus. This surgery is preferred over manipulations that induce further esophageal trauma and has a favorable prognosis for first-intention healing.

Dehiscence and Stricture

The key to handling breakdown of a sutured esophageal incision is early recognition and treatment. For this reason, a suction drain placed next to the esophagus at the time of surgery serves a second function in addition to drainage of serum and blood from the surgical site; it provides a method to detect salivary leakage. Not all incisions that leak saliva will dehisce, especially if saliva is removed from the periesophageal tissues. However, if extreme amounts of saliva are produced through the incision or complete dehiscence occurs, the initial incision should be completely opened and lavaged on a daily basis to remove any ingesta or saliva. Dissection planes ventrally along the trachea should be drained to the outside to prevent development of mediastinitis or pleuritis. Dissecting infections can occur following esophagostomy as well, and inadvertent replacement of a dislodged feeding tube into a tissue plane or the thorax would obviously have an unfavorable outcome. The patient may be permitted to drink, which in many cases will lavage the wound. Nutritional requirements may be met by oral feeding or placement of a feeding tube into the esophagus at the point of dehiscence or distally through a separate esophagostomy. The outcome of this complication from this point will depend on management of water and electrolyte balance. The most common complication following treatment of an annular lesion is stricture. This complication is the bane of the esophageal surgeon and its successful treatment is limited in case reports (see Chapter 55).

Acid-Base and Electrolyte Alterations

In the face of adequate nutrition, daily losses of large amounts of saliva in horses result in hyponatremia, hypochloremia, and transient metabolic acidosis followed by progressive metabolic alkalosis. The alkalosis probably results from renal compensation of electrolyte imbalances. Oral administration of sodium chloride daily will reverse the electrolyte imbalance and the alkalosis will be corrected through renal mechanisms. Potassium requirements are adequately met in the feed.

Laryngeal Hemiplegia

Manipulative procedures and/or diseases of the esophagus in the cervical area can very easily result in laryngeal hemiplegia because of the close proximity of the recurrent laryngeal nerves. The surgeon should be aware that apparently minor manipulations of these nerves can have deleterious effects on their function.

BIBLIOGRAPHY

DeBowes RM, Grant BD, Sande RD: Esophageal obstruction by antibiotic boluses in a Thoroughbred filly: A case report. *J Equine Vet Sci* 1982;2:23–26.

Freeman DE, Naylor JM: Cervical esophagostomy to permit extraoral feeding of the horse. *J Am Vet Med Assoc* 1978;172:314–320.

McIlwraith CW, Turner AS: Esophagotomy for removal of an esophageal foreign body, in *Equine Surgery Advanced Techniques*. Philadelphia, Lea & Febiger, 1987, pp 264–267.

Stick JA: Diseases affecting the esophagus, in Mayhew IG, Merrit AM, Colahan PT, Moore JN (eds): *Equine Medicine and Surgery*, ed 4. (in press).

Stick JA: Esophageal disease, in Robinson NE (ed): *Current Therapy in Equine Practice*, ed 2. Philadelphia, WB Saunders Co, 1987, pp 12–15.

Stick JA, Derksen FJ, Scott EA: Equine cervical esophagostomy: Complications associated with duration and location of feeding tubes. *Am J Vet Res* 1981;42:727–732.

Stick JA, Krehbiel JD, Kunze DJ: Esophageal healing in the pony: A comparison of sutured vs non-sutured esophagotomy. *Am J Vet Res* 1981;42:1505–1513.

Stick JA, Robinson NE, Krehbiel JD: Acid-base and electrolyte alterations associated with salivary loss in the pony. *Am J Vet Res* 1981;42:733–737.

Stick JA, Slocombe RF, Derksen FJ, Scott EA: Esophagotomy in the pony: Comparison of surgical techniques and form of feed. *Am J Vet Res* 1983;44:2123–2132.

55
Esophageal Stricture

John A. Stick

Narrowing of the esophageal lumen because of stricture formation is usually an annular lesion and can be classified into three types, depending on the anatomic location of induration and fibrosis: (*a*) mural lesions that involve only the adventitia and muscularis, (*b*) esophageal rings or webs that involve only the mucosa-submucosa, and (*c*) annular stenosis that involves all layers of the esophageal wall. Stenosis of the esophagus usually is acquired as a result of external or internal trauma to the esophageal walls (especially following impactions that produce circumferential ulceration or following surgical treatment of annular lesions). In most instances, strictures are less likely to occur when traumatic insults involve only a portion of the circumference of the esophagus. For this reason, mobilization of the esophagus from its fascial attachments during surgery should be avoided whenever possible.

DIAGNOSIS

Presenting Signs

The signs of esophageal stricture are produced by secondary feed impaction proximal to the constricted segment. Therefore, the clinical manifestations of stricture mimic those of other esophageal obstructions. Occasionally, the signs of "choke" will be observed periodically during the development of a stricture as feed becomes impacted and then is spontaneously passed.

Confirmatory Tests

Strictures usually impede complete passage of the nasogastric tube and are best demonstrated by positive pressure contrast esophagograms (Fig 55–1). Esophageal rings or webs can be observed endoscopically (Fig. 55–2).

Medical Management

Conservative management of a stricture is aimed at dilatation of the stenotic segment. Bougienage or pneumatic or hydrostatic dilators have limited practical value in horses because of the inaccessibility of special equipment and chronicity of the problem. In early cases, such as postsurgical strictures or those following circumferential ulceration, the esophagus can be dilated by feeding small quantities of soft food over a period of several months. In seven horses that developed stricture following esophageal impaction, medical management over 2 months revealed that the esophageal lumen was maximally reduced (strictured) 30 days after circumferential ulceration was observed, after which lumen diameter increased to normal by 60 days. This also has been documented following experimental resection and anastomosis. Therefore, it is recommended that a low-bulk diet, nonsteroidal anti-inflammatory drugs, and antimicrobial therapy be used and surgical intervention be delayed for 60 days from the original insult. It is important to impress upon horse owners that several episodes of "choke" may occur up to 40 days following the original obstruction.

SURGERY

Strictures more than 50 days old usually have matured to the point where the cicatrix is too firm to yield to dilation through feeding and therefore may be classified as chronic. Chronic strictures of the esophagus may be corrected by esophagomyotomy, partial or complete resection and anastomosis, or patch grafting. All of these surgical treatments are associated with complications and the surgeon should take care to pick the most conservative therapy that will meet the aim of treatment. Leakage of luminal contents and reformation of the stricture requiring prolonged medical management are to be expected following resection and patch grafting.

Esophagomyotomy

Strictures that are mural in origin will respond to myotomy and have the best prognosis for recovery without restricture. Three successful reports appear in the literature, and I have had similar experience with two additional horses. The surgery should be performed with the horse under general anesthesia. A nasogastric tube is passed to the level of the stricture to permit easy identification of the involved area. The approach for esophagotomy or esophagostomy is at the surgeon's discretion. Normally, it is on the left side of the neck

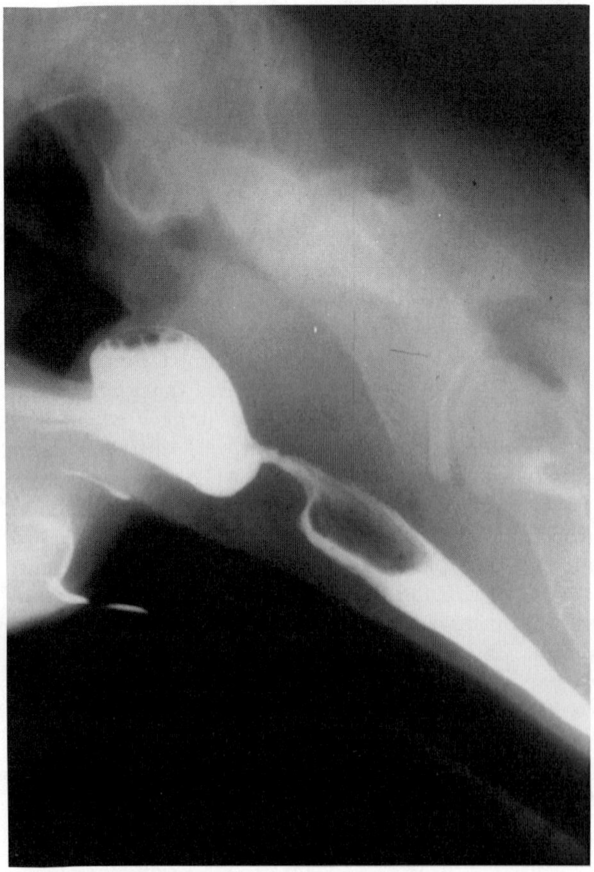

Figure 55–1. Barium liquid administered through a nasogastric tube under pressure demonstrates the typical appearance of an esophageal stricture. Note the pre- and poststenotic dilatations.

and uses fascial separation to maintain muscular continuity and avoid damaging the jugular vein or carot:.d sheath.

The esophagus is incised longitudinally to the level of the mucosa, through the stricture, and 1 cm caudal and cranial to it. The nasogastric tube may be passed through the stenotic area at this point. From this single incision the muscularis is separated by sharp dissection from the mucosa around the entire circumference of the esophagus (Fig. 55–3). When the mucosa is freed in this manner, it makes removal of a portion of the muscularis or multiple myotomy incisions necessary in only a few cases. The myotomy is not sutured and the approach incision is closed and drained in a routine manner. If the mucosa is inadvertently opened, it should be immediately closed with 3–0 polypropylene sutures in a simple interrupted pattern.

Recurrence of postsurgical cicatricial stricture after esophagomyotomy is slow to develop, with clinical signs occurring weeks or months after the operation. Conservative treatment (a change from hay to a complete pelleted diet) may be all that is necessary to resolve recurrent obstructions. A postsurgical stricture that occurs long after the original operation is usually due to mature, nonresilient cicatrix and may not respond to dilatation. If surgery is necessary, the surgeon should not hesitate to perform a second esophagomyotomy; however, early surgical reintervention in a stenotic area of the esophagus prior to allowing the acute inflammation of the previous surgery to subside greatly increases the propensity for restricture. If such is the case, a more hazardous procedure may have to be selected to eventually correct the problem.

Partial Resection

Longitudinal esophagomyotomy combined with mucosal resection will provide relief of stricture caused by esophageal rings or webs and annular stenosis of all muscle layers. Performed under general anesthesia, this procedure is indicated when the cicatrix involves the mucosa and prevents passage of a nasogastric tube

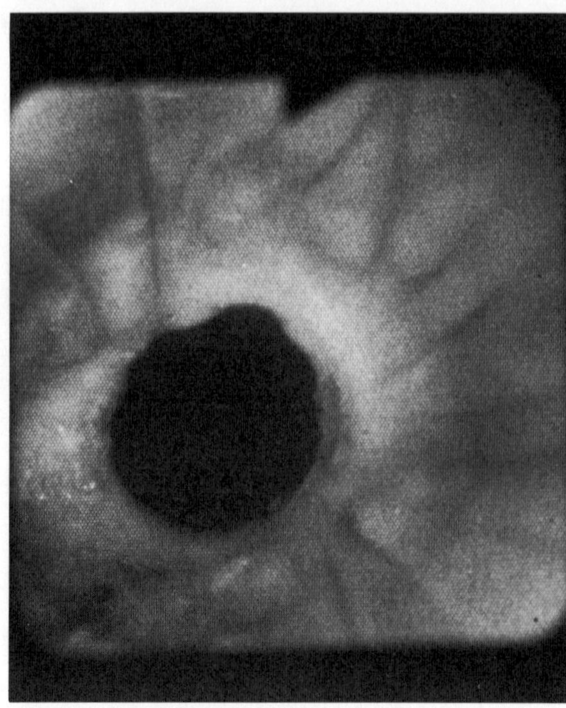

Figure 55–2. Endoscopic appearance of an esophageal web (stricture) that developed after feed impaction that had caused a circumferential ulcer.

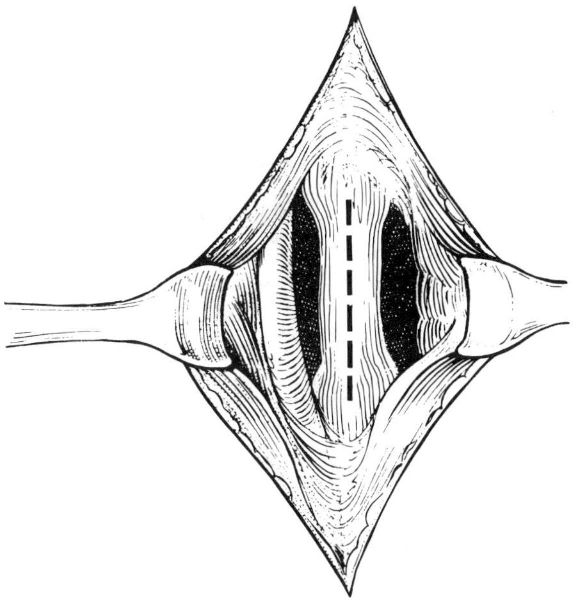

A

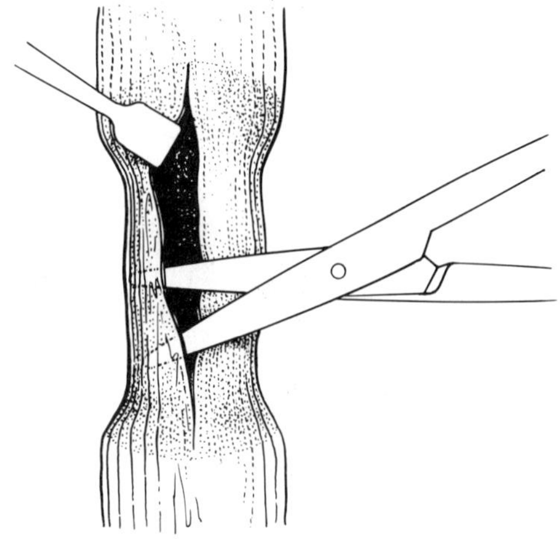

B

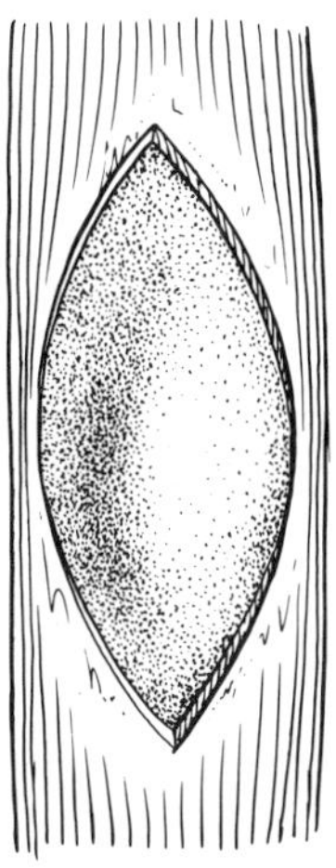

C

Figure 55–3. Esophagomyotomy. **A.** The ventral wall of the esophagus in the area of the stricture is exposed after abaxial retraction of the trachea (right). The *dashed line* represents the direction of the incision, which is made only through the stricture to the level of the mucosa. **B.** The outer muscular layer (which may in fact be only firm scar tissue in the area of the stricture) is separated from the mucosa around the entire circumference of the esophagus using scissors. **C.** The release of the mucosa from the strictured external layer should result in near-normal diameter of the esophagus. Sutures are not placed in the esophagus.

following myotomy. Antibiotics should be initiated preoperatively and maintained for 6 to 10 days after surgery.

The esophagus is exposed and incised as previously described for esophagomyotomy. A longitudinal incision is made through the mucosa that is long enough to permit identification of the diseased segment. The mucosal scar is separated by sharp dissection from normal or diseased muscle layers. Circumferential incisions are made at the cranial and caudal edges of the mucosal cicatrix and it is removed, leaving the muscular tube intact (Fig. 55–4).

If the cut edges of the mucosa can be brought into apposition without undue tension, they are apposed by three 3–0 polypropylene simple continuous sutures with the knots tied in the lumen. When mucosal rings or webs are the cause of the stenosis, the normal esophageal muscle should be apposed over the mucosal anastomosis, but in the case of an annular stenosis that involves the entire esophageal wall, the muscularis

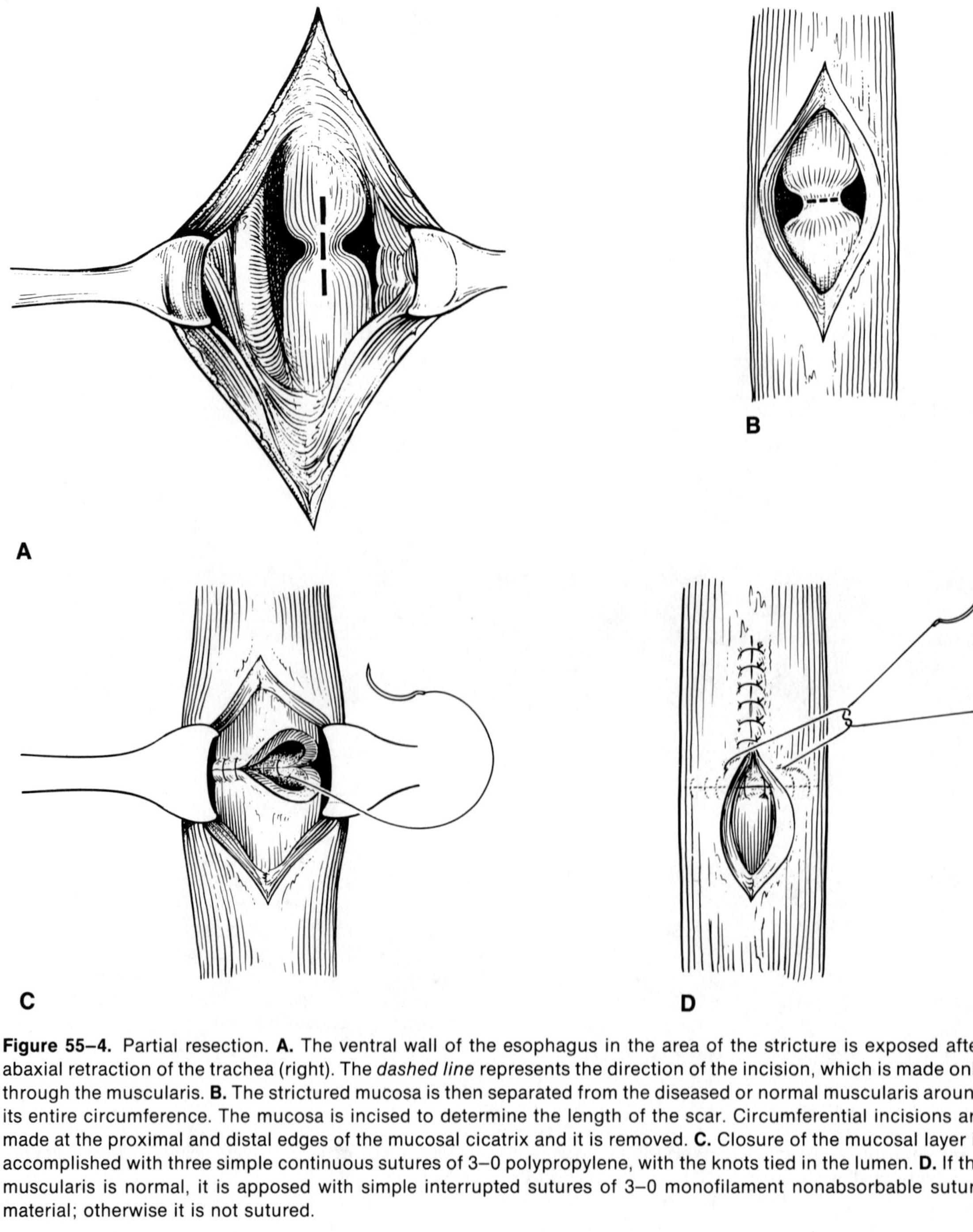

Figure 55–4. Partial resection. **A.** The ventral wall of the esophagus in the area of the stricture is exposed after abaxial retraction of the trachea (right). The *dashed line* represents the direction of the incision, which is made only through the muscularis. **B.** The strictured mucosa is then separated from the diseased or normal muscularis around its entire circumference. The mucosa is incised to determine the length of the scar. Circumferential incisions are made at the proximal and distal edges of the mucosal cicatrix and it is removed. **C.** Closure of the mucosal layer is accomplished with three simple continuous sutures of 3–0 polypropylene, with the knots tied in the lumen. **D.** If the muscularis is normal, it is apposed with simple interrupted sutures of 3–0 monofilament nonabsorbable suture material; otherwise it is not sutured.

should not be sutured. A drain is placed next to the esophagus and the approach incision is closed.

If space permits, tube feeding through an esophagostomy placed through a separate incision caudal to the stricture is ideal. When this is not possible, frequent feeding of small quantities of soft food may begin 48 hours after surgery and should be continued for 10 days before normal roughage is offered to the patient.

When the stricture is extensive and the mucosa cannot be sutured, regeneration within the muscle tube will readily occur. The muscularis may be sutured if it is healthy or left open if only scar tissue remains. Spontaneous healing will be aided if esophagostomy tube feeding (located closer to the stomach than the operative site) is used. When the stricture is located too close to the thoracic inlet to permit placement of a separate esophagostomy incision, the tube may be inserted directly through the stricture site. Recurrence of stricture following this procedure may be an indication for esophagomyotomy or an esophagostomy tube placed through the stricture.

Patch Grafting

An extensive cervical esophageal stricture produced by annular stenosis of the entire wall may preclude successful repair by techniques previously described. The diameter of the equine esophageal lumen can be increased by using a graft of the sternocephalicus muscle.

Antibiotics should be given preoperatively and maintained for 6 to 10 days after surgery. Under general anesthesia, a ventral midline or lateral approach to the esophagus is made, and depending on location of the defect and the approach used, the brachiocephalic or sternocephalic muscle will serve as donor for the graft. With a nasogastric tube passed to the level of the stenosis, a longitudinal incision is made through the muscularis from a point 3 cm caudal to and extending 3 cm cranial to the stricture. The mucosa-submucosa is sharply incised and the nasogastric tube is passed into the stomach. A caudal portion of the muscle belly of the brachiocephalicus or sternocephalicus is mobilized by blunt separation of muscle fibers. The strip of muscle should maintain its cranial and caudal attachments and should be freely movable so as not to exert tension on the closure when the patient's head and neck are moved. The graft should be wide enough to appreciably increase the lumen of the esophagus.

The edges of the mucosa-submucosa are sutured to the muscle graft using 3–0 interrupted through-and-through polypropylene mattress sutures, and the edges of the muscularis are sutured to the graft with 3–0 simple interrupted sutures of monofilament polypropylene. Preplacement of mattress sutures and closure of both layers on one side of the esophageal defect at a time will facilitate the repair. The nasogastric tube should be removed before the second edge is closed. Suction drains are placed next to the esophagus and the approach incision is closed.

POSTOPERATIVE CARE

When an esophagomyotomy has been performed without entering the esophageal lumen, frequent feeding of small quantities of soft feed may be necessary if a prestenotic dilatation is present prior to surgery. When this dilatation is no longer recognized radiographically, normal feeding may be resumed.

Following resection with primary closure or patch grafting, extraoral alimentation is preferred for 10 days (by esophagostomy if space allows, or by intravenous feeding), but soft foods may be given as early as 48 hours if salivary leakage has not occurred. An indwelling nasogastric tube should be avoided because it will provide a stimulus for salivation and increase the incidence of fistula formation. Endoscopic and radiographic examinations of the esophagus should be performed 30 and 60 days after surgery.

PROGNOSIS AND SPECIAL CONSIDERATIONS

Esophagomyotomy has a favorable prognosis for successful treatment and is seldom life threatening. The procedure may even be repeated with success if restricture develops. However, the second esophagomyotomy should be delayed for 45 days after the initial surgery, if possible. This delay may permit enough dilation to occur from feeding to make the second surgery unnecessary.

When the esophageal lumen is entered surgically during correction of a stricture (i.e., resection or grafting), some dehiscence and its associated complications are to be expected (see Chapter 54). Most certainly, some early stricture formation will occur. If possible, this should be treated medically as previously described (with nonsteroidal anti-inflammatory drugs and a soft diet following removal of the esophagostomy tube) for at least 60 days. Any indication of a developing phlegmon should be aggressively treated by opening the approach incision and lavaging the periesophageal tissues.

The prognosis for life when the esophageal lumen is invaded to correct a stricture is guarded. The surgeon should expect complications and be willing to pursue multiple surgeries and intensive aftercare.

BIBLIOGRAPHY

Craig D, Todhunter R: Surgical repair of an esophageal stricture in a horse. *Vet Surg* 1987;16:251–254.

Derksen FJ, Stick JA: Resection and anastomosis of esophageal stricture in a foal. *Equine Pract* 1983;5:17–20.

Hoffer RE, Barber SM, Kallfelz FL, et al: Esophageal patch grafting as a treatment for esophageal stricture in a horse. *J Am Vet Med Assoc* 1977;171:350–354.

Nixon AJ, Aanes WA, Nelson AW, Messer NT: Esophagomyotomy for relief of an intrathoracic esophageal stricture in a horse. *J Am Vet Med Assoc* 1983;183:794–796.

Steward KA, Reinertson EL: Congenital esophageal stricture in a pony foal. *Mod Vet Pract* 1983;64:753–754.

Stick JA: Diseases affecting the esophagus, in Mayhew IG, Merritt, AM, Colohan PT, Moore JN (eds): *Equine Medicine and Surgery,* ed 4. (in press).

Stick JA: Surgery of the esophagus. *Vet Clin North Am Large Anim Pract* 1982;4:33–59.

Todhunter RJ, Stick JA, Slocumbe RF: Comparison of three feeding techniques after esophageal mucosal resection and anastomosis in the horse. *Cornell Vet* 1986;76:16–29.

Todhunter RJ, Stick JA, Trotter GW, Boles C: Medical management of esophageal stricture in seven horses. *J Am Vet Med Assoc* 1984;185:784–787.

Wagner PC, Rantanen NW: Myotomy as a treatment for esophageal stricture in a horse. *Equine Pract* 1980;2:40–45.

56 Esophageal Diverticulum

John A. Stick

Diverticula of the esophagus in horses only occasionally cause esophageal dysfunction. These diverticula are usually acquired lesions that result either from contraction of periesophageal fibrous scar tissue, causing outward traction and tenting of all layers of the esophageal wall (traction or true diverticulum), or from the protrusion of mucosa and submucosa through a defect in the esophageal musculature (pulsion or false diverticulum).

A traction diverticulum commonly develops at the site of an esophagostomy or of a surgical or traumatic wound of the esophagus that is allowed to heal by second intention. A traction diverticulum may also follow penetration of the esophageal lumen (traumatic or surgical) where leakage of saliva has caused inflammation or an abscess. Pulsion diverticula are reportedly caused by fluctuations in esophageal intraluminal pressure and overstretch damage to esophageal muscle fibers by impacted feedstuffs. A more probable cause in the horse is external trauma to the cervical area.

DIAGNOSIS

Diverticula in the cervical esophagus should be considered whenever there is enlargement in the neck that results in dysphagia and the nasogastric tube can be passed. On barium swallow esophagograms, traction diverticula are spherical and have a wide neck (Fig. 56–1), whereas pulsion diverticula will be flasklike in configuration, with a narrow neck (Fig. 56–2). Differentiation of these two types of diverticula can be aided by additional contrast techniques that distend the esophageal lumen and outline the opening into the evagination. Esophagoscopy will also define the relative size of the opening of a diverticulum (Fig. 56–3).

A traction diverticulum, even when quite large, produces few clinical symptoms and seldom requires treatment. A pulsion diverticulum, however, has a tendency to enlarge progressively so that risk of obstruction and rupture increases with time. Surgical repair is indicated.

SURGERY

Repair of pulsion diverticulum can be accomplished by: (*a*) diverticulectomy with resection of the mucosal-submucosal sac followed by reconstruction of the mucosa-submucosa and muscularis, or (*b*) inversion of the mucosal-submucosal sac with reconstruction of the muscular layer. Diverticulectomy should be used when the mucosal sac is very large and the neck of the diverticulum very narrow. There is a single report of the repair of an apparently congenital esophageal diverticulum using this technique. However, mucosal inversion is the preferred technique because it decreases the chance of postoperative leakage, infection, or fistula and does not appear to predispose to postoperative obstruction.

Mucosal Inversion

The esophagus is exposed and the diverticulum and defect in the muscularis are identified by careful dissection (Fig. 56–4). Inadvertent perforation of the mucosa-submucosa should be immediately repaired. The

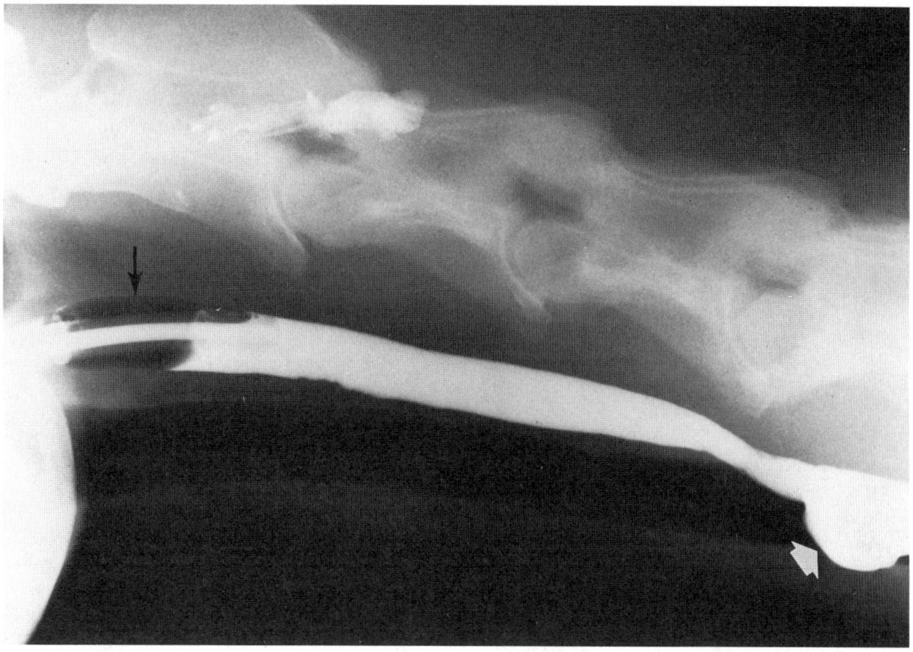

Figure 56–1. Lateral contrast radiograph demonstrates a traction diverticulum (*white arrow*). Barium is administered under pressure through a cuffed nasogastric tube (*black arrow*) used to prevent reflux of barium into the pharynx. Note the wide neck characteristic of a traction diverticulum.

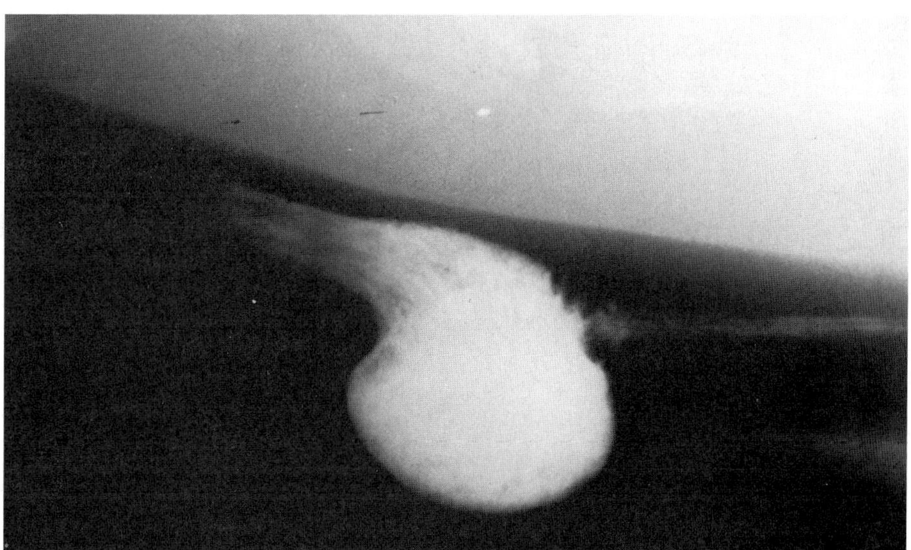

Figure 56–2. Barium swallow (grain mixed with barium powder) demonstrates a pulsion (false) diverticulum. Note the narrowing at the neck of the diverticulum resulting in a flasklike configuration. (Photograph courtesy of R.P. Hackett, Cornell University.)

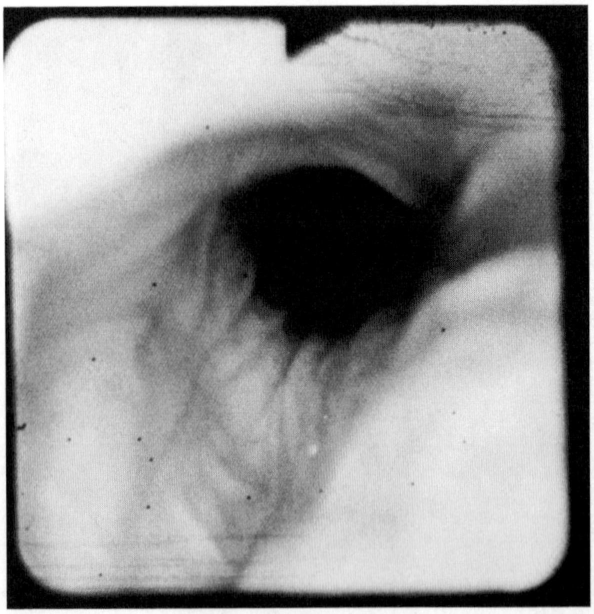

Figure 56–3. Endoscopic photograph of the esophageal lumen demonstrates the wide neck of a traction diverticulum (ventral). This horse did not have signs of "choke."

edges of the muscular defect should be débrided back to healthy-appearing tissue (Fig. 56–4). The sac is inverted and the edges of the muscularis are apposed with simple interrupted sutures of 3–0 polypropylene in a manner designed to avoid undue tension on the closure and prevent stenosis of the esophageal diameter.

POSTOPERATIVE CARE

Postoperatively, feeding should consist of soft foods for 4 to 6 days. Antibiotic therapy is left to the discretion of the surgeon.

PROGNOSIS

The prognosis for surgical repair of a pulsion diverticulum is favorable and should not become life threatening, unless the mucosal sac becomes so large that diverticulectomy is necessary.

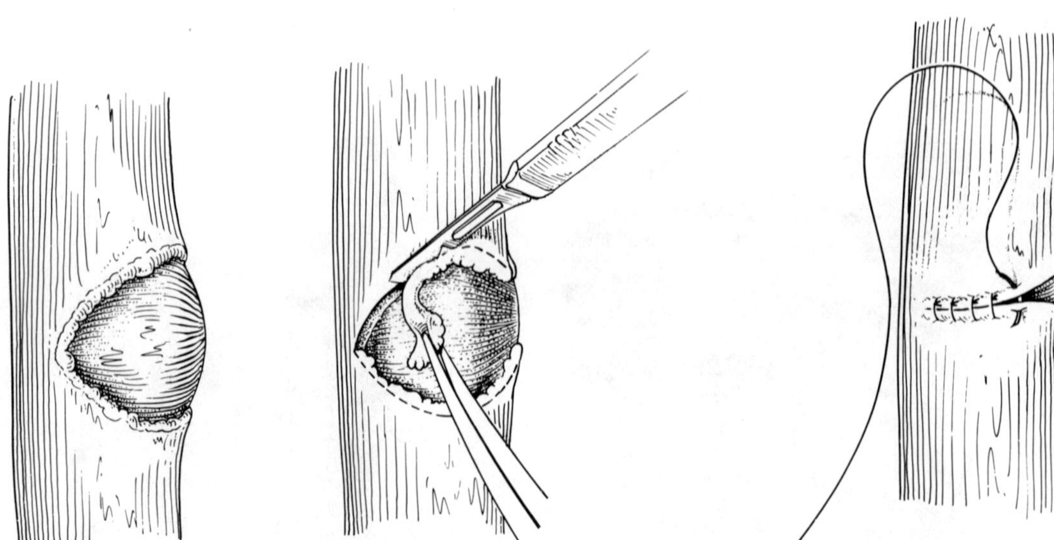

A B C

Figure 56–4. Mucosal inversion. A. The pulsion diverticulum of the esophagus is exposed and the muscular defect is identified using careful dissection to avoid entering the lumen. Shown is a small mucosal sac after food had been massaged from the lumen. B. The edges of the muscularis are débrided back to healthy-appearing tissue. C. The mucosal sac is inverted and the edges of the muscularis are apposed with simple interrupted sutures of 3–0 monofilament nonabsorbable suture material.

BIBLIOGRAPHY

Aanes WA: The diagnosis and surgical repair of diverticulum of the esophagus. *Proc Am Assoc Equine Pract* 1975; pp 211–221.

Haasjes C: Esophageal diverticulum. *J Am Vet Med Assoc* 1945;109:278.

Hackett RP, Dyer RM, Hoffer RE: Surgical correction of esophageal diverticulum in a horse. *J Am Vet Med Assoc* 1978;173:998–1000.

57 Abdominal Approaches and Complications of Celiotomy

Susan L. Fubini

APPROACHES TO THE ABDOMEN

Access to the abdomen of the horse is provided by ventral, flank, and vaginal incisions (Fig. 57–1). When deciding on the best approach, considerations include: the probable location of the surgical problem; the facilities, personnel, and equipment available; the nature of the patient; and the surgeon's preference.

Ventral approaches to the abdomen require general anesthesia, and, therefore, specialized equipment and facilities. It is desirable, although not essential to have a mechanical ventilator. Speed and efficiency are crucial when performing surgery on the anesthetized horse with an acute abdominal problem. Good technical support is a tremendous asset. In general, equine surgeons are most familiar with the ventral midline celiotomy because it provides the best opportunity for manipulative and therapeutic procedures. However, a standing flank celiotomy is possible in the tractable adult horse, and provides access for abdominal exploration and limited manipulative procedures. This approach should be considered in large-breed horses that are difficult to anesthetize and position and that are prone to develop postoperative myositis.

Ventral Approaches

Ventral Midline Celiotomy. The ventral midline incision provides the greatest exposure and access to most of the abdominal viscera. The horse is positioned in dorsal recumbency. In males, the penis is replaced in the prepuce so it is excluded from the surgical field. A laparotomy sponge is packed into the prepuce and the preputial orifice is closed either with sutures or with towel clamps.

The ventral abdomen is widely clipped and prepared for aseptic surgery. A skin incision is made starting at the umbilicus and extending craniad. The length of the incision will vary with the surgical lesion but will usually range from 25 to 30 cm. This can be extended if necessary (e.g., to exteriorize the distended large colon). The subcutaneous tissues are sharply incised and hemostasis is established, either with electrocoagulation or ligation. The linea alba, a narrow fibrous raphe extending from xiphoid to pubis, is carefully incised. The incision is best started at the umbilicus, where the linea alba is easily palpable. The surgeon should carefully avoid deviation from the linea alba as the incision is extended. Retroperitoneal fat is dissected bluntly or removed. The peritoneum is grasped with thumb forceps and a small hole is made with scissors. The round ligament that runs in the peritoneum is usually just beneath the incision and is easily identified, elevated, and incised. The incision in the peritoneum is extended bluntly or with scissors.

At the conclusion of surgery, the peritoneum may or may not be closed. Advantages of closure include retention of intestines during closure of the abdominal tunic and the formation of a seal to prevent leakage of peritoneal fluid into the incision postoperatively. Closure is by a simple continuous suture pattern with a synthetic absorbable suture. However, the peritoneum will heal without closure.

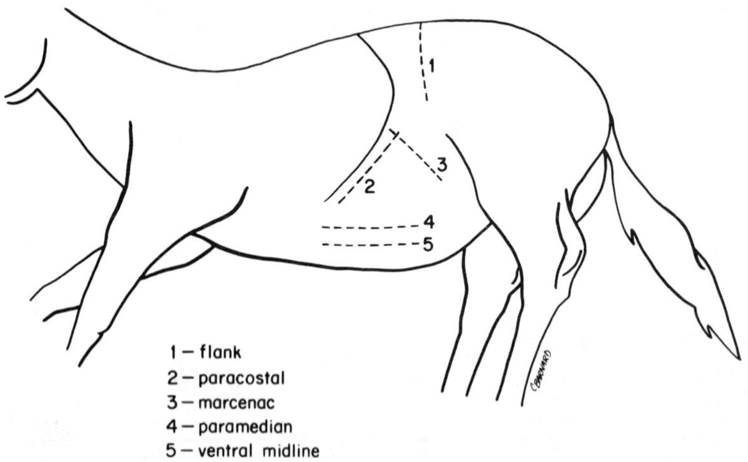

Figure 57–1. A schematic diagram identifying the commonly used approaches to the abdomen of the horse.

The incision in the linea alba can be closed with any acceptable suture pattern, including simple interrupted, simple continuous, and near-far–far-near patterns. Absorbable or nonabsorbable suture material can be used. The latter maintains its strength for longer periods of time but runs more of a risk of forming suture sinuses. This is particularly a problem with multifilament or braided nonabsorbable sutures. Subcutaneous tissues are closed in a continuous pattern using an absorbable suture. Skin can be apposed with a nonabsorbable suture or with skin staples. Popular current absorbable suture material for abdominal closure includes polyglactin 910 (Vicryl; Ethicon Inc), polyglycolic acid (Dexon; Davis and Geck, Inc) and polydioxanone (PDS; Ethicon Inc). Monofilament nonabsorbable sutures that are commonly used include polypropylene (Prolene; Ethicon Inc) and nylon (Ethicon Inc).

A stent bandage may be useful to keep the incision dry during recovery. After surgery the horse should be confined to a stall for 2 weeks. Controlled walking can begin at this time, and the horse can be turned out 8 to 12 weeks after surgery.

The greatest advantage of the ventral midline incision is that the majority of the mobile intestinal tract can be exteriorized. This includes the jejunum and the majority of the ileum, cecum, right and left colon, and small colon. The pylorus, duodenum, ileocecal junction, base of the cecum and right dorsal colon, and transverse colon can be palpated in situ but cannot be exteriorized. The ventral midline incision also can be readily extended past the umbilicus and cranially up to the xiphoid if additional exposure is necessary. A ventral midline celiotomy has been combined with median sternotomy and incision of the diaphragm to achieve access to an obstruction at the cardia in a foal.

Some authors suggest that there is a greater risk of herniation with this incision compared to a flank or paramedian incision. Their hypothesis is that because the fibers within the linea alba are continuations of the sheaths of the three abdominal muscles, transverse tension is placed upon the linea alba sutures.

Ventral Paramedian Approach. The ventral paramedian approach can be performed either to the right or to the left of the linea alba. The horse is anesthetized and positioned in dorsal recumbency. A 20- to 25-cm skin incision is made parallel to and 6 to 8 cm lateral to the linea alba. Subcutaneous tissues are incised, exposing the external sheath of the rectus abdominus muscle. This is incised and the rectus muscle fibers are separated by dissection. The internal rectus sheath is incised, retroperitoneal fat is dissected, and the peritoneum is opened.

To close the paramedian incision, the internal rectus sheath is sutured with an interrupted or continuous pattern. This layer is thin and easily tears. The rectus muscle is apposed to decrease dead space. The external rectus sheath is the strongest component of the closure and should be closed with absorbable or nonabsorbable suture with a simple interrupted or simple continuous suture pattern. Subcutaneous tissues and skin are closed as described for the ventral midline incision.

The caudal ventral paramedian approach is useful for removing retained abdominal testicles and to provide access to the caudal abdomen, especially in the male horse. It has been suggested that healing of a paramedian incision is superior to that of a ventral midline incision. Intact fibers of the rectus abdominus muscle act as a "sling" to support the viscera and dissipate tension on the external rectus sheath. However, the approach and closure of paramedian incisions are more time consuming than those of the ventral midline celiotomy. There may also be considerable hemorrhage encountered when incising the rectus muscle, the exposure is limited to one side of the abdomen, and it is difficult to extend the incision.

Inguinal Approach. An approach over the inguinal canal is used for cryptorchidectomy and to repair inguinal or scrotal hernias. Again, general anesthesia and positioning of the horse in dorsal recumbency are required. The abdomen is prepared as previously described.

An 8- to 10-cm skin incision is made over the superficial inguinal ring. The subcutaneous tissues are sharply incised and, in an effort to avoid the large external pudendal artery and vein, blunt dissection is used to expose the superficial inguinal ring. When a hernia is present, the hernial sac (parietal vaginal tunic) is carefully incised, the contents inspected, and the appropriate procedures performed. Closure will depend on the surgeon's preference. Commonly, the spermatic cord is twisted, ligated, and transfixed to the borders of the inguinal canal. The superficial inguinal ring is closed with size 2 suture in an acceptable pattern. Subcutaneous tissues and skin are closed as previously described, being careful to avoid major vessels.

The inguinal approach permits very limited access to the abdomen. If there is strangulated bowel present in an inguinal hernia, it is usually necessary to perform a ventral midline celiotomy to manipulate the affected bowel.

Transverse Abdominal Approach. A transverse abdominal approach is used occasionally for exposure of viscera located within the pelvic cavity, such as for direct repair of a rectal tear. The horse is anesthetized and placed in dorsal recumbency. Because of the interference of the viscera with visualization of the caudal abdomen, it is helpful to elevate the horse's hindquarters.

The incision is centered approximately 3 cm caudal to the umbilicus and is contained laterally by the fold of the flank. The incision is extended through the subcutaneous tissue and the external sheath of the rectus abdominus muscle. The fibers of the rectus abdominus muscle are then incised transversely to their long axis. Because of the numerous tendinous intersections uniting the rectus muscle to its sheath, the muscle does not retract from the surgeon's view. Incision of the muscle does result in significant hemorrhage that must be controlled. The incision is then continued through the internal rectus sheath into the abdomen. Closure is achieved by first applying traction on the horse's tail to relieve tension on the incision. The internal sheath and the rectus abdominus muscle are closed in separate layers using a simple continuous pattern. The external rectus sheath is apposed with a simple continuous or interrupted pattern. The remainder of the incision is closed as previously described. Limited experience with this procedure suggests that the possibility of incisional hernias is greater than with the ventral midline incision.

Flank Approaches

Flank Approach. A right or left flank incision can be performed on the standing animal using local anesthesia or with the animal in lateral recumbency using general anesthesia. If a standing approach is chosen, the area is desensitized with local anesthetic administered in an "inverted *L*" pattern. A 20-cm skin incision is made 6 cm distal to the transverse processes of the lumbar vertebrae and between the last rib and the tuber coxae. The incision can be confined to the paralumbar fossa, or extended into the midflank region if necessary. To perform a "grid" incision, the external and internal abdominal oblique muscles and the transversus abdominus muscle are divided in the direction of their fibers. To create a larger incision, the external abdominal oblique muscle can be incised and the deeper muscles divided in the direction of their fibers ("modified grid" incision). The retroperitoneal fat is bluntly separately and the peritoneum incised.

Each muscle layer is closed individually. It is not necessary to close the peritoneum. If the external abdominal oblique muscle is incised, it may be advantageous to close it in a simple interrupted pattern. The subcutaneous tissues and skin are closed routinely. A stent bandage is secured in place for 48 to 72 hours. This may help to dissipate some of the tension on the skin sutures. After surgery, the horse should be confined to a stall for 2 weeks. At that time, controlled walking can be initiated. After 1 month, the horse can be turned out.

This approach permits removal of abdominal cryptorchid testicles and ovariectomy using an ecraseur. It will allow a limited exploration of the abdomen. The approach through the right flank allows palpation of the terminal duodenum, the jejunum, the ileocecal junction, the cecum, and the middle parts of the right ventral and small colon. A left flank approach exposes the jejunum, ileum, spleen, pelvic flexure, and part of the small colon and rectum.

The flank approach is useful, especially for diagnostic purposes, when there is reluctance to subject the patient to general anesthesia. However, exposure and room for manipulation are limited, and fractious or painful horses are reluctant to remain standing. The anatomy from this approach is less familiar to most equine surgeons, and these incisions are prone to seroma formation, which may delay wound healing.

Marcenac Approach. The Marcenac approach is a low oblique flank incision that is popular in Europe for cesarean sections. Use of this approach in the standing animal has been reported. More frequently the horse is anesthetized and positioned in lateral recumbency. The skin is incised on the right or left side of the abdomen from the costal arch in a caudoventral direction to reach the inside of the fold of the flank. The abdominal tunic is transected and the external abdominal oblique muscle is split in the direction of its fibers. The internal abdominal oblique muscle, which is aponeurotic at this level, and the transverse abdominus muscles are incised. The rectus muscle is retracted ventrally, the retroperitoneal fat is bluntly separated, and the peritoneum incised. Each layer is closed individually.

Paracostal Approach. The paracostal incision also provides access to the abdomen through the low flank. This incision traverses the flank in the cranioventral direction, and parallels the costal arch. The skin incision is made 10 cm from the last rib. At this site, the external abdominal oblique muscle is primarily aponeurotic, whereas the internal abdominal oblique is muscular dorsally and aponeurotic ventrally. These muscles are incised and the incision is extended through the transversus abdominis, retroperitoneal fat, and peritoneum. Each layer is closed individually. Abdominal exposure is limited. A right paracostal celiotomy has been used to perform a cecotomy or cecal resection.

Seventeenth or Eighteenth Rib Resection. Access to the ileocecal region, the base of the cecum, and the right dorsal colon can be achieved by a right-sided 17th and/or 18th rib resection. The animal is anesthetized and restrained in left lateral recumbency. A 25-cm incision extending from just below the epaxial musculature to the costochondral junction is made over the rib to be excised. The incision is continued through subcutaneous tissues, intercostal muscles, and the periosteum of the rib. The periosteum is elevated, and the rib is transected proximally with the use of a Gigli wire; distally it is sharply disarticulated at the costochondral junction. The peritoneum is incised as described previously. Closure involves apposition of the periosteum and intercostal muscles in one layer, followed by each muscle layer, subcutaneous tissues, and skin.

This approach has the advantage of allowing access to the ileocecal junction and base of the cecum and right dorsal colon. However, opening and closing the abdomen is more difficult and time consuming. Furthermore, the gastrointestinal anatomy from this approach is less familiar to most equine surgeons.

Transthoracic Approach. There is one report in the literature of using a transthoracic approach to gain access to the gastric cardia. This approach is similar to the 17th or 18th rib resection except that the left tenth rib is removed. The pleura is incised and a rib retractor used to aid visualization of the area. It is necessary to incise the left crus of the diaphragm to gain access to the stomach.

A transthoracic approach using a 16th rib resection has also been used to perform a splenectomy in horses. The approach is similar to a 17th or 18th rib resection except that, with resection of the 16th rib, the periosteum on the medial aspect of the rib is incised along with the endothoracic fascia and costal pleura. The edges of this incision are sutured to the underlying muscular part of the diaphragm using a 2–0 absorbable suture. This suture seals the pleural cavity from the surgical site. The diaphragm is then incised caudal and parallel to this suture line. Large (size 2) absorbable sutures are used to close the diaphragm and costal periosteum. The remainder of the closure is as described above for the 17th and 18th rib resections.

Transthoracic approaches have the disadvantage of invading another body cavity. Intermittent positive pressure ventilation is essential with this technique.

VAGINAL APPROACH

A dorsal colpotomy has been used to manipulate the small colon and pelvic flexure, but most commonly it is used to perform an ovariectomy (see Chapter 138).

COMPLICATIONS OF CELIOTOMY

Incisional complications of ventral midline celiotomy include swelling, suture sinuses, drainage, incisional infection, dehiscence, acute failure with evisceration, herniation, and hematoma within the rectus muscle. Some of these are of minor consequence while others are life threatening. Regardless, complications can result in increased postoperative care and delayed return of the horse to its normal function. Complications of the other abdominal incisions are similar. Flank incisions have a high incidence of seroma formation, which would need to be treated appropriately with drainage and local wound care. Careful wound closure with obliteration of dead space or use of negative pressure drains immediately postoperatively will avoid most of these fluid accumulations.

Patient Factors

Causative factors of wound disruption include those related to the patient and those related to the surgical procedure. Patient factors include metabolic state, nutritional status, duration of illness, and degree of intraabdominal pressure. Anemia and vitamin deficiency can delay wound healing, although these are rare in the horse with an acute abdominal crisis. More often horses will be treated with drugs such as flunixin meglumine, which can cause reduction in wound strength early in the postoperative period (7 to 10 days). Although not proven in horses, the combination of shock and inadequate nutrition during the postoperative period is suspected to cause poor wound healing and inadequate wound strength.

Surgical Factors

Surgical factors include the type of incision, the selection of suture material, the method of closure, the length of the surgery, and the degree of surgical trauma. Excess surgical trauma will cause increased incisional complications. Multiple procedures are more likely to result in incisional problems. Kobluk et al. reported that 28.6% of horses (20 of 70) that had undergone one celiotomy developed incisional problems, whereas 87.5% of horses (seven of eight) that had undergone two abdominal surgeries developed problems with the surgical wound.

Some of these problems can be prevented by careful surgical technique. It is important to avoid deviating from the midline when incising the linea alba so that there is no muscle interposed in the closure, and strict attention to hemostasis and proper placement of sutures will avoid unwanted seroma formation and tearing of the abdominal tunic, respectively. The type of suture material used can affect wound healing. Nonabsorbable materials are more likely to result in suture sinuses, particularly if there is contamination during the surgical procedure. Removal of the offending suture is usually necessary to resolve draining tracts. If it is difficult to appose the linea alba, penetrating towel clamps and/or mattress sutures may be useful, but the added stress and trauma to the abdominal tunic should be avoided whenever possible.

Most ventral abdominal incisions will swell to some degree, but most swelling is due to subcutaneous edema. Abdominal support bandages or corsets may help to control postoperative edema but are difficult to keep in place. They must be changed frequently to prevent drainage from being trapped next to the incision, and they often become saturated with urine when used on geldings and stallions. Swelling can usually be managed conservatively with exercise. The edema normally gravitates cranially on the abdomen and is absorbed over 2 to 3 weeks.

Incisional Drainage. Incisional drainage usually originates in the subcutaneous tissues. Most subcutaneous infections drain a thick, yellow-tinged exudate and will resolve after local treatment of drainage or skin suture removal. This includes removal of the most ventral skin sutures or staples. It may be necessary to establish several areas where the incision can drain. Flushing should be reserved for subcutaneous incisions only, carefully avoiding deeper tracts that may enter the abdominal cavity. Even though most of the drainage will resolve with local treatment, culture and sensitivity tests of drainage fluid should be performed. Antibiotic therapy may be necessary as indicated by fever, painful swelling, or continued drainage with increased inflammation despite local treatment. Most cases of incisional infection will resolve with drainage and use of broad-spectrum antibiotics or antibiotic combinations.

If there is a steady drip of clear yellow or serosanguinous fluid from the incision, this may be peritoneal fluid. A localized peritonitis could be present as a result of retrograde infection at the drainage site. Alternatively, peritonitis from the original lesion or the surgical procedure could be present, causing fluid to leak through the incision. In either case the peritonitis should be treated (see Chapter 74). Once drainage of peritoneal fluid is confirmed, incisional dehiscence must be suspected. The incision should be cleaned and palpated with a sterile gloved hand for any indication of dehiscence of the entire body wall closure. If there is dehiscence, reoperation should not be delayed. Although bandages or a corset can be used to support the incision, they will not prevent evisceration if the incision is failing acutely.

At surgery, the incision should be evaluated to determine the reason for the dehiscence. The four most common reasons are weakening of absorbable sutures, the suture breaking as a result of increased abdominal pressure or violent recovery, knot slippage, or tearing of the abdominal tunic as a result of infection or inflammation. If the abdominal tunic is not infected, and the sutures have not torn through the tissue, reapposing the linea alba may be adequate to promote primary healing. A secondary closure of infected abdominal incisions using through-and-through stainless steel is usually the most appropriate method of repair in cases of acute dehiscence. This technique allows adjustment of suture tension by untwisting the wires as the incision swells.

Herniation. Herniation of the abdominal wall (with subcutaneous and skin closures intact) is most commonly related to incisional infection, but other suggested causes include early strenuous postoperative exercise, suture material failure, failure to properly appose tissues, reduction of tissue strength as a result of infection or delayed rate of healing, and a violent recovery. Hernia formation is not usually evident until 1 to 2 months after surgery. The time frame for hernia repair will vary with each case. In most instances it is desirable to allow for maturation of the hernial ring prior to repair (3 to 6 months). Most hernial defects can be closed primarily by suturing. However, very large body wall defects may require the use of a prosthetic mesh, and repair should be delayed until the abdominal tunic is strong enough for the repair. Mesh should not be used unless absolutely necessary because of the problems that may be encountered with infection, prosthesis rejection or failure.

BIBLIOGRAPHY

Gibson KT, Curtis CR, Turner AS, McIlwraith CW, Aames WA, Stashak TS: Incisional hernias in the horse: incidence and predisposing factors. *Vet Surg* 1989;18:360–366.

Kobluk CN, Ducharme NG, Lumsden JH, Pascoe PJ, Arighi M, Horney FD, Hurtig M: Incisional complication rates in colic surgery and factors associated with their occurrence, in *Proceedings of the Second Equine Colic Research Symposium.* Veterinary Learning Systems, 1986;2:313–316.

McIlwraith CW: Complications of laparotomy incisions in the horse. *Proc Am Assoc Equine Pract* 1978; pp 209–218.

Peterson FB, Donawick WJ, Merritt AM, Raker CW, Reid CF, Rooney JR: Gastric stenosis in a horse. *J Am Vet Med Assoc* 1972;160:328–332.

Rigg DL, Reinertson EL, Buttrick ML: A technique for elective splenectomy of equidae using a transthoracic approach. *Vet Surg* 1987;16:389–391.

Schneider HL, McClure JR, Cho DY, Crawford MP: The effects of flunixin meglumine on early wound healing of abdominal incisions in ponies (abstr). *Vet Surg* 1987;16:101.

Swanick RA: The non-suturing of parietal peritoneum in abdominal surgery of the horse. *Vet Rec* 1973;93:328–335.

Tulleners EP, Donawick WJ: Secondary closure of infected abdominal incisions in cattle and horses. *J Am Vet Med Assoc* 1983;182:1377–1379.

Vaughan JT: Surgical management of abdominal crisis in the horse. *J Am Vet Med Assoc* 1972;161:1199–1212.

58 Upper Gastrointestinal Obstructions in Foals

James A. Orsini

Although gastric ulcers, duodenitis, and obstructions of the upper gastrointestinal tract occur with some regularity in foals, the specific etiology for these clinical problems remains unclear. A number of possibilities have been proposed, including stress and/or the use of nonsteroidal anti-inflammatory drugs. The vast majority of foals with signs compatible with "gastric ulcers" respond to symptomatic treatment with no recurrence of the disease. In some foals, however, the disease progresses and may ultimately result in esophageal obstruction, stomach wall abscessation, pyloric stenosis, and/or localized or generalized duodenal stricture complicated by obstruction of the common bile duct.

The cause of the gastroduodenal obstruction is believed to be gastritis and duodenitis, with chronic inflammation or wound contraction leading to fibrosis and stricture. No specific cause for the ulceration has been identified, although the action of gastric acid may play a role in sustaining inflammation.

DIAGNOSIS

Foals with signs of gastroduodenal obstruction are generally 4 days to 4 months old. Typically, a few days to several weeks before admission, affected foals were noted to exhibit fever, anorexia, depression, and diarrhea, and may have had elevated total white blood cell counts and/or high plasma fibrinogen concentrations. A number of these foals may have been treated with nonsteroidal anti-inflammatory drugs (phenylbutazone, flunixin meglumine) as part of the treatment for this initial episode of gastrointestinal disease. These drugs have often been administered for more than 1 day. Response to therapy for the initial gastrointestinal complaint is considered to be good.

Signs of gastroduodenal obstruction may include weakness, depression, anorexia, odontoprisis, salivation, frothing at the mouth, protrusion of the tongue, and spontaneous reflux of milk from the nares. Abdominal pain is most commonly noted after nursing. Passage of a nasogastric tube frequently results in reflux of milk, which at times may be sour and fetid. If the obstruction has been present for several days, megaesophagus containing milk and saliva, and aspiration pneumonia have been seen on survey radiographs taken of the caudal thorax and cranial portion of the abdomen. The plasma fibrinogen concentration is frequently elevated, but mean total white blood cell counts and serum sodium, potassium, calcium, chloride, and bicarbonate concentrations are usually within normal limits.

A tentative diagnosis of gastroduodenal obstruction is based on history, presenting signs, physical examination, and peritoneal fluid analysis, but the diagnosis is confirmed by contrast radiography. Peritoneal fluid, when obtained for analysis, should be within normal limits unless perforation of the stomach or duodenum has occurred.

Standing right lateral survey radiographs of the caudal thorax and cranial abdomen should be taken first. These will help to determine the location of the obstruction (cardia versus pylorus and duodenum). When obstruction has occurred at the cardia an enlarged and fluid-filled esophagus will be seen on the survey radiographs, and the stomach and intestines will be free of excessive gas and fluid. When an obstruction of short duration occurs at or distal to the pylorus, the stomach will be greatly distended with fluid and gas but the intestines will be empty. With a long-standing pyloric or duodenal obstruction, megaesophagus will be present as well.

After the stomach and, if necessary, the esophagus are drained of fluid and gas, a stomach tube is positioned in the caudal thoracic esophagus and barium sulfate (E-Z-Pake; E-Z-EM Co, Inc) (10 mL/kg) is administered. Sequential radiographs should be taken during the barium administration and at 10, 20, 30, and 60 minutes following barium administration.

If the obstruction is at the level of the cardia, there will be dilatation of the esophagus and retention of the barium in the thoracic esophagus. When the obstruction is at or beyond the pylorus, stomach motility will be present, but at 60 minutes no barium will be seen to have passed from the stomach. Because no barium passes the pylorus, it is impossible to differentiate obstruction of the pylorus from obstruction in the duodenum or both.

Great care is required in interpreting contrast radiographs. Retention of barium in the esophagus or stomach 1 hour after administration, especially if accompanied by fluid- or gas-filled intestines, does not necessarily indicate gastric or duodenal obstruction. Obstruction at the ileum can cause failure of passage of barium if the small intestine is already filled. Megaesophagus does not always indicate obstruction at the cardia. Chronic stomach distention and pyloric and duodenal obstruction is associated with megaesophagus as well.

Gastritis, gastric abscessation, and ulcers may be present at the time of admission and are often of sufficient severity to contribute to the obstruction. Cholangitis and cholangiohepatitis can be presumed to be present on admission based on clinical evidence at surgery and upon laboratory assessment of hepatic function (total bilirubin, direct bilirubin, aspartate aminotransferase, gamma glutamyl transferase). Additional evidence of cholangiohepatitis can be based on the clinical evidence seen at surgery and the finding of barium-stained bile ducts observed during the postoperative standing right lateral contrast abdominal radiographs. Pancreatitis can be recognized at surgery by edema, swelling, and discoloration of the pancreas. Aspiration pneumonia may be present on admission, especially if the obstruction has been present for a sufficient period of time to cause megaesophagus and gastroesophageal reflux.

SURGERY

Before surgery, feed and access to the dam for nursing are withheld for several hours. A nasogastric tube is passed as required to relieve stomach distention. Based on serum electrolyte concentrations, hemogram, and total protein values, intravenous crystalloids containing dextrose are administered and continued into the postoperative period. In anticipation of peritoneal contamination during surgery and to treat aspiration pneumonia when present, foals are treated prophylactically with parenteral penicillin (Pen G Potassium, 22,000 U/kg twice daily) and gentamicin (2.2 mg/kg four times a day) or amikacin (6.6 mg/kg three times a day). Antibiotic therapy is continued until physical and laboratory findings indicate no further need for antimicrobial administration or signs of toxicity become apparent. A nasogastric tube is positioned before anesthesia is induced.

Induction of anesthesia is preceded by the preoperative administration of xylazine (1.1 mg/kg intramuscularly), meperidine hydrochloride (3.3 mg/kg intramuscularly), or acetylpromazine (0.04 to 0.05 mg/kg intravenously). Anesthesia is usually induced in these young foals by inhalation of halothane, enflurane, or isoflurane in oxygen through a face mask.

In the older foal, 5% guaifenesin combined with thiopental or ketamine can be used for induction. Foals are generally maintained on halothane or isoflurane and oxygen delivered by a semi–closed circle system anesthesia apparatus. Ventilation is assisted with a pressure-sensitive, volume-limited ventilator.

A cranial ventral midline celiotomy is performed and the stomach and duodenum are examined. To provide for additional exposure of the cranial abdomen, the large colon is exteriorized as completely as possible and covered with moist towels. One of the seven following surgical procedures may be required, depending on the site of the gastroduodenal obstruction (Fig. 58–1).

Esophagogastrostomy

Esophagogastrostomy is used to bypass an obstruction at the cardiac sphincter. Median sternotomy and transection of the diaphragm are performed. Dorsal and ventral branches of the vagus nerve are dissected free, and the thoracic esophagus is occluded with a Doyen intestinal clamp. The esophagus is transected just proximal to a stapled closure of the terminal esophagus. A disposable curved EEA (end-to-end anastomosis) Auto-Suture instrument (United States Surgical Corp) is inserted through a stab incision located cranial to the origin of the greater omentum in the stomach. The instrument is advanced until it is firmly in place against the mucosal surface of the stomach at the planned gastric stoma site (approximately 6 to 8 cm to the right of the cardia). A stab incision is made over the tip of the instrument to permit attachment of the anvil nose cone, which is advanced into the esophagus. A purse string is placed on the distal end of the esophagus and tied tightly around the center rod (Fig. 58–2). The EEA instrument is discharged to complete the end-to-end inverting circular esophagogastrostomy. The donor ring, removed from the EEA instrument after discharging, is checked for a complete mucosal ring. If the anastomotic ring lacks mucosa-to-mucosa contact in its entirety, the stapled anastomosis should be oversewn with interrupted Lembert sutures of 2–0 surgical gut (Chromic gut; Ethicon Inc). After removal of the EEA stapling instrument, the gastric stab incision is closed with a TA-55 Auto-Suture stapling instrument (United States Surgical Corp) and the wound is oversewn with 2–0 surgical gut in an interrupted Lembert pattern.

Gastroduodenostomy

Gastroduodenostomy is performed for correction of pyloric stenosis. A side-to-side gastroduodenostomy is performed on the greater curvature of the stomach using 2–0 surgical gut in a three-tier method of anastomosis (Fig. 58–3). The anastomosis is begun with a

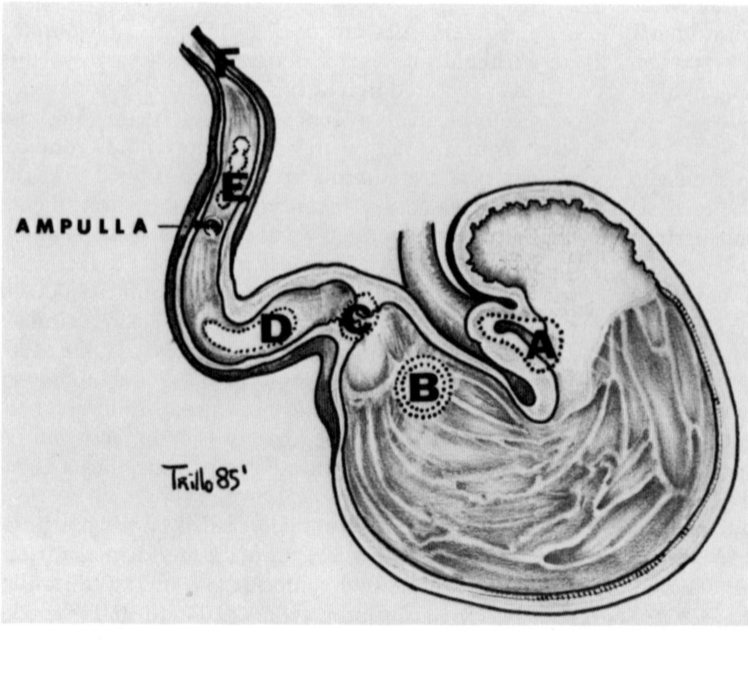

Figure 58–1. Sites of primary gastroduodenal obstruction. *A*, esophageal obstruction at cardia; *B*, antral abscess; *C*, pyloric stenosis; *D*, duodenal stenosis above hepaticopancreatic ampulla; *E*, duodenal stenosis beyond ampulla; *F*, generalized duodenitis.

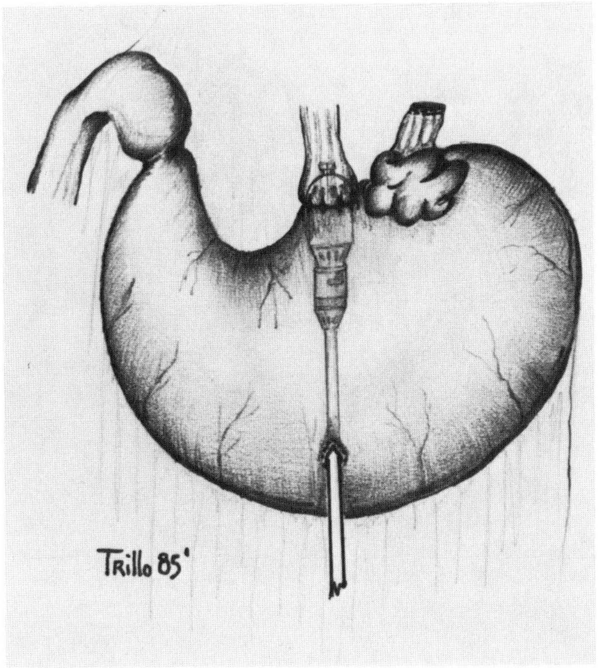

Figure 58–2. Relocation of the esophagus by esophagogastrostomy with the EEA Auto-Suture stapling instrument. The esophagus is transected, a purse string is placed on the distal end around the anvil of the EEA, and the center rod of the EEA is placed through a gastrotomy and attached to the anvil through a small stab incision at the new site of attachment.

dorsal row of continuous sutures, slightly longer than the proposed anastomotic opening, that approximates seromuscular layers of the stomach and duodenum. A second row of continuous sutures is placed, following an incision down to the mucosa of the stomach and duodenum, approximating the seromuscular layers. A third dorsal row of continuous sutures is placed to approximate the incised mucosa of the stomach and duodenum. The suture used for the third row is continued as the first row of ventral sutures. The second ventral row of sutures is a continuation of the second row of dorsal stitches and the third ventral row of sutures is the continuation of the first dorsal row of sutures. This three-tiered hand-sutured technique should be used in all procedures other than the esophagogastrostomy and jejunojejunostomy.

Partial Gastrectomy and Gastroduodenostomy

Partial gastrectomy and side-to-side gastroduodenostomy (modified Billroth I procedure) are performed to bypass an abscess or chronic fibrosis at the pyloric antrum. Mobilization and excision of the pyloric antrum, pylorus, and duodenum is accomplished using stapling instruments. The vascular supply is divided close to affected portions of the stomach and duodenum with the LDS Auto-Suture stapler (United States Surgical Corp). The TA-90 Auto-Suture stapling instrument (United States Surgical Corp) is applied sufficiently proximal to the lesion to permit placement of a Payr intestinal clamp (Sklar Products) adjacent to the stapler distally. The TA-90 stapler is discharged and then used as a guide to transect the stomach between the clamp and the stapler. The GIA Auto-Suture stapler (United States Surgical Corp) is used to transect the duodenum, completing the pyloric resection. The remaining stomach is anastomosed to the duodenum in a side-to-side fashion using either a hand-sutured technique as described for the gastroduodenostomy or the GIA stapling instrument.

The GIA Auto-Suture technique has been implicated as a cause of late stricture of anastomotic stoma, especially when used to create gastroenterostomies. The size of the jejunojejunostomy stomas created with the GIA stapler does not seem to be related to the development of this late stricture.

Duodenojejunostomy and Jejunojejunostomy

Duodenojejunostomy and jejunojejunostomy are used to bypass a duodenal obstruction distal to the hepatopancreatic ampulla. A duodenojejunostomy is performed by creating a 5-cm stoma using the previously described three-tier technique (Fig. 58–3). This is created between the cranial part of the normal duodenum proximal to the hepatopancreatic ampulla and a segment of jejunum distal to the duodenocolic fold. Following completion of the duodenojejunostomy a stapled side-to-side adjunctive jejunojejunostomy, with one segment being the bypassed jejunal segment, is performed using the GIA stapler to prevent jejunoduodenal reflux proximal to the duodenojejunostomy.

Gastrojejunostomy and Jejunojejunostomy

Gastrojejunostomy and jejunojejunostomy are performed to bypass extensive duodenal disease and stricture beginning immediately distal to the pylorus and extending to the caudal flexure of the duodenum. The stomach and a loop of proximal jejunum are approximated without tension, with either traction sutures or Babcock clamps (Sklar Products). Side-to-side anastomosis is performed using a three-tiered hand-sutured method. After completion of the jejunostomy, a side-to-side adjunctive jejunojejunostomy is performed with a GIA stapling instrument.

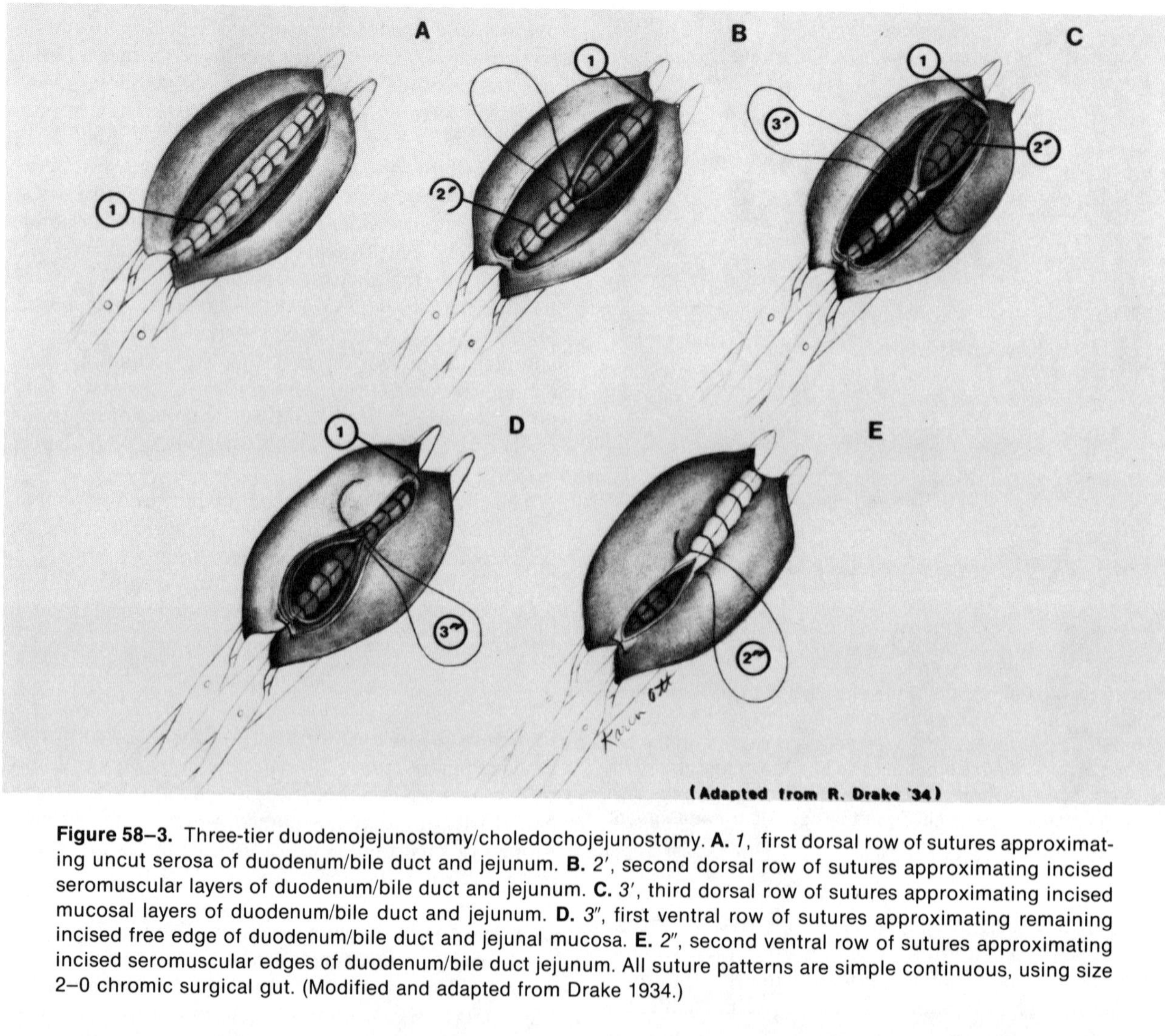

Figure 58–3. Three-tier duodenojejunostomy/choledochojejunostomy. **A.** *1*, first dorsal row of sutures approximating uncut serosa of duodenum/bile duct and jejunum. **B.** *2′*, second dorsal row of sutures approximating incised seromuscular layers of duodenum/bile duct and jejunum. **C.** *3′*, third dorsal row of sutures approximating incised mucosal layers of duodenum/bile duct and jejunum. **D.** *3″*, first ventral row of sutures approximating remaining incised free edge of duodenum/bile duct and jejunal mucosa. **E.** *2″*, second ventral row of sutures approximating incised seromuscular edges of duodenum/bile duct jejunum. All suture patterns are simple continuous, using size 2–0 chromic surgical gut. (Modified and adapted from Drake 1934.)

Choledochojejunostomy

Choledochojejunostomy, duodenojejunostomy, and jejunojejunostomy are used for a duodenal obstruction found at the hepatopancreatic ampulla with obstruction of the common hepatic (bile) duct. A side-to-side choledochojejunostomy 2 cm distal to the previously described duodenojejunostomy is performed to bypass a common bile duct obstruction. An approximately 1.2-cm stoma is created using a three-tiered hand-sutured method of anastomosis (Fig. 58–3).

Jejunojejunostomy

Adjunctive side-to-side jejunojejunostomy is routine in foals in which a duodenojejunostomy or gastrojejunostomy is performed. The site of anastomosis is 25-cm proximal and distal to the duodenojejunostomy or gastrojejunostomy. Stay sutures and Babcock clamps are used to align the segments of jejunum at the planned site of anastomosis, and the GIA stapler is used to create a side-to-side 5-cm stoma. A reinforcing row of continuous Lembert sutures of 2–0 surgical gut is placed around the staple lines.

The rationale for performing a jejunojejunostomy in addition to the duodenojejunostomy or gastrojejunostomy is to prevent stagnation of intestinal contents in the loop of jejunum proximal to the anastomosis. Without a jejunojejunostomy, any secretions or ingesta in the proximal loop of jejunum must enter or reenter the stomach or duodenum before it can pass distally. Creation of a jejunojejunostomy makes it possible for intestinal contents to proceed aborally without reentering the stomach or duodenum. No adverse effects of creating this jejunojejunostomy have been observed.

POSTOPERATIVE CARE

To maintain normothermia, the foals are given supplemental heat with a heating pad and blankets during recovery. The empirical use of histamine H_2 antagonists (i.e., cimetidine [Tagamet; SK&F], ranitidine [Zantac; Glaxo, Inc]) and sucralfate (Carafate; Marion Laboratories) has been proposed for prophylaxis and treatment of gastroduodenal ulceration. Generally, all foals requiring surgery receive this medication. Dosages and treatment intervals are still under investigation.

As soon as it is practical, the foals are reintroduced to their dams and allowed to suckle for short periods. If no regurgitation or abdominal discomfort occurs, the frequency of feeding is returned to normal over 24 to 48 hours. Intravenous fluid administration is discontinued as soon as practical depending on correction of acid-base and electrolyte abnormalities. Generally, antimicrobial therapy is continued for 3 to 5 days.

Follow-up contrast radiographs are taken 24 hours after surgery. A standing right lateral thoracic radiograph is used to locate the previously administered barium. Barium sulfate (5 mL/kg) is then given by nasogastric tube in the thoracic esophagus. A radiograph is taken during and 2 and 5 minutes after administration. When the obstruction has been successfully bypassed, there is rapid movement of barium into and out of the stomach, although the stomach is still larger than normal and contains gas and fluid. In foals with cholangitis without obstruction of the hepatopancreatic ampulla, barium may be seen within dilated bile ducts.

Approximately a 50% recovery rate can be expected using the above-described techniques. Foals with pyloric stenosis have the best prognosis, whereas those foals with generalized duodenitis extending beyond the hepatopancreatic ampulla have the poorest prognosis.

Recovery may be complicated by conditions other than the gastroduodenal obstructions that are present on admission, as well as by disease conditions that develop after surgery. The improvement in hepatobiliary function as demonstrated by a return to normal of total, direct, and indirect bilirubin, aspartate aminotransferase, and gamma glutamyl transferase levels following performance of a choledochojejunostomy is important in supporting the presumption that cholangiohepatitis is reversible if the obstruction of the common bile duct is surgically bypassed. If pneumonia develops after surgery it is generally not associated with aspiration of gastric contents and saliva but may be related to a nosocomial agent that has reached the alveoli via the airway in droplets of mucous or saliva.

BIBLIOGRAPHY

Acland HM, Gunson DE, Gillette DM: Ulcerative duodenitis in foals. *Vet Pathol* 1983;20:653–661.

Elliott TE, Albertazzi VJ, Danto LA: Stenosis after stapler anastomosis. *Am J Surg* 1977;133:750.

Morris DM: Chronic pancreatitis, in *Current Therapy in Equine Medicine.* Philadelphia, WB Saunders Company, 1983, p 253.

Orsini JA, Donawick WJ: Surgical treatment of gastroduodenal obstructions in foals. *Vet Surg* 1986;15:205.

Orsini JA, Donawick WJ: Choledochojejunostomy for treatment of common bile duct obstructions associated with duodenal stenosis in foals. *Vet Surg* 1988;18:34–38.

Rehbun WC, Dill SG, Power HT: Gastric ulcers in foals. *J Am Vet Med Assoc* 1982;180:404–407.

Rooney JR: Gastric ulceration in foals. *Pathol Vet* 1964;1:497–503.

United States Surgical Corporation: *Stapling Techniques in General Surgery,* ed 2. Norwalk, CT, United States Surgical Corporation, 1980.

59
Gastric Surgery in Adult Horses

William P. Barclay

Access to the stomach during abdominal surgery is difficult in the adult horse. The stomach is bounded cranially and dorsally by the diaphragm, on the right by the liver, and on the left by the spleen. The large colon lies ventral to the stomach and the pancreas and small intestine lie caudad. The area encompassed by the stomach and surrounding organs is bounded by the 11th to the 17th ribs. The stomach varies in volume depending on feeding practices and disease processes, but generally can hold 8 to 15 L. Internally the stomach is divided by the margo plicatus into a glandular part (fundus and pyloric regions) and an aglandular (squamous) part (pars esophagea). The cardia has numerous folds of mucosa that tend to occlude the orifice. The pyloric sphincter is a thick ring of muscle readily palpable during laparotomy or at necropsy.

DIAGNOSTIC PROCEDURES

Endoscopic examination of the stomach of an adult horse is possible if a sufficiently long flexible fiberoptic instrument is available (2 to 3 m). Feed should be withheld from the horse for 18 to 24 hours. Insufflation of air into the esophagus aids in passing the endoscope through the esophagus into the stomach. Mucosal lesions may be masked by retained solid ingesta. Biopsy instruments are available for retrieval of small tissue specimens. Cervical esophagostomy can be done to pass a shorter endoscope, but may create additional problems for the horse, such as an esophageal fistula, abscess, or electrolyte imbalances.

Contrast radiography of the stomach of an adult horse is usually not feasible. Small, thin-bodied horses or yearlings can be imaged standing with radiographic units capable of 200 mA/100 kv using rare earth screens. A barium mixture (250 to 500 g/500 to 1,000 mL of H_2O w/v) can be administered by a nasogastric tube. The normal horse or foal should show movement of some barium into the small intestine in 10 minutes, and almost all barium should leave the stomach within 35 to 60 minutes. Retention of barium in the stomach indicates mechanical or functional obstruction of the pylorus or small intestine. The dorsal gastric wall can be visualized by a double-contrast technique. Air is pumped into the stomach to stretch the wall and aid in identifying thickened areas.

Gastric lavage and examination of the retrieved gastric fluid is clinically the easiest and fastest way to assess gastric and function. Retrieval of fluid is aided by establishing a siphon. Water (300 to 400 mL) is pumped into the stomach and the end of the tube is lowered below the level of the stomach. The pH of gastric contents is normally 3 to 4, but may vary with diet or when the pH is measured in relation to eating. Reflux of small intestinal secretions into the stomach may raise the pH to 6 to 8. Assessment of the odor and color of the fluid often provides the most meaningful information. Fluid from a normal stomach is usually light green in color and smells sweet. A sour or rancid smell of fatty acids indicates stasis, and blood-tinged, necrotic-smelling fluid is usually associated with small intestine inflammation, obstruction, or gastritis. Large quantities of fluid in the stomach, particularly bile, indicates small intestine obstruction from any of a variety of causes.

SURGICAL APROACHES TO THE STOMACH

A ventral midline or paramedian incision extended to the xiphoid or costal arch usually gives sufficient exposure for palpation and limited visual inspection of the stomach within the abdomen. Extension of the incision caudally to the level of the umbilicus allows wide retraction of the body wall for visualization of the greater curvature of the stomach and possibly the pylorus. The large colon should be exteriorized to aid both palpation and visualization. If the stomach is greatly distended, as is the case with small intestine obstruction or pyloric obstructive diseases, the greater curvature may approach the cranial end of a ventral midline incision so that a gastrotomy or gastrojejunostomy may be performed.

Transthoracic approaches to the stomach have been reported. This is the best method of attempting to empty the stomach, since the stomach can be brought to the incision to minimize spillage. A left thoracotomy is performed and one or two ribs, between the tenth and 17th, are removed from the costochondral junction dorsally 20 to 30 cm. The lung is packed off cranially and ventrally with sterile moistened towels and the diaphragm is incised. The spleen and small colon may protrude through the diaphragmatic incision. The parietal surface of the stomach can be grasped with vulsellum forceps or stay sutures and gently pulled through the incision. Care must be taken to avoid spillage in the pleural cavity if a gastrotomy is done. The diaphragm should be closed with synthetic absorbable sutures (polyglycolic acid, polyglactin 910, or polydioxanone) in sizes 0 to 2 depending on the size of the horse. A simple continuous suture pattern is the most suitable to perform in this area. The lung is reinflated and the body wall is closed with synthetic absorbable sutures in the intercostal muscles. The adjacent ribs can be approximated with size 2 monofilament nonabsorbable suture if necessary to maintain chest closure. The remaining air should be evacuated from the pleural cavity with an indwelling suction drain placed dorsally and tunneled subcutaneously at least one rib space. The drain is removed 4 to 6 hours after the last positive aspiration of air.

DISEASES REQUIRING SURGICAL TREATMENT

Diseases of the stomach in the adult horse that require surgical intervention are rarely encountered. The stomach is often secondarily involved with other intestinal emergencies, however, and should be evaluated along with the rest of the bowel at laparotomy. Decompression of gas with a needle is the most common procedure, and should be done if the stomach is dilated. A 12- or 14-gauge needle attached to a suction hose can be introduced through the incision and angled through the stomach wall so as to tunnel a short distance in the gastric submucosa. Care should be taken to guard the needle from penetrating other viscera. Overlying omentum need not be removed from the needle puncture site. To prevent leakage of stomach contents, the puncture site should be pinched off after the needle is withdrawn. Suturing the puncture site is not necessary unless leakage is apparent. Spillage from the needle and tube can be prevented by continuing suction or completely occluding the tube as the needle is withdrawn from the abdominal cavity.

Gastric impaction can occur as a primary problem or secondary to other intestinal diseases. The diagnosis is made at surgery because the clinical signs are nonspecific, usually intermittent but unrelenting abdominal pain. The stomach is distended with compressed and dehydrated ingesta. Fluid passed through a nasogastric tube usually will not penetrate the mass sufficiently, even with massage, to soften it enough to pass into the duodenum. A 12-gauge 3-in needle attached to a fluid administration set can be placed through the stomach wall as described above and sterile water or saline injected by gravity flow or a fluid pump into the center portion of the mass. Gentle massage starts the softening process, although there is no way to move the ingesta out of the stomach at surgery. The mass will often clear from the stomach within 48 hours after this massage process. The horse should be fed small amounts of feed frequently for 2 to 3 days only after the stomach is known to be cleared of the impaction. Maintenance of systemic hydration is important in maintaining gastric secretion and saliva production, both of which are helpful in hydration of the dehydrated mass.

Obstructive diseases of the pylorus are rarely encountered in the adult horse. Gastric tumors such as squamous cell carcinoma and lymphomas are more often associated with weight loss and inappetance than with colic from a pyloric obstruction. Diagnosis of gastric tumors can be made from peritoneal fluid cytology in some cases if the gastric peritoneum is involved, or at laparotomy, or with gastric endoscopy. Tumor inva-

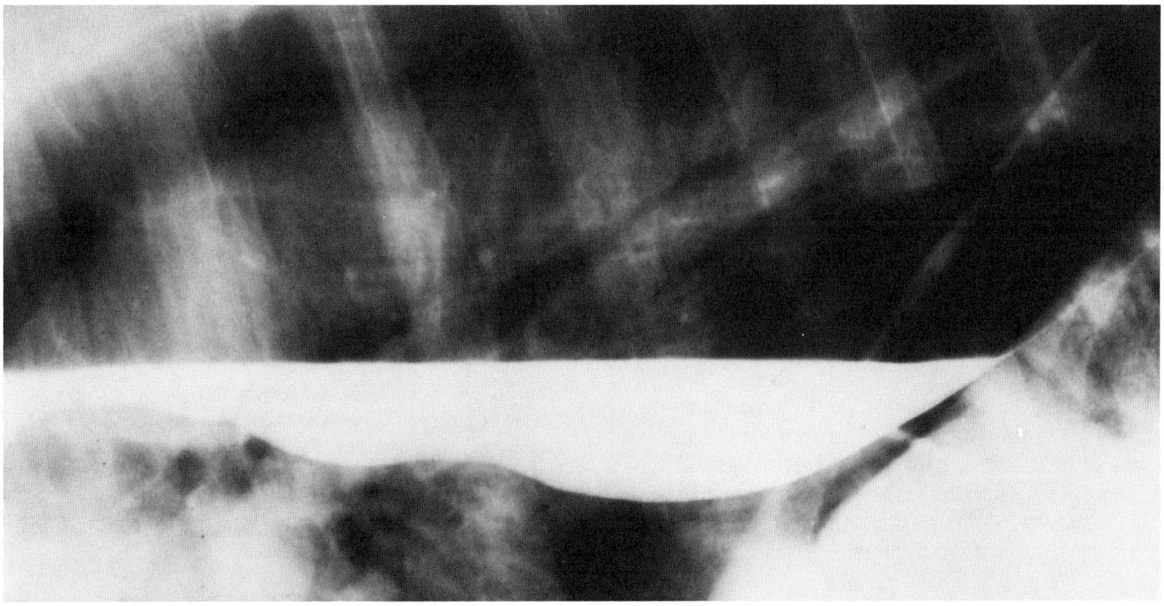

Figure 59–1. Barium esophagogram of a mature horse with chronic gastric ulceration showing a dilated atonic thoracic portion of the esophagus secondary to obstruction of the cardia.

sion and metastasis usually prevent consideration of surgical therapy. Pyloric hypertrophy has not been reported as a definitive disease in the horse. Pyloromyotomy has been performed, although not reported, with successful outcomes in suspected cases. The pylorus normally feels thickened in the adult horse and this makes determination of muscular hypertrophy difficult. Gastric ulcers can cause pyloric and cardiac sphincter obstruction, more often in foals. Endoscopic examination of the affected area usually reveals swollen, raw areas in the stomach wall. Biopsy of the area would differentiate ulcers from tumors. Obstruction of the cardia presents as achalasia with dilation or hypertrophy of the thoracic esophagus (Fig. 59–1). Pyloric obstruction by an ulceration of the pylorus or duodenum presents as recurrent colic and weight loss in foals and young horses. Bruxism and salivation have also been reported. Delayed emptying of the stomach can usually be demonstrated with a barium gastrogram or by repeated reflux of gastric contents with nasogastric intubation. Treatment includes changing the feeding practices to facilitate esophageal and gastric emptying. Moistened pellets rather than course roughage seem to pass from the stomach more rapidly. A gastrojejunostomy can be done for pyloroduodenal obstruction if medical therapy is unsuccessful. Relief of a cardiac sphincter obstruction by surgery would be very difficult, particularly in the adult horse, but can be considered in the foal (see Chapter 58). Recent experience with histamine H_2 receptor antagonists indicates that medical therapy may be the treatment of choice once a definitive diagnosis of gastric ulcers is made. Most cases will resolve if the diagnosis is made early.

Foreign bodies rarely lodge in the stomach of the horse. Sharp objects usually perforate the small intestine and fibrous objects tend to lodge in the transverse or small colon. Larger solid objects that can be swallowed tend to lodge in the cervical or thoracic esophagus. Removal of a foreign body from the stomach would best be accomplished through a transthoracic approach unless the stomach was very distended and could be isolated and held with stay sutures from a ventral midline incision.

Fluid distention and rupture of the stomach occur secondary to small intestine obstruction or proximal enteritis. Acute gastric rupture can occur without any other reported signs, and usually occurs shortly after feeding. Once the stomach has ruptured and the contents are in the peritoneal cavity, treatment is futile. Muscular and serosal tears can be sutured via a cranial ventral midline celiotomy. The tears usually occur on the greater curvature. Simple continuous or continuous Lembert pattern using synthetic absorbable suture should be placed along the length of the tear to prevent complete rupture. The primary disease or obstruction should also be treated and the stomach should be decompressed regularly after surgery. A small (1- to 2-cm) duodenocecal or proximal jejunocecal fistula can be made to facilitate gastric emptying if ileus of the small intestine is present. This fistula will usually close in 3 to 7 days. If a larger fistula is created between the duodenum and cecum, a second surgery is usually required to close the fistula to prevent chronic weight loss and a potential internal incarceration between the cecum and duodenum. This can be done 7 to 14 days after the first surgery through the same incision. Metoclopramide 0.1 to 0.5 mg/kg/h in an intravenous drip seems to be effective in facilitating gastric emptying and small intestine motility after surgery, although results are variable and neurologic derangements have been observed at higher dosages.

BIBLIOGRAPHY

Barclay WP, Foerner JJ, Phillips TN, MacHarg MA: Primary gastric impaction in the horse. *J Am Vet Med Assoc* 1982;181:682–683.

Brown CM, Slocombe RF, Derksen FJ: Fiberoptic gastroduodenoscopy in the horse. *J Am Vet Med Assoc* 1985;186:965–968.

Church S, Baker JR, May SA: Gastric retention associated with acquired pyloric stenosis in a gelding. *Equine Vet J* 1986;18:332–334.

Greet TRC, Whitwell KE: Barium swallow as an aid to the diagnosis of grass sickness. *Equine Vet J* 1986;18:294–297.

Hammond CJ, Mason DK, Watkins KL: Gastric ulceration in mature thoroughbred horses. *Equine Vet J* 1986;18:284–287.

Hunt JM Gerring EL: A preliminary study on the effects of metoclopramide on equine gut activity. *J Vet Pharmacol Ther* 1986;9:109–112.

McGill CA, Bolton JR: Gastric retention associated with a pyloric mass in 2 horses. *Aust Vet J* 1984;61:190–191.

Steenhaut M, Vlaminck K, Gasthuys F: Surgical repair of a partial gastric rupture in a horse. *Equine Vet J* 1986;18:331–332.

Todhunter RJ, Erb HN, Roth L: Gastric rupture in horses: A review of 54 cases. *Equine Vet J* 1986;18:288–293.

60
Small Intestinal and Colonic Obstruction in Foals

Rolf M. Embertson

INTESTINAL OBSTRUCTIVE DISEASES

Simple Obstruction of the Small Intestine

Simple obstructions are those that obstruct the intestinal lumen with minimal or no vascular compromise.

Small intestinal impactions occur infrequently in foals. Ascarid impactions may be seen shortly after deworming in foals infested with large numbers of the parasite. The obstruction may be severe enough to require abdominal surgery for removal of the roundworms via small intestinal enterotomy. This disease is rarely seen in the foal from a well-managed farm.

Discrete, short, midjejunal impactions with concomitant distention and mild inflammation of the small intestine cranial to the lesion is infreqently seen in older sucklings and weanlings. Surgical correction of the impaction generally involves softening the impaction and advancing the material from the small intestine into the cecum. Injecting the impaction with saline or mixing it with intestinal fluid oral to it is helpful in manually breaking down the impaction. If the impacted ingesta cannot be easily reduced, removal via an enterotomy is indicated. These foals generally recover well from surgery unless affected by adhesions postoperatively.

Abdominal adhesions causing obstruction of the small intestine are generally associated with previous intraperitoneal inflammation. This is most commonly due to previous abdominal surgery, but has also resulted from severe infection of the umbilical remnants. Depending on the degree of obstruction (partial to complete) the foal may show mild to severe colic. This disease usually has a very poor prognosis because adhesions tend to reform in areas where they have been surgically removed or broken down. Resection of all involved tissue is ideal; however, the extent and location of the adhesions usually make this difficult.

Paralytic ileus is most often associated with enteritis and is seen in severely ill neonates. These foals tend to be depressed, show mild abdominal pain, and have gas-distended intestines (primarily small intestine) as seen radiographically. These foals are not candidates for abdominal surgery.

Strangulation Obstruction of the Small Intestine

Strangulation obstructions are those that obstruct the intestinal lumen and compromise the venous return and/or arterial supply.

Intussusception of the small intestine causes an initial partial simple obstruction, but as the tissues become edematous, the vasculature is compromised, leading to strangulation of the involved segment. The location of the intussusception may be jejunal, ileal, or ileocecal. In the early stages an intussusception may be surgically reducible, and if the tissue is viable, some intussusceptions will remain reduced. However, there is a substantial risk of recurrence in the foal. Therefore, resection of the affected tissues is advisable. An exception to this is an early ileocecal intussusception. If the ileum is viable, a simple side-to-side ileocecostomy and suturing of the ileum to the cecum will prevent recurrence. An in-depth discussion of this disease is presented in Chapter 63.

Small intestinal volvulus (twisting of the small intestine on its mesentery) is the most common intestinal obstruction in foals encountered at our hospital that require abdominal surgery. Volvulus characteristically affects foals less than 3 months of age and most commonly occurs at the distal jejunum and ileum. The reason for this consistent location of small intestinal volvulus may be twofold: the mesentery is longer than in the proximal small intestine and the ileum is fixed at the ileocecal junction, around which it can twist. Rather than twisting on its own mesentery, the small intestine may twist around a persistent Meckel's diverticulum, which is the rarely encountered remnant of the omphalomesenteric duct. The prognosis for small intestinal volvulus is fair in the early stages, when no resection and little handling of the intestine are necessary. The prognosis is guarded to poor in foals when resection and anastomosis are necessary, primarily because of subsequent adhesion formation.

Hernias have the potential for incarceration with strangulation of intestines. Internal hernias (those not involving the abdominal wall) include rents in the omentum, gastrosplenic ligament, mesentery, and mesodiverticular bands. These rents are uncommon in foals. The most common defect responsible for small intestinal incarceration is a rent in a mesodiverticular band. This band of tissue is infrequently present and is formed from a persistent vitelline artery, resulting in an extra sheet of mesentery, continuous with that of the jejunum, that attaches to the antimesenteric side of the jejunum, thus creating a mesenteric pocket. Surgical repair consists of reduction of the incarcerated intestine, resection of nonviable intestine, and surgical closure of the rent.

External hernias are considered to be those involving the abdominal wall. Incarceration of small intestine in an umbilical hernia is rare but usually leads to strangulation of the involved segment. This generally results in acute heat, pain, and swelling at the umbilicus, in addition to signs of strangulation obstruction of the small intestine. Ultrasonography is a useful adjunct to the physical examination in determining the presence of incarcerated intestine in an umbilical hernia. Incarceration and strangulation of a section of the wall of the intestine (parietal or Richter's hernia) does not cause a complete intestinal obstruction. Thus, local pain and edema are present at the umbilicus, but other signs of small intestinal obstruction disease may not be present. The incarcerated small intestine may infrequently free itself from the hernia, but generally surgical correction of the lesion is necessary. The abdomen is entered cranial to the umbilicus to evaluate the extent of intestinal involvement from within the abdomen and to prevent an inadvertent incision into incarcerated intestine. The hernial ring is then carefully opened to exteriorize incarcerated intestine and to resect any devitalized intestine. Occasionally, the hernial ring will be adhered to necrotic friable intestine, which requires en bloc resection of the fascial edge of the hernial ring and its contents.

Congenital inguinal hernias in male foals generally resolve shortly after birth. Scrotal hernias usually resolve during the first few months of life, and rarely does intestine become incarcerated. Incarceration and obstruction of intestine in an inguinal or scrotal hernia requires surgical correction. This involves an approach to the inguinal area, occasionally combined with a ventral midline celiotomy and evaluation of and reduction or resection of involved bowel. This is discussed in depth in Chapter 62.

Diaphragmatic hernias are infrequently encountered in foals and may be congenital or acquired. Congenital defects are the result of incomplete fusion of the embryonic components of the diaphragm. Acquired defects are usually the result of trauma and may result during foaling. Thoracic radiographs are necessary in the preoperative diagnosis of this lesion. Surgery involves reduction of any herniated bowel. The diaphragmatic hernia is then closed if possible by apposition of the edges of the hernia or suturing a mesh implant over the rent.

Simple Obstruction of the Large Intestine

Atresia of the intestine is an occasional cause of intestinal obstruction seen in neonates. The diagnosis is suggested by the history (onset of abdominal pain 2 to 3 days after birth), routine diagnostic workup, and abdominal radiographs (plain film and barium enema). However, the definitive diagnosis is usually made at surgery or necropsy. The most common segment of the intestine missing is the distal large colon and proximal small colon. Creating a patent functional intestinal tract by anastomosis of the proximal and distal intestine ends in foals with atresia coli is usually unsuccessful. Atresia of the rectum and anus may also be seen, and may be successfully repaired if the atretic segment is short.

Impaction of the cecum or large colon is rare in the foal. These can be insidious in nature and may perforate before an indication for exploratory surgery is recognized. The prognosis tends to be poor due to lack of early surgical intervention and to the frequent presence of other debilitating disease.

Small colon impactions are relatively common in foals. The most frequent of these is meconium impaction in the neonate. These are generally successfully treated medically, primarily with enemas, and rarely need surgery. If surgery is needed, fluid is injected into the mass or an intraoperative enema is given to allow the mass to soften and be broken up manually. Removal of the mass through an enterotomy is rarely necessary. Enema tubes should not be passed beyond the pelvic inlet to minimize the risk of perforation of the small colon.

Displacements of the large colon requiring surgical correction are most often seen in older foals (weanlings). Left dorsal displacement of the large colon (over the renosplenic ligament) is the most common form of displacement. The foal tends to exhibit more abdominal pain than the adult horse does with this same lesion. If diagnosed early, so that there is minimal intestinal compromise, these are not difficult to correct and have a good prognosis.

Paralytic ileus with severe gaseous distention of primarily the large intestine seen radiographically is encountered occasionally in foals less than 3 months of age. These foals tend to present depressed, show mild to severe abdominal pain, usually have diarrhea, and thus are treated for enteritis. Rotavirus infection has been confirmed in some of these foals. Severe abdominal pain unresponsive to medication has led to an exploratory celiotomy in a few of these foals. This reveals distention of the large intestine but no mechanical obstruction. Decompression of the gas from the intestines results in less colic postoperatively. The prognosis is good with appropriate medical therapy and if septicemia or other infective complications do not become a problem.

Another form of paralytic ileus is ileocolonic aganglionosis. This disease occurs in white offspring of overo spotted parents, and has been diagnosed in the Belgian breed. Although the intestinal tract is patent, lack of normal peristalsis prevents movement of ingesta through the affected region. These foals present with a clinical picture similar to that of foals with atresia coli. There is no known treatment, and euthanasia is indicated.

Strangulation Obstruction of the Large Intestine

Incarceration and strangulation of the large intestine through an internal or external hernia is rare in the foal. Large intestinal intussusception is also rare in the foal. Large colon volvulus is occasionally encountered in the older weanling. The clinical signs, anatomic abnormality (dorsolateral-ventromedial rotation near the base of cecum), surgical decisions, and postoperative course tends to be similar to those of adult horses. The earlier the surgical correction is performed the better the prognosis. The surgery is discussed in Chapter 66.

Nonstrangulating Necrosis of the Small and Large Intestines

Nonstrangulating necrosis of the intestine, may have different causes, including thromboembolism with infarction, clostridial enteritis, necrotizing enterocolitis, and unknown etiologies. Thromboembolism due to migrating larva of *Strongylus vulgaris* may produce an infarctive lesion with extensive or focal necrosis. Foals fortunate enough to have focal lesions amenable to resection and anastomosis have a fair prognosis. Extensive lesions warrant euthanasia. This disease can occur in foals as young as 2 to 3 months of age. Foals with severe clostridial enteritis may show clinical signs suggesting the need for exploratory celiotomy. The extensive intestinal involvement usually necessitates euthanasia. This disease tends to occur during the first few days of life. Necrotizing enterocolitis in two neonatal foals has been reported. This disease as encountered in the human infant is caused by periparturient ischemia of the intestine with bacterial colonization of the intestinal wall. Intramural intestinal gas seen radiographically is apparently pathognomonic for this disease. Surgical repair of bowel perforations is necessary in some human infants. The disease in the foal has a poor prognosis.

DIAGNOSIS

Evaluation of the foal with colic should proceed in a fashion similar to that for the adult horse, with a few differences. Evaluation of the clinical and laboratory data will suggest the probable location and type (e.g., strangulation versus simple obstruction) of lesion. However, the definitive diagnosis is generally not determined until the abdomen is explored. The important question is whether or not exploratory surgery is indicated. The following considerations are most important in determining the probable lesion and the need for surgery. One should keep in mind, however, that these are general guidelines, and often, as in the adult horse, surgery is used as a diagnostic technique as well as the mode of therapy.

The foal tends to be less tolerant of pain than the adult horse, hence pain is a more sensitive indicator of mild abdominal disease in the foal. Acute severe abdominal pain, with little to no abatement in response to analgesic medication (e.g., xylazine and flunixin meglumine, usually indicates a strangulation obstruction or an infarctive lesion. After the acute severe pain, foals with these lesions generally enter a period of depression, and later become quite painful again. Initial mild abdominal pain progressing to severe pain may result from a simple obstruction of the small or large intestine as distention increases over time. Identical signs of mild intermittent pain, occasionally with depression, may be caused by a partial simple obstruction, gastric or intestinal ulceration, or enteritis.

The presence and character of intestinal sounds, the amount of gastric reflux, and the degree of abdominal distention provide useful information in evaluation of the foal. Auscultation of the abdomen may reveal normal to hypermotile intestinal sounds in the early stages of a simple obstruction. These sounds gradually diminish over time. Intestinal sounds subside rapidly in foals with a strangulation obstruction or an intestinal infarction. Gastric fluid obtained through a nasogastric tube generally indicates an obstruction of the small intestine, although inhibition of gastric emptying by gastric or duodenal ulcers can mimic this type of gastric reflux. Usually, the more proximal the obstruction the greater the quantity of fluid obtained. Infrequently, displacement with distention of the large intestine may occlude the duodenum, causing increased gastric fluid volume. Gross abdominal distention results from small and large intestinal distention more frequently in the foal than in the adult horse.

Rectal examination is either not possible or of minimal use in evaluation of a colicky foal. Digital rectal examination may reveal a meconium impaction in the neonate. A limited manual rectal examination extending just past the brim of the pelvis can be performed in the large weanling. This may reveal gaseous distention of the small intestine or large colon. The increased risk of a rectal tear in this size animal must be balanced against the information possibly gained from this procedure.

Abdominocentesis to obtain peritoneal fluid from a foal can be difficult and is not without risk. Puncture of the intestinal wall with a sharp needle is of concern, because punctures or small lacerations in the thin intestinal wall may allow leakage of ingesta into the abdomen. Fatalities due to linear bowel lacerations have been described. In the standing foal, severe intestinal distention leaves little area for peritoneal fluid to accumulate ventrally between the intestine and the body wall. Obtaining abdominal fluid from a painful recumbent foal is often difficult. Peritoneal fluid values are generally within normal limits in foals with simple obstructive lesions of the small and large intestine. However, with increasing duration, the protein values become elevated. Strangulation obstruction and infarctive lesions usually have normal peritoneal fluid in the early stage, but become rapidly abnormal (initially an increased protein level, then increased red and white blood cell values).

In foals up to approximately 500 lb abdominal radiography can yield information useful in determining the site and type of lesions. Standing lateral radiographs of the abdomen are ideal; however, in foals that are unable to stand, lateral recumbent radiographs can be useful. The radiographic technique used at our hospital varies from 5 to 28 mAs with 75 to 95 kVp, depending on body weight. Fast rare earth screens, long latitude film, and a 103-line focus grid are used with a 40-in film-focal distance. Abdominal radiographs may not be diagnostic of the type of obstruction; however, they do allow one to recognize what parts of the intestinal tract are gas and/or fluid distended. Matched with other findings, this allows tentative classification of the abdominal lesion. Prior knowledge of normal radiographic anatomy of the foal abdomen is of obvious benefit.

Gaseous distention of the small intestine is seen radiographically in all foals with small intestinal obstructive lesions. This finding is also present in some septicemic neonates and in foals with enteritis or peritonitis, but is uncommon in foals that have large intestinal obstruction. Multiple intraluminal gas-fluid interfaces associated with small intestinal distention (Fig. 60–1) are quite common with small intestinal obstructive lesions and are rarely seen with other abdominal problems. Vertical, inverted, *U*-shaped loops of distended small intestine, seen on the standing lateral radiograph, in our experience have only been seen in foals with small intestinal obstructive lesions. However, this last finding is not present in all foals with small intestinal lesions. During enteritis, large intestinal distention is seen concomitant with small intestinal distention, and the loops of small intestine are not as enlarged; often the distended loops of intestine are of variable size. Gas-filled small intestine appears in the ventral abdomen as well as the dorsal regions. Also, stomach distention is greater with small intestinal obstruction than with enteritis, although this sign is variable. Gaseous distention of the large intestine is seen radiographically in most foals with large intestinal obstruction. Although seen with enteritis and/or peritonitis, as a result of generalized ileus, the distention is not as severe. Displacement of the large intestine (Fig. 60–2) has been diagnostic for large intestinal obstruction. Pneumoperitoneum seen on abdominal radiographs usually indicates intestinal perforation.

SURGERY

Many of the specific facets of perioperative care, especially of the neonate, are not discussed in this paper. However, the following are some useful considerations for surgical management of intestinal obstruction in the foal.

Preoperative Care

The foal should be in the best metabolic condition possible prior to surgery. This includes administering appropriate fluids to rehydrate the foal, balancing serum electrolytes, and correcting any acid-base abnormalities. Preoperative antibiotics consisting of penicillin and gentamicin (amikacin in the neonate) or ticarcillin are indicated. The abdomen should be surgically scrubbed in a manner that will allow a surgical approach anywhere from the xiphoid process of the sternum to the pubis. Chlorhexidene acetate (Nolvasan; Aveco Co, Inc) or chlorhexidene gluconate (Hibiclens;

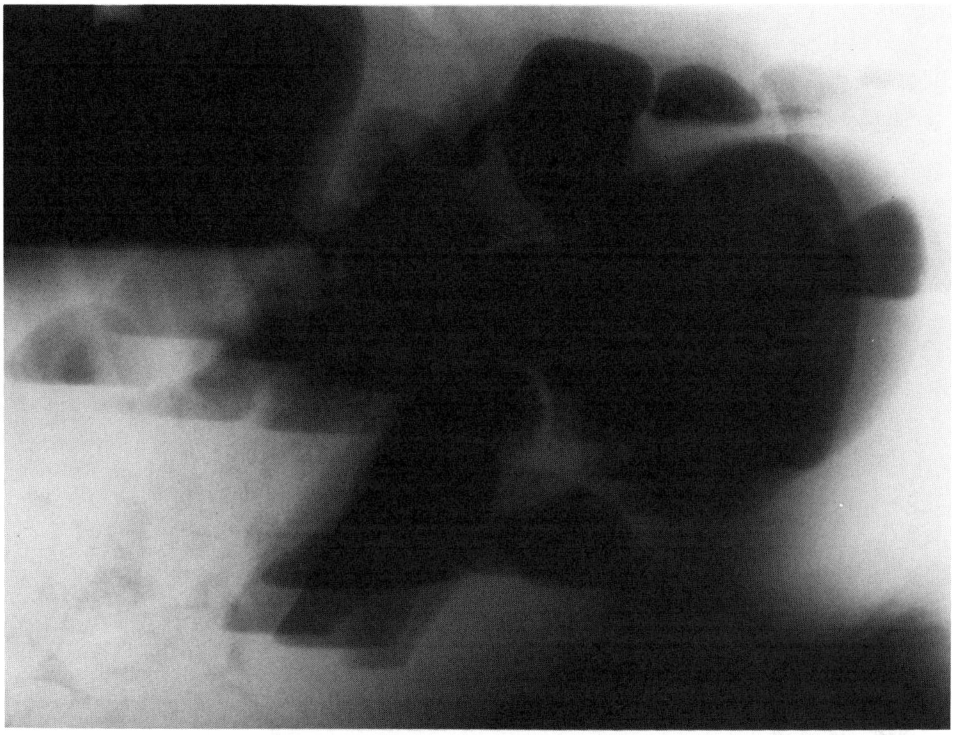

Figure 60–1. Small intestinal distention with multiple intraluminal gas-fluid interfaces. (From Cudd TA, Toal RL, Embertson RM: The use of clinical findings, abdominocentesis, and abdominal radiographs to assess surgical vs. nonsurgical abdominal disease in the foal. *Proc Am Assoc Equine Pract* 1987; pp 41–53.)

Stuart Pharmaceuticals) scrub preparations for the skin preparation tend to be less irritating to the skin of the foal than poloxamer-iodine (Prepodyne; West Argo). If the umbilicus is open it should be oversewn prior to the skin preparation to lessen the risk of contamination of the surgical field.

Intraoperative Care

A ventral midline approach to the abdominal cavity is made with an incision starting at the umbilicus and extending cranial approximately 20 cm. If a gastric or duodenal lesion is found, the incision can be extended cranial to the xiphoid. If a caudal abdominal lesion is found, the incision can be extended caudad past the umbilical structures to the pubis. The umbilical vein, present along the ventral midline cranial to the umbilicus, and the urachus, umbilical arteries, and bladder, found caudal to the umbilicus, will be encountered in the abdominal approach in the young foal. If examination of these structures reveals sepsis and thickening, resection is indicated.

Surgical instrumentation is essentially the same as that used for abdominal surgery in the adult horse. An additional useful instrument is the Balfour retractor, used to retract the edges of the abdominal incision to provide better visualization of deep abdominal structures. Exploration of the foal's abdominal cavity is done in a manner similar to that in the adult; however, the structures are much more fragile. The mesentery will tear with rough handling. The serosa tends to be much more reactive to handling in the foal than the adult, as evidenced by a more rapid reddening of and exudation of fibrinous material from the serosa. Constant lavage of serosal surfaces with a balanced electrolyte solution is recommended during the surgery. Resection and anastomosis techniques are similar to those used in the adult horse. For intestinal anastomosis, a two-layer closure, first closing the mucosa and then the seromuscular layer, using 3–0 polyglactin 910 (Vicryl; Ethicon Inc) in a continuous pattern has been reliable. A similar two-layer closure is used for enterotomies.

The abdominal wall at the linea alba is closed in three layers using a continuous suture pattern in each. In foals weighing less than 300 lb, size 1 polyglactin 910 is placed in the linea alba, 3–0 polyglactin in the subcutaneous tissue, and 3–0 polyglactin 910 in the

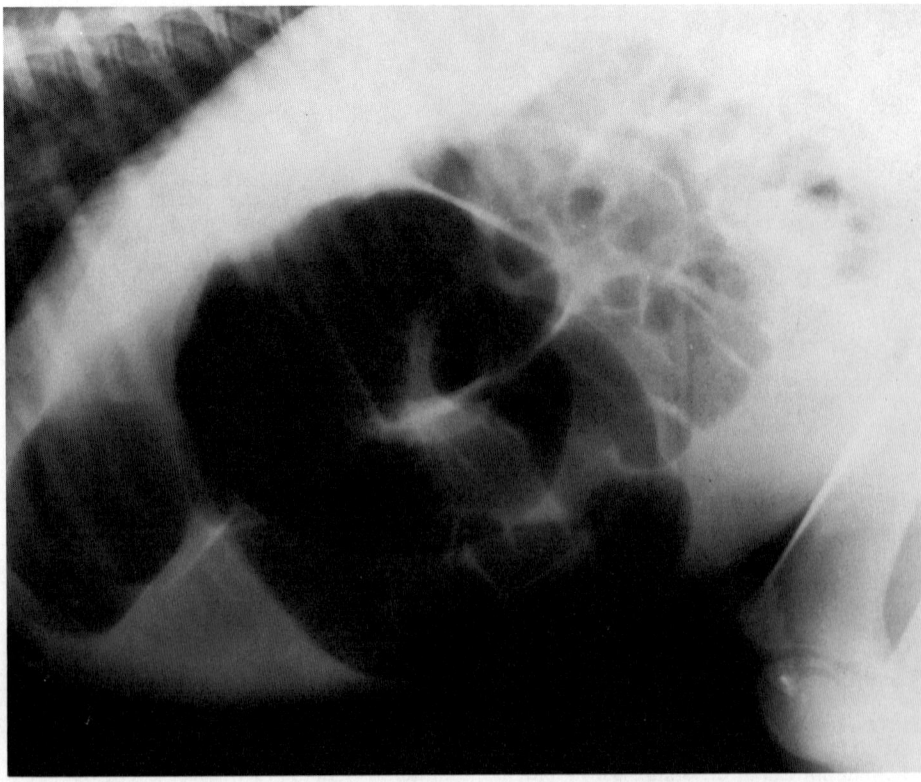

Figure 60–2. Large intestinal distention and displacement cranial in the abdomen. (From Cudd TA, Toal RL, Embertson RM: The use of clinical findings, abdominocentesis, and abdominal radiographs to assess surgical vs. nonsurgical abdominal disease in the foal. *Proc Am Assoc Equine Pract* 1987; pp 41-53.)

skin. In foals weighing greater than 300 lb, size 2 polyglactin is placed in the linea alba, 2–0 polyglactin 910 in the subcutaneous tissue, and 2–0 polyglactin 910 in the skin. If incisional contamination is a possibility, the use of monofilament polydioxanone (PDS; Ethicon Inc) in place of polyglactin 910 is recommended. Absorbable sutures in the skin ideally should be removed at about 2 weeks, but allow one the option of not removing them from uncooperative foals.

Postoperative Care

Maintenance of hydration postoperatively is critical. Antibiotics are continued for approximately 72 hours postoperatively, or longer if there was a major break in sterile technique or if septicemia was also present in a neonate. Because of the stress and the potential for gastroduodenal ulceration, ranitidine (Zantac; Glaxo Laboratories, 2 mg/kg orally twice daily) is administered to the foal during its stay in the hospital. Flunixin meglumine (0.25 mg/kg intravenously four times a day) is used for a few days postoperatively for its anti-inflammatory and antiendotoxic effects, bearing in mind that long-term usage could potentiate gastric ulceration. Heparin (60 USP u/kg subcutaneously twice daily) is used for four days in selected foals in an attempt to decrease the formation of fibrinous peritoneal adhesions. The use of heparin in foals with small intestinal lesions appears to have resulted in fewer foals developing subsequent peritoneal adhesions that lead to abdominal pain. In comparison, the incidence of postoperative peritoneal adhesions in foals that had large intestinal lesions has been minimal whether or not heparin was used.

As auscultable intestinal motility gradually returns to normal, the suckling foal is allowed to nurse more frequently. The weanling is gradually allowed to eat hay as auscultable intestinal motility returns, and grain is introduced a few days later. As is true in the adult horse, the return to normal intestinal motility generally takes longer with small intestinal lesions than with large intestinal lesions.

Mild exercise is important in the postoperative period. Fifteen-minute walks, three to four times per day, starting the day after surgery seems to brighten a foal's attitude and stimulate intestinal motility, and may possibly help prevent adhesions by increasing movement of the abdominal contents. The foal and its mare are generally turned out in a small paddock by 1 to 2 weeks postoperatively and then turned out with other mares and foals or weanlings approximately 4 weeks postoperatively.

Complications

Postoperative complications depend on the abdominal lesion. Prolonged ileus with gastric reflux tends to be a problem with small intestinal lesions. Intravenous fluid therapy to replace fluid loss and balance the electrolyte and acid-base status, and occasionally the use of metoclopramide (0.1 mg/kg in 500 ml saline, given over 1 hour intravenously four times a day) has helped resolve this problem. The value of metoclopramide in these cases is empirical, and its use is indicated by poor gastric emptying. Other forms of therapy, including total parenteral nutrition, are often more beneficial since metoclopramide can have adverse neurologic effects in the foal.

Postoperative diarrhea is occasionally encountered, generally associated with large intestinal lesions. Diarrhea is treated with oral electrolyte solutions and intravenous fluids to replace fluid loss and a bismuth subsalicylate preparation (Corrective Mixture; Beecham) as an intestinal protectant. Discontinuing all oral intake and relying on parenteral nutrition is helpful in severe cases. Septic peritonitis is a possible but rare complication of abdominal surgery in the foal. Incisional infections are occasionally encountered and these generally respond to local hydrotherapy and drainage. Incisional hernias are rare.

Postoperative peritoneal adhesions are more of a concern in the foal than they are in the adult horse. In my experience, if peritoneal adhesions do cause colic in the foal, this will generally occur between 2 and 6 weeks postoperatively. Peritoneal adhesions tend to be much more of a problem in foals with small intestinal than large intestinal lesions. In addition. the younger the foal the greater the chance for postoperative peritoneal adhesions that produce clinical problems.

PROGNOSIS

In our practice area, foals with a surgical intestinal obstructive disease carry a worse prognosis than do adults. However, one must recognize that common lesions encountered in the foal are different than those in the adult. Foals with large intestinal lesions have a slightly better prognosis than foals with small intestinal lesions, but the type of lesion is more important for prognostication than its location. Foals with simple obstructions such as a meconium impaction have a better prognosis than foals with strangulation obstructions. Nonstrangulated necrotic lesions have the worst prognosis of the three types.

BIBLIOGRAPHY

Becht JL: Physical examination of the horse with colic, in Robinson NE (ed): *Current Therapy in Equine Medicine,* ed 2. Philadelphia, WB Sanders Co 1987, pp 19–22.

Becht JL, Semrad SD: Gastrointestinal diseases of foals. *Compend Contin Educ Pract Vet* 1986;8:S367–S373.

Campbell ML, Ackerman N, Peyton LC: Radiographic gastrointestinal anatomy of the foal. *Vet Radiol* 1984;25:194–204.

Cudd TA, Pauly TH: Necrotizing enterocolitis in two equine neonates. *Compend Contin Educ Pract Vet* 1987;9:88–92.

Cudd TA, Toal RL, Embertson RM: The use of clinical findings, abdominocentesis, and abdominal radiographs to assess surgical vs. nonsurgical abdominal disease in the foal. *Proc Am Assoc Equine Pract* 1987; pp 41–53.

Fischer Jr AT, Kerr LY, O'Brien TR: Radiographic diagnosis of gastrointestinal disorders in the foal. *Vet Radiol* 1987;28:42–48.

Robertson JT: Conditions of the stomach and small intestine: Differential diagnosis and surgical management. *Vet Clin North Am Large Anim Pract* 1982;4:105–127.

Ross MW, Martin BB, Donawick WJ: Cecal perforation in the horse. *J Am Vet Med Assoc* 1985;187:249–253.

Thanks to Dr. Tim Cudd for his contributions to this chapter.

61
Ileal Impaction

Douglas Allen

Impactions of the small intestine in horses most commonly involve the ileum. Ileal impaction is seen predominantly in the southeastern United States, a geographic incidence possibly associated with the feeding of Bermuda grass hay. Spasmodic contraction of the ileum around this type of feedstuff is thought to lead to impaction. Other less common causes of ileal impaction include ileal muscular hypertrophy, thrombotic mesenteric vascular disease, and ascarid impaction in foals.

DIAGNOSIS

Horses presented with ileal impactions are usually adults. There is no sex predisposition for the condition. Vaccination and deworming are usually current. If vascular thrombosis or ascarid impaction are the predisposing insults, feed type is not important and an inadequate deworming program is a common history.

The clinical signs associated with ileal impactions are variable and relate to the duration of impaction. Therefore, the history elicited from the client must be carefully considered in conjunction with clinical signs and physical findings at initial presentation. Immediately after impaction of the ileum, the horse will show signs of severe abdominal pain because of focal intestinal distention and spasmodic contraction around the impaction. The effectiveness of analgesics during this time may be short lived. If a rectal examination is performed during this phase of the disease, the impacted ileum can often be palpated as a 5- to 8-cm diameter, firm, smooth-surfaced tube originating at the cecal base and extending from right of midline obliquely downward to the left ventral abdomen. This initial episode of severe colic may subside after a few hours and the horse may become depressed.

During this quiescent phase, small intestinal distention develops as the aboral flow of intestinal contents is prevented. Approximately 8 to 10 hours after the initial onset of colic, the horse may again show signs of severe pain because of proximal small intestinal and gastric distention. The horse may appear anxious and become dehydrated. On rectal examination, multiple loops of distended small intestine are evident. It is unusual to be able to definitively locate and identify the impacted ileum during this period because of displacement and concealment by other loops of distended small intestine.

Abdominal auscultation and nasogastric intubation findings are again dependent on the duration of the disease. Normal borborygmi may initially be auscultated equally around the abdominal perimeter, only to diminish as time progresses. Similarly, nasogastric intubation will yield little fluid early in the disease course. However, with continued development of gastrointestinal filling, up to 5 to 6 L of fluid with a neutral pH may eventually be removed at 1.5- to 2-hour intervals.

The systemic signs and laboratory changes associated with ileal impactions reflect the duration of the disease. Initially, an elevated heart rate (>50 beats/min) and respiratory rate may be noticed in response to pain. The packed cell volume and plasma protein concentration will be normal, whereas the white blood cell count may reflect a stress leukogram. Electrolyte, blood gas, and peritoneal fluid analysis values are usually within normal ranges. As the disesase progresses, fluid losses from both decreased intake and increased intestinal secretion into the proximal small intestine begin to change cardiovascular homeostasis. Increases in packed cell volume and plasma protein concentration (>45% and 8 mg/dL, respectively) are detected. The heart and respiratory rates further increase in response to reduced cardiac output secondary to hemoconcentration and as a result of pain from gastrointestinal distention. If the lesion remains uncorrected for longer than 20 to 24 hours, marked metabolic changes consistent with acidemia can be identified on blood gas analysis.

Peritoneal fluid analysis is perhaps the most helpful in differentiating a simple impaction from a strangulation obstruction. As the animal's systemic condition deteriorates and the stomach and small intestine distend, degenerative changes begin to occur in these organs. Increased accumulation of interstitial fluid caused by intestinal distention coupled with microvascular endothelial damage secondary to the reduced splanchnic blood flow in shock contribute to increased peritoneal fluid protein and cellular concentrations. An increase in the peritoneal total protein concentration usually occurs prior to changes in peritoneal cell numbers or type. These values are usually lower in an animal with a simple obstruction than in one with a stangulating obstruction. Additionally, diapedesis of erythrocytes into the peritoneal cavity, commonly found with strangulating lesions, is rarely observed with ileal impactions.

MEDICAL MANAGEMENT

Initial therapy of horses with ileal impaction is supportive and should include analgesics, intravenous fluids, and gastric decompression. Definitive therapy usually includes surgical reduction of the impaction with or without bypassing the ileum. In our experience, the occasional horse may respond to conservative therapy and reduce the impaction spontaneously. All horses with diagnosed or suspected ileal impactions should be considered as surgical candidates. Preoperative therapy includes cardiovascular stabilization of the patient, gastrointestinal decompression, and administration of broad-spectrum antibiotics. During the initial 1 to 2 hours of therapy, the horse should be monitored very closely with continual reevaluation of its physiologic and clinical status. Changes may be noted in temperature, pulse rate, pulse character, capillary refill time, abdominal sounds, volume of nasogastric reflux, respiratory rate, and degree of clinical pain with rapid administration of intravenous fluids.

One of the most clinically apparent changes after initiation of therapy will be the improvement of the horse's cardiovascular status. Pulse character will usually improve and the capilliary refill time will decrease, but changes in heart rate are variable and may depend on the animal's response to pain. With rapid rehydration, many horses will become increasingly painful, due in part to changes that are occurring in the intestine during this period of therapy.

Work performed in humans, dogs, and cats indicates that, as rapid hemodilution occurs with a balanced crystalloid solution, an increased small intestinal capillary filtration of fluid will occur. This happens as the plasma protein concentration approaches 4.5 to 5.0 g/dL, thereby reducing the intravascular osmotic pull of endogenous proteins. Once the intestitium and lymphatics become saturated, the excessive fluid is then secreted into the intestinal lumen as a secondary mechanism to prevent the formation of edema in the small intestine. In horses suspected of having a simple small intestinal obstruction, large volumes of a crystalloid solution may be given rapidly intravenously, at the rate of 10 to 12 L/h, to rehydrate and hemodilute the animal. Thus, the plasma protein concentration will decrease (approximately 5.0 mg/dL) and the volume of fluid that is secreted into the intestines will increase. Following intravenous fluid therapy, those animals that become increasingly painful, have increasing small intestinal distention, and produce increased amounts of gastric reflux will definitely require surgical intervention. Conversely, if the horse shows reduced pain, less-distended intestinal loops on rectal examination, and a decrease in gastric reflux, conservative management may be successful.

SURGERY

Surgery is best performed with the horse in dorsal recumbency under general anesthesia. Upon entrance into the abdominal cavity through a ventral midline celiotomy, multiple loops of distended small intestine are usually encountered. The cecum and colons may be mildly displaced from their normal locations because of the distended small bowel filling the abdominal cavity.

The ileum is usually located in the left caudal abdomen and courses from left to right at the level of the third or fourth lumbar vertebra. Depending on the amount of ileum involved in the impaction, the typical firm, sausage-like impacted small intestine is easily located against the cranial-medial cecal base adjacent to the dorsal abdominal body wall. Careful palpation will reveal a dramatic demarcation between the impacted ileum and the cecum at the ileocecal orifice. The small intestine proximal to the obstruction is usually fluid filled, with little palpable solid ingesta.

Reduction of the impaction usually requires rehydrating the impacted ingesta. This can be accomplished most easily by one of two methods. The first technique is to break the impaction down by manual massage and move it orally into the more fluid-filled small intestine. Once mixed with the fluid, the impaction can be reduced by gently massaging the contents of the distal small intestine into the cecum. This procedure may have to be repeated several times because the contents have a tendency to reimpact during the aboral massage. Almost all impactions can be reduced in this manner given enough manipulation and patience. However, damage to the intestine is a consideration with extensive impactions. Excessive small intestinal manipulation will predispose to intraabdominal adhesion formation that may ultimately result in luminal obstruction. Therefore, in those cases requiring excessive manipulation, direct infusion of the impaction with saline will help relieve the obstruction. The saline is infused with a 12- to 14-gauge needle directly into the midpoint of the impaction. Approximately 2 to 3 L are usually required to rehydrate the ingesta in extensive lesions. Again, gentle massage is used to mix and extrude the ingesta into the cecal lumen. Once this impaction is reduced, the majority of the contents of the proximal small intestine should be gently evacuated into the cecum. Excessive manipulation of the small intestine, however, may cause serosal damage and predispose to adhesion formation.

Once the ileal contents have been moved into the cecum, the ileum should be evaluated for excessive thickenings or stenotic areas. If any of these changes are present, the ileum should be resected or bypassed. The bypass procedure is performed to create a shunt between the small intestine and the cecum. A normal segment of either distal jejunum or proximal ileum is placed side to side against the cecum between the dorsal and medial bands. An anastomosis of approximately 10 cm should be made, using either surgical staples or a hand-sewn technique. If ileal resection is required, a part of the diseased ileum can be excised and a side-to-side anastomosis of the blind-ended distal small intestine to the cecum can be performed. Since the terminal ileum is inaccessible, approximately 10 to 15 cm of the ileum must be blind ended and left attached at the ileocecal orifice. This remaining segment usually causes little problem, will atrophy, and may spontaneously invaginate into the cecum.

POSTOPERATIVE CARE

Postoperative ileus is a common problem after successful correction of ileal impaction. A nasogastric tube should be passed, and left in situ, and the stomach actively decompressed every 2 to 3 hours. Ileus can last from a few hours to 4 to 5 days depending on the severity of the impaction, the amount of manipulation required for reduction, and, perhaps most importantly, the interval between the onset of the condition and surgical correction. Neostigmine (2 to 3 mg intravenously or subcutaneously every 30 to 60 minutes) has been recommended to enhance intestinal motility and decrease the attending postoperative ileus. Although its effectiveness has been challenged experimentally, it is routinely used in some surgical referral centers. Broad-spectrum antibiotics can be administered perioperatively and should be included in the postoperative regimen in horses that have required a resection or bypass procedure. The horse must be supported with intravenous fluids to replace the accelerated fluid losses from the intestinal tract and the insensible losses during this period. As the quantity of reflux declines, the horse should be offered small amounts (<1 L) of water every 1 to 2 hours. The horse should be carefully monitored for pain or heart rate elevation, which may herald a return of ileus. If there are no adverse effects encountered, free access to water can then be allowed.

Once the gastric reflux has abated and the horse is maintaining its hydration with oral water, small handfuls of hay (preferably alfalfa or timothy) can be offered every 1 to 2 hours over the next 2 to 3 days. Frequent short intervals of grazing can also be encouraged, and small amounts of alfalfa pellets can be offered. Normal forage feeding can then be resumed in 5 to 7 days. Because of the potential for developing impactions with Bermuda grass, our clients are advised to consider an alternative source of hay.

Stall rest should be imposed, especially in active animals, for the first 2 months postoperatively, with exercise being limited to controlled walking. The animal may be put back into work after 3 to 3.5 months using an escalating exercise regimen.

PROGNOSIS

The postoperative course appears to relate more to the severity of the horse's metabolic and cardiovascular status before surgical intervention than to the specific technique used to correct the impaction. In those animals that have a prolonged preoperative course (>15 hours), an increased incidence of abdominal adhesions, enteritis, laminitis, and gastric reflux is apparent clinically. This is probably a result of the intestinal ischemia that results from prolonged reduction of splanchnic blood flow during hypovolemia. Experimental studies performed in dogs, cats, and horses indicate that a reduction of small intestinal perfusion pressure for 1 hour or more followed by rapid reperfusion will result in mucosal epithelial necrosis, thus potentially exposing the systemic circulation and peritoneal cavity to intestinal microflora and/or toxins. This may explain why horses with a longer duration of obstruction have a poorer prognosis for long-term survival and return to work (even though this is not a strangulating condition). With proper postoperative rest and dietary management, the prognosis for life and athletic soundness is good in uncomplicated cases.

BIBLIOGRAPHY

Embertson RM, Colahan PT, Brown MP, et al: Ileal impaction in the horse. *J Am Vet Med Assoc* 1985;186:570.

Gabella G: Hypertrophy of smooth muscle. *J Physiol* 1975;249:183.

Jones RS: Intestinal obstruction, in Sebastion VC (ed): *Textbook of Surgery*. Philadelphia, WB Saunders Co, 1977, p 1002.

Lundgren O: Studies on blood flow distribution and countercurrent exchange in the small intestine. *Acta Physiol Scand Suppl*, 1967;303:1.

Robertson JT: Conditions of the stomach and small intestine. *Vet Clin North Am* 1982;4(1):105.

Parks DA, Granger DN: Oxygen radicals and ischemia induced tissue injury, in Greenwald RA, Cohen G (eds): *Oxyradicals and Their Scavenger Systems, vol II, Cellular and Medical Aspects*. New York, Elsevier Science Co, Inc, 1983, p 135.

62 Inguinal Hernia

Michael A. Livesey

The term "inguinal hernia" is used to describe the passage of abdominal contents from the abdominal cavity into the inguinal canal. If the contents pass through the external inguinal ring and descend into the scrotum, the condition may be described as a scrotal hernia; however, the term "inguinal hernia" is frequently used to describe either condition. The hernial contents are usually omentum or coils of small intestine, although herniations of the small colon, the bladder, and the pelvic flexure of the large colon have been observed. Inguinal herniation may occur in either sex but is most commonly seen as an acquired condition in the adult stallion and as a congenital condition in male foals. A predisposition to inguinal herniation has been reported in the Standardbred and the draft breeds and has been observed commonly in Tennessee Walking Horses and American Saddlebreds.

Inguinal hernias may be described as either indirect or direct. Indirect hernias occur most commonly in the horse. In this form, abdominal viscera pass through the vaginal ring to enter the hernial sac formed by the tunica vaginalis. The herniated structures thus share the same space as the testis and its associated structures (Fig. 62–1). A variation of this form occurs when the hernial sac ruptures, allowing the intestines to lie subcutaneously. Direct inguinal hernias, although the most common form in humans, only occasionally occur in the horse. In this type of hernia, abdominal viscera enter the inguinal canal through a defect in the peritoneum close to the vaginal ring (Fig. 62–2). Protruding intestine lies in a hernial sac lined by peritoneum, outside the tunica vaginalis. This type of hernia is more often the result of a traumatic incident, and the peritoneum is also ruptured.

In the mare and gelding the cavity of the tunica vaginalis is narrowed or closed, making herniation a rare event. When herniation does occur in the mare, it presents as a soft hemispherical swelling in the region of the udder. The differential diagnosis should include ventral abdominal herniation and mastitis.

INGUINAL OR SCROTAL HERNIA IN THE FOAL

Diagnosis

Inguinal or scrotal hernias are usually observed in male foals at birth, or within the first few days of life. The problem, which is considered an inherited defect, may be unilateral or bilateral. The presenting sign is swelling in one or both halves of the scrotum. The history often indicates that an enlargement was first noticed after the foal was observed straining to pass meconium. The size of the swelling may range from that of a hen's egg to a large grapefruit, although rarely, the swelling may be large enough to cause edema and apparent closure of the prepuce. Fluid sounds are frequently audible on auscultation of the scrotum, because of the presence of fluid-filled intestinal loops. Palpation reveals a soft, fluctuant mass that can be readily reduced, although in the standing animal the reduction may be only temporary, because the coils of intestine soon reherniate when manual pressure is removed. Strangulation of bowel within the hernial sac in foals is extremely rare.

Most congenital inguinal and scrotal hernias will spontaneously resolve by the time the foal is 3 to 4 months of age. The recommended treatment is daily manual reduction of the hernia to ensure that incarcer-

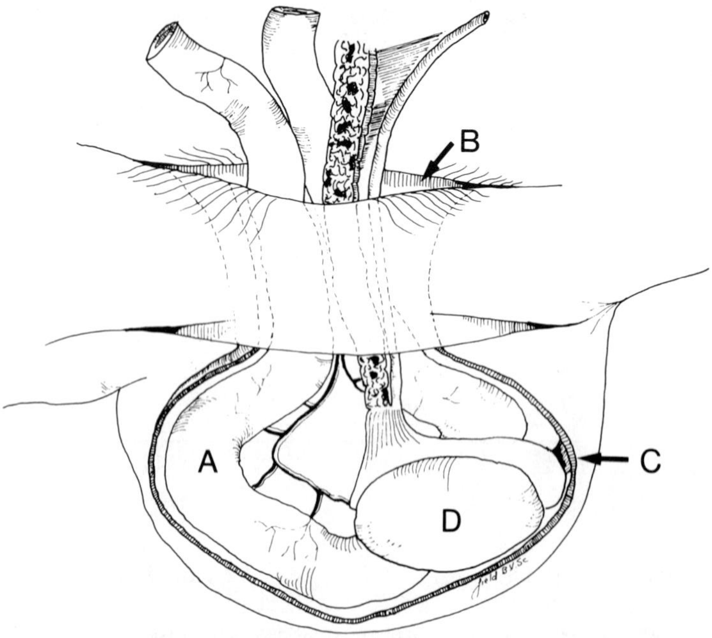

Figure 62–1. Indirect inguinal hernia. The herniated loop of bowel (*A*) has passed through to the vaginal ring (*B*) to enter the hernial sac lined by the tunica vaginalis (*C*), and lie adjacent to the testis (*D*).

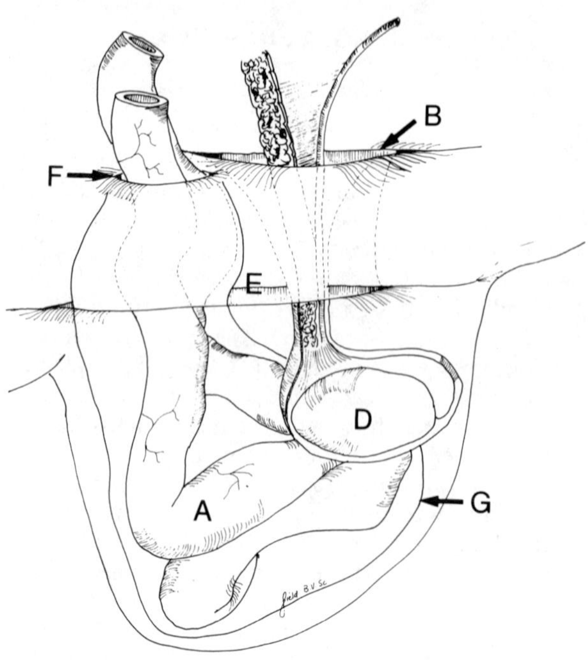

Figure 62–2. Direct inguinal hernia. The herniated loop of bowel (*A*) enters the inguinal canal (*E*) through a defect in the body wall (*F*) close to the vaginal ring (*B*). Intestine lies in a hernial sac lined by peritoneum (*G*) adjacent to the testis (*D*).

ation of the bowel will not go undetected. Often in neonates a supportive bandage can be applied to maintain reduction. Herniation in most of these foals will be spontaneously corrected after 72 hours from birth. Surgery is indicated if the hernia becomes incarcerated or the foal exhibits signs of colic. Very large hernias and those that have not spontaneously resolved by 4 months of age should be surgically repaired.

Bilateral closed castration is recommended at the time of surgical correction of the hernia. Routine open castration of an animal with an inapparent hernia may lead to evisceration, regardless of whether the procedure is performed with the animal in the recumbent or standing position.

Surgical Repair

Inguinal herniorrhaphy, the surgical repair of an inguinal hernia, is performed with the foal in dorsal recumbency under general anesthesia. The scrotal and inguinal regions are finely clipped, prepared for sterile surgery, and draped in a routine manner.

A 10-cm straight skin incision is made in an oblique manner over the external inguinal ring (see Chapter 57). Large hernias may require elongation of the incision caudally to achieve adequate exposure. Using a scalpel, the skin, tunica dartos, and subcutaneous tissues are incised to expose the scrotal fascia and common vaginal tunic. The incision must be made carefully because loops of small intestine may have ruptured through the tunica vaginalis and be lying subcutaneously.

The flask-shaped common vaginal tunic is freed from the surrounding fascia by blunt dissection, then grasped around the testis. While traction is applied, the structure is twisted several times about its longitudinal axis, until the contents of the hernia are squeezed back into the abdominal cavity. A transfixation ligature of absorbable suture material is then placed at the level of, and secured to, the external inguinal ring (Fig. 62–3). The spermatic cord is emasculated distal to the ligature and the testis removed (closed castration). The limb on the affected side should be adducted slightly as the suture is tied, to bring the edges of the ring closer together and facilitate closure. If the transfixation ligature is not secured to the external inguinal ring, the longitudinal twist applied to the remaining spermatic cord is rapidly lost, and a potential space exists that may permit the prolapse of bowel into the remaining vaginal tunic. However, the risk of complications from this eventuality is low. This method of herniorrhaphy should only be employed where there is no evidence of bowel incarceration and the animal is less than 1 year of age. Beyond this age, there is the risk that the testicular artery and vein will not be adequately occluded by the transfixation ligature or the emasculation.

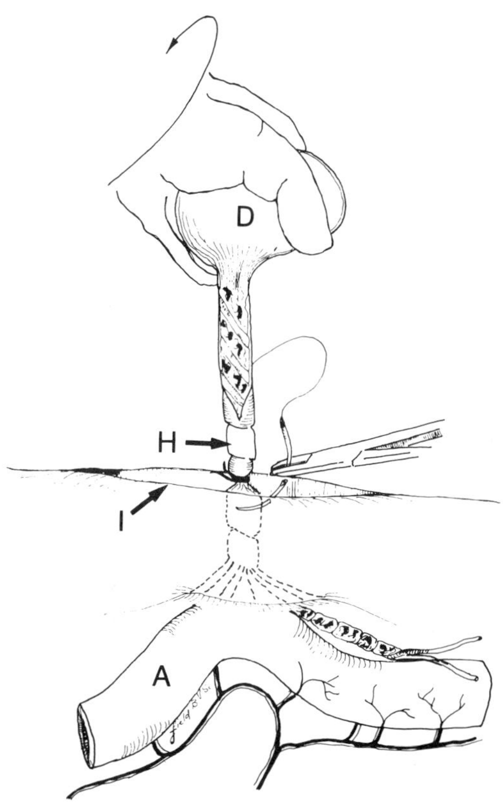

Figure 62–3. Surgical repair of an inguinal hernia. The testis (*D*), contained within the common vaginal tunic, is grasped and twisted about its longitudinal axis, until the bowel (*A*) is squeezed into the abdominal cavity. A transfixation ligature is then placed through the cord (*H*) at the level of the external inguinal ring (*I*).

In a modification of the technique, the common vaginal tunic is opened by incising in a longitudinal direction to expose the herniated bowel and the testicle (Fig. 62–4). The bowel is inspected for evidence of damage prior to reduction into the abdominal cavity. A transfixation ligature is placed around the testicular artery and vein close to the external inguinal ring, the spermatic cord is emasculated distal to the ligature, and the testicle is removed (open castration). The cord is allowed to retract after hemostasis is ensured, and the vaginal tunic is closed with a transfixation ligature close to the vaginal ring. The tunic distal to the ligature is then emasculated and removed.

The subcutaneous tissues are apposed with two layers of absorbable suture in a continuous pattern, taking care to avoid perforating the large external pudendal artery and vein. Although placing a Penrose drain through the wound and then closing the skin edges in a subcuticular pattern using synthetic absorbable material has been advocated, primary closure without a drain is recommended. Because of the suspected heritable nature of the condition, the opposite testicle should be removed in a routine manner.

INGUINAL OR SCROTAL HERNIA IN THE ADULT

Diagnosis

Acquired inguinal and scrotal hernias in the stallion may be divided into three types: (*a*) reducible, (*b*) nonreducible, and (*c*) evisceration of intestine or omentum following castration.

Reducible Inguinal or Scrotal Hernias. Reducible inguinal or scrotal hernias occur infrequently in the adult. They may present as a unilateral or bilateral soft reducible swelling in the inguinal or scrotal region, from which fluid sounds are audible on auscultation (Fig. 62–5). The history may include mild recurrent bouts of colic or hind limb lameness on the affected side.

Reducible hernias, and incarcerated hernias that have recently occurred, may sometimes be reduced by either external manipulation, traction applied to the herniated bowel per rectum, or a combination of these

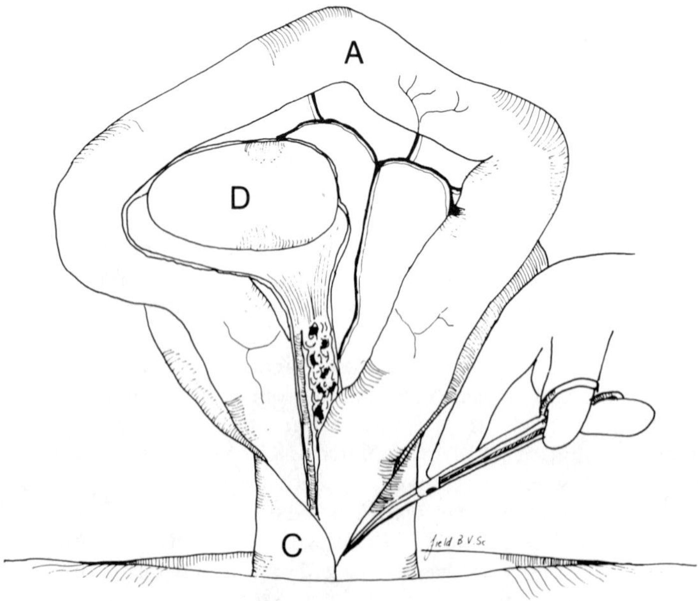

Figure 62–4. Surgical repair of an inguinal hernia. The common vaginal tunic (*C*) is incised in a longitudinal direction to expose the herniated bowel (*A*) and testes (*D*).

techniques. Both techniques may be attempted in the standing sedated animal. External manipulative reduction is performed by grasping the testicle on the affected side in one hand and applying traction downward and laterally from the abdomen of the horse. The other hand is placed proximal to the testicle, and the spermatic cord is compressed manually to reduce edema and venous congestion. While maintaining traction on the testicle, the bowel is pushed proximally in the vaginal tunic and back through the vaginal ring into the abdominal cavity. Traction on the testicle is necessary to narrow and straighten the vaginal tunic and thus prevent the intestine from folding upon itself during the reduction process.

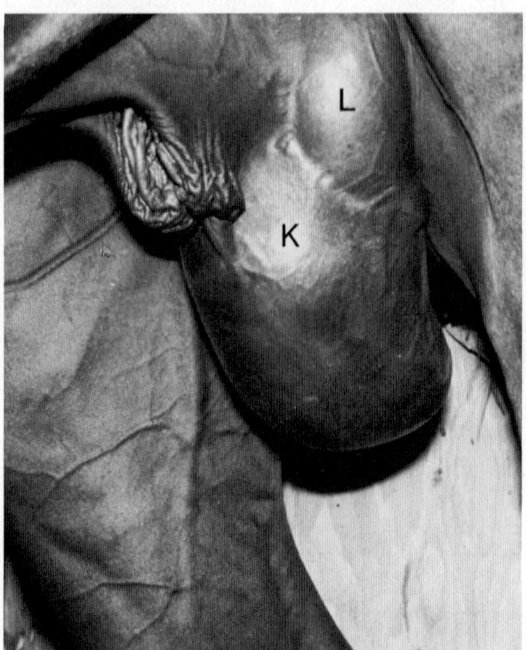

Figure 62–5. An acquired reducible scrotal hernia in the stallion. The right half of the scrotum (*K*) is enlarged, and the left half of the scrotum (*L*) is normal.

A well-lubricated, gloved arm should be used when attempting reduction by traction per rectum. The herniated loop of bowel is gently grasped close to the vaginal ring, and traction is applied. The process is aided by having an assistant perform simultaneous external manipulation. Although the technique is sometimes effective, persistent attempts to free bowel by this manner should not be made because there is a significant risk of rectal perforation or bowel rupture. In addition, both techniques described have the disadvantage that irreversible damage may have occurred to the herniated section of bowel, which initially may go unnoticed. Animals in which reduction is successful should therefore be closely observed for several days in the immediate post-reduction period.

Nonreducible Inguinal Hernia. Nonreducible inguinal herniation is the most common form of the condition in the stallion and produces an acute strangulation obstruction of the small intestine. Nonreducible scrotal herniation occurs infrequently. Most hernias are unilateral and indirect. Although a cause has not been clearly demonstrated, conditions said to predispose to herniation include those that increase the intraabdominal pressure and stretch the vaginal and internal inguinal rings. Inguinal herniation is commonly seen in stallions shortly after breeding a mare, after strenuous exercise, or after a traumatic incident, such as being cast in a stall or caught over a fence.

When bowel has become strangulated, the presenting sign is colic. The scrotum and inguinal region may be swollen, depending on the position and length of herniated intestine. Frequently the only finding on palpation of the scrotum is a cool, firm testis with a slight thickening at the neck of the scrotum on the affected side. In animals with these presenting signs, the differential diagnosis should include testicular torsion and thrombosis of the testicular artery. A definitive diagnosis is made by palpation per rectum of intestine entering the vaginal ring on the affected side. The bowel proximal to the obstruction is usually mildly to moderately distended, and distal bowel is flaccid and empty. This examination is essential in all stallions exhibiting signs of colic, unless the horse is too small. The treatment of choice is the immediate surgical correction of the condition.

Evisceration of Intestine or Omentum following Castration. Herniation and evisceration of small intestine has been observed up to 144 hours following castration. Once intestine has entered the inguinal canal, peristalsis rapidly creates further prolapse. The mesenteric attachments of the jejunum and ileum and the size of the vaginal ring usually restrict the amount of intestine that prolapses to between 20 and 100 cm. Stretching of the mesentery and vascular compromise of the bowel rapidly produce severe colic and shock. Herniation and prolapse of omentum occur in a similar manner, at or shortly after castration. Frequently, however, this may not be observed for up to 24 hours postoperatively. The presenting sign is the prolapse of a fatty structure, variable in length and approximately 4 cm in diameter, from one of the scrotal incisions. Most animals do not respond to this condition with pain. Confirmation of the diagnosis is obtained by palpation per rectum of a structure passing through the vaginal ring on the affected side.

Surgical Repair

Inguinal herniorrhaphy, the surgical repair of an inguinal hernia, is performed with the horse in dorsal recumbency under general anesthesia. In those animals with acute intestinal obstruction, changes in hydration and acid-base status must be corrected prior to induction of anesthesia. Stomach decompression should be attempted before surgery. When bowel has become strangulated or eviscerated, it is necessary to perform a ventral midline exploratory celiotomy to help return the bowel to the abdominal cavity, perform an intestinal resection, and examine the abdomen for other lesions. To avoid contamination of both surgical areas, the penis is placed in the prepuce and the orifice is closed by drawing the skin edges together with a simple continuous suture pattern using a monofilament, nonabsorbable material. Both regions are then prepared for sterile surgery in a routine manner and draped in preparation for using both approaches. In two recent reports, 7 of 13 and 14 of 24 horses presenting with acquired inguinal hernias required a ventral midline celiotomy in addition to an inguinal approach.

Reducible Nonstrangulating Inguinal or Scrotal Hernia. Surgical repair is similar to that previously described for the foal.

Nonreducible Inguinal Hernia. Nonreducible inguinal hernias usually contain a strangulated section of bowel. The surgical approach to the inguinal region is identical to that described for the foal. A longitudinal incision is made in the common vaginal tunic to the level of the external inguinal ring, allowing the bowel to be exteriorized and inspected. Necrotic or devitalized bowel must be resected and an anastomosis performed. The devitalized segment of bowel is frequently distended and edematous and must be decompressed prior to manipulation. This is achieved by means of suction via an 18-gauge, 1.5-in needle introduced obliquely through the bowel wall. Bowel resection and anastomosis may be performed via the inguinal canal, by pulling additional viable intestine from the abdomen. To ensure proper alignment of the proximal and distal segments of bowel, and to avoid the creation of a mesenteric defect through which an internal herniation may occur, bowel examination and alignment during the resection-anastomosis should be done through a ventral midline incision. Similarly, decompression of the proximal small intestine cannot be accomplished solely by the inguinal approach, and requires manipulation through the ventral midline.

Frequently the affected segment of bowel is the distal small intestine, and it may not be adequately exteriorized by the inguinal route. In these cases, the bowel must be returned to the abdominal cavity and exposed through a ventral midline approach. When the devitalized section of bowel is jejunum or proximal ileum, an end-to-end jejunojejunal or jejunoileal anastomosis is performed. If the distal ileum is involved, a jejunocecal anastomosis may be required.

Excessive pressure or traction should not be applied to a devitalized section of bowel or one having a recently performed anastomosis. Therefore, in some cases it is necessary to enlarge the cranial margin of the vaginal ring with scissors and additionally to apply traction to the bowel from within the abdominal cavity, before reduction of the hernia can be achieved. The enlargement is minimized since closure of the internal inguinal or vaginal rings may prove difficult and time consuming.

An alternative approach is to deliver additional bowel from the abdomial cavity until healthy tissue is exteriorized. The devitalized bowel is then resected and the clean bowel returned to the abdominal cavity after closure of both ends. Anastomosis is then performed via the ventral midline approach. Contamination of the abdominal cavity and the difficulties associated with replacing edematous and congested bowel through the vaginal ring are thus avoided.

Strangulated hernias frequently result in impaired testicular venous return with resultant degenerative changes in the testis. To facilitate adequate closure of the vaginal and external inguinal rings, unilateral castration should be performed. If the stallion has no value for breeding, the opposite testicle should be removed. Inguinal hernioplasty techniques, designed to save the testis while preventing recurrence of the hernia, have been described, but are not recommended. These involve suturing the common vaginal tunic and the external inguinal ring sufficiently to prevent intestine entering the vaginal cavity, while leaving enough space for passage of the spermatic cord. If an insufficient opening is left, ischemic orchitis will result, whereas if an excessive opening remains reherniation may ensue.

Evisceration following Castration. The treatment of postcastration bowel evisceration is dependent upon the presence of devitalized tissue and contamination, the length of prolapse, and the availability of surgical facilities. If there is extensive prolapse of intestine with evidence of devitalization, the animal should be referred to a surgical facility immediately. The use of a testicular support may help to minimize further prolapse and pain associated with stretching of the mesentery. Animals will frequently become very agitated with intestine hanging between their hind legs, and appear more calm when the tissues have been supported.

If a small segment of devitalized tissue is present in the scrotal region, it is prudent to attempt to close the scrotum with sutures or to pack the inguinal canal prior to referral to a surgical facility. In acute evisceration with no evidence of bowel devitalization, the animal should be immediately restrained in dorsal recumbency under general anesthesia. The prolapsed intestine should be lavaged with sterile saline and replaced into the abdomen via the vaginal ring, and then the common vaginal tunic should be closed with a transfixation ligature. If the surgeon is unable to return the bowel to the abdominal cavity and has limited equipment and anesthetic capabilities, he or she has to decide whether to perform an inguinal incision and enlarge the vaginal ring in order to replace the bowel or to merely contain the intestine by closure of the scrotum, recover the animal from anesthesia, and then refer to a surgical facility. Enlargement of the vaginal ring may enable the intestine to be replaced into the abdominal cavity and thus avoid the problems associated with bowel resection. If this is done, the external inguinal ring must be closed rather than attempting closure of the vaginal ring.

The surgical repair of eviscerated omentum may be performed in the standing sedated animal, or with the animal restrained in dorsal recumbancy under general anesthesia. In both instances, the prolapsed omentum and scrotal incisions are surgically prepared. Traction is applied to the prolapsed omentum until clean tissue is exposed. The omentum is then ligated close to the skin edges using an absorbable suture material, and the tissue distal to the ligature is emasculated and removed. In the standing animal the proximal portion is allowed to retreat into the wound. It is then usually an easy matter to reduce the hernia by traction per rectum. Nonabsorbable skin sutures are placed in the edges of the scrotal incision to prevent the possibility of eventration. The vaginal ring on the affected side is checked twice daily by palpation per rectum for 2 days, to determine if intestinal adhesions or further herniation has occurred. If not, the skin sutures may be removed at this time and exercise permitted. In this technique no attempt is made to close the vaginal tunic. The risk of reherniation is therefore greater than if repair was accomplished under general anesthesia with closure of this structure.

Alternatively, with an animal restrained under general anesthesia, the proximal portion of omentum is replaced into the abdominal cavity. The edges of the common vaginal tunic are grasped and twisted, and a transfixation ligature of synthetic absorbable suture material is placed close to the vaginal ring. If the vaginal ring is small and closure has been achieved, closure of the external inguinal ring is not required. However, if the closure of the common vaginal tunic is incomplete, closure of the external inguinal ring is recommended.

POSTOPERATIVE CARE

Animals that have undergone the surgical repair of an incarcerated or strangulated inguinal hernia should receive intensive monitoring in the immediate postoperative period, with special attention to their hydration, electrolyte, and acid-base status. Those animals large enough to permit palpation per rectum should be examined by this method daily for 4 to 5 days following the surgery to ensure adequate reduction of the hernia and to examine for the presence of intestinal adhesions. Herniation may recur following a traumatic recovery from anesthesia, with subsequent disruption of the sutures closing the vaginal tunic or external inguinal ring. If closure of the external inguinal ring has been adequate, bowel may then lie in the inguinal canal and not be palpable externally, although this is rarely a problem.

Following surgery, nasogastric intubation should be performed for gastric decompression. If signs of ileus develop, gastric decompression should be repeated at regular intervals until the condition resolves. Pre- and postoperative broad-spectrum antibiotics are recommended in all cases, and are especially important when an intestinal resection and anastomosis has been performed, or eviscerated viable intestine has been returned to the abdominal cavity.

Extensive postoperative edema may develop in the inguinal and preputial regions after surgery. In the adult, postoperative edema may be controlled by controlled walking for 30 minutes two to three times daily for 3 weeks. In the foal, normal activity within the stall will often help to minimize the swelling. After 1 week of stall rest, the mare and foal may be walked in a confined area for a further 2 weeks, before allowing free exercise. Those animals having undergone a ventral midline celiotomy should have stall rest with controlled walking exercise for at least 4 weeks, with restricted exercise for a total of 8 weeks. Free exercise prior to these times may cause disruption of the suture line and incisional herniation. In the absence of signs of ileus, adult horses may be gradually returned to feed 24 hours postoperatively. Foals are allowed to suckle immediately following the surgery.

PROGNOSIS

There appear to be no published reports detailing the outcome of the surgical repair of congenital inguinal or scrotal hernias. The prognosis for uneventful recovery is good in those cases with reducible hernias. Foals appear to have a greater tendency to develop intestinal adhesions than do adults. The prognosis for uncomplicated recovery is therefore guarded in foals with strangulated hernias that require bowel resection and anastomosis.

The reported mortality rates for stallions undergoing the surgical correction of an acquired strangulated inguinal hernia range from 25.9 to 76%. One important factor would appear to be the mean interval between strangulation and surgical intervention. The more protracted the disease course the more likely the development of irreversible shock or profound ileus. The postoperative development of intestinal adhesions at the anastomotic site or to the vaginal ring may result in an acute obstruction of the lumen of bowel, or chronic bouts of low-grade abdominal pain.

BIBLIOGRAPHY

Ashdown RR: The anatomy of the inguinal canal in the domesticated animals. *Vet Rec* 1963;75:1345–1351.

Hutchins DR, Rawlinson RJ: Eventration as a sequel to castration of the horse. *Aust Vet J* 1972;48:288–291.

Noone JP: Scrotal herniation of the urinary bladder in the horse. *Irish Vet J* 1966;2:11.

Sembrat RF: The acute abdomen in the horse: Epidemiologic considerations. *Arch Am Coll Vet Surg* 1975;4:34–39.

Schneider RK, Milne DW, Kohn CW: Acquired inguinal hernia in the horse: A review of 27 cases. *J Am Vet Med Assoc* 1982;180:317–320.

van der Velden H: Surgical treatment of acquired inguinal hernia in the horse: A review of 51 cases. *Equine Vet J* 1988;20:173–177.

Vasey JR: Simultaneous presence of a direct and an indirect inguinal hernia in a stallion. *Aust Vet J* 1981;57:418–421.

Vaughan JT: Surgery of the male equine reproductive system, in Jennings P (ed): *Textbook of Large Animal Surgery*. Philadelphia, WB Saunders Co, 1984, pp 1101–1102.

Weaver DA: Acquired incarcerated inguinal hernia: A review of 13 horses. *Can Vet J* 1987;28:195–199.

White NA, Moore JN, Cowgil LM, Brown J: Epizootiology and risk factors in equine colic at university hospitals, in *Proceedings of the Second Equine Colic Research Symposium*. Veterinary Learning Systems, 1986, 2:26–29.

63
Ileocecal Intussusception

Richard P. Hackett

ETIOLOGY

Intussusception of the distal ileum into the cecum is the most common form of small intestinal intussusception in horses. The etiology of intussusception is unknown in most cases. It has been suggested, however, that most cases of intussusception in young horses are related to verminous arteritis. Localized bowel hypoxia allows a segment of hyperperistaltic bowel to push distally into a dilated, atonic segment of bowel. It has also been suggested that intussusception is related to induration of the intestinal wall and to abrupt changes in bowel diameter. Intramural polyps, neoplasms, and granulomas have been recognized causes of small intestinal intussusception in many species, including horses. Intramural lesions due to tapeworm (*Anoplocephala perfoliata*) infestation have been observed in a number of young horses with ileocecal intussusception. Acariasis, enteritis, treatment with anthelmintics, previous intestinal surgery, and dietary changes have also been linked to intussusception.

Ileocecal intussusception is diagnosed most frequently in young (<3 years) animals but may be seen in older horses. There is no apparent breed or sex predisposition for this disease.

Two forms of ileocecal intussusception are recognized in horses. Acute ileocecal intussusception results in strangulation obstruction of the intussusceptum and leads to acute abdominal crisis. Chronic ileocecal intussusception is a cause of incomplete, simple ileal obstruction and leads to chronic, intermittent colic. Acute ileocecal intussusception is associated with intussusception of a long segment (usually >50 cm) of ileum into the cecum. Interference with venous and lymphatic return from the intussusceptum results in edema and eventual necrosis. Swelling of the intussusceptum rapidly results in complete intestinal obstruction. Chronic ileocecal intussusception occurs when a short segment (<10 cm) of ileum invaginates into the cecum. The vascular integrity of the ileum remains intact and partial obstruction is due to the presence of the extra thicknesses of bowel at the ileocecal orifice.

ACUTE ILEOCECAL INTUSSUSCEPTION

Diagnosis

Horses with acute ileocecal intussusception demonstrate clinical signs characteristically associated with small intestinal obstruction. An acute onset of signs of severe abdominal pain is typical. After 12 to 24 hours, signs of pain will be overridden by those of depression. The heart and respiratory rates are elevated. Deterioration of the cardiovascular and metabolic status is typically slower than that encountered with other forms of strangulation obstruction of the small intestine. Intestinal borborygmi may be normal or reduced. Palpation per rectum, if permitted by the size of the animal, will usually reveal multiple loops of fluid-distended small intestine, thus strongly suggesting a diagnosis of small intestinal obstruction. Only rarely is it possible to palpate the intussusception as a firm, painful mass in the right dorsal quadrant of the abdomen. If the disorder is of several hours' duration, reflux of small intestinal content into the stomach will be apparent if a nasogastric tube is passed. Peritoneal fluid cellularity and total solids concentration may increase with time. It should be kept in mind that, because the involved segment of bowel is enclosed within the intussuscipiens, peritoneal fluid abnormalities are not often observed.

Surgery

A clinical diagnosis of small intestinal obstruction is the basis for surgical exploration of affected horses. A ventral midline celiotomy should be used. Numerous loops of fluid-distended small intestine confront the surgeon when the abdomen is opened. The cecum is identified and the ileocecal fold is traced from the cecum onto the ileum. The ileum is followed distad to the ileocecal junction. A cleft palpated between the ileocecal junction and the intussusceptum confirms a diagnosis of ileocecal intussusception. The length of the intussusception can be determined by palpation through the wall of the cecum. The goals of surgery are removal or isolation of devitalized intestine, restoration of intestinal continuity, and decompression of distended small intestine. The relative inaccessibility of the distal ileum and ileocecal junction makes it difficult to accomplish the first of these goals.

Moderate traction should be applied to the ileum in an effort to reduce and examine the intussusceptum and to assess its viability. In most cases, either reduction is not possible or the intussusceptum is so obviously devitalized that reduction is unwarranted. If the intussusception cannot be reduced, the ileum is transected and the distal end is closed as close to the ileocecal orifice as possible. This may be done by a Parker-Kerr oversew or, if bowel thickness permits, with either the GIA or TA-90 Auto-Suture stapling devices (United States Surgical Corp). If small intestinal distention is marked, the small intestine should be decompressed before the anastomosis is performed. The small intestine proximal to the point of transection is freed from its mesenteric attachments for a distance of approximately 1 m. This transected end of this segment of bowel is placed over the edge of the surgical table and used as a conduit so that small intestinal contents. may be emptied into a receptacle on the floor. It is important that the small intestine be emptied as completely as possible. The small intestine is then closed by hand suturing or by stapling and the portion that had been freed of mesenteric attachments is transected and discarded.

A side-to-side enterocecal anastomosis is performed (ileocecostomy or jejunocecostomy) (Fig. 63–1). A site

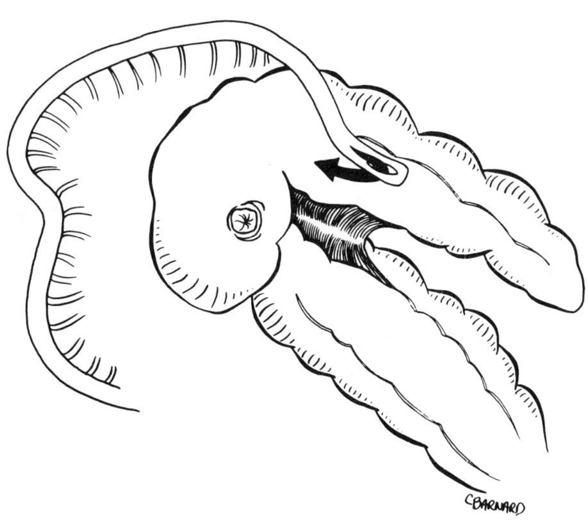

Figure 63–1. Enterocecal anastomosis as treatment for acute ileocecal intussusception (as seen with the horse in dorsal recumbency). The ileum has been transected and the distal stump has been prolapsed into the cecum. A side-to-side anastomosis between the small intestine and the cecum has been completed.

is chosen on the cecum on either side of the dorsal band as close to the cecal base as exposure permits. The small intestine is apposed to the cecum with stay sutures and a side-to-side anastomosis is performed. Either a hand-sewn two-layer inverting (standard) anastomosis or two applications of the GIA stapling instrument are used to create an approximately 10-cm stoma. End-to-side enterocecal anastomosis is an alternative to side-to-side anastomosis, but it is generally accepted that the former is more likely to result in signs of obstruction after surgery, presumably related to kinking at the anastomosis site or swelling of the stoma.

The problem of the distal stump then must be addressed. Intussusception disrupts blood flow through the right ileal mesenteric artery, which supplies the ileum from distal to proximal. At the time of surgery there is adequate mural flow and flow from smaller mesenteric ileal and jejunal arteries to supply exposed small intestine proximal to the intussusception. It must be emphasized, however, that this blood supply is exclusively proximal to distal. The portion of small intestine between the intussusception and the point of bowel transection (the "stump") usually appears normal at the time of surgery. Vascularity to this area, however, is disrupted by transection of the small intestine and mesenteric vessels preparatory to the side-to-side anastomosis. Hence, even a stump that appears viable at the time of surgery will usually undergo devitalization after surgery. Every effort should be made to preserve the blood supply to the stump. Visual criteria for determining viability of the stump are not reliable since the duration of ischemia is short. Objective indicators may be of more value. Unless there is clear objective evidence that the stump is viable, it should be assumed that the stump will undergo devitalization. It is important, therefore, that the stump is not left exposed in the abdomen.

If the intussusception is not reduced, the only option to achieve this goal is to further prolapse the stump into the intussuscipiens (the cecum) and hence isolate it from the abdomen. In most cases, especially those horses with shorter intussusceptions, the stump can be intussuscepted into the cecum manually or with the aid of a long sponge or cervical forceps. An alternative technique is to use umbilical tape to secure the stump to a length of stomach tubing that has been passed through the stump into the cecum. The tubing is then delivered via the cecal incision made during the side-to-side anastomosis. Traction is applied to the umbilical tape to aid in complete intussusception of the stump. In animals weighing less than 500 kg in which the small intestine has been completely decompressed, it is usually possible to place sutures across the ileocecal orifice to maintain the stump within the intussuscipiens.

If the stump cannot be advanced into the cecum, a problem apparently due to mesenteric tension in horses with very long intussusceptions, it is necessary to shorten the stump. Using the TA-90 stapler, the jejunum is closed immediately adjacent to the ileocecal orifice and the shortened stump is advanced into the cecum. A preferred technique is to apply traction to the stump so that the stapling instrument can be applied to the intussusceptum itself. It could be argued that application of the stapler to the devitalized intussusceptum is inappropriate technique, but this segment will readily retract into the cecum when the bowel is transected and, in truth, the stump has no better blood supply than does the intussusceptum in most cases. In either case, every effort should be made to oversew the ileocecal orifice. The mesenteric defect created by the entero-cecostomy is closed by suture of the small intestinal mesentery to itself and to the ileocecal fold.

Generally, efforts should be made to reduce the intussusception only in the rare case in which it appears that the intussusception may still be viable. If reduction is accomplished, the viability of the intussusceptum must be confirmed not only by visual criteria but also by objective means. If ileal viability is confirmed, a side-to-side ileocecostomy is performed without ileal transection. Simple reduction is not adequate therapy. Even if the ileum is viable, there will probably be sufficient mural edema to interfere with the flow of ingesta through the site. Additionally, an ileocecal anastomosis will act to fix the ileum to the cecum and potentially prevent recurrence of intussusception.

It is possible to close the ileocecal orifice in many horses with ileocecal intussusception. It is a relatively easy technique in immature horses but also can be performed in many adults. The nature of the disease is such that the cecum and large colon are virtually empty at the time of surgery. If the small intestine is thoroughly emptied, reasonable exposure of the area can be obtained. Closure of bowel at this level is readily achieved using the TA-90 stapling instrument. Long instruments are useful for hand suture of the ileocecal orifice, especially in adult horses. If it is not possible to adequately invert or resect the distal stump, an alternative is to perform a celiotomy using a right 16th or 17th rib resection. This approach will provide sufficient access to the ileocecal junction to resect the stump flush with the orifice and to close the ileocecal orifice.

Prognosis

The prognosis for life after surgical treatment of acute ileocecal intussusception is guarded. Necrosis of the distal stump is responsible for most fatalities, but shock, ileus, anastomosis failure, and other typical complications of colic surgery contribute to the mortality rate. Even if the stump is isolated from the abdomen, many horses will exhibit moderate pain for several days after surgery, presumably as a result of ongoing necrosis of the intussusception and traction on the mesentery of the intussuscepted segment. The fate of the intussuscepted portion of bowel is unclear. Obstruction of the cecocolic orifice by the inverted stump has been observed as a long-term complication in horses in which the small intestine was inverted into the cecum.

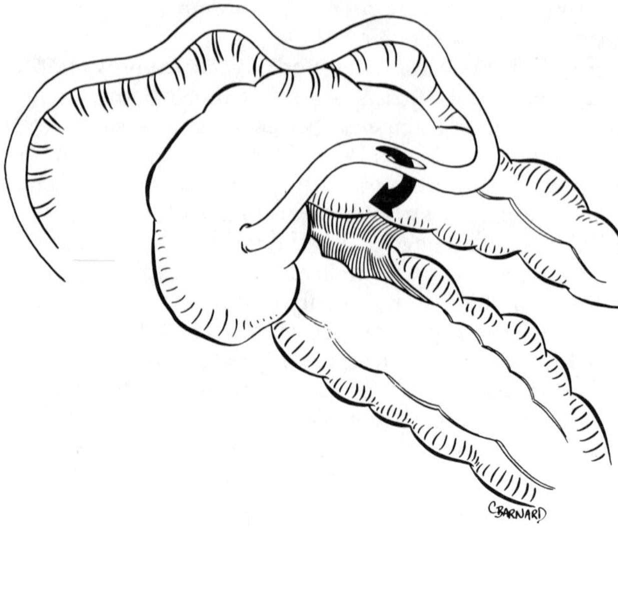

Figure 63–2. Enterocecal anastomosis as treatment for chronic ileocecal intussusception (as seen with the horse in dorsal recumbency). A side-to-side anastomosis between the small intestine and the cecum has been completed. The ileum is not transected.

CHRONIC ILEOCECAL INTUSSUSCEPTION

Diagnosis

Intussusception of a short segment of ileum into the cecum results in a very different clinical picture. Most animals with this disorder are yearlings, but it can occur in older horses. Poor general physical condition, signs of intermittent or continual mild abdominal pain, depression, and poor appetite are common clinical findings. Bouts of colic are readily managed with analgesic therapy. The duration of signs may range from several days to many months. It is often possible to palpate large, relatively flaccid loops of small intestine per rectum. Laboratory findings are not remarkable. Surgical exploration is usually performed electively in an attempt to make a diagnosis when chronic colic and poor physical condition are present.

Surgery and Prognosis

Chronic ileocecal intussusception is readily diagnosed upon surgical exploration. Palpation of the ileocecal area reveals a short intussusception (usually 3 to 5 cm). The intussusception is usually readily reducible. Dilation and hypertrophy of ileum and distal jejunum proximal to the intussusception are often marked. The ileum should be left intact and a side-to-side enterocecostomy performed (Fig. 63–2). No problems have been encountered after leaving grossly abnormal small intestine intact. The prognosis for complete recovery after surgery is good.

BIBLIOGRAPHY

Barclay WP, Phillips TN, Foerner JJ: Intussusception associated with *Anoplocephala perfoliata* infection in five horses. *J Am Vet Med Assoc* 1982;180:752–753.

Edwards GB: Surgical management of intussusception in the horse. *Equine Vet J* 1986;18,313–321.

Hackett MS, Hackett RP: Chronic ileocecal intussusception in horses. *Cornell Vet* 1989;79:353–361.

Peterson FB, Stewart JV: Experimental ileocecal anastomosis in the horse. *J Equine Med Surg* 1978;2:461–464.

Vasey JR, Julian RJ: Elective inversion of the distal ileal stump into the caecum of the horse. *Equine Vet J* 1987;19:223–225.

64
Cecal Impaction

Richard P. Hackett

ETIOLOGY

Cecal impaction is a relatively uncommon cause of colic in horses. There are no apparent sex or breed predispositions for the disease, but it is more common in aged horses than in juvenile animals. The etiology of cecal impaction in horses is obscure, but evidence suggests that the problem is functional rather than mechanical. Ingesta in the cecum in affected horses is typically normal in consistency, and evidence of physical obstruction at the cecocolic orifice is rare. These findings, coupled with the observation that many affected horses have concurrent medical problems, strongly suggest that cecal impaction in most horses results from accumulation of an excessive amount of ingesta in the cecum secondary to impaired cecal motility. Poor dentition, low-quality feedstuffs, and thromboembolic bowel disease have been suggested as predisposing factors. Of particular concern, however is the recognition that this disease may occur in horses undergoing treatment for unrelated gastrointestinal or other systemic disease or as a postoperative complication of horses undergoing either elective surgery or colic surgery. Fasting, general anesthesia, and surgery may possibly have a temporary adverse effect on cecal motility, as may antimicrobial or analgesic drug therapy.

Cecal perforation may occur either secondary to cecal impaction or as a primary event. Primary cecal perforation is not associated with overfilling of the cecum and has been observed primarily as a periparturient event in mares. Many, if not most, cases of cecal perforation in periparturient mares are secondary to cecal impaction. The cause of primary cecal perforation in broodmares is unknown, although excessive intraabdominal or intracecal pressures at parturition, positional relationships between the fetus and cecum at parturition, and postparturient cecal tympany have all been suggested. Generally, there is no evidence of preexisting disease of the cecal wall. However, in a few cases of primary cecal rupture, a relationship between cecal injury from tapeworm (*Anoplocephala perfoliata*) infestation and cecal perforation has been suggested.

CLINICAL SIGNS

Clinical signs of cecal impaction in horses may be subtle. The capacity of the cecum coupled with the anatomic proximity of the ileocecal and cecocolic orifices are such that a large amount of ingesta can accumulate in the cecum and yet the horse does not exhibit typical signs of intestinal obstruction. Typically, gas and some ingesta will pass through the cecum so that distention proximal to the impaction (in the small intestine) is not a feature of the disease. Most horses therefore exhibit signs of only mild abdominal pain, although the occasional horse may show evidence of more severe pain. Affected animals usually are depressed and have a reduced appetite. Intestinal hypomotility and passage of a reduced amount of soft or loose manure are common. These vague signs may be overlooked, especially in animals with other medical problems. In a number of hospitalized patients subtle signs of cecal impaction either were not observed or were not properly interpreted, and the impaction was not diagnosed until cecal perforation or even sudden death had occurred.

There is an apparent association between the use of nonsteroidal anti-inflammatory drugs and secondary cecal perforation. There is no evidence to suggest that these drugs contribute to cecal dysfunction. It appears that their effect is merely to mask the clinical signs associated with cecal impaction and thus delay recognition of the problem.

The natural course of horses affected with cecal impaction tends to be somewhat prolonged. Often, the horse will appear to respond well to analgesic therapy and may remain fairly stable for several days. In many affected horses, however, cecal perforation will occur and there will be a dramatic deterioration of the animal's condition. Clinical signs in horses with cecal perforation include severe depression, mild colic, trembling, sweating, tachycardia, dehydration, reduced or absent borborygmi, and severe dehydration. Death occurs within several hours.

DIAGNOSIS

A diagnosis of cecal impaction is made by rectal palpation of a cecum distended with ingesta. The cecal base is readily palpable in the right upper abdominal quadrant. An appropriate "index of suspicion" is important and dictates that a rectal examination be performed on any hospitalized horse that shows signs of even mild abdominal pain. Laboratory determinations are of no value in confirming the diagnosis, but analysis of peritoneal fluid is recommended to rule out cecal perforation in particularly ill horses. A complete blood count and determination of acid-base and electrolyte status are indicated so that supportive therapy may be tailored to the patient's needs.

Perforation of a viscus leads to abrupt, dramatic clinical deterioration of affected horses. A diagnosis of cecal perforation is confirmed by rectal palpation and by abdominocentesis. In most cases, the cecum is readily palpable as a firm, enlarged viscus in the right upper quadrant of the abdomen. In many patients, a distinct grittiness is appreciated as the hand is moved across serosal surfaces. The detection of plant material, bacteria, and degenerative neutrophils on examination of peritoneal fluid confirms the diagnosis of bowel perforation.

SURGERY

It is generally agreed that a diagnosis of cecal impaction warrants a recommendation for surgical intervention. Although medical therapy (analgesics, fluid therapy, and laxatives) has been successful in some horses, there is a substantial (over 50%) risk that horses undergoing medical therapy for cecal impaction will develop lethal cecal perforation. For this reason, medical therapy should be reserved for only those cases in which financial constraints prohibit surgical therapy.

A number of surgical options are available. These include massage, typhlotomy and evacuation, partial or complete typhlectomy, cecocolic anastomosis, and ileocolic anastomosis. Massage of the impaction, with or without transmural injection of fluid or surfactants, may enhance passage of ingesta from the cecum and has the advantage that an enterotomy is not performed. Both massage and typhlotomy may be performed in standing animals but, in most cases, ventral celiotomy is used. The cecum may be emptied by a typhlotomy performed near the cecal apex. Great care should be taken during manipulation of the heavy, impacted cecum to minimize the risk of its rupture; nonetheless, the cecal apex and body should be exteriorized as completely as possible so that the apex may be isolated from the sterile field over the side of the horse. The cecal contents may be evacuated manually or preferably be lavaged out by use of a large volume of water delivered by a hose. The cecum is closed either with sutures (Connell with Lembert oversew) or with staples. Although either massage or typhlotomy may be successful methods for management of cecal impaction, both techniques assume that cecal motility is normal. In horses treated only by massage, ingesta is not removed from the cecum and may inspissate to again form an impaction. This procedure, therefore, is associated with an unacceptably high incidence of postoperative cecal perforation and cannot be recommended.

Evacuation of the cecum by typhlotomy has been a highly successful procedure in some reports. Campbell et al. reported survival of seven of eight horses (88%) with cecal impaction treated by typhlotomy and cecal evacuation. Other authors, however, have indicated that this is an unacceptable procedure because of a high incidence of postoperative recurrence of impaction and perforation. A difference in etiology (perhaps related to forages in different geographic areas) may account for the difference. If cecal function is normal, evacuation of the cecum followed by appropriate dietary management after surgery should be curative. However, if cecal function is abnormal, a recurrence of impaction and risk of perforation would be expected after this procedure.

Huskamp described successful treatment of chronic cecal impaction by typhlectomy in two horses. A celiotomy that included resection of the 18th rib was used to gain access to the base of the cecum. After resection of the cecum, a side-to-side anastomosis between the ileum and the right ventral colon was performed to restore intestinal continuity. Although this procedure quite effectively negates possible recurrence of an impaction, the approach, regional anatomy, and techniques are unfamiliar to most surgeons and consequently the procedure has not gained popularity.

Ross et al. recommended cecocolostomy in recognition of the fact that cecal motility is impaired in many horses with cecal impaction. It was reasoned that creation of a stoma between the cecum and the right ventral colon would enhance movement of ingesta from the cecum and avert recurrence of impaction and perforation (Fig. 64–1). Experience with 14 horses was reported. A 15- to 20-cm side-to-side anastomosis was created between the cecum (between the lateral and dorsal teniae) and the right ventral colon (between the lateral and medial free teniae) using either sutures (five horses) or the GIA Auto-Suture stapling instrument

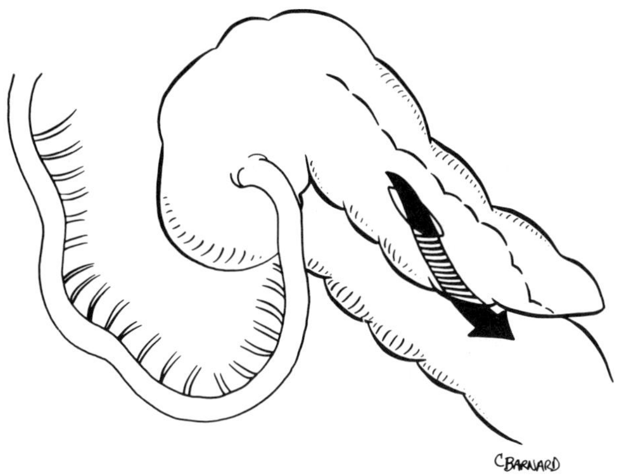

Figure 64-1. Cecocolostomy as viewed from a ventral midline incision with the horse in dorsal recumbency. Flow of ingesta out of the cecum is enhanced by creation of a stoma between the cecum and the right ventral colon.

(United States Surgical Corp) (nine horses). Cecocolic anastomosis was preceded by typhlotomy and evacuation of the cecum in nine horses and by injection and massage in two horses, and was the sole procedure in three horses. Following surgery, two horses succumbed

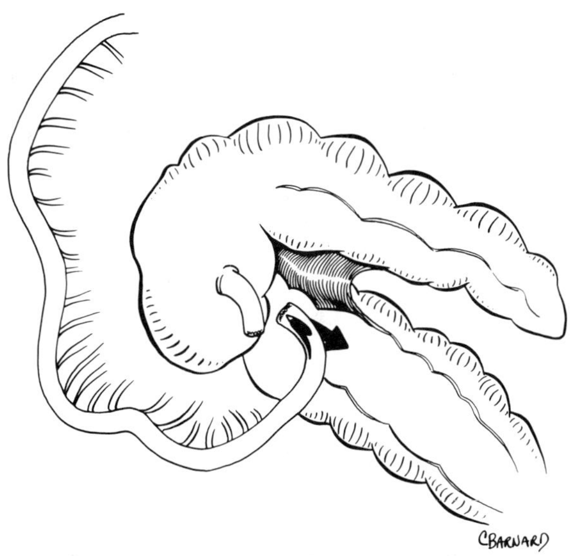

Figure 64–2. Ileocolostomy. The cecum and colon are drawn as they would be seen with the horse in dorsal recumbency. The cecum is excluded from the flow of ingesta by creation of a stoma between the ileum and the right ventral colon.

to acute peritonitis, one died of mesenteric volvulus 3 months after surgery, and one was euthanized for an unrelated disease. The long-term survival rate (12-month follow-up) was 71%. Four of the ten long-term survivors experienced chronic, intermittent, mild abdominal pain apparently associated with gaseous distention of the cecum. It was postulated that either the cecocolic anastomosis did not permit gas to exit the cecum or it allowed reflux of gas from the right ventral colon into the cecum. Further investigation of this procedure is warranted, but its usefulness in clinical patients appears limited because of this complication.

In 1987, Craig et al. advocated complete cecal bypass for treatment of cecal impaction. It was believed that diversion of all ingesta from the ileum into the right ventral colon would satisfactorily address the problem of recurrence of impaction in horses with impaired cecal motility (Fig. 64–2). The ileum was transected and closed with stapling instruments and the GIA stapling instrument was used to perform a 10-cm side-to-side anastomosis between the ileum and the right ventral colon (between the lateral and medial free teniae). Experience with complete cecal bypass in five horses was reported. Ileocolostomy was preceded by typhlotomy and cecal evacuation in four cases. All horses survived the procedure, but one horse was euthanized 2 months after surgery with colic due to adhesions from a previous abdominal procedure. The long-term survival rate (6-month follow-up), therefore, was 80%. Chronic postoperative colic was not observed in this small group of horses. Apparently, maintenance of a competent cecocolic orifice prevented reflux of gas from the right ventral colon into the cecum. No nutritional consequences of complete cecal bypass were recognized in these horses or in five ponies in which an identical procedure was experimentally performed. Results from this study are quite encouraging, but it is apparent that a greater number of clinical cases must be evaluated before the procedure can be give unreserved recommendation. Incomplete cecal bypass (ileocolic anastomosis without ileal transection) also was investigated in this study but was not recommended since it did not appear to appreciably change the amount of ingesta entering the cecum.

PREVENTION

Since the etiology of cecal impaction is obscure, specific recommendations cannot be made to prevent the problem. General recommendations would include a good parasite control program, appropriate routine dental care, and feeding high-quality forages. In patients undergoing surgery, it has been observed that a gradual introduction of feed after surgery and administration of mineral oil after anesthesia appear to reduce the incidence of postoperative ileus, which presumably contributes to the development of impaction. The routine use of analgesic medication in postsurgical horses should be avoided when possible so that subtle signs of cecal impaction are not masked.

BIBLIOGRAPHY

Campbell ML, Colahan PC, Brown MP, Grandstedt ME, Peyton LC: Cecal impaction in the horse. *J Am Vet Med Assoc* 1984;184:950–952.

Craig DR, Pankowski RL, Car BD, Hackett RP, Erb HN: Ileocolostomy: A technique for surgical management of equine cecal impaction. *Vet Surg* 1987;16:451–455.

Huskamp B: Some problems associated with intestinal surgery in the horse. *Equine Vet J* 1977;9:111–115.

Platt H: Caecal rupture in parturient mares. *J Comp Pathol* 1983;93:343–346.

Ross MW, Martin BB, Donawick WJ: Cecal perforation in the horse. *J Am Vet Med Assoc* 1985;187:249–253.

Ross MW, Tate LP, Donawick WJ, Richardson DW: Cecocolic anastomosis for the surgical management of cecal impaction in horses. *Vet Surg* 1986;15:85–92.

65
Cecocolic and Colocolic Intussusception

James T. Robertson

Cecocolic and colocolic intussusceptions are uncommon causes of intestinal obstruction. Similar factors predispose to both conditions and they include parasitism, changes in diet, impaction, intramural abscessation, and drug-induced alterations in motility. Intussusception of the colon has been reported to occur most frequently in horses less than 3 years of age.

CECOCOLIC INTUSSUSCEPTION

Diagnosis

Cecocolic intussusception is preceded by an invagination of the apex of the cecum into the body of the cecum. This invagination may stop at this stage or may progress, with the cecal apex passing though the cecocolic orifice into the right ventral colon. Ultimately, the entire cecum invaginates into the colon and the distal portion frequently becomes strangulated (Fig. 65–1A). Cecocolic intussusception can produce signs of acute colic, or the colic may be subacute and protracted, with associated weight loss and the passage of scant amounts of soft feces. This variability of clinical signs is likely related to the stage of cecal invagination and the degree of cecal swelling and resultant obstruction. On rectal examination, the intussusception may be palpable as a large mass in the right dorsal quadrant of the abdomen. Occasionally small intestinal obstruction with palpable distension occurs if the ileum is drawn into the intussuception. Inflammation of the invaginated cecum produces changes in the peritoneal fluid that suggest peritonitis, but this change is slow to occur since the affected tissue is often isolated from the abdominal cavity. In one reported case, the white blood cell count was markedly elevated. Failure of medical therapy with recurrence of abdominal pain usually leads to surgical exploration.

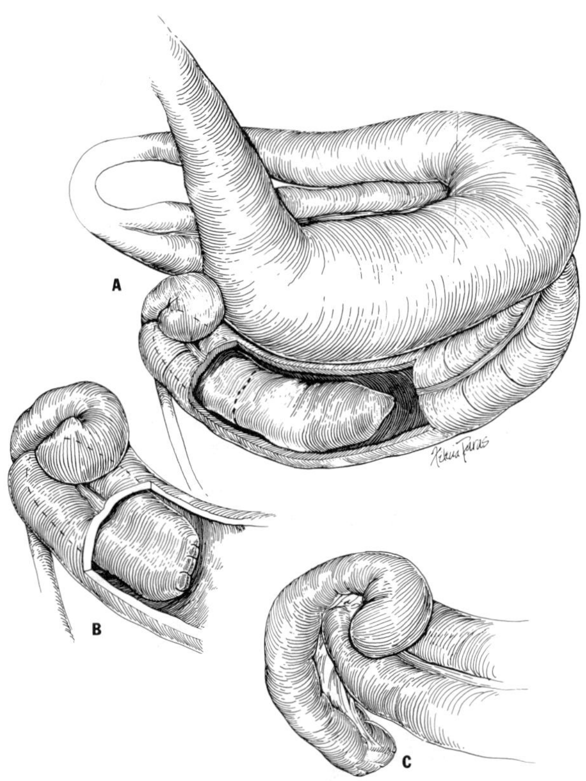

Figure 65–1. A. A cutaway of the right ventral colon showing a complete cecocolic intussusception. The dotted line across the cecum indicates the level of cecal resection. **B.** Amputated stump of the cecum prior to reduction of the intussusception. **C.** Intussusception has been reduced and the amputated stump of the cecum oversewn to ensure integrity of the suture line.

Surgery

A ventral midline celiotomy is performed. If the cecum cannot be located and a mass is palpable in the right ventral colon, a cecocolic intussusception should be suspected. The diagnosis can be confirmed by palpating the base of the cecum and feeling the invagination. The distal ileum and ileocecal junction are usually drawn into the intussusception. In my experience, attempts to reduce this form of intussusception have been unsuccessful. The combination of adhesions that develop between the serosal surfaces of the cecum and edema in the wall of the cecum make attempts at manual reduction unsuccessful.

The large colon is exteriorized as completely as possible. The right ventral colon is packed off and a 40-cm longitudinal incision is made through the ventral tenia, exposing the intussusceptum. Although the entire cecum is edematous, the mucosa of the distal portion of the cecum usually appears more devitalized. Further attempts can be made to manually reduce the intussusception, but amputation of the apex and a portion of the body of the cecum is usually necessary to allow reduction. Because of the thickness of the cecal wall, intestinal clamps or mechanical stapling devices cannot be utilized for the cecal resection. Large mattress-type sutures of a size 2 absorbable suture material are placed across the cecum prior to amputation. Alternatively, the cecum is transected, the cecal vessels are transfixed, and the seromuscular and mucosal layers are then sutured (Fig. 65–1B). The intussusception is reduced through the enterostomy by pushing the amputated stump of the cecum out of the ventral colon and having an assistant apply gentle traction to the distal ileum (Fig. 65–1C). After reduction, interrupted inverting sutures are placed in the seromuscular layers, across the line of amputation, to reinforce the cecal closure. The enterotomy in the tenia of the right ventral colon is then closed.

Postoperative Care and Prognosis

Following surgery, broad-spectrum antibiotic therapy should be maintained for at least 1 week. The horse can resume eating hay within 24 hours of surgery, providing there is good intestinal motility and an absence of abdominal pain. Following successful surgery, the horse will have a good appetite, maintain its weight, have normal feces, be free of abdominal pain, and ultimately be able to return to work. This is possible providing the horse is in good preoperative condition, there is minimal contamination during surgery, and the distal ileum and base of the cecum are viable and remain so following correction. There is an increased risk of developing peritonitis or an incisional infection if there is peritoneal contamination associated with the enterotomy or manipulation of the intussuscepted cecum.

Infarction of the base of the cecum or strangulation of the entire cecum and distal ileum is possible. In such a case a total typhlectomy is necessary and the prognosis is poor. Fortunately, in each of the horses with cecocolic intussusception that I have surgically treated, only the apex and a portion of the body of the cecum were devitalized.

COLOCOLIC INTUSSUSCEPTION

Diagnosis

Colocolic intussusception is likely to involve the left ventral, pelvic flexure, or the left dorsal segments of the large colon. Initially, there are episodes of mild to moderate abdominal discomfort and clinical signs that are similar to those seen with an impaction or a simple colonic displacement. As the disease progresses (24 to 48 hours), moderate abdominal pain persists despite analgesic therapy. There is an increased heart rate (>60 beats/min), decreased fecal production, and intestinal hypomotility. Mild dehydration will develop. On rectal examination, the intussusception may be palpable as a firm viscus and the large colon proximal to the obstruction will be distended with gas and ingesta. Progressive abdominal and large bowel distention are indicators of large bowel obstruction. Complete obstruction produces ileus and nasogastric reflux. In more advanced cases, the abdominal fluid may have an elevated white blood cell count and a high protein content. The decision to perform exploratory surgery is based on a persistence of abdominal pain, tachycardia, and evidence of a large bowel obstruction.

Surgery

A ventral midline celiotomy is performed, the large colon is decompressed, and the intussusception is exteriorized and packed off. Manual reduction of the intussusception should be attempted and may be successful. If reduction of the intussusception is not possible or the reduced bowel appears devitalized, resection and anastomosis are necessary. Several techniques for large colon resection and anastomosis have been described. The use of mechanical stapling devices helps to reduce surgical time and minimize the amount of contamination. An end-to-end anastomosis is possible if the ends of the large colon are of similar diameter, whereas a side-to-side anastomosis is advantageous if the two segments have different luminal diameters. The side-to-side anastomosis should create a generous stoma that is situated at the end of each blind segment. This prevents the formation of blind pouches that could promote impaction.

Postoperative Care and Prognosis

Postoperative management is similar to that described following a cecocolic intussuception. Long-term follow-up of these horses revealed that they had normal appetites, maintained their weight, were free of abdominal pain, and had resumed normal activity.

Reports of surgical correction of large colon intussusception would indicate that the prognosis is good following either manual reduction or surgical resection and anastomosis. Success is dependent upon minimizing peritoneal contamination if resection and anastomosis are performed.

BIBLIOGRAPHY

Allison CJ: Invagination of the cecum into the colon in a Welsh pony. *Equine Vet J* 1977;9:84–86.

Bertone AL, Stashak TS, Sullins KE: Large colon resection and anastomosis in horses. *J Am Vet Med Assoc* 1986;188:612–617.

Cowles RR Jr, Bunch SE, Flynn DV, Schmidt GR: Cecal inversion in a horse. *Vet Med Small Anim Clin* 1977;72:1346–1348.

Dyson S, Orsini J: Intussusception of the large colon in a horse. *J Am Vet Med Assoc* 1983;182:720.

Hackett RP: Colonic volvulus and intussusception, in Robinson NE (ed): *Current Therapy in Equine Medicine*, ed 2. Philadelphia, WB Saunders Co, 1987, pp 66–68.

Pearson H, Messervy A, Pinsent PJN: Surgical treatment of abdominal disorders in the horse. *J Am Vet Med Assoc* 1971;159:1344–1352.

Robertson JT, Johnson FM: Surgical correction of cecocolic intussusception in a horse. *J Am Vet Med Assoc* 1980;176:223–224.

Robertson JT, Tate LP Jr: Resection of intussuscepted large colon in a horse. *J Am Vet Med Assoc* 1982;181:927–928.

Wilson DG, Wilson WD, Reinertson EL: Intussusception of the left dorsal colon in a horse. *J Am Vet Med Assoc* 1983;183:464–465.

66
Large Colon Volvulus

James A. Orsini

Large colon volvulus, also known as large colon torsion, is the most severe colonic disease causing a strangulation obstruction and is often fatal. Because of the rapid progression of signs and intestinal degeneration, it is vital that large colon volvulus be recognized in its early stages to have a chance at reducing the high mortality rate. Most cases of large colon volvulus occur at the origin of the large intestine (excluding the cecum; Fig. 66–1), or at the cecocolic mesentery (including the cecum). When the volvulus is limited to the colon, the dorsal and ventral portions of the large colon rotate on the mesocolon, and since they are in close opposition they also rotate around each other. The direction of the rotation is usually a lateral-dorsal movement of the ventral colon and a medial-ventral movement of the dorsal colon, which is a clockwise rotation of the right colons (Figs. 66–2 and 66–3).

There is substantial variation in the degree of rotation of the large colon. Rotation of 90 degrees or less is considered to be within normal physiologic limits; those rotations between 90 and 180 degrees may correct spontaneously; and a rotation in excess of 180 degrees is considered pathologic and will not correct spontaneously. Rotations of the large colon in excess of 360 degrees (up to 720 degrees have been encountered. The most frequent clinical finding is a 360-degree rotation just cranial to the cecocolic ligament. This presentation involves almost the entire large colon and sometimes the cecum. The loops of colon are spirally wrapped around each other at the point of volvulus. A rotation of 180 degrees results in luminal narrowing, and rotation greater than 270 degrees causes total occlusion.

DIAGNOSIS

Signalment

All ages of horses and breeds are affected by large colon volvulus, but mares are more often affected than stallions or geldings. Two reasons have been hypothesized for the occurrence of large colon volvulus in horses. First, when there is a change from a high-fiber diet (hay and straw) to a low-fiber, high-carbohydrate diet (such as grain or grass), increased fermentation occurs. This is believed to cause an intensive production of volatile fatty acids that cause a decrease in motility of the large colon. Second, after foaling, the abdominal musculature of the mare is stretched and permits freer movement of the large colon within the abdominal cavity. The potential for a large colon volvulus is thus enhanced.

History

Historic information obtained by the veterinarian should include the duration of the present illness, the number and frequency of recurrences, and the severity of the clinical signs. Environmental or management portions of the history may include dietary, exercise, and stabling changes that may be associated with the onset of colic. In most cases mares will have foaled recently and will be lactating. Other commonly affected horses are those in work that are kept in stalls most or part of the day and have a high proportion of the diet as concentrate.

Presenting Signs

The disease may start with signs of low-grade pain due to luminal narrowing from a 180-degree rotation of the large colon, and then gradually progress in severity. If total obstruction occurs, there is a sudden onset of very severe, unrelenting abdominal pain. Affected animals may initially demonstrate evidence of pain by pawing, lying down, and then standing. Rolling may also be observed; these animals generally drop to the ground, roll uncontrollably, and then jump up only to fall to the ground again. Affected horses are unpredictable and can be dangerous to the assistants and veterinarians trying to manage them. Consequently, thorough physical examination is usually not possible. Horses with large colon volvulus seem to prefer lying on their back for pain relief. Analgesics tend to provide only a very short period of pain relief, and in many cases, are totally ineffectual. Sweating, tachycardia, tachypnea, and abdominal distention are consistent findings. As the disease progresses, abdominal distention becomes so severe that the paralumbar fossae are not identifiable. In advanced stages of the disease, pain may be diminished or, in some cases, absent and replaced by depres-

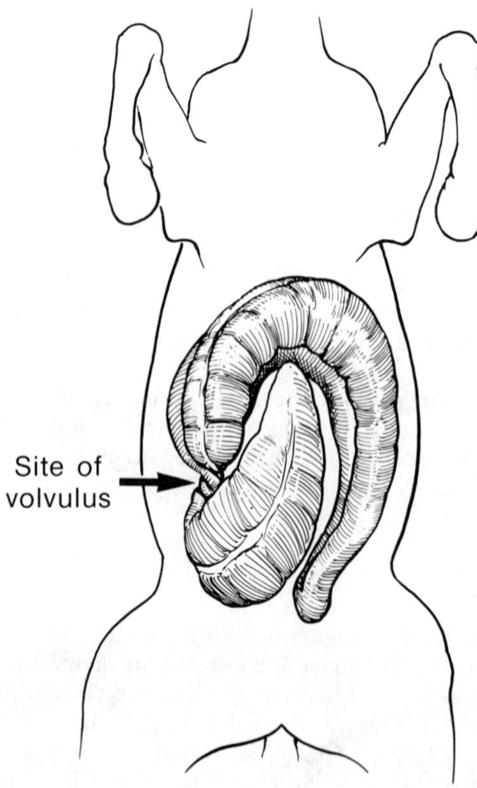

Figure 66–1. A ventral view of the horse's abdomen illustrating the most common site for a volvulus of the large colon.

sion. The horse may be apathetic, prefering to lie in dorsal recumbency and resist any form of movement.

Physical Examination and Confirmatory Tests

The clinical diagnosis of volvulus of the large colon relies heavily on the clinical picture of a dramatic and rapidly progressive colic that leads to a state of depression and severe shock. Rectal examination, an essential part of the examination, reveals horizontally positioned tympanitic loops of large colon palpable at the pelvic inlet. There is characteristically a large amount of gas distention within the strangulated portion of colon. Palpation of thickened colonic walls is considered almost pathognomonic for this disease. This thickening is due to intramural edema typical of a strangulated large colon. The specific site of the obstruction cannot be determined by rectal examination. If the torsion is 360 degress, the orientation of tenia is often normal, which can be misleading in the early stages prior to marked colon distention.

Colon volvulus of 180 degrees will often have an insidious onset of signs and a mild course of disease over a few days. On rectal examination, there may be a relatively empty colon, as a result of the lack of gas production from the small amount of ingesta within the bowel. The intraluminal pressure will only be slightly increased, especially if no strangulation of the bowel wall has occurred. Despite marked intramural edema, this rather chronic form of volvulus leads to episodic attacks of colic. There are few systemic effects from this type of disease. This form of large colon volvulus can be diagnosed by rectal examination. The clinician should feel carefully for edema of the bowel wall and mesocolon, confirmed by the fleshy, rigid feel of the bowel loops. Gastric reflux may be part of the presenting signs even though small bowel disease is not present. This is believed to occur secondary to increased tension on the duodenocolic ligament, resulting in occlusion of the duodenum and prevention of gastric emptying.

SURGERY

Anatomy

Surgical treatment of large colon volvulus is the only successful method of therapy. The horse is positioned in dorsal recumbency and a ventral midline celiotomy is performed. A long incision frequently is required to exteriorize the large colon. The midline incision is preferred over the paramedian approach because it provides greater exposure of the abdominal organs. The incision begins just cranial to the umbilicus and extends craniad; its length is generally 30 to 40 cm. The bands and sacculations of the large intestine are valuable aids in identifying the different segments of the colon. The cecum is sacculated and has four bands. The dorsal and medial bands extend to the apex. The lateral band may or may not reach the apex. The ventral band joins the medial. The medial and lateral bands are accompanied by the medial and lateral cecal arteries. The cecocolic fold connects the lateral band of the cecum with the lateral free band of the right ventral colon. The entire ventral colon is sacculated and has four bands, two of which are free of the mesocolon on the ventral surface, the lateral and medial free bands. On the dorsal surface are the lateral and medial mesocolic bands, which are concealed, but can be palpated. At the pelvic flexure, only the medial mesocolic band is continued to the left dorsal colon, and the sacculations are no longer present. Therefore, the left dorsal colon has only one mesocolic band and no sacculations. A marked decrease in diameter occurs from the left ventral colon to the pelvic flexure. Near the diaphragmatic flexure, the dorsal colon acquires two free (dorsal) bands, so that the diaphragmatic flexure and the right

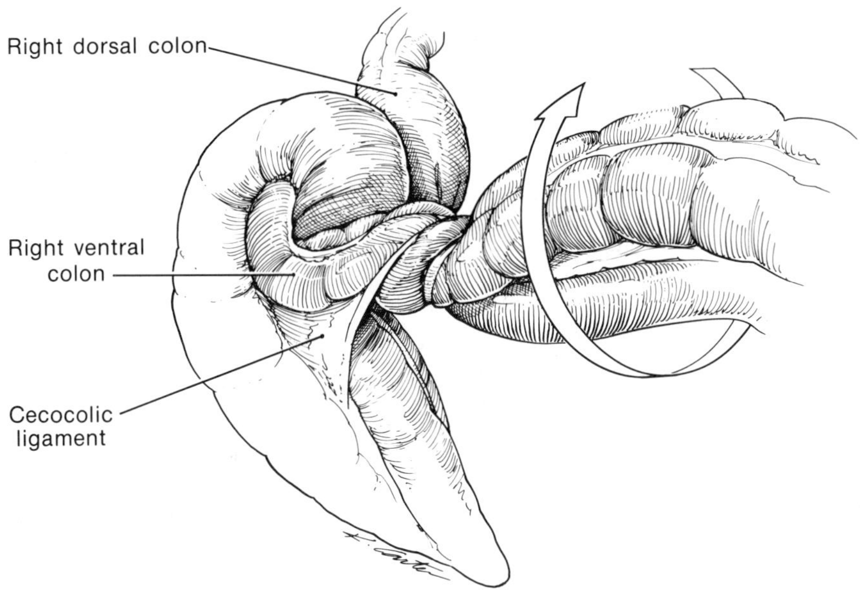

Figure 66–2. A diagrammatic sketch depicting a clockwise volvulus of the large colon near the junction of the right ventral colon with the cecum. The right dorsal colon, right ventral colon, and cecocolic ligament are identified.

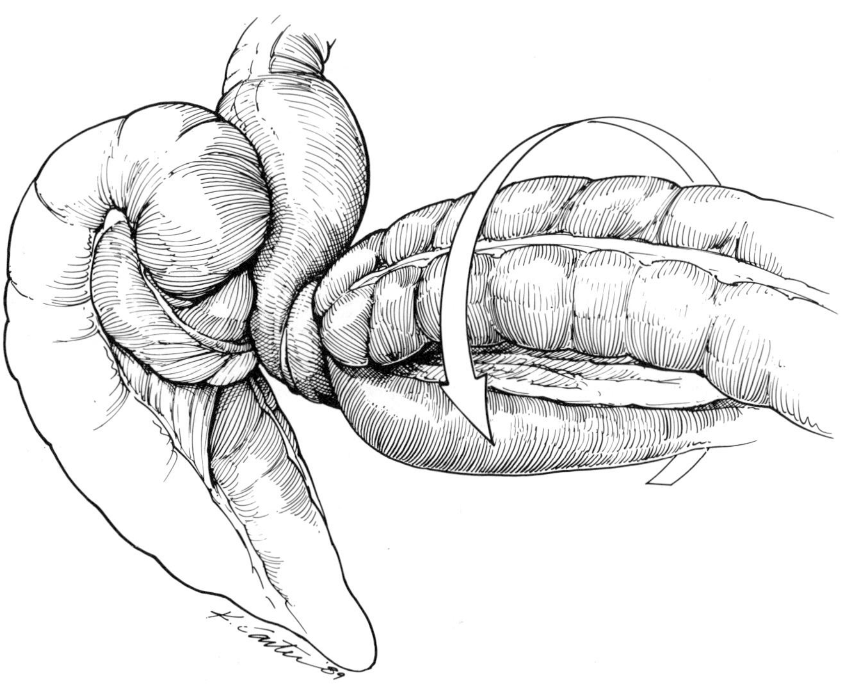

Figure 66–3. A diagrammatic sketch depicting a counterclockwise volvulus of the large colon near the junction of the right ventral colon with the cecum.

dorsal colon have three bands. There are no sacculations in the dorsal colon, except some indistinct ones in the terminal portion. The right dorsal colon is the largest portion of the colon. It turns to the left and decreases markedly in diameter as it joins the transverse colon.

Technique and Special Concerns

On entering the abdominal cavity, tremendous distention of the large colon is usually present. If there is a volvulus of 360 degrees the colon will appear to be in a normal position with the exception that the cecum is often displaced dorsally. The serosal surface of the large bowel will be pale white to dark blue and generally is very edematous. The tip of the apex may be the only portion of the cecum that can be exteriorized. This is true when the volvulus occurs at the origin of the entire large intestine. If the volvulus occurs more craniad in the right colon, the cecum can be exteriorized and followed to the cecocolic ligament. Repositioning of the large colon requires a combination of manipulation, decompression, and delicate handling. Because of the vascular embarrassment, the bowel wall is friable and very susceptible to rupture during manipulation.

Decompression and/or evacuation are essential preludes to attempted reduction. Evacuation will decrease the weight of the large intestine and may remove some of the toxins from the lumen that may be absorbed once the volvulus is corrected. If evacuation is deemed necessary, the pelvic flexure and left colons are exteriorized and suspended over the edge of the table or on an enterotomy tray. A large incision is made in the pelvic flexure region and ingesta is flushed from the colon with water. A hose is used to introduce water into the bowel lumen that will mix with the intestinal contents. The bowel can thus be almost completely emptied. Both the ventral and dorsal portions of the colon should be emptied in a similar fashion. The serosal surface of the bowel is rinsed thoroughly with saline and the enterotomy is closed. Before closing the enterotomy site, the colonic mucosa is evaluated. If the mucosa is pink, the prognosis is favorable; if it is dark red in color the prognosis is guarded; and if it is black, the prognosis is poor.

Before colonic reduction is attempted, the direction of the volvulus should be determined. In the majority of cases, the volvulus will start by the ventral colon, rotating dorsolateral (Fig. 66–2). It is important to remember that because of the *U*-shaped nature of the large intestine, the left colon must be moved in the opposite direction of the desired rotation of the right colon while in the abdomen. Therefore, the colon is exteriorized and straightened to ease reduction. Correction is confirmed by: (*a*) return of the cecum and colon to their normal anatomic positions, and (*b*) an inability to palpate the point of strangulation obstruction. The reduction is started at the pelvic flexure and carried around to the right colon. Intraabdominal handling is greatly eased by the introduction of sterile saline solution warmed to body temperature. Generally, 5 to 10 L of this solution will reduce the frictional effects and enable the surgeon to manipulate the suspended bowel loops with greater ease.

Partial colonic resection may be an option in horses with large colon volvulus that excludes the cecum and in which necrosis has developed (Chapter 67). Resection of up to 95% of the length of large colon has been tolerated without difficulty and with few signs of intestinal malabsorption. Resection and anastomosis is performed with either stapling instruments or hand placed sutures to close the transected stumps of the dorsal colon and ventral colon, followed by a side-to-side anastomosis. If a small portion of the left ventral and dorsal colon is the primary site of the volvulus, successful resection and anastomosis can be performed with minimal contamination.

A procedure reported to prevent a recurrence of a large colon volvulus is colopexy of the ventral colon to the ventral abdominal wall. Additional experience is needed before this procedure can be recommended.

POSTOPERATIVE CARE

Appropriate postoperative care of horses following surgical treatment of large colon volvulus is essential. This is particularly true when there has been compromise of the vascular integrity in the strangulated portion of large bowel, since there will be marked loss of protein into the extravascular space and lumen of the intestine. Therefore, the total plasma protein needs to be monitored closely during the postoperative period. While fluid administration requirements during the postoperative period may be large, it is important that the total plasma protein not be allowed to fall below 4.0 g/dL. Should this occur, a plasma transfusion is necessary.

Additionally, the release of endotoxins from the strangulated portion of bowel plays an important role in the collapse of the circulatory system in these patients. Endotoxemia will result in arterial hypoxemia, reduced arterial blood pressure, poor capillary refill, leukopenia, colic, diarrhea, and systemic lactic acidosis. Endotoxins may reach the systemic circulation by transperitoneal absorption, thereby bypassing the hepatic reticuloendothelial system. Consequently, signs of circulatory shock may ensue. Therefore, patients recovering from large colon volvulus should be closely monitored for signs of endotoxemia and treated aggressively for fluid, electrolyte, and acid-base abnormalities.

Antimicrobial administration is recommended in patients that have had an enterotomy or resection performed. Because of the large number of gram-negative aerobic and anerobic bacteria, particularly *Escherichia coli* and *Bacteroides fragilis*, the administration of appropriate antimicrobials (i.e., gentamicin and metronidazole) should be considered during the postoperative period. Nonsteroidal anti-inflammatory agents are widely used for their analgesic properties, and have been used to prevent some of the early deleterious effects of endotoxemia.

PROGNOSIS AND SPECIAL CONSIDERATIONS

The prognosis following surgical correction of large colon volvulus is directly dependent on the severity and duration of the vascular embarrassment to the large colon. Hypoproteinemia and the development of endotoxic shock are the primary reasons for a poor rate of survival. The principal cause of high morbidity and mortality in large colon volvulus is a transmural leakage and subsequent peritoneal absorption of toxic substances and bacteria. For this reason, surgery should be undertaken immediately after recognition of this problem.

BIBLIOGRAPHY

Bertone AL, Stashak TS, Sullins KE: Large colon resection and anastomosis in horses. *J Am Vet Med Assoc* 1986;188;612–617.

Donawick WJ: Metabolic management of the horse with acute abdominal crisis. *Arch Am Coll Vet Surg* 1975;5:39.

Foerner JJ: Diseases of the large intestine: Differential diagnosis and surgical management. *Vet Clin North Am Large Anim Pract* 1982;4:129–146.

Harrison, IW: Equine large intestinal volvulus, a review of 124 cases. *Vet Surg* 1988;17:77–81.

Huskamp B: Torsion of the large colon in the horse (torsio colic ascendentis), in Pfeiffer CJ (ed): *Animal Models for Intestinal Disease.* Boca Raton, FL, CRC Press, 1985, pp 197–204.

Kohn CW: Preparative management of the equine patient with an abdominal crisis. *Vet Clin North Am Large Anim Pract* 1979;1:289.

Markel MD, Meagher DM, Ford TS: Abstract: Colopexy of the equine large colon. *Vet Surg* 1986;115:128.

Meagher DM: Obstructive disease in the large intestine of the horse: Diagnosis and treatment. *Proc Am Assoc Equine Pract* 1972;pp 269–380.

Orsini JA: Large bowel obstruction, in Robinson NE (ed): *Current Therapy in Equine Medicine.* Philadelphia, WB Saunders Co, 1983, pp 231–236.

Robertson JT: Obstructive diseases, In Mannsman, RA, McAllister ES, Pratt PW (eds): *Equine Medicine and Surgery,* ed 3 Santa Barbara, CA, American Veterinary Publishing, 1982, pp 559–579.

Robertson JT, Tate LP: Resection of intussuscepted large colon in a horse. *J Am Vet Med Assoc* 1982;181:927–928.

67 Large Colon Resection

Norm G. Ducharme

Advances in veterinary surgery, medicine, and anesthesia over the last 20 years have markedly increased the survival rate of horses with acute abdominal crisis. However, treatment of large colon strangulation or nonstrangulating infarction is still associated with a high mortality rate. In a recent survey of horses with colic presented to 14 teaching hospitals, the mortality rate of large colon volvulus was 73%. Large colon resection has gained popularity in the last 5 years in an attempt to increase survival rate of horses affected with various disease involving the large colon.

SURGICAL ANATOMY

Viscera

The equine colon is subdivided into three components: the ascending or large colon, the transverse colon, and the descending or small colon. The large colon commences at the cecocolic orifice and terminates at the transverse colon. The average length of the large colon is 3 to 3.7 m and the large colon has a capacity of 55 to 130 L. The large colon can be subdivided into two parallel parts, the ventral and dorsal colon, both of which have right and left components. The three flexures connecting these parts are named according to their adjacent anatomic structure in the abdominal cavity, that is the sternal flexure, the pelvic flexure, and the diaphragmatic flexure. The muscular bands of the colon on these different parts vary in number. The ventral colon has four bands, the pelvic flexure one, and the left dorsal colon one to three depending on the site examined. In addition, the ventral colon has alternate constrictions and sacculations called haustra coli.

The large colon is fixed in the abdominal cavity to the cecum and to a short area of the body wall in the right sublumbar region. Many authors have suggested that the large colon of the horse is predisposed to volvulus or torsion because of its relatively long unfixed portion.

The large colon up to the level of the cecocolic ligament can be exteriorized through a ventral midline incision. Resection requiring access to the very proximal aspect of the ventral colon and the most distal part of the dorsal colon would necessitate a surgical approach involving removal of the 17th or 18th ribs.

The Vascular Supply

The cranial mesenteric artery divides into the jejunal vessels, the ileocecocolic vessels, the middle colic artery, and the right colic artery. The ileocecocolic artery yields the ileal artery, the medial and lateral cecal arteries, and a colic branch (Fig. 67–1). These blood vessels are located on the medial aspect of the large colon in what has been termed the vascular mesocolon (Fig. 67–2). The blood supply of the cecum is obtained from the two cecal arteries. The large colon is perfused by the right colic artery and the colic branch, which have, up to the level of the diaphragmatic and sternal flexure, many anastomotic branches (Fig. 67–1). The transverse colon and the proximal half of the small colon are vascularized by the middle colic artery. The blood supply

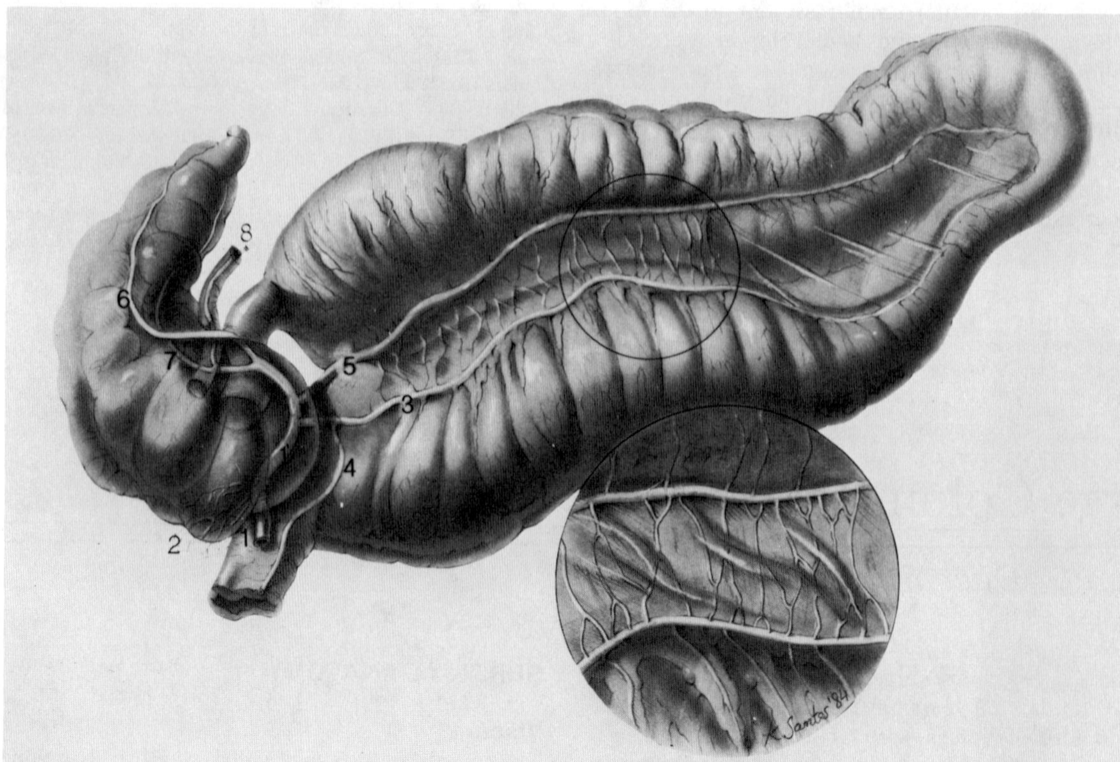

Figure 67–1. Blood supply to the cecum, large colon, and ileum: *1*, cranial mesenteric artery; *1′*, ileocecocolic artery; *2*, jejunal artery; *3*, right colic artery; *4*, middle colic artery; *5*, colic branch; *6*, lateral cecal artery; *7*, medial cecal artery; *8*, ileal artery. The enlarged view illustrates the many anastomotic branches between the right colic artery and the colic branch of the ileocecocolic artery. (From Ducharme NG, Horney FD, Baird JD, Arighi, M, Burton JH: Extensive large colon resection in the pony. 1 Surgical procedures and clinical results. *Can J Vet Res* 1987;51:66–75.)

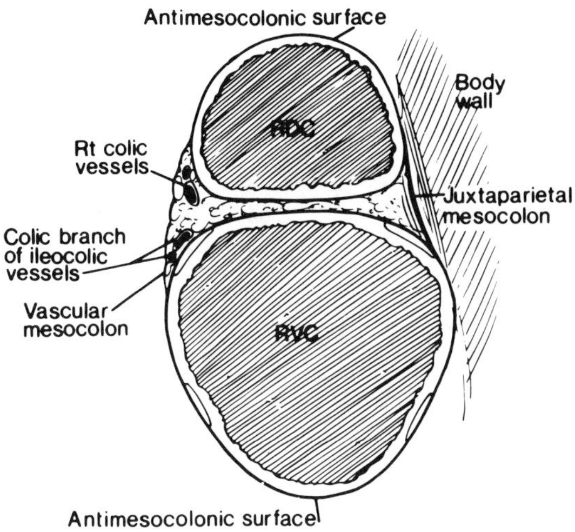

Figure 67–2. Cross-section of the colon demonstrating the anatomic position of the vascular mesocolon and the juxtaparietal mesocolon. *RDC*, right dorsal colon; *RVC*, right ventral colon. (From Bertone AL, Stashak TS, Sullins KE, Ralston SL: Experimental large colon resection at the cecocolic ligament in the horse. *Vet Surg* 1987;16:5–12.)

of the distal half of the small colon and the rectum comes from the cranial rectal artery, a branch of the caudal mesenteric artery.

Innervation

Cecal and colonic innervation is derived from the sympathetic and parasympathetic nervous systems. The splanchnic nerves from the iliac, cranial, and caudal mesenteric ganglia are responsible for the sympathetic innervation, which tends to decrease the contractility of the intestinal muscle while increasing sphincter tone. The vagal nerve supplies the parasympathetic innervation, which has the opposite effects. The large intestine is also under local reflex control through the Auerbach's and Meissner plexi. In addition, the presence of a "pacemaker" in the midcolon area near the pelvic flexure has been demonstrated. The electrical activity in this area originates in the circular smooth muscle and spreads axially bidirectionally through both the longitudinal and circular muscle layers of the colon.

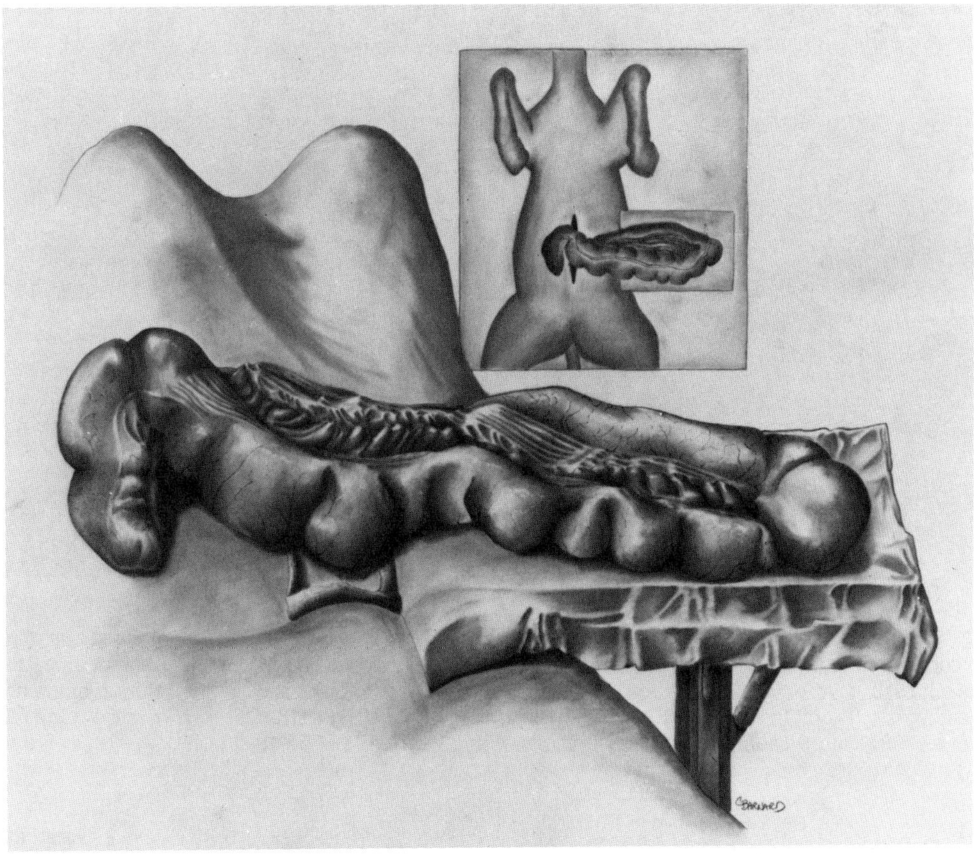

Figure 67–3. The colon is exteriorized and placed on a colon tray.

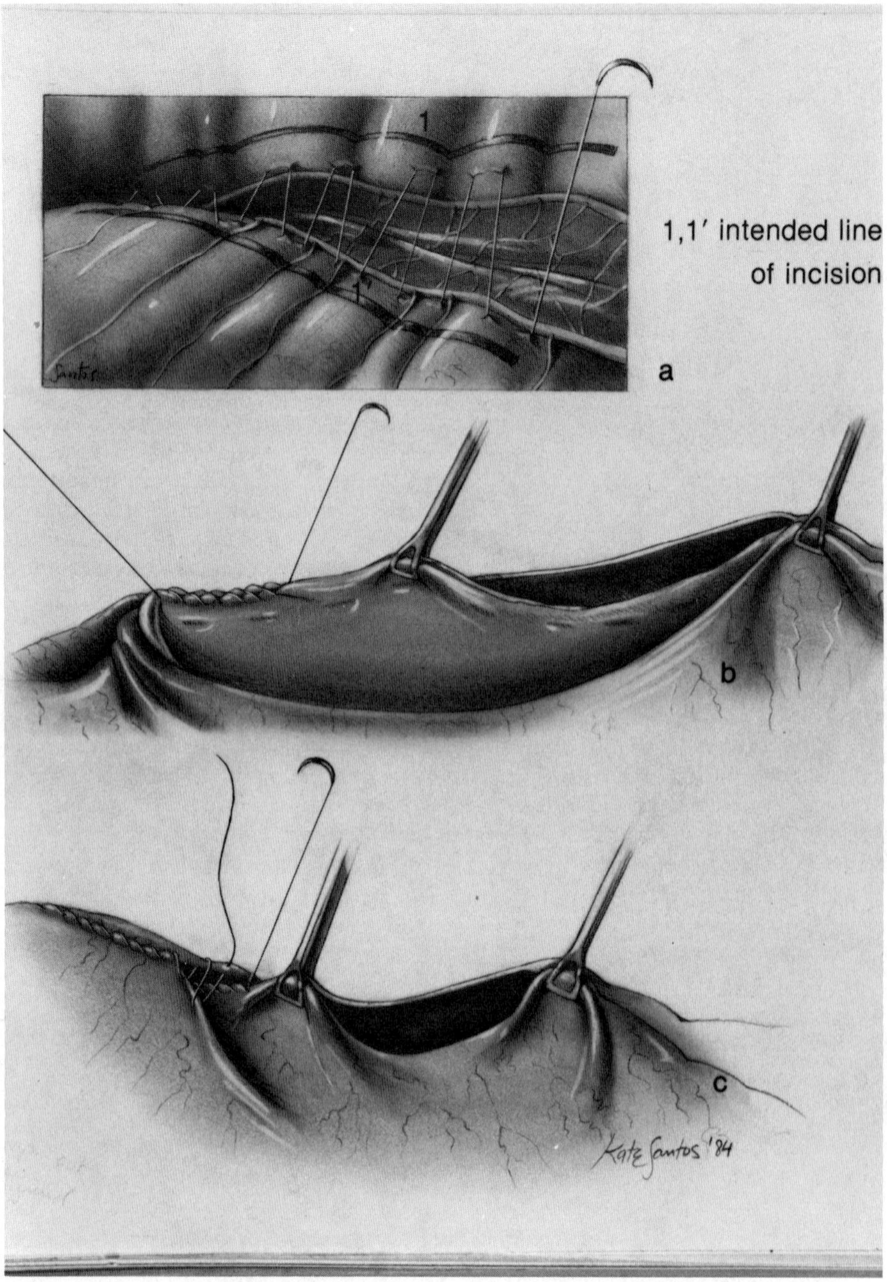

Figure 67–4. First hand-sutured technique. **A.** Placement of anastomosis in relation to the intended line of transection. The seromuscular layers of the ventral and dorsal colons are apposed using a simple continuous pattern with 2-0 polyglactin 910. **B.** After incising the bowel, the far side of the anastomosis is sewn. **C.** Suturing of the near side of the anastomosis. (From Ducharme NG, Horney FD, Baird JD, Arighi M, Burton JH: Extensive large colon resection in the pony. 1 Surgical procedures and clinical results. *Can J Vet Res* 1987;51:66–75.)

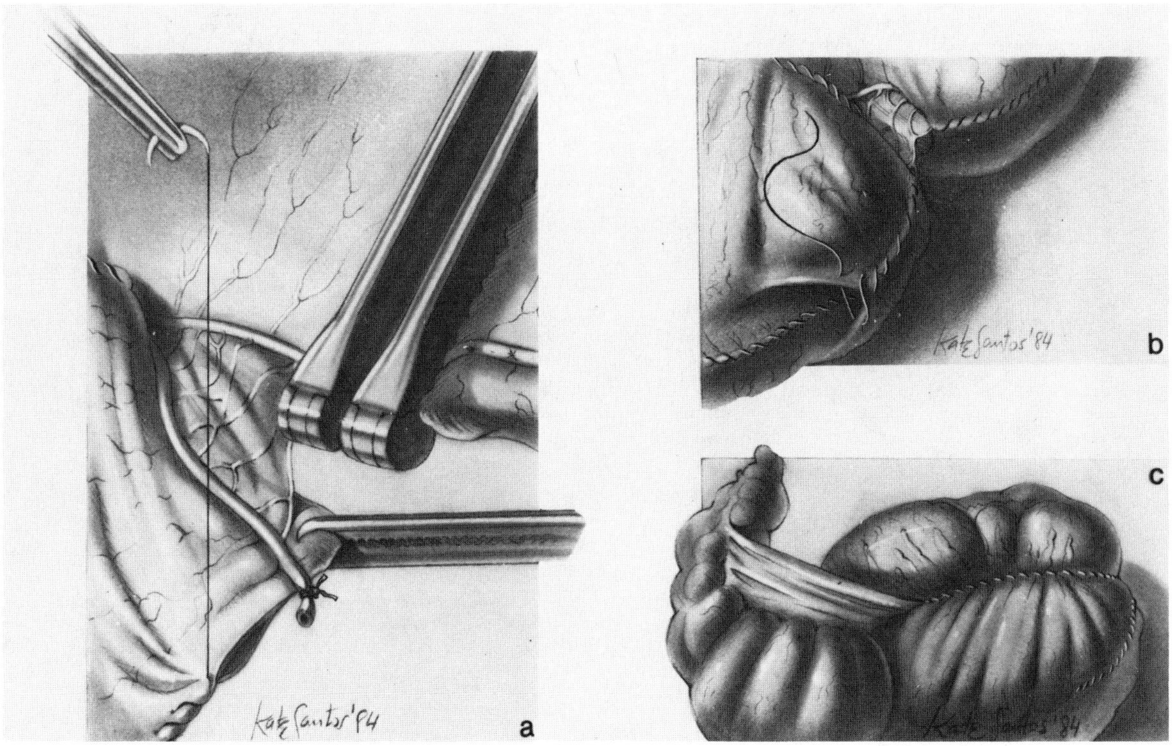

Figure 67–5. First hand-sutured technique. **A.** The transected extremity of the ventral colon is being sutured while the intestinal clamp is still on the dorsal colon. **B.** Closure of the ventral colon with second row of sutures. The dorsal colon has been sutured. **C.** Appearance of the large colon at termination of the procedure. (From Ducharme NG, Horney FD, Baird JD, Arighi M, Burton JH: Extensive large colon resection in the pony. 1 Surgical procedures and clinical results. *Can J Vet Res* 1987;51:66–75.)

The presence of this pacemaker in the intended area of resection raises the question as to whether coordination and motility of the remaining large intestine would be disturbed following extensive large colon resection. Experimental and clinical trials have not resulted in apparent motility disturbance following resection of this pacemaker.

SURGERY

Preoperative Preparation

When elective large colon resection is intended, preoperative fasting of 24 to 36 hours greatly decreases the bulk of the content of the large colon. This facilitates large colon resection and decreases the potential for spillage of intestinal contents into the abdominal cavity.

Prophylactic antibiotics are indicated. Because the source of contamination is the colonic flora (both gram-negative and gram-positive bacteria), broad-spectrum antibiotics such as sulfonamide-trimethoprim combination or aminoglycosides combined with penicillin are recommended.

Surgical Techniques

Because of technical difficulty in performing end-to-end anastomosis in the large colon, a side-to-side anastomosis is generally performed.

A 30- to 40-cm ventral midline or paramedian incision is made starting at the umbilicus and extending toward the xiphoid. The large colon is exteriorized and placed on a colon tray on the left side of the horse (Fig. 67–3). The large colon is placed so that its medial surface with the vascular mesocolon is facing the surgeon. At the intended transection site, the colic branch of the ileocecocolic artery and the right colic artery are located using blunt dissection and are double ligated and transected. The procedure is repeated for their associated veins. The right ventral and dorsal colons are sepa-

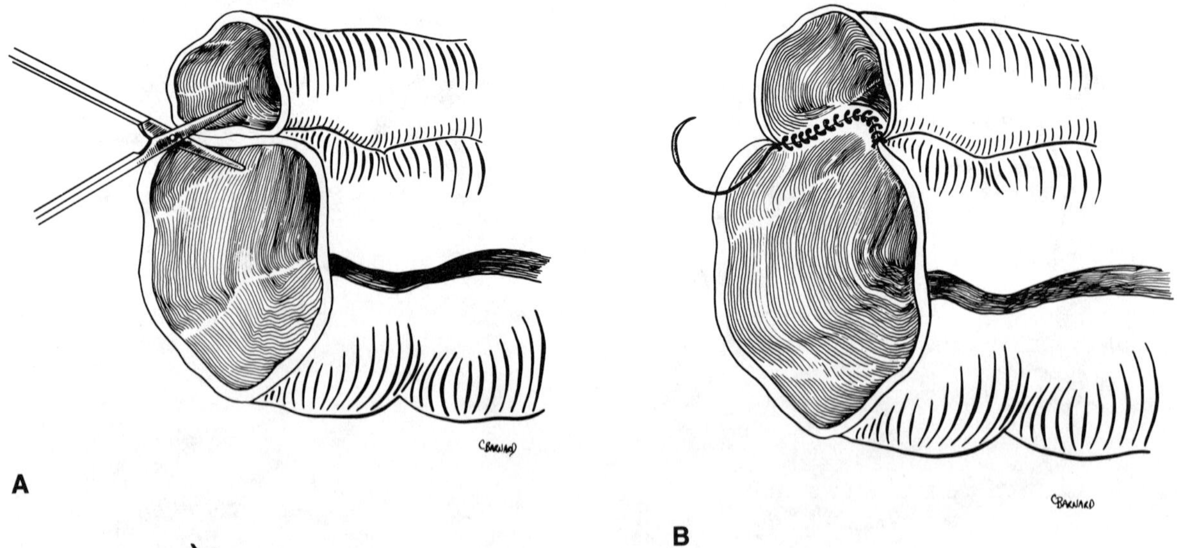

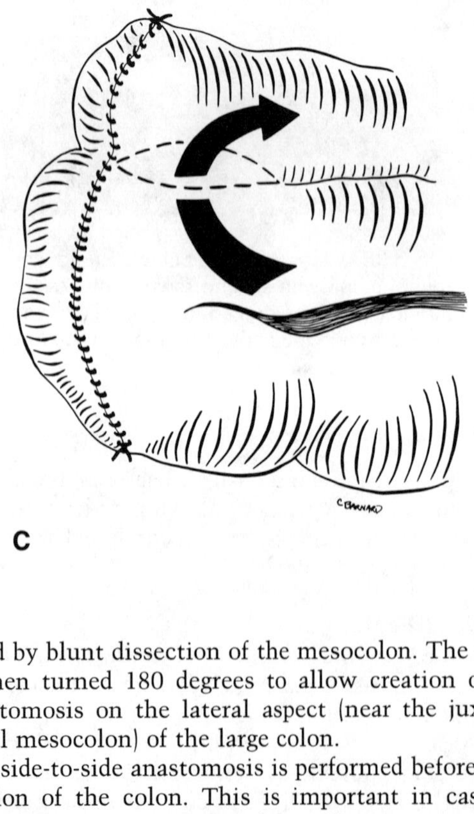

Figure 67–6. Second hand-sutured technique. **A.** A 12- to 15-cm incision is made in the area of mesenteric attachment between left dorsal and ventral colons. **B.** Mucosal edges of the ventral and dorsal colons are being reapposed with a simple continuous pattern. **C.** The completed anastomosis with oversewn dorsal and ventral colons. (Redrawn from Boening KJ and Von Saldern F CH: Resection of the left parts of the large colon in horses, in *Proceedings of the Equine Colic Research Symposium.* 1986, pp 337–340, 1986.)

rated by blunt dissection of the mesocolon. The colon is then turned 180 degrees to allow creation of the anastomosis on the lateral aspect (near the juxtaparietal mesocolon) of the large colon.

A side-to-side anastomosis is performed before transection of the colon. This is important in cases in which extensive resection of the colon is required. Exteriorization of the large colon allows the surgeon to perform the anastomosis at the level of the laparotomy incision instead of within the abdomen. If fasting was not possible preoperatively, a pelvic flexure enterotomy is performed to permit decompression and evacuation of the large colon prior to performing the anastomosis.

Three surgical techniques have been described, two using a hand-sutured anastomosis and one using the autosuture equipment. For the first technique the anastomosis should start 2 cm from the transection site and extend toward the base of the cecum and the transverse colon. A large self-retaining intestinal clamp is placed on a fold of the ventral colon and another is placed on the dorsal colon. Two stay sutures uniting the dorsal and ventral colon are placed 2 cm from the intended line of transection. The seromuscular layers of the ventral and dorsal colon are apposed using a simple continuous pattern with 2–0 polyglactin 910 (Vicryl; Ethicon Inc) (Fig. 67–4A). Approximately 3 mm lateral to the sutured line on the antimesenteric side, an intestinal incision of 15 cm is made (Fig. 67–4A) in both the dorsal and ventral colons. The far side of the anastomosis is sutured using a simple continuous pattern, again with polyglactin 910 (Fig. 67–4B). The near side is then sutured in a similar fashion and oversewn using a Lembert pattern (Fig. 67–4C), again using polyglactin 910. Two large self-retaining intestinal clamps are placed on the right ventral colon at the intended level of transection. The right ventral colon is then sharply incised between the clamps and the colon is closed with a double inverting pattern (a Cushing pattern oversewn with a Lembert pattern) using an absorbable suture material (Fig. 67–5). This procedure is then repeated for transection and closure of the left dorsal colon.

To complete the second technique, two stay sutures are placed on the antimesenteric surfaces of the ventral and dorsal colons. A large intestinal clamp is placed on the pelvic flexure side of the intended transection line. The ventral and dorsal colon are transected. A 12- to 15-cm incision is then made between the left dorsal and ventral colon where they attach within the mesentery (Fig. 67–6A). The edges of this incision are then apposed with a simple continuous pattern (Fig. 67–6B). The open end of the ventral and dorsal colon are closed as previously described (Fig. 67–6C).

If the tissue thickness allows, a third technique using stapling instruments is advised. It is more rapid and minimizes contamination of the abdominal cavity (see Chapter 2). The procedures are performed in the same chronologic order as in the first technique described. The colotomy is performed at the same level but four stay sutures are required, as illustrated in Figure 67–7A. Two 1-cm colostomies are made in the right ventral and dorsal colons and the arms of the stapling

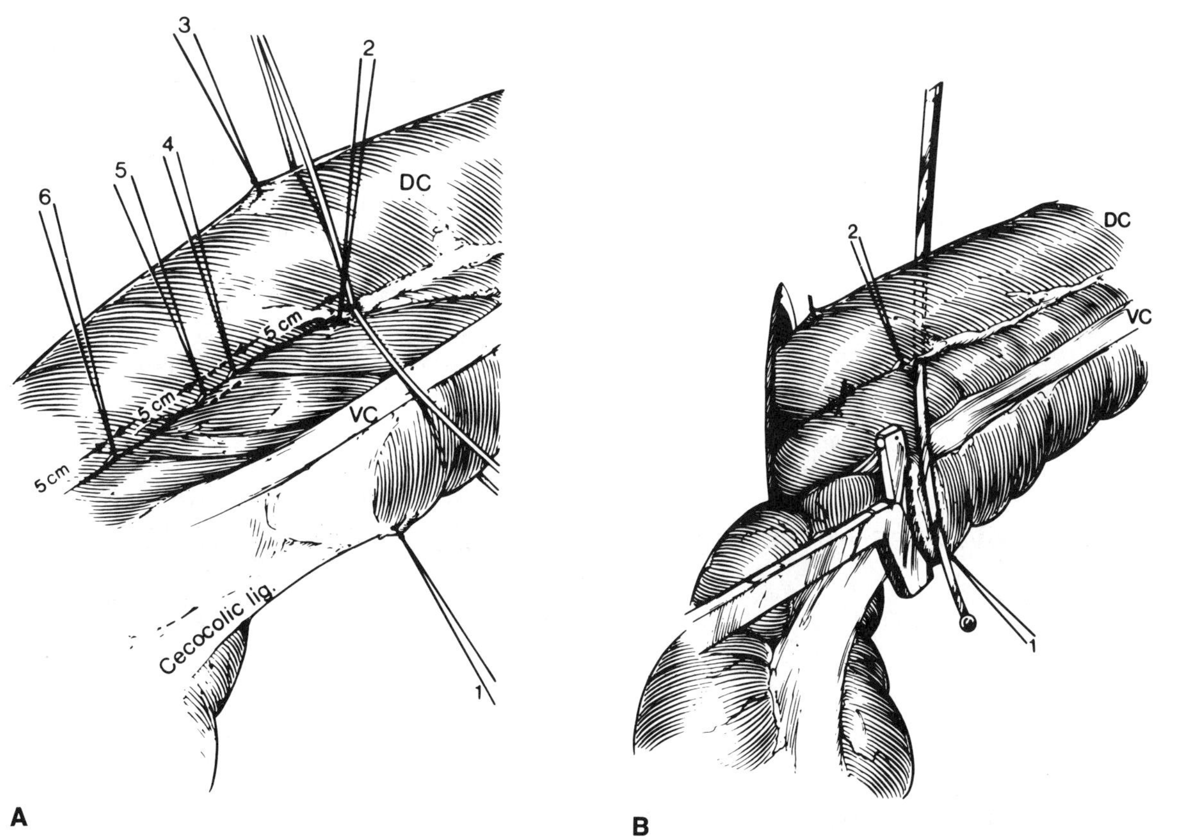

Figure 67–7. Stapling technique. **A.** Juxtaparietal surface of the colon at the level of the transection. The stay sutures are placed to mark the transection level (1, 2, and 3) and the side-to-side anastomosis (2, 4, 5, and 6). The *dotted lines* represent the stab incision into the right ventral (*VC*) and dorsal (*DC*) colons for insertion of the anastomosing device. **B.** Placement of the intestinal clamp and the stapling instrument. The transection is performed along the *dotted line.* (From Bertone AL, Stashak TS, Sullins KE, Ralston SL: Experimental large colon resection at the cecocolic ligament in the horse. *Vet Surg* 1987;16:5–12.)

TABLE 67–1. OUTCOME OF HORSES UNDERGOING LARGE COLON RESECTION

	>50% Resection		<50% Resection	
Reference	No. of Horses	Survival Rate	No. of Horses	Survival Rate
Arighi et al. (1987)	12	42%	0	—
Bertone et al. (1986)	5	80%	6	83%
Boening and Von Saldern (1986)	0	—	5	100%
Total	17	53%	11	92%

device (GIA Premium; United States Surgical Corp) are inserted toward the intended transection line (Fig. 67–7A). The device is then discharged two more times toward the base of the cecum, creating a 15-cm anastomosis. The colotomy site is closed with a double inverting suture pattern of absorbable suture material. The stay sutures are left in place to support the staple line.

The transection of the ventral and dorsal colons is performed with the multiple use of another stapling device (TA-90 Premium; United States Surgical Corp), followed by sharp transection (Fig. 67–7B). All staple lines must be inspected after each use. It appears preferable to oversew the everted edge of the transection site because of reported staple failure. Although this enclosed contaminated, everted tissue may potentially lead to abscess formation; in clinical use this has not been a problem and is recommended.

Following the performance of one of these three types of anastomosis, the drapes isolating the colon are removed. The surgeon and assistants change into new gloves and gowns, and the incision is closed routinely.

POSTOPERATIVE CARE AND PROGNOSIS

Postoperative care includes fasting for 24 hours followed by feeding a laxative diet (grass, good-quality hay, and bran mash). The diet is intended to keep the feces soft for 7 to 10 days.

Normal digestive function is observed by 5 to 6 months postoperatively. Dietary modification may be required to maintain adequate energy intake for performance animals. The overall survival rate of clinical patients that have undergone large colon resection is presented in Table 67–1.

BIBLIOGRAPHY

Argenzio RA: Functions of the equine large intestine and their interrelationship in disease. *Cornell Vet* 1975;65:303–330.

Arighi M, Ducharme MC, Horney FD, Livesey MA: Extensive large colon resection in 12 horses. *Can Vet J* 1987;28:245–248.

Bertone AL: *Large colon resection in horses,* PhD thesis. Colorado State University, 1987.

Bertone AL, Stashak TS, Sullins KE: Large colon resection and anastomosis in horses. *J Am Vet Med Assoc* 1986;188:612–617.

Bertone AL, Stashak TS, Sullins KE, Ralston SL: Experimental large colon resection at the cecocolic ligament in the horse. *Vet Surg* 1987;16:5–12.

Boening KJ, Von Saldern FCH: Resection of the left parts of the large colon in horses, in *Proceedings of the Equine Colic Research Symposium.* Veterinary Learning Systems, 1986, pp 337–340.

Ducharme MC, Horney FD, Baird JD, Arighi M, Burton JH: Extensive large colon resection in the pony. 1 Surgical procedures and clinical results. *Can J Vet Res* 1987;51:66–75.

Schummer A, Nickel R, Sack WO: Alimentary canal of the horse, in Schummer A, Nickel R, Sack WO (eds): *The Viscera of Domestic Animals.* New York, Springer-Verlag, 1979, p 188.

Sellers AF, Lowe JE, Drost CJ, Rendano WT, Georgi JR, Robert S: Retropropulsion-propulsion in the equine large colon. *Am J Vet Res* 1982;43:390–396.

Sullins KE, Stashak TS, Ralston SL: Experimental large intestinal resection in the horse: Technique and nutritional performance. *Proc Am Assoc Equine Pract* 1985;pp 497–503.

68 Enterolithiasis

Andrew T. Fischer, Jr.

Enterolithiasis in the horse has been documented for several hundred years. Enteroliths are composed primarily of magnesium ammonium phosphate and often form around a central nidus. Surgical treatment of enterolithiasis was reported in the last century. Advances in equine anesthesia and surgery coupled with early diagnosis have made the surgical management of enteroliths very successful. Current research is geared at the understanding of the pathogenesis and possible prevention of enterolithiasis.

DIAGNOSIS

Enterolithiasis is most frequently diagnosed in middle-aged animals. All breeds are affected but there appears to be overrepresentation of the Arabian breed. Of animals undergoing abdominal surgery for enterolithiasis in the last 2 years at Chino Valley Equine Hospital 42% ($n = 40$) were Arabians or Arabian crosses, 21% Quarter horses, and 13% Thoroughbreds. Although the percentage of Arabians appears to be high, Arabian owners tend to be more willing than the general horse-owning public to pursue the economic involvement that colic surgery entails. Both sexes are evenly represented. The age of reported cases ranges between 4 and 30 years. The mean age of affected animals at our hospital is 10.5 ± 5.5 years. Enterolith formation around a fibrous foreign body has been reported in horses 3 years of age and older. In our practice, the youngest horse operated on for enteroliths was 3 years of age. In southern California enterolithiasis is an important diagnostic rule-out in any horse with colic that is over 4 years of age.

Affected horses present either with recurren that has been increasing in frequency or with severe colic. Some of these horses will have beer to pass enteroliths in pasture. Behavioral chang tability) have been noticed in some horses months prior to presentation for exploratory s The horse will frequently not pass feces during hours before presentation or will pass only amounts of mucus-covered feces.

There are no pathognomonic findings on phys amination unless one can palpate the enterol rectum. This is an extremely rare occurrence. A nal palpation per rectum will demonstrate eit abnormality or distention of the large or small Frequently, only a few mucus-covered fecal ba be found. The severity of the pain is directly rel the amount of intestinal distention proximal obstruction. Many affected horses presenting hospital are bloated and painful, and their hea are generally elevated. The presence of nasogas flux is a variable finding but tends to be pre animals that have been obstructed for several d some horses, administration of mineral oil or sodium sulfosuccinate may enable passage of fe cated in the large colon, indicating lack of to struction. Fluid obtained by abdominocentesis mal early in the disease, but protein concentrati cell counts typically increase over time. The m curate method to diagnose enterolithiasis is by a nal radiography. Early diagnosis of enterolithi

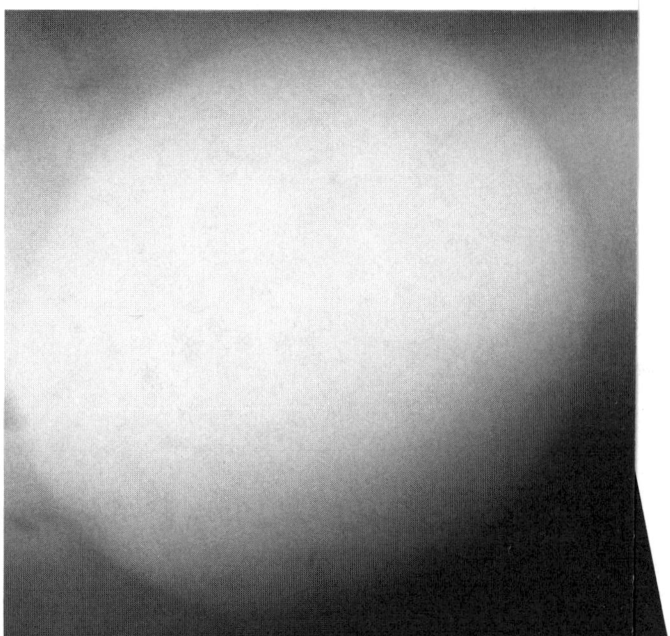

Figure 68–1. Standing lateral abdominal radiograph with an enterolith in the right dorsal colon. The technique for this 800-lb Arabian was 450 mAs at approximately 100 kVp using an 8:1 grid and fast-screen-film cassette.

t colic
acute
noted
es (irri-
in the
urgery.
the 24
small

cal ex-
ith per
bdomi
her n
colo
ls w
ated
to
to
t
tr

justifies earlier surgical inter-
ie presence of a demonstrable
hs, increasing pain, absence of
ioration indicates the need for

tient preparation and broad-spec-
rophylaxis (Chapter 5), the patient
placed in dorsal recumbency. A
tomy is performed and the abdom-
natically explored. Obstructing en-
ntly found in the transverse colon
moval of small colon enteroliths is
orizing and isolating the affected
he incision, if possible. An antime-
ıy (through the muscular band) is
to easily extract the enterolith and
ie bowel. The enterotomy must fre-
med in compromised bowel because
move the enterolith. Stay sutures are
he assistant to maintain good control
ing closure of the enterotomy and to
ıces of contamination. A two-layer in-
(simple continuous pattern oversewn

with a Lembert patten) using 3–0 polyglactin 910 (Vicryl; Ethicon Inc) is used to close the enterotomy. Cushing-type sutures are not used because they frequently cut through the muscular band of the small colon because of the normal fiber alignment.

Enteroliths in the proximal small colon or transverse colon can usually be removed by evacuation of ingesta from the left dorsal and right dorsal colons by a pelvic flexure enterotomy. A hose is then passed per rectum to flush (using warm water) the enterolith back into the transverse or right dorsal colon. It is much easier to move the enterolith orally if the contents have been evacuated previously. Small enteroliths may be milked back to a pelvic flexure enterotomy incision and removed. Larger enteroliths are removed from the right dorsal colon by a separate enterotomy (Fig. 68–2). The enterotomy should be closed by two inverting suture layers. The bowel is lavaged and returned to the abdomen.

It is extremely important to check the rest of the large colon and small colon for other enteroliths. If there is a flat side on an enterolith or the enterolith has the shape of a polyhedron, there is at least one more enterolith present. Systematic exploration is always indicated; I have operated on a horse with an enterolith that also had a small intestinal incarceration within the epiploic foramen. Abdominal closure is routine (see Chapter 57).

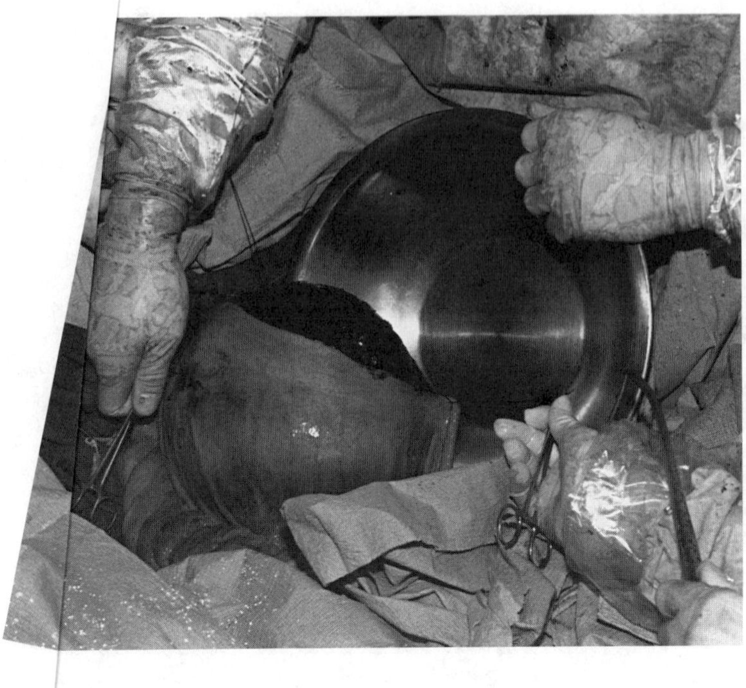

Figure 68–2. Removal of an enterolith from the right dorsal colon (note stay sutures). The surgeons are manipulating the colon with stay sutures to remove the enterolith into the sterile stainless steel bowl.

POSTOPERATIVE CARE

Postoperative care of the patient is geared toward early return to a normal diet. Feeding starts when the animal passes manure and there is no evidence of continued nasogastric reflux. Systemic antibiotics and nonsteroidal antiinflammatory drugs (flunixin meglumine) are used routinely for 48 hours after surgery. Intravenous fluids are used on an as-needed basis but are not routine for horses with uncomplicated enterolith removal. For more information on postoperative care, see Chapter 73).

Box stall confinement with controlled walking is used for the first 30 days. No strenuous exercise is permitted until 3 months after surgery.

PROGNOSIS AND COMPLICATIONS

The prognosis for survival in an uncomplicated enterolith removal is very good. In the last 2 years over 85% of animals operated on for enterolithiasis were discharged alive from our hospital. As long as the horse presents in good cardiovascular status, a successful outcome is anticipated. Although peritonitis was a complication in 26% of the horses described in an earlier study by Evans et al., we have not recognized this complication. Incisional drainage, however, was a complication in 18% of our cases operated on for enteroliths.

It is of concern that devitalized bowel may be left in place when removing enteroliths from the transverse or proximal small colon. It is impossible to directly assess the viability of the transverse colon. Rupture of the colon may occur in these areas either during or after surgery and necessitate the animal's destruction. Recurrence of enteroliths following surgical treatment has been encountered.

BIBLIOGRAPHY

Blue MG: Enteroliths in horses—a retrospective study of 30 cases. *Equine Vet J* 1979;11:76–84.

Blue MG, Wittkopp RW: Clinical and structural features of equine enteroliths. *J Am Vet Med Assoc* 1981;179:79–82.

Boles CL, Herthel DJ: Enteroliths and small colon obstructions, in Robinson NE (ed): *Current Therapy in Equine Medicine*, ed 2. Philadelphia, WB Saunders Co, 1987, pp 68–70.

Evans DR, Trunk DA, Hibser NK, Everman T, London CA: Diagnosis and treatment of enterolithiasis in equidae. *Compend Cont Educ Vet Pract* 1981;3:S383-S390.

Lloyd K, Hintz HF, Wheat JD, Schryver HF: Enteroliths in horses. *Cornell Vet* 1987;77:172–186.

Rose JA, Rose EM, Sande RD: Radiography in the diagnosis of equine enteroliths. *Proc Am Assoc Equine Pract* 1980; pp 211–219.

69
Small Colon Obstruction

Michael A. Livesey

Small colon obstruction occurs relatively infrequently when compared to obstruction of the small intestine or the large colon. Causes of obstruction that may necessitate surgical intervention can be classified as congenital abnormalities, simple obstructions, vascular lesions, strangulating obstructions, and ruptures of the small colon (Table 69–1).

The small or descending colon, a continuation of the short transverse colon, forms the distal segment of the horse's gastrointestinal tract. The small colon is approximately 3.5 m in length, has a diameter of between 7.5 and 10 cm, and is continued distally as the peritoneal rectum at the pelvic inlet. The small colon is attached to the sublumbar region by the mesocolon, and to the terminal duodenum by the duodenocolic fold. The mesenteric attachment of the small colon is short at its origin but lengthens to between 80 and 90 cm as the rectum is approached. Coils of intermingled small intestine and small colon occupy the left dorsal quadrant of the abdomen. The small colon is distinguished from the small intestine by two longitudinal muscular bands (tenia): the mesocolic band concealed in the attachment of the mesocolon and a wider antimesenteric band. Contractions of the bands result in the formation of two rows of sacculations (haustra) in which the feces are divided into characteristic balls.

TABLE 69–1. SMALL COLON OBSTRUCTION

Congenital Abnormality
- Atresia coli
- Colonic aganglionosis

Simple Obstruction
- Impaction
- Foreign body
- Enterolithiasis
- Fecoliths
- Phytobezoars
- Trichobezoars
- Retained meconium
- Adhesions
- Neoplasms—leiomyoma, polyps

Vascular Lesions
- Intramural hematoma
- Mesocolic rupture
- Edema of the terminal small colon

Strangulating Obstruction
- Internal herniation
- Volvulus
- Lipoma

Small Colon Tears

The small colon receives arterial blood supply from both the cranial and caudal mesenteric arteries. The majority of the small colon is supplied by the caudal mesenteric artery, which gives off the left colic artery and is continuous as the cranial rectal artery. These arteries give off branches that form anastomosing arcades, becoming narrower distally. The middle colic artery, a branch of the cranial mesenteric artery, passes along the dorsal aspect of the transverse colon to the origin of the small colon, enters the mesocolon, and anastomoses with the left colic artery. Terminal arteries arise from the vascular arcades, enter the bowel wall, and give rise to three intramural plexuses (serosal, intermuscular, and submucosal). The mesocolon contains a considerable quantity of fat that makes visual identification of vessels difficult.

CLINICAL FINDINGS AND DIAGNOSIS

Horses with small colon obstruction demonstrate a variety of clinical signs that vary according to whether the obstruction is partial or complete. If the obstruction is complete, there is absence of the passage of feces and the gradual onset of mild abdominal pain that develops because of tympany in more proximal segments of the bowel. If the obstruction is incomplete, a reduced quantity of fecal material may be passed, tympany may or may not develop, and the signs of colic will be mild and slow in onset. In an experimental study of small colon obstruction, horses survived 36 hours after complete obstruction and showed signs of mild intermittent colic. Blood pH, bicarbonate, partial pressures of oxygen and carbon dioxide, urea nitrogen, and plasma protein levels remained within normal limits. Serum electrolytes showed little deviation from normal and hematologic values were only slightly above normal.

Gaseous distention of the cecum and colon may be detected on percussion of the abdomen. When the size of the animal permits, palpation per rectum may reveal the obstructed segment of the small colon. However, because of the variable position of this segment of bowel, it may be impossible to reach the site of the obstruction and, instead, empty coils of small colon and/or distended cecum and colon may be palpated.

Abdominocentesis is a useful diagnostic test when dealing with suspected obstructions of the small colon. Alterations in the leukocyte count and protein content are indicative of degenerative changes occurring in the bowel wall. Elevations in these values may assist in differentiating between a simple impaction and one resulting in ischemic necrosis of the bowel.

SIMPLE OBSTRUCTION

Feed-Related Impactions

Impaction of the small colon with inspissated fecal material occurs less frequently than in the large colon. In one report, an unusually high incidence of the condition was seen in ponies in the fall and winter. Broodmares in their third trimester of pregnancy appear predisposed to develop impaction. Factors that may precipitate the condition include the ingestion of poor-quality roughage, inadequate mastication of food because of poor dentition, decreased water intake, lack of exercise, and parasitism.

Most horses with feed impactions of the small colon will respond to conservative medical therapies, which include enemas and the oral administration of lubricants, laxatives, or cathartics. Commonly employed medical treatments include the administration of mineral oil (4 L/450 kg) by nasogastric intubation. Dioctyl sodium sulfosuccinate is frequently given orally with water or mineral oil. One disadvantage associated with the use of mineral oil is its ability to channel around an obstruction and thus fail to penetrate or break up the fecal material. However, mineral oil does provides an excellent marker, and its presence on the perineum and tail provides evidence that the obstruction is incomplete. Hydration and softening of a fecal mass may be enhanced by the chronic parenteral administration of large volumes of balanced electrolyte solutions. An alternate approach is hydration by the administration of water with or without an ionic cathartic via nasogastric tube.

The administration of hypertonic solutions of magnesium sulfate, sodium sulfate, or sodium chloride (500 g in 4 L water/450 kg) has been recommended for the treatment of impactions. These compounds draw fluid into the lumen of the bowel and soften the fecal mass. These solutions are contraindicated unless it has first been established that the digestive tract is patent. These solutions may be responsible for causing disturbances of the serum electrolyte values, and in the event that a misdiagnosis has been made, severe dehydration and/or bowel rupture may occur. Frequent enemas have been recommended, these exercising their effect by stimulation of peristalsis and local softening of the feces. Nonsteroidal anti-inflammatory drugs may be used for pain control, if indicated.

Foreign Body Impactions

Small colon obstruction may occur as a result of the ingestion of nondigestible foreign material. The problem, which occurs most commonly in foals and young horses, has been observed following the ingestion of braided ropes, baling twine, and nylon-based cording from tires, conveyor belts, rubberized fencing, and hay nets. The impacting material usually consists of concretions of fecal material surrounding the foreign substance. Such objects may remain asymptomatically in the large colon for substantial periods of time. Up to 5 years have been known to elapse between exposure to the material and the development of clinical signs. Obstruction typically occurs at the junction of the right dorsal colon and the transverse colon, or in the proximal small colon. The clinical signs are similar to those exhibited by a horse with a simple impaction. Intermittent colic may develop if the obstruction is incomplete or if the material periodically falls back into the right dorsal colon. More commonly, the offending material produces an acute complete obstruction of the small colon, with subsequent cessation of the passage of feces. Colic signs that develop are mild initially, but gradually increase in intensity with distention of bowel proximally.

Intestinal Concretions

Obstruction of the small colon may also result from a variety of concretions that develop in the lumen of the large colon. These include enteroliths (see Chapter 68), fecoliths, and combinations of plant fibers (phytobezoars) or animal hair (trichobezoars) with magnesium ammonium phosphate. These objects develop and may remain asymptomatically in the large colon for long periods of time. Clinical signs develop as with a foreign body when the mass is transported from the right dorsal colon into the transverse colon or proximal small colon, where it becomes lodged, causing a complete or partial obstruction. Spherical masses frequently cause complete obstruction, whereas irregularly shaped or coarse masses may produce an incomplete obstruction, allowing the passage of gas and liquid. The cranial location of the intraluminal mass usually prevents detection by palpation per rectum. Because of the nondegradable nature of the impacting masses, medical therapy is of no value. The recommended treatment is therefore the surgical removal of the obstructing material.

Adhesions

Adhesion of the small colon and rectum to other structures in the pelvic canal may result in the development of constricting bands that reduce the luminal size of the bowel or cause sufficient deviation to produce a site for impaction. Adhesions of the small colon most commonly develop following inflammatory pelvic disease or previous small colon surgery. Inflammation within the pelvic canal may result from damage incurred during a traumatic parturition or from perforation of the rectum or cranial vagina during natural breeding. Diagnosis of pelvic inflammation is made on palpation per rectum of the pelvic viscera. Treatment is aimed at treating the inflammatory process and maintaining soft fecal production.

Vascular Lesions

Vascular lesions may cause obstruction of the small colon. Those described include transmural and intramural hematomas, submucosal edema, and mesocolic rupture secondary to segmental ischemic necrosis of the bowel.

Intramural hematomas have been reported to be as large as 60 cm in length and primarily affect older horses. The condition produces more severe pain than is usually associated with small colon obstruction, the pain probably arising from intramural distention of the bowel wall. Chronic ulceration and iatrogenic tears have been postulated as possible causes of the condition. Diagnosis is usually made at the time of exploratory celiotomy. Treatment involves resection of the affected segment of bowel and anastomosis of healthy tissue.

Submucosal edema usually develops at the junction of the small colon and the rectum, producing a circumferential luminal obstruction of varying length. The obstruction, which is usually incomplete, produces signs of mild intermittent colic. Diagnosis can usually be made by palpation per rectum. The mucosa of the affected segment of bowel appears swollen and edematous and has lost its normal plication. Attempts by the animal to pass fecal material result in the affected mucosa becoming abraded and roughened. Hemorrhage may occur secondarily. Impacted coils of small colon may be palpated proximally. The etiology of the condition is unknown, although verminous arteritis of the caudal mesenteric artery has been suggested. Conservative medical treatment of horses with this condition is often successful. Food is withheld from the animal and the fecal mass proximal to the obstruction is softened by oral laxatives and enemas. Treatment is continued until the swelling is reduced and spontaneous defecation is resumed.

Mesocolic rupture with segmental ischemic necrosis of the small colon has been recognized as a rare complication of parturition in the mare and as a complication of type III or IV rectal prolapse. Rectal prolapse may be caused by any condition that causes tenesmus, including urethral obstruction, enteritis, and dystocia. The parturient mare is predisposed to rectal prolapse because of pelvic ligament laxity and the increased intraabdominal pressure and forceful expulsive efforts associated with parturition. Intussusception of the small colon through the rectum results in stretching of the mesocolon and possible disruption of vascular arcades. The risk of vascular damage increases with the tension placed on the mesentery and therefore the length of the intussusception. Mesocolic rupture and ischemic necrosis of the small colon may occur when more than 30 cm of small colon and rectum have prolapsed. The mesocolon, although short at its origin, lengthens to 80 to 90 cm as the rectum is approached. Exploratory celiotomy is recommended in those cases in which more than 30 cm of rectum and small colon has prolapsed. The celiotomy is performed to reduce the intussusception and assess the vascular supply to the bowel.

Mesocolic rupture has been observed both in mares that foaled normally and in those requiring manual assistance. It is suspected that increased intraabdominal pressure tears the mesocolon and disrupts vascular arcades, resulting in segmental ischemic necrosis of the bowel. The condition has been observed in aged (mean 14 years old) pluriparous mares. Affected mares will demonstrate signs of colic within 24 hours of parturition, the signs worsening with the gradual onset of tympany. Because the signs are often mild initially, some of the delay in recognition may be accounted for by the difficulty in differentiating between the pain of postpartum uterine contractions and that originating from colonic obstruction. A consistent finding is the failure of mares to pass feces following parturition. The findings on palpation per rectum are inconsistent and may vary from an absence of detectable abnormalities to impaction of the small colon. The differential diagnosis should include simple impaction of the small colon and rupture of the middle uterine artery, cecum, right ventral colon, uterus, or urinary bladder. Abdominocentesis reveals consistent elevations of the protein level and leukocyte count in horses with mesocolon rupture and ischemic necrosis of the small colon. Exploratory celiotomy is recommended in those cases in which the condition is suspected. The treatment involves resection of devitalized tissue and end-to-end anastomosis of the small colon.

Strangulating Obstruction

Strangulating obstruction of the small colon may occur when a segment of the bowel becomes involved in either an internal or an external hernia. Sites for internal herniation include the omentum, the mesentery of the small or large bowel, and tears in the broad ligament of the uterus, the uterus, or the vagina. Sites of external herniation include the umbilicus and the inguinal ring. Small colon volvulus is not common but is occasionally associated with adhesions to internal abscesses, other organs or abdominal incisions.

The mesocolon, because it contains a considerable amount of fat in most animals, is a common site for the development of pedunculated lipomas. These are frequently incidental findings on postmortem examination or exploratory celiotomy in older horses. The suspended lipomatous mass does, however, have the potential to twist around a loop of bowel, producing obstruction or strangulation. This occurs most frequently in the small intestine or small colon of older horses. Strangulating obstructions of the small colon are rarely identifiable per rectum; exploratory celiotomy is usually required for definitive diagnosis. The treatment involves resection of the compromised bowel and end-to-end anastomosis.

Small Colon Tears

Many rectal tears actually occur in the terminal small colon, in the region of the pelvic inlet. This subject is dealt with in more detail in Chapter 70.

SURGICAL CONSIDERATIONS

The investigation of small colon obstruction is complicated by the difficulty in exposing sections of the bowel. Lesions frequently occur in the proximal and distal sections, which have a short mesentery and fixed extremities. Surgical intervention in these regions carries the risk of spillage of intestinal contents into the abdominal cavity.

The mesocolon contains a large amount of fat in most animals, making identification of vessels and surgical procedures more difficult than in other sections of bowel. Healing of the small colon is poor compared with that of the small intestine. This is because of the presence of solid fecal material with high bacterial concentration, a relatively poor blood supply, and strong muscular activity. Postoperative ileus and dehydration of ingesta proximal to an enterotomy incision or bowel anastomosis may contribute to wound breakdown.

SURGICAL REPAIR

The small colon may be exposed either by a standing left flank approach or by ventral midline celiotomy. The ventral midline approach provides optimum surgical access to the small colon and is the preferred approach in those cases in which mesocolic rupture is suspected. The standing left flank approach may provide suitable access if a lesion involving the middle or distal small colon can be identified on palpation per rectum.

When a distal small colon obstruction is suspected, the ventral midline celiotomy incision is made more caudal than that made for routine abdominal exploration. In the male, this may require reflection of the penis and prepuce. Alternatively, a paramedian approach may be used.

Obstruction of the small colon may be conveniently divided into three anatomic sections: (*a*) the proximal, (*b*) the middle, and (*c*) the distal sections of the bowel.

Proximal Small Colon

The proximal small colon, having a short mesocolon and a fixed position at the duodenocolic fold, cannot be totally exteriorized via either ventral midline or left flank celiotomy. To relieve an obstruction at this site or one in the transverse colon, the object or material must be moved retrograde or broken up by external manipulation. If at all possible, the bowel should be visualized prior to manipulation to permit assessment of its viability. Extreme caution must be observed during any manipulative procedures because the distended, possibly ischemic bowel is easily ruptured. Intestine proximal to the obstruction is frequently distended and should be decompressed prior to manipulation. Attempts are made to gradually move the obstruction in a retrograde manner into the right dorsal colon by gentle digital manipulation. This may be aided by the intraluminal infusion of lubricants, saline, or water, because the colonic mucosa frequently becomes adherent to the surface of the obstruction. Water may be flushed in a retrograde manner using a stomach tube passed per rectum into the small colon. This technique is useful but should be used with great caution, because rupture of weakened ischemic bowel may occur if excessive pressure is applied. An alternate approach is to inject water or saline into the ingesta proximal to the obstruction. By then massaging this region, the mass may be softened and a foreign body or enterolith moved in a retrograde manner.

If the obstruction cannot be moved by external manipulation, the large colon is isolated from the abdominal cavity with sterile impervious drapes and an enterotomy is performed in the right dorsal colon close to the diaphragmatic flexure. The surgeon's arm is introduced into the lumen of the bowel through the enterotomy incision and the right dorsal colon is followed down to the origin of the transverse colon. Impacted fecal material is removed through the enterotomy incision, allowing the obstructing mass to be grasped and removed. Great care should be taken to isolate the enterotomy site from the abdominal cavity, to prevent contamination.

Middle Small Colon

The relatively long mesentery permits the majority of the small colon to be exteriorized from the abdomen. Surgical management consists of careful external massage to break up an obstructing mass, evacuation through an enterotomy incision, or resection and end-to-end anastamosis. Retrograde flushing with water or the intraluminal injection of saline or laxatives as previously described, is usually successful in breaking up impactions.

Evacuation of the small colon through an enterotomy incision is performed after the bowel has been exposed and adequately isolated from the abdominal cavity. The enterotomy incision should be made proximal or distal to the intraluminal obstruction and the mass then moved to the incision. It is thus possible to avoid suturing a section of bowel that may have undergone a degree of ischemia sufficient to impair healing. The incision is made directly over the mass if this movement is impossible.

The incision is typically made parallel to the long axis of the bowel, through the antimesenteric tenial band. There are conflicting views as to whether the incision should be made through this band or adjacent to it. It has been suggested that the increased muscular activity associated with the band is not conducive to optimal wound healing. Others have suggested, however, that incisions made parallel to the band through the sacculations may compromise the blood supply to the antimesentric border and lead to dehiscence. Recent experimental evidence in ponies has demonstrated that incisions made through the antimesenteric

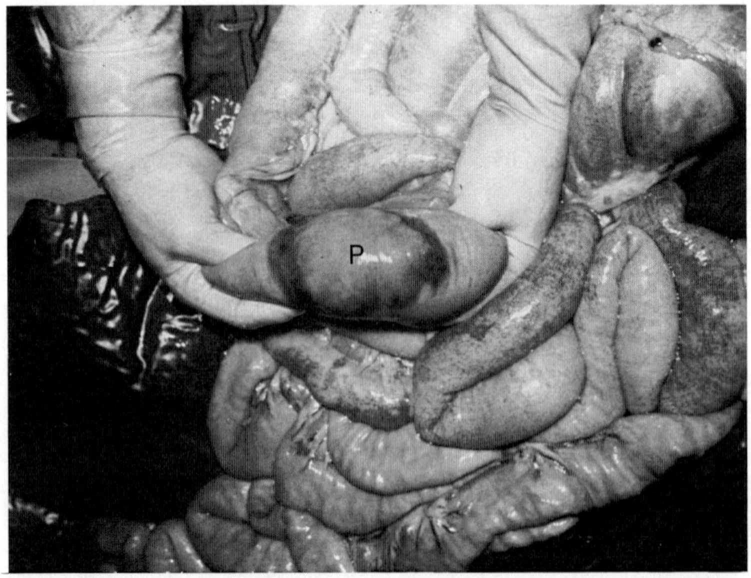

Figure 69–1. Focal Ischemic necrosis of the small colon (*P*) subsequent to foreign body impaction.

tenial band were associated with less intraoperative hemorrhage and were quicker to perform. Tissues were more accurately apposed and the wounds were stronger at 96 hours than were incisions made through the haustra.

When evacuation of the bowel has been completed, the enterotomy site is lavaged with sterile polyionic fluids. Two-layer closures using a continuous inverting pattern are recommended. The synthetic absorbable suture materials polyglactin 910 (Vicryl; Ethicon Inc) and polydioxanone (PDS; Ethicon Inc) are preferred.

Bowel resection and end-to-end anastomosis are indicated if the small colon is devitalized (Fig. 69–1). Additional bowel is delivered from the abdominal cavity until healthy tissue is exteriorized. If possible, the intestinal contents are milked from the segment to be resected, which is then isolated with intestinal clamps or Penrose drains encircled around the small colon through the mesentery. The mesocolon is divided and the devitalized small colon transected and removed. End-to-end bowel anastomosis is performed with a synthetic absorbable suture. A recent report compared single appositional, double appositional, and double inverting closures. The double appositional closure technique, consisting of a full-thickness simple interrupted layer oversewn with a continuous Cushing pattern, resulted in the lowest incidence of postoperative peritonitis, impaction, and adhesion formation.

The TA stapling device (United States Surgical Corp) has been advocated for end-to-end anastomosis of the small colon. However, the triangulation technique employed with this instrument is harder to perform in the small colon than on the small intestine because the abundant fat in the mesocolon makes identification of vessels more difficult. There are conflicting reports of intestinal adhesions subsequent to the use of the stapling device. One study comparing the staple device technique with a double appositional suturing technique reported a lower incidence of intestinal adhesions, whereas a more recent study demonstrated more extensive adhesion formation and narrower lumen size, with the stapling method.

Following completion of the intestinal anastomosis, the mesenteric defect is closed in a routine manner. If the defect resulted from mesocolic rupture at parturition or prolapse of intestine, it may extend to the root of the mesentery. Complete closure of the mesentery may then be impossible, and a defect will remain through which internal herniation and strangulation may later develop. It is important, prior to closure of the abdominal cavity, that thorough examination of the bowel proximal and distal to the obstruction be made. This may prevent the possibility of further intestinal masses causing obstruction at a later date. If firm ingesta has accumulated proximal to an enterotomy or anastomotic site in the small colon, this should be removed rather than assuming that normal bowel function will resume immediately postoperatively. If the integrity of the anastomosis of the small colon is in question, evacuation of the large colon should also be considered to prevent immediate passage of large amounts of ingesta past the sutured intestine.

Distal Small Colon

The short mesocolon and mesorectum prevent adequate exposure of this segment of bowel. Ventral midline or paramedian incisions must be used for optimal exposure. Intraluminal exposure through the rectum should be considered as an alternative.

POSTOPERATIVE CARE

Animals that have undergone surgery of the small colon should receive intensive monitoring in the immediate postoperative period. Food is withheld for at least 24 hours or until signs of ileus have resolved. In cases of small colon anastomosis, feed is withheld for 7 to 10 days or a low-bulk pelleted ration is fed in small quantities, slowly increasing the fecal output. Small amounts of food material may then be introduced, gradually increasing the quantity while carefully monitoring fecal production. Intestinal lubricants are administered via nasogastric tube for 3 to 4 days to maintain soft feces. Palpation per rectum is conducted daily to examine for the presence of intestinal adhesions or impaction.

Pre- and postoperative broad-spectrum antibiotics are recommended in those horses having bowel of questionable viability and those in which an enterotomy or intestinal resection has been performed.

PROGNOSIS

There are few reports that document the outcome of cases that have undergone the surgical correction of a small colon problem. A success rate of 47% was recorded for 30 cases of enterolithiasis and only one of five horses with mesocolic rupture was successfully treated. These figures reflect the difficulty in reaching a definitive diagnosis or decision that exploratory celiotomy is indicated. The frequently mild colic signs and incomplete nature of the obstruction often lead to a protracted disease course and greater likelihood of bowel ischemia.

BIBLIOGRAPHY

Archer RM, Lindsay WA, Smith DF, Wilson JW: Vascular anatomy of the equine small colon. *Am J Vet Res* 1989;50:893–897.

Archer RM, Parsons JC, Lindsay WA, Wilson JW, Smith DF: A comparison of enterotomies through the antimesenteric band and the sacculation of the small (descending) colon of ponies. *Equine Vet J* 1988;20:406–413.

Hanson RR, Nixon AJ, Calderwood-Mays M, Gronwall R: Evaluation of three techniques for end to end anastomosis of the small colon in horses. *Am J Vet Res* 1988;49:1613–1620.

Hanson RR, Nixon AJ, Calderwood-Mays M, Gronwall R, Pendergast JF: Comparison of staple and suture techniques for end to end anastomosis of the small colon in horses. *Am J Vet Res* 1988;49:1621–1628.

Huskamp B: Diseases of the stomach and intestine, in Dietz O, Wiesner E (eds): *Diseases of the Horse* 2/1. Basle, S. Karger, 1984, pp 198–199.

Keller SD, Horney FD: Diseases of the equine small colon. *Compend Contin Educ Pract Vet* 1985;7:S113-S122.

Livesey MA, Keller S: Segmental ischemic necrosis following mesocolic rupture in postparturient mares. *Compend Cont Educ Pract Vet* 1986;8:763–768.

Ramey DW: Healing in the small colon of the pony. Stapling vs. Suturing. In *Proceedings of the Second Equine Colic Research Symposium*. Veterinary Learning Systems, 1986;2:166–167.

70
Rectal Surgery

Dennis M. Meagher

RECTAL TEARS

Diagnosis

Rectal tears are usually iatrogenic, although it is recognized that they occasionally occur spontaneously, as the result of a breeding accident when the stallion's penis accidentally enters the rectum or as an idiopathic rupture. Regardless of etiology, they should be considered as an emergency and evaluated to determine the extent of the tear.

Rectal tears have been classified as grades 1 through 4 according to the number of tissue layers that have been perforated. Grade 1 tears involve only the mucosa, or mucosa and submucosa. In grade 2 tears only the muscularis has been separated. This results in the development of a mucosal-submucosal diverticulum that rarely progresses to rupture. Grade 2 tears are often not identified until the horse is presented for rectal impaction or straining to defecate, or at the time of rectal examination for some other reason. The diverticulum is identified when the fecal material is manually removed from the rectum. These horses can often be managed by keeping them on a laxative diet such as lush green pasture or good-quality alfalfa hay. Grade 3 tears perforate the mucosa, submucosa, and muscularis, leaving only serosa (or serosa and mesentery) between the rectal lumen and peritoneal or pelvic cavities intact. All layers are perforated in grade 4 tears, so that there is communication between the rectal lumen and the peritoneal or pelvic cavity.

Rectal tears usually occur during rectal examination and often with very little warning. In most cases, the examiner is not aware that a tear has occurred until the arm is withdrawn and fresh blood is seen on the sleeve. A sudden release of rectal wall tension against the pronated hand may have been experienced, but that is usually assumed to have been the passage of a peristaltic wave. Although this accident is more common among inexperienced palpators, it also happens to the very experienced. It appears that certain horses may have a predisposition to rectal tearing since manual attempts at creating rectal tears in horses experimentally have been unsuccessful.

The diagnosis can be confirmed by careful manual and digital examination of the rectum with the bare hand and visual inspection via a glass vaginal speculum and flashlight. Tranquilization with acetylpromazine (0.06 mg/kg intravenously) or xylazine (0.5 mg/kg intravenously) and caudal epidural anesthesia, using 6 to 10 mL of 2% lidocaine hydrochloride administered into the first intercoccygeal space facilitates the examination. Propantheline bromide (Probanthine Powder; G.D. Searlet Co. 0.014 mg/kg intravenously) can be used to induce relaxation of the rectal wall and a 2% lidocaine hydrochloride enema (25 mL mixed with lubricant or water) will help to desensitize the rectum. Fecal material in the area should be removed. Once identified, the tear must be accurately assessed for depth of penetration, size, position, and distance from the anus.

Management

Most tears occur on the dorsal aspect of the rectum between 10 and 2 o'clock in or near the area of the mesenteric attachment. Rectal tears that occur more than 15 to 20 cm proximal to the anus are at a level beyond the peritoneal reflection, and therefore may extend into the peritoneal cavity. Examination of peritoneal fluid will give an indication of extent of abdominal contamination.

If the hemorrhage presents as a few flecks of blood or a small amount of blood-tinged fluid, most likely it is a mild mucosal irritation that will not cause a serious problem. However, it is wise to evaluate these cases either by a very careful bare-armed rectal examination or with a glass speculum. Small mucosal or mucosal-submucosal tears will usually heal spontaneously. The horse should be monitored for 3 to 5 days and placed on a laxative diet. Additionally, flunixin meglumine (Bananine; Schering Corp) at the rate of 1 mg/kg twice daily and broad-spectrum antimicrobial drugs should be administered for 3 to 5 days. Occasionally, a horse with a mild grade 1 tear will have a reduction of intestinal motility and will be anorexic for a few days without other signs of systemic illness. More severe grade 1 and grades 3 and 4 rectal tears need to be considered as emergencies, and immediate plans should be made to transport the horse to a surgical facility. Following epidural anesthesia, cotton soaked in a nonirritating disinfectant such as dilute povidone-iodine solution should be packed into the rectum beyond the site of the tear. This will help prevent fecal balls from becoming packed into the tear during transportation and preparation for surgery.

A number of surgical procedures have been utilized for the management of rectal tears. These include one-handed blind suturing of the defect, suturing the defect via ventral midline laparotomy with or without enterotomy into the small colon, direct suturing utilizing one or two Caslick's speculums and stay sutures to retract the tear into view, and a diverting colostomy. A rectal liner that is held in place by a rigid ring sutured into the small colon via laparotomy has also been used. The feces pass out through the plastic tube, thus preventing contact with the tear, which heals by second intention. An expandable rectal speculum of adjustable length combined with modified long surgical instruments (Adjustable rectal speculum; Robert N. Roland, Davis, CA) has been developed to allow direct visualization and suturing of the rectal tear with the horse in the standing position.

The technique selected depends on the equipment and facilities available, the experience of the surgeon, the location and severity of the tear, and the temperament of the horse. If severe abdominal contamination has occurred, lavage of the abdomen with large volumes (6 to 12 L twice daily for 2 to 4 days) of isotonic fluids may be beneficial. It is important that the tear be repaired as soon as possible. Grade 1 tears may be closed with a simple continuous suture pattern utilizing chromic catgut or polyglactin 910 (Vicryl; Ethicon Inc) with size 0 or 1 suture material. If the mucosal tear is large and has extended through the submucosa, the addition of a submucosal suture layer with the same material will add strength to the repair. Grades 3 and 4 tears should be sutured by apposing each layer if adequate exposure can be gained.

Surgical Techniques

One-handed suturing of rectal tears has been done successfully with the horse sedated in a standing stocks combined with epidural anesthesia. This has been done using a large, curved, swaged-on taper needle and a long strand of absorbable suture material. The technique is very difficult and frustrating for the surgeon, and requires a great deal of manual dexterity. There is a danger of making the tear worse or causing excessive tissue trauma as the result of excessive manipulation. It is often difficult to suture the wound edges without incorporating adjacent folds of rectal mucosa. It then becomes difficult to determine when the tear is completely closed. Incomplete closure usually results in breakdown of the suture line because of continued fecal contamination of the wound.

Rectal tears that are in the caudal two thirds of the rectum may be repaired with the horse in lateral recumbency under general anesthesia. One or two Caslick speculums are used to dilate the rectum, and long stay sutures are placed at each end of the tear and used for traction. The rectum is inverted or partially prolapsed to bring the tear into direct view. The tear is then sutured with a single layer of a simple continuous suture utilizing size 0 or 1 chromic catgut or polyglactin 910 suture on a large, swaged-on, half-round, tapered needle. If the tear can be positioned in such a way to allow good visualization, this technique can be very effective. There is considerable difference in the mobility of the rectum between horses. Generally, thin, older horses tend to have very moveable rectums, whereas the rectums in young horses and those that have a lot of pelvic fat tend to be very difficult to mobilize. With this technique, there is also difficulty getting adequate visualization in some horses. This may result in inadvertently suturing adjacent mucosal folds, which can reduce the lumen size or fail to completely suture the tear.

A diverting colostomy, by either a loop (Fig. 70–1) or

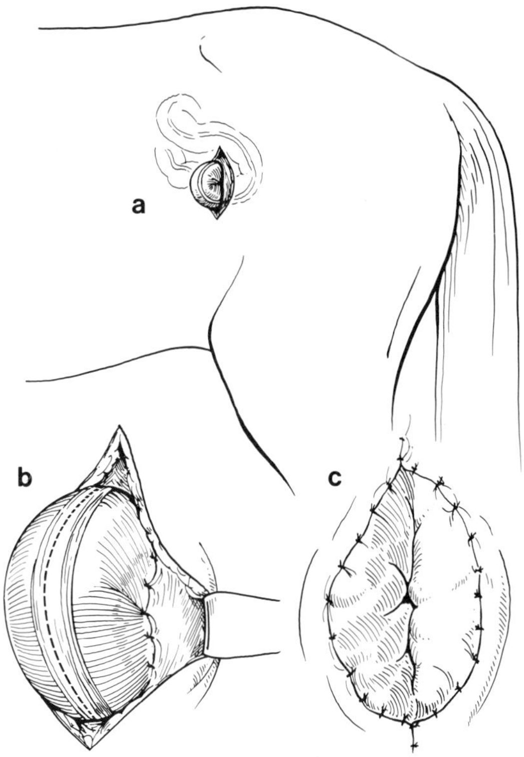

Figure 70–1. Loop colostomy. **A.** Flank incision with a loop of small colon exteriorized. **B.** Small colon sutured to the muscle in layers; sutures do not penetrate the mucosa. **C.** Small colon is incised and the incised edges, including the mucosa, are sutured to the skin.

end-on (Fig. 70–2) technique, has been used to avoid continued contamination and allow the rectal tear to heal by second intention. This technique requires careful planning and attention to detail. If the colostomy is placed too far dorsally, the fecal material will not pass freely. If it is positioned too far ventrally, spontaneous prolapse of the small colon may occur. At the time of colostomy, the large colon should be evacuated to reduce the volume of dry ingesta that has to be passed through the fresh colostomy. This technique can be very useful in severe grades 3 and 4 tears. It has the advantage of completely bypassing the site of injury, but has the disadvantage of requiring a second surgical procedure to close or rejoin the colon. Closure of the colostomy can be a very demanding and time-consuming procedure. It is best done as early as possible (3 to 5 weeks after the initial surgery) to avoid excessive mature adhesions. There may be fewer adhesions with the end-on technique, but it has the disadvantage that the distal segment of colon tends to atrophy resulting in

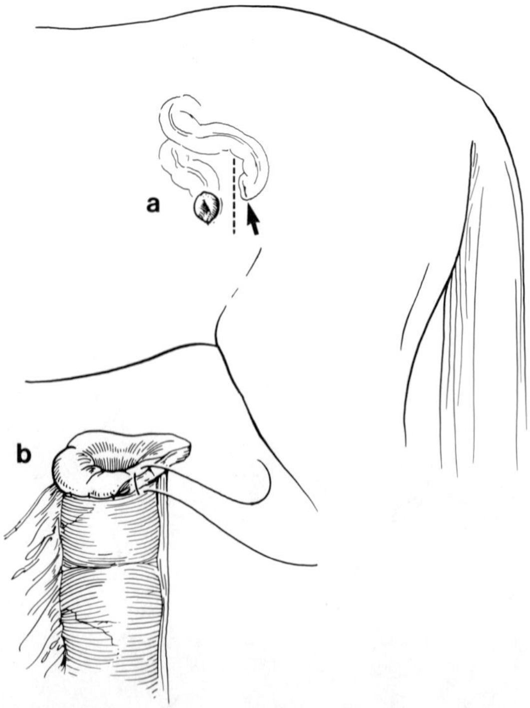

Figure 70–2. End-on colostomy. **A.** The *heavy dotted line* represents the major flank incision. The proximal end of the colon has been brought to the outside through a small adjacent incision and the colon has been sutured to the muscle in layers. The distal end of the colon has been sutured to produce a blind stump (*arrow*). **B.** The mucosa is sutured to the serosa to form the open end of the colostomy.

difficulty of anastomosis because of the large difference in lumen size between the distal and proximal segments of small colon. The loop colostomy avoids this problem, but does allow some fecal material to pass the colostomy site and thus become a source for continued contamination for the rectal tear.

The use of a rectal liner is another means of protecting the rectal tear from contamination during healing. The large colon is evacuated through a ventral midline celiotomy, and a rigid plastic ring is sutured in the lumen of the colon proximal to the rectal tear. The plastic liner, which is attached to the ring, protects the tear from contamination. The fecal material passes through the ring and into the plastic liner, which extends to outside the anal sphincter. Some difficulty has been encountered getting the fecal material to pass the ring, or with the ring and liner sloughing out prematurely.

Some surgeons have preferred a direct approach to repair of rectal tears via a ventral midline celiotomy made as far caudal as possible. Although this technique has been successful, visualization is often poor and in some instances the tear simply cannot be exposed by this approach. Since the majority of rectal tears occur dorsally in the area of the attachment of the mesorectum, this location may completely obscure them from a ventral midline approach. To overcome this problem a technique has been developed whereby an enterotomy incision is made in the antimesenteric side of the small colon as far caudally as can be visualized. Then, using traction on the colon and elevating the horse's hind quarters, the tear is brought into view and sutured directly through the enterotomy incision in the small colon. The enterotomy is closed and the large colon is evacuated. If the tear can be brought into view, this technique can work well; the problem lies in the fact that a significant number of rectal tears are positioned in such a way that they are still inaccessible via this approach.

Surgical instruments designed specifically for the repair of rectal tears have been developed. These include an expandable rectal speculum of adjustable length (Fig. 70–3); a light that attaches to the speculum intrarectally, and curved Kelly forceps, needle holder, Allis tissue forceps, and curved scissors with long handles (Figs. 70–4 and 70–5). The surgical instruments were modified to a 64-cm length and operate on a pistol grip principle (Fig. 70–6). The speculum can be collapsed for insertion and positioning (Fig. 70–3A). The light metal rods are rotated independently to expand the rectum by bringing the speculum into the open position (Fig. 70–7). The rods can be positioned in such a way that the tear is located between two rods but the rectal wall is tight enough to prevent mucosal folds from obscuring the tear. Although these instruments have been very effective for repair of grades 1 and 3 tears experimentally, they have only been used on a limited number of clinical cases. Tears that are near the rectal-colonic junction may be difficult to bring into view with this speculum because it may not be possible to position the plastic cone beyond the tear. The use of a stay suture to retract the area of the tear during speculum placement may overcome this difficulty.

Although this speculum provides very good rectal exposure if properly placed, considerable dexterity and experience is needed to effectively and efficiently use surgical instruments that employ a pistol grip principle and are 64-cm in length.

Postoperative Care

Regardless of the method of repair, horses with rectal tears require careful postoperative care. The use of fe-

Figure 70–3. A. Expandable rectal speculum collapsed for insertion into the rectum. Small wrench facilitates rotation of the metal rods to expand and collapse the speculum. B. The expandable rectal speculum in the open position.

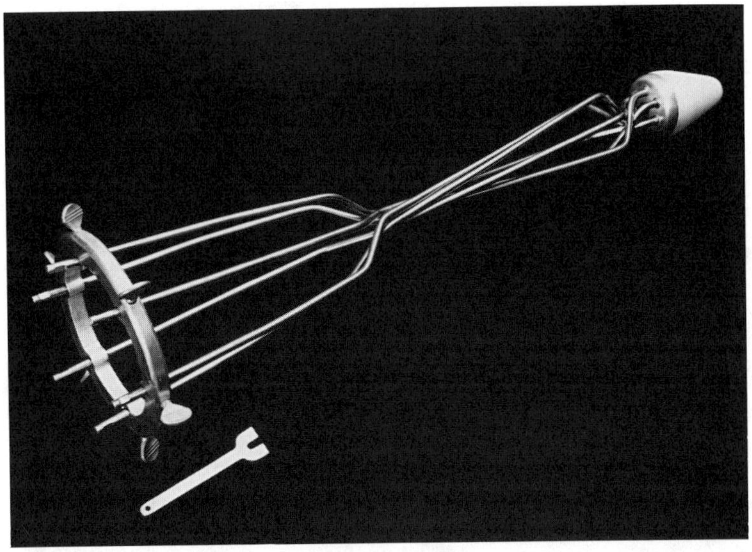

A

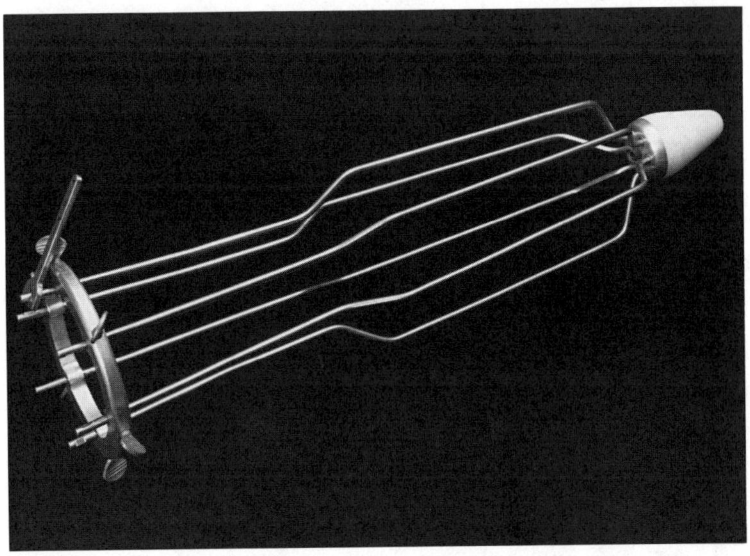

B

cal softeners combined with a laxative diet is important. If lush green pasture is available, the horse may be turned onto it immediately postoperatively. The lush grass combined with the exercise seems to be one of the most effective means of promoting regular defecation with the least discomfort. The horse should be monitored carefully and treated with antibacterial drugs and flunixin meglumine.

Occasionally, partial-thickness rectal tears will go undetected for several days and a dissecting necrotic tract will develop from the site of the tear. If the defect into the mesorectum (grade 3) causes compromise of the blood supply, necrosis of the rectal wall similarly will allow tearing or rupture. If this tract ruptures into the abdominal cavity the horse will usually die rapidly of shock and sepsis. If the tract becomes walled off, it may persist while causing peritonitis. The horse is usually presented for a mild to moderate illness with fever, anorexia, and occasional straining. These tracts may be managed by gently cleaning and lavaging the tract, fol-

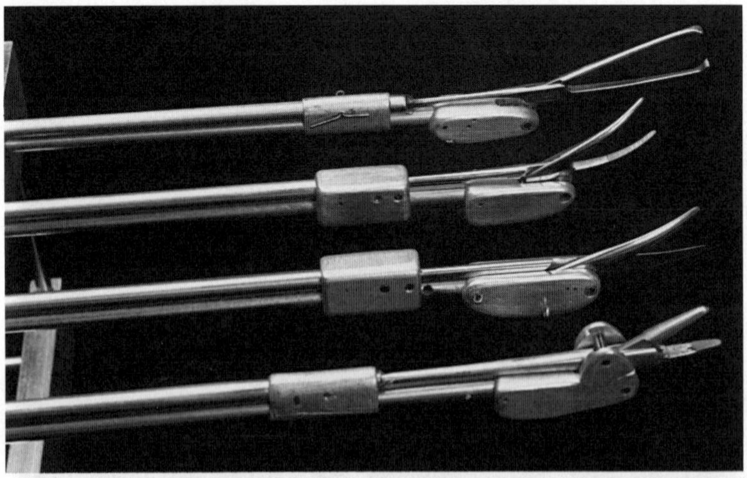

Figure 70–4. Modified Allis tissue forceps, Kelly forceps, scissors, and needle holder (top to bottom).

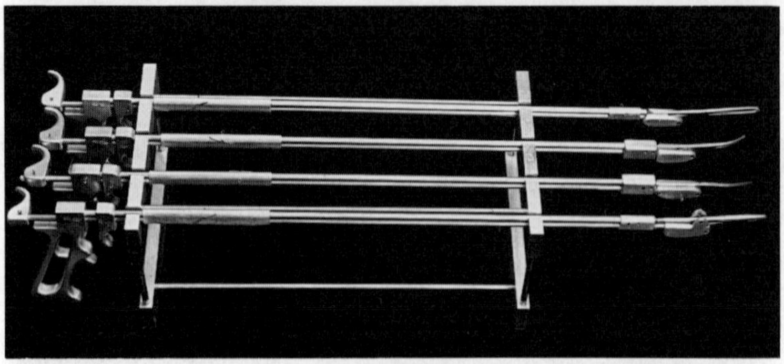

Figure 70–5. Modified instruments 64 cm long held in sterlizing rack.

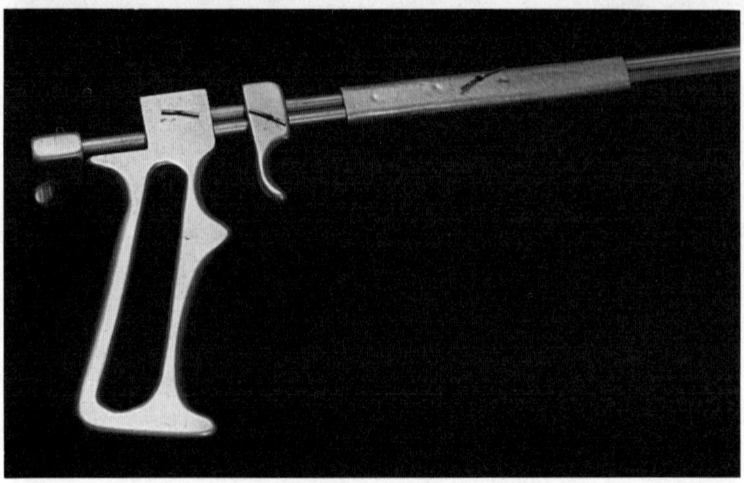

Figure 70–6. Pistol-grip handle of modified instruments.

lowed by daily packing of the tract with gauze soaked in povidone-iodine until it has granulated to the surface of the rectal wall.

Complications relating to rectal tears and surgery for their repair include breakdown of the suture line, peritonitis, pelvic abscesses, impactions, prolapse of the colon (with colostomy), and laminitis. The prognosis for mucosal irritations and grade 1 tears is generally good, but for grades 3 and 4 tears it is guarded to poor. In most instances with grade 4 tears there is gross con-

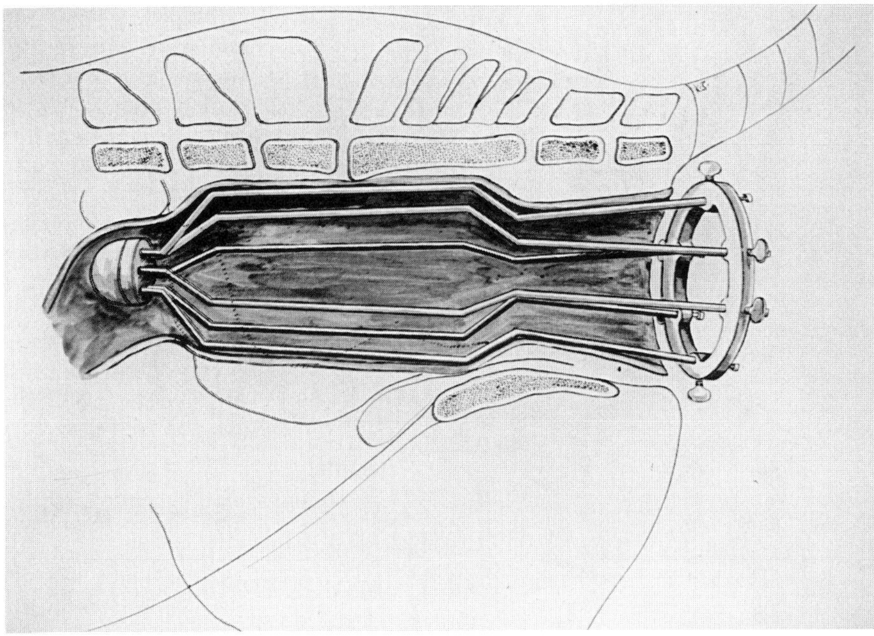

Figure 70–7. Diagram showing the position of the speculum inserted into the rectum and expanded.

tamination, which occurs rapidly, making case management extremely difficult.

RECTAL PROLAPSE

Diagnosis

Any condition that results in prolonged tenesmus, such as parturition, dystocia, diarrhea, constipation, or rectal irritation, can lead to prolapse of the rectum. The classification of rectal prolapse is based on the anatomic structures involved. The four types, in increasing degree of severity, include: (*a*) prolapse of mucosa or mucosa and submucosa to form a doughnut-shaped protrusion; (*b*) prolapse of all layers of the rectum; (*c*) prolapse of the rectum with small colon evagination; and (*d*) prolapse of a small colon or rectal intussusception.

Treatment

In all cases of rectal prolapse, the inciting cause must be attended to and the reason for continued tenesmus relieved. If the prolapse is small, manual reduction may be successful. Application of a demulcent, such as glycerin, to the tissue may facilitate replacement. Tranquilization, a lidocaine enema, caudal epidural anesthesia, colonic laxatives, and the feeding of mashes or green pasture will help to reduce recurrence.

Prolapses that are larger and of longer duration may be more difficult to reduce, and the rectal swelling and edema may persist for several hours or days. These animals should be kept standing if possible, be maintained on fecal softeners, and have glycerin placed in the rectum every few hours. A purse-string suture placed around the anus tight enough to prevent prolapse but loose enough to allow the passage of soft feces may be needed. If tenesmus persists, continuous epidural anesthesia can be provided by placing an indwelling intravenous-type catheter into the epidural space so that local anesthetic can be administered on an as-needed basis.

Surgical treatment may become necessary if the prolapsed tissue becomes necrotic or conservative management has failed (Fig. 70–8). These animals should be given tetanus toxoid and started on broad-spectrum antibiotic therapy. After tranquilization, caudal epidural anesthesia, and thorough cleaning of the prolapse, submucosal resection can be performed. Two 6- or 8-inch spinal needles or steel pins are placed perpendicular to each other through the anal sphincter to fix the prolapse in place. Two circumferential mucosal incisions are made at the junctions of viable and nonviable tissue at the apex of the prolapse and at the anus. These two incisions are joined by a longitudinal incision and the tissue is removed by blunt and sharp scissor dissection in a plane between the mucosa and submucosa (Fig. 70–8B). The two mucosal edges can be brought

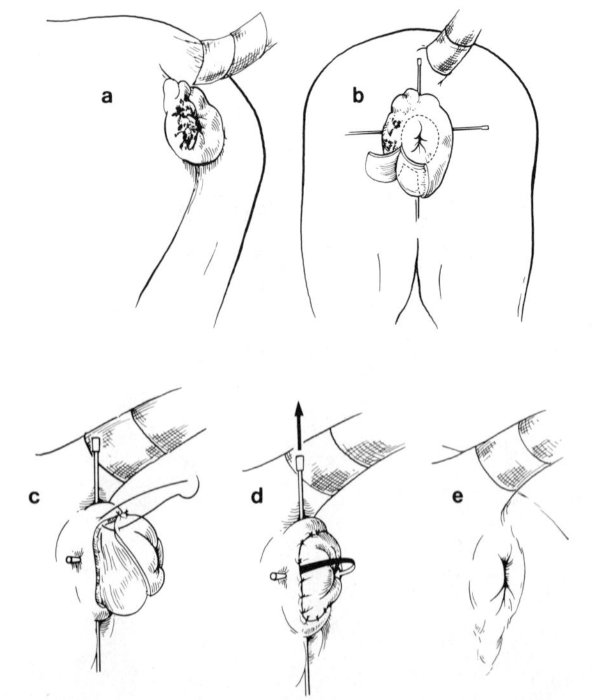

Figure 70–8. Submucosal resection for rectal prolapse. **A.** Rectal prolapse with mucosal damage. **B.** Needles in place to stabilize the prolapse and incisions made to resect the affected mucosa. **C.** Suturing of the edges of the normal mucosa after the affected section has been removed. **D.** Needles are removed and rectal tissue replaced (*arrow*). **E.** Normal appearance of anus after repair and reduction.

together because of the mobility of rectal tissue. They are sutured together with a simple interrupted pattern using size 0 or 1 chromic gut or polyglactin 910 (Fig. 70–8C). The retention needles are removed and the remaining portion of rectum is reduced (Fig. 70–8D and E).

Complete ablation may be performed if the prolapsed rectal tissue is damaged beyond the mucosa (Fig. 70–9). This is done by dividing the necrotic prolapse into quadrants and employing repeated resection and suture of one section at a time. This is most easily done by transfixation to a tube using long needles or pins (Fig. 70–9B and C). Long suture ends help stabilize the rectal tissue during the proceedure (Fig. 70–9D). The suture ends are cut short and the retention pins removed, allowing the sutured rectal tissue to retract through the anus. Glycerin enemas combined with a laxative diet are used for 3 to 5 days to promote defecation. If straining persists a purse-string suture and or epidural anesthesia may be needed during the postoperative period.

When large prolapses occur, the distal small colon is prolapsed with the rectum. This usually results in major disruption of the blood supply to the distal colon, which prevents successful management. Therefore, humane destruction is warranted. These severe prolapses occur more often in association with dystocia in the mare than from other causes. Once the distal small colon starts to prolapse, the vasculature in the mesocolon is torn off, with resultant ischemic necrosis. Although the prolapse may be reduced, the distal colon usually will not survive. Resection and colostomy may provide a means of salvage. However, the area of loss of blood supply may extend caudally to very close to the anus, making complete resection difficult and precluding anastomosis of the colon to the rectum.

PERIRECTAL ABSCESS

Perirectal abscesses are usually the result of a rectal tear or iatrogenic puncture through the rectal wall.

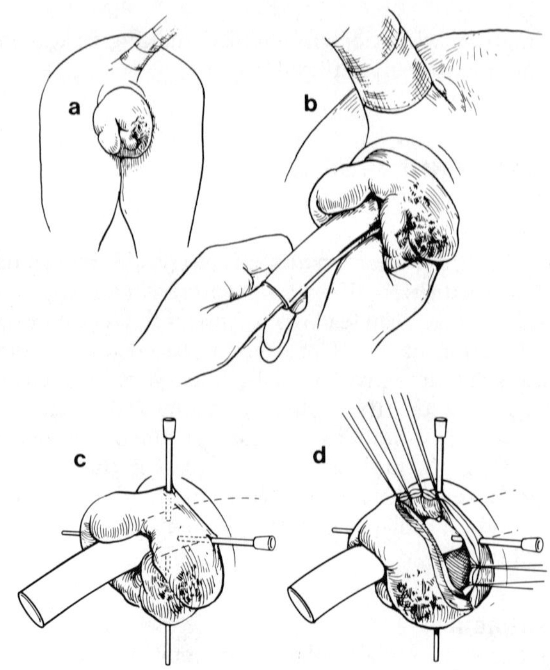

Figure 70–9. Complete ablation of a rectal prolapse. **A.** Tissue damage that extends deeper than the mucosa. **B.** Rubber or plastic tube is inserted into the rectum. **C.** Two needles are placed through the rectum and the tube for retention. **D.** Resection and suturing done in quadrants by excising the abnormal tissue and then suturing the nonprolapsed rectal wall to the rectal wall adjacent to the anal sphincter.

They are often identified on rectal palpation as an asymmetric swelling in the rectal wall or lateral to it. Alternatively, there may be chronic drainage noted from the rectum, perineum, or vagina. Diagnostic ultrasound may be useful to determine the location and size of the abscess. Pelvic abscesses also may result from postcastration infections or septicemia.

Pelvic abscesses are best drained via a perianal incision with daily lavage of the abscess cavity until healing by second intention occurs. If an open communication with the rectal lumen is already established, daily packing with povidone-iodine—soaked gauze after gentle cleaning and flushing may be sufficient. If not, drainage can be established through the perineum, and the cavity flushed and packed. The evacuation of the abscess cavity may be facilitated with a surgical suction unit, particularly if the abscess is draining into the rectum or vagina. Granulation tissue should be encouraged to fill the cavity before allowing the entrance site to close. Horses should be protected with tetanus prophylaxis, given fecal softeners, and maintained on a laxative diet. Antibiotics are needed only if sepsis or peritonitis is present.

Sometimes, an abscess cavity will remain chronically infected and persist as a source of drainage and septicemia. These may require surgical extirpation. Scar tissue in the rectal wall may be a cause of intramural thickening and cause stenosis and stricture of the rectum. Fecal consistency should remain soft to prevent obstruction.

RECTAL POLYPS

Rectal polyps or fibromas in the horse are usually inconsequential and of little concern. They may be seen as small, smooth, pedunculated masses with a pink or reddish hue. If they become large and polypoid, they may be a source of intraluminal obstruction, impaction, or rectal irritation.

Surgical removal is facilitated by tranquilization, caudal epidural anesthesia, a Caslick's or expandable lighted rectal speculum, and long-handled instruments. The masses are superficial, but can bleed extensively when cut. Simple mucosal apposition using chromic catgut or polyglactin 910 is required following removal. The entire base or area of attachment of the polyp to the mucosa needs to be removed to avoid recurrence. Tetanus prophylaxis and a laxative diet are required. Although postoperative hemorrhage and perirectal abscessation are potential sequelae, there are usually no complications.

BIBLIOGRAPHY

Arnold JS, Meagher DM: Management of rectal tears in the horse. *J Equine Med Surg* 1978;2:55.

Arnold JS, Meagher DM, Lohse CL: Rectal tears in the horse. *J Equine Med Surg* 1978;2:64.

Azzie MAJ: Temporary colostomy in the management of rectal tears in the horse. *J S Afr Vet Assoc* 1975;46:121.

Levine SB: Surgical treatment of recurrent rectal prolapse in a horse. *J Equine Med Surg* 1978;2:248.

Meagher DM: Discussion of DM Witherspoon's paper: Exploration of the abdominal cavity by digital manipulation. *Proc Am Assoc Equine Pract* 1977;p 20.

Slone DE, Humburg JM, Jagar JE, Powers RD: Noniatrogenic rectal tears in three horses. *J Am Vet Med Assoc* 1982;180:50.

Speirs VC, Christie BA, VanVeenendaal JC: The management of rectal tears in horses. *Aust Vet J* 190;56:313.

Spensley MS, Meagher DM, Hughes JP: Instrumentation to facilitate surgical repair of rectal tears in the horse: A preliminary report. *Proc Am Assoc Equine Pract* 1985;p 553.

Stashak TS, Knight AP: Temporary diverting colostomy for the management of small colon tears in the horse: A case report. *J Equine Med Surg* 1978;2:196.

Taylor TS, Watkin JP, Schumacher J: Temporary indwelling rectal liner for use in horses with rectal tear. *J Am Vet Med Assoc* 1987;191:677.

Turner TA, Fessler JF: Rectal prolapse in the horse. *J Am Vet Med Assoc* 1980;177:1020.

Vaughan JT: Discussion of DM Witherspoon's paper: Exploration of the abdominal cavity by digital manipulation. *Proc Am Assoc Equine Pract* 1977;p 24.

Witherspoon DM: Exploration of the abdominal cavity by digital manipulation. *Proc Am Assoc Equine Pract* 1977;p 13.

71
Biliary Calculi

Elizabeth P. Boulton
Conrad H. Boulton

Biliary calculi are uncommon in the horse. They have been identified most often by postmortem examination. Affected horses have ranged in age from 5 to 23 years and no sex or breed predilections have been identified. No particular diet has been incriminated. Suspected etiologies include bile stasis, biliary or intestinal bacterial infection, and changes in bile composition.

DIAGNOSIS

Cholelithiasis should be considered when a horse has weight loss, intermittent fever, recurrent colic, or jaundice. Concurrent liver disease may produce additional clinical signs of lethargy, depression, ataxia, and intermittent diarrhea. Diagnostic aids useful in supporting a diagnosis of cholelithiasis include serum biochemistries, liver function tests, nuclear scintigraphy, ultrasonography, and liver biopsy and histopathology. Differentiation of cholelithiasis from hepatitis is difficult because horses with cholelithiasis have concurrent hepatitis as a result of the toxic effects of retained bile acids.

Determination of serum bile acids provides a sensitive indicator of acute cholestasis. Prolonged increases of up to 17 times the normal levels of 5.94 ± 2.72 μmol/L have been reported following ligation of the bile duct in ponies. A tenfold increase in bile acids has been reported in animals with carbon tetrachloride–induced hepatocellular necrosis. Minor increases in serum bile acid levels are not useful in supporting a diagnosis of cholelithiasis because increases of up to three times normal may be seen in healthy fasting horses. Gamma glutamyl transpeptidase (GGT) is a better indicator of chronic cholestasis since it is membrane bound in biliary epithelium. Prolonged increases in plasma GGT may reflect the proliferation of biliary ductules. In cholestasis, there is a more pronounced, and progressive increase in GGT than that observed in hepatitis alone, where GGT values tend to plateau at four times normal. Alkaline phosphatase and both total and direct bilirubin increase markedly during cholestasis. Measurement of liver-specific enzymes, such as arginase and sorbital dehydrogenase, is used to assess the severity of concurrent hepatitis, as are measures of blood urea nitrogen, aspartate aminotransferase, and blood ammonia.

Prolonged cholestasis in humans and dogs causes an increase in abnormal lipoproteins. The most prominent is lipoprotein X. Although quantitation of this lipoprotein may be available in the future, its present value in the horse is unknown.

Liver function tests can be performed to assess hepatobiliary transport. Sulfobromophthalein (Bromsulphalein; BSP) excretion is the most popular test utilized. BSP is a dye that the liver clears in a manner similar to bilirubin. Because of the increasing difficulty in obtaining BSP, indocyanine green may become a viable alternative.

Recently a technique for nuclear scintigraphy of the equine hepatobiliary system has been described using technetium 99–labeled Disofenin. This is a sophisticated liver function test with the added dimension of visualizing the hepatobiliary system. Excretion of the Disofenin is independent of fasting or feeding. Washout curves have been established for both the liver and biliary system.

Mechanical sector or linear array scanners with 3.0-MHz crystals are recommended for ultrasonographic imaging of the liver. The liver is located ventral to the lung and dorsolateral to the right dorsal colon between the right ninth and 16th intercostal spaces. Hepatomegaly secondary to extrahepatic cholestasis is easily appreciated as an increase in liver mass in relation to lung mass. In severe cases, dilated bile ducts may appear as cystic structures deep in the liver parenchyma. Choleliths may either cast echogenic shadows or be sonolucent, depending upon their composition.

A liver biopsy can be collected percutaneously either blindly or using ultrasound guidance. Either a Franklin-modified Silverman needle or a Tru-cut biopsy needle is employed. Prothrombin and partial thromboplastin times should be obtained before using either technique to identify possible coagulopathies. Samples should be swabbed for bacterial culture and sensitivity before they are placed in formalin. Histopathologic examination of liver biopsies in horses with cholestasis often reveal portal fibrosis with chronic inflammation, bile duct hyperplasia, and distention of biliary canaliculi with bile stasis.

Although not contributory to a diagnosis of cholelithiasis, additional diagnostic procedures should be performed to detect other causes of weight loss, intermittent fever, recurrent colic, and jaundice. These include a complete blood count, urinalysis, abdominocentesis, and Coggins test for equine infectious anemia. The reader is referred to an appropriate medical text for a complete discussion of the diagnostic approach for each of these presenting problems.

SURGERY

Preoperative considerations include assessment of hydration, acid-base, and electrolyte imbalances and treatment with appropriate intravenous fluids. Perioperative prophylactic antibiotic therapy is indicated because the bile is likely contaminated with bacteria. A trimethoprim-sulfamethoxazole combination is a good choice because of its broad-spectrum activity against known bile contaminants, including gram-negative bacilli, enterococci, *Escherichia coli,* and *Klebsiella* species, and because it is highly concentrated in bile. Although penicillin in combination with an aminoglycoside yields a broad spectrum of action, neither antibiotic is concentrated in bile.

In prolonged complete bile duct obstruction, the lack of bile salts results in faulty fat absorption and thus poor vitamin K absorption. Secondarily, deficiencies of vitamin K–dependent factors (II, VII, IX, and X) develop. These may be treated with vitamin K_1 (40 to 50 mg/450 kg body weight subcutaneously) or by plasma transfusions (1 to 2 L/100 kg).

Induction of general anesthesia should be performed with xylazine and ketamine hydrochloride. Barbiturates are inadvisable because of their hepatic-dependent metabolism and associated splenic engorgement, which complicates the surgery. Anesthesia is continued with a halogenated ether. Halothane is acceptable, but isoflurane undergoes less hepatic biotransformation and, therefore, is recommended.

Biliary calculi in humans may be treated either medically with chenodeoxycholic acid to dissolve the calculi or by surgical removal. Chenodeoxycholic acid is not used in horses because 6 to 22 months are required to dissolve calculi. Surgical removal is the most common treatment in humans but is rarely reported in horses. The size of the equine abdomen and location of the common hepatic duct make surgery difficult. The hepatic ducts unite to form a common hepatic duct that exits the liver between the caudal and right lobes. The common hepatic duct then passes between the two layers of the mesoduodenum and opens with the pancreatic duct 12 to 15 cm distal to the pylorus on the major duodenal papilla. During surgery, the duct is slightly to the right of midline, with the portal vein and hepatic artery located deeper and more axial (Fig. 71–1).

The horse should be positioned in dorsal recumbency with provision to raise the front half of the animal. Access from both sides of the horse is required so that at least one and possibly two assistants may be positioned for retraction. A 40-cm ventral midline skin incision is made beginning at the xiphoid cartilage and extending caudad. Large abdominal retractors (Balfour or Finochietto) are positioned in the cranial aspect of the incision and attached to the skin with towel clamps to prevent slippage. The majority of the large colon and cecum are removed from the abdomen and placed in a waterproof bag to prevent dessication.

An assistant is positioned to retract the stomach and duodenum caudally and the spleen caudally and laterally. The visceral surface of the liver is exposed and the mesoduodenum identified and isolated from the remainder of the abdomen with multiple towels. Care-

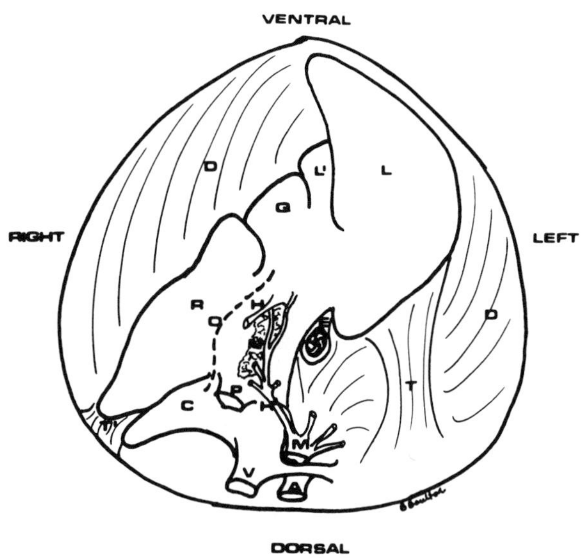

Figure 71–1. Visceral surface of equine liver. *A*, aorta; *C*, caudate process; *D*, diaphragm; *E*, esophagus; *H*, common hepatic duct; *H'*, hepatic artery; *L*, left lateral lobe; *L'*, left medial liver lobe; *M*, cranial mesenteric artery; *N*, hepatic lymph nodes; *O*, cut edge of lesser omentum; *P*, portal vein; *Q*, quadrate liver lobe, *R*, right liver lobe; *T*, left triangular ligament; *T'*, right triangular ligament; *V*, caudal vena cava.

ful dissection into the mesoduodenum exposes the greenish-colored common hepatic duct. Identification is confirmed by palpation of choleliths or by aspiration of bile with a 21-gauge needle and syringe. Bile samples should be submitted for culture and sensitivity testing.

Preferably, choleliths should be manually fragmented without incising the duct. If the choleliths will not fragment, the duct may be stabilized with stay sutures and incised longitudinally to remove the calculi. Multiple calculi are more common than solitary stones. Suction is required at the time of choledocholithotomy to recover spilled bile and irrigation fluid.

The duct is closed using 3–0 absorbable suture material in either a continuous or simple interrupted pattern, avoiding suture placement within the bile duct lumen. Because postoperative stricture is a possible complication, an effort should be made to maintain maximal duct lumen. Because of the depth of the surgical field and limited exposure, the right-handed surgeon will find it easier to stand on the horse's right side during closure. The security of closure may be confirmed by injection of saline into the duct. Closure of the mesoduodenum is optional. The surgery site is lavaged and simultaneously fluid is removed from the abdomen by suction. The large colon and cecum are repositioned within the abdomen and the abdominal incision closed.

POSTOPERATIVE CARE

Postsurgical treatment is similar to that used for horses recovering from abdominal surgery (Chapter 73) in which there exists the possibility of bile-induced or bacterial peritonitis and the management of concurrent hepatitis. Intravenous fluids are administered to maintain intravascular volume, electrolyte balance, blood pH, and glucose. A trimethoprim-sulfamethoxazole combination is administered unless a specific microorganism and its sensitivity indicate differently. Pain is controlled with nonsteroidal anti-inflammatory drugs (flunixin meglumine, 0.5 mg/kg). Plasma transfusions are indicated if excessive bleeding or hypoproteinemia develop. In horses manifesting hepatoencephalopathy with increased blood ammonia levels, neomycin (10 g/450 kg body weight) and lactulose (200 mL/450 kg body weight) can be administered by mouth every 6 hours for 2 days. The purpose of these treatments are to reduce bacterial production of ammonia and to acidify colonic contents, thus encouraging production of nonabsorbable ammonium instead of ammonia. Xylazine (0.5 to 1.0 mg/kg) or diazepam (0.05 to 0.4 mg/kg) can be used to control secondary neurologic abnormalities. The dosage of both drugs may have to be decreased because of their increased serum half-lives in patients with liver disease.

Exposure to sunlight should be limited to alleviate the risk of photosensitization. Fecal cultures are indicated in the event of postoperative enteritis. *Salmonella* species has been isolated from the bile duct during cholelith removal and may be present in the feces. The diet should provide 30 to 40 kcal/kg kilogram of body weight in the form of low-protein, high-energy feeds such as sorghum, beet pulp, and milo, which are rich in branched-chain amino acids. Branched-chain amino acids compete with the abnormally increased aromatic amino acids, which may cross the blood-brain barrier to form false neurotransmitters. Parenteral administration of B vitamins is also indicated.

The horse is confined to a box stall and exercise is limited to controlled walking for 30 days followed by 60 days of paddock rest. During convalescence, response to therapy can be monitored with repeated laboratory determinations (hematology, serum biochemistries, and abdominocenteses) and by assessment of weight gain/loss. The presence of urinary urobilinogen acids is indicative of a patent common hepatic duct.

PROGNOSIS

Without surgical intervention, horses with biliary calculi have a poor prognosis. The prognosis for horses requiring choledocholithotomy is dependent upon the severity of concurrent liver disease and the size of the horse. The surgical technique is difficult in larger horses. Bile contamination and resultant peritonitis, dehiscence, bile duct stricture, cholelith reformation, and enteritis can prevent a successful outcome. The procedure is technically demanding because of the limited exposure and poor visibility of the common hepatic duct. The prognosis improves if choledocholithotomy can be avoided and the calculi gently fragmented within the duct and manipulated into the duodenum.

BIBLIOGRAPHY

Blass CE: Surgery of the extrahepatic biliary tract. *Compend Cont Educ Pract Vet* 1983;5:801–808.

Byars TD: Chronic liver disease, in Robinson NE (ed): *Current Therapy in Equine Medicine,* ed 2. Philadelphia, WB Saunders Co, 1987, pp 112–113.

Divers TD: Acute hepatic failure, in Robinson NE (ed): *Current Therapy in Equine Medicine,* ed 2. Philadelphia, WB Saunders Co, 1987, pp 110–112.

Hoffman WE, Baker G, Rieser S, Dorner JL: Alterations in selected serum biochemical constituents in equids after induced hepatic disease. *Am J Vet Res* 1987;48:1343–1347.

Hornof WJ, Baker DG: Biliary kinetics of horses as determined by quantitative nuclear scintigraphy. *Vet Radiol* 1986;27:85–88.

Johnston JK, Divers TJ, Reef VB, Acland H: Cholelithiasis in horses: Ten cases (1982–1986). *J Am Vet Med Assoc* 1989;194:405–409.

McDole MG: Cholelithiasis in a horse. *Equine Prac* 1980;2:37–40.

Meyer DJ, Chiapella AM: Cholestasis. *Vet Clin North Am Small Anim Pract* 1985;15:215–227.

Roussel AJ, Becht J, Adams SB: Choledocholithiasis in a horse. *Cornell Vet* 1984;74:166–171.

Scarratt KW, Fessler RL: Cholelithiasis and biliary obstruction in a horse. *Compend Cont Educ Pract Vet* 1985;7:5428–5431.

Traub JL, Grant BD, Rantanen NW, McElwain T, Wagner PC, Bayly W: Surgical removal of choleliths in a horse. *J Am Vet Med Assoc* 1983;182:714–716.

Traub JL, Rantanen N, Reed S, Schecter L: Cholelithiasis in four horses. *J Am Vet Med Assoc* 1982;181:59–62.

72
Determination of Intestinal Viability

Kenneth E. Sullins

Intraoperative assessment of intestinal viability in all species continues to frustrate surgeons. Clinically observable criteria have been reported to allow correct identification of 36 to 75% of nonviable intestine. Excessive resection of questionable segments is acceptable in some instances, but overestimation of viability can lead to fatal peritonitis or adhesions. Bowel of questionable viability has been examined by relaparotomy in humans; however, the possibility of adhesions from disturbing an irritated peritoneal surface, stress to the patient, and economics cause the equine surgeon to more often avoid routine reliance upon a second abdominal procedure. Because the physiologic limit of equine small intestinal resection (length that the horse can lose without nutritional consequences) is approximately 45% of the total length, determination of viability becomes important in deciding whether euthanasia is elected at surgery. Similarly, correct assessment of large colon viability is critical, because it is sometimes impossible to expose intestine capable of surviving after resection. With limitations, the surgeon's experience and visual assessment provide the first estimate of bowel viability and affect interpretation of ancillary methods described below.

PHYSICAL SIGNS OF BOWEL NONVIABILITY

The appearance of the compromised bowel depends upon the type of ischemia. The most common type is strangulation obstruction, in which the bowel rapidly becomes thickened and blackened as a result of sequestration of blood within the affected segment because arterial flow persists while venous drainage is occluded. Infarction can also occur from compression of the mural vasculature during increased intraluminal pressure from solid masses or fluid/gas distention. With total arterial obstruction, seen with nonstrangulating infarction, the bowel wall is not thickened and becomes cyanotic, dark red, or green. After a longer period, thinning or perforation of the wall may occur depending on the degree of compromise in arterial perfusion.

Obstructed intestine becomes distended and is subjected to tremendously increased intraluminal pressures. In one series, horses with small bowel intraluminal pressures greater than 15 cm H_2O did not survive. Accurate prediction of viability in such cases is imperative, since lengths of bowel involved usually exceed the resection limit. Complicating the situation, the severity of the ischemic lesion can progress following decompression due to reperfusion injury. Peritoneal adhesions can also follow nonlethal ischemia and/or significant luminal distention. It is hoped that bowel destined to develop such adhesions would be selected as nonviable, yet this determination has not always been possible.

Return of normal color has been shown to be an unreliable indicator of intestinal viability; however, it should be considered a favorable sign. Obvious lack of viability is indicated by greenish or darkened discoloration retained after reperfusion. When strangulation obstruction has produced a blackened visceral surface, the serosa becomes dull or dry and unable to remain wet after moistening. This should be considered evidence of nonviability. Unfortunately, return of pink color is not always indicative of survival, particularly in the small intestine.

Spastic contractions of the intestine frequently appear when perfusion is reestablished. Smooth muscle may contract when pinched; however, general anesthesia has been shown to abolish all but basal slow wave activity of the distal jejunum and ileum in ponies. Although the presence of apparently progressive motility can probably be considered encouraging, the physiologic significance of such activity at surgery should be questioned.

The appearance of the mucosal surface is useful for determining the severity of ischemia. Normal mucosa is velvety pink. With strangulation, the mucosa rapidly thickens and blackens with hemorrhage, indicating a poor chance of maintaining viability. Less congested but infarcted mucosal surfaces appear granular rather than smooth, and ulcerations may be found. As the lesion progresses, the mucosal surface may be absent, particularly in the colon.

TECHNICAL METHODOLOGY

The above criteria (color, texture, motility, and mucosal appearance) more accurately estimate bowel viability as experience is gained. However, since these signs can be inaccurate, technical means of improving prediction of viability have been investigated. Most clinically useful methods of evaluating intestinal viability measure tissue perfusion. These include intravenous injection of dye (particularly sodium fluorescein), Doppler ultrasound, oximetry of the serosal surface, and thermography. The first two techniques have been the most frequently reported methods of detecting local perfusion of segments of bowel. Experience is needed to use either method, and one should remember that perfusion indicated by these methods does not always predict future viability.

The variation among reports can be attributed to differences in species or ischemia models, or, perhaps most significantly, to differences in definitions of viable bowel. Most reports have used histologic evaluation within 24 to 48 hours to determine viability, but some used clinical follow-up only. Accurate prediction of the fate of an ischemic segment of bowel based upon its histologic appearance is difficult and may not be possible.

Injection of Dye

Fluorescein dye injected intravenously (11 mg/kg) is distributed to all perfused tissues. Normal serous surfaces rapidly become yellow-green and emit a yellow fluorescence when illuminated with long-wave ultraviolet light. Fluorescent patterns have been correlated to histologic lesions in cats and rabbit and their application has been reported in humans. Differences reported indicate species variation in pattern of ischemia and resiliency of the bowel. Further variation was noticed in the horse, in which small bowel segments survived after fluorescing with patterns considered to be nonviable in the cat. Moreover, rabbit intestine subjected to severe ischemia survived with no stricture or complications, whereas shorter periods of ischemia resulted in eventual adhesion formation in the horse. Following identical ischemia, such complications were not observed when horses received anti-inflammatory and antimicrobial therapy. One must remember that failure of the published criteria to predict outcome of experimental small intestinal lesions in the horse stemmed from determinations based on work from other species.

Clinically, horses with small intestine totally lacking fluorescence have survived. These have been horses with tightly distended bowel or with reduced total perfusion. It is important to compare the segment in question to unaffected small intestine or colon. When reduced fluorescence is generalized, little credence can be placed upon the procedure.

Large colon viability may be more accurately evaluated with fluorescein; however, variations must be recognized. Finer grained disruptions are observed commonly following nonstrangulating displacements or volvulus of short duration and generally are predictive of a favorable outcome. Blotchy patterns following venous obstruction are generally compatible with survival as long as there is no deterioration of fluorescence toward the pelvic flexure. When the fluorescence reverses, and the bright areas become the "blotches" and the nonfluorescent bowel is the predominant background, necrosis is likely. The patterns may vary considerably throughout the colon, but the fluorescence generally decreases toward the pelvic flexure. With volvulus of the large colon, such a distribution can be seen with the progression being blotchy, reversed, or lack of fluorescence. These guidelines represent my experience. As with most procedures, there is a questionable gray zone between those intestinal segments that will obviously survive and those that are obviously nonviable. When colon resection does not seem feasible but viability appears possible, I encourage recovering the horse for 2 to 3 days of observation. Support with fluids, antibiotics, and flunixin meglumine will be required, but the colon may survive when the mucosal epithelium has regenerated. If persistent toxemia indicates bowel necrosis, relaparotomy can be considered with the possibility of the colon being in better condition for resection. The decision to reoperate the horse can be difficult, because some horses with viable colon will be affected by diarrhea and/or endotoxemia for several days postoperatively.

Edema of the colon is commonly present in early cases of volvulus or nonstrangulating displacement. Even severe edema with no associated hemorrhage has minimal clinical consequences in the large colon. The fluorescent appearance is uniformly "washed out," with areas of reduced intensity rather than well-demarcated nonfluorescent blotches. Granulomatous plaques occur in the colon that are capable of causing luminal obstruction and usually require resection. Fluorescein will demonstrate the margins of such lesions, which may be obscure when the colon is distended or impacted with ingesta.

Fluorometric evaluation of ischemic bowel is a more recent technique involving quantitation of fluorescent intensity at levels even below the visual threshold. This device can demonstrate fluorescein clearance rates following the peak fluorescence. Stolar and Randolph showed by reoperation that bowel retaining fluorescence 24 hours after injection was nonviable because insufficient vasculature for clearance was present. Similarly, acutely affected bowel that clears fluorescein more slowly than normal can be considered to have compromised vasculature allowing leakage of dye into the interstitium. In addition to detecting perfusion, a measure of vascular integrity is afforded by this method. Although not grossly perceivable, fluorescein normally has a short-lived peak and rather rapid clearance. The fluorometer (Perfusion Fluorometer; Diversatronics, Inc) allows serial administration of the dye if desired, overcoming a major disadvantage of the routine visual technique. Results in rats have been favorable, and have been similarly promising in the horse.

Ultrasound

The Doppler probe senses the passage of blood through vessels within the intestinal wall. The detection of arterial flow signals is thought to indicate viable bowel with reasonable accuracy. A limitation is that the probe must be placed in the exact area to be evaluated. Since the problem is to identify questionable sites, some ischemic foci could be missed. Compared to sodium fluorescein fluorescence, the Doppler technique is generally no better in detecting nonviable segments. Where differences have been shown, Doppler ultrasound was more accurate in evaluating segments suffering venous occlusion. However, in other studies it was much less accurate when compared to fluorescein, most particularly when evaluating venous occlusion. In ponies, Doppler ultrasound was inferior to surgeons' observations and a visual fluorescein test for detection of viable segments subjected to total ischemia; however, significantly more viable segments suffering venous occlusion were detected by the Doppler technique than by the other methods. The notion of Doppler ultrasound superiority with venous occlusion is logical since fluorescence is obscured by intramural hemorrhages, which should not affect viability of bowel. Patchy changes are more easily noticed with fluorescein since the entire bowel wall can be visualized at once. Although it is not deceived by mural hemorrhages, it remains to be established that the Doppler technique is equally accurate in detecting marginal but nonviable segments for which there are no concrete criteria for histologic identification. The laser Doppler is a sensitive measure of tissue blood flow but has not proven any more useful than other Doppler instruments or fluorometry in evaluation of tissue viability. Again, perfusion does not always equal viability.

Oximetry

Surface oximetry measures the oxygen tension (PO_2) where the electrode contacts the tissue surface. The PO_2 on the surface of the bowel (P_sO_2) depends upon diffusion distance from the nearest vessel, local oxygen consumption, arterial oxygen tension (P_aO_2), and local blood flow. Measurement of P_sO_2 gives a quantitative estimate of tissue oxygenation beneath the 3-mm electrode. Applied to ischemic bowel, values are compared to normal bowel and the P_aO_2. These ratios have been correlated to viability via anastomotic integrity in the dog.

Snyder et al. have established the normal P_sO_2 value for horse intestine to be approximately 55 mm Hg (±20%). When the technique was applied to ischemic colon, dramatic decreases in P_sO_2 were observed, although the decrease observed during a 2-hour ischemia period proved inconsequential to the horses. Snyder et al. have applied the technique to horses with large colon volvulus and observed that those with P_sO_2 less than 20 mm Hg have not survived. When the P_sO_2 is more than 30 mm Hg, the horses have survived. Cases falling between 20 and 30 mm Hg represent the cases that could respond either way. Two horses studied by Snyder et al. survived in spite of having bowel which visibly appeared nonviable but was predicted to be viable by oximetry. In another case, the bowel appeared viable but was predicted by oximetry to be nonviable; the horse did not survive. An average reading is taken between the antimesenteric surfaces of the dorsal and ventral colons and the pelvic flexure; however, little variation in P_sO_2 values among those segments is observed. The surface oxygen readings have been found to be less consistent in the small intestine and cecum.

Thermography

Reactive hyperemia is generally defined as increased blood flow in the previously ischemic bowel segment when compared to adjacent normal tissue. This has been determined by surface temperature increase, relatively increased radioactivity after injected radionuclide-labeled microspheres, or infusion of silicone elastomer to form casts of patent vessels. This collection of research and clinical methods strives to demonstrate microvascular patency as well as retention of autoregulation of blood flow. Reactive hyperemia following release of occlusions indicated viability in some reports; however, others have shown less consistent results. Care must be taken to avoid missing focal areas of impending necrosis when the determination depends upon application of a probe or instrument. Reactive hyperemia has been shown to be precluded in ischemic muscle when the animals were maintained in hyperbaric oxygen. Since no report describes monitoring of Po_2 and most animals were maintained without respiratory support, significant variation in results is to be expected. Species differences in vascular patterns and resistance to ischemia make transfer of data between species inadvisable.

Tetrazolium Dye

Inconsistencies in methods described that largely evaluate perfusion make additional functional evaluations seem desirable. Tetrazolium dye (MTT) has been used to evaluate viability of transplant tissue. Carter et al. investigated the technique for evaluation of intestinal viability in the rat and dog. The MTT is reduced by dehydrogenase enzymes found in living cells. When this occurs, the color changes from yellow to dark blue. The rate at which this change occurs becomes slower as tissue degenerates. Correlation to viability appeared encouraging in earlier work; however, the technique has not been applied to the horse.

CONCLUSION

In summary, intraoperative evaluation of bowel viability remains a dilemma. Standard clinical criteria (and surgeon's experience) employed with the emerging techniques will gradually improve accuracy of the evaluation, but a recipe for predicting outcome of questionable intestine is not yet available.

BIBLIOGRAPHY

Brusie RW, Sullins KE: Fluorometric evaluation of large and small intestinal ischaemia in the horse. *Equine Vet J* 1989;21:358–363.

Carter K Jr, Halle M, Cherry G, Myers MB: Determination of the viability of ischemic intestine. *Arch Surg* 1970;100:695–701.

Cooperman M, Martin EW, Carey LC: Evaluation of ischemic intestine by doppler ultrasound. *Am J Surg* 1980;139:73–77.

Lundin C, Sullins KE, White NA, et al: Induction of peritoneal adhesions with small intestinal ischaemia and distention of the foal. *Equine Vet J* 1989;21:451–458.

Purohit RC, Hammond LS, Rossi A, Pablo LS: Use of thermography to determine intestinal viability, in *Proceedings of the 1st Equine Colic Research Symposium.* University of Georgia, 1982, pp 75–87.

Silverman DG, Hurford WE, Cooper HS, Robinson M, Brousseau DA: Quantification of fluorescein distribution to strangulated rat ileum. *J Surg Res* 1983;34:179–186.

Snyder JR, Pascoe JR, Holland M, Kupershoek CJ: Surface oximetry of healthy and ischemic equine intestine. *AJVR* 1986;47:2530–2535.

Stolar CJH, Randolph JG: Evaluation of ischemic bowel viability with a fluorescent technique. *J Pediatr Surg* 1978;13:221–225.

Sullins KE, Stashak TS, McChesney AE: Clinical significance of ischemia of the equine large colon and use of fluorescein to evaluate colonic viability. *Vet Surg* 1986;15:136.

Sullins KE, Stashak TS, Mero KN: Evaluation of fluorescein dye as an indicator of small intestinal viability in the horse. *J Am Vet Med Assoc* 1985;186:257–261.

Wheaton LG, Strandberg JD, Hamilton SR, Bulkley GB: A comparison of three techniques for intraoperative prediction of small intestinal viability. *J Am Anim Hosp Assoc* 1983;19:897–902.

73
Intensive Care after Abdominal Surgery

Andrew T. Fischer, Jr.

The improvements in techniques for treating equine gastrointestinal disease have increased the survival rate following surgery. Advances in perioperative supportive therapy, anesthesia, and monitoring of the severely compromised patient with acute abdominal disease have further served to reduce operative mortality. With more animals surviving surgery, the next challenge is improved postoperative care. It is hoped that, with further experience, careful monitoring, and hemodynamic stabilization of the postoperative acute abdominal patient, improved survival rates can be achieved. For the purpose of this chapter, intensive care of the horse after abdominal surgery has been divided into the following areas: necessary equipment, nursing care, fluid therapy, drugs, exercise, other therapies, and complications.

EQUIPMENT

Most of the required equipment for postoperative care of the acute abdominal patient is necessary for patient assessment and for administration of intravenous fluids. A microhematocrit centrifuge and refractometer are required to assess the patient's packed cell volume and plasma total protein concentration. A microscope with a counting chamber is needed for performing manual white blood cell counts and cytology. A quick staining set is useful for staining of peripheral blood and body fluids for cytologic study. Facilities should be available for the determination of serum enzymes and electrolytes. This may consist of a large central lab or currently available benchtop analyzers. The increased inhouse testing in the human medical field has spawned the evolution of reasonably priced serum chemistry and electrolyte analyzers that may be affordable to the veterinarian. Advantages of in-house testing include rapid turnaround time and an increased ability to economically follow serial samples to assess the patient's condition 24 hours a day.

Other necessary equipment items are those required to allow the rapid administration of intravenous (IV) fluids. Standing stocks or another means of comfortably restraining the animal while administering IV fluids is mandatory. Large containers (e.g., 20-L carboys) facilitate the rapid administration of large quantities of fluid. Coiled IV lines allow the patient some mobility but require observation to ensure patency and that the patient has not dislodged the system. Intravenous fluids may be obtained commercially or made in hospital. Commercially available fluids have the advantages of rigorous quality control, convenience, and decreased technician time in preparation. Their major disadvantage is an approximate doubling of cost compared to in-hospital preparation.

NURSING CARE

Nursing care of the postoperative colic patient is probably the most important part of postoperative care and is also the most time consuming. The individuals administering this care must be well trained, observant, attentive to detail, and trained to record appropriate data. As soon as the animal has regained a standing position and is able to stand unassisted, the abdomen may be wrapped with a sterile compress held in place with adhesive elastic bandages or a reusable corset. The abdominal wrap helps support the incision, minimizes periincisional edema, and keeps the incision clean. This wrap is changed as needed (at least every several days) and then removed when sutures are taken out. Some clinicians believe the frequency of incisional drainage is less when the abdomen is wrapped although the efficacy of this technique is frequently debated with no proven conclusion.

The postoperative patient requires rigorous monitoring to evaluate fluid therapy and progression from surgery, and to assess the need for any possible changes in therapy. Temperature, heart rate, pulse quality, respiratory rate, nasogastric reflux, gastrointestinal motility, pain, attitude, and digital pulses should be serially monitored. A specific intensive care record should be part of the medical record since it facilitates the recording and monitoring of this information. These evaluations should be done every 1 to 4 hours during the early postoperative period.

Gastric decompression is one of the most important procedures necessary after surgery. A nasogastric tube should be passed immediately after surgery if the stomach was felt to be at all distended during surgery. Postoperatively, the nasogastric tube is passed every 3 to 4 hours until there is no further reflux. If the patient shows signs of discomfort or if its heart rate increases, nasogastric decompression should be performed. Patients may have low heart rates (below 45 beats/min) but large accumulations of gastric fluid. In fractious patients or patients requiring frequent decompression, the nasogastric tube may be secured in place. It is important to flush this tube regularly or it will become plugged with ingesta; also, it must be checked for fluid accumulation that has not been drained by simple tube placement. Flushing of the tube allows the establishment of a siphon effect to facilitate emptying the stomach. It is recommended that gastric decompression be performed every 2 to 4 hours if a significant volume of fluid (>2 L) is removed from the stomach. The need for adequate gastric decompression cannot be overemphasized. Some animals will proceed to the point of gastric rupture before showing any signs of discomfort. Other animals have ruptured their stomachs because the distal end of the nasogastric tube was placed in the esophagus rather than the stomach or because the tube became plugged with ingesta. In animals requiring small intestinal resection and anastomosis, nasogastric reflux is common for 48 hours postoperatively but has been observed for up to 10 days. The animal should not be allowed any food or water until intestinal borborygmi are heard, defecation occurs, and nasogastric reflux ceases. Most animals can be gradually returned to feed (a small quantity of a laxative diet) at 24 to 48 hours after surgery.

FLUID THERAPY

Intravenous fluids are administered to replace the fluid deficit encountered during the development of the disease, to offset ongoing fluid losses, and to provide adequate circulatory volume to counter the effects of endotoxemia. Many horses that present in stable cardiovascular status and remain off feed for 24 hours or less postoperatively do not require intravenous fluids. For instance, it is rare for horses that are operated on for simple colon displacements or enteroliths to require IV fluids after surgery, provided they do not have ileus and can drink water immediately. The horse that presents in compromised cardiovascular status with a severe fluid deficit will require extensive fluid therapy during surgery and postoperatively. Other indications for postoperative fluid therapy include ileus with its concomitant nasogastric reflux, diarrhea, shock, and oral fluid restriction secondary to enterotomy or resection and anastomosis.

Intravenous fluids are administered through aseptically placed, secure catheters in the jugular vein. The catheter should be flushed every 2 to 4 hours with heparinized saline. Polyethylene and Teflon catheters should be automatically changed every 48 to 72 hours, whereas polyurethane or silicone catheters may be able to be left in place for longer periods. Should jugular thrombosis occur, consideration should be given to using other peripheral veins (e.g., median or lateral thoracic) rather than taking the risk of thrombosis in the opposite jugular. Bilateral jugular thrombosis will cause a swollen head, discomfort, and possibly dyspnea. Although clinical evidence of thrombosis is an indication for heparin therapy, considerable controversy exists about the dosage and treatment schedule to be used.

Assessment of fluid losses should be made by serial determinations of the packed cell volume, total plasma protein concentration, and electrolyte values. The most common electrolyte abnormalities encountered postoperatively are hypokalemia combined with mild hyponatremia and hypochloremia, and slight metabolic acidosis. In these cases, the intravenous fluid of choice is lactated Ringer's solution supplemented with 10 to 30 mEq of potassium chloride/L. This solution will provide replacement of the depleted electrolytes and act as a source for buffer. Obviously, the rate of administration should be sufficient to replace the patient's preexisting deficits and to provide maintenance fluid requirements. Hypochloremic metabolic alkalosis may occur as a result of loss of fluid rich in chloride and hydrogen ion from the stomach. If it occurs, these animals should be supplemented with physiologic sterile saline and potassium chloride.

The most accurate way to assess electrolyte deficiencies is by serial electrolyte determinations. Fluid therapy can then be customized by calculating deficits and selecting the appropriate fluid or supplementation necessary. Sodium and chloride are primarily extracellular ions considered to have a volume of distribution of one third of the body weight. The Na^+ and Cl^- deficits and resultant necessary supplementation can be calculated as follows:

$$\text{Deficit (mEq)} = (\text{normal (mEq)} - \text{measured (mEq)}) \times \left(\frac{\text{body weight (kg)}}{3}\right)$$

The number of liters of fluid necessary to provide this deficit is calculated by the following formula:

$$\text{Liters required} = \frac{\text{Deficit (mEq)}}{\text{mEq/L of replacement fluid}}$$

Since potassium is primarily an intracellular ion, the total body deficit cannot be accurately determined by measurements of plasma or serum potassium. It can, however, be assessed by determining red cell potassium. Hypokalemia results from lack of ingested potassium and ongoing renal excretion of potassium. As previously mentioned, addition of 10 to 30 mEq of potassium chloride/L of IV fluid can be used to replace losses. Potassium chloride should always be administered slowly intravenously (0.2 to 0.3 mEq/kg/h maximum) since it can affect cardiac rhythm.

The base deficit is calculated by applying the first formula to measured bicarbonate or total CO_2 levels. These values can be obtained by using a total CO_2 apparatus or serum electrolyte machines. Blood pH can also be used to determine the presence of acidosis. A pH of less than 7.3 or base deficit of greater than 10 mEq/L are indications for sodium bicarbonate administration, provided there is no evidence of respiratory acidosis. Sodium bicarbonate should not be administered in greater than a 5% solution. One half to two thirds of the calculated deficit can be administered rapidly. The rest of the calculated deficit should be slowly administered over several hours. Rapid administration of sodium bicarbonate has been associated with hyperosmolarity, hypokalemia, impaired oxygen release from hemoglobin, and cerebrospinal acidosis.

The daily fluid requirement for a 500-kg horse that is not eating or drinking has been estimated at 25 to 30 L/day. This should be considered a baseline to which other losses resulting from endotoxemia, diarrhea, or reflux are added. Serial assessment of the patient's packed cell volume and total plasma protein concentration may indicate that more or less fluid is required. Efforts should be made to maintain the packed cell volume below 45%. Plasma protein concentrations should be maintained greater than 4.0 g/dL to decrease the possibility of pulmonary and peripheral edema. If the patient's plasma protein concentration cannot be maintained above this value and there is evidence of fluid retention, the administration of plasma or colloid agents such as dextrans is warranted. Disadvantages to be considered include expense and the possibility of reactions to either the plasma or dextrans.

DRUGS

Antibiotics

Antibiotics should be administered preoperatively and continued 24 to 48 hours after surgery. Broad-spectrum combinations of bactericidal antibiotics such as penicillin and gentamicin are recommended. Longer courses of antibiotic administration are indicated if there is evidence of infection or significant intraoperative contamination. Disadvantages associated with overuse of antibiotics postoperatively include colitis, nephrotoxicity, potentiation of neuromuscular blockade, and injection reactions. Renal function of patients on prolonged courses of aminoglycoside antibiotics should be monitored by serial blood urea nitrogen and serum creatinine determinations and by evaluation of urinary gamma glutamyl transpeptidase values. The patient's temperature, white blood cell count and differential, and fibrinogen level should be assessed prior to the discontinuation of antibiotics to screen for subclinical problems of peritonitis or enterocolitis.

Nonsteroidal Anti-inflammatory Drugs

Nonsteroidal anti-inflammatory drugs are used to decrease the effect of endotoxic shock by interrupting the production cycle of prostaglandins. Flunixin meglumine is currently used for this purpose. Flunixin has been shown in multiple trials to abate the effects of endotoxins, particularly when administered prior to challenge. Recent experimental work has shown that protective effects are obtained with doses of 0.25 mg/kg using a shorter dosage interval of 6 to 8 hours. Clinical use at these levels, which are lower than the manufacturer's recommended dose, has confirmed the benefit of this dosage schedule for the postoperative colic patient. The lower dose is used in an attempt to avoid the side effects of these drugs, especially nephrotoxicity and gastrointestinal ulceration. Adequate hydration is extremely important to prevent the possible nephrotoxicity associated with the use of these substances in combination with aminoglycosides. Flunixin meglumine is routinely administered in our hospital for 48 hours after surgery. Other nonsteroidal anti-inflammatory drugs have not been utilized as effectively after abdominal surgery. Phenylbutazone can be used but is not as effective in reducing the effects of endotoxemia.

EXERCISE

Exercise in the postoperative period is restricted to controlled walking for the first 21 to 30 days after surgery. Subjectively, exercise appears to improve the animal's attitude and encourage the reestablishment of normal intestinal motility. Grazing of green grass is permitted during this period. Animals are turned out into a small paddock area for the second month following surgery and then to pasture for the third month. Depending on the size of the incision, return to training is not recommended until 2 to 3 months after surgery.

OTHER THERAPIES

Attention to electrolyte levels is important in the prevention of ileus. Both hypokalemia and hypocalcemia have been associated with ileus in humans. Ileus can best be treated by thorough decompression of the bowel at surgery, attention to electrolyte balance, exercise, and adequate gastric decompression postoperatively. When postoperative ileus is refractory to the above treatments, pharmacologic intervention is indicated in the form of neostigmine or metoclopramide. Experimental evidence has not supported the use of neostigmine with small intestinal disease, but clinical improvement has resulted from its use. Metoclopramide (0.1 to 0.5 mg/kg in 30-minute IV infusion or 0.22 mg/kg by mouth three times a day) primarily affects gastric emptying and speeds transit through the proximal small intestine.

Heparin, dimethylsulfoxide (DMSO), and plasma are but a few of the other treatments used in the postoperative patient. Heparin, an anticoagulant, is used to combat disseminated intravascular coagulopathy, venous thrombosis, and laminitis, and to prevent abdominal adhesions. There are few experimental data to support the use of this compound, but clinical improvement is occasionally noted following administration. The optimum dosage and treatment schedules have not been established, but many clinicians presently administer heparin at 40 U/kg subcutaneously two to three times a day.

DMSO is a clear, hydroscopic solvent that has been recently investigated for its ability to function as a free radical, specifically hydroxyl ion, scavenger. Following resumption of blood flow in bowel that has suffered from ischemia, the intestine undergoes reperfusion injury. DMSO administered prior to reperfusion experimentally has protected against these effects in other species. DMSO may be helpful when administered intravenously (in concentrations less than 10% to avoid hemolysis) at a dosage of 0.1 to 1.0 mg/kg twice daily when reperfusion injury is suspected.

Plasma administration is helpful in some postoperative patients. Plasma is used to help replace protein lost from compromised bowel segments following strangulating obstruction. Plasma should be harvested from donors that lack Aa and Qa alloantigens and have no serum alloantibodies. The patient is supplied with protein, immunoglobulins, and clotting factors from the transfused plasma. Another product, hyperimmune antiendotoxin serum, may help patients deal with postoperative endotoxemia.

COMPLICATIONS

Possible complications following abdominal surgery include peritonitis, laminitis, pleuritis, pneumonia, venous thrombosis, ileus, diarrhea, adhesions, hernias, and myositis. The best treatment for any of these is prevention or early detection and appropriate therapy. Most of these complications can be diagnosed or predicted in the postoperative period if careful postoperative care and monitoring are being practiced.

BIBLIOGRAPHY

Arden WA, Stick JA, Chou CC: Effects of ischemia-reperfusion on the equine jejunum: Evaluation of the protective effects of dimethylsulfoxide (abstr). *Vet Surg* 1986;15:111–112.

Becht JL, Gordon BJ: Blood and plasma therapy, in Robinson NE (ed): *Current Therapy in Equine Medicine,* ed 2. Philadelphia, WB Saunders Co, 1987, pp 317–322.

Donawick WJ: Fluid, electrolyte, and acid-base therapy in large animal surgery, in Jennings PB (ed): *The Practice of Large Animal Surgery.* Philadelphia, WB Saunders Co, 1984, pp 99–128.

Ewert KM, Fessler JF, Templeton CB, et al: Endotoxin induced hematologic and blood chemical changes in ponies: Effects of flunixin meglumine, dexamethasone, and prednisolone. *Am J Vet Res* 1985;46:24–30.

Gerring EEL, Hunt JM: Pathophysiology of equine postoperative ileus: Effect of adrenergic blockade parasympathetic stimulation and metoclopramide in an experimental model. *Equine Vet J* 1986;18:249–255.

Gunson DE: Renal papillary necrosis in horses. *J Am Vet Med Assoc* 1982;182:263–266.

Moore JN, Hardee MM, Hardee GE: Modulation of arachadonic acid metabolism in endotoxic horses. Comparison of flunixin meglumine, phenylbutazone, and a selective thromboxane synthetase inhibitor. *Am J Vet Res* 1986;47:110–113.

Parker JE, Fubini SL, Carr B, et al: The use of heparin in preventing intra-abdominal adhesions secondary to experimentaly induced peritonitis in the horse (abstr). *Vet Surg* 1987;16:98.

Semrad SD, Hardee GE, Hardee MM, et al: Flunixin meglumine given in small doses: Pharmacokinetics and prostaglandin inhibition in healthy horses. *Am J Vet Res* 1985;46:2474–2479.

Stover SM: Pre- and post-operative management of the colic patient, in Robinson NE (ed): *Current Therapy in Equine Medicine,* ed 2. Philadelphia, WB Saunders Co, 1987, pp 33–38.

74
Peritonitis and Peritoneal Drainage

Karl Frederick Bowman

Peritonitis is defined as inflammation of the mesothelial lining of the peritoneal cavity. In horses, pathologic changes of the peritoneum are usually secondary to other diseases; however, the systemic responses elicited during peritonitis are often life threatening. Peritonitis may be described as primary or secondary, acute or chronic, and localized or diffuse. Primary peritonitis (i.e., bacterial infection without an obvious intraperitoneal source) is less common than peritonitis secondary to another disease process involving the abdominal organs. Secondary peritonitis may be caused by external trauma, parasitism, breeding and foaling injuries, diseases of the gastrointestinal tract, postoperative infection, and inflammatory disease of the internal organs, especially the liver, kidneys, and urogenital organs. Inadvertent bowel puncture during abdominocentesis, rectal tears during palpation of abdominal contents, and laceration of distended bowel during percutaneous bowel decompression may cause peritonitis. Intraoperative factors contributing to peritonitis include excessive trauma, hemorrhage, manipulation of devitalized bowel, contamination during gastrointestinal procedures, and frank peritoneal soilage. The most important postoperative factor contributing to peritonitis is leakage from an enterotomy or anastomosis site.

ANATOMY AND PHYSIOLOGY

The peritoneum is the mesothelial lining of the peritoneal cavity, which is responsible for maintaining surface integrity of the intraabdominal organs and for providing a smooth, lubricated surface for their free movement. The peritoneum consists of flat mesothelial cells, basement membrane, and an underlying network of vessels, lymphatics, nerves, and connective tissue. Visceral peritoneum covers the intraabdominal organs, mesentery, and omentum, and parietal peritoneum lines the abdominal walls, pelvis, and diaphragm. The peritoneal surface is continuous in males; in females, it communicates with the external environment via the fallopian openings. The visceral peritoneum is supplied and drained by the splanchnic vasculature. The parietal peritoneum is supplied by arterial branches within the abdominal wall and diaphragm, and is drained by veins emptying into the caudal vena cava. The parietal peritoneum is innervated by branches of the spinal nerves supplying the abdominal wall. The visceral peritoneum lacks pain receptors and afferent stimuli are conducted centrally via the visceral sympathetic nervous system. The diaphragmatic peritoneum is innervated centrally by the phrenic nerve and peripherally by branches of the intercostal nerves.

The peritoneum, especially its visceral portions, is a semipermeable barrier to the bidirectional diffusion of water and solutes. Solutions administered into the peritoneal cavity equilibrate rapidly with plasma. Consequently, intraperitoneal administration of drugs has an absorption profile similar to an intramuscular injection. Peritoneal clearance of water and solutes can be reduced in shock and altered with injury, temperature, inflammation, and vasoactive substances. The diaphragmatic peritoneal lymphatics have a major role in the removal of particulate matter and solutions from the peritoneal cavity. Diaphragmatic lymphatic drainage is aided by respiration, resulting in the cranial flow of peritoneal fluid and rapid clearance of fluids and particulate matter from remote portions of the peritoneal cavity. This one-way process, limited by lymphatic valves, appears to be the first line of defense following peritoneal contamination; however, it does contribute to the systemic spread of bacteria and their toxins.

The cellular defenses of the peritoneal cavity are provided primarily by the peritoneal macrophages and mesothelial cells. Peritoneal macrophages have antimicrobial activity as a result of their complement receptors, phagocytic function, and participation in the T cell–dependent immune responses. In addition, they participate in the processes of neutrophil chemotaxis and induction of clotting which aids bacterial entrapment. Peritoneal mesothelial cells, a rich source of plasminogen activators, are responsible for normal fibrinolytic activity on the surface of the peritoneum.

PATHOPHYSIOLOGY

Inflammatory stimuli cause immediate and nonspecific inflammatory reactions within the peritoneal cavity. Peritoneal macrophages and mast cells release prostaglandins and histamine, which leads to vasodilatation and increased vascular permeability. Transudation of fluid containing clotting factors, immunoglobulin, and complement occurs to localize the inflammatory insult, seal defects, and opsonize bacteria. Concurrently, mesothelial cell fibrinolytic activity is reduced, which aids formation of fibrin adhesions and localization of infection. Stimulation of the sympathetic nervous system causes ileus, which inhibits dissemination of the inflammatory insult. Within 4 to 6 hours, an influx of neutrophils occurs in response to chemotaxins generated by the peritoneal macrophages, mast cells, neutrophils, and complement activation. The stomata of the diaphragmatic peritoneal lymphatics enlarge to hasten clearance of particulate matter.

If the inflammatory response is overcome and cellular repair begins, the fibrinolytic activity of the peritoneal mesothelial cells returns, initiating removal of the fibrin clots. However, prolonged inflammation causes continued fibrin production followed by fibroblast proliferation and migration, resulting in fibrous scarring and adhesions. Many peritoneal injuries can heal without fibrous adhesions unless infection, adjuvants, and ischemia are associated with the inflammatory result.

Secondary bacterial peritonitis is usually the result of intestinal degeneration and transmural passage of bacteria into the peritoneal cavity. Gram-negative, gram-positive, and anaerobic bacteria are commonly present in the intestinal contents. Anaerobes have been shown to enhance the pathogenicity of aerobic organisms, probably through suppression of neutrophil function. The combination of facultative organisms and anaerobes, especially *Bacteroides fragilis*, promotes peritoneal abscess formation in many species. In horses, peritoneal abscess formation associated with secondary bacterial peritonitis is not encountered frequently, probably because of the low survival rate in horses with acute peritonitis and because of the diffuse distribution of the infection.

Adjuvants enhance the virulence of intraperitoneal bacteria. Important adjuvants include hemoglobin, excess intraperitoneal fluid, fibrin, bile, necrotic tissue, and fecal matter. Presence of hemoglobin has been shown to increase the growth rate of intraperitoneal *Escherichia coli*. Excess peritoneal fluid dilutes the opsonic proteins (complement, immunoglobulin) and floats phagocytic cells away from bowel and peritoneal surfaces that are utilized for entrapment of bacteria. Fibrin is important for localizing bacteria, but excessive amounts prevent phagocytes from reaching the bacteria and cause neutrophils to degranulate prematurely in their attempt to digest fibrin. Necrotic tissue, fecal matter, and the surgical procedure itself affect the ability of the body to control and eradicate peritonitis.

DIAGNOSIS

Signalment and History

Peritonitis may occur in horses of all ages; however, internal abdominal abscesses due to disseminated *Streptococcus equi* or *S. zooepidemicus* infection are frequently found in patients less than 5 years of age. Colic, fever, diarrhea, and weight loss (chronic peritonitis or internal abdominal abscess) are typically noted by owners of affected horses. Trauma, surgical procedures, or respiratory infections may have preceded onset of peritonitis.

Presenting Signs

Typically, horses with peritonitis are depressed and anorexic, and sweating may be observed. The rectal temperature, heart rate, and respiratory rates are elevated. Clinical signs of endotoxemia and circulatory collapse may be present. Low-grade abdominal pain and tenderness may be detected. Because ileus accompanies peritonitis, intestinal motility and fecal output will usually be diminished. Diarrhea may also be observed. Accumulated gastric fluid due to ileus may need evacuation by nasogastric intubation. Horses with marked intestinal distention and gastric reflux are usually very painful. Palpation per rectum of the abdominal contents often elicits pain, and if adhesions are present moderately distended bowel may be felt. Internal abdominal or perirectal abscesses can be palpated in many cases and may cause mechanical obstruction of the bowel. In cases in which ruptured bowel has occurred, a roughened peritoneal surface can be palpated, and in some cases palpation of crepitus is an indication of gas release or the presence of gas-producing bacteria. A urogenital examination should be performed because it may reveal vaginal, cervical, or uterine tears in mares, or infected castration wounds extending to the peritoneal cavity in geldings.

Confirmatory Tests

Peritoneal fluid should be collected and examined for abnormalities; Table 74–1 lists the "normal" alterations of peritoneal fluid following surgical procedures. Hematologic values will normally represent hemoconcentration, neutropenia, degenerative left shift, decreased total plasma protein values, and elevated fibrinogen levels (up to 1,000 mg/dL) in acute peritonitis. Chronic peritonitis and internal abdominal abscesses have greater variation in the laboratory values but are often characterized by neutrophilia, monocytosis, and elevated total plasma protein values as a result of increased immunoglobulin production.

TABLE 74–1. SELECTED PERITONEAL FLUID VALUES FROM NORMAL HORSES, FROM HORSES WITH INTERNAL ABDOMINAL ABSCESS OR PERITONITIS, AND FOLLOWING SURGICAL PROCEDURES

		Peritoneal Fluid Values*					
Reference	Disease/ Procedure	Color	Appearance	Nucleated Cell Counts (/μL)	Neutrophil (%)	Proteins (g/dL)	Comments
Nelson (1979)	Normal values	Pale yellow	Clear	<10,000	24–60	1.0–2.3	Normal cytologic appearance of leukocytes, peritoneal mesothelial cells, peritoneal macrophages.
Rumbaugh et al. (1978)	Internal abdominal abscesses (data from 14 of 25 cases)	Yellow	Cloudy	8,000–436,000	>80	>2.5	All fluids classified as exudates, tended to clot; abnormal lymphoid or mesothelial cells not seen; bacteria engulfed when present.
Dyson (1983)	Peritonitis (n = 30)	Variable	Cloudy	11,000–385,000	52–99	1.8–5.9	Toxic changes in neutrophils; bacteria observed in 8 of 30 cases (all cases treated for bacterial infection).
Schumacher et al. (1985)	Multiple abdominocentesis (n = 6, q24h × 5 d)	WNL	WNL	WNL	WNL	WNL	
	48 h after enterocentesis (data from 6 of 9 horses)	ND	ND	113,333 ± 87,532†	>90	ND	Toxic changes common in neutrophils, but bacteria not seen; 8 of 9 horses without systemic signs of disease.
Schumacher et al. (1988)	5 d after open castration (n = 24)	Red	ND	30,177 ± 18,363†	>85	ND	By day 7, mean nucleated cell counts approaching normal; no toxic or degenerative changes in neutrophils or bacteria seen at any time.
Santschi et al. (1988)	4 d after exploratory laparotomy (n = 10 ponies)	ND	ND	199,800 ± 28,001†	>84	4.3–5.3	Degenerative neutrophils seen in 2 ponies on day 1, and 1 pony on day 3.

* Key: WNL, within normal limits; ND, not done.
† Mean value plus/minus standard error of mean.

Secondary bacterial peritonitis can be caused by any of the bacteria found in the gastrointestinal tract; therefore, aerobic and anaerobic cultures of the peritoneal fluid should be done. Gram's stain of peritoneal fluid will indicate the presence of bacteria and guide the initial antibiotic treatments. Microbiologic culture is performed to identify the aerobic and anaerobic bacteria, and antibiotic susceptibility testing is done to select the definitive antibiotic therapy. Serial cultures of peritoneal fluid are important for detection of emerging bacterial populations, especially anaerobes, and antibiotic resistance. The presence of multiple bacterial species during microscopic examination, or following culture, usually indicates intestinal leakage or rupture. Ultrasonography may detect fluid, fibrin tags, or ingesta within the ventral peritoneal cavity.

It appears that the best indicators for diagnosis of peritonitis are increased neutrophils, elevated protein concentration, and the presence of degenerative cells, bacteria, or ingesta in peritoneal fluid accompanied by compatible clinical signs, especially persistent fever in the face of antibiotic therapy.

TREATMENT

Horses with peritonitis usually require antimicrobial therapy, intravenous fluid infusion, antiendotoxin and analgesic medications, and peritoneal lavage and drainage. Surgical intervention may be indicated in selected cases in which bowel degeneration is the original source of infection and continues to cause a systemic problem.

Medical Treatment

Presumptive antibiotic therapy should be initiated immediately. A combination of potassium penicillin (20,000 to 50,000 IU/kg intravenously [IV] every 6 hours) and gentamicin sulfate (2.2 mg/kg IV every 8 hours and 3.3 mg/kg IV every 12 hours) achieves adequate concentrations of these antibiotics in peritoneal fluid. These antibiotics are effective against most aerobic bacteria. I routinely employ therapeutic drug monitoring of horses and foals receiving aminoglycoside antibiotic therapy to assure adequate peak serum concentrations and minimum persistent trough levels thereby assuring efficacy and safety, respectively. Although many anaerobes are susceptible to penicillin therapy, an important exception is *B. fragilis*, which will require treatment with metronidazole. The dosage for metronidazole in horses is 15 to 25 mg/kg by mouth every 6 hours. Antibiotic therapy should be continued until clinical signs have resolved, and the peripheral white blood cell count and characteristics of the peritoneal fluid are normal.

Horses with internal abscesses due to *S. equi*, *S. zooepidemicus*, or *Corynebacterium pseudotuberculosis* require long-term (2- to 3-month) antibiotic therapy with procaine penicillin G. Sodium iodide infusions (0.4 mL/kg of the 16% solution IV twice weekly for 4 weeks) for treatment of peritonitis complicated by fibrosis and adhesions has been recommended although its efficacy is not proven.

Diffuse peritonitis characterized by massive peritoneal effusion leading to dehydration and cardiovascular collapse should be treated with intravenous fluid therapy to correct hypovolemia, metabolic acidosis, electrolyte imbalance, and protein loss. Monitoring the packed cell volume, total plasma protein, blood gases, and electrolytes as frequently as every 4 to 6 hours should be done to assure satisfactory replacement therapy (see Chapter 73). Intravenous fluid therapy should be continued until gastrointestinal motility returns and fluids can be taken orally. Specific replacement of potassium or plasma protein may be indicated.

Flunixin meglumine treatments (0.25 mg/kg IV every 8 hours) diminish the effects of endotoxemia, peritoneal inflammation, and the potential for adhesion formation. Affected horses often require analgesics to control pain. Xylazine (100 to 200 mg IV) or flunixin meglumine (0.5 to 1.0 mg/kg IV) are usually adequate and may be used as necessary. Severe abdominal pain should prompt passage of a stomach tube to remove gastric reflux secondary to ileus.

Peritoneal Lavage and Drainage

Peritoneal lavage and drainage is performed to dilute and evacuate bacteria, ingesta, and inflammatory byproducts in the peritoneal fluid. Its use in horses has been questioned because the procedure has not been proven effective clinically, and lavage fluid may be distributed unequally within the peritoneal cavity. This latter concern is especially true if fibrin and adhesions are present. Currently, peritoneal lavage and drainage is considered to be beneficial in horses with acute peritonitis, systemic illness, and a purulent effusion. Peritoneal lavage and drainage is performed two to three times daily for 3 to 4 days. Satisfactory response to peritoneal lavage and drainage is indicated by improvement in the clinical signs and reduction of degenerate white blood cells in the peritoneal fluid. Use of peritoneal lavage and drainage may avoid the morbidity and expense of exploratory laparotomy; however, incomplete response may indicate need for surgery.

The site for drain insertion is on the ventral midline at the most dependent part of the abdomen, which is prepared aseptically and anesthetized. A 1-cm incision, extending through skin, subcutaneous tissue, and muscle fascia, is made to allow introduction of the abdominal drain. The selected drain, either a mushroom drain, size 16 to 20 French thoracic cannula with trocar (Argyl Trocar Catheter; Sherwood Medical, St. Louis, MO), or sterilized segment of nasogastric tubing, is inserted and secured. The mushroom drain should be stretched over a female canine or Chambers mare catheter to aid its insertion. Preference is expressed for the thoracic cannula with trocar because of its multiple fenestrations and tendency to remain patent for up to 5 days. If bowel is punctured during insertion, the drain should not be disturbed until repair of the injury can be accomplished surgically with the horse under general anesthesia.

Using the drain as an ingress cannula, the peritoneal cavity is filled with 9 to 12 L of warmed lavage solution. Antimicrobial activity in peritoneal lavage solution is probably not needed provided broad-spectrum, systemic antibiotic treatments are administered. Furthermore, the presence of these substances may cause problems. Intraperitoneal infusion of povidone-iodine cannot be recommended because solutions as dilute as 3% will cause chemical peritonitis, and intraoperative peritoneal lavage with povidone-iodine has been associated with increased mortality rates. Intraperitoneal administration of 0.2% nitrofurazone in polyethylene glycol causes hypovolemia, hyperosmolarity, and acidosis in healthy horses and is therefore contraindicated. Presently, I use balanced polyionic fluid for peritoneal lavage solution.

If abdominal discomfort due to rapid filling is encountered, the infusion rate should be adjusted and xylazine administered. The horse is walked for 10 to 15 minutes to promote distribution of lavage fluid, which is subsequently drained. The abdominal drain should be filled with heparinized saline, sealed, and protected by a sterile bandage between treatments.

An alternate method of peritoneal lavage and drainage involves placement of ingress catheters in the paralumbar fossae. Insertion of the egress cannula at the ventral midline is delayed until lavage solution is instilled; the distended abdomen facilitates placement of the egress cannula. Perforation of the cecal base by an ingress catheter has been reported when the right paralumbar fossa is used; however, rectal manipulation of the viscera during catheter placement avoids this complication. It is unclear which location for catheters is preferred for peritoneal lavage and drainage.

Horses treated by peritoneal lavage and drainage are susceptible to hemoconcentration, additional protein losses (up to 0.5 to 1.0 g/dL daily), and electrolyte disturbances; therefore, frequent monitoring of these parameters and replacement therapy are mandatory.

Surgical Treatment

Surgical therapy for secondary bacterial peritonitis is done to eliminate the source of contamination, which is usually a leaking or perforated viscus, and to remove septic material. Unfortunately, my experience with a limited number of horses with acute, diffuse peritonitis has not been encouraging. When peritoneal soilage is extensive, repair or resection of the lesion is difficult, and exposure of the contaminated surfaces limits débridement. Drainage of internal abdominal and perirectal abscesses may be attempted surgically; however, the procedure is made difficult by the need to evacuate exudate without additional peritoneal contamination. Many abscesses are not removeable and may rupture during handling. Marsupialization or aspiration of contents and long-term antimicrobial therapy may be viable alternatives for treatment. Bypass enteroenterostomy of obstructed bowel may be indicated in complicated intraabdominal abscessation.

Open peritoneal drainage for treatment of contaminated peritoneal cavity and septic peritonitis has improved results in affected dogs and cats. The method, which involves intraoperative lavage and open packing of a loosely apposed incision extending from the xiphoid to the pubis followed by secondary wound closure, is probably not applicable to the horse. However, a smaller incision sutured with monofilament stainless steel retention sutures as described for secondary closure of infected abdominal incisions has been used successfully for open peritoneal drainage in three horses.

PROGNOSIS

Based upon the results described in three case series, the mortality rate for peritonitis in horses ranges from 25 to 67%. No individual laboratory parameter in affected horses can be used for determining prognosis; however, rapid response to therapy is considered a favorable prognostic sign. Patients with diarrhea or intestinal perforation generally have unfavorable outcomes. Internal abdominal abscesses due to unusual or metastatic infection with *S. equi*, *S. zooepidemicus*, and *C. pseudotuberculosis* have a recovery rate of 68% following long-term penicillin therapy. The prognosis for perirectal abscess is good if surgical drainage is effective and no complications occur. When peritonitis accompanies perirectal abscess, the prognosis is worsened. Adhesions from severe peritonitis may adversely affect the long-term prognosis.

PREVENTION

Peritonitis associated with surgical procedures is prevented by use of accepted surgical methods. Prophylactic antibiotic therapy should be initiated prior to emergency abdominal surgery, because the extent of disease and need for gastrointestinal procedures cannot be predicted prior to exploration. Atraumatic surgery should be performed rapidly, including frequent moistening of bowel and use of impermeable drapes and sleeve covers. Everting patterns for intestinal anastomosis should not be used because of the increased prevalence of peritonitis and adhesion formation. I routinely perform intraoperative peritoneal lavage with 5 to 10 L of warmed, balanced polyionic fluid following enterotomy or anastomosis procedures to dilute and evacuate bacteria and debris. Suctioning of the abdomen is aided by use of a Poole abdominal suction tip. Maximum removal of debris and fluid is done, because residual blood clots and fluid have negative effects on the normal peritoneal host defense mechanisms. Although most abdominal drains are ineffective for prolonged drainage of the peritoneal cavity, the author has found closed suction wound drains to be useful for short-term (2- to 4-hour) evacuation of residual irrigation fluids postoperatively.

BIBLIOGRAPHY

Crowe DT, Bjorling DE: Peritoneum and peritoneal cavity, in Slatter DH (ed): *Textbook of Small Animal Surgery*. Philadelphia, WB Saunders Co, 1985, pp 571–595.

Dyson S: Review of 30 cases of peritonitis in the horse. *Equine Vet J* 1983;15:25–30.

Gossett KA, McCoy DJ, Jowett PLH, Kearney MT: Hypovolemia, hyperosmolality, and acidosis associated with intraperitoneal infusion of nitrofurazone solution in healthy horses. *Am J Vet Res* 1988;49:1601–1604.

Maddaus MA, Ahrenholz D, Simmons RL: The biology of peritonitis and implications for treatment. *Surg Clin North Am* 1988;68:431–443.

Markel MD: Prevention and management of peritonitis in horses. *Vet Clin North Am Equine Pract* 1988;4:145–156.

Nance FC: Diseases of the peritoneum, mesentery, and omentum, in Berk JE (ed): *Bockus Gastroenterology*, ed 4. Philadelphia, WB Saunders Co, 1985, pp 4177–4198.

Nelson AW: Analysis of equine peritoneal fluid. *Vet Clin North Am Large Anim Pract* 1979;1:267–274.

Rumbaugh GE, Smith BP, Carlson GP: Internal abdominal abscesses in the horse: A study of 25 cases. *J Am Vet Med Assoc* 1978;172:304–309.

Sanders-Shamis M: Peri-rectal abscesses in six horses. *J Am Vet Med Assoc* 1985;187:499–500.

Santschi EM, Grindem CB, Tate LP, Corbett WT: Peritoneal fluid analysis in ponies after abdominal surgery. *Vet Surg* 1988;17:6–9.

Schneider RK, Meyer DJ, Embertson RM, Gentile DG, Buergelt CD: Response of pony peritoneum to four peritoneal lavage solutions. *Am J Vet Res* 1988;48:889–894.

Schumacher J, Scrutchfield WL, Martin MT: Peritonitis following castration in 3 horses. *Equine Vet Sci* 1987;7:220-221.

Schumacher J, Spano JS, McGuire J, Scrutchfield WL, Feldman RG: Effects of castration on peritoneal fluid in the horse. *J Vet Intern Med* 1988;2:22-25.

Schumacher J, Spano JS, Moll HD: Effects of enterocentesis on peritoneal fluid constituents in the horse. *J Am Vet Med Assoc* 1985;196:1301–1303.

Tulleners EP, Donawick WJ: Secondary closure of infected abdominal incisions in cattle and horses. *J Am Vet Med Assoc* 1983;182:1377–1379.

Valdez H, Scrutchfield WL, Taylor TS: Peritoneal lavage in the horse. *J Am Vet Med Assoc* 1979;175:388–391.

Vaughan JT: Peritonitis and acute abdominal diseases, in Anderson NV (ed): *Veterinary Gastroenterology*. Philadelphia, Lea & Febiger, 1980, pp 651–673.

75 Intestinal Adhesions

Susan L. Fubini

Adhesions are an important cause of gastrointestinal obstruction in the horse. Retrospective data indicate that adhesions are responsible for 10% of the small intestinal obstructions in horses at our hospital. In another study of 51 horses that had relaparotomy following surgery for a small intestinal obstruction, 13 (25%) suffered from adhesions. There is no definitive evidence to date that there is an age, sex, or breed predilection for adhesion formation in horses. However, "clinical impression" indicates that adhesions are a greater problem in foals than in adults.

Adhesion formation is part of the normal response to peritoneal injury. Scarring occurs both within and on the surface of the serosa. These scars may contract the mesentery or the bowel lumen, or cause adherence of bowel to bowel or bowel to abdominal wall. Simple loss of the mesothelium or serosa does not result in adhesions. Rather, release of vasoactive substances following peritoneal injury results in increased capillary permeability and extravasation of fibrinogen-rich plasma and inflammatory cells. Peritoneal injury also results in activation of the extrinsic and intrinsic pathways of coagulation. Sequential activation of clotting factors results in activation of factor X. Factor X catalyzes the conversion of prothrombin to thrombin, which converts fibrinogen to fibrin. Fibroblasts subsequently migrate into the inflamed tissue and fibrin, initiating capillary ingrowth, collagen deposition, and the formation of mature fibrous tissue. Adhesions can form during this process if an appropriate stimulus, such as tissue anoxia or bacterial contamination, is present.

Fibrin formation can be prevented or fibrin can be removed naturally by mechanisms that involve antithrombin III and plasmin. Under controlled circumstances, plasminogen is converted to plasmin, a specific fibrinolytic enzyme, by the catalytic activity of plasminogen activators released by peritoneal macrophages, mesothelial cells, and endothelial cells. Consequently, lysis of fibrin occurs in balance with fibrin deposition. However, uncontrolled peritoneal injury reduces the fibrinolytic activity, which shifts the balance in favor of fibrin deposition.

The fibrinolytic system can modify adhesion formation. Thus, it is the balance between fibrin deposition and fibrinolysis that determines the number and severity of adhesions that remain following peritoneal injury. Adhesions have been reproduced experimentally by production of intestinal ischemia or mechanical abrasion. Other peritoneal insults that can cause adhesions include foreign bodies, peritonitis, intestinal anastomoses, enterotomy, and drying of serosa in association with the presence of blood.

DIAGNOSIS AND TREATMENT

Intestinal adhesions may cause either a simple or strangulating intestinal obstruction and typically affect the small intestine (Fig. 75–1). Simple obstructions are characterized by decreased fecal output, moderate to severe, intermittent, abdominal pain, palpable distention of loops of fluid-distended small intestine, nasogastric reflux, and eventually hypovolemic shock. Strangulation obstruction of the small intestine by adhesions is characterized by a rapidly deteriorating clinical course, endotoxic shock, rectally palpable fluid distention of the bowel, and peritoneal fluid changes characteristic of bowel injury and vascular leakage. The large colon and small colon can be obstructed by adhesions, but this is much less common.

Following abdominal surgery in the horse, adhesions can cause obstruction at different time intervals. Most horses will develop abdominal pain within 3 months of surgery, but it can also be several years before a problem occurs.

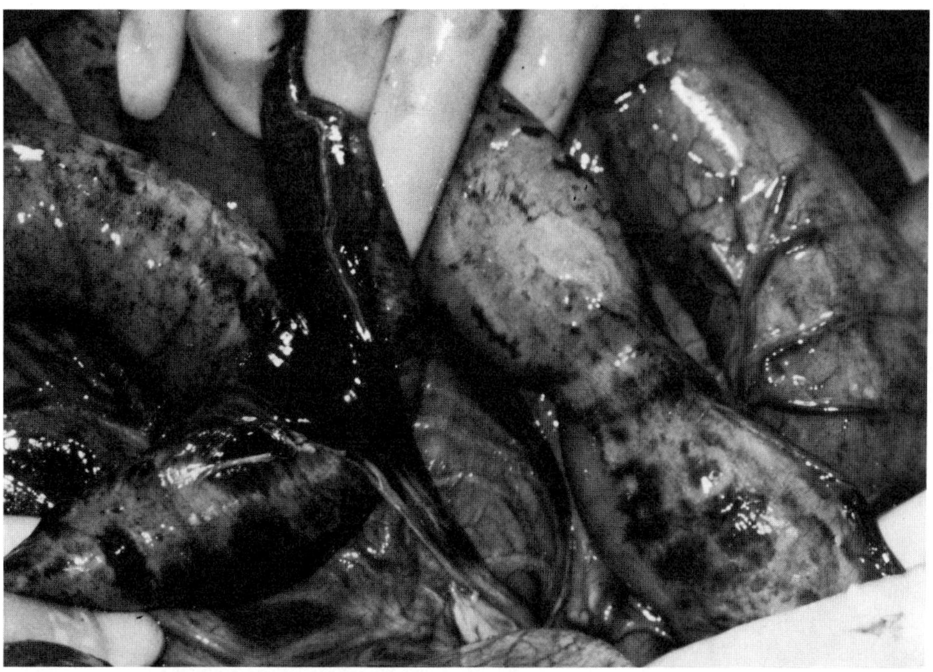

Figure 75–1. An example of an intestinal adhesion that caused a strangulating small intestinal obstruction.

One surgical option is to transect the adhesive fibers and free the occluded intestine. It may be necessary to ligate these structures prior to transection because they are often vascular in nature. In some instances it is better to bypass obstructive adhesions rather than cause increased peritoneal damage by breaking down or removing adhesions. There must be no compromise of the blood supply to the involved intestines. Generally a side-to-side anastomosis is performed. This is particularly useful for broad-based adhesions or those that cannot be exteriorized. If there is vascular compromise of the intestinal tract, a resection and anastomosis must be performed. Once again, this is more typically a problem in the small intestine.

PREVENTION

Many prophylactic modalities have been used in an attempt to decrease postoperative adhesion formation. These agents act in one or more of the following ways: (*a*) reduction of the initial inflammatory response and subsequent exudate release, (*b*) inhibition of coagulation of this exudate, (*c*) promotion of the removal of deposited fibrin, (*d*) mechanical separation of fibrin-covered surfaces, or (*e*) inhibition of fibroblast proliferation. Unfortunately, experimental methods have lacked uniformity. Most studies have used laboratory or small animals and a variety of different models. Grading of adhesions has varied, as have the therapeutic modalities and the routes of administration used.

Those agents that are currently being used clinically in human surgery or are under active investigation include:

1. *Corticosteroids and nonsteroidal anti-inflammatory drugs* (with or without antihistamines)—act to reduce the initial inflammatory response.
2. *Progesterones*—used because of their immunosuppressive action.
3. *Colchicine*—used for its anti-inflammatory action.
4 *High-molecular-weight dextrans, sodium carboxymethylcellulose*—employed to mechanically separate fibrin-covered surfaces while mesothelial healing occurs.
5. *Anticoaclulants*—act to prevent or decrease fibrin deposition.

Heparin sulfate (40 USP U/kg) given intravenously at surgery and subcutaneously twice daily for 48 hours was effective in decreasing the formation of adhesions in ponies following experimentally induced intestinal ischemia. Further investigation of heparin and other drugs is needed. Much is not known about the specific indications for each (i.e., to prevent adhesions or adhesion reformation). The effect of the different therapies on intestinal anastomosis, wound healing, and hemostasis has not been satisfactorily evaluated in many species. Finally, information concerning the pharmacokinetics, appropriate dosage, and route of administration are incomplete in many instances in the horse.

Perhaps the most effective techniques available to equine surgeons to date are surgical techniques that minimize adhesion induction. These include strict aseptic technique, precise hemostasis, atraumatic tissue handling, and prevention of drying of serosal surfaces. Minimal foreign tissue should be left in the abdomen, tissue ischemia should be prevented, and as much devitalized tissue as possible should be removed. Finally, although the literature is extensive and controversial, perioperative prophylactic antibiotics and nonsteroidal anti-inflammatory drugs are indicated in any abdominal surgery in which small intestine is distended or compromised or in which enterotomy or anastomosis is performed.

BIBLIOGRAPHY

Buckman RF, Woods M, Sargent L, Gervin A. A unifying pathogenetic mechanism in the etiology of intraperitoneal adhesions. *J Surg Res* 1976;20:1–5.

Davidson RK, Cardenas A, Busuttil RW: The effects of heparin and low molecular weight dextran on survival after fibrinopurulent peritonitis. *Surg Gynecol Obstet* 1981;153:327–331.

Ducharme NG, Hackett RP, Ducharme GR, Long S: Surgical treatment of colic: Results in 181 horses. *Vet Surg* 1983;12:206–209.

Ellis H: The cause and prevention of postoperative intraperitoneal adhesions. *Surg Gynecol Obstet* 1971;133:497–511.

Fischbach DP, Fogdall RP: *Coagulation: The Essentials.* Baltimore, Williams & Wilkins, 1982.

Henderson RA: Controlling peritoneal adhesions. *Vet Surg* 1982;11:30–33.

Holtz G: Prevention and management of peritoneal adhesions. *Fertil Steril* 1984;41:497–507.

Huskamp B, Bonfig H: Relaparotomy as a therapeutic principle in postoperative complications of horses with colic, in *Proceedings of the 2nd Symposium on Equine Colic Research.* Veterinary Learning Systems, 1986;2:317–321.

Parker JP, Fubini SL: The use of heparin in preventing intra-abdominal adhesions resulting from experimentally induced intestinal ischemia in the horse. *Vet Surg* 1987;16:459–462.

Perry JF Jr, Smith GA, Yonehiro EG: Intestinal obstruction caused by adhesions: A review of 388 cases. *Ann Surg* 1955;142:810–816.

76
Nutritional Considerations for Digestive Tract Surgery

Norm G. Ducharme

The digestive tract has multiple functions, including feed intake, nutrient digestion and absorption, and maintenance of acid-base and electrolyte status. Intestinal obstructive and ischemic diseases as well as bowel resection have the potential to have a negative effect upon a horse's nutritional balance. Thus, dietary management may be required in the acute or chronic care of many horses following surgical treatment of digestive disorders.

Negative imbalance in nutritional status may be a result of morphologic or functional abnormalities of any part of the intestinal tract, including the hepatobiliary and pancreatic systems. In addition, abnormality of one component of the digestive tract may influence function at another level. For example, small intestinal malabsorption syndrome may result in carbohydrate overload of the large intestine. This may cause increased volatile fatty acid production, leading to impaired motility and possible osmotic diarrhea. It is possible, however, that the large colon would compensate for the small intestinal malabsorption such that no change in quantity or quality of feces would be observed.

SMALL INTESTINE

Digestive and Absorptive Function

In horses, the proximal small intestine is the main site of digestion and absorption of soluble carbohydrates, fat, protein, and several minerals and vitamins. Soluble carbohydrates and proteins first undergo mild enzymatic hydrolysis by pancreatic enzymes (α-amylase for the α-1,4 interior linkage of carbohydrates, and endopeptidases and exopeptidases for protein) and then are degraded mainly to monosaccharides by saccharidase and oligopeptidases in the brush border of intestinal epithelial cells. These monosaccharides and amino acids are then absorbed by an active process with or without a carrier mechanism. The percentage of soluble carbohydrate absorbed by the small intestine varies from 40 to 75 depending on the percentage of fiber in the diet and the amount of intake. It appears that the high fiber content of the diet protects the soluble carbohydrate from hydrolysis such that a larger proportion reaches the large intestine. It may also be possible that the fibrous material is moved more rapidly through the small intestine as a result of the stimulation of motility by the increased bulk. The quantity of intake can also be an influence, because high levels of concentrates in the diet lead to a higher concentration of soluble carbohydrates reaching the large intestine.

Most of the dietary fat is in the form of water-insoluble triglycerides. These are first emulsified in the stomach. Lipid digestion is a result of the action of pancreatic lipase and yields β-monoglycerides and free fatty acids. These products are then solubilized by bile salts, creating micelles that act as transport vehicles to the brush border of the intestinal epithelium. In addition, certain minerals such as calcium, phosphorus, and magnesium are absorbed in the small intestine.

Implications of Small Intestinal Resection

Experimental studies in ponies and experience in clinical patients have shown that resection of 40% or less of the small intestine or bypass of the ileocecal valve is unlikely to significantly interfere with digestive function. Although small intestinal absorption as evaluated by the D-xylose absorption test is reduced, this does not appear to warrant modification of the diet. However, resection or bypass of 60% or more of the small intestine results in significant weight loss. It has been suggested, therefore, that resection of 60% or more of the small intestine is not compatible with life.

Pathophysiology of Malabsorption in Small Intestinal Resection

Experimental evidence in ponies revealed that, following either bypass of the ileocecal valve or resection of 40% or more of the small intestine, a decreased absorptive and digestive capacity occurs. Digestibility of minerals that are absorbed in the small intestine, such as calcium, phosphorus, and magnesium, is also decreased following nearly complete small intestinal bypass. The loss of digestive and absorptive surface is the most obvious cause of loss of body weight following nearly complete small intestinal bypass. It has also been postulated that some of the decreased digestion and absorption is a result of decreased intestinal transit time. In humans and presumably in horses, the ileocecal valve acts to prolong intestinal transit time. Thus, resection involving a bypass of the ileocecal valve may result in decreased small intestinal transit time, decreasing the time available for digestive and absorptive functions. Bypass of the ileocecal valve may also result in colonization of the small intestine by the colonic flora. This may lead to microbial rather than host digestion of nutrients. Colonization of the small intestine may also result in mucosal cell injury that can impede absorption.

Second, in addition to resulting in loss of body weight, lack of absorption leads to passage of larger quantities of soluble carbohydrate and protein into the large intestine. The end products of carbohydrate digestion are not hexoses but instead volatile fatty acids (VFAs). The VFAs are usually rapidly absorbed by the epithelium of the large colon and cecum. However, excess VFA production increases the buffer required in the large intestine. When the buffer system is overloaded, the content of the large intestine becomes more acidic. This leads to increased microbial production of lactic acid, which is absorbed far more slowly than other VFAs. Increased osmotic pressure results, which, in combination with acidification, leads to osmotic flow of water from blood to lumen, effecting systemic acidosis and dehydration. In addition, luminal acidification may cause mucosal damage.

A third and perhaps the most important effect of extensive small bowel resection is decreased feed intake. In ponies with jejunoileal bypass, a decrease in feed intake of nearly 60% was noted. Increasing the palatability of the diet with molasses failed to increase the appetite. This is a similar consequence to extensive small bowel resection in humans. The reason for this decreased feed intake is unknown in horses, but in humans there is a decreased generation of a signal at the oral, gastrointestinal, and postingestional levels. There is a change in taste (the sweet taste of glucose becomes less pleasant) apparently due to decreased copper and zinc absorption, which decreases signals at the oral cavity that lead to continued eating. At the gastrointestinal level, factors such as mechanical distention, direct effects of glucose, fatty acids, amino acids, and glycerol, and indirect effects such as release of cholecystokinin, gastrin, enteroglucagon, and neurotensin are associated with modulation of eating habits. Following intestinal absorption, factors such as glucose, fatty acids, amino acids, glycerol, and chylomicrons act at the postingestional level and may modulate feeding. Insulin, glucagon, pancreatic polypeptide, steroid hormones, and growth hormone may all play a role in the control of eating habits and appetite.

LARGE INTESTINE

Digestive and Absorptive Function

The main functions of the large intestine (cecum and colon) in the horse include microbial digestion and the storage and absorption of fluid. These functions are achieved by mechanisms that regulate the passage of digesta, ensure optimum conditions for microbial digestion, and allow efficient transport of water and solutes.

There are four requirements for microbial digestion in the large intestine:

1. Neutralization of acidic end products released by microbes into the luminal fluid. The two buffer systems of the large intestine are bicarbonate and phosphate. The pancreas and the ileum are the sources of bicarbonate and intestinal phosphate is both dietary in origin and secreted by the colon.
2. Long retention time of digesta to permit cellulose hydrolysis. The mean transit time in the cecum is 5 hours compared to 50 hours in the large colon.
3. A fluid environment to dilute the released end products to prevent feedback inhibition.
4. Continuous removal of end products by absorption.

The large intestine of the horse contains approximately 75% of the total gastrointestinal water, and each day a volume of water equal to or greater than the total extracellular fluid volume is reabsorbed. Sodium is actively absorbed and is the major ion associated with large intestinal water absorption. Chloride is freely diffusible across the mucosa and is guided by transmucosal electrochemical potential differences and therefore mainly follows sodium transport.

Both soluble and insoluble carbohydrates are degraded by microbial enzymes, yielding VFAs, which, after absorption, serve as an energy source. However, soluble carbohydrate is degraded much more rapidly than insoluble carbohydrate. Carbohydrate digestion leads to the production of lactate, acetate, propionate, and butyrate, whose proportion varies depending on the relative amount of soluble versus insoluble carbohydrate. In addition, it appears that the insoluble carbohydrates are digested in the distal part of the large intestine as opposed to soluble carbohydrates, which are digested in the cecum.

The fate of the protein reaching the large intestine is far less clear. The microbial digestion of dietary protein results in production of amino acids and peptides, from which microbial proteins are resynthesized. It is doubtful, however, that this protein is absorbed because the nutritional value of microbial protein is low. During microbial digestion, some urea is produced but it is rapidly converted to NH_3, which keeps the urea concentration in the large colon at a low value.

Implications of Large Intestinal Resection

Removal of the cecum results in a mild decrease in the digestibility of organic substrate and fiber and an increase in water content of the feces. Digestion of sodium and, to a lesser extent, of magnesium is reduced. However, from experimental studies and experience in clinical patients, it is known that the cecum can be resected or bypassed without apparent side effects.

Resection of the ventral and dorsal colon from the pelvic flexure to the cecocolic ligament leads to a decrease in digestion of crude protein, crude fiber, and phosphorus for at least 3 to 6 weeks after surgery. Ischemic injury of the colon may lead to similar disturbances in nutrient digestion. All present evidence suggests that digestibility is normal 6 months after resection or ischemic insult to the large colon, except perhaps for phosphorus absorption. One year following resection it was determined in horses that adaptation occurred by altering compartment turnover (increasing fractional rate of passage) and by expansion of the remaining cecum and colon. Resection of the cecum or large colon may also lead to decreased absorption of water.

Pathophysiology of Cecum or Large Colon Resection

Removal or functional loss of a significant portion of the large intestine may interfere with digestion of insoluble carbohydrate. This may result in loss of a source of energy, leading to loss in body weight. The soluble carbohydrate that does reach the large colon will rapidly be metabolized to VFAs. This would lead to an increased need for luminal buffers, resulting in increased secretion of phosphate. If there is not enough colonic surface for reabsorption of phosphorus, hypophosphatemia may result. In experimental studies, lower digestibility of zinc, copper, sodium, magnesium, and manganese was observed but was temporary and/or of questionable significance.

Although the major site of protein digestion is the small intestine, it has been suggested that surgical trauma leads to a catabolic response and to a loss of protein. Therefore, resection of the cecum or large colon or loss of function may lead to hypoproteinemia.

DIAGNOSIS OF MALABSORPTION SYNDROME

The known history of the extent of intestinal resection will help assess the likelihood of a malabsorption syndrome. For instance, resection of less than 40% of the length of the small or large intestine makes the diagnosis of malabsorption syndrome unlikely. In such cases, a history of weight loss, chronic colic, or recurrent fever postoperatively may suggest adhesions or intraabdominal abscess rather than malabsorption. Information regarding quantity of feed intake is important. A history of intermittent or persistent diarrhea may support a diagnosis of malabsorption, although the presence of normal feces has no diagnostic value. The overall health care program, especially the nature of ration and vaccination and deworming programs, should be carefully assessed. Finally, it is important to determine the history of previous drug administration (particularly nonsteroidal anti-inflammatory drugs) so that the possibility of toxicity can be evaluated.

Clinical examination reveals nonspecific signs such as poor condition, weight loss, depression, and decreased appetite. Oral examination is indicated to rule out dental pain or impaired mastication. The surgical incision should be evaluated for presence of chronic inflammation. Palpation per rectum may identify the presence of an abscess or of a thickened intestinal wall indicative of chronic partial intestinal obstruction. The presence of abdominal distention may reflect abnormal fermentation in the colon.

Initial laboratory examination should be directed toward confirming a low protein concentration and eliminating more common causes of poor condition, such as abscessation or parasitic infestation. A complete blood count, fibrinogen, and determination of the concentration of gamma globulin, albumin, and total protein are part of the initial laboratory workup. Fecal examination for parasites is also recommended. When laboratory results indicate a low albumin concentration, investigation of possible sources of protein loss is indicated. Urinalysis, peritoneal fluid analysis, and serum biochemical profile of renal and hepatic functions are indicated. Occult fecal blood may indicate inflammation of the intestinal tract.

Specific evidence of malabsorption syndrome is obtained by the D-xylose absorption test. This test is based on extrapolation from human studies where the xylose is absorbed in the small intestine by active transport utilizing a glucose carrier and by facilitated diffusion. Following a fast of 8 hours, D-xylose (0.5 to 1.0 g/kg of body weight) is administered orally as a 10% solution. Blood is collected in heparinized tubes at 30-minute intervals for 3 hours. Peak levels (70.60 mmol/L) are generally noted at 60 to 90 minutes.

Digestibility studies determine feed intake and fecal and urine output over a 5- to 7-day period, and thus the percentage of nutrient absorbed may be calculated. By using radiolabeled albumin, one can also identify and quantify enteric protein loss. Both of these evaluations are cumbersome and consequently they are rarely used in clinical patients.

TREATMENT AND PROGNOSIS

Because of the paucity of specific information in the equine literature, some of the following recommendations are based upon only limited experience with clinical patients. Others are based entirely upon extrapolation of information from the literature on similar problems in other species.

In cases of malabsorption syndrome originating from loss of function of the small or large intestine, there is evidence of an adaptive mechanism as shown by improved D-xylose absorption and digestibility studies with time. This suggests that, if the animal can be maintained temporarily on an alternate diet, then resumption of a regular diet may be possible 3 to 6 months after extensive intestinal resection.

Specifically, following extensive small intestinal resection, it is important to feed the most palatable diet available since decreased intake may be an important reason for loss of body weight. For example, young grass or fresh, leafy hay is more palatable than old stemmy hay. Dividing the diet into many small meals and providing a companion animal may encourage increased feed consumption. If feed intake cannot be increased, then the prognosis is grave.

Horses with malabsorption problems due to abnormalities of the small intestine may benefit from increased amounts of concentrates. Small amounts (no more than 0.5 g/kg) of concentrates are given several times daily until body weight is maintained. Close observation is required since carbohydrate overload may result from this diet modification. Good-quality hay should be fed but not at the same time that the concentrates are offered. If this approach fails to improve the horse's condition, one may consider removing or greatly reducing the concentrate from the diet. Since horses and ponies may derive 70% of their total digestible energy from products of fermentation in the cecum and large colon, a diet high in fiber (with little or no concentrate) should be considered in horses with malabsorption after small intestinal resection. Removing the concentrate from the diet would reduce the amount of soluble carbohydrate reaching the colon. This should allow more normal digestive function of the large intestine.

Horses with malabsorption due to an abnormality of the large intestine should not be fed grass because this may lead to diarrhea as a result of decreased water absorption. These horses may also benefit from a ration richer in phosphorus. Although increasing concentrate may correct the hypophosphatemia, it may also result in carbohydrate overload. If the colon proves intolerant to excessive soluble carbohydrate, a diet free of concentrate has been successful in some cases. An easily digestible source of insoluble carbohydrates, such as hay cubes or pellets, may increase the amount of energy available to the horse.

NONVOLUNTARY NUTRITION

Nonvoluntary alimentation is required in horses that fail to eat a sufficient quantity and quality of feed because of appetite suppression. Also, in the period following esophageal or soft palate surgery, it is sometimes advisable to withhold feed. Similarly, in cases of persistent ileus (e.g., proximal enteritis), prolonged fasting may be necessary.

TABLE 76–1. COMPLETE DIET FOR ORAL ALIMENTATION OF THE ADULT HORSE (450 kg)*

	Day						
Nutrient (g)	**1**	**2**	**3**	**4**	**5**	**6**	**7**
Dextrose	300	400	500	600	800	800	900
Dehydrated† cottage cheese	300	450	600	750	900	900	900
Dehydrated alfalfa meal	2,000	2,000	2,000	2,000	2,000	2,000	2,000

* Adapted from Naylor et al. (1984). These allowances should be divided and administered in 3 feedings daily.

† Dehydrated cottage cheese—82% crude protein with less than 2% β-lactose (American Nutritional Laboratory) or casein (Sigma Chemicals).

TABLE 76–2. DAILY INFUSION SOLUTION* FOR TOTAL PARENTERAL NUTRITION IN ADULT HORSES (450–500 kg) SUPPLYING 16,000 CALORIES

Nutrients	Dose/24 h	Volume (mL)
50% dextrose	5 g/kg	4,800
8.5% amino acid	0.75 g/kg	4,000
10% lipid emulsion	1.25 g/kg	6,000

* Added to 11.2 L of polyionic solution and 500 ml of calcium gluconate (23%).

Partial or complete nutritional support can be given in these instances either through intranvenous therapy or gastric intubation. Gastric intubation is not appropriate in horses affected with ileus, however.

Enteral Alimentation

Nasogatric intubation may be used to deliver nutrients to the stomach in horses that fail to eat sufficient quantities of feed. In certain cases, an esophagostomy is required to protect the oral cavity, pharynx, or esophagus following surgical intervention. Feed in such cases is delivered into the stomach by a tube passed through an esophagostomy placed distal to the surgical site.

Foals are fed a commercial milk replacer preparation by bottle or by gastric intubation. It is important to pay strict attention to the specific manufacturer's recommendations to avoid overfeeding.

Adults are fed through a large-diameter tube. One of two diets is divided into four to six meals daily. The first diet consists of soaking a complete horse feed in water to form a slurry. The amount of feed offered is based on the manufacturer's recommendations. The second diet (Table 76–1) is rich in highly digestible protein. It is diluted in 20 L of water and added to an oral electrolyte solution containing sodium chloride (10 g), sodium bicarbonate (15 g), potassium chloride (75 g), potassium phosphate (dibasic anhydrous) (60 g), calcium chloride (45 g), and magnesium oxide (25 g).

With either of these diets, there may be a problem with passing the slurry through the feeding tube. In addition, diarrhea and laminitis are possible complications that would require either discontinuance of the diet or decreasing the amount fed.

Parenteral Alimentation

When exposure of nutrients to the alimentary tract is impossible, impractical, or contraindicated, intravenous parenteral nutrition is an alternative. The cost of implementation of such therapy may be prohibitive. Complications of this form of alimentation reside in catheter-related problems such as occlusion or phlebitis and in metabolic derangements associated with hyperglycemia and hyperosmolality. Large quantities of glucose given intravenously bypass normal homeostatic mechanisms. Hyperglycemia may result, leading to urinary loss of glucose and osmotic diuresis. Therefore, blood and urine levels of glucose should be monitored and the rate of infusin adjusted if either hyperglycemia or hypoglycemia occurs. Tolerance of the infusion is observed with blood glucose near 150 mg/dL. Monitoring of acid-base and electrolyte status is essential to adjust the fluid and electrolyte therapy to meet the patient's needs.

Intravenous infusion is accomplished through a 16-gauge catheter placed in the jugular vein or in the cranial vena cava. If long-term parenteral nutrition is thought to be necessary a central venous catheter is best to prevent venous irritation and thrombosis from the hypertonic glucose solution. Fat emulsions are also used because they can provide increased caloric density compared to glucose and without vein irritation and can be used to provide up to 60% of the nonnitrogen calories. Protein hydrolysates and amino acid solutions are used as the protein sources. The recommended infusions are based on energy requirement of 35 kcal/kg for the adult horse and approximately 120 kcal/day for

TABLE 76–3. INFUSIONS FOR PARENTERAL NUTRITION FOR 50-kg FOALS

	Preparation A*		Preparation B†	
Nutrients	Dose/24 h	Volume (mL)	Dose/24 h	Volume (mL)
50% dextrose	12 g/kg	1,200	15 g/kg	1,500
8.5% amino acid	3 g/kg	1,500	3 g/kg	1,500
10% lipid emulsion	2 g/kg	1,000	3 g/kg	1,500

* Caloric intake of 3,700 cal.
† Caloric intake of 4,700 cal.

the neonate. To help replace loss of nitrogen levels the parenteral formulation should have approximately 100 to 200 cal/g of nitrogen. Recommended infusions (administered over 24 hours) are listed in Tables 76–2 and 76–3.

Hydration and electrolyte supplementation are maintained by administering a balanced electrolyte solution as needed. If long-term total parenteral nutrition is to be administered (>10 days) electrolyte, vitamin, and trace mineral requirements can be calculated and added to the mixture.

Partial parenteral nutrition may be helpful for animals that require only short-term supplementation. This can often be accomplished easily with dextrose and amino acid solutions giving 50% of the total needed energy requirement.

Discontinuation of parenteral nutrition is done once the animal is consuming a satisfactory oral diet. Parenteral nutrition may also be reduced gradually over a 3-day period. The intravenous diet can be decreased in volume each day while monitoring blood glucose levels for hypoglycemia. There is normally no need to change the contents of the diet during the reduction period.

BIBLIOGRAPHY

Argenzio RA: Digestion and absorption of carbohydrate, fat and protein, in Swenson MJ (ed): *Duke's Physiology of Domestic Animals,* ed 10. Ithaca, NY, Cornell University Press, 1984, pp 301–310.

Bertone AL, Stashak TS, Sullins KE, Ralston SL: Experimental large colon resection at the ceco-colic ligament in the horse. *Vet Surg* 1987;16:5–12.

Bertone AL, Van Soest PJ, Johnson D, Ralston SL, Stashak TS: Large intestinal capacity, retention times and turnover rates of particulate ingesta associated with extensive large colon resection in horses. *Vet Surg* 1989;50:1621–1627.

Ducharme NG, Horney FD, Baird JD, Arighi M, Burton JH: Extensive large colon resection in the pony. I Surgical procedures and clinical results. *Can J Vet Res* 1987;51:66–75.

Ducharme NG, Burton JH, van Dreumel AA, Horney FD, Baird JD, Arighi M: Extensive large colon resection in the pony. II Digestibility studies and post mortem findings. *Can J Vet Res* 1987;51:76–82.

Hansen TO: Parenteral nutrition in foals. *Proc Am Assoc Equine Pract* 1986;pp 153–156.

Hansen TO, White NA, Kemp DT: Total parenteral nutrition in horses, *Am J Vet Res* 1988;49:122–124.

Naylor JM, Freeman DE, Kronfeld DS: Alimentation of hypophagic horses. *Compend Cont Educ Pract Vet* 1984;6:S93–S99.

Ralston SL, Sullins KE, Stashak TS: Digestion in horses after resection or ischemic insult. *Am J Vet Res* 1986;47:2290–2293.

Roberts MC: Malabsorption syndromes in the horses. *Compend Cont Educ Pract Vet* 1984;7:S637–S646.

Tate LP, Ralston SL, Koch CK, Everitt JI: Effects of extensive resection of the small intestine in the pony. *Am J Vet Res* 1983;44:1187–1191.

77 Prognosis for Acute Abdominal Diseases

Martin O. Furr
Nathaniel A. White II

Many variables, including clinical (physical) examination and hematologic parameters, have been applied to prognosticate equine colic. The findings of numerous studies indicate that, in general, variables that evaluate, either directly or indirectly, cardiovascular status have the most prognostic merit. Prognosis of the surgical case can be difficult. When the abdomen is open and a diseased segment is discovered, the surgeon faces the perplexing problem of determining if the horse has a chance to survive. Unfortunately, the lesion or its apparent severity cannot be used as the sole determining factor. Horses with severe infarction causing devitalization of segments of the small intestine have survived after resection with few after effects. Other horses with simple obstruction of the intestine suffer from ileus and/or circulatory shock, which can be fatal even though the lesion appeared relatively mild. The common denominator is the effect of the disease on the cardiovascular system. This effect is similar in all types of colic and, with some additional parameters, may be utilized in the surgical case to help determine the outcome.

Although many of the physical signs normally recorded during the examination—such as the degree of skin tenting, duration of colic, amount of nasogastric reflux, and absence of intestinal sounds—are important in evaluating the need for surgical treatment, individually these have little value in predicting outcome. Information that can be applied to prognosis can be gained from specific physical signs and selected laboratory tests.

PHYSICAL EXAMINATION

Physical examination findings that are useful in forecasting the outcome in cases of equine colic are those that relate to the severity of pain, the cardiovascular status of the patient, and rectal examination.

Pain associated with colic arises through a limited number of mechanisms. Pain receptors within viscera are stimulated by distention, ischemia, chemical irritation, and stretching of the mesentery. Hypoxia, resulting from vascular compromise, enhances the sensitivity of pain receptors. Pain that is continuous and uncontrollable is associated with a poor prognosis. When the degree of pain was rated as mild, moderate, or severe in a recent study, horses had probable survival rates of 90, 50, and 25%, respectively.

Examination of the cardiovascular system should include heart rate, pulse quality, capillary refill time, and mucous membrane color. The heart rate in horses with colic is frequently elevated as a result of pain and/or circulatory collapse. The degree of increase in the heart rate is proportional to both the intensity of pain and the severity of cardiovascular compromise; hence, evaluation of the heart rate gives an estimate of the severity of the condition.

Heart rate has been used prognostically. A heart rate of greater than 100 beats/min is considered a grave prognostic sign and was associated with a probable survival rate of less than 30% in a recent study. This value is similar to those found in other surveys in which increasing heart rates were associated with decreasing survival rates (Table 77–1).

TABLE 77–1. RELATIONSHIP OF HEART RATE TO SURVIVAL IN EQUINE COLIC*

Heart Rate (bpm)	Survival Rate (%)
<40	100
41–60	83
61–80	76
81–100	54
101–120	29
>120	20

* From Parry B: Use of clinical pathology in evaluation of horses with colic. *Vet Clin North Am Equine Pract* 1987;3:529–542.

While an increased heart rate implies a significant degree of pain or vascular collapse, heart rate alone cannot be used to prognosticate equine colic. This is because of the many variables that can alter heart rate but not necessarily survivability (fear, excitement, or nervousness). Therefore, the heart rate must be evaluated along with other values such as membrane color, capillary refill time, and pulse quality to assess the true circulatory status of the animal.

Pulse quality (taken via the great metatarsal artery or the facial artery) varies directly with the systolic and pulse pressures. A weak, thready pulse, or no pulse, indicates inadequate blood pressure, and is associated with a poor prognosis. In one survey, 92% of horses with a systolic pressure of less than 80 mm Hg (coccygeal uncorrected values) died. Decreasing blood pressure was associated with decreased survival (Table 77–2).

In field situations, digital palpation can give a relative evaluation of systolic pressure. The arterial pressure must be greater than 65 mm Hg and the pulse pressure greater than 25 mm Hg to be palpable. The prognostic value of pulse quality will be enhanced if it is reevaluated following volume expansion in animals with a weak arterial pulse. Poor response to volume expansion is usually associated with a high mortality rate.

Mucous membrane color and capillary refill time are measures of peripheral perfusion. Hypovolemia, secondary to fluid sequestration or dehydration, results in a compensatory vasoconstriction. This will produce pale mucous membranes and a prolonged capillary refill time. When the mucous membranes are pale, the prognosis is still favorable. When the color of the mem-

TABLE 77–2. RELATIONSHIP OF BLOOD PRESSURE TO SURVIVAL RATE IN CASES OF EQUINE COLIC*

Systolic Pressure†	Survival Rate (%)
50	5
80	24
110	69
140	94

* From Parry B: The use of clinical pathology in evaluation of horses with colic. *Vet Clin North Am Equine Pract* 1987;3:529–542.
† Coccygeal uncorrected values.

branes progresses to dark red to purple, it reflects venous pooling and cyanosis and is associated with a poor prognosis. Venous pooling arises because the postcapillary sphincters remain functional under lower oxygen tensions than do the precapillary sphincters. This imbalance in capillary blood flow further decreases cardiac output and perpetuates the cellular hypoxia. Horses with red and cyanotic mucous membranes were found to be 5 and 38 times, respectively, more likely to die than those with normal mucous membranes.

TABLE 77–3. RELATIONSHIP OF PACKED CELL VOLUME TO SURVIVAL RATE IN EQUINE COLIC*

Packed Cell Volume (%)	Survival Rate (%)
<35	>86
36–45	64–79
46–50	64
51–60	20–52
>60	10–25

* Combined data from Parry (1987) and Poutenen-Reinert (1986).

RECTAL EXAMINATION

Rectal examination is a valuable part of the examination of the colic patient. The value of information gained from the examination is variable, however, based upon the skill and experience of the operator and the location of the lesion. In a recent study of colic 42 of 350 horses (12%) with a normal rectal exam died, whereas 194 of 812 horses (24%) with an abnormal rectal exam died. Abnormal rectal findings that indicate a poorer prognosis are distended small intestine, severe gas distention, strangulating displacements of the large colon, or a "gritty" feel or crepitus within the peritoneal cavity (indicating possible peritonitis).

The value of clinical evaluation in prognosticating equine colic is demonstrated in a recent study by Pascoe et al in which clinical exam findings correctly identified 68% of nonsurvivors and 74% of survivors. This study utilized 13 parameters and predicted that the animal would not survive if any four were abnormal.

LABORATORY EVALUATION

Several clinicopathologic values have been evaluated for their value in the prognosis of equine colic, including cases requiring surgery. Factors that have proven to be of value are packed cell volume (PCV), blood lactate, anion gap, blood glucose, peritoneal fluid total protein concentration, and various coagulation abnormalities. The PCV is frequently elevated in patients with abdominal disease and has been used as a prognostic indicator: The higher the PCV the lower the corresponding survival rate (Table 77–3). Using PCV alone as a prognostic indicator, however, 30% of horses were classified into the incorrect group. Therefore, PCV is a valuable indicator of the probability of survival in horses with abdominal disease, but cannot be used alone.

Blood lactate is often elevated in horses with abdominal distress. The accumulation of lactate in the peripheral circulation reflects poor tissue perfusion associated with hypovolemia or endotoxemia. As tissue perfusion and oxygenation deteriorate, cells convert to anaerobic metabolism to survive. The liver is responsible for removal of lactate from the blood; however, when hepatic blood flow is decreased (as in hypovolemic shock), lactate accumulates in the circulation. The degree of cardiovascular compromise correlates with the elevation of blood lactate concentration, and this clinicopathologic value has proven to be a valuable aid in the prognosis of equine colic. It has been reported that blood lactate levels of less than 75 mg/dL are associated with a survival probability of 93%. However, as blood lactate levels exceed 75 mg/dL, there is a precipitous decline in survival rates (Table 77–4).

The anion gap is a reflection of the unmeasured anions in blood and is closely related to elevations in blood lactate. In one report, 82% of the change in anion gap could be attributed to lactate. The remaining portion was postulated to be due to volatile fatty acids absorbed from the bowel. Increases in the anion gap ($AG = [Na^+] - \{[Cl^-] + [HCO_3^-]\}$) were associated with decreasing survival rates (Table 77–5). In the field situation or at the time of surgery, calculation of anion gaps may be preferable to lactate measurement, be-

TABLE 77–4. RELATIONSHIP OF BLOOD LACTATE TO SURVIVAL IN CASES OF EQUINE COLIC*

Blood Lactate (mg/dL)	Survival Rate (%)
50	98
75	90
100	32
>100	25

* From Moore JN, Owen RR, Lumsden JH: Clinical evaluation of blood lactate levels in equine colic. *Equine Vet J* 1976;8:49–54.

TABLE 77–5. RELATIONSHIP OF ANION GAP TO SURVIVAL IN CASES OF EQUINE COLIC*

Anion Gap (mEq/L)	Survival Rate (%)
<20	81
20–24.9	47
>25	0

* From Gosset KA, Cleghorn B, Martin GS, Church GE: Correlation between anion gap, blood lactate concentration and survival in horses. *Equine Vet J* 1987;19:182–187.

cause sample handling is simpler and plasma or serum electrolyte determinations are more likely available. Although helpful, this can also be misleading when chloride concentration is low as a result of small intestinal obstruction. An exceptionally high anion gap created by fluid sequestration is not always an accurate reflection of the prognosis.

Severe hyperglycemia (>300 mg/dL) and hypoglycemia (<60 mg/dL) are grave prognostic indicators in horses with colic. In one survey, all colic patients with a blood glucose in these ranges died. Glucose levels between these two extremes, however, are difficult to interpret and have little prognostic value when used alone.

Elevations in peritoneal fluid protein concentration result from peritoneal inflammation or compromise of the intestinal vasculature. In more advanced cases of intestinal compromise, there are progressively higher peritoneal fluid protein concentrations. It is thought, therefore, that peritoneal fluid protein levels help to indicate the severity of an intestinal lesion, which is potentially related to the amount of endotoxin absorbed. Peritoneal protein concentrations are related to mortality and are significantly different in survivors and nonsurvivors of surgical intervention for abdominal diseases. However, the values are so variable that prediction of the outcome is not accurate on an individual case basis. As with other indices, the peritoneal fluid protein concentration must be used with other values to predict the outcome. Generally, concentrations exceeding 4.5 g/dL in small intestinal disease requiring surgical intervention and 3.5 g/dL in large colon diseases requiring surgery correspond with low survival rates.

Other laboratory evaluations that have been proposed for use as prognostic indicators in equine colic include measurement of serum phospholipase A_2 and various coagulation parameters. In a recent report evaluating hemostatic testing as a prognostic indicator in equine colic, certain types of abnormalities were more frequently associated with nonsurvivors. Specifically, reduced numbers of platelets (<100,000/μL), reduced antithrombin III activity (85%), prolonged prothrombin time, prolonged total clotting time, and elevated levels of fibrin degradation products were found more frequently in nonsurvivors than survivors. The presence of fibrin degradation products in a greater than 1:20 dilution for latex agglutination in horses taken to surgery was indicative of a poor chance of survival. These values indicate a condition of disseminated intravascular coagulopathy associated with endotoxic shock and are a very poor prognostic sign in any disease process.

At surgery, there are few criteria that help prognosticate the acute abdomen. Most of the decisions are subjective. For example, extensive small intestinal infarction and necrosis when the small intestine has a 360-degree volvulus would be associated with a poor prognosis since it is not possible to surgically remove the great majority of the small intestine and expect the horse to survive. In horses with small intestinal obstruction or strangulation, the intraluminal pressure can be measured easily with a needle placed in the distended bowel, which is outside the abdomen, just proximal to the site of the obstruction. The needle is attached to a water manometer or a blood pressure transducer and the intraluminal pressure is measured. Horses with small intestinal intraluminal pressures greater than 15 cm H_2O (11 mm Hg) have a poor prognosis, whereas horses with pressures less than 10 cm H_2O (7.4 mm Hg) have a good prognosis.

INTEGRATED CASE PROGNOSIS

No one single clinical or pathologic parameter exists that can accurately predict survival or death in equine colic. Several parameters must be evaluated together to enhance the accuracy of prediction of outcome. Logistic regression analysis of pulse rate, peritoneal total protein, total plasma protein, PCV, and peritoneal white blood cells together improved success in predicting survival in a retrospective study of horses treated surgically. This technique improved the overall prediction of survival by 15%, however, there was still considerable error (32%) when attempting to predict the outcome in individual cases. The best predictive model reported by Orsini et al for surgical cases used lactate and PCV together and was very accurate in predicting survival but less accurate in predicting nonsurvival. This model has a combined accuracy of 76%, indicating the usefulness of these two parameters in estimating a prognosis. Another method used blood pressure,

TABLE 77–6. SURVIVAL (SI) AND DEATH (DI) INDEX FORMULAS*

SI = 0.180 (systolic pressure [mm Hg]) + 0.213 (lactate [mg/dL]) + 0.164 (BUN [mg/dL]) + 0.486 (PCV) − 27.0

DI = 0.132 (systolic pressure [mm Hg]) + 0.330 (lactate [mg/dL]) + 0.582 (PCV) − 31.7

* From Parry B: Use of clinical pathology in evaluation of horses with colic. *Vet Clin North Am Equine Pract* 1987;3:529–542.

blood lactate, blood urea nitrogen, and PCV and correctly classified 93% of all types of cases into the correct group (survivor versus nonsurvivor). A survival index and a death index may be calculated from the laboratory data. If the death index is larger the animal will most likely die, whereas if the survival index is larger it will most likely live (see formulas given in Table 77–6).

We have devised a "scoring table" for prognosis of equine colic that is particularly applicable to horses about to undergo surgery for acute abdominal disease (Table 77–7). To provide a simple, usable system, three grades are used to presurgically quantitate an animal's chances of survival. Most cases will fall into one of these groups. The guarded group has the widest range, being the most difficult to predict. This table can be used with individual values, but, as has been demonstrated with heart rate, PCV, peritoneal protein concentration, and glucose, the importance of individual values is variable, particularly for the "guarded" group. The accuracy will increase as more values fall in the same group. When values differ widely, the accuracy of the colic scoring table is diminished and the formulas listed in Table 77–6 become the best way to presurgically predict the outcome. In fact, the accuracy is not good enough to assure the surgeon that the horse will not live, and a subjective decision must be made based on the viability of the intestine and the amount of intestine that may have to be removed. In some cases, the economic value of the animal will often have to be considered.

TABLE 77–7. COLIC SCORING TABLE

	Prognosis (Anticipated Survival)		
	Good (>90%)	**Guarded (50%)**	**Poor (<20%)**
Heart rate (bpm)	40–60	60–100	>100
PCV (%)	<45	45–64	>65
Peritoneal protein (g/dL)	<2.5	2.6–6.5	>6.5
Glucose (mg/dL)	80–100	100–299	>300
Anion gap (mEq/L)	<15	16–30	>30
Blood urea nitrogen (mg/dL)	14	42	>70

BIBLIOGRAPHY

Allen D, White NA, Tyler DE: Factors for prognostic use in equine obstructive small intestinal disease. *J Am Vet Med Assoc* 1986;189:777–780.

Gosset KA, Cleghorn B, Martin GS, Church GE: Correlation between anion gap, blood lactate concentration and survival in horses. *Equine Vet J* 1987;19:182–187.

Johnstone IB: The prognostic value of hemostatic testing in horses with colic, in *Proceedings of the 2nd Equine Colic Research Symposium.* Veterinary Learning Systems, 1986;2:186–188.

Moore JN, Owen RR, Lumsden JH: Clinical evaluation of blood lactate levels in equine colic. *Equine Vet J* 1976;8:49–54.

Orsini J, Elser AH, Galligan DT, Donawick WJ, Kronfeld DS: Prognostic index for equine acute abdominal crisis (colic). *Am J Vet Res* 1988;49:1969–1971.

Parry B: Use of clinical pathology in evaluation of horses with colic. *Vet Clin North Am Equine Pract* 1987; 3:529–542.

Pascoe PJ, et al: Accuracy of clinical examination in the prognosis of abdominal pain in the horse, in *Proceedings of the 2nd Equine Colic Research Symposium.* Veterinary Learning Systems, 1986;2:149–152.

Puotenen-Reinert A: Study of variables commonly used in examination of equine colic cases to assess prognostic value. *Equine Vet J* 1986;18:275–277.

White NA, Lessard P: Risk factors and clinical signs associated with cases of equine colic. *Proc Am Assoc Equine Pract* 1986;pp 637–644.

UNIT VII

Musculoskeletal Disorders of the Feet and Tendons

78
Abscesses and Punctures of the Foot

Tracy A. Turner

DIAGNOSIS

History and Signalment

Abscesses and punctures can affect any age, breed, or sex of horse. The majority of these horses will present with an acute onset of moderate to severe lameness. The most important historic information to obtain is the immunization status against tetanus. If the animal has not been vaccinated within the previous 6 months, standard doses of tetanus toxoid and antitoxin should be administered.

In chronic cases, the history becomes much more important. One must establish the duration of the condition and response to previous treatments. Draining tracts or lesions of long duration that have failed to resolve often indicate the presence of necrotic bone or cartilage. Inappropriate treatment with caustics or vesicants may delay epithelialization of the wound or even destroy normal tissue, causing prolongation of wound morbidity.

Physical Examination

Because abscesses and punctures can involve the sole, frog, hoof wall, or coronary band, careful and systematic examination of the foot is essential. In the case of punctures, swelling may be present proximal to the coronary band. The swelling may be localized, involve the deep digital flexor tendon sheath, involve the area between the bulbs of the heel, or be a diffuse cellulitis that may extend proximal to the carpus or tarsus. If more than 24 to 48 hours have elapsed since the initial injury, exudate may be draining from the coronary band.

When a foreign object such as a nail or piece of wire is identified, its location, depth, and direction of penetration must be evaluated. If possible, radiographs of the foot should be taken with the foreign body in place. If a foreign body is not present or cannot be identified, the entrance site can often be located by the horse's response to percussion or application of pressure with hoof testers. Often when the injury is more than 12 hours old, the entire foot is sensitive because of sepsis or generalized inflammation. Careful, gentle examination usually reveals the most sensitive area, which is usually at the entrance portal.

Proper preparation of the hoof is necessary for a thorough examination of the foot. Horseshoes should be removed, the hoof trimmed, and the sole, sulci, and frog pared to expose fresh underlying horn. All discolored areas should be pared out. These spots often signify the entry site of a foreign object or the opening into an abscess. Hoof testers should be used over all areas of the foot, including nail holes. In most cases, regional anesthesia will aid physical examination by further defining the exact source of pain in the foot and by permitting subsequent examination of tracts. A palmar digital nerve block is useful for injuries of the caudal hoof, and an abaxial sesamoid nerve block will be necessary for injuries to the remaining sole. After the puncture site is identified, a blunt probe should be introduced into the site to determine the depth and direction of the tract. It may be useful to take radiographs of the foot with the probe in place to determine the extent of the tract.

Confirmatory Tests

Radiographic examination of the foot is a very useful diagnostic aid to define the location and depth of punctures. At least two views (lateral and dorso–45-degree–proximopalmarodistal) should be evaluated. Punctures through the caudal aspect of the foot should be further assessed by a tangential view (palmaroproximodorsodistal), which permits evaluation of the flexor surface of the navicular bone. Even though osseous radiographic changes may not be evident for 1 to 2 weeks following injury or the onset of infection, the radiographs must be assessed carefully for evidence of gas that might indicate pockets of infection. Because nonmetallic foreign objects will not be identifiable by radiographic evaluation, a fistulogram (contrast radiography) in these cases may help determine the presence of these objects, the extent of the tract, or the specific structures involved.

If sepsis of the deep digital flexor tendon sheath or navicular bursa is suspected, centesis of these structures is indicated. Centesis of the deep digital flexor tendon sheath is most easily accomplished by surgically preparing a site over the most fluctuant aspect of the tendon sheath. After surgical preparation of the skin, a 20-gauge 1- to 1.5-inch needle is inserted into the fluctuant area. Gentle aspiration with a syringe will usually permit retrieval of sufficient fluid for analysis. Unfortunately, fluid within the navicular bursa is not always as easy to obtain. There are two effective techniques for entry into the navicular bursa. One involves surgical preparation of the area between the bulbs of the heels. A 20-gauge 3-inch needle is inserted along the midline through the fossa between the heels in a line paralleling the angle of the coronary band. When the needle encounters bone, it is in the navicular bursa. If the needle is not angled properly it can go above the navicular bone into the palmar/plantar pouch of the distal interphalangeal joint. The second method is performed by surgically preparing the lateral aspect of the pastern at the level of the collateral cartilages of the hoof. A 20-gauge 1.5-inch needle is inserted at that point proximal to the collateral cartilage, dorsal to the deep flexor tendon, and palmar to the middle phalanx. The needle is directed toward the ground surface of the medial hoof wall. This method is usually easier to perform and more successful because it takes advantage of the bursa's width rather than its depth. Because the bursa only holds a small volume of fluid, lavage of the bursa confirms this site versus the palmar or plantar pouch of the distal interphalangeal joint. If a tract is open, fluid injected into the navicular bursa will exit from the wound, indicating the involvement of the bursa. If cytologic evaluation of the fluid or lavage indicates increased numbers of neutrophils or degenerative changes of the neutrophils, sepsis should be suspected. This fluid should be cultured to try to identify the organism or organisms involved.

SURGERY

Anatomy

The hoof wall is divided into three distinct layers. The most superficial layer is the periople or stratum tectorium. The middle layer (stratum medium) forms the bulk of the hoof wall and is composed of tubular and nontubular horn. The stratum medium is the most dense part of the hoof wall. The deep layer (stratum lamellatum) forms from the epidermal laminae. This layer consists of about 600 thin primary laminae. The laminae cover the distal phalanx circumferentially and align along the vertical axis of the bone. Each primary lamina bears about 100 secondary laminae. This layer forms the bond between the hoof wall and the bone. Because infections in the hoof wall follow paths of least resistance, they will usually invade along the primary laminae. Hence, infections tend to break out at the coronary band directly above a lesion that has formed in the hoof wall.

The ground surface of the foot consists of the bars, frog, and sole. The bars are hoof wall that at the heels of the foot turn dorsally and axially and converge while paralleling the collateral sulci of the frog. The bars eventually blend into the sole after traveling about two thirds the length of the frog. The frog is a wedge-shaped structure in the palmar/plantar portion of the foot. The sole is similar to the hoof wall except it has a higher moisture content. The sole is composed of tubular and nontubular horn. The tubules parallel the hoof wall. The tubules curve near the ground surface, which accounts for the self-limiting growth and shedding of the sole. The white line is the junction of the sole and hoof wall. It follows the circumference of the wall but it is not a secreted structure. The white line serves as a landmark between sensitive and insensitive tissue. Any tissue deep to the white line has neurovascular supply.

The digital cushion is one of several accessory structures of the hoof. It is a fibroelastic network containing masses of fat and islands of cartilage. The cushion is bounded distally by the frog and proximally by the middle phalanx and deep digital flexor tendon. It is relatively avascular.

In general, the hoof is a well-vascularized structure with excellent collateral circulation. Consequently, the hoof heals rapidly, providing infection is controlled or removed. The main arterial supply is via the medial and lateral digital arteries, which are formed by the bifurcation of the common digital artery in the forelimbs and greater metatarsal artery in the hind limbs. The arteries diverge and pass over the abaxial surface of the proximal sesamoid bones and descend parallel to the borders of the deep digital flexor tendon. The vessels bifurcate near the collateral cartilage; the superficial branch passes through the dorsal longitudinal canal of the distal phalanx, and the more distal branch surrounds the distal edge of the bone. The deepest branch enters the volar foramina and forms the terminal arch of the artery. The veins ascend the limb just dorsal to the artery.

The nerve supply to the front feet is via the median and ulnar nerves. The hind feet are innervated by the superficial fibular and tibial nerves. These nerves combine to form the digital nerves. The first branch just proximal to the metacarpophalangeal/metatarsophalangeal joint innervates the dorsum of the foot and pastern region. The second branch at the distal portion of the proximal sesamoids innervates the dorsal half of the sole and middle third of the foot. The third branch, the palmar digital nerve, innervates the palmar/plantar one third to one half of the foot.

The deepest structures of the foot are the bones, ligaments, and tendons. Two tendons attach to the distal phalanx. The common extensor tendon attaches over the extensor process. The deep digital flexor tendon likewise has a broad aponeurosis that inserts on the inner circumference of the solar surface of the distal phalanx. The insertion is just distal to the volar foramina. The most distal aspect of the tendon sheath is located at about the middle of the middle phalanx. Just deep to the deep flexor tendon is the navicular bursa. This structure extends proximally 1 cm above the navicular bone; distally it extends to the insertion of the deep flexor tendon, and side to side it extends to the collateral cartilages of the distal phalanx.

The foot consists of the proximal and distal interphalangeal joints and the associated structures. The proximal interphalangeal joint is formed by the distal portion of the proximal phalanx and proximal portion of the middle phalanx. The distal interphalangeal joint is a ginglymus joint formed by the articulation of the middle phalanx, distal phalanx, and navicular bone (distal sesamoid). The navicular bone makes up about one third of the distal articular surface of the distal interphalangeal joint. The bone lies in the palmar/plantar aspect of the joint and is supported by strong ligamentous structures. The proximal suspensory ligament (collateral sesamoidean ligament) originates on the dorsum of the distal extremity of the proximal phalanx and is inserted on the medial and lateral proximal extremities of the navicular bone. The ligament then branches to the collateral cartilages and angles of the distal phalanx. Distally, the navicular bone is attached to the distal phalanx via the ungulosesamoidean or impar ligament. Because of the close proximity of the synovial sheath, navicular bursa, and distal interphalangeal joint, all may be involved during infection in this area.

Surgical Technique

Treatment of superficial puncture wounds of the sole necessitates the removal of horny tissue overlying the damaged soft tissue. Opening the abscess cavity and providing drainage alleviates the pain in most cases. Although this procedure is often done without regional anesthesia, anesthesia does facilitate the thorough débridement of the affected area. The use of a tourniquet is not necessary. The key to débridement is to avoid disrupting the sensitive layers (stratum germinativum and corium). If these layers are damaged, the wound must heal by granulation and epithelialization rather than cornification. Another important aspect of proper débridement is to remove enough horn overlying the abscess. The margin of the cavity should be removed until only healthy horn surrounds the abscess cavity and there is no separation from the sensitive lamina. On occasion the area that must be removed is extremely large, sometimes the entire sole or frog. If the surgeon is unsure of how much to débride, the procedure can be performed in stages over a few days.

Puncture wounds require more extensive débridement than do subsolar abscesses. Punctures through the sole and quarter region should have 1 to 2 cm of horn débrided from around the puncture site. The horny bar should be removed if the puncture site is in the heel region. When the wound penetrates the solar corium but does not contact other structures, then the corium should be débrided by sharp dissection. If the distal phalanx is involved, abnormal bone should be removed by curettage. Portions of the affected tissue should be submitted for bacterial culture and antibiotic sensitivity.

Wounds that penetrate the frog or bar have a high probability of affecting other vital structures such as the deep flexor tendon, distal flexor tendon sheath, navicular bursa, navicular bone, distal interphalangeal joint, or distal phalanx. For these reasons, the veterinarian must make a determination of the depth of injury within the first 48 hours. Conservative medical therapy consisting of soaking the foot and systemic antibiotics will invariably fail if these structures are involved unless early lavage and antimicrobial therapy is initiated or sufficient surgical débridement is performed early to allow for drainage of these tissues. Any delay in the assessment of the response to conservative therapy only worsens the prognosis.

The surgical procedure for deep punctures should involve cutting a larger window around the puncture site and removing tissue in a conical shape to the depth of the wound. The depth of the wound can be determined by inserting a sterile probe into the tract. Alternatively, methylene blue dye may be injected into the tract and followed until it terminates at the end of the tract or dyes other structures. If there is a question whether the joint, navicular bursa, or distal flexor tendon sheath are involved, a needle can be inserted into the synovial sac in question and sufficient sterile saline injected to pressurize the joint. If the saline leaks into the débrided tract, one must assume communication exists between the tract and the synovial sac. Consequently, the sac is assumed to be infected. However, if fluid does not leak, the puncture may still have entered the bursa and subsequently sealed.

Punctures penetrating the deep flexor tendon should be treated by removing one half to two thirds of the central frog and underlying digital cushion (Fig. 78–1). This exposes the deep flexor tendon, which is charac-

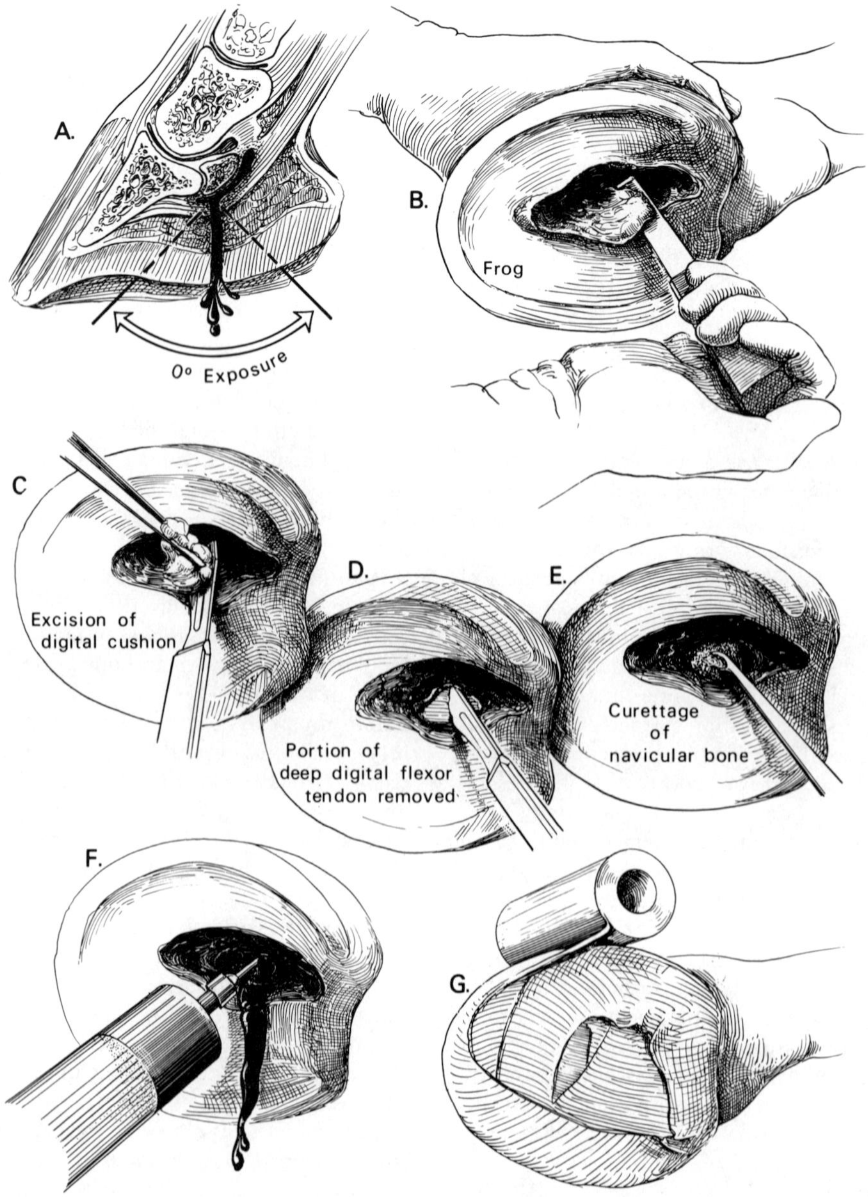

Figure 78–1. Resection of the frog, digital cushion, and a portion of the deep flexor tendon during a navicular bursotomy (Street nail operation). **A.** The puncture wound through the frog, digital cushion, and deep flexor tendon must be totally removed by wide excision. **B.** The tract is identified and resection of the frog around the tract is done initially with a sterilized hoof knife. **C.** A portion of the digital cushion is removed directly over the deep flexor tendon. **D.** A portion of the deep flexor tendon approximately 2 × 3 cm is removed to expose the flexor surface of the navicular bone. **E.** If the fibrocartilage or any portion of the bone is necrotic, a curette is used to débride the bone. **F.** The navicular bursa is flushed with povidone-iodine diluted in saline. If there is a question about communication with the distal interphalangeal joint a needle is placed in the distal interphalangeal joint above the coronary band and a sterile flush is initiated through the joint. If the fluid can be flushed through the joint out the navicular bursa, this proves there is a communication with the distal interphalangeal joint. **G.** The foot is packed with sterile gauze to soak up exudate from the navicular bursa, and the foot is wrapped with a waterproof bandage. (Courtesy of Dr. N. A. White.)

terized by a firm appearance with a linear orientation of fibers. An opening should be cut through the tendon to expose the flexor surface of the navicular bone. If the bone has been damaged, then it should be débrided by currettage. To determine if the infection communicates with the distal interphalangeal joint, arthrocentesis should be performed and saline injected to test for communication into the navicular bursa. If communication exists, joint lavage should be utilized as adjunctive therapy. Further affected deep tissue should be evaluated by bacterial culture and antibiotic sensitivity testing.

POSTOPERATIVE CARE

Careful postoperative management is necessary for a successful outcome. Cleanliness and care of the postoperative bandages are imperative. Packing of the affected tissue with antiseptics is recommended by some authors, whereas others recommend dry dressings. The object should be to maintain a proper wound environment. Waterproof materials should be used for the outer layer of the bandage. The dressings should be changed on a daily basis to protect against soilage of the bandages, maintain cleanliness of the hoof, and remove excessive exudate. Bandaging should continue until the wound is covered with horn. Alternatively, a treatment plate shoe can be used and the wound packed with a dressing. Soaking the foot in water saturated with magnesium sulfate can aid in drawing out any residual infection in the tissues. Where deep wounds are present, foot soaking is not appropriate until granulation tissue has covered the regions susceptible to reinfection.

Antibiotic therapy is not necessary unless there are deep puncture wounds. Antibiotic therapy should be based on the results of culture and sensitivity tests. Phenylbutazone is useful for decreasing pain associated with débridement. A dose of 2 to 4.4 mg/kg daily is usually adequate. In severe cases 8.8 mg/kg daily may be required to make the horse comfortable. The dose should be reduced as soon as feasible to avoid possible toxicity. In all cases tetanus prophylaxis is necessary and is best administered for abscesses and punctures even if a history of tetanus protection has been recorded.

The horse should be kept in a clean, dry stall until the wound is covered by horn. Exercise should be minimized to prevent trauma to the surgical area. However, for injuries involving the navicular bursa, exercise is cautiously encouraged after the wound is healed to reduce the severity of adhesions between the deep flexor tendon and the navicular bone. Exercise may cause increased pain and necessitate larger doses of phenylbutazone for the comfort of the animal.

PROGNOSIS

Once normal horn covers the surgical area, the problem is resolved in most cases. Horn will usually not cover an area of infection. Horn that does not look normal is another indicator that infection or inflammation is present. Accurate prognostication for return to function is difficult prior to surgical intervention, especially in chronic cases. For most superficial injuries the prognosis is excellent for return to function. In the case of punctures, prognosis is based on the structures involved and duration of the injury. In the case of navicular bursal injuries, the prognosis worsens markedly with each day's delay before a deep flexor tenotomy (Street nail procedure) is performed. The infection spreads into the surrounding tissues, making it more difficult to eliminate. Furthermore, the infection and associated inflammation destroy the fibrocartilage of the flexor surface, exposing the subchondral bone to infection. When not controlled, navicular osteomyelitis has a poor prognosis. Pathologic fractures of the navicular bone are a common sequela to osteomyelitis. As with most diseases, accurate and early diagnosis is imperative for the most favorable outcome.

BIBLIOGRAPHY

Richardson GL, Pascoe JR, Meagher D: Puncture wounds of the foot in horses: Diagnosis and treatment. *Compend Cont Educ Pract Vet* 1986;8:S379–S388.

Steckel RR: Puncture wounds, abscesses, thrush and canker, in Robinson NE (ed): *Current Therapy in Equine Medicine.* Philadelphia, WB Saunders Co, 1987, p 266.

Steckel RR, Fessler JF: Surgical management of seven hoof wounds in the horse: A retrospective study of 30 cases. *Compend Cont Educ Pract Vet* 1983;5:S435–S443.

79
Hoof Wall Lacerations

Tracy A. Turner

Lacerations to the hoof causing loss of germinal tissue and either partial or complete avulsions of the hoof wall are not common injuries to the horse. When these injuries do occur, however, their management can be perplexing for the veterinarian.

EVALUATION

Complete examination of the wound is necessary to determine the extent of the injury. Although the foot has as great a capacity for healing as any other tissue, the prognosis for return to full function is dependent on the severity of tissue destruction and the tissues involved. In most cases, adequate collateral circulation develops following injury. Because ischemia will impair healing and predispose the wound to infection, permanent loss of blood supply necessitates surgical removal of the ischemic portions of the wound.

Complete denervation of the foot by extensive damage to the digital nerve trunks may result in neurogenic degeneration and sloughing of the foot. Ironically, transection of the nerve, where damage has not been extensive, may aid recovery by reducing chronic pain associated with the injury.

Injuries that involve the corium of the foot should be inspected carefully. The corium is modified vascular tissue similar to the dermis, and is responsible for nutrition to the horny layers of the hoof. Damage to these structures often results in permanent defects in the coronary band and hoof. Injuries that cause avulsion or necrosis of corium will cause changes in horn production around the hoof. Many times one must wait for the regrowth of the hoof to assess these changes and how they may affect the horse.

Deep wounds that extend to the middle or distal phalanges cause additional complications. Hoof avulsions may involve all or part of the wing of the distal phalanx. In these cases, it is usually easiest to simply remove the fractured portion of the bone. However, wounds that damage the periosteum or collateral ligaments surrounding these bones may cause permanent lameness as a result of excessive calcification of soft tissues or joint instability. Associated soft tissue injuries such as these will not be apparent on initial radiographic examination and can only be anticipated after close examination of the wound. Once soft tissue support is damaged the veterinarian may have to wait 3 to 4 months to evaluate the final consequences of this type of deep injury.

Although wounds that enter a joint may appear to have a poor prognosis, they can respond quite well if appropriate therapy is initiated immediately. Small wounds into a joint may not be readily apparent, the only sign being synovial fluid leaking into the wound. Occasionally, serum is mistaken for joint fluid or vice versa. If any doubt exists whether a joint has been entered, saline is injected under pressure into the joint and the wound examined for the leakage of fluid. Another method of testing for joint involvement is to perform an arthrogram and see if leakage of contrast media from the joint is evident on a radiograph.

Other criteria that must be considered when evaluating these wounds are the horse's age, value, and function. Immature horses tend to heal more readily, and growth may help resolve some deformities. Wounds of the foot usually heal over an extended period, resulting in increased expense and residual lameness due to the injury; permanent deformity is a distinct possibility.

SURGERY

The foot should be prepared for aseptic surgery. In addition, the hoof wall, sole, and frog should be trimmed, pared, and rasped in order to remove any contamination that may be in cracks or crevices. The hair from the fetlock distally should be clipped to allow surgical preparation of the entire foot and pastern area with an antiseptic soap. Exposed tissues should be cleansed and irrigated with a physiologic saline solution. Harsh antiseptics or irritating cleansers should not be used on exposed tissues because these chemicals may cause further damage. After thorough cleansing, the wound should be covered with a sterile, nonadherent dressing and the entire foot bandaged. The outer layer of the bandage should be impervious to water.

Surgery may be performed on either a standing or an anesthetized patient. Standing surgery should be performed with sedation and local anesthesia. However, this should be reserved for the most tractable of horses. It will also often require one person to hold the leg or to tie the leg up for surgery to be performed. General anesthesia provides optimal conditions to establish and maintain aseptic techniques, as well as optimizing the surgeon's ability to inspect the wound.

The principle goals of surgery are to optimize conditions for wound healing and to achieve the most favorable cosmetic and functional result. The horse's hoof is not amenable to suturing and therefore wounds must heal by second intention. The most important factor in the management of these wounds is adequate débridement. Necrotic or severely damaged tissues and all foreign materials provide media for bacterial growth and impede wound healing. However, vital tissues such as nerves, arteries, and tendons should be salvaged, if possible. Complete wound excision is the simplest, most effective means of débridement. If this is not feasible, simple débridement of obviously devitalized tissue and foreign material combined with wound irrigation should be performed. Pulsating lavage is the most effective type of irrigation system.

If a synovial structure is opened or if it is suspected that a synovial cavity has been entered, the structure should be lavaged with copious amounts of physiologic saline solution so that the lavage flows out through the wound. The foot is a highly vascular structure and hemostasis is difficult. Ligation and electrocautery are usually not adequate. A temporary pressure bandage is usually necessary and will stop bleeding if left in place for 12 hours. The initial bandage applied after surgical débridement should be moistened with sterile saline, or an antimicrobial dressing over the wound and covered with an outer waterproof bandage.

Wounds of the hoof generally heal slowly, due in part to the high incidence of contamination of these wounds. This problem can be minimized by proper cleaning, appropriate bandaging, and ensuring that enough help is available when changing the dressing (this usually requires two people). Contraction of hoof wounds is also minimal because of the inelasticity of the epithelial tissues and the fact that they are all attached to bone or rigid connective tissue. Thus, healing is the result of epithelialization and regeneration of connective tissue. All portions of corium can migrate and cover a healthy bed of granulation tissue. This process will be slow and may take 3 to 5 months.

POSTOPERATIVE CARE

Immobilization and protection of the wound are important considerations in order to maintain the same tissue environment achieved at surgery. A short limb cast that encases the hoof is usually the most effective method (Chapter 25). The cast will not only immobilize the tissues and protect them from excess motion but will also serve as protection for the hoof from moisture and fecal contamination. On a long-term basis, a cast can be a much less expensive method of immobilization than daily bandage changes.

Ten to 14 days is the minimum duration suggested for cast maintenance. The cast should be maintained as long as necessary to provide a good initial healing (4 to 6 weeks if necessary). The cast needs to be monitored daily. If lameness, excessive heat, or odors develop, the cast should be removed. After cast removal, bar shoes with clips can be effective in immobilizing the hoof. The glue-on shoe is also effective at immobilizing the hoof. This can also be used with less severe wounds of the foot when combined with aseptic dressings and water-impervious bandaging.

Antibiotics are advocated during the acute phase of wound healing and are indicated with traumatic wounds, when deep structures are involved, or when there has been severe tissue damage and loss. However, antibiotics should not be used in lieu of adequate surgical débridement, or without appropriate bacterial cultures and antibiotic sensitivity testing. Often the contamination in these cases involves multiple organisms, so the débrided deep tissues should be used for the culture.

Pain relief may be necessary postoperatively, particularly for 48 to 72 hours. Nonsteroidal anti-inflammatory drugs are recommended to reduce inflammation and to minimize the effects of unequal weight bearing on the unaffected limbs. Pain relief may also be provided by soaking the hoof in warm or hot water. This aids the wound healing by reducing surface contamination and stimulating reflex hyperemia with increased blood flow. If a wound is immersed in water, the water must be clean to prevent contaminants from contacting the wound through the water bath. Wounds involving the joints, tendon sheaths, or bursae are not soaked until healing is adequate to prevent secondary contamination.

As healing progresses, the hoof should be trimmed to remove excess horn. The hoof should have excess wall removed, the sole should be pared of scales, and the horn surrounding the wound should be kept even with the wound until complete keratinization of the wound has occurred.

The horse should not be allowed free exercise until keratinization is complete. Follow-up examination at 2- to 4-week intervals is usually adequate. Once keratinization is complete, corrective shoeing, acrylic remodeling, or simply cessation of bandaging is in order. Corrective shoeing and/or acrylic remodeling are often necessary for complete soundness. This will have to continue until the hoof completely grows out. Usually this takes about 8 to 12 months.

PROGNOSIS

The prognosis for these injuries is generally good for soundness. However, a prognosis should be withheld until after adequate inspection of the wound has been made. The prognosis should be based on the duration of injury, the structures involved, the temperament of the horse, how adequately débridement can be achieved, and the structural integrity of the hoof after débridement. In one study of 30 cases reported by Steckel and Fessler, 22 horses were athletically sound, 2 were pasture sound, 4 were euthanized as a result of the injury, and 1 died of other causes. These represented a variety of injuries. The most common reason for destruction was osteomyelitis. This emphasizes the need for early surgical intervention and proper wound care before infection is established.

BIBLIOGRAPHY

Fessler Jr: Surgical management of equine foot injuries. *Mod Vet Pract* 1971;52:41–46.

Henninger RW, Owen DL: Management of hoof wall disease in horses part I: Diagnosis and surgical treatment. *Mod Vet Pract* 1986;67:141–146.

Nickels FA: Hoof wall lacerations and avulsions, in Robinson NE (ed) *Current Therapy in Equine Medicine*. Philadelphia, WB Saunders Co, 1983, pp 275–277.

Steckel RR, Fessler JF: Surgical management of severe hoof wounds in the horse: A retrospective study of 30 cases. *Compend Cont Educ Pract Vet* 1983;5:S435-S443.

80
Repair of Hoof Wall Defects

Tracy A. Turner

Hoof defects or interruptions in the continuity of the hoof wall may be described as cracks, clefts or crumbling. A *hoof crack* is a split in the wall that runs parallel to the horn tubules. A crack can start from the ground surface and extend proximally or can originate from the coronary band and extend distally. *Hoof clefts* are defects that run perpendicular to the horn tubules, and can be located anywhere on the hoof. *Hoof crumbling* involves the large segment of hoof wall that breaks away from the hoof starting at the weight-bearing surface.

The defects are classified as to location on the hoof (toe, quarter, heel), by their length, and by their depth. A defect is complete if it extends from the coronary band to the weight-bearing surfaces and incomplete if it does not. A simple defect is one in which only the horn is involved, whereas a complicated defect involves the sensitive tissue.

EVALUATION

There are numerous causes of defects in the hoof. Careful examination of the hoof can often identify the probable cause, which must be eliminated before therapy will be effective. The first consideration is moisture; either excessive dryness or excessive moisture can result in defects. Dryness usually results in a brittle hoof that tends to crack when it is stressed. If the hoof is unprotected, large portions (1 or 2 cm^2) of hoof wall may break away at the edge of the weight-bearing surface. A common complication to this problem is excessive hoof length. Because the hoof wall becomes less resilient the further it grows from the coronary band, there is a greater tendency for it to break off when it becomes long. This problem is compounded if the hoof wall is dry. This type of hoof is very difficult to cut with a hoof knife or hoof nippers. Conversely, excessive moisture can cause the hoof wall to crumble. This is probably due to a combination of a decay process caused by microorganisms, a disruption of the normal horn tubules by the moisture, and stress on the hoof wall. This problem has several popular names depending on the area of the country in which it is seen. It may be called "dew poisoning" in the West and is referred to as "yeast infection" in the South. Both problems are characterized by hoof wall crumbling starting at the weight-bearing surface. Examination of the wall reveals a hoof wall that is soft in nature at the area of crumbling. The wall can easily be dislodged for several millimeters around the defect. The wall that is affected has little normal architecture and crumbles into a fine powder when pressure is applied.

The next consideration for evaluating the cause of the defects is hoof conformation, balance, or improper shoe application. These problems can cause overloading of a portion of hoof wall and result in disruption of the integrity of the horn. Defects resulting from speed work or work on uneven surfaces are also due to similar abnormal stresses.

Infection or foreign bodies in the hoof may also result in defects. Clefts and crumbling are the most common results of these factors. Clefts may result from either a separation of horn from the coronary band, as occurs with "gravel," or from splitting of the hoof wall as a result of the inflammation associated with infection. This can also be a cause of crumbling. The inflammation caused by the infection disrupts the normal architecture of the hoof sufficiently to cause the wall to break and crumble under normal stress and usage.

Defects should always be examined to determine their depth and size. Depth can usually be determined by probing the defect. The examiner needs to determine if sensitive tissues are involved. If pain is elicited by probing of the defect, then the defect involves sensitive tissue. A percussion hammer is useful in determining the size of a defect that is not readily visible. Normal percussion of the hoof results in a crisp resonance. If the hoof wall is separated from its deeper structures, the resonance is dull. The percussion hammer is also useful in locating infection, foreign bodies, or inflamed areas in the hoof wall. In these cases, gentle percussion causes the horse discomfort over the involved area. Radiography is very useful in these cases in identifying gas under the hoof wall, which indicates either infection or undermined hoof wall.

Defects at or near the coronary band should have the hair clipped from the coronary band. The coronary band should then be examined for injuries, wounds, splits, or other defects that would account for the abnormal hoof growth.

SURGERY

The first objective and most important goal of treatment is to eliminate or correct the problem that caused the hoof defect in the first place. In most cases, if this is achieved the defect will simply grow out. Adjunctive therapy will usually make it possible to return the horse to work faster. If the underlying problem is not corrected recurrence should be expected.

It must be remembered that healing of these injuries is based on growth of new horn. These tissues do not heal side to side; therefore healing is slow and will take 5 to 10 months. The first goal in the treatment of the cracks should be to immobilize and prevent spreading of the defect. Immobilization of the crack can be accomplished by application of a bar shoe that relieves pressure on the affected wall. The bar may be a full bar or a diagonal bar. The objective is to relieve pressure, which causes movement at the area of the defect. In addition to the full bar, clips placed on either side of the crack will help prevent hoof expansion and, therefore, will immobilize the crack (Fig. 80–1). To further immobilize the crack it can be sutured or wired. In some cases a small metal plate can be screwed into the wall over the crack.

Further changes in the hoof wall must be made to prevent a crack from lengthening. The simplest method to prevent lengthening of a crack involves removing the affected wall from the weight-bearing surface (Fig. 80–1). Whenever this technique of "easing" is performed, it must be followed by daily cleaning of the space created so that it does not fill with dirt and subsequently apply pressure to the wall. "Grooving" the hoof wall perpendicular to the crack has the effect of deflecting stress away from the crack. Cracks that originate from the weight-bearing surface should be grooved at the most proximal aspect of the crack. The groove should be made deeper than the crack. Cracks that originate from the coronary band should be

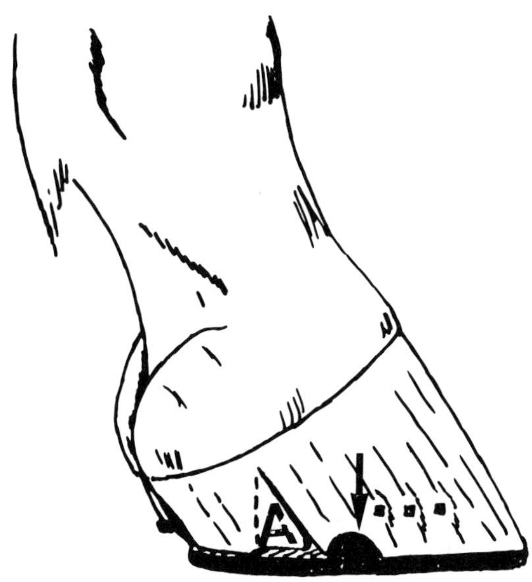

Figure 80–1. Quarter clip (arrow) is applied dorsal to the defect to prevent movement of the wall. All hoof wall under the defect (A) is removed to prevent weight bearing.

grooved at the distal aspect of the crack and in the shape of a *V*. Grooving will only work if the crack does not extend to the sensitive tissues. Grooving is not cosmetic. Bonding or acrylic repair of the crack is a cosmetic and very successful method used to obliterate the crack. This technique of repair will be described later.

Because of their horizontal orientation hoof clefts do not lengthen as do cracks. However, clefts are much more likely to involve sensitive layers and cause lameness. The horn around the cleft should be removed to the depth of the cleft. Sufficient horn should be removed so there is no undermined horn. In many cases this may require a resection of the hoof wall from the cleft to the weight-bearing surface. A rotary burr does an excellent job of performing this task. After sufficient hoof wall is débrided, the underlying tissue should be inspected carefully.

Hoof crumbling may require wide débridement of hoof wall. As for a cleft, all undermined hoof wall should be removed. The hoof wall should be removed until intact hoof wall is present around the edge of the débrided area. Again the deep tissues must be carefully examined for necrotic tissue or contaminated debris.

POSTOPERATIVE CARE

The goal of postoperative therapy is to make the horse usable as soon as possible. In most cases this will require some type of repair to restore the integrity of the hoof wall. However, before any repair can be performed the hoof must be properly prepared. First, the area must be free of hemorrhage or sepsis. Controlling hemorrhage requires packing the bleeding area with gauze and wrapping the foot. Approximately 1 week is required to dry the hemorrhagic area and allow some new horny growth over the area. Application of a 1% tincture of iodine to the horn in and around the defect will usually dry the area without dessicating it. If sepsis has occurred or a foreign body has penetrated the hoof wall, it is necessary to soak the foot in a saturated magnesium sulfate–tamed iodine solution to eliminate the infection. It may be necessary to soak the foot for 7 to 10 days before the septic area is healed. This treatment is followed by application of tincture of iodine solution. A helpful hint to determine if infection is still present is to examine the area 24 hours after application of iodine. The presence of moisture or exudate in or around the defect indicates infection is still present. Soaking should continue until the infection is resolved.

The hoof wall can be repaired only after the defect has been adequately débrided and the hemorrhage/sepsis has been controlled. The hoof should be properly trimmed and balanced. In most cases, a bar shoe with clips should be applied. The hoof should be dry. Acetone or alcohol are excellent agents to remove debris from the surface and help to dry the outer layers of horn. The hoof wall around the defect should be beveled inward (undermined) for one-quarter inch using a rotary hand burr (Fig. 80–2). This technique will help the retention of the repair material. Some defects can be wired or laced across the defect. This not only helps immobilize the area, but also adds substrate to which the repair material can bond. If the defect is not sutured, holes should be drilled through the hoof from the normal wall into the undermined area. The holes should be 0.5 to 1 cm apart. This will further aid retention of the repair material. There are numerous agents that are available for repair, including fiberglass, rubber, thin metal sheets, leather, and acrylic/epoxy materials. The most popular materials used presently are the acrylic/epoxies. There are numerous agents available (10x, Farriers, Inc; Technovit, Jorgeson Lab; Kwik-Poly, Anvil Brand Shoe Co; Hoof Repair Compound, Pegasus Products), and all have the advantage that they actually bond to the terminal hydroxyl radical of the keratin molecule, so they will become more like a prosthetic hoof wall when they cure. The acrylic/epoxy is mixed and applied to the defect and surrounding hoof wall. It is usually helpful to cover the hoof wall with a nonstick material such as aluminum foil to facilitate molding the acrylic to the shape of the hoof. Once suffi-

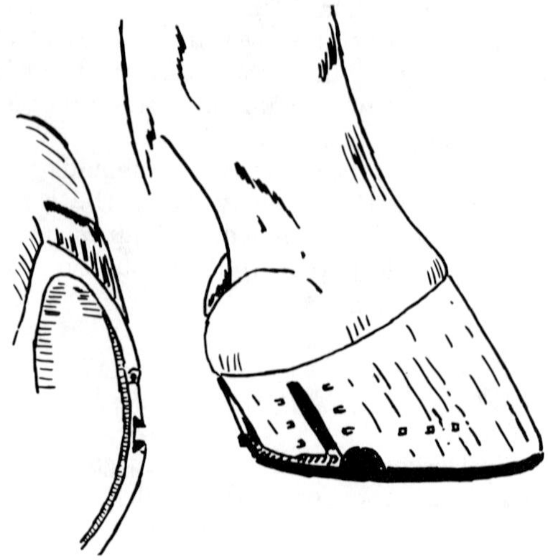

Figure 80–2. The defect is débrided to remove all abnormal horn. The edges are beveled inward to aid retention of acrylic.

cient time is elapsed to allow hardening of the material (10 to 15 minutes), excess acrylic is rasped away and a cosmetic repair is left.

In all cases, exercise of these animals should be minimized until the defect can be sufficiently protected and immobilized. Otherwise, exercise may worsen the condition. Once a shoe is applied and the crack protected, work can resume. When large amounts of hoof wall have been lost, it may be necessary to complete the entire repair process before the horse can be exercised. On rare occasions I have had to completely rebuild the hoof before a shoe could be applied. The acrylic/epoxies are too hard to nail a shoe to, but with glue-on shoes the ability to completely rebuild a foot is possible. The horse can go back to a normal routine once a repair has been completed.

Since healing of the defect is dependent on growth of new hoof, the horse must be reexamined at 4- to 8-week intervals. The shoe will need to be reset and in most cases the repair repeated until the hoof grows out. If the animal is active/competitive, the constant trauma to the repair may cause the acrylic/epoxy repair to loosen. If this occurs the material should be removed and the repair repeated. Under no circumstances should new acrylic be applied over the top of old acrylic. This can trap bacteria and cause an abscess with new hoof wall defects.

PROGNOSIS

For small defects that do not involve the sensitive structures the prognosis is excellent. For all other defects the prognosis is good to excellent. Given proper hoof care, adequate time, and follow-up, the defect will heal. The hoof wall will usually grow one-quarter inch per month. Large defects that have resulted from an underlying inflammatory cause may have a tendency to recur because of damage to the laminae and loss of hoof wall bonding between the layers. However, if the hoof is kept shod and protected, further problems can be avoided.

BIBLIOGRAPHY

Evans LH, Jenny J, Raker CW: The repair of hoof cracks with acrylic. *J Am Vet Med Assoc* 1966;148:355–359.

Krpan MK, Crawley GR: Management of hoof-wall disease in horses Part 2: Repair of hoof-wall defects. *Mod Vet Pract* 1986;67:147–151.

Moyer W: Repairing hoof cracks in horses: A review and report of a new technique. *Compend Cont Educ Pract Vet* 1983;5:S495-S500.

Nickels FA: Hoof cracks, in Robinson NE (ed): *Current Therapy in Equine Medicine.* Philadelphia, WB Saunders Co, 1987, pp 272–274.

81
Laminitis

Tracy A. Turner

Acute laminitis always must be considered an emergency. Laminitis causes severe lameness and, if untreated or nonresponsive to treatment, can cause permanent loss of function or even necessitate euthanasia. Laminitis simply means inflammation of laminae within the hoof. Although "founder" is a lay term considered to be synonomous with laminitis, more correctly the term refers to the changes that occur in hoof appearance as a result of laminitis. Laminitis is the result of a systemic metabolic syndrome with a complex pathophysiology. The disease manifests itself as congestion, ischemia, and necrosis of the laminae, which causes lameness.

DIAGNOSIS

Laminitis occurs most often in ponies but affects all breeds of horses. The disease has increased incidence during spring with the early growth of pasture. Horses that are overweight are more predisposed to develop the condition. Grain overload is probably the single most common cause of laminitis and is used reliably to reproduce the disease experimentally. Endotoxemia secondary to gastrointestinal disease and retained placenta also is associated with laminitis. Corticosteroid-induced laminitis occurs occasionally, as does "support laminitis," which develops when one limb must bear excessive weight during convalescence from an injury to the contralateral limb. Similarly, traumatic laminitis ("road founder") can occur when a horse is worked excessively on a hard surface. Laminitis can also occur after excessive consumption of water immediately after exercise.

Once a horse has had laminitis, the condition tends to recur. Presumably, prior damage to the laminae makes it easier for the circulatory changes to recur. Laminar damage can occur not only from previous episodes of laminitis but also from sole abscesses, submural abscesses, punctures, or even severe pedalosteitis.

The disease can be divided into three phases: developmental, acute, and chronic. Each phase is characterized by specific pathologic changes and clinical signs. The developmental phase begins when the horse comes into contact with the inciting agent and ends with the first sign of lameness. During this phase there is vascular constriction resulting in reduced blood flow in the laminar region. A coagulopathy also occurs, causing further ischemia of the secondary laminae. There are no clinical signs referable to the feet during this phase. The veterinarian must suspect that this phase of laminitis exists whenever the systemic or physical abnormalities are present. In other words, in cases of severe gastrointestinal disease or systemic toxemia one should assume that laminitis is in the developmental phase.

The acute phase of laminitis begins when clinically apparent alterations occur in the horse's feet. A bounding digital pulse will become palpable and heat can be detected over the hoof wall. Hoof tester examination of the feet will indicate sensitivity over the entire sole, especially at the toe. The horse assumes a "camped in front" stance and is lame. Lameness due to laminitis is divided into four grades. Grade I lameness is characterized by the horse constantly shifting its weight from leg to leg. The horse's gait is stiff and stilted at the trot but not at the walk. A horse with grade II laminitis has a stiff and stilted gait at both the walk and the trot and is not willing to bear full weight on one foreleg, although either foreleg can still be held up. Grade III lameness is characterized by a stiff and stilted gait at the walk and trot. Most characteristic of grade III laminitis, however, is the horse's refusal to allow either of its forelegs to be held up. Horses with grade IV laminitis will move only with strong encouragement and most will be recumbent. An important fact to remember is that permanent morphologic changes occur in the laminae within 12 hours after the onset of grade III lameness. These changes can also occur more insidiously in horses showing less severe lameness.

The pain associated with acute laminitis is presumed to be due to ischemia and necrosis of the secondary laminae caused by poor capillary perfusion. Systemic changes, including hypertension, tachycardia, and mild metabolic acidosis also occur during the acute phase. Although many of these changes can be related to pain, they are also consistent with circulatory shock. Generally, the acute phase of laminitis ends 48 hours after the onset of lameness or when rotation of the distal phalanx occurs. Therefore, it is very important to take lateral radiographs of the foot as soon after the onset of lameness as possible. Radiopaque markers to indicate the dorsal hoof wall and most proximal aspect of the hoof are helpful guides when evaluating the radiographs.

The chronic phase of laminitis begins with the separation of the distal phalanx from the hoof wall. In the normal hoof there are supporting and distracting biomechanical forces. The supporting forces include the pull of the extensor tendon, support from the ground to the sole and frog, and interdigitation of the sensitive and insensitive laminae. The opposing forces include the horse's weight transmitted via the distal phalanx to the sole, the pull of the deep digital flexor tendon against the attachments of the distal phalanx to the hoof wall, and a force exerted as leverage at the toe just prior to breakover of the foot. When the forces promoting the attraction of the laminae are lost as a result of damage due to laminitis, the distracting forces on the foot disrupt the normal hoof–distal phalanx attachment and allow rotation (Fig. 81–1). Careful clinical examination of the foot can help the clinician determine if rotation is occurring. Normally, the coronary band fits like a cuff over the hoof. If a depression is palpated at the toe of the coronary band or the edge of the hoof wall is more easily palpable around the circumference of the coronary band, one should suspect that rotation exists. Similarly, if the sole of the foot changes shape from concave to flat, one should suspect rotation.

Radiographs are absolutely necessary to confirm that rotation or distal displacement of the distal phalanx exists. Rotation of the distal phalanx is usually quite obvious on a lateral radiographic projection because the distance between the hoof wall and bone is greater distally than proximally. "Sinking," or distal displacement of the distal phalanx, is more difficult to diagnose and has a poorer prognosis. Sinking indicates the laminar separation is occurring in all parts of the hoof and the horse's weight is literally forcing the bone through the sole. Thus, this condition is indicative of more severe damage to the laminae than occurs during rotation. Because radiographically the hoof wall and

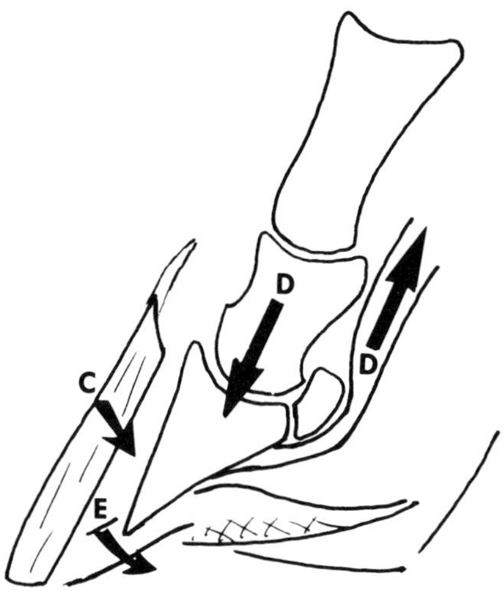

Figure 81–1. Mechanics of distal phalanx rotation. When the laminae are severely damaged (*C*), the horse's weight (*D*) and the pull of the deep flexor tendon (*D*) tear the distal phalanx from the hoof wall, which results in rotation (*E*).

the distal phalanx remain parallel during total separation, the radiographic diagnosis may be obscured. One of the earliest signs evident on radiographs is a widening of the space between the hoof wall and the bone. I consider this sign as pending rotation and/or sinking and treat the horse accordingly. Another early indicator is a change in the position of the coronary band. On a lateral radiograph of a normal foot the coronary band is positioned over the hoof wall. With rotation or sinking, however, a soft tissue depression appears on the radiograph at the previous site of the coronary band. Radiographs should also be assessed for the presence of gas between the hoof wall and the bone. Gas indicates either gas-producing bacteria are present or there is a communication between the separated hoof wall and the air. The damage from ischemia and tearing of the laminae makes this a prime location for infection.

TREATMENT/SURGERY

Therapy during each phase of the disease is designed to counteract systemic changes and lesions produced during that phase and prevent further changes.

Developmental Laminitis

Treatment during the developmental phase is directed at the potential cause of laminitis and at preventing the vascular lesions in the foot. A common finding in horses with acute laminitis is endotoxemia. Flunixin meglumine has excellent efficacy against the early systemic changes attributable to endotoxins. There has also been an effort to develop an effective toxoid and antisera directed against endotoxins. To prevent laminitis, the vascular shunting/coagulopathy lesion must be minimized. Phenoxybenzamine, an α-adrenergic blocker, has been used to improve circulation to the foot. The hoof is modified skin and is thought to have only α-adrenergic receptors in the microvasculature. Phenoxybenzamine has been effective in preventing laminitis when administered at 2 mg/kg in two doses 12 hours apart. The drug has a long half-life and is effective up to 72 hours. This drug causes hypotension, however, and can cause depression or even fainting. Other α-adrenergic blockers that may have use in treatment of developmental laminitis are acetylpromazine and promazine. Like phenoxybenzamine, these compounds increase capillary circulation via α-adrenergic receptor blockade; however, the duration of action of the promazine tranquilizers is much shorter and they must be dosed as dictated by the clinical situation. One must be sure not to administer any of these drugs to a horse in circulatory shock.

Therapy during this phase of the disease should also be directed toward preventing coagulation within the microvasculature. One drug that has been used commonly is heparin. Heparin has been used at a variety of dosages, with the most common ranging between 40 and 70 U/kg administered twice daily, subcutaneously, or three times daily intravenously. A disadvantage of heparin is that it causes agglutination of erythrocytes. To monitor for this effect, the hematocrit must be measured routinely during treatment. A precipitous drop in the hematocrit is evidence of agglutination. Once this decrease in volume is observed, the drug is normally discontinued. The efficacy of heparin in laminitis is unknown. There appears to be benefit from using heparin early in the developmental stage to prevent the clinical signs of laminitis.

Although antihistamines have been used widely in the treatment of laminitis, the efficacy of these drugs has been questioned. If used, these drugs should be administered during the developmental phase. Another aspect of therapy that is controversial is exercise. Exercise increases the digital circulation, yet during laminitis should be used with discretion. The animal should not be walked for long periods of time, but may be turned out for free-choice exercise in a sand paddock or on another soft surface. On the other hand, forcing a horse with severe pain and marked rotation to walk may cause more physical damage and is therefore contraindicated.

Acute Laminitis

If lameness ensues despite treatment, therapeutic measures must be taken to counteract inflammation, as well as the vascular shunt/coagulopathy. It must be remembered that laminitis is a dynamic disease. The main objective of therapy during this phase is to prevent rotation or displacement of the distal phalanx. This goal is achieved by circulation modification, anti-inflammatory drug therapy, and foot care.

Circulatory Drugs. Drugs used to improve circulation are the same as those used during the developmental phase. Isoxsuprine hydrochloride (0.6 mg/kg by mouth twice daily) is a β-adrenergic agonist that has been recommended for navicular disease. The drug causes dilation of the digital arteries and increases blood flow to the hoof. However, it has not been shown to increase capillary circulation within the foot. During laminitis, circulation to the hoof is increased but the capillary circulation within the secondary laminae is decreased. It would seem unlikely that isoxsuprine would have any beneficial effects during laminitis, but more studies are needed to determine its efficacy.

Anti-inflammatory Drugs. Anti-inflammatory drug treatment is important to decrease inflammation of the laminae, decrease swelling, ease pain, and indirectly aid circulation. Phenylbutazone (2.2 to 4.4 mg/kg) can be administered intravenously or orally and is the most popular of the anti-inflammatory agents for laminitis. Aspirin is another potent nonsteroidal anti-inflammatory drug that has been used in selected clinical cases. Because of its profound effect on platelet activity, aspirin may be given every 2 to 3 days at 20 mg/kg. Flunixin meglumine (1.1 mg/kg) administered intravenously is a potent nonsteroidal anti-inflammatory agent. These inhibitors of cyclooxygenase activity can cause renal and gastrointestinal damage. Although all nonsteroidal anti-inflammatory drugs are highly protein bound, presently there are no reports to indicate whether the toxic effects of these drugs are increased or decreased when the drugs are used in combination. Therefore, the dosage of each of these drugs should be titrated to the lowest effective dose.

Dimethylsulfoxide is a potent anti-inflammatory agent that can be used in combination with the nonsteroidal agents. The drug can be administered topically or intravenously. When given intravenously, the most commonly used dosage is 0.25 to 0.5 g/kg twice daily. Dimethylsulfoxide should be diluted to 20% in saline or dextrose and administered over a 30-minute period (too rapid a rate of administration can cause hemolysis). The drug's ability to decrease swelling, relieve pain, and combat endotoxemia by scavenging hydroxyl radicals is well documented, although its efficacy is not proven for treatment of laminitis. Corticosteroids are the one class of anti-inflammatory drugs that are absolutely contraindicated in the treatment of laminitis. They enhance the vasoconstrictive effects of catecholamines and in some cases have caused laminitis.

Foot Care. Care of the foot is of utmost importance, because the entire objective of treatment is to prevent rotation or displacement of the distal phalanx. The key to foot care is support of the skeletal column. Normally the hoof supports the skeletal column, but with damage to the laminae this basic structural support is lost. To maintain the normal hoof–distal phalanx configuration, the remaining supporting forces must be increased or the distracting forces decreased. The only supporting force that can be increased is the ground support of the foot. Standing the horse in sand is one of the best methods to support the foot during the acute phase. Sand more evenly distributes pressure across the bottom of the foot. Packing the sole with resilient material, such as silicone, tar and oakum, orthoplast, unvulcanized rubber, gauze, and cast material, is also a popular way to increase the sole support. Regardless of the material used, it must be placed so it distributes pressure evenly. Uneven pressure may cause areas of sole necrosis. Extra care must be taken with the less resilient materials because it is like putting the sole between a "rock and hard spot." Frequent examinations of the sole each day are necessary when packing the sole. If sole tenderness is increased or the sole starts to drop, the support should be modified to cover only the frog.

Trimming and shoeing of the hoof is occasionally performed during the acute phase of laminitis. The hoof should be trimmed so it is balanced and level. It is also helpful to roll the toe of the hoof so the toe is not directly weight bearing. This has the dual effect of removing the most painful area of the foot from ground contact and eliminates the distracting force caused during hoof breakover. Dorsal hoof wall resection is sometimes done during acute laminitis when the pain cannot be relieved. If shoes are placed on the foot during this stage yet the pain is not relieved or worsens, a dorsal hoof wall resection should be considered. Some authors have recommended decreasing the heel length of the foot to increase frog pressure and improve circulation. However, this will also increase the tension on the deep flexor tendon and could potentiate rotation. Other authors have recommended raising the heels of the hoof to decrease the pull of the flexor tendon. However, this also has the effect of angling the distal phalanx and the lamina more toward the ground and could potentiate penetration of the sole. It is my opinion that neither of these should be done; the feet should be trimmed to an angle normal for the horse and the toe shortened and rolled. Shoeing is often recommended to help support the skeletal column. Several techniques have been described, and all can be effective depending on the severity of the laminar damage. An important factor to remember is that the sole must be able to be examined for signs of penetration while giving extra support to the ground surface. A disadvantage of shoeing is the hammering of nails into the hoof, which may exacerbate the inflammation. The advent of glue-on shoes should help eliminate this disadvantage.

Other Treatments. Some veterinarians have used nerve blocks therapeutically. The sensory blockade of the pain will encourage the horse to walk. Presumably this will improve circulation to the laminar region and will help break the sympathetic reflex to pain. This type of treatment must be used cautiously during this phase, as is the case with exercise. While some exercise has definite advantages, excessive exercise can promote rotation of the distal phalanx if there is severe laminar damage. If one assumes the horse's pain corresponds to the amount of ischemic damage, then the horse provides the best guide to the amount of exercise to be used. I prefer to turn the horse out into a sand pen large enough to allow the horse free exercise but small enough to keep it from trotting or running. At the first clinical sign of rotation or sinking, exercise should be discontinued.

Chronic Laminitis

The chronic phase of laminitis offers a new set of therapeutic challenges. The first goal of treatment is to support the skeletal system. This requires corrective trimming to realign the hoof wall with the new position of the distal phalanx. Shoeing is generally required to give the foot sufficient support. There are several different types of shoes and shoeing methods that can be used. These are covered in Chapter 83. The basic principle is that solar support of the distal phalanx is imperative but there should not be any pressure on the sole itself, because direct pressure on the sole can lead to necrosis. Pressure should be applied only to the frog, bars, and angles of the sole. Because the position of the distal phalanx is altered by the mechanical forces acting on it, the laminar attachments are literally stretched and torn apart. This causes hemorrhage and necrosis and makes these feet very prone to infection. The key to treatment of the infection is drainage.

Hoof Wall Resection. Hoof wall resection is performed to remove the hoof wall (stratum media) to the depth of the laminae for the purpose of exposing necrotic tissue and/or allowing drainage of infected laminae. There are two criteria for performing a hoof wall resection during the chronic phase of laminitis: (*a*) serous or purulent drainage with complete separation of the hoof wall from the skin at the coronary band, and (*b*) the presence of a gas density between the hoof and distal phalanx on a lateral radiograph. Generally, the resection is begun to include the entire toe. The resection can be made wider if necessary, as dictated by the presence of necrotic debris. A complete hoof wall resection (coronary band to the ground surface) should be performed if there is separation of the hoof wall from the coronary band; otherwise, the resection should extend to include the most proximal extent of gas as seen on radiography. Some veterinarians recommend complete hoof wall resection in all cases because they believe it relieves pressure on the coronary band and because the bone can be pushed back into normal position if the hoof wall is removed. Neither of these theories has been proven. However, in some cases pain that is refractory to other treatments or corrective shoeing can be relieved by dorsal hoof wall resection. The hoof wall resection can be performed with hoof nippers and hoof rasp, a rotary burr power tool (probably the most popular method), or an oscillating cast saw. As the stratum medium is cut through with the cast saw, there is a distinct texture change that can be felt, and in this manner one can avoid cutting too deep. In performing an incomplete resection the wall must be cut longitudinally on the medial and lateral sides, then cut transversely to connect the medial and lateral cuts. The wall can then be peeled away. To perform a complete hoof wall resection only the medial and lateral longitudinal cuts are necessary. Once these cuts are made, the hoof wall is peeled from the laminae and gently peeled off the coronary band. This action takes very little effort. Care must be taken to avoid trauma to the coronary band.

Proper care of the foot and leg after hoof wall resection is essential. The hoof should be cleaned and bandaged in an aseptic manner on a daily basis. The daily cleansing will remove any necrotic debris that tends to accumulate over the wound. For the first 1 to 2 weeks, twice-daily bandage changes may be necessary depending upon the extent of necrotic laminae. This wound should heal like any open wound. Areas that have had necrosis or severe infection will heal by granulation after débridement. Corium will cover the granulation tissue and new horn will be produced from that tissue. At the same time, new horn will begin to grow immediately from the coronary band (0.5 cm/month). During the initial stages after hoof wall resection, soaking the feet in a saturated solution of magnesium sulfate with povidone-iodine added as an antiseptic may be beneficial in treating infection of the laminae. Daily bandaging should continue until horn covers the wound. During this healing phase, exercise should be confined to movement within a stall.

Desmotomy/Tenotomy. Tendon releasing procedures are recommended to decrease the pull of the deep flexor tendon on the bone. Inferior check desmotomy will decrease the tension of the deep flexor tendon without disrupting the muscle-tendon-bone complex. The greatest disadvantage to this procedure is the variable response and the requirement of general anesthesia. It is also difficult to determine when the procedure is indicated. Since relief is variable, it is best to perform this surgery on less severely affected horses. In severe cases, inferior check desmotomy fails to provide sufficient relief and a more drastic procedure is required. Deep digital flexor tenotomy will completely eliminate that distracting force from the foot. In many cases, some pain relief is immediate after the procedure is performed. However, this surgery should be used as the last stage in therapy. Surgery is indicated when rotation of the distal phalanx is progressing and other measures have failed to stop rotation, or in chronic refractory laminitis where it is necessary to release the tendon to allow the bone to be realigned to a more normal position by shoeing. Generally, the chance for an athletic career after tenotomy is slim, but the animal can be salvaged for breeding or light pleasure riding.

Two surgical techniques for tenotomy of the deep digital flexor have been described. One is performed at the level of the midmetacarpus/metatarsus and the other at the level of the pastern. The midmetacarpal approach is the easiest and can be performed under local anesthesia or with short-acting general anesthesia, such as xylazine-ketamine. Following aseptic preparation of the limb, a 3- to 4-cm incision is made over the deep flexor tendon in the middle third of the tendon (distal to the check ligament attachment and proximal to the tendon sheath). The paratenon is bluntly dissected and the neurovascular structures are freed from the deep flexor tendon. With the fetlock in flexion, the deep flexor tendon can be easily exteriorized and transected. The skin is closed in a routine manner. Some controversy has existed about the preferable technique of tendon transection (*Z*-plasty, diagonal). It has been my experience that the technique did not change the postoperative course of these cases. The single transverse transection, which is the fastest and requires the least dissection, is preferred. The tenotomy technique at the pastern requires that the horse be under general anesthesia. Following aspetic preparation, a 3-cm skin incision is made along the palmar midline of the pastern 1 cm proximal to the heel bulbs. The subcutaneous tissues are dissected to expose the deep digital flexor tendon sheath. The sheath is incised to expose the deep flexor tendon. A curved hemostat is placed under the tendon and the tendon is transected. The tendon sheath is closed with 2–0 absorbable monofilament suture in a continuous pattern. Skin is closed in a routine fashion. The pastern approach is best used as an alternative if disease prevents the midmetacarpal approach. The pastern approach is also useful as a site for repeat tenotomy procedures.

Horses undergoing tenotomy procedures should have their distal limbs (carpus or hock distally) wrapped aseptically and supported by a heavy cotton wrap. These bandages should be changed every 3 to 5 days until suture removal 10 to 14 days after surgery. Although elevation of the toe is a common complication after traumatic disruption of the deep flexor tendon, it has not been a complication of this procedure. The reason it is not seen in these cases is not fully understood, but this may be related to contracture of the palmar distal interphalangeal joint capsule or the type of shoe used for these cases. As a result, bandaging of the limb for support after the skin sutures are removed is not necessary. Shoeing to realign the hoof wall around the distal phalanx should be performed just before the tenotomy or as soon after as feasible. If the deep flexor tendon is cut at the level of the pastern the release of the proximal segment of tendon causes swelling behind the third metacarpal bone like a "bowed tendon." This is normal and will diminish with healing.

POSTTREATMENT MANAGEMENT/PROGNOSIS

Several changes should be made in the overall management of horses with laminitis. The content of grain and legume hay in the horse's ration should be reduced. The horse should receive mostly grass hay and receive only enough grain or legume to maintain its ideal weight. In many cases, laminitic horses should be on a weight-reducing diet. Some veterinarians empirically recommend the use of D,L-methionine to help the horse grow a better hoof. Likewise, others recommend that the total daily sodium intake be lowered (i.e., free-choice salt removed). The value of these treatments has not been proven.

It may take 2 days to 2 weeks for a horse with laminitis to respond to therapy. Successful management should be judged on the basis of progressive daily improvement. If rotation or sinking does not occur, the chances of full recovery are excellent. However, the horse may be more prone to additional episodes of laminitis in the future. For horses that do suffer rotation, measurement of the degree of rotation can be used prognostically. Horses with rotation of 5.5 degrees or less usually can be returned to athletic function with corrective trimming and shoeing. Horses with more than 11.5 degrees of rotation are the most difficult to restore to normal and are usually lost as performance animals. Many of these animals need additional therapy besides corrective trimming/shoeing to return them to pasture soundness. These are the cases in which tenotomy is useful. In one report, 38% of the horses having tenotomies (5 of 13 cases) returned to limited athletic endeavors. Based on the data presently available, this surgery should be considered a salvage procedure and pasture soundness accepted as the long-term benefit.

Horses undergoing hoof wall resection have increased morbidity from hoof infection. Increased time must be given these horses to grow a new hoof; approximately 6 months to 1 year to grow out a complete hoof resection. Persistent hoof infection due to necrosis, chronic osteomyelitis, or focal ischemia from laminitis is probably the most common cause necessitating euthanasia of the chronic laminitic horse. Hoof wall resection and débridement is the only viable means of dealing with these cases if complete resolution is expected. Six to 8 months are also required for healing of the deep flexor tendon after tenotomy. Regrowth of a normally shaped hoof will be seen during this time if laminar reattachment has occurred. Exercise should be restricted during the first 2 to 3 months after tenotomy to prevent tendon damage during initial healing.

Successful treatment of laminitis requires daily care and attention to the horse. It is the culmination of teamwork between the owner, veterinarian, and farrier. The daily care of the horse and its feet requires a real dedication to the horse on the part of the owner. With people who are willing to spend the time and effort, treatment of these cases can be very rewarding. However, without their dedication treatment is frustrating and usually ends with the destruction of the animal.

BIBLIOGRAPHY

Allen D, White NA, Foerner JF, Gordon BJ: Surgical management of chronic laminitis in horses: 13 cases (1983–1985). *J Am Vet Med Assoc* 1986;189:1604–1606.

Anderson GF: Laminitis in horses: A practitioner's approach. *Mod Vet Pract* 1986;67:605–607.

Goetz TE: Anatomic, hoof, and shoeing considerations for the treatment of laminitis in horses. *J Am Vet Med Assoc* 1987;190:1323–1332.

Hood DM, Stephens KA: Physiopathology of equine laminitis. *Compend Cont Educ Pract Vet* 1981;3:S454-S460.

Redden RF: Minimizing complications of laminitis in horses. *Mod Vet Pract* 1986;67:446–450.

Stick JA: Laminitis, in Robinson NE (ed): *Current Therapy in Equine Medicine.* Philadelphia, WB Saunders Co, 1987, pp 277–281.

82 Navicular Disease

Tracy A. Turner

DIAGNOSIS

Navicular disease is a complex syndrome causing lameness in the horse. It has been estimated to be the cause of one third of the chronic lameness in horses. Horses that develop navicular disease are performance horses. Although the syndrome affects all types of performance horses, there is a distinct breed predisposition. In the United States, Quarter Horses and Thoroughbreds have a higher incidence of navicular disease than any other breed. The now-popular warmbloods also appear to be predisposed to navicular disease. Geldings are more commonly affected with the disease, but this is probably a reflection of the type of horse preferred for performance rather than a true sex predilection. The diagnosis is most commonly made in horses between 7 and 14 years of age. Horses less than 3 years or older than 15 years of age are three to five times less likely to develop the disease.

The diagnosis of navicular disease is not easy, because many other conditions causing lameness mimic signs of the disease. The diagnosis should be based on history and clinical signs. Generally, the history indicates either an intermittent lameness or inconsistent performance. In the earliest stages of navicular disease, lameness is usually not noted but a change in performance or behavior is a common complaint. The rider may complain that the horse is unwilling or difficult to work. The most common complaints are that the horse refuses leads and loses suppleness. This causes many riders to mistakenly believe the problem is in the horse's shoulder. Often the horse is presented to the veterinarian for examination of a shoulder injury.

Navicular disease is characterized as chronic in nature but may be seen as an acute disease. The lameness is often more noticeable after heavy work, will usually improve with rest, and will return when hard work is resumed. The horse will usually perform poorly on hard or rough surfaces. These surfaces will also accentuate the lameness.

In most cases, navicular disease is a bilateral lameness. The horse's gait is short and choppy, and the horse has a tendency to land on its toe, although this is not always apparent. The lameness can be accentuated by turning the horse in a tight circle at the trot, which causes the horse to be lame on the inside leg. Because of its bilateral nature, it is often difficult to observe lameness on a straightaway. Lounging the horse in tight circles may be the only way to visualize the lameness.

Diagnostic Tests

Diagnostic tests for navicular disease include examination with a hoof tester, wedge tests, and flexion tests. Pain caused by application of the hoof testers from the collateral sulci to contralateral hoof wall, central sulcus to toe, and across the heels is consistent with navicular disease. If the reponse is due to navicular disease, it should be uniform and consistent. However, lack of a painful response to application of the hoof testers does not rule out navicular disease. Careful examination of the remaining portions of the foot with hoof testers must be made and the responses evaluated relative to the pain in the navicular area. Thus, the veterinarian must make sure the horse does not have another problem, such as bruising, that accounts for the painful response to the hoof testers.

Two types of wedge tests help in the diagnosis of navicular disease. The hyperextension test consists of placing the horse's foot on one end of a board and raising the opposite end of the board. This technique effectively raises the toe 1 to 1.5 in while the heel of the foot stays in contact with the ground. A positive response is recorded if the horse shows discomfort by jumping off the board, or if the lameness is excerbated when the horse is trotted. The second test, the frog pressure test, is performed by placing a block of wood directly under the caudal two thirds of the frog. The opposite limb is held off the ground, forcing the horse to stand on the block. A positive response is characterized by an exacerbation of the lameness when the horse is trotted. Although positive responses to these tests are consistent with the existence of navicular disease, negative responses do not rule out navicular disease.

Flexion of the joints in the distal limb (metacarpophalangeal, proximal interphalangeal, and distal interphalangeal joints) also provides useful additional information regarding navicular disease. Because positive response to joint flexion (exacerbation of lameness when trotted after flexion) could be expected for conditions involving the distal interphalangeal joint, collateral sesamoidean ligaments, and deep digital flexor tendonitis, a positive response is not pathognomonic for navicular disease. Furthermore, a negative response to these flexion tests does not rule out the existence of navicular disease. Each test provides important information that must be evaluated in comparison with the horse's response to the same tests using regional anesthesia.

Regional nerve blocks are invaluable in determining the location of lameness. Typically, a horse with navicular disease will improve at least 90% following a medial and lateral palmar digital nerve block. Important exceptions to this rule are horses with navicular disease that have secondary lamenesses. Two notable causes are pedal osteitis and suspensory desmitis. In addition to the palmar digital blocks, distal interphalangeal and navicular bursa anesthesia adds useful additional information relative to the diagnosis. Distal interphalangeal anesthesia can be expected to alleviate lameness associated with conditions involving the distal interphalangeal joint. Navicular bursa anesthesia could be expected to block those structures in direct contact with the navicular bursa, but this does not completely block out all the possible structures that could be involved with navicular disease.

Radiographic, Scintigraphic, and Thermographic Evaluation

After a diagnosis of navicular disease is made based on history and clinical signs, imaging of the navicular bone by radiography and scintigraphy and evaluation of the local circulation by thermography are useful tools to help confirm the diagnosis. There are five radiographic changes associated with navicular disease. These include marginal osteophytes, remodeling, enlarged synovial fossae, cysts, and flexor cortex changes. While none are pathognomonic, the radiographic changes provide insight into the possible inciting injury. Three radiographic projections are needed to completely assess the navicular bone—a dorsopalmar, lateral, and palmaroproximal-palmarodistal (PP-PD) projection. The dorsopalmar projection provides the most useful interpretive information regarding the presence of marginal osteophyte formation (osseous metaplasia of the wings of the navicular bone), remodeling of the proximal and distal borders of the navicular bone (enthesophytosis), cyst formation, and enlarged synovial fossa ("lollipops"). The PP-PD view is most useful for evaluating the flexor cortex. A lateral view is helpful in confirming the presence of any of these changes.

Marginal osteophyte formation is ossification (in all three cites) of the collateral sesamoidean ligaments along the wings of the navicular bone, whereas remodeling along the proximal border of the bone is of the same ligament. Remodeling changes are also seen as of the impar ligament or as possible chip fractures off the distal border of the navicular bone. Evidence of these changes on radiographs may indicate a primary injury to one of the ligaments of the navicular bone. Enlarged synovial fossae ("lollipops") may indicate an inflammatory process in the distal interphalangeal joint. The presence of cysts tends to indicate a primary navicular bone lesion, and flexor changes may indicate an injury to the tendon.

While radiographs confirm the presence of lesions in the navicular bone, they cannot be used alone to diagnose navicular disease. Scintigraphy is a technique that evaluates the rate of bone turnover and relative tissue vascularity. This information can be useful in determining if the cause of the disease is ischemia, high bone remodeling rate, or soft tissue trauma. Most cases of navicular disease show high bone remodeling rates scintigraphically. Thermography provides information regarding skin temperature that gives insight into the presence of local inflammation and the adequacy of tissue perfusion. Horses with navicular disease have decreased skin temperatures in the palmar aspect of the foot after exercise, indicating reduced perfusion. Ultrasound examination of the soft tissues around the navicular bone would be useful to evaluate tendon and ligament injuries, but to date has not been completely successful or consistent because of the difficulty in positioning the ultrasound head.

TREATMENT

Treatments for navicular disease are as varied and controversial as any other aspect of the disease. Treatment can be divided into three categories: shoeing, medicinal, and surgical. Shoeing for navicular disease is discussed in Chapter 83.

Medicinal Therapy

Medicinal therapy involves anti-inflammatory/analgesic and vascular-altering drugs. The use of anti-inflammatory/analgesic drugs such as phenylbutazone is the most common treatment, but the use of warfarin and isoxsuprine hydrochloride is becoming more popular. Warfarin is administered to slow thrombosis and decrease blood viscosity. Warfarin is given at 0.018 mg/kg daily and is increased in increments of 20% until the stage one-prothrombin time is increased by 2 to 4 seconds. The efficacy of this therapy has been 40 to 80% depending on the report. The most serious disadvantage of this therapy is that warfarin interacts with many drugs, among which are phenylbutazone and protein-binding antibiotics. This interaction can lead to increased plasma concentrations of warfarin and fatal hemorrhage. There has been a 1% death loss associated with this treatment. Isoxsuprine hydrochloride increases distal limb circulation. Effective doses range between 0.6 and 1.2 mg/kg administered orally twice daily. Long-term efficacy has varied between 40 and 87%. The only disadvantage at this time is that the drug is considered a forbidden substance by the American Horse Show Association. The drug must be withdrawn 96 hours prior to any competition.

Surgical Treatment

Four surgical techniques have been used in the treatment of navicular disease. *Palmar digital neurectomy* is the most common surgery performed for treatment of this disease. The surgery is described in Chapter 26. It is important to bear in mind that the surgical procedures do not treat the disease. The effects of surgery are palliative, in that only the pain is eliminated. Further, palmar digital nerve anesthesia should be performed 2 weeks prior to surgery to assess how much pain relief will be achieved by transecting the nerves. Overall, the surgery can be expected to be effective for 6 months to 6 years depending on the technique used. Care must be taken postoperatively to protect the horse's feet from inadvertent damage from sharp objects or bruising. Painful neuroma formation is the most common cause of neurectomy failure, but vascular necrosis of the hoof and rupture of the deep flexor tendon are catastrophic causes of failure that have been reported.

Distal check desmotomy is a procedure that has been discussed as a possible treatment for navicular disease. Some veterinarians are presently using this procedure on horses with navicular disease. Horses that have upright pastern conformation and/or have steep hoof angles are the types of horses in which the surgery is being used. The surgery is performed as described in Chapter 93. The theory in these cases is that the desmotomy should allow the pastern and hoof to assume a more ideal angle. This would allow the horse to be shod in a more ideal fashion. To date, there is not a thorough follow-up study of the surgery and its efficacy relative to navicular disease.

An interesting procedure that has recently been developed in Europe is *palmar digital fasciotomy.* Damage to the palmar digital nerves has been proposed as a possible inciting cause of navicular disease. Although the evidence for neuronal damage as a cause of navicular disease is not without some question, palmar digital fasciotomy and neurolysis was recommended as a method of treatment. With the horse under general anesthesia and the distal limb prepared for aseptic surgery, a skin incision extending from the level of the proximal sesamoid to the middle of the first pastern bone is made directly over the palmar digital nerve. Fascia surrounding the nerve is dissected free and any adhesions to the nerve are transected atraumatically. The incision is closed routinely. The wounds are managed under bandages, as would be routine for any surgical incision. The horses are exercised by controlled walking daily for 5 weeks. At 5 weeks after surgery, the horse is gradually worked back into training. Although long-term follow-ups were not available on the treated horses, the report indicated the authors considered navicular flexor surface changes as a poor prognostic sign. They further recommended that the surgery was most successful when performed early in the clinical course of the disease. More long-term follow-up is necessary before this procedure can be recommended. It is important to recognize that most veterinarians agree that any appropriate treatment for navicular disease is most successful when undertaken early in the clinical course.

Another procedure that has been used first in Europe is the *desmotomy of the collateral sesamoidean ligaments.* These ligaments are also called the proximal suspensory ligaments of the navicular bone. They originate from the medial and lateral distal dorsal depression of the first phalanx. The ligaments are intimately associated with the deeper collateral ligaments of the proximal interphalangeal joint. The collateral sesamoid ligaments run obliquely from their origin across the dorsal medial and lateral aspects of the joint, continue across the palmar medial and lateral aspects of the middle phalanx, and insert on the border of the navicular bone. Desmotomy is performed at the level of the pastern joint. Two oblique skin incisions, 3 to 4 cm in length, are made starting from the medial and lateral eminences of the distal first phalanx and extending in a dorsal and distal direction toward the common digital extensor tendon. The ligament runs perpendicular to the skin incision. A hemostat can be bluntly dissected under the ligament. The ligament is elevated and transected. Care must be taken not to cut the collateral ligaments of the pastern joint, which could disrupt the stability of that joint. Closure is routine. The wounds are cared for under bandages in a routine manner. The horses are exercised by controlled walking for 2 weeks following surgery and then are gradually reintroduced to full work by 3 months after surgery. Follow-up on 43 horses from 6 to 12 months following surgery indicated 30 of the 43 horses (70%) were able to work without lameness. My experience with the surgery has been limited to six cases. Two horses have shown improvement but no horse has been able to return to previous use as a result of the surgery.

PROGNOSIS

One of the basic problems in dealing with navicular disease is the fact that it is a syndrome that appears to have more than one cause. Successful results reported by one veterinarian are occasionally difficult for others to repeat. Further improvement in our diagnostic capabilities will be necessary to make a specific diagnosis as to the type of navicular disease. Once this is determined, therapy specific for that problem can be initiated. Therapy will obviously vary depending on the cause and will utilize one or all of the treatment modalities; shoeing, medicinal, or surgery. When specific treatments can be matched to the proper disease, there will be an improvement in the consistency of therapeutic success rates.

BIBLIOGRAPHY

Fricker CL, Hugelshofer J, Attinger P: Fasziotomie/neurolyse zks therapie der strahlbeinahmheit (podotrochlose) des pferdes. *Schweiz Arch Tierheilk* 1986;128:87–91.

Turner TA: Management of navicular disease in horses: An update. *Mod Vet Pract* 1986;67:24–27.

Turner TA, Fessler JF: The anatomic, pathologic and radiographic aspects of navicular disease. *Compend Cont Educ Pract Vet* 1982;4:5350–5355.

Wright IM: Navicular suspensory desmotomy in the treatment of navicular disease. Technique and preliminary results. *Equine Vet J* 1986;18:443–446.

83 Corrective Shoeing

Tracy A. Turner

Corrective trimming and shoeing are important therapeutic aspects of the treatment of lameness in horses. Unfortunately, these are often overlooked and left to the farrier's judgment. This is probably because veterinary curricula usually do not cover farriery in depth. As a result, many veterinarians are not comfortable in prescribing corrective shoeing.

FUNDAMENTALS

Trimming and shoeing are designed to properly align and balance the hoof. Corrective trimming and shoeing are performed to realign or rebalance the hoof because (*a*) changes in either the alignment or balance of the foot cause problems and (*b*) their correction will help resolve lameness. The hoof performs several functions; it bears weight, absorbs concussion, and aids in moving blood through the distal aspect of the leg. These functions are most efficient when the foot is properly aligned and balanced. Proper alignment includes having the pastern and hoof aligned in the same plane. Futhermore, the plane of the angle at the toe and heel is parallel to the plane of the pastern and hoof (Fig. 83–1). This is a subjective evaluation and must be made when the horse is standing square and bearing weight evenly. In the past, many texts have described the normal hoof angle to be between 45 and 50 degrees in the forelimbs and between 50 and 55 degrees in the hind limbs. This led many people to assume that the hooves should be trimmed to these angles. Actually the "normal" hoof angle is dependent on the individual horse. In fact, the normal forelimb hoof angle for most horses falls between 50 and 55 degrees, with a normal angle for some horses of between 55 and 60 degrees.

Hoof balance is a difficult concept. It may be defined as the manner in which an individual hoof contacts and leaves the ground, or as the manner in which the horse loads the limb during weight bearing. A hoof is balanced when the medial and lateral aspects of the hoof (heel to toe) are loaded evenly (although not always simultaneously) and hoof breakover occurs at the center of the toe. Ideally, during weight bearing the load on the leg would be axial so that medial and lateral load on the skeleton would be equal. The balanced hoof absorbs the loads on the limb, disperses the load evenly, and allows maximal dissipation at takeoff. To observe for balance, the hoof is held up and viewed from the heels toward the toe. The hoof wall and bars should be perpendicular to a line bisecting the foot. The hoof should also be symmetric. Finally, the horse must be observed in motion, to determine if it is landing on the hoof properly.

Once proper alignment and balance have been established, the remainder of corrective shoeing is technical. The branches of the shoe should be fit so they are slightly wider than the hoof. Generally, one sixteenth to one eighth of an inch of shoe outside the hoof wall is adequate to allow for hoof expansion. Expansion of the hoof is necessary for the hoof to absorb concussion and for normal blood flow. The horseshoe nails should not be placed caudal to the widest portion of the hoof because nails placed too far caudally inhibit hoof expansion. Proper paring of the sole is also important to permit adequate expansion. The normal sole should be concave. This shape allows the sole to expand by flattening slightly when the hoof contacts the ground.

SHOEING

Farriery is as much an art as it is a science. There are many techniques used to create a desired effect on the hoof. Careful consideration must be given to the advantages and disadvantages of any technique before it is used.

A bar shoe refers to a shoe that has no open end. Although there are many variations of the bar shoe, the full bar, egg bar, and heart bar shoes are those most commonly used. The bar shoe can be used to protect an area of hoof, to apply pressure to a specific area of the hoof, to give additional support to the hoof, and to stabilize the hoof. The full bar and diagonal bar shoes are generally used to protect and stabilize an area of hoof. The bar reinforces the shoe and accepts stresses that normally would have been applied to the hoof. The bar increases the weight of the shoe, which is a disadvantage. Although there has been speculation that bar shoes cause hoof contraction, there is no scientific evidence to support this idea. The egg bar shoe helps sup-

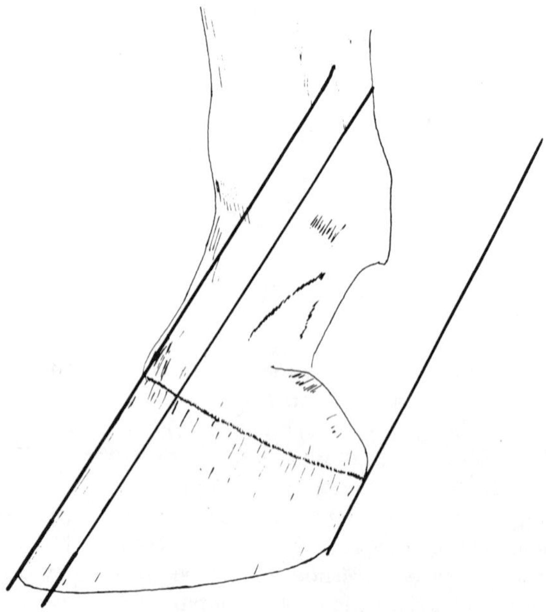

Figure 83–1. Schematic diagram of proper hoof alignment. The toe and heel are parallel to a straight line through the pastern and hoof.

port the caudal aspect of the hoof by extending behind the heels of the hoof. The shoe also increases the ground surface contact of the hoof. The major disadvantage of this shoe is that it may be torn off by interfering or overreaching. The heart bar shoe is designed to apply pressure to the frog and is most commonly used in the treatment of laminitis.

The shoe may be modified at the toe to improve, ease, or cause breakover of the hoof. A square toe, rolled toe, or rocker toe can be used. Each technique effectively shortens the hoof wall length, reducing the leverage and easing the breakover at that point. The square toe simply eliminates the circular portion of wall and causes hoof breakover along the straight surface. This can be modified so the hoof will break over either the medial or lateral aspect of the toe by changing the position of the straight part of the shoe. A rolled toe shoe is produced by grinding the shoe down at the desired point of breakover. This is the simplest means to ease breakover. The rocker toe shoe is made by forging the shoe so that the toe is bent up. The hoof wall must be trimmed shorter at that point so the shoe fits properly. Although this is the most effective method to encourage breakover, it is also the most technically difficult method. These techniques can be used (*a*) to

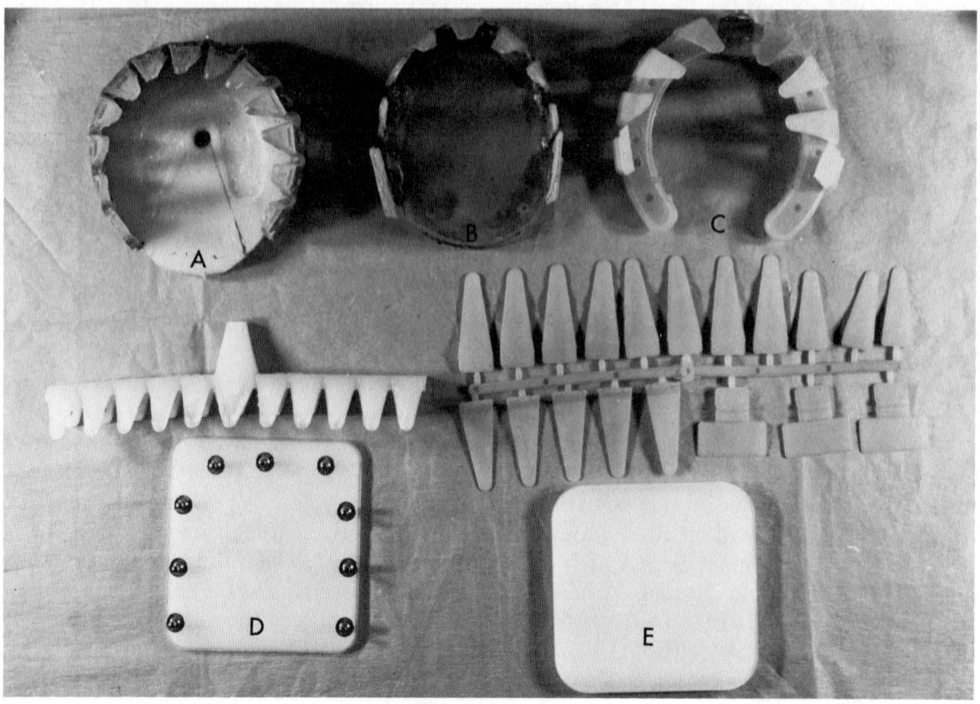

Figure 83–2. The five variations of Mustad's glue-on shoes: **A.** Glu-Strider. **B.** Glu II. **C.** Easy Glu. **D.** Baby Glu. **E.** Baby Glu II.

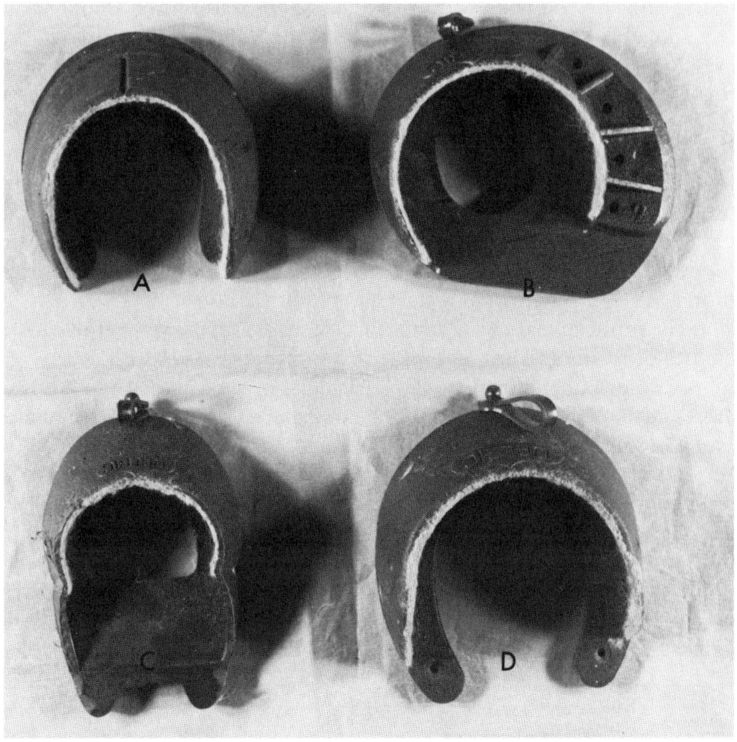

Figure 83–3. Variations of Advance Equine Productions' glue-on shoes. **A.** Toe extension, for flexural deformity. **B.** Lateral extension for rotational deformity. **C.** Heel extension for weak flexors. **D.** Standard glue-on.

treat conditions such as osteoarthritis or navicular disease, in which it is desirable to ease breakover, and (*b*) to correct gait abnormalities such as paddling, winging in, or forging.

Gait abnormalities such as paddling and winging in may result from rotational limb deformities as the horse rotates its hoof to the high side. In other words, nonsymmetric wear of the hoof wall will cause the horse to deviate its hoof placement. For instance, excessive wear of the medial hoof wall will make the horse rotate its feet laterally. Consequently, the horse will toe out. In addition to the use of roller toe shoes, the length of the hoof wall can be modified. Trimming of the lateral wall so it is level with the medial wall will correct the problem. Similarly, if a horse is toed out, the lateral wall can be shortened to force the hoof to rotate inward. Unfortunately, this can also unbalance the hoof and cause more problems. The best rule of thumb is to trim the hoof so it is level and then use a roller toe technique to encourage breakover to occur centrally. This prevents the hoof from becoming unbalanced and negates the worry about how the foot will rotate if the lateral or medial hoof wall is trimmed.

Trailers or heel extensions have also been used to alter the flight of the foot. Trailers are used most often to widen the horse's gait when the horse travels close

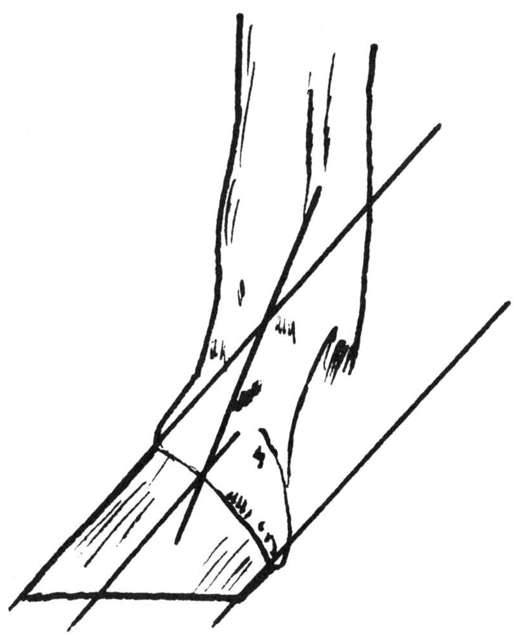

Figure 83–4. Schematic representation of "broken back" hoof conformation.

behind. In these instances, the trailer is applied to the lateral heel so it will make contact first and cause enough drag to turn the foot outward. Trailers can also be used to support the hoof in cases of a damaged or severed deep flexor tendon. For these horses, the trailers should extend 7 to 10 cm behind from both the medial and lateral heels. Generally, if two trailers are used it is helpful to join then by a bar. As the horse puts weight on the hoof, the trailers keep the foot flat on the ground instead of allowing the toe to raise off the ground, as is typical of deep flexor tendon injuries. There is some disparity of opinion as to any further benefits of trailers. Some veterinarians contend that a lateral trailer is beneficial in the treatment of tarsitis, whereas others suggest that trailers exacerbate the disease. There is little scientific evidence to support either hypothesis. If a trailer is to be used, it should extend straight behind the heel. If the trailer is bent to the lateral side, it will inhibit the foot's sliding motion as it lands and could increase the shear stress on the joints.

ADVANCES

Recently there has been a renewed interest in farrier science. Several advances have been made in shoe technology, pad technology, and hoof science. The advances in shoe technology have been in the area of nailless shoes. The glue-on shoe technology has been pioneered by three companies. Mustad Inc., Bloomfield, CT, Advance Equine Productions, Versailles, KY, and Shoe Bond Systems Inc., Hyannis, MA, have each marketed different variations of glue-on shoes. Each system uses tabs that glue to the outer layer of the hoof wall. By attaching the shoe in this manner, the glue bonds to the wall but does not have the stress of wall movement applied to it. The earliest glue-on shoes literally were glued to the bottom of the horse's foot. Unfortunately, these shoes did not stay on very well because the constant expansion/contraction of the hoof caused the glue bond to break. The new glue-on shoes make it possible to apply a shoe to a hoof where previously, because of wall damage, it would have been impossible to nail a shoe to the hoof.

Mustad's system has five different variations, Glu-Strider, Glu II, Easy Glu, Baby Glu, and Baby Glu II (Fig. 83–2). The Glu-strider is a custom-made system consisting of a pad and metal profile with hoof attachment tabs. The metal profile attaches to a pad that is cut into the particular shape and form that is needed. It can be cut into the shape of a heart bar pad or into a shape that will compress the hoof. In the latter case, the shoe is excellent for treatment of fractures involving the distal phalanx. The Glu II system is similar except that the metal profile has been deleted. The hoof attachment tabs are secured directly to the pad after it is shaped. The Easy Glu is essentially a regular shoe that attaches to the hoof with the tabs. The Baby Glu and Baby Glu II are pad and tab systems designed for young horses that would be difficult to shoe. This system is available only to farriers and veterinarians who take an instructional course from Mustad. This procedure prevents the system from being used improperly.

The Advance Equine Production glue-on shoe, the Dallmar series, consists of a variety of made-to-order glue-on shoes (Fig. 83–3). The shoes are designed as a glue-on regular shoe for those horses having an insufficient amount of hoof wall to accept a nail. There is also an excellent series of glue-on shoes designed for the foal to treat angular and flexural limb deformities as well as tendon laxity. The only disadvantage to this system is that the glue is somewhat slow to set up, which can be frustrating with a fractious animal. Shoe Bond System's glue-on shoe (SBS 100) is essentially a standard shoe made of space-age plastic that is bonded to the hoof using techniques adapted from human dentistry. The shoe is lighter and supposedly stronger than

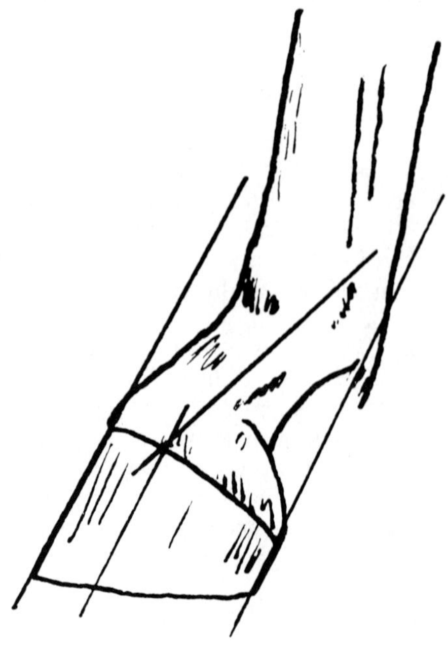

Figure 83–5. Schematic representation of "broken forward" hoof conformation.

steel. The glue-on shoes are the future of farriery. As improvements are made and the shoes are refined, these will become the standard for horse shoeing.

The new viscoelastic plastics that are being used in the running shoe market are finding their way into the shoe pads. These materials have excellent shockabsorbing properties and are being used in many new designs. Some designs apply pressure to the frog while others protect areas of the foot. Often these products are backed by empirical claims, even though there is little scientific evidence to support some of these claims. Unfortunately, some of the substances have not been able to withstand the forces commonly applied to the horse's foot.

Recent studies on the manipulation of hoof angle have shown that changing the hoof angle will effectively manipulate only those structures directly attached to the distal phalanx. For instance, the deep flexor tendon strain should change as the hoof angle is changed. However, the previously held theory that raising the hoof angle would cause the metacarpophalangeal joint to drop has been proven to be untrue. Similarly, decreasing the hoof angle does not significantly increase the stride length. Decreasing the hoof angle does cause the horse to land toe first and increase the support phase of foot flight. Because landing toe first can cause stumbling, this change in hoof angle could subsequently lead to injuries to ligaments or tendons. The increase in support phase of the stride affects the timing of leg movements and increases the chances of a hind leg hitting a foreleg. The actual foot flight of a hoof with an acute angle was not appreciably altered from that of a normal angle, disproving the time-honored theory that lowering hoof angle would increase stride length. Therefore, the hoof should be shod normally whenever possible because no benefits can be gained from changing the angle from what is normal. As more studies are completed, our understanding of the hoof and how to properly manipulate it should improve.

COMMON HOOF PROBLEMS

There are five common hoof problems that have been associated with lameness. These problems are broken hoof axis, run-under heels, contracted heels, shear heels, and mismatched hoof angles. *Broken hoof axis* occurs whenever the hoof and pastern are not in alignment. If the hoof is too acute and the pastern too steep, a "broken back" posture exists (Fig. 83–4). This conformation has been associated with increased strain on the deep digital flexor tendon, proximal suspensory ligament of the navicular bone, and navicular bursa. This problem is corrected by either raising the heels of the foot with a wedge pad or reducing the length of the toe sufficiently to realign the hoof and pastern. Some horses require a compromise since the pastern angle is so high that increasing the hoof angle to match the pastern will cause abnormal hoof balance, lack of frog pressure, and abnormal foot loading. The opposite conformation, "broken forward" or too steep a hoof angle and too low a pastern angle (Fig. 83–5), has been associated with injury to the extensor process of the distal phalanx, osteoarthritis of the distal interphalangeal

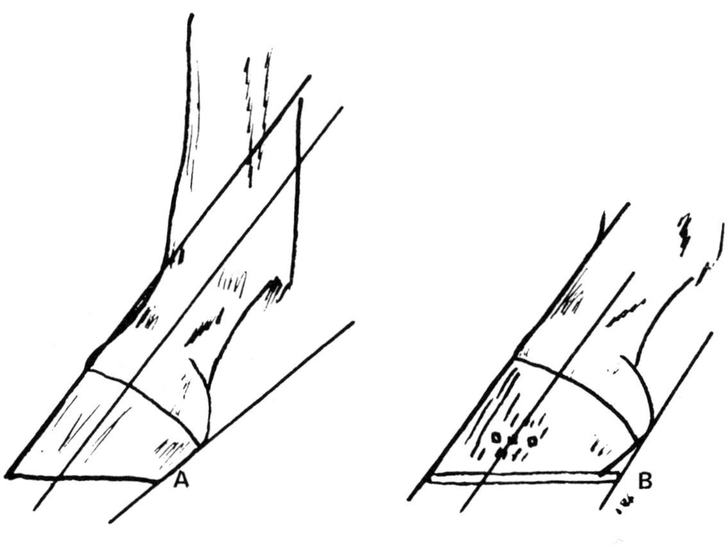

Figure 83–6. A. Schematic representation of run-under heels. **B.** Schematic illustration of how the shoe should be extended back to the point where the heels should be.

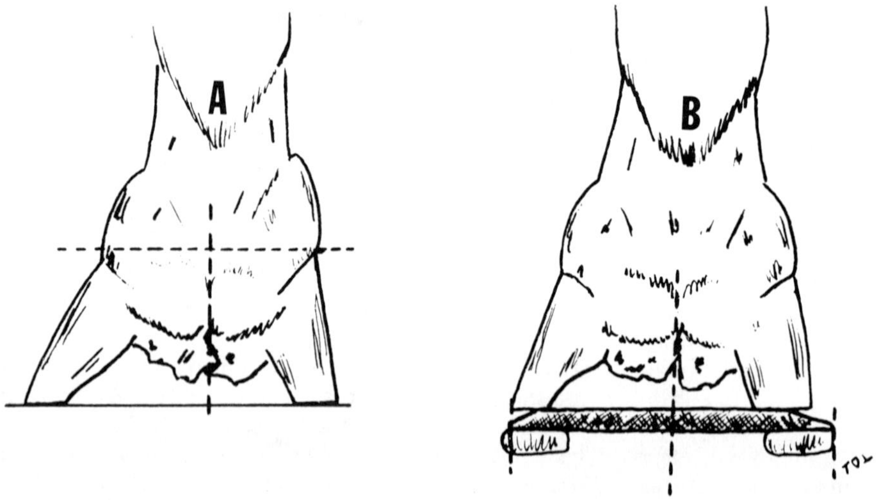

Figure 83–7. A. Schematic representation of shear heels. The coronary band is not level and the hoof wall is flared to one side. **B.** Schematic representation of the shoe applied to rebalance the foot.

joint, and pedal osteitis. This problem can be corrected by removing heel or shimming the toe to add length.

Run-under heels exist when the angle of the heel is 5 degrees less than that of the toe. This condition positions the heels further under the foot than would be ideal (Fig. 83–6A). This problem can be caused by trimming the heels of the hoof too low or using too small a shoe. I have observed this problem in 77% of a group of horses with navicular disease. Run-under heels can be corrected using a variety of shoes. Basically, the heels of the shoe should extend behind the heels of the hoof to the point where the heels of the hoof normally would have been (Fig. 83–6B). This has been estimated to be the level of the bulbs of the heels.

Although *contracted heels* are usually diagnosed by subjective evaluation, the condition was well characterized in one study comparing frog length and width. A hoof was considered to be contracted if the frog width was less than two thirds its length. This condition is thought to increase concussion to the hoof and to be associated with reduced perfusion. In the past, mechanical devices such as a Chadwick spring have been used to forcefully expand the hoof. Unfortunately, this may cause separation of the hoof wall from the laminae. Slippering the heels is a more physiologic means of spreading the heels. The portions of the pad or shoe that will be in contact with the heels of the hoof are filed to taper down and out so when the hoof hits the ground the heels will slide along the filed surface and expand laterally. Other important factors in treating this condition are to keep the heel and toe in proper relationship and to allow for hoof expansion by using a shoe that is slightly wider than the hoof at the quarters and heels.

Shear heels involve an imbalance in the heel region. This condition refers to the asynchronous striking of

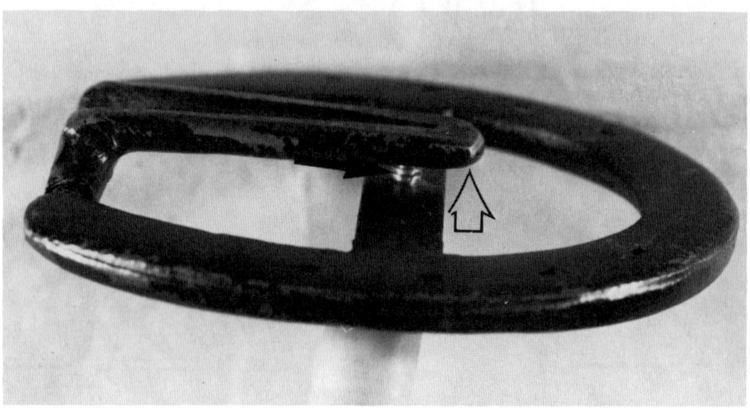

Figure 83–8. The adjustable heart bar, which utilizes an Allen screw to adjust the point (*arrow*) of the heart bar.

one heel before the other to the extent that shearing takes place between the medial and lateral heel. This leads to a loss of structural support in the heels of the hoof, allowing the heels to be displaced in opposite directions. The "overused" heel will usually be displaced proximally and that portion of the hoof wall will be steep. The wall of the "underused" heel will be flared (Fig. 83–7A). The central sulcus is usually quite deep and will often extend to the hairline. To treat this problem the hoof must be rebalanced. The shoe should be centered on the hoof so the forces are equal medially and laterally (Fig. 83–7B). Care must be taken to ensure that the lengths of the hoof walls are symmetric. This may mean that the overused heel initially will not touch the shoe. The heel will drop into normal position with use. This is one of the few cases in which the hoof is shaped to the shoe. The application of the shoe in a balanced fashion will allow the hoof to return to a balanced configuration.

Mismatched hoof angles or the horse having hoof angles that are not equal can be likened to a person wearing shoes with one heel on and one heel off. Although this may not directly cause any problems, fatigue and discomfort are likely consequences. The problem is easily corrected by trimming the feet so the hoof angles match. Care should be taken when measuring the hooves because one hoof often has a dish at the toe. Visually the feet appear symmetric when in fact the hoof with the dish in it is more upright. The hoof wall should be dressed so the dish is removed and the hoof wall is straight before the feet are compared. Occasionally, a horse with mismatched hoof angles also has a flexural deformity. In these instances the deformity must be treated (see Chapters 93 through 95).

TREATMENT OF SPECIFIC LAMENESSS

Laminitis

Shoeing therapy for the laminitic horse is aimed at the chronic case with rotation of the distal phalanx. The objectives of trimming and shoeing are to place the bone in a more normal position relative to the ground and to provide skeletal support. The foot is trimmed by lowering the heels, shortening the toe, and rasping the dorsal hoof wall so it is more parallel with the distal phalanx. This allows the horse to stand on the caudal aspect of the hoof and removes the toe from any major weight bearing. The purpose of shoeing is to further protect the sole from direct contact with the ground while maintaining support of the horse's weight. There are several techniques of shoeing that have been used successfully.

The oldest method involves the use of a wide web shoe and pad. A full bar is often added to the wide web to provide further support of the caudal portion of the hoof. The sole surface of the shoe is beveled so as to prevent pressure from being applied to the sole. The wide web allows for a wider base of support from the shoe. The pad can be used as a rim, thus further elevating the sole from the ground, or as a full pad. The disadvantage of the full pad in horses with laminitis is that the sole cannot be examined and the full pad may apply pressure to the sole and cause pressure necrosis of the sole beneath the distal phalanx. The shoes should be reset every 3 to 5 weeks and adjustments made as dictated by examination (including radiographs).

Because controversy exists about whether the wide web shoe provides enough support to the skeletal column, other methods to increase support have been devised. Most popular among these techniques is the use of a heart bar shoe. The shoe works by supporting the hoof wall in normal fashion, but the point of the heart bar is bent proximally so that when the shoe is applied, the point of the bar exerts pressure near the point of the frog. The exact location of the point of the bar should be determined by radiographs. Pressure should be applied at or slightly dorsal to the insertion of the deep digital flexor tendon. The theory behind the shoe is that the pressure on the frog will stabilize the distal phalanx. With stabilization of the bone, the horse will be more comfortable and healing will occur more readily. In most cases, the pressure point is approximately 1 cm palmar to the apex of the frog. Enough pressure should be exerted by the point of the bar that the horse exhibits mild discomfort when the shoe is applied. Conversely, evidence of too much pain would indicate that excessive pressure is being applied and the horse is likely to be more painful after application of the shoe. If no discomfort is noted, the shoe is probably not providing any support to the distal phalanx. Care must be taken to ensure that the bar exerts pressure only on the frog. If the bar contacts or applies pressure to the sole, solar necrosis will most likely occur. The main disadvantage of this shoe is the skill that is required to make the shoe and then properly apply it to the hoof.

To overcome some of the technical aspects of the heart bar shoe an adjustable shoe was devised (Fig. 83–8). This shoe has the heart bar hinged at the heels so it is freely movable. A support bar is then welded across the shoe near the apex of the frog. A hole is drilled in the center of the bar and the hole is tapped to accommodate an Allen screw. The screw contacts the apex of the hinged heart bar and pushes the heart bar into position. This shoe is then applied to the hoof, and the Allen screw is adjusted to exert pressure on the frog

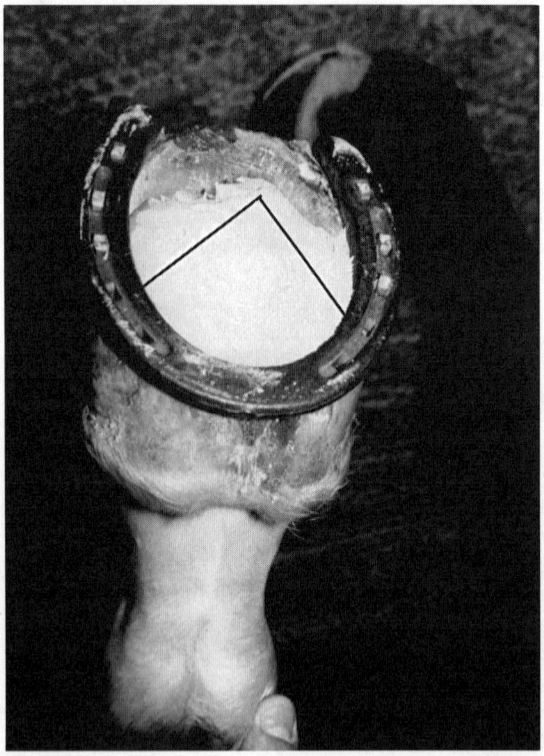

Figure 83–9. The reverse shoe with acrylic poured in the caudal hoof. The acrylic should be trimmed (above *solid line*) so as not to apply pressure to the sole.

via the heart bar. Enough pressure is exerted so the horse is mildly uncomfortable with the pressure. This shoe has the advantage that the pressure exerted by the heart bar can be changed instantaneously for the comfort of the horse. Unfortunately, the adjustable heart bar is even more difficult to construct.

Because of these difficulties, veterinarians have searched for simpler methods of accomplishing the same goal. The reverse shoe has the advantage of not requiring any special welding or shaping of the shoe. New nail holes may have to be punched to allow for proper nail placement. The shoe is applied to the hoof backward and the toe is left open so pressure is not applied to it. Full pads may be used with this shoe but have the same problem as previously discussed. If the shoe is applied without sole or frog support, further rotation or sinking may occur. To overcome these problems, I have poured acrylic over the frog to make a heart bar—like support. After the reverse shoe is applied, a mold of tape is placed on the sole. An acrylic/epoxy compound (Kwik-Poly; Anvil Brand Shoe Co) is poured into the mold over the frog, bars, and angles of the sole. It is poured so it is at or above the level of the shoe. The acrylic sets up in seconds to a very firm consistency but remains soft enough to cut. The acrylic is cut and shaped such that pressure is applied to the acrylic and then only to the frog and bars when the horse steps on its foot. This has been used clinically with good success. It is simple, easy to construct, and can be done by any farrier (Fig. 83–9). It has the further advantage of having the toe open, which makes performing dorsal hoof wall resections, if necessary, much easier. The acrylic can be very messy, and on occasion it may take multiple attempts to get the acrylic poured onto the frog in the desired fashion.

Applying shoes to the hoof with nails is often painful to the horse with laminitis. In response to this problem, the Glu-Strider or Glu II is an excellent alternative (Fig. 83–10). The pad can be cut into the shape of a heart bar support. The shoe is then glued onto the foot. Although this method has obvious advantages, the pad does not provide frog support as rigid as the other methods. To alleviate this, the metal profile of the Glu-Strider can be welded to a heart bar or reverse metal shoe and the shoe then glued to the hoof.

There are also innovations with pads that give additional frog support. Among these are the Poly Hoof

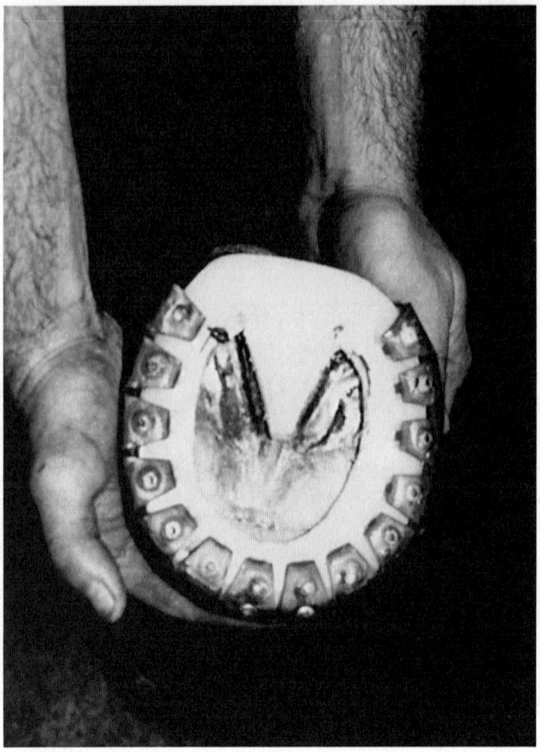

Figure 83–10. A Glu-Strider shoe that has been designed for heart bar support.

(Eques-Tech Inc), Thera-Flex (Thera-Flex Inc), and Lily Pad (Advance Equine Productions). These pads are designed to increase frog support. Thus, their addition to more traditional routine shoeing regimens would probably help support the skeletal system. Many times in the treatment of these cases the therapy is enhanced by the imagination and resourcefulness of those working on the case.

Navicular Disease

Shoeing that is recommended for navicular disease can be divided into formula shoeing and shoeing based on individual case needs. The classic textbook form of shoeing recommends raising the heels by 2 to 4 degrees. This is thought to reduce tension on the deep flexor tendon and ease hoof breakover. A full bar or full pad shoe is recommended to protect the frog from trauma. In addition, a rolled toe is suggested because it further aids hoof breakover. This type of shoeing could be expected to be most beneficial in horses with "broken back" hoof conformation. One study estimated that this problem occurred in 25% of horses with navicular disease. Follow-up studies of 1 year or more after treatment have indicated that this shoeing formula is successful in 10 to 25% of cases.

The use of an egg bar shoe as the only means of treatment has also been recommended for navicular disease. The egg bar supports the caudal aspect of the hoof because it extends well behind the heels of the hoof. This formula also suggests the use of a rolled toe. This shoeing method would be most beneficial in treating horses with run-under heels. It is estimated that 77% of the horses with navicular disease have run-under heels and that in 56% run-under heels is the only hoof abnormality present. Egg bar shoeing for navicular disease has resulted in 57% of the horses treated remaining sound for periods of 12 to 40 months.

It has been suggested that formula shoeing be abandoned in lieu of shoeing each horse with navicular disease based on its own individual needs. The horse should be shod to correct any preexisting hoof abnormalities such as a broken hoof axis or run-under heels. The objective is to obtain a balanced and properly aligned hoof. Next, steps must be taken to ensure proper hoof expansion. This may require a slippered heel technique, thinning the hoof wall in the quarters to make them more pliable, or more simply not placing nails caudal to the bend in the quarters and properly cupping the sole of the hoof. Others have found that by just giving enough support to the caudal aspect of the hoof, including the frog, the horse will begin landing on the hoof more naturally, which stimulates normal expansion. Finally, the work of moving the foot should be decreased. This is most easily accomplished by use of the rolled toe. This method of shoeing has been most successful when used early in the disease. In one report, 29 of 30 horses treated within 10 months of the first sign of lameness remained sound for up to 54 months, whereas only 7 of 13 horses that had been lame for 1 year or longer remained sound. That study emphasizes the need for early recognition and treatment of problems involving the caudal aspect of the foot.

BIBLIOGRAPHY

Butler KD: The prevention of lameness by physiologically sound horseshoeing. *Proc Am Assoc Equine Pract* 1985; pp 465–475.

Goetz TE: Anatomic, hoof, and shoeing consideration for the treatment of laminitis in horses. *J Am Vet Med Assoc* 1987;190:1323–1331.

Moyer W: The basics of corrective shoeing. *Compend Cont Educ Pract Vet* 1980;2:S193—S199.

Moyer W, Anderson JP: Lameness caused by improper shoeing. *J Am Vet Med Assoc* 1975;166:47–52.

Turner TA: Navicular disease management: Shoeing principles. *Proc Am Assoc Equine Pract* 1986; pp 625–633.

84
Ultrasonic Evaluation of Tendons and Ligaments

Virginia B. Reef

Horses of all ages, breeds, and sex can be affected with tendon or ligament injuries. The most common injury to the flexor tendons or suspensory ligament is associated with highspeed work and is therefore more commonly seen in racehorses or other groups of horses that work at near-maximal speed. Horses that race on the flat, such as Thoroughbreds, Standardbreds, Arabians, and Quarter Horses, tend to be younger than horses that race over fences, compete in combined training, or are used as barrel racers, cutting horses, or polo ponies. Other occupations for horses with a lower incidence of these problems include show hunters, dressage horses, endurance horses, and pleasure horses. Lacerations or other traumatic injuries to the tendinous or ligamentous structures may occur in any age horse and are less common.

The frequency of injuries to the various tendinous and ligamentous structures varies with the breed of the horse and type of work performed. The left foreleg of Thoroughbred and Standardbred racehorses is more commonly injured in the United States, whereas injuries occur with equal frequency to the left and right foreleg in horses used for steeplechase, jumping, three-day eventers, and other types of performance. Injuries to the superficial digital flexor tendon are most common in all types of horses performing at speed. These injuries are more common in Thoroughbred racehorses when compared to the Standardbred racehorse. Although bowed tendons are the most common tendon or ligament injury in the Standardbred racehorse, suspensory ligament injuries occur frequently in both the fore and hind limbs.

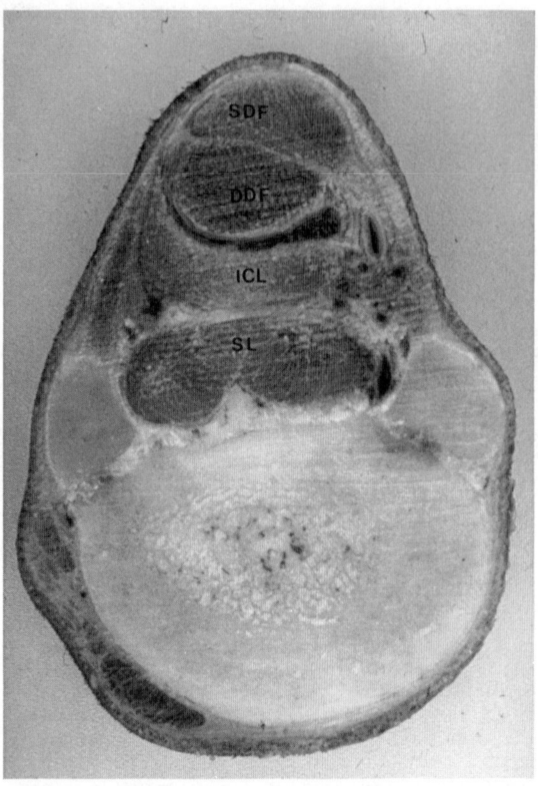

Figure 84–1. Cross-section through the proximal metacarpus (zone 1A) from a normal horse showing the anatomy and interrelationships of the superficial digital flexor tendon (*SDF*), deep digital flexor tendon (*DDF*), inferior check ligament (*ICL*), and suspensory ligament (*SL*). The origin of the suspensory ligament is bilobed in this zone.

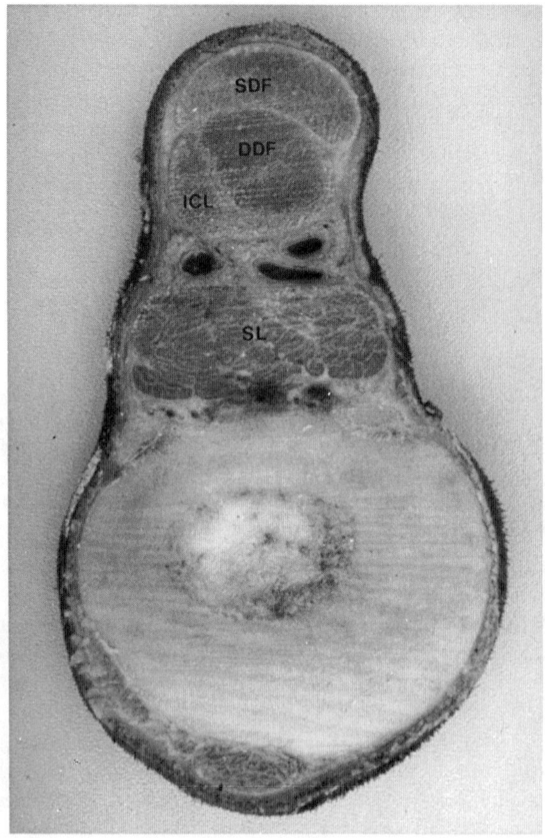

Figure 84–2. Cross-section of the limb of a horse taken near the junction of the proximal and midmetacarpal region in zone 2B. Notice the anatomy and interrelationships of the superficial digital flexor tendon (*SDF*), deep digital flexor tendon (*DDF*), inferior check ligament (*ICL*), and suspensory ligament (*SL*). Note that the inferior check ligament inserts into the deep digital flexor tendon at this level.

DIAGNOSIS

The majority of horses with injuries of the flexor tendons or suspensory ligament have a history of having completed a fast workout, competition, or race within the previous 48 hours. The most consistent complaint is swelling in the area of the tendon or ligament, fol-

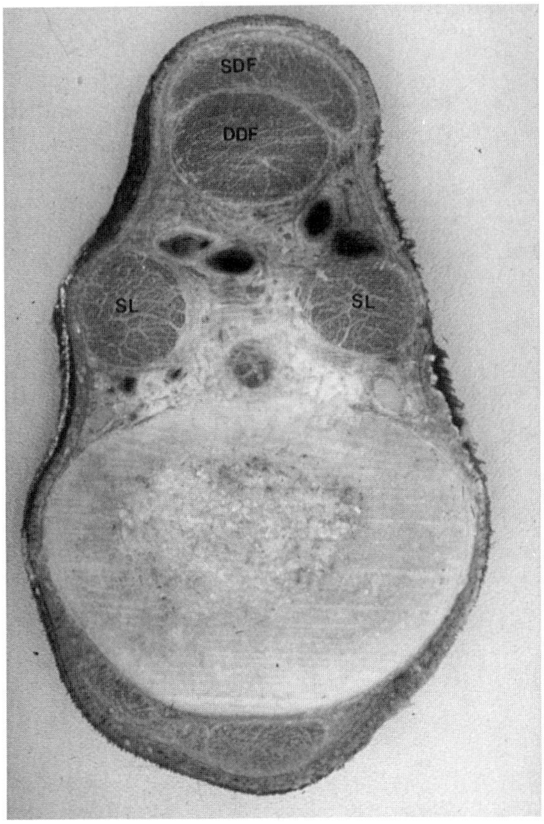

Figure 84–3. Cross-section of an equine limb taken near the junction of the mid- and distal third of the metacarpus. Notice the anatomy and interrelationships of the superficial digital flexor tendon (*SDF*), deep digital flexor tendon (*DDF*), and suspensory ligament (*SL*) in zone 3B. The inferior check ligament has already inserted into the deep digital flexor tendon and the suspensory ligament has split into medial and lateral branches.

lowed by heat and sensitivity on palpation of the affected area. Historically, lameness has been present in only slightly less than 50% of the cases at the time that the injury occurred or in the days that followed. A rapid response to aggressive local therapy, including cold water hydrotherapy, poulticing, anti-inflammatory drugs, and stall rest with controlled walking, often results in a dramatic improvement in these signs. Lameness is present in less than 50% of the horses when they are presented for evaluation. Abnormal angulation of the limb (dropped fetlock, subluxation of the pastern) may be present with severe damage to the tendinous or ligamentous structures. In most cases, however, abnormal limb configuration will not be one of the historic or presenting signs.

Prior to the advent of ultrasonography the diagnosis of bowed tendons, suspensory ligament desmitis, or other tendon and ligament injuries in the horse was based on historic and physical examination findings. The response of the affected area to topical or systemic therapy was also used in assessing the severity of the injury. Diagnostic ultrasonography has provided the clinician with an accurate and reliable means of confirming a diagnosis in horses in which tendon or ligament disease is suspected. Diagnostic ultrasonography should be considered in all horses in which swelling has been noted in the tendon or ligament region or in which heat or sensitivity to palpation of these structures was noted. Lameness, in the absence of tendon or ligament swelling, is unlikely to be associated with tendon or ligament damage. However, ultrasonography should be considered in horses in which lameness is the primary presenting complaint when other diagnostic modalities, such as diagnostic nerve blocks and ra-

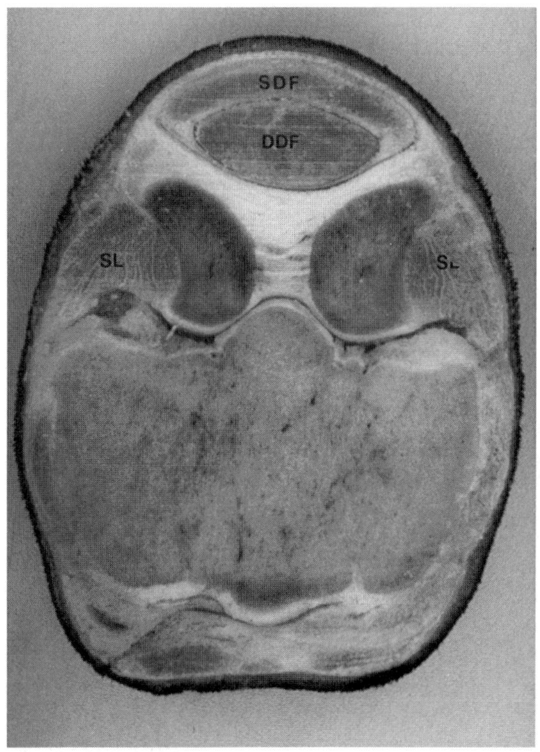

Figure 84–4. Cross-section of the distal metacarpal region in a normal horse at zone 3C. Notice the anatomy and interrelationships of the superficial digital flexor tendon (*SDF*), deep digital flexor tendon (*DDF*), and suspensory ligament (*SL*). Here the medial and lateral branches of the suspensory ligament insert on their respective sesamoid bones.

diology, have been employed and suggest a possible tendon or ligament injury.

ULTRASONOGRAPHIC ANATOMY

Thorough knowledge of the normal anatomy of the tendinous and ligamentous structures and their interrelationships to one another is essential for the interpretation of the sonogram. Each tendinous or ligamentous structure has its own characteristic appearance and changes shape from its origin to its insertion. The palmar surface of the limb is routinely scanned from the proximal-most portion of the metacarpus below the accessory carpal bone to the metacarpophalangeal joint. This region is often divided into six zones approximately 4 cm in length, which have been labeled lA, 1B, 2A, 2B, 3A, and 3B. An additional zone, 3C, has been added to incorporate the distal-most portions of the superficial and deep digital flexor tendons as they cross over the palmar aspect of the fetlock joint. The site being examined can also be measured in centimeters from the point of the accessory carpal bone so that the precise location of an injury can be reproduced on subsequent examinations.

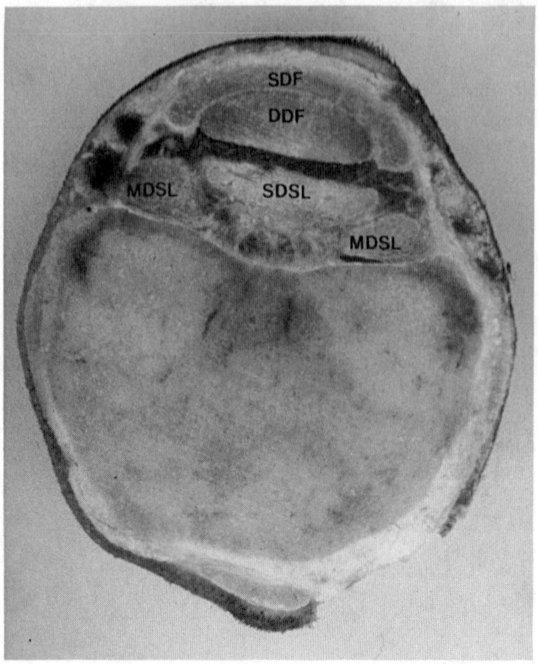

Figure 84–5. Cross-section of a normal equine limb taken in the proximal pastern region. Notice the relationship of the superficial digital flexor tendon (*SDF*), deep digital flexor tendon (*DDF*), middle distal sesamoidan ligament (*MDSL*), and straight distal sesamoidean ligament (*SDSL*).

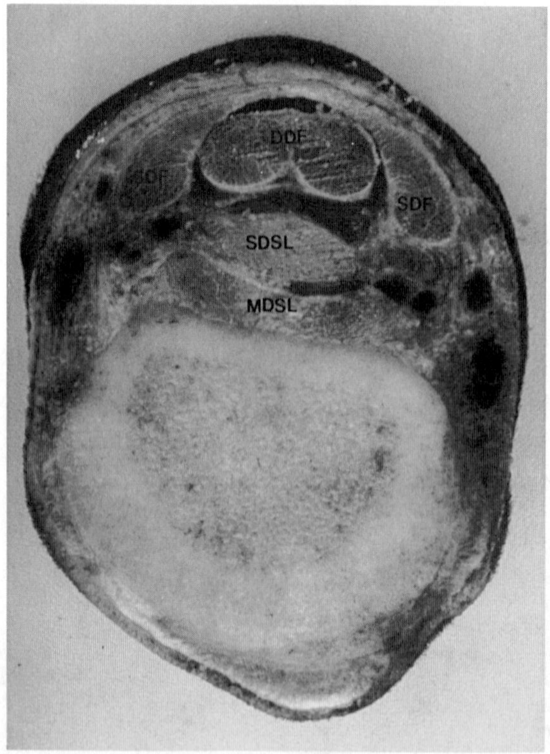

Figure 84–6. Cross-section through the midpastern region in a normal horse. Notice the superficial digital flexor tendon (*SDF*), deep digital flexor tendon (*DDF*), straight distal sesamoidean ligament (*SDSL*), and middle distal sesamoidean ligament (*MDSL*).

The superficial digital flexor tendon begins as an oval structure in zone lA and measures approximately 0.7 cm in a palmar-to-dorsal direction and 0.9 cm in a medial-to-lateral direction. The deep digital flexor tendon at this level is adjacent to the thin, triangular-shaped carpal sheath, which is located immediately dorsal to it. The inferior check ligament is located dorsal to this and is attached to the carpal sheath. The inferior check ligament normally measures 0.4 to 0.7 cm in a palmar-to-dorsal direction and 1.4 to 1.6 cm in a medial-to-lateral direction. The origin of the suspensory ligament is in this region, and it often begins as a bilobed structure (Fig. 84–1). The palmar surface of the third metacarpal bone can then be seen immediately dorsal to the suspensory ligament. As one proceeds into zone 1B the suspensory ligament widens and becomes rectangular (0.8 to 0.9 cm in a palmar-to-dorsal direction; 1.7 to 1.9 cm in a medial-to-lateral direction). The superficial digital flexor tendon becomes more flattened in a palmar-to-dorsal direction while the deep digital flexor tendon becomes more rounded. In zone 1B the inferior check ligament begins to narrow in a palmar-to-dorsal direction and the space between the inferior check ligament and suspensory ligament begins to increase in size.

In zones 2A and 2B there is continued flattening of the superficial digital flexor tendon in a palmar-to-dorsal direction, whereas the deep digital flexor tendon continues to appear more rounded. The inferior check ligament lies immediately dorsal and lateral to the deep digital flexor tendon and the carpal sheath is no longer visible in zone 2B (Fig. 84–2).

In zone 3A the superficial digital flexor tendon continues to become more narrow and crescent shaped, with the inferior check ligament beginning to insert into the deep digital flexor tendon. A gradual splitting of the body of the suspensory ligament into medial and lateral branches occurs. In zone 3B the superficial digital flexor tendon continues to narrow to 0.4 cm in a palmar-to-dorsal direction and widens in a medial-to-lateral direction to 3 cm. The deep digital flexor tendon widens and becomes more oval in shape (1.1 cm in a palmar-to-dorsal direction; 2.6 cm in a medial-to-lateral direction); the inferior check ligament is not visualized at this level (Fig. 84–3). The suspensory ligament is now visualized as two distinct branches (a medial and lateral suspensory ligament branch), and ultrasonographic examination of these structures should be performed with careful scanning over each individual suspensory ligament from the medial and lateral aspects of the limb. In zone 3C continued narrowing and widening of the superficial digital flexor tendon occurs and the deep digital flexor tendon is more oval. The suspensory ligaments insert on the medial and lateral sesamoids and the intersesamoidean ligament can be visualized from the palmar surface of the leg (Fig. 84–4).

The visualization of the structures along the palmar surface of the pastern is more difficult. The superficial digital flexor tendon can be visualized as a thin rim surrounding the deep digital flexor tendon along its palmar, lateral, and medial aspects (Fig. 84–5). The deep digital flexor tendon begins to appear as a bilobed structure and can be seen until the level of the bulbs of the heel where it passes distally toward the distal phalanx. At this level the medial and lateral branches of the superficial digital flexor tendon have inserted. Just

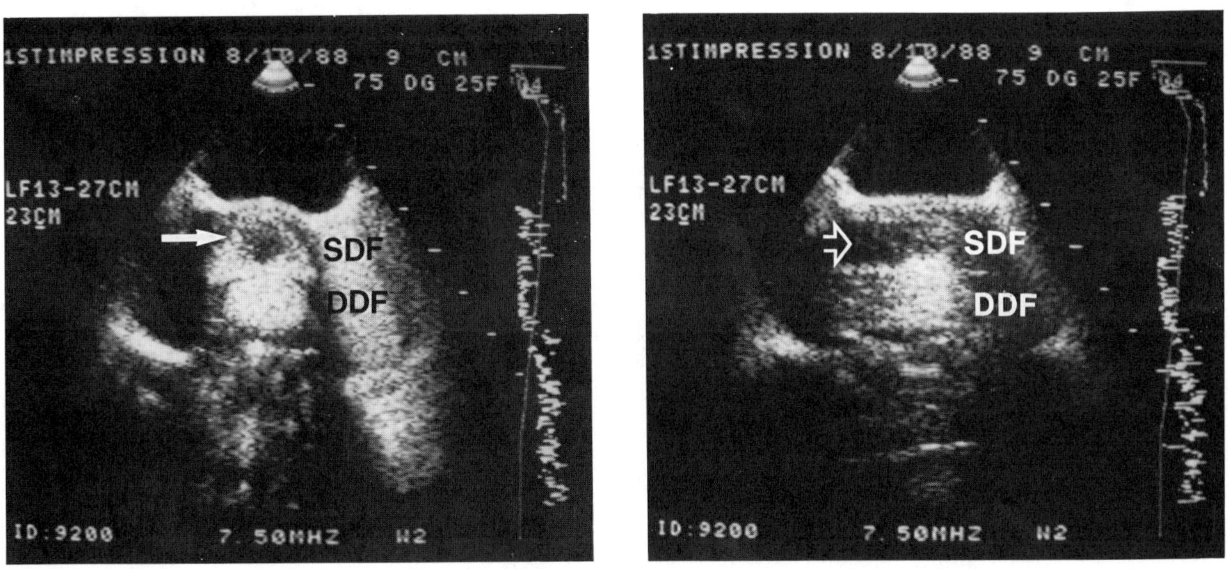

A B

Figure 84–7. Sonogram from a 3-year-old Thoroughbred gelding who sustained a superficial digital flexor tendon injury during training. These sonograms were obtained 1 week after the injury occurred. **A.** Short-axis sonogram (horizontal cross-section) of the superficial digital flexor tendon obtained 23 cm distal to the accessory carpal bone (zone 3B) demonstrating a central hypoechoic to anechoic core lesion (*arrow*) in the superficial digital flexor tendon (*SDF*). *DDF*, deep digital flexor tendon. **B.** Long-axis sonogram (sagittal section) of the superficial digital flexor tendon 23 cm distal to the accessory carpal bone (zone 3B). Notice the lack of parallel fiber alignment (*arrow*) in the central portion of the superficial digital flexor tendon (*SDF*). *DDF*, deep digital flexor tendon.

distal to the metacarpophalangeal joint the medial and lateral branches of the middle distal sesamoidean ligaments can be visualized, as can the straight distal sesamoidean ligament dorsal to the deep digital flexor tendon. At the midpastern level the middle distal sesamoidean ligament inserts on the proximal phalanx as its medial and lateral branches converge at this point. This insertion is located immediately dorsal to the straight distal sesamoidean ligament (Fig. 84–6). The straight distal sesamoidean ligament subsequently inserts on the second phalanx.

PATIENT PREPARATION

Adequate patient preparation is essential for imaging the tendinous and ligamentous structures with diagnostic ultrasound. The leg should be clean and closely clipped to remove any hair from the area to be scanned. Shaving the hair over the affected area may be necessary on occasion. The excess hair and debris should be removed from the skin with water or alcohol prior to liberal application of ultrasound transmission gel to provide an air-free interface between the skin and the transducer.

EQUIPMENT

Because higher frequency ultrasound transducers provide a superior image, a 7.5-MHz transducer is optimal to obtain a superior image of the tendinous or ligamentous structures along the palmar aspect of the distal limb. An offset, either hand held or built into the transducer, is necessary to see structures immediately under the skin surface without a superimposed transducer artifact. The scanner head must be held so that the structure under investigation is perpendicular to the ultrasound beam to maximize the returning echoes and the image.

NORMAL ULTRASONOGRAPHIC APPEARANCE

The ultrasonographic appearance of the tendinous and ligamentous structures varies with composition and fi-

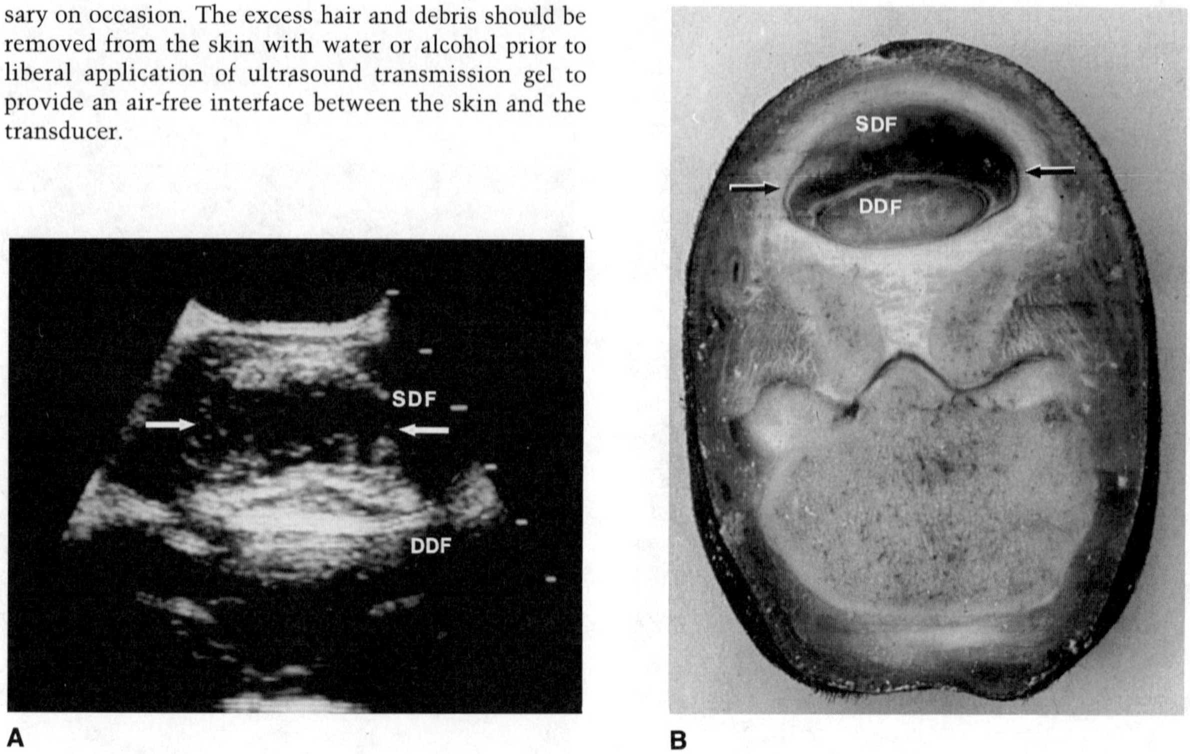

Figure 84–8. Sonographic and actual cross-section of a 5-year-old Thoroughbred gelding with an acute bowed tendon that occurred 2-days earlier. **A.** Short-axis sonogram of the acute superficial digital flexor tendon injury in zone 3B. Notice the large central anechoic lesion involving the majority of the superficial digital flexor tendon (*SDF*). The *arrows* point to the large anechoic lesion along the palmar, central, medial, and lateral aspects of the tendon. *DDF*, deep digital flexor tendon. **B.** Photograph of a cross-section taken at the same level as the sonogram in A at level of zone 3B. The *arrows* point to the large area of hemorrhage, fluid accumulation, and fiber disruption in the palmar portion of the superficial digital flexor tendon (*SDF*). *DDF*, deep digital flexor tendon.

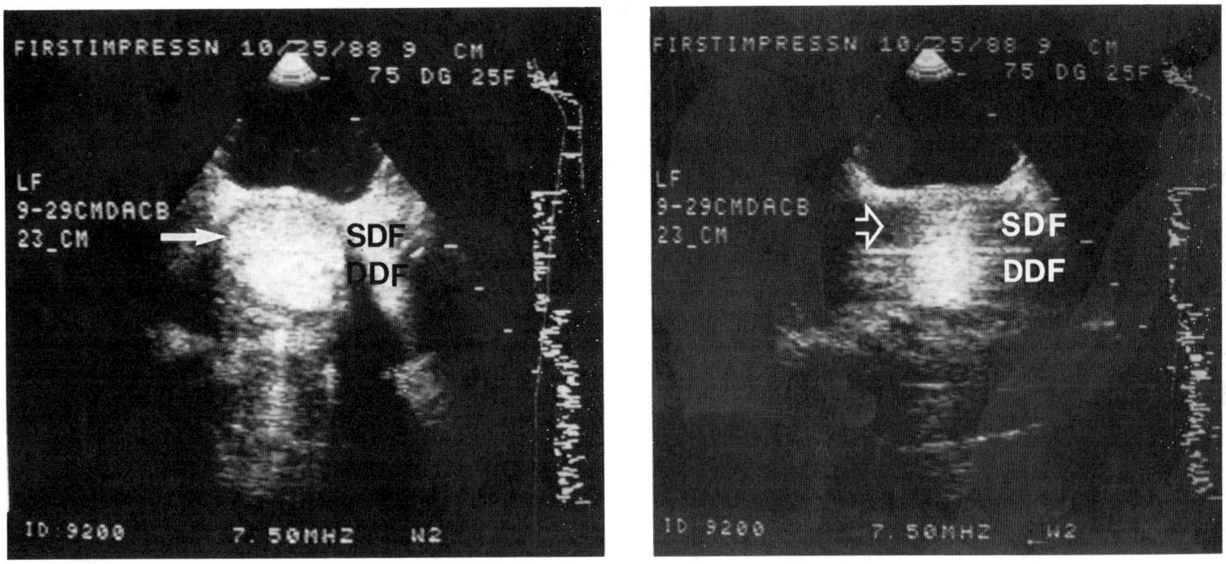

A B

Figure 84–9. Healing injury in the superficial digital flexor tendon of the same 3-year-old Thoroughbred gelding as in Figure 84–7. These sonograms were taken 2 months after the initial scan and show significant increase in echogenicity in the area of the lesion and an increase in the amount of fiber alignment visualized. **A.** Short-axis sonogram of the superficial digital flexor tendon 23 cm distal to the accessory carpal bone in zone 3A. Notice that the original core lesion in the superficial digital flexor tendon (*SDF*) can no longer be visualized (*arrow*), although there is a slight decrease in echogenicity along the palmar surface of the superficial digital flexor tendon. *DDF*, deep digital flexor tendon. **B.** Long-axis sonogram 23 cm distal to the accessory carpal bone showing the increased fiber alignment 2 months after the injury in the superficial digital flexor tendon (*SDF*). The *arrow* points to the area of previous injury, and increased alignment of fibers can now be seen in this portion of the superficial digital flexor tendon. *DDF*, deep digital flexor tendon.

ber alignment. The tendinous and ligamentous structures are routinely scanned in a horizontal plane, perpendicular to the long axis of the limb, and in a vertical plane, parallel to the axis. The tendinous and ligamentous structures appear as a relatively uniform distribution of echoes, which are seen as white dots in the short axis or horizontal cross-section of the structure and white linear echoes in the vertical or long axis section. The superficial digital flexor tendon has a uniform echogenicity that is slightly less than that of the deep digital flexor tendon. Its fibers are seen as parallel linear echoes throughout the length of the tendon. The deep digital flexor tendon is slightly more echogenic than the superficial tendon and has a uniform appearance with parallel linear echoes throughout its length. Immediately dorsal to the deep digital flexor tendon is a hypoechoic to anechoic space that is the carpal sheath. The inferior check ligament has the greatest echogenicity and is composed of linear echoes that subsequently insert into the deep digital flexor tendon. The suspensory ligament has a less uniform and more mottled appearance, with both echogenic and hypoechoic fibers visualized. The suspensory ligament contains muscle fibers, which are less echogenic than collagen fibers. The amount of these fibers varies with the age of the horse and decreases with age. Parallel linear echoes are also visible in the normal suspensory ligament. Both the middle and straight distal sesamoidean ligaments appear as relatively uniform echogenic ligaments with parallel linear fibers.

ULTRASONOGRAPHIC APPEARANCE OF LESIONS

Any change in the echogenicity of the tendon, the uniformity of the ultrasonographic appearance of a structure, or the linearity of the structure corresponds to a change in the affected tendon or ligament. The length of the segment of tendon or ligament affected and the change in its shape or cross-sectional area should be noted. The size of the lesion should also be measured if

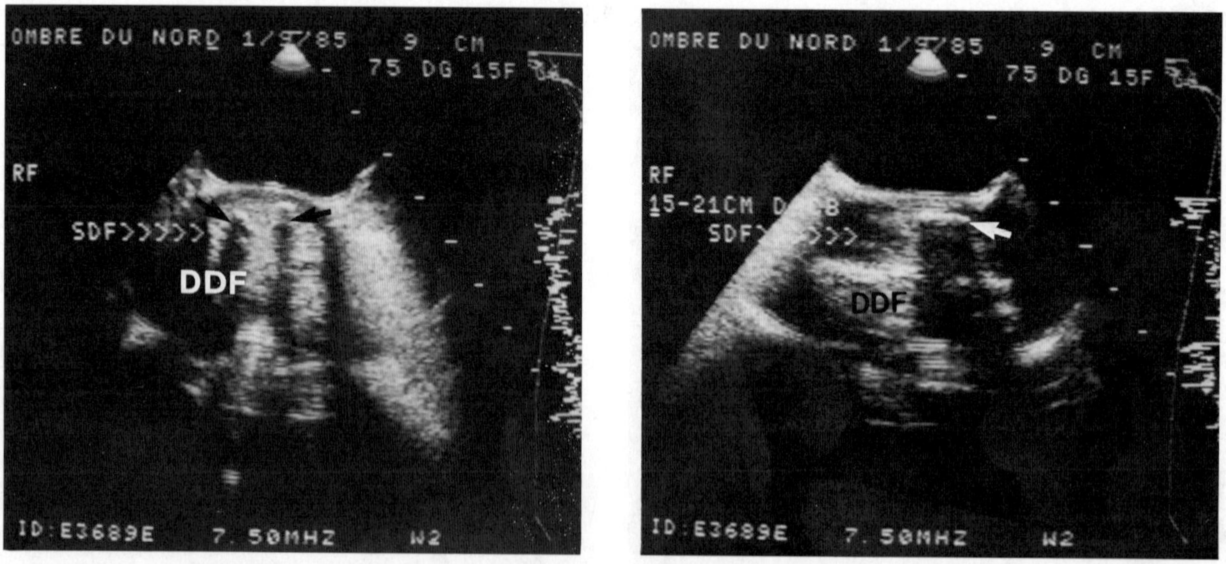

A B

Figure 84–10. Sonograms obtained from a 5-year-old Thoroughbred gelding that show calcification in the superficial digital flexor tendon in zones 2B and 3A. **A.** Short-axis sonogram demonstrating hyperechoic areas with acoustic shadowing (*arrows*) representing calcification in the superficial digital flexor tendon (*SDF*). *DDF*, deep digital flexor tendon. **B.** Long-axis sonogram showing the hyperechoic areas (*arrow*) in the superficial digital flexor tendon (*SDF*) casting acoustic shadows consistent with areas of calcification within the superficial digital flexor tendon. *DDF*, deep digital flexor tendon.

a discrete lesion is visualized. Thus, characterization of the tendon or ligament injury as it heals is possible, with reassessment of the same area on subsequent examinations.

The most common lesion visualized ultrasonographically in the tendons or ligaments is an anechoic core (circular) lesion (Fig. 84–7). This lesion is most typically located in the central portion of the tendon or ligament, but may be seen less frequently along either the medial or lateral aspect. Involvement of the palmar or dorsal surface of the structure is less frequently seen. In most horses only a single area of injury can be visualized; however, on occasion multiple anechoic cores may be dispersed throughout the tendon.

These anechoic cores represent areas of fiber disruption and hemorrhage in an acute injury. Gross postmortem evaluation of these areas confirms the disruption of tendon fibers and the presence of hemorrhage in this region (Fig. 84–8). Histologic evaluation confirms the shredding of tendon fibers at the proximal- and distal-most extremities of the core lesion, with hemorrhage and fibrin in the center. These lesions are graded on the lack of echogenicity from I to IV. Type I lesions are mostly echogenic, with a diffuse decrease in echogenicity compared to normal tendons or ligaments. Type II lesions are half anechoic and half echogenic. Type III lesions are mostly anechoic, and type IV lesions are completely anechoic and represent complete fiber disruption and hemorrhage in the affected portion of tendon or ligament. As the tendon heals, the core lesion becomes hypoechoic, corresponding to the development of granulation tissue in this region. The lesion becomes more echogenic with the presence of immature and maturing fibrous tissue (Fig. 84–9). The echogenicity of the normal tendon may be regained or the area of original injury may remain mottled with hyperechoic, echogenic, and hypoechoic areas. The presence of mature fibrous tissue with collagen is represented by an echogenicity approaching that of the normal tendon, and such tissue may be hyperechoic when the collagen is densely packed. Calcification may be seen in some tendinous and ligamentous structures as bright hyperechoic echoes with acoustic shadowing due to the high acoustic impedance of bone relative to that of soft tissue, resulting in reflection of the majority of the ultrasound beam (Fig. 84–10).

The linearity of the affected tendon or ligament also provides information relative to the type of damage and subsequent healing that has taken place in the tendon. A diffusely hypoechoic tendon or ligament without a discrete lesion and normal fiber alignment is consistent with a tendinitis, swelling and inflammation of the tendon in the absence of fiber disruption. Loss of linearity of the tendon and ligament fibers is consistent with previous fiber disruption and repair of this area with granulation tissue and immature and maturing fibrous tissue. In some horses a discrete lesion cannot be visualized but the tendon is markedly enlarged, with variable echogenicity consistent with areas of hemorrhage and intermittent fiber disruption (Fig. 84–11). Loss of the normal linearity of the tendon will be noted in these cases as well, both in the acute phase and during the healing process. Thus, diagnostic ultrasonography provides an accurate method of diagnosing tendon or ligament injury and characterizing the tissue in the damaged area.

The severity of the injury to the affected tendon or ligamentous structure is described by the type of lesion, the size of the lesion, the extent or length of the lesion, and the percentage of the tendinous or ligamentous structure affected. The more severe injuries are the larger lesions, involving the majority of the tendon or ligamentous structure in its cross-sectional area, and extending for the entire length of the affected structure from its origin to insertion. Horses with these injuries are readily differentiated from those in which the tendinous and ligamentous structures are normal but

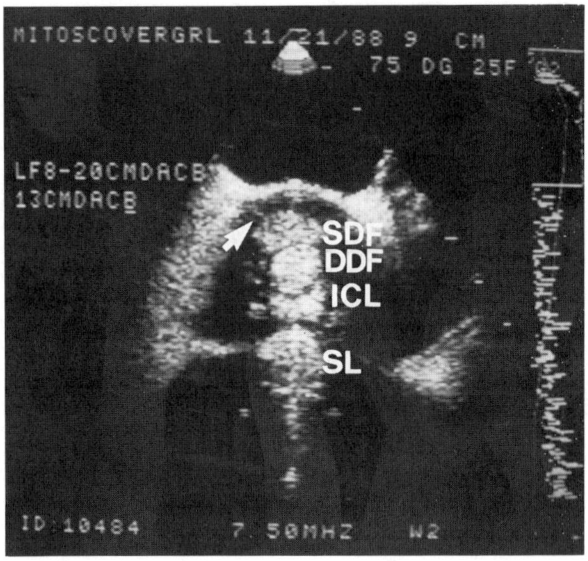

Figure 84–12. Short-axis sonogram taken from a 5-year-old Quarter Horse mare with a bandage bow and peritendonous fluid accumulation but no evidence of tendon injury. The *arrow* points to the peritendinous fluid accumulation surrounding the superficial digital flexor tendon (*SDF*), deep digital flexor tendon (*DDF*), inferior check ligament (*ICL*), and suspensory ligament (*SL*).

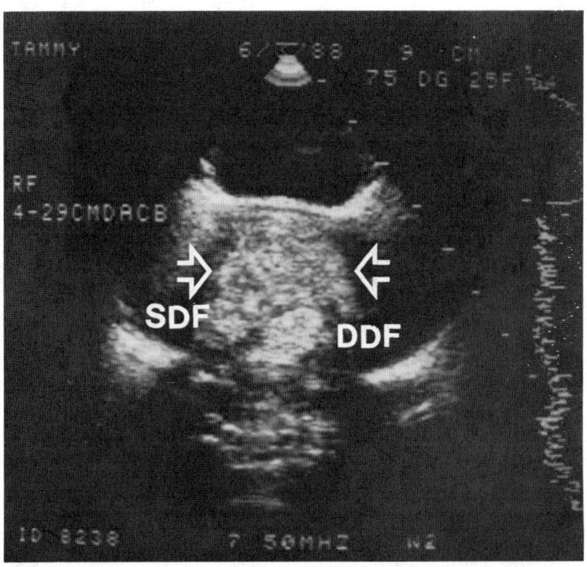

Figure 84–11. Short-axis sonogram of a 10-year-old Thoroughbred mare with an acute superficial digital flexor tendon (*SDF*) injury with intermittent fiber disruption and no discrete core lesion visible (*arrows*). *DDF*, deep digital flexor tendon.

there is peritendinous fluid accumulation (Fig. 84–12) or fluid accumulation within the digital or carpal sheath (Fig. 84–13). In these horses the ultrasonographic appearance of the tendons and ligaments is normal, as is their fiber alignment. A large anechoic space is visualized between the tendons and ligaments and the overlying skin (Fig. 84–12) or within the digital or carpal sheath (Fig. 84–13).

TREATMENT

Treatment of the acute tendon or ligament injury should include cold water hydrotherapy, anti-inflammatory drugs, poulticing and stall rest with controlled walking. This should continue until the heat and sensitivity have disappeared or no additional improvement is seen for 5 to 7 days. Continued bandaging of the leg with a dry bandage is indicated after discontinuing topical therapy. Stall rest with controlled walking is recommended for 8 to 10 weeks until the lesion is filling in and appears hypoechoic to echogenic ultrasonographically. The controlled walking is gradually increased from 5 to 40 or 45 minutes twice daily. The horse can then begin a controlled exercise program

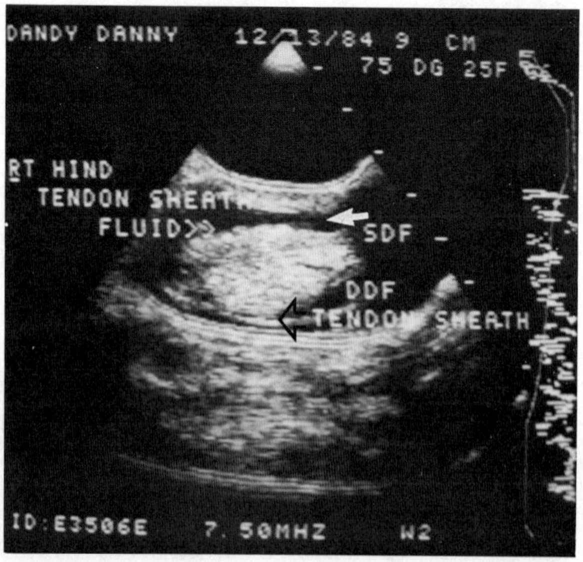

Figure 84–13. Short-axis sonogram taken from a 5-year-old Standardbred gelding with a digital sheath tenosynovitis in his right hind leg. Notice the effusion within the digital sheath with no evidence of tendon damage. The *arrows* point to the fluid accumulation within the digital sheath. The superficial (*SDF*) and deep digital (*DDF*) flexor tendons are normal.

with gradually prolonged perids of trotting or be turned out. Tranquilization is often needed with initial turn out. The horse should not be returned to fast training or racing until the original injury is no longer discernible ultrasonographically; there should be a return to normal fiber density or the lesion should have been filled in with echogenic fibrous tissue. This may take anywhere from 4 months to greater than 1 year depending upon the severity of the initial injury.

Surgical treatments such as tendon splitting and superior check ligament desmotomy have been recommended by some clinicians for the treatment of the acute type III or IV lesions. Tendon splitting surgery is considered to be most successful when performed in the first 2 weeks after injury. Superior check ligament desmotomy is recommended in the type III or IV core lesion that does not involve the entire length of the tendon or its entire cross-sectional area. Tendon splitting surgery can be combined with this (see Chapter 86).

PROGNOSIS

The prognosis for a horse returning successfully to work following a tendon or ligament injury varies with the type of work performed by the horse, the breed of the horse, and the severity of the original injury. Appropriate treatment, including an adequate length of time off from fast work before returning the horse to training or racing, is essential in comparing the outcomes of horses with tendon or ligament injuries.

In our hospital population the majority of Standardbreds with bowed tendons were able to return to racing successfully, as were the steeplechasers. Conversely, the Thoroughbred racehorses were less likely to do so. Furthermore, the majority of Thoroughbreds that returned to racing competed at a level inferior to that prior to the injury, whereas the Standardbreds, steeplechasers, and three-day eventers were equally likely to return to their prior performance level. Thoroughbreds with bilateral bowed tendons were less likely to return successfully to racing than those with unilateral bowed tendons. There was no significant difference in the subsequent performance of Standardbred horses between those with unilateral and those with bilateral bowed tendons. Recurrences were most common in horses with enlarged superficial digital flexor tendons and an intermittent fiber disruption pattern with no discrete lesion visible. Recurrences were more common in Standardbred racehorses with bowed tendons or suspensory ligament injuries when compared to Thoroughbred racehorses.

Although the percentage of the suspensory ligament affected was an important predictor of subsequent success in both Thoroughbred and Standardbred racehorses, this was not the case in horses with bowed tendons. However, the extent or length of the lesion in the superficial digital flexor tendon was associated with the subsequent performance of the horse, whether Thoroughbred or Standardbred. The horses with longer lesions were more likely to perform at a level inferior to that prior to incurring the injury. The horses with the smaller lesions and smaller total cross-sectional area of the tendon that were able to successfully return to performance were more likely to compete at a level equal to that prior to the injury than were those with larger lesions and enlarged tendons or ligaments. Recurrences of bowed tendons were also more likely in those horses with larger lesions.

CONCLUSIONS

Diagnostic ultrasonography is an accurate means of confirming a diagnosis of a tendon or ligament injury, and of describing the type and the extent and severity of the injury. Diagnostic ultrasonography can be successfully used to monitor the healing of the affected tendon or ligament and assess when the horse is ready to return to fast work. The findings on the ultrasonographic examination coupled with the breed and type of work performed by the horse can be used to determine the likelihood of the horse returning to perform successfully.

BIBLIOGRAPHY

Genovese RL, Rantanen NW, Hauser ML, Simpson BS: Diagnostic ultrasonography of equine limbs. *Vet Clin North Am Equine Pract* 1986;2:145–226.

Hauser ML: Ultrasonographic appearances and correlative anatomy of the soft tissues of the distal extremities in the horse. *Vet Clin North Am Equine Pract* 1986;2:127–144.

Hauser ML, Rantanen NW: Ultrasound appearance of the palmar metacarpal soft tissues of the horse. *J Equine Vet Sci* 1983;3:19–22.

Hauser ML, Rantanen NW, Genovese RL: Suspensory desmitis: Diagnosis using real-time ultrasound imaging. *J Equine Vet Sci* 1984;4:258–262.

Hauser ML, Rantanen NW, Modransky PD: Ultrasound examination of distal interphalangeal joint, navicular bursa, navicular bone and deep digital flexor tendon. *J Equine Vet Sci* 1982;2:95–97.

Pharr JW, Nyland TG: Ultrasonography of the equine palmar metacarpal soft tissues. *Vet Radiol* 1984;25:265–273.

Rantanen NW, Hausner ML, Genovese RL: Superficial digital flexor tendonitis: Diagnosis using real-time ultrasound imaging. *J Equine Vet Sci* 1985;5:115–119.

Silver IA, Rossdale PD (eds): A clinical and experimental study of tendon injury, healing and treatment in the horse. *Equine Vet J* 1983;IS:1–42.

Spaulding K: Ultrasonic anatomy of the tendons and ligaments in the distal metacarpal-metatarsal region of the equine limb. *Vet Radiol* 1984;25:155–166.

Watkins JP, Over JA, Gay S, Morgan SJ: Healing of surgically created defects in the equine superficial digital flexor tendon: Collagen-type transformation, and tissue morphologic reorganization. *Am J Vet Res* 1985;46:2091–2096.

85 Annular Ligament Constriction

Alan J. Nixon

Annular ligament constriction is a relatively frequent syndrome in horses and has several different causes. Original descriptions implicated swelling due to tendinitis of the superficial or deep digital flexor tendons within the inelastic canal bounded by the volar annular ligament and sesamoid bones. Alternatively, inflammation and subsequent fibrous thickening of the annular ligament could result in pressure and continued irritation of the tendons within the so-called "fetlock" canal. Recently, the tendon sheath itself has been implicated as an additional or sole source of pressure and pain.

The mechanisms involved in causing the condition may vary, but all result in restriction of the free movement of the flexor tendons within the fetlock canal. Secondary changes include tenosynovitis with effusion of the tendon sheath, resulting in pain and lameness. Subsequent fibrous thickening of the synovial sheath often develops in chronic cases, obscuring the original injury to the tendon and exacerbating the cycle of compression occurring within the fetlock canal.

DIAGNOSIS

Although the pathogenesis of annular ligament constriction is obscure, the clinical signs exhibited by the horse are consistent and characteristic. A history of chronic lameness exacerbated by flexion of the fetlock, and findings of tendon sheath effusion and thickening, and a notching of the sheath over the width of the volar annular ligament are highly suggestive of annular ligament constriction (Fig. 85–1). Most horses are affected in only one limb, with an equal chance of fore and hind limb involvement. Many horses have a history of decreased effusion and lameness with rest and return of signs with exercise.

In younger horses in training an obvious acute tendinitis (low bow) may have developed, but healing of the lesion and return of the horse to work are delayed by constriction of the lesion by the normal annular ligament. Some authors advocate sectioning the annular ligament 4 to 8 weeks following a substantial tendinitis of either the superficial or deep digital flexor

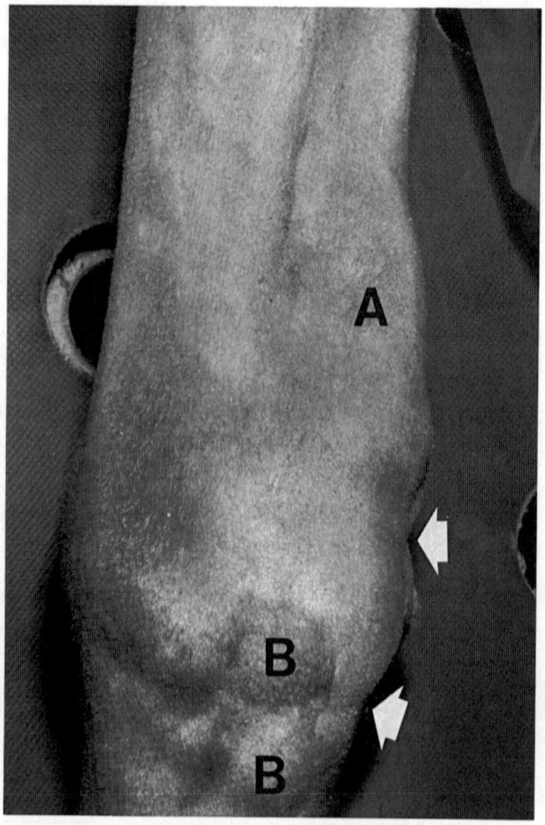

Figure 85–1. Constriction of the annular ligament results in a notching on the palmar or plantar aspect of the fetlock. Considerable tendon sheath effusion is present, resulting in distension of the proximal portion of the sheath (*A*) and distal pouches (*B*) on either side of the proximal digital annular ligament (*white arrows*).

tendon within the fetlock canal. This procedure hastens the recovery of the damaged tendons by eliminating any restriction to intrinsic blood flow or tendon movement.

Ultrasonographic evaluation of the tendons within the canal is useful to determine the extent of tendon lesions, and to assess the thickness of the synovial tendon sheath and annular ligament. Central core lesions of the flexor tendons detected by ultrasonography can be treated at surgery (Fig. 85–2). Adhesions resulting from chronic tenosynovitis can also be evaluated by this method, thereby allowing a more accurate plan for surgical correction and postoperative medication (Fig. 85–3).

Intrasynovial anesthesia is rarely necessary to establish the diagnosis and often does not completely eliminate the lameness. Regional perineural anesthesia of the volar nerves at the level of the distal extremity of the splint bones may be required to assist in the diagnosis if other more proximal limb problems compound the condition and interfere with isolating the lameness to the digital sheath region.

SURGICAL TREATMENT

The most effective treatment for the clinical syndromes associated with annular ligament constriction is division of the ligament. Depending on the presence of tendon core lesions or peripheral adhesions, other surgical procedures such as tendon splitting or adhesiolysis are performed as indicated. Preoperative planning is important to determine the degree of exposure of the tendons required to optimize treatment. If only the annular ligament is involved, severing the ligament can be performed in the standing animal with a curved, blunt-nosed bistoury introduced through a 1-cm incision made proximal to the ligament. In the majority of cases, however, other structures are involved and a larger incision provides access to evaluate and surgically treat these components. Original descriptions of the surgical division of the annular ligament called for incision of the skin over the entire proximodistal length of the annular ligament. This provided access to allow sectioning of the annular ligament and subsequent division of adhesions under direct view. Currently, where ultrasonograms reveal persisting tendon core lesions, this extensive approach also permits splitting of the affected flexor tendon (generally the deep digital flexor) to hasten tendon healing. Flexor tendons having a uniform fiber density are not routinely split, and the exposure required for division of the annular ligament can be reduced to a 2-cm skin incision made over the proximal border of the annular ligament.

The horse is anesthetized, positioned in lateral recumbency with the affected limb uppermost, and prepared for aseptic surgery. For an extensive dissection, an 8-cm skin incision is made parallel and 1 cm caudal to the lateral palmar neurovascular structures on the abaxial surface of the lateral sesamoid bone. The incision extends beyond the obvious proximal and distal limits of the tense annular ligament (Fig. 85–4A). The skin incision should avoid the palmar or plantar midline to allow penetration of the annular ligament and tendon sheath cranial to the normal attachment of these structures to the superficial surface of the superficial digital flexor tendon. The lateral palmar or plantar vessels and nerves are identified and the incision is deepened through the dense fibers of the annular ligament and underlying tendon sheath. The tendon sheath is initially penetrated on the proximal border of

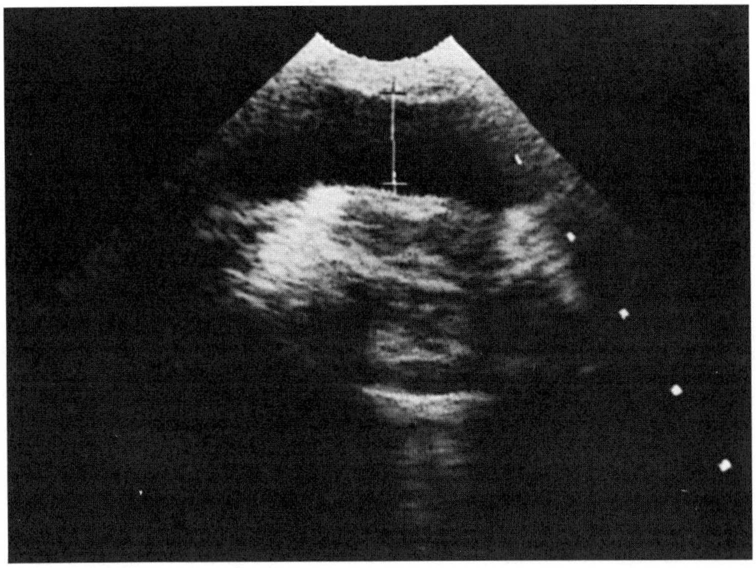

Figure 85–2. Sonogram showing a central core lesion of the deep flexor tendon occurring simultaneously with constriction of the palmar annular ligament. This transverse ultrasound scan was recorded 2 cm distal to the distal edge of the annular ligament.

the annular ligament and the incision is enlarged when a satisfactory plane of dissection is verified. The initial aim of the procedure is to sever the entire width of the ligament (Fig. 85–4B). Care is necessary to avoid inadvertently incising the tendons within the fetlock canal or to extend the division of the annular ligament distally and section the proximal digital annular ligament. Adhesions of the tendon to the sheath are divided and small adhesions between the flexor tendons are transected. The superficial digital flexor tendon normally completely envelopes the deep digital flexor tendon within the fetlock canal and is firmly attached to the tendon sheath along its axial palmar or plantar border. Difficulty can arise attempting to separate the tendons in this region because of this anatomic relationship, although in chronic cases the ring of the superficial digital flexor tendon is frequently disrupted, exposing the deep digital flexor tendon (Fig. 85–5). After freeing the deep digital flexor tendon and dorsal aspects of the superficial digital flexor tendon, a longitudinal tendon

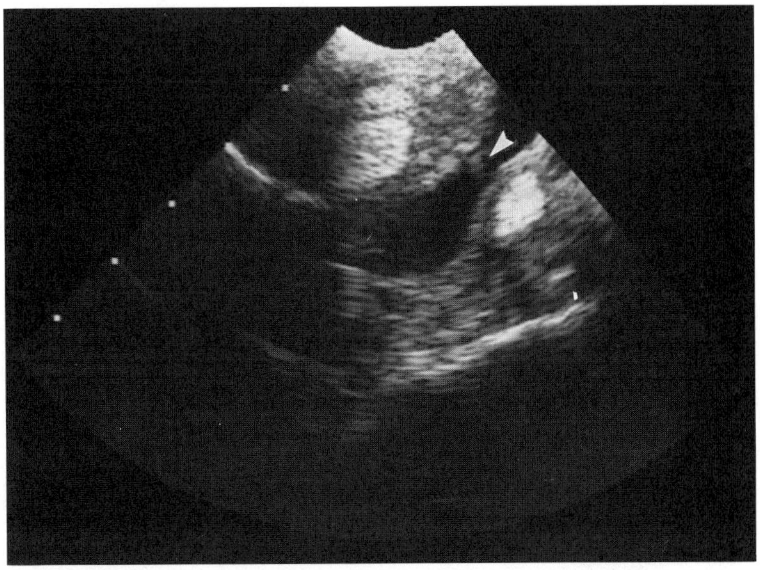

Figure 85–3. Sonogram of a peritendinous soft tissue mass attached to the lateral aspects of both the superficial and deep digital flexor tendons, 1 cm proximal to the apex of the sesamoid bones. An adhesion (*arrowhead*) connects the mass to the tendon sheath near the lateral branch of the suspensory ligament.

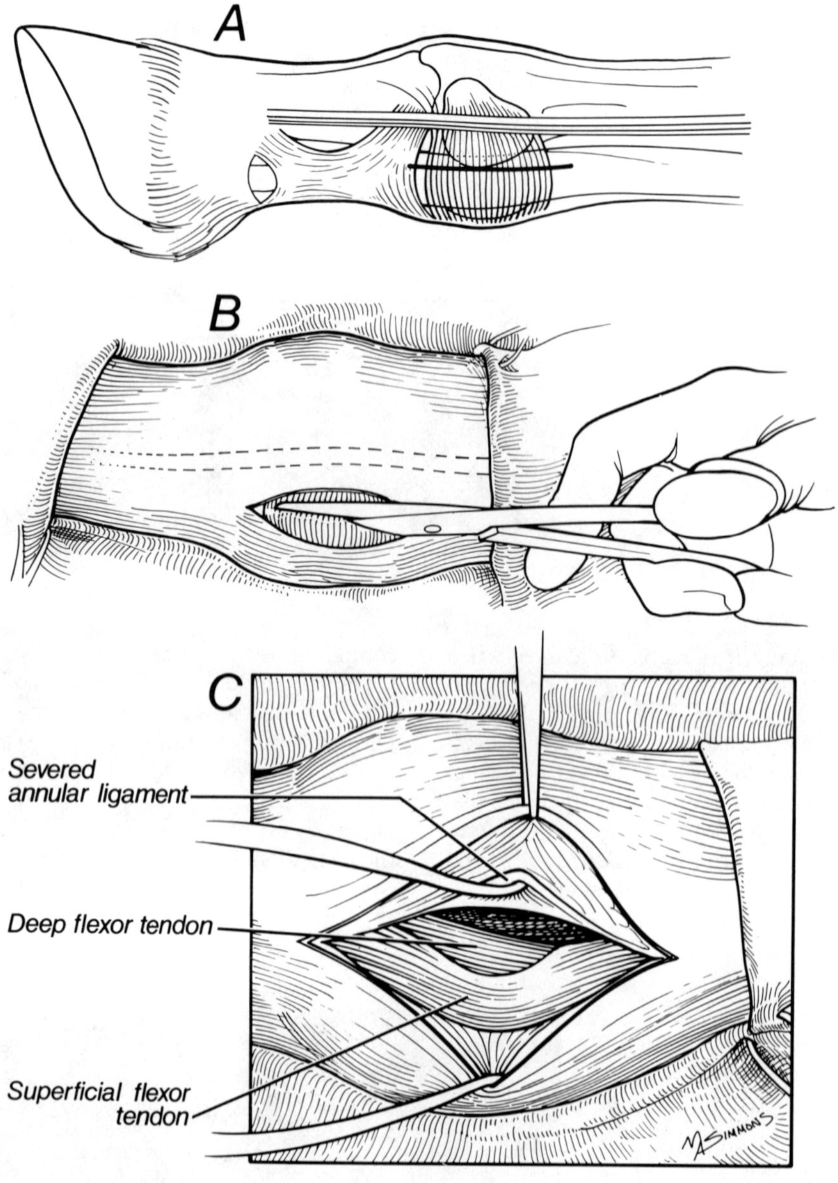

Figure 85–4. Annular ligament section. **A.** The skin incision is made parallel and 1 cm caudal to the palmar neurovascular structures. It extends 2 cm beyond the proximal and distal limits of the annular ligament. **B.** The entire proximodistal width of the annular ligament is severed. **C.** The superficial and deep digital flexor tendons within the fetlock canal are exposed and evaluated.

stabbing of the deep digital flexor tendon can be performed if a core lesion has been previously identified. The superficial digital flexor tendon is not usually affected.

After copious lavage of the tendon sheath, the subcutaneous tissues are firmly apposed with 2–0 synthetic absorbable suture material placed in a simple continuous pattern. No attempt is made to close the tendon sheath or the annular ligament. The skin is closed using 2–0 monofilament nylon and a sterile dressing is applied, followed by a padded cotton bandage to maintain firm, even pressure on the wound.

If the preoperative ultrasonographic assessment reveals limited or no adhesions and normal tendon fiber structure, the exposure required is considerably reduced. The horse is prepared for surgery and draped as previously described. A 2-cm skin incision is made parallel to and 1 cm behind the lateral palmar neurovascular structures. This incision is centered over the proximal border of the annular ligament. The incision is extended into the tendon sheath and the tendon sheath fluid is removed by suction to allow inspection of the flexor tendons within the fetlock canal. If the exposure is adequate, a subcutaneous tunnel is bluntly formed over the desired path of annular ligament transection. The skin is not incised over the annular ligament. A scissor is then inserted, maintaining one blade of the scissors superficial and one deep to the annular ligament, and the annular ligament is severed blindly (Fig. 85–6). Further inspection and resection of tendon adhesions can then be performed as necessary. Following copious lavage of the tendon sheath cavity, the subcutaneous tissues and skin are sutured as previously described.

Sodium hyaluronate (40 to 120 mg) is injected into the tendon sheath at the time of wound closure. Research in horses and experimental animals indicates hyaluronate reduces the formation and reformation of tendon adhesions in the sheath area and may enhance intrinsic tendon healing. A concentrated form of sodium hyaluronate (Synoflex, 30 mg/mL; Chesapeake Biological Laboratories) is viscous and may provide a space-occupying effect to maintain separation of the tendon and tendon sheath in the early phases of healing.

POSTOPERATIVE CARE

The incidence of synovial fistulae associated with the extensive skin incision can be reduced by utilizing the simplified exposure. Maintenance of a firm bandage with careful wrap changes and sterile nonadhesive padding is important. The limb is usually bandaged for 3 to 4 weeks postoperatively.

Antibiotics such as procaine penicillin (22,000 U/kg intramuscularly) are commenced prior to surgery and continued for 3 to 4 days postoperatively. Although some horses undergoing extensive tendon adhesion resection are painful postoperatively, the majority of horses undergoing simple annular ligament transection do not require extensive analgesia. Nevertheless, phenylbutazone at a dose of 2.2 mg/kg by mouth is

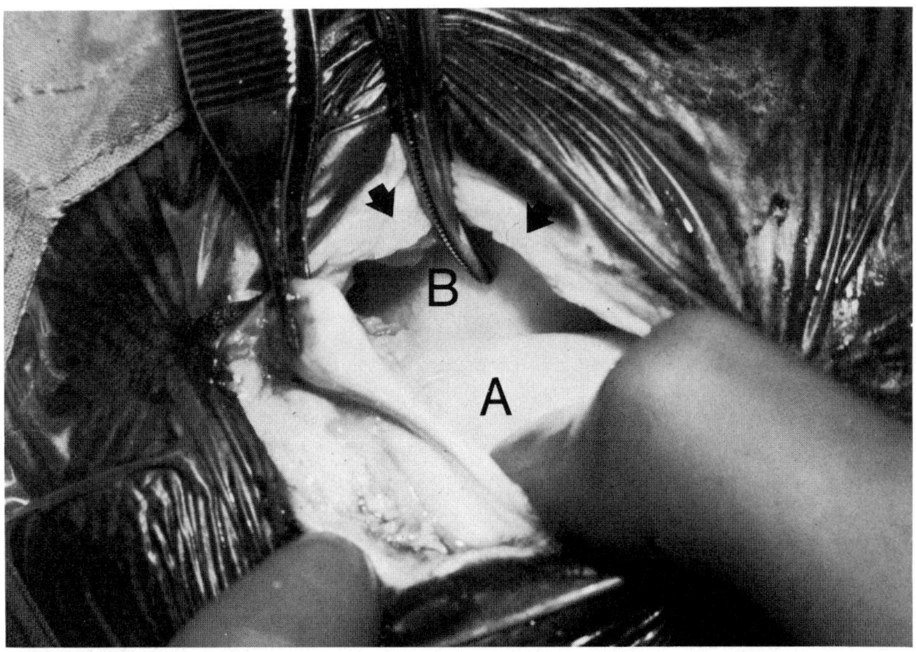

Figure 85–5. Chronic annular ligament constriction has resulted in disruption of the normal ring of superficial flexor tendon around the deep flexor tendon within the fetlock canal. The remnants of the superficial flexor are elevated in the tissue forcep. The cut edge of the annular ligament (*arrows*), deep flexor tendon (*A*), and intersesamoidean ligament (*B*) are also evident.

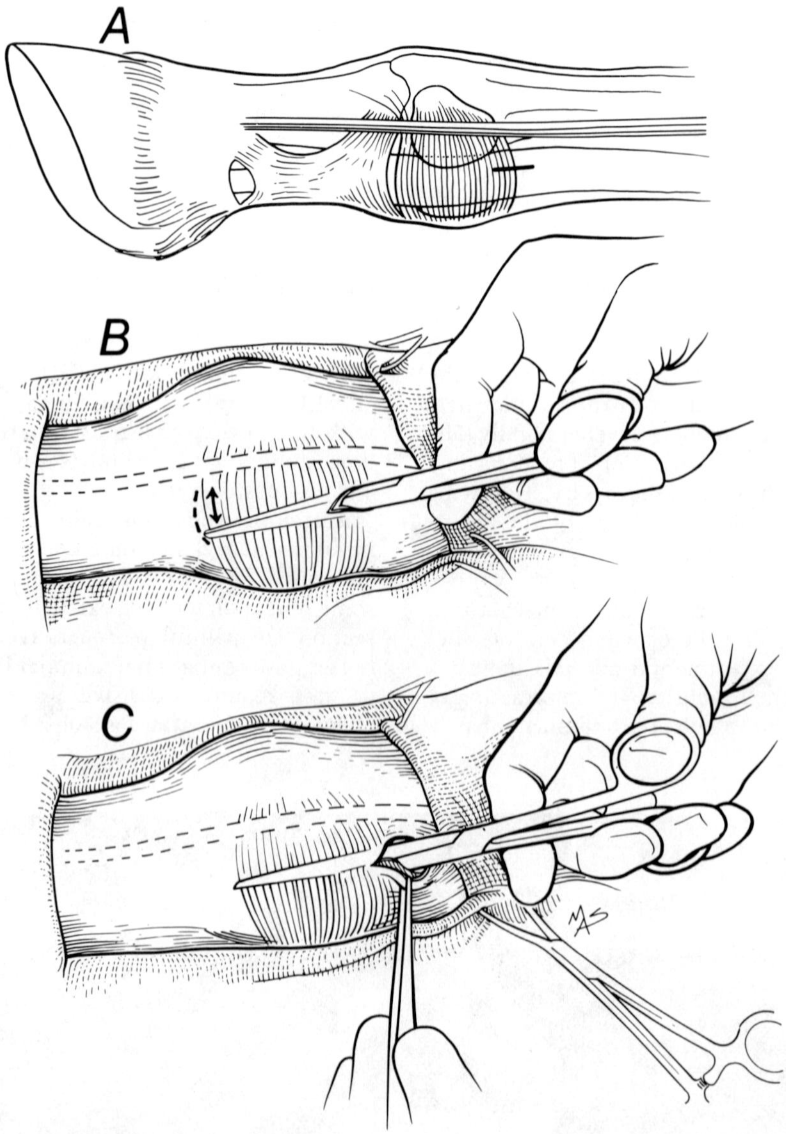

Figure 85–6. Modified annular ligament transection procedure. **A.** A limited skin incision is made over the proximal aspect of the annular ligament. **B.** Scissors being used to undermine the skin over the proximodistal width of the annular ligament. **C.** Scissors being used to blindly transect the ligament across its entire width. Care is needed not to also sever the proximal digital annular ligament.

usually administered for 7 to 10 days to minimize tissue inflammation and swelling.

Stall confinement without exercise is recommended initially, but controlled walking can be instituted for increasing periods of time after 10 days. Long periods of walking exercise are particularly helpful if tendon adhesions were present at surgery. A compromise between the tenuous healing of the incision and the beneficial effects of early exercise should be determined on a case-by-case basis. Use of mechanical walkers, swimming, and passive flexion and extension exercises are encouraged 2 weeks after surgery.

If adhesiolysis was performed at surgery a follow-up injection of sodium hyaluronate is recommended 2 weeks postoperatively. Injection of the digital sheath is generally easiest to perform in the space between the proximal digital annular ligament and the remnants of the volar annular ligament.

PROGNOSIS

Horses with simple constrictive syndromes due to a wound or desmitis of the annular ligament or chronic fibrosing synovitis of the tendon sheath have a good prognosis for return to work after sectioning of the annular ligament. The outlook is guarded if extensive tendon adhesions were resected, because there are often residual adhesions which obliterate the tendon sheath cavity in the proximal and distal limits of the sheath.

Constriction due to tendinitis of the flexors in the fetlock canal is readily relieved by annular ligament division; however, return to work is governed by the tendon healing rate. A guarded prognosis should be offered and extended periods of sedentary activity are generally recommended. Follow-up ultrasonograms are useful to evaluate the repair of tendon lesions, particularly if core lesions were incised at the time of annular ligament transection. A minimum of 6 months and often 9 months is required before the horse is returned to work. Horses with simple annular ligament constrictive syndromes can be returned to work within 4 months of surgery.

BIBLIOGRAPHY

Adams OR: Constriction of the palmar (volar) or plantar annular ligament of the fetlock in the horse. *Vet Med Small Anim Clin* 1974;69:327–329.

Churchill EA: Treating tendinitis with sodium hyaluronate. *J Equine Vet Sci* 1985;5:240–242.

Gerring EL, Webbon PM: Fetlock annular ligament desmotomy: A report of 24 cases. *Equine Vet J* 1984;16:113–116.

Spurlock GH, Spurlock SL, Parker GA: Evaluation of hylartin-V therapy for induced tendonitis in the horse. *J Equine Vet Sci* 1989;9:242–246.

Stashak TS: Constriction of or by the palmar (volar) or plantar annular ligament, in Shashak TS (ed): *Adams' Lameness in Horses*, ed 4. Philadelphia, Lea & Febiger, 1987, pp 593–595.

Thomas SC, Jones LC, Hungerford DS: Hyaluronic acid and its effect on postoperative adhesions in the rabbit flexor tendon. *Clin Orthop* 1986;206:281–289.

Verschooten F, Picavet TM: Desmitis of the fetlock annular ligament in the horse. *Equine Vet J* 1986;18:138–142.

86
Superficial Flexor Tendinitis

Alan J. Nixon

Tendinitis of the superficial digital flexor tendon is usually caused by external trauma or mechanical overload. In the region of the tendon sheaths, tendinitis is usually referred to as tendosynovitis or tendovaginitis because the tendon sheath is also inflamed. The inflammatory swelling and subsequent fibrosis after severe tendinitis results in the classic "bowed" tendon appearance, especially when the flexor tendons in the midmetacarpal region are affected.

Tendinitis of the superficial digital flexor tendon is particularly common in Thoroughbred racehorses. The tendons of the forelimbs are more frequently involved than those of the hind limbs, largely because of the increased weight bearing of the forelimbs. Standardbreds have a markedly different gait, and the tendons of the hind limb are also occasionally affected.

There is general agreement that tendinitis results from excessive stress on the tendon that stretches and ruptures the tendon fiber bundles. Controversy remains concerning the state of the tendon before tendon fiber rupture. Although there is no question that momentary extraordinary stress can rupture a tendon, the majority of tendinitis cases are thought to result from previous low-grade tendon fiber disruption that results in an accelerating cycle of inflammation, edema, hydrolytic enzyme production, and further tendon weakening and disruption. The cycle can only be broken by reduced tendon stress during a rest from race training. The same cycle can be initiated by external blunt trauma, resulting in inflammation and edema. The possibility that primary degeneration of the tendon can lead to fiber disruption under conditions of normal stress has been proposed, but not adequately proven. Several regions of the flexor tendons are known to have reduced blood supply, especially the midmetacarpal region of the superficial digital flexor and the fetlock region of the deep digital flexor tendons. These areas are also the common sites for tendinitis of each tendon respectively. However, an additional predisposing factor may be the reduced cross-sectional area at these sites. Furthermore, one study recorded a relative acellularity in the superficial tendon at the midmetacarpal level, although a relationship between cell population, collagen turnover, and tendon fiber strength has not been established.

More obvious factors that are implicated in flexor tendinitis include increased tendon stresses from uneven and deep track surfaces, muscle fatigue from poor training, excessively long toes and long sloping pasterns, and poorly placed bandages or boots.

DIAGNOSIS

Clinical signs such as heat, swelling, and lameness are prominent when moderate or severe tendon fiber disruption has occurred. However, tendon damage and associated symptoms can be so slight that the only detectable abnormality is pain on firm palpation. Unfortunately, many of these early lesions go undetected, and the fiber disruption results in minor hemorrhages within the tendon substance, leakage of edema fluid, and separation and weakening of the remainder of the tendon cross-section. Normal tendon loads at this stage can lead to much greater fiber disruption with loss of normal tendon architecture, hemorrhage, fibrin accumulation, and ischemia. With time, central necrosis of the tendon may develop as a result of tendon ischemia. Subsequently, the clinical signs are quite prominent and the horse may be reluctant to bear weight, preferring to rest the limb in a partially flexed position. Palpation of the affected tendon reveals a soft, very enlarged tendon with considerable peritendinous edema and occasionally free fluid. Pain on palpation is usually marked. Distinguishing between involvement of the superficial and deep digital flexor tendons may be difficult during this acute stage.

With treatment and time, the disrupted tendon begins to heal by fibrosis, but remains enlarged and often slightly painful on palpation. Horses with chronic tendinitis frequently reinjure the affected tendon and superimpose acute injury and pain on a chronically enlarged, but relatively quiescent state. The end result is an enlarged, fibrotic tendon.

Involvement of the superficial flexor tendon within the digital tendon sheath is less common than in the midmetacarpal region. When these so-called low bows occur, additional clinical signs include effusion of the sheath cavity and fibrosis of the tendon sheath, resulting in enlargement and distention proximal and distal to the fetlock region (Fig. 86–1). Notching due to the inelastic volar annular ligament can occur and may signal the need for surgical release of the annular ligament (see Chapter 85).

Radiography of the affected tendon region is useful to assess mineralization in a chronic bowed tendon. The technique of negative contrast tendinography using air has been described by Verschooten and de Moor and provides additional information about the surface and thickness characteristics of the bowed tendons and associated annular ligaments. By introducing air into the digital sheath and surrounding paratenon and subcutaneous tissues, the tendons can be delineated and adhesions between the tendons and the sheath can be seen. Additionally, soft tissue masses within the sheath can be detected and constriction of the fetlock canal by the annular ligament can be assessed. Although not rou-

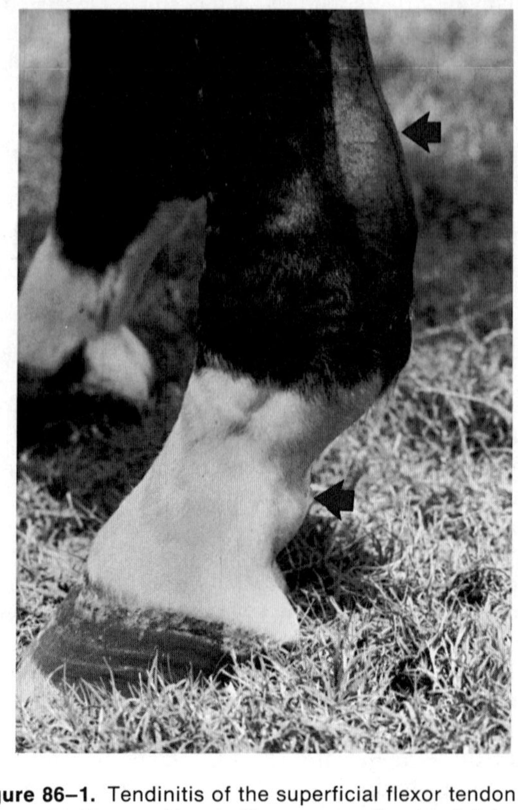

Figure 86–1. Tendinitis of the superficial flexor tendon in a 3-year-old Thoroughbred. The surrounding digital tendon sheath is also distended (*arrows*), increasing the deformity.

tinely used, the technique is useful, especially if ultrasound equipment is unavailable.

The most useful diagnostic tool for tendon examination is ultrasound (see Chapter 84). Its use in evaluation of flexor tendon or suspensory ligament strain has become commonplace. Detection and differentiation of tendinitis from peritendinous swellings and subcutaneous fibrosis markedly changes the treatment and prognosis associated with a swelling in the flexor tendon region. Separation of tendinitis involving the superficial digital flexor tendon from that of the deep digital flexor tendon allows a more accurate diagnosis, treatment, and prognosis to be established. Furthermore, the healing response and early recurrence of tendon damage can be monitored and training altered accordingly. Ultrasonography provides a more critical ability to identify horses that may need surgery and provides a means of assessing the response following surgery. Moreover, it provides a means of detecting early damage before a major recurrence of the injury takes place.

TREATMENT

Therapy for acute tendinitis includes complete rest; application of cold by ice baths, cold packs, or cold water hosing; antiphlogistic wraps; administration of systemic nonsteroidal anti-inflammatory agents such as phenylbutazone; and firm pressure by heavy bandages. Cold therapy is usually maintained for 3 to 5 days, keeping the limb bandaged between treatments. Where severe tendon separation is suspected and supported by ultrasonography, application of a fiberglass cast for 2 weeks and a fetlock support shoe for 4 weeks may be indicated.

Four weeks after injury, the acute inflammatory response has generally dissipated and the immature repair tissue within the damaged tendon is beginning to remodel. At this stage, experimental studies by Gelberman and others have demonstrated that the repair rate and the efficiency of the final product is enhanced by frequent passive motion or mild exercise. Increasing periods of controlled walking exercise are used to improve the collagen turnover in remodeling. The arrangement of collagen within the repair tissue is generally disoriented at 4 weeks. A combination of stall rest with frequent and increasing lengths of controlled walking exercise periods is useful in this remodeling and strengthening phase. Swimming is an excellent form of therapy that more closely resembles experimental continuous passive motion. Return to work or continued turnout is determined by the healing response as seen on ultrasound (see Chapter 84). Most Thoroughbred horses with substantial tendinitis resulting in at least moderate tendon enlargement will require 8 to 12 months before reentering training. Many severely affected horses are retired from racing immediately. Standardbred horses generally have a slightly better chance of returning to work after tendinitis of the superficial digital flexor tendon because of their more even gait and symmetric weight distribution.

Reduced rest times may be obtained by less pasture turnout and a more controlled regular exercise program. Two months after injury, a combination of swimming for a further 2 months followed by light ridden exercise for a further 3 to 4 months has been recommended to hasten the restrengthening of a bowed tendon. A critical requisite for any early active exercise program is regular ultrasonographic evaluations to monitor the return of regular tendon architecture and detect any damage that develops with increased exercise. Modulation of the entire rehabilitation program is generally done using ultrasonography.

Surgical therapy for tendinitis has not achieved notable success. Many techniques have been used for several years, but in the final analysis were determined to be little better than rest alone. However, several current surgical procedures appear to have substantial rationale in the treatment of tendinitis.

Tendinitis of either flexor tendon within the confines of the volar annular ligament often heals slowly because of the restrictive action of the annular ligament on tendon motion, vascular access, and circulation of tendon sheath fluid. Compromise of the fetlock canal also results in persisting tenosynovitis of the tendon sheath, which later fibroses, further narrowing the canal. Although not all "low bows" heal in a compromised manner, sufficient problems can develop that release of the annular ligament 3 to 6 weeks after acute tendinitis in this area is often warranted (see Chapter 85). The improved rate of tendon healing and more expeditious relief of pain are cited as indications for surgery.

In recent years, attention has been directed toward promotion of early return to work. A critical deficiency of the superficial digital flexor tendon muscle unit after moderate to severe tendinitis is the loss of elasticity in the chronically fibrosed tendon. The loss of the regular crimped and co-crimped wave pattern of the tendon fiber bundles results in an increased susceptibility to reinjury, especially at the junction of normal and abnormal tendon tissue. A unique characteristic of the flexor tendons in horses is the check ligaments attaching their substance to the long bones, thereby forming the stay apparatus. Unfortunately, this bone-tendon-check ligament–bone unit relies critically on its intrin-

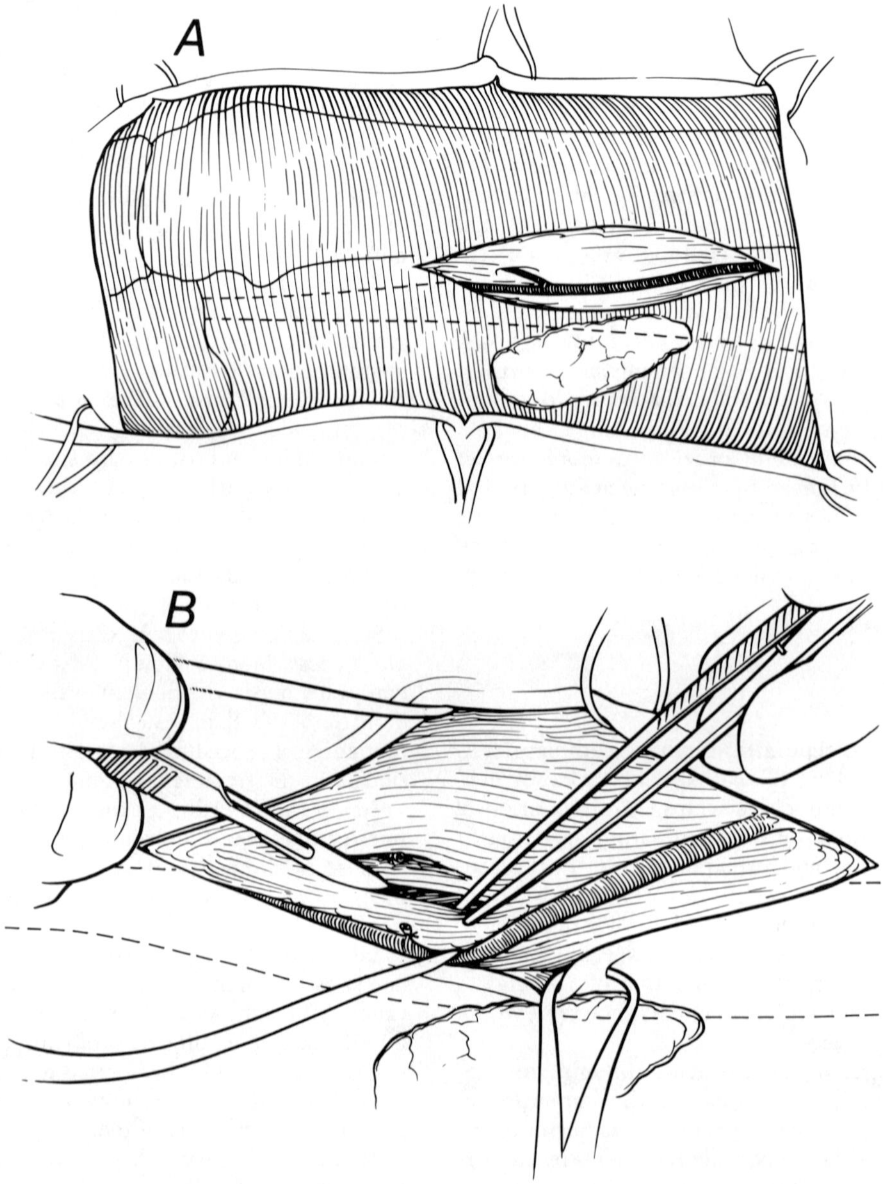

Figure 86–2. Proximal check desmotomy for superficial flexor tendinitis. **A.** Skin incision between the cephalic vein and radius. The vascular foramen in the antebrachial fascia and the communicating branch of the cephalic vein are exposed. **B.** The communicating branch of the cephalic vein is ligated and divided and the cephalic vein retracted caudad. The exposed antebrachial fascia and tendon sheath of the flexor carpi radialis muscle are incised directly over the myotendinous junction. (*Figure continues.*)

sic elasticity for physiologic function and survival. Disruption of tendon fiber architecture results in reduced elasticity within this bone-tendon-bone system and consequently increases the likelihood of reinjury. Bramlage has speculated that by releasing the proximal check ligament, the loss of elasticity in the superficial digital flexor tendon can be overcome to some extent by recruiting the muscle belly into the strain path. Proximal check desmotomy is indicated immediately after the peracute phase of tendon injury has passed, usually at 3 to 6 weeks. More than half of 36 Thoroughbred racehorses undergoing proximal check desmot-

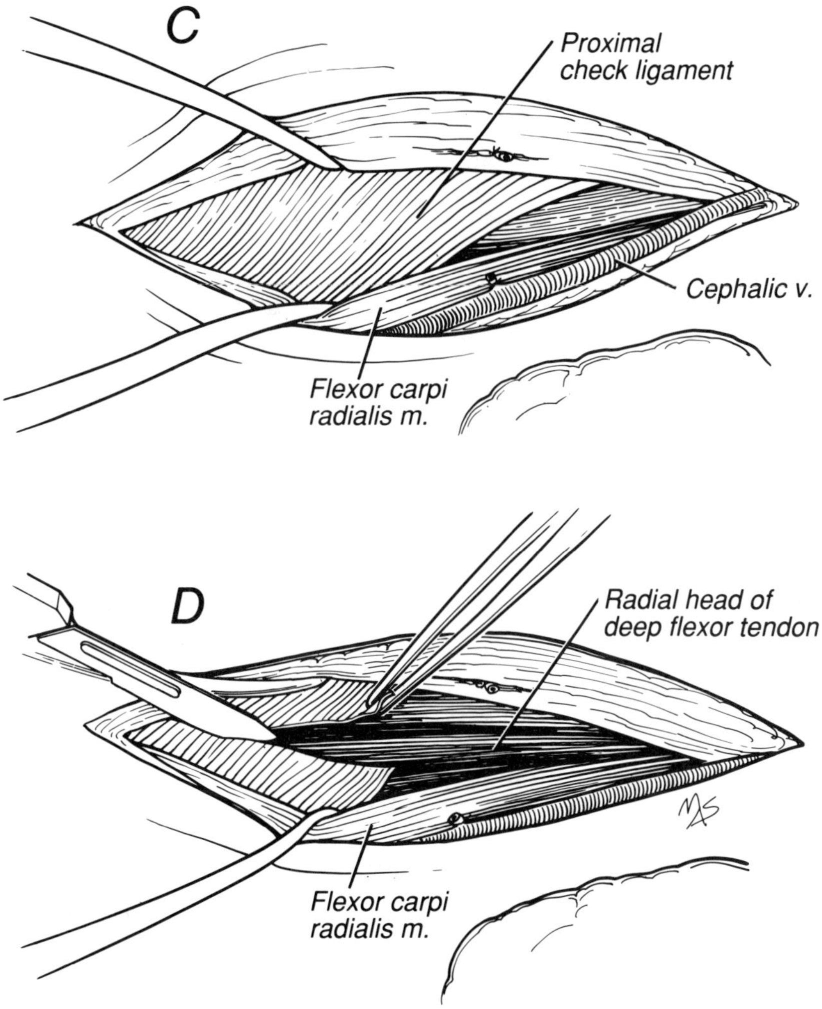

Figure 86–2. (*continued*) **C.** The flexor carpi radialis muscle and tendon are retracted caudad, exposing the combined deep (lateral) aspect of the tendon sheath and proximal check ligament. **D.** The proximal check ligament is carefully incised, exposing the radial head of the deep flexor tendon.

omy had been presented for surgery because they had recently injured the superficial digital flexor tendon for the second time.

SURGICAL TECHNIQUE

Proximal check desmotomy has previously been described in the treatment of contracture deformity of the fetlock joint. The horse is anesthetized and placed in lateral recumbency with the affected limb down or in dorsal recumbency with the affected limbs extended. The medial aspect of the limb is prepared and draped from midmetacarpus to midradius. A 10-cm skin incision is made between and parallel to the cephalic vein and radius (Fig. 86–2A). This incision begins at the level of the proximal aspect of the chestnut and extends distally, overlying the tendon of the extensor carpi radialis. The subcutaneous tissues are divided and retracted to expose the antebrachial fascia. In the center of the wound, a perforating foramen allowing a branch of the cephalic vein to exit and course caudally to the main cephalic trunk is identified by palpation and enlarged with scissors. The cephalic branch is ligated and divided allowing the main trunk of the cephalic vein to be mobilized and retracted caudally. The exposed antebrachial fascia over the flexor carpi radialis tendon, and myotendinous junction is identified along the caudal aspect of the dissection. The antebrachial fascia and the median veins and superficial aspect of the tendon sheath of the flexor carpi radialis tendon are incised longitudinally for 6 cm and the tendon retracted caudally (Fig. 86–2B). The exposed deep aspect of the tendon sheath is thin and blends imperceptibly with the proximal check ligament adjacent to the junction of the check ligament with the superficial digital flexor tendon. The proximal and distal borders of the check ligament are readily apparent and the entire ligament can be severed (Fig. 86–2C). The median veins and radial head of the deep digital flexor muscle are apparent through the divided check ligament (Fig. 86–2D). The proximal reflection of the carpal synovial sheath of the flexor tendons can also be observed in the distal extremity of the dissection, and care is taken to avoid penetrating this sheath. By isolating the check ligament toward its junction with the superficial digital flexor tendon, the thin indiscrete origin of the ligament on the radius is avoided, thereby simplifying the procedure and avoiding the vessels of the palmar carpal rete.

The superficial (medial) entry into the flexor carpi radialis sheath and the antebrachial fascia are apposed using size 0 synthetic absorbable suture placed in a simple interrupted pattern. The subcutaneous tissues and skin are closed routinely and the limb is bandaged up to the midradius for recovery from anesthesia.

If preoperative ultrasonography reveals lesions in the core of the tendon, tendon splitting by the percutaneous tendon stab technique may be combined with proximal check desmotomy (Fig. 86–3). The entire medial aspect of the limb is prepared and draped from the fetlock to the elbow joints. Following proximal check desmotomy, the enlarged tendon is stabilized between thumb and forefingers and a no. 15 scalpel blade is fully inserted through the skin to penetrate to the center of the affected tendon at a 45-degree angle to the perpendicular (Fig. 86–4). Without enlarging the skin incision, the scalpel blade is fanned through approximately 90 degrees of the longitudinal tendon structure and removed. This incision can be guided by ultrasound to make sure the core lesion is opened. The procedure is repeated at 1-cm intervals along the medial edge of affected tendon until all involved tendon has been incised. The skin incisions do not require suture; however, a sterile padded dressing is applied to control hemorrhage and minimize swelling.

On occasion, percutaneous tendon stabbing is employed as a solitary procedure and can be performed with the horse standing or under general anesthesia depending on the surgeon's preference and availability of facilities. Perineural anesthesia of the palmar nerves at the proximal metacarpal level usually is sufficient to allow a tendon stabbing procedure; however, local infiltration is occasionally also necessary to allow an unhurried and careful placement of the tendon stab wounds.

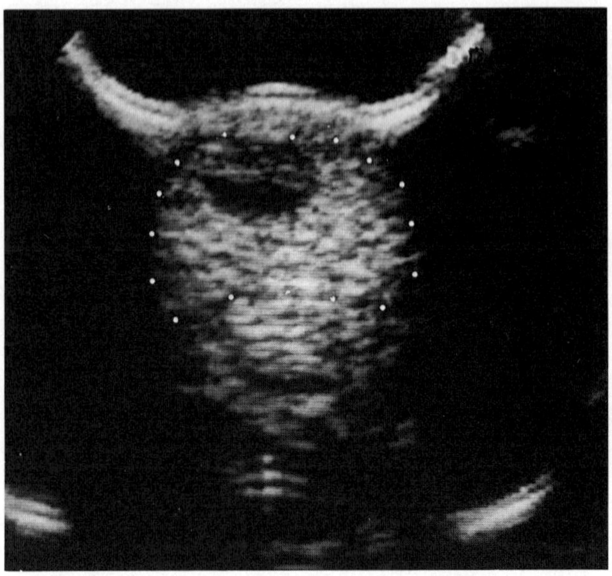

Figure 86–3. Ultrasound scan of the flexor structures at the midmetacarpal level of a 3-year-old Thoroughbred with superficial flexor tendinitis of 3 weeks' duration. The tendon (outlined with *white dots*) is three times normal size and contains an anechoic core lesion.

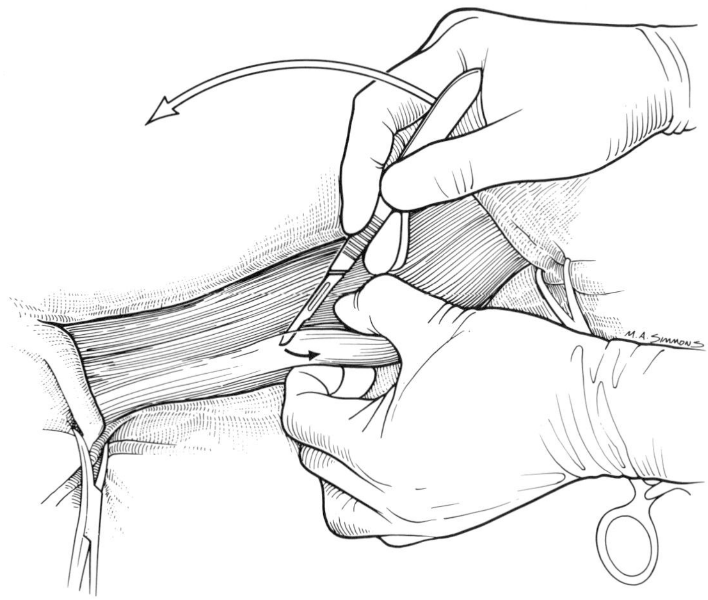

Figure 86–4. Percutaneous tendon stab procedure using a no. 15 scalpel blade inserted at 1-cm intervals along the affected superficial flexor tendon.

POSTOPERATIVE CARE

Perioperative antibiotics such as procaine penicillin are administered at the time of either surgical procedure. Continuation of antibiotic use beyond 24 hours postoperatively is not generally indicated. Nonsteroidal antiinflammatory agents, usually phenylbutazone, are administered for 3 to 5 days or longer if there is extensive swelling at the sites of tendon stabbing. Bandaging of the proximal check desmotomy surgical incision is maintained until the sutures are removed. Because of the extra support needed and slower healing of tendon tissues, bandaging of the lower limb is maintained for 3 to 4 weeks after these procedures, and stall rest is similarly recommended for 4 weeks after either procedure. Early controlled walking is encouraged, commencing 3 to 4 weeks postoperatively and slowly increasing to 30 minutes twice daily by 8 weeks after surgery. After evaluating the healing response by ultrasonography, horses are turned out to a 2- to 3-acre pasture for increasing exercise and can be placed in a larger paddock by 4 months postoperatively. The minimum time out of training is usually 6 months. Earlier return to training may be possible if more intensive swimming, unridden trotting exercise (accompanying exercise horse), and careful monitoring by physical examination and ultrasonography are used. Healing of tendon lesions is most accurately assessed by ultrasonography, and this modality has become an integral part of the diagnostic, prognostic, and rehabilitation programs. Nevertheless, tendon tissue is extremely slow to heal and early return to work increases the likelihood of reinjury, usually at the junction of a previous lesion and more normal tendon.

PROGNOSIS

The chances of return to a competitive race career depend upon the severity and type of tendon lesion and the treatment used. Generally, horses with mild to moderate tendinitis respond well to rest alone and can be returned to work within 6 months with a fair to good outlook. Horses with moderate lesions with obvious tendon enlargement benefit from proximal check desmotomy, in that some can recommence training within 90 days of surgery. However, under circumstances of financial constraint, these horses occasionally respond reasonably well to rest alone. Horses with more severe tendinitis, and those with bilateral lesions, need a proximal check desmotomy and usually 1 year of rest before reentering work. Bramlage recently surveyed 51 Thoroughbred horses treated by proximal check desmotomy, and 36 were available for long-term follow-up. Of these 36 horses, 83% had no recurrence of tendinitis after a minimum of three starts, with 43% improving in class and 34% remaining in the same class. This is considerably better than the results of other surgeries and particularly better than those treated by rest alone. Moreover, more than half of the horses in that study had tendinitis recur at least once prior to surgery and only 17% developed a recurrence after surgery. The total time wasted in convalescence appears to be reduced by as much as 30% following the desmotomy procedure.

The prognosis is poorest for horses with enlarged tendons with ultrasonographic evidence of multiple diffuse lytic areas. These horses respond poorly to any form of therapy, including percutaneous tendon stabbing and proximal check desmotomy, and are at greatest risk of recurrence. A minimum of 12 months rest from training is essential.

The outlook for Standardbreds with tendinitis of the superficial digital flexor tendon is better than that for Thoroughbred horses. In a follow-up study by Bramlage, eight of nine affected Standardbreds treated by proximal check desmotomy returned to racing and successfully started on numerous occasions.

Seemingly, the use of proximal check desmotomy has improved an otherwise poor outlook for many horses. Although the precise mechanism of action remains speculative, an early reduction of load on the tendon and improvement in elasticity by recruitment of the superficial digital flexor muscle belly are considered important. Although the desmotomy site ultimately heals, it may result in a longer ligament, effectively decreasing the shortening of the bone-tendon–check ligament—bone pathway that results from tendon fibrosis and secondary collagen contracture. Therefore, there may be a sparing of the susceptible area at the transition zone adjacent to the original tendon disruption. Watkins et al. have shown that this area retains more type III collagen than the central tendon lesion, which may explain its predisposition to reinjury.

The tendon stab procedure was largely discarded as the only treatment modality for flexor tendinitis. However, it is currently still recommended if a persistent central tendon core lesion has been documented. Such lesions are typically recalcitrant to conservative methods of treatment, and a combination of percutaneous tendon stab and proximal check desmotomy is recommended to improve the tendon fiber organization and assist in preventing reinjury of the entire tendon unit.

BIBLIOGRAPHY

Bramlage LR: Superior check ligament desmotomy as a treatment for superficial digital flexor tendinitis—follow-up results, in *Proceedings of the Veterinary Orthopedic Society*, Breckenridge, CO, 1988, p 10.

Cannon JH: Results of tendon splitting in Thoroughbred racehorses. *J Equine Vet Sci* 1981;1:77–79.

Fackelman GE: The nature of tendon damage and its repair. *Equine Vet J* 1973;5:141–149.

Gelberman RH, Vande Berg JS, Lundborg GN, Akeson WH: Flexor tendon healing and restoration of the gliding surface. *J Bone Joint Surg [Am]* 1983;65:70–80.

Genovese RL, Rantanen NW, Hauser ML, Simpson BS: Clinical application of diagnostic ultrasound to the equine limb. *Proc Am Assoc Equine Pract* 1985; pp 701–721.

Knudsen O: Percutaneous tendon splitting—method and results. *Equine Vet J* 1976;8:101–103.

Riemersma DJ, de Bruyn P: Variations in cross-sectional area and composition of equine tendons with regard to their mechanical function. *Res Vet Sci* 1986;41:7–13.

Stromberg B, Tufvesson G: Lesions of the superficial flexor tendon in race horses. A microangiographic and histopathologic study. *Clin Orthop* 1969;62:113–123.

Verschooten F, de Moor A: Tendinitis in the horse: Its radiographic diagnosis with air-tendograms. *J Am Vet Radiol Soc* 1978;19:23–30.

Watkins JP, Auer JA, Gay S, Morgan SJ: Healing of surgically created defects in the equine superficial digital flexor tendon: Collagen-type transformation and tissue morphologic reorganization. *Am J Vet Res* 1985;46:2091–2096.

Webbon PM: A postmortem study of equine digital flexor tendons. *Equine Vet J* 1977;9:61–67.

87 Suspensory Desmitis

Alan J. Nixon

Suspensory desmitis is a relatively common condition of racehorses, especially Standardbreds. Other types of horses occasionally can be affected, including the hunter-jumper classes and polo ponies. Suspensory desmitis can involve any portion of the suspensory ligament but is most common in the branches and midbody regions. Proximal desmitis and avulsion fractures involving the origin of the suspensory ligament are much less common.

Excessive momentary or repetitive tension from acute trauma, overextension of the fetlock and carpus, or blunt injury are generally implicated in the etiology of suspensory desmitis. Avulsion fractures of the origin of the ligament are also due to overload of the suspensory apparatus; however, the exact mechanism resulting in avulsion rather than tearing of the ligament fibers is not known. Unequal loading of the suspensory branches as a result of conformational abnormalities, poor foot balance or shoeing, and uneven and deep track surfaces can result in sudden overload and tearing of one suspensory branch. This form of suspensory desmitis is common in Standardbred racehorses, presumably as a result of the extended cranial weight-bearing phase of their stride. Fractured splint bones and callus developing from periostitis of the splint may exert pressure on the midbody portion of the suspensory ligament, resulting in a secondary desmitis. This type of injury occurs in most breeds, particularly Thoroughbreds, and is one of the few serious consequences of enlarged splint bones.

DIAGNOSIS

Desmitis of the body and branches of the suspensory ligament is easily recognized by visualization and palpation. Generally, primary desmitis involves either the medial or lateral branch and extends a variable distance proximally into the conjoined body of the ligament. Occasionally both branches of the suspensory ligament are simultaneously affected. Although suspensory desmitis is most often a problem in the forelimbs, Standardbred horses are often affected in the hind limbs. Palpation with the limb in the non-weight-bearing position permits separation of the suspensory ligament from the flexor tendons and the splint bones. This procedure is especially important when palpating deep to an enlarged splint bone. Detecting ligament swelling and painful regions in the proximal suspensory ligament is more difficult and is complicated by the surrounding structures and depth of the ligament. Very firm localized pressure with the limb elevated and the carpus partially flexed generally elicits a withdrawal response. The pathologic process of proximal desmitis is confined to the core of the ligament and consequently there is little external swelling.

The degree of pain and swelling varies with the stage of the inflammatory reaction. In the early phase of ligament damage the only signs may be pain on palpation and mild lameness. With continued exercise, however, increased fiber disruption results in inflammatory edema and periligamentous swelling with obvious ligament enlargement. Acute suspensory desmitis can result in a severe lameness for several days, which diminishes with treatment and time but takes several weeks to dissipate. Even then, residual swelling and obvious pain on palpation remain. The lameness can be exacerbated by digital pressure on the suspensory ligament, forced flexion of the fetlock and/or carpus, or stretching the ligament by standing the horse on a wedge block to elevate the toe. Diagnostic local infiltration or perineural anesthesia is generally not required unless a proximal desmitis is suspected. Even then it is not easy to specifically block only the proximal suspensory ligament without also desensitizing the inferior check ligament, portions of the splints, and often the carpometacarpal joint. Ultrasound examination is important to define the extent of the ligament damage and provide an accurate prognosis for return to work (Fig. 87–1). Generally, the greater the lesion area within the body of the ligament, the more extended is the rehabilitation that is required. Radiography is recommended to detect mineralization within the substance of the ligament and is essential for diagnosing avulsion fractures occurring at the origin of the ligament (Fig. 87–2). Mineralization of the insertion of the suspensory ligament onto the proximal sesamoid bones

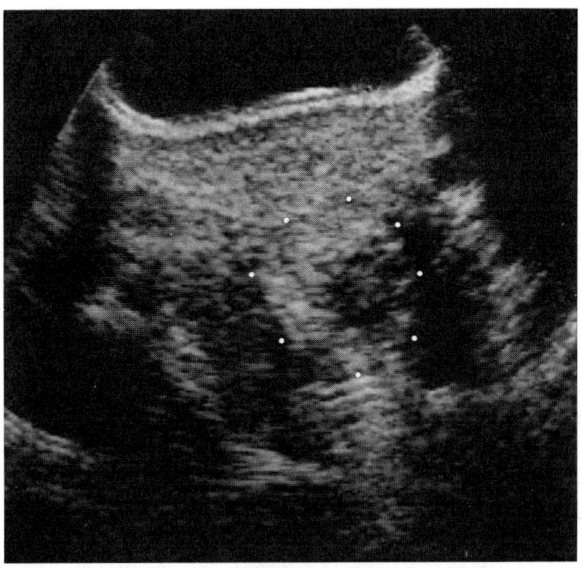

Figure 87–1. Ultrasound examination showing suspensory desmitis of the medial branch of the suspensory ligament (outlined with *white dots*). A central hypoechoic region is present. (Courtesy of Dr. Amy Dietze.)

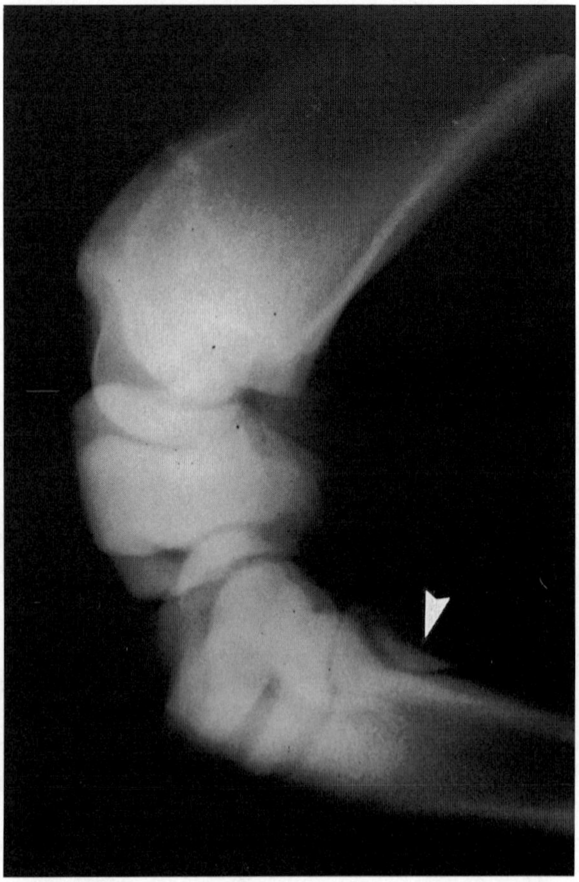

Figure 87–2. Avulsion of the origin of the suspensory ligament (*arrow*).

and "sesamoiditis" are important complications and make radiographic analysis of the entire suspensory ligament necessary.

TREATMENT

Medical and surgical therapy for suspensory desmitis generally parallels that used for tendinitis of the digital flexors in the horse. Immediate care for acute desmitis is the most critical aspect governing the long-term rehabilitation of the horse, and includes immobilization by strict stall rest and heavy padded bandages. Casts and splints are not required unless almost total disruption of the suspensory ligament has occurred. Cold therapy with ice "boots," chilled wraps, or simply cold hosing is important to reduce soft tissue swelling. Nonsteroidal anti-inflammatory agents such as phenylbutazone are frequently administered to relieve the pain and further reduce the tissue inflammation. The suspensory ligament is slow to heal and, like disruptions of the flexor tendon, the uniform collagen structure and final strength rarely return to normal. Permanent enlargement is found where repeated ligament injuries have occurred. An extended period of rest is necessary in the treatment of suspensory desmitis. Following therapy during the acute stage of approximately 1 month, many horses can commence brief but increasing periods of walking exercise. Bandaging and stall rest with controlled walking is continued for 6 to 10 weeks. Swimming is particularly helpful after this time to gradually reintroduce exercise while increasing fitness. Most horses cannot enter training sooner than 4 months following the injury, and more extensive suspensory damage generally results in a 6- to 10-month lay-up. This may be shortened by swimming and controlled work increasing in intensity over time rather than paddock turnout.

The rationale for surgical intervention has not been adequately defined. Procedures used to treat chronic tendinitis, such as tendon splitting, percutaneous tendon stabbing, carbon fiber implantation, and injection of sclerosing agents, corticosteroids, or sodium hyaluronate, have all been used in the suspensory ligament. None have shown clearly defined advantages over rest alone, although the percentage of horses responding to these treatments is greater than that recorded for horses with involvement of the flexor tendons treated similarly. Horses with acute suspensory desmitis are not candidates for surgery. Although many horses with suspensory desmitis heal satisfactorily with rest alone, horses with recurring desmitis and/or an obvious anechoic core may need surgical intervention (Fig. 87–1). Although many surgical techniques in the literature result in reasonable success, percutaneous ligament splitting is generally preferred and is less invasive than open ligament splitting.

SURGICAL TECHNIQUE

Percutaneous suspensory ligament splitting can be done with the horse tranquilized and the area desensitized with perineural anesthesia. However, more precise insertion and control over the blade path can be achieved in the anesthetized horse. The horse is placed in lateral recumbency with the affected suspensory branch uppermost. If only the body of the ligament is affected, the procedure can be performed from either the medial or lateral aspect of the ligament. After sterile skin preparation and draping, a no. 15 scalpel blade is inserted through the skin to penetrate to the center of the affected ligament. Without expanding the skin wound, the blade is fanned parallel to the ligament's fibers, effectively splitting a 5- to 7-mm length. The skin stab and ligament splitting procedure is repeated at 1-cm intervals until the entire affected portion of the ligament has been split. The skin incisions do not require sutures. Bandages are applied to control hemorrhage, prevent contamination, and minimize swelling in the recovery phase. Antibiotics are usually not necessary; however, nonsteroidal anti-inflammatory agents are administered for 2 to 3 days. The procedure is generally not as painful as flexor tendon splitting.

Postoperatively, the bandages are changed every 2 days and maintained for 3 to 4 weeks. Stall rest and controlled walking exercise are allowed as for horses with more acute suspensory desmitis. A very gradual return to exercise is critical for effective recovery. Ultrasonography is used to evaluate the improvement in ligament structure, size, and consistency. Recurrence of ligament fiber disruption may be detected before swelling or lameness return, thereby signaling the need for extended rest before further attempts at increasing exercise.

PROGNOSIS

The prognosis for suspensory desmitis and the likelihood of a successful return to racing are better than with flexor tendinitis. A fair prognosis for athletic work can generally be offered. Many horses with unilateral branch desmitis heal well and have a good prognosis. Recurrence of suspensory desmitis is the most common complication during return to work, although sesamoiditis and ongoing splint problems are often also involved. Removal of enlarged splints up to and including the level of the suspensory body should be done as early as possible after the initial injury. Proximal suspensory desmitis carries a good prognosis, with one report indicating 91% of horses returning to previous work following 8 weeks of stall rest.

Conservative therapy is always recommended at the initial presentation. Failure of more conservative treatment methods and unresolving ligament core lesions are the two occasions where surgery may be useful. Reports by Knudsen and by Nilsson and Bjorck from Sweden evaluating percutaneous ligament splitting in 142 and 285 horses respectively, revealed that 73% and 88% of the treated horses raced at least once and that over 55% of the horses competed more than ten times. The prognosis for lesions involving the suspensory ligament is generally not markedly improved by surgery except in the circumstances previously outlined.

BIBLIOGRAPHY

Bramlage LR, Gabel AA, Hackett RP: Avulsion fractures of the origin of the suspensory ligament in the horse. *J Am Vet Med Assoc* 1980;176:1004–1010.

Fackelman GE: The nature of tendon damage and its repair. *Equine Vet J* 1973;5:141–149.

Knudsen O: Percutaneous tendon splitting—method and results. *Equine Vet J* 1976;8:101–103.

McIlwraith CW: Diseases of joints, tendons, ligaments and related structures, in Stashak TS (ed): *Adams' Lameness in Horses*. Philadelphia, Lea & Febiger, 1987, pp 469–470.

Moyer W, Raker CW: Diseases of the suspensory apparatus. *Vet Clin North Am Large Anim* 1980;2:61–80.

Nilsson G, Bjorck G: Surgical treatment of chronic tendinitis in the horse. *J Am Vet Med Assoc* 1969;155:920–926.

Personett LA, McAllister ES, Mansmann RA: Proximal suspensory desmitis. *Mod Vet Pract* 1983;64:541–545.

88 Septic Tenosynovitis

Alan J. Nixon

Septic tenosynovitis is a debilitating and often permanently disabling condition predominantly involving the digital sheath and occasionally the tarsal and extensor tendon sheaths. Although primary septic tenosynovitis can arise as a result of hematogenous localization within the tendon sheath, tenosynovitis secondary to a penetrating injury or injection is far more common. Local involvement of a tendon sheath adjacent to a septic joint has also been described in foals.

DIAGNOSIS

Septic tenosynovitis usually results in the sudden onset of marked lameness, with severe effusion of the tendon sheath and associated heat, pain, and swelling. Occasionally a moderate fever will develop. Sepsis secondary to penetrating wounds often results in a draining wound over the tendon sheath. Insertion of a sterile metal probe, hemostat, or teat cannula will usually confirm communication of an external wound to the sheath cavity. The diagnosis of hematogenous tenosynovitis or sepsis secondary to injections may require needle centesis and aspiration of suppurative synovial fluid. Laboratory analysis can be performed to confirm an elevated white blood cell count and an elevated protein content, both present with infection. White blood cell counts higher than 40,000 cells/mm^3 in the affected synovial fluid are common, with the majority of cells being degenerate neutrophils. Normal laboratory values for tendon synovial fluid parallel those for joint fluid; however, the hyaluronate content is lower than in most joints (normal 0.5 to 0.7 mg/mL). Intracellular and extracellular bacteria are not commonly observed.

Routine aerobic and anaerobic cultures are performed in an attempt to identify the infective organism. Positive cultures are difficult to obtain except in severely contaminated wounds secondary to penetrating foreign bodies. Hematogenous tenosynovitis is generally caused by the same bacteria that are commonly isolated from septic arthritis in foals (e.g., *Rhodococcus equi, Escherichia coli, Streptococcus species, Actinobacillus equuli,* and *Salmonella species*). Several reports of septic tenosynovitis in foals describe the infection as having spread from locally adjacent joints, and the same organism was isolated from both synovial environments. In adult horses, hematogenous septic tenosynovitis is rare, and *Streptococcus* and *Klebsiella* species have been isolated.

SURGICAL TREATMENT

Prompt treatment of punctures and lacerations penetrating a tendon sheath is important in preventing intractable sepsis. Immediate exploration of a wound over a tendon sheath is indicated. This can usually be achieved under tranquilization and local anesthesia; however, if an obvious entry point to the intrathecal space is established, further aggressive treatment usually requires general anesthesia. The affected area is

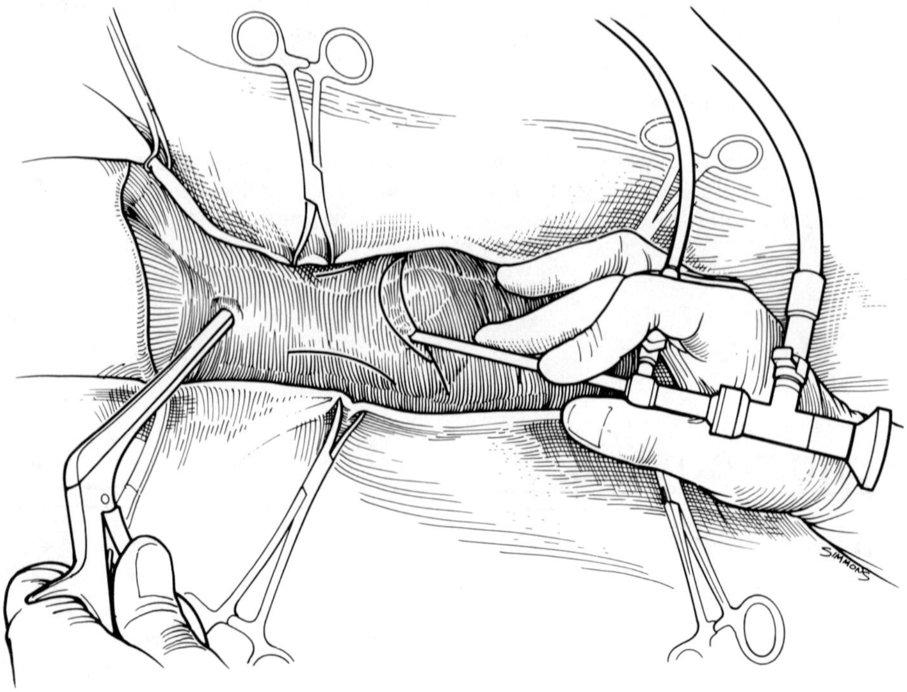

Figure 88–1. Tenoscopic examination of the digital flexor tendon sheath. The standard entry portal is between the annular ligament and the proximal digital annular ligament.

prepared and draped with impervious draping materials. The wound is then surgically explored to meticulously remove debris, necrotic tissue, and fibrin. Contaminated and devitalized portions of tendon, tendon sheath, and more superficial tissues should be débrided. Continuous lavage of the tendon sheath with sterile saline or lactated Ringer's solution is indicated. A series of large-bore needles or catheters placed in the proximal and distal extremities of the sheath may be used to achieve a thorough lavage. If the wound is fresh and very clean, partial or complete suture closure can be performed. Broad-spectrum antibiotics are commenced prior to surgery, and local instillation of additional quantities at the time of wound closure achieves high intrathecal concentrations.

Acute hematogenous tenosynovitis is treated similarly to hematogenous septic arthritis. Aspiration of synovial fluid for culture is followed by extensive tendon sheath lavage using sterile lactated Ringer's solution. Systemic antibiotics are commenced following aspiration for culture, and antibiotics may be added to the lavage fluid.

Severely contaminated and early infected tendon sheath wounds are irrigated and débrided but are not closed unless an ingress and egress drainage system is installed. Small penetrating wounds such as pitchfork injuries are not sutured and may even be further opened by débridement. They can then be bandaged and allowed to heal by second intention.

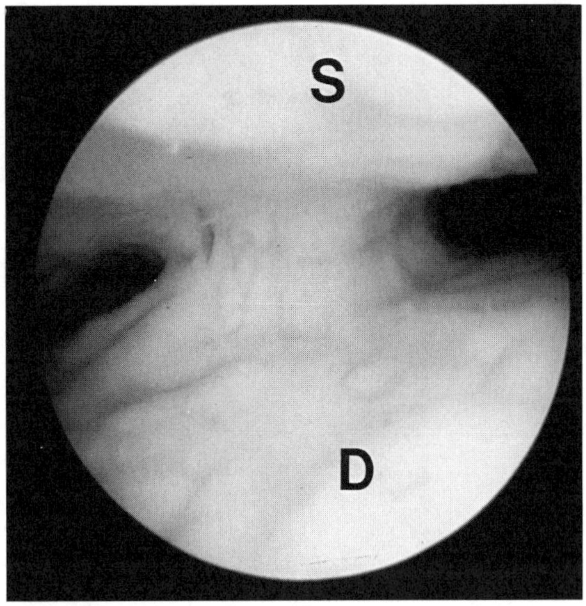

Figure 88–3. Broad adhesions between the deep (*D*) and superficial (*S*) digital flexor tendons of a horse with septic tenosynovitis of 4 weeks' duration. The roughened surfaces of the tendons are typical of chronic active inflammation.

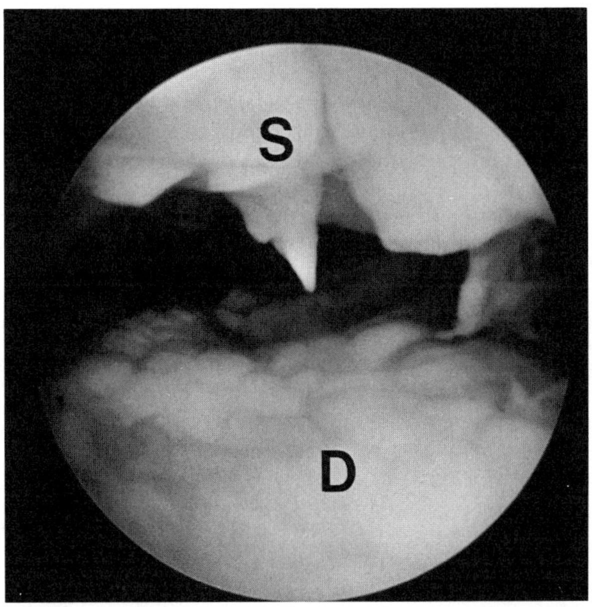

Figure 88–2. Chronic septic tenosynovitis with free fibrin and inspissated purulent material between the deep (*D*) and superficial (*S*) flexor tendons 4 cm proximal to the annular ligament. Note the typical cobblestone appearance of the surface of the deep flexor tendon.

Chronically infected tendon sheath cavities are extremely difficult to resolve, and careful evaluation of the cost: benefit ratio of extensive treatment is important. Seemingly, chronic intrathecal infections are more recalcitrant than are septic joints, respond less satisfactorily to lavage, and result in more permanently crippling lameness. The development of extensive tendon adhesions appears to be a feature in the poor overall response. Where treatment is elected, general anesthesia is necessary. After sterile preparation of the draining wound, the area is draped and septic material is collected from the tendon sheath for culture. This can be followed by initiation of broad-spectrum antibiotics. Procaine penicillin G (22,000 IU/kg), gentamicin (2.2 mg/kg) and metronidazole (15 mg/kg orally) provide broad-spectrum activity and may be used pending the culture results. Extensive lavage of the tendon sheath is performed and as much of the fibrin and inspissated material as possible is removed with forceps. Adhesions are often well developed and tend to loculate areas of purulent material, making exposure and drainage difficult. Examination of the sheath cavity

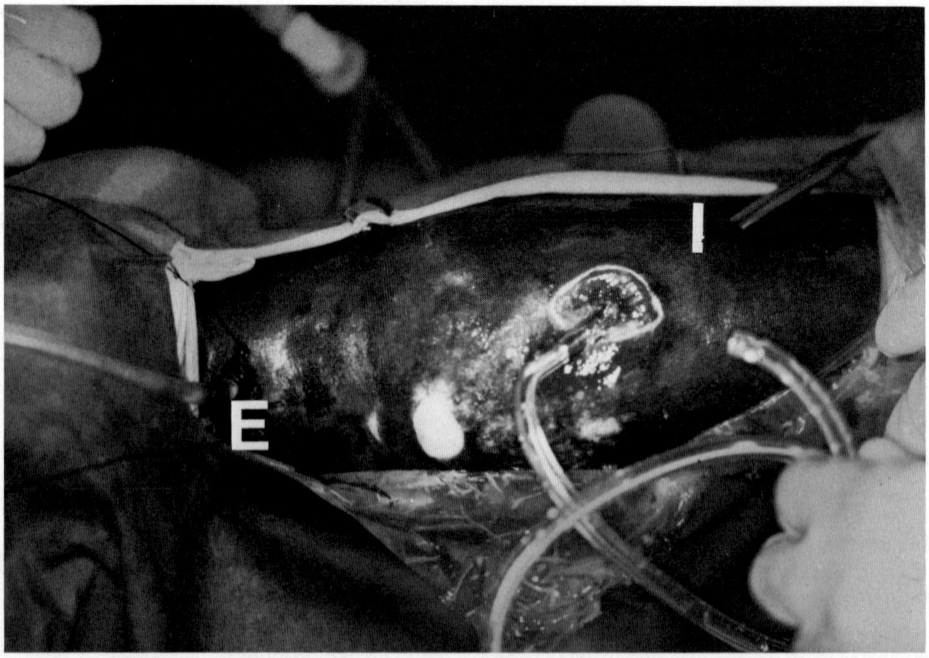

Figure 88–4. Insertion of an ingress and egress drainage apparatus into the digital sheath following tenoscopic débridement and lavage. The egress drain (*E*) is exteriorized on the palmar midline immediately distal to the bifurcation and insertion of the superficial flexor tendon. The ingress drain (*I*) is inserted through the original wound and exits near the proximal reflection of the tendon sheath. Once the drains are placed, the original penetrating wound can then be débrided and closed.

(tenoscopy) and resection of adhesions (tenolysis) is facilitated by use of an arthroscope or other rigid medical endoscope. The original wound makes a convenient entry portal in most instances. If the wound has closed or sepsis originated without a wound, the arthroscope is inserted on the lateral or medial surface of the tendon sheath, 1 cm caudal to the volar neurovascular structures and between the annular ligament and proximal digital annular ligament (Fig. 88–1). This entry point allows examination, lavage, and débridement of most areas of the tendon sheath cavity (Fig. 88–2). Adhesions can be severed with a guarded scalpel (Zimmer), biopsy forceps, or laser (Pfizer) inserted through a second portal, giving convenient access to the adhesions (Fig. 88–3). Synovectomy of hypertrophic synovial tissue and attached fibrin is performed to a limited extent; however, hemorrhage generally is profuse and the benefits are not known with certainty. Following copious lavage, ingress and egress drains are inserted in the tendon sheath proximally and distally (Fig. 88–4). Perforated polyvinyl chloride drains (OEC Drain; Orthopedic Equipment Company) or silicone drains (Blake Fluted Drain; Johnson & Johnson Inc) are suitable for egress under suction, but Penrose drains can be used for passive drainage. Ingress drains are useful for continuous or intermittent lavage of sterile lactated Ringer's solution through the tendon sheath following surgery. Resection of the wound edges and closure of the original wound is generally successful and allows maintenance of negative pressure in the tendon sheath.

After resection of adhesions, instillation of 40 to 120 mg sodium hyaluronate gel (Hylartin, Pharmacia; Synoflex, Chesapeake Biological Laboratory) assists in preventing their reformation. Repeated doses can be used in the convalescent period.

POSTOPERATIVE TREATMENT

Except under circumstances of acute laceration or injury to the tendon sheath, appropriate antibiotics are continued for 2 to 4 weeks after surgery. Intermittent lavage via the drainage apparatus is performed twice daily using sterile lactated Ringer's solution or saline.

Additional antibiotics can be added to the flush solution; however, there are no definitive data to support the use of local antibiotics in addition to the same drugs administered parenterally. The affected limb is bandaged to reduce edema, limit the free space within the tendon sheath, reduce pain, and protect the drains and sutured wounds. Rebandaging is necessary as frequently as the tendon sheath is flushed. If continuous lavage of the tendon sheath is used, a bandage is difficult to keep dry and an open drain exteriorized from the bandage allows constant egress. Postoperative pain is usually severe, and phenylbutazone at doses up to 8.8 mg/kg by mouth may be needed for several days. This dose should be reduced to 6.6 mg/kg after 7 days. Long-term anti-inflammatory agents are generally needed to maintain pain at a tolerable level. Follow-up doses of sodium hyaluronate are used after the lavage drainage system is removed.

Controlled walking exercise is commenced 4 to 7 days after surgery. Although walking exercise does not represent a form of continuous passive motion, it is still considered beneficial in reducing adhesion formation and reformation, and is instituted early and increased in frequency quickly. Elevation of the heel with a wedge pad or shoe relieves tension on the flexor tendons and often reduces the pain associated with septic digital sheaths, allowing early exercise. The elevation of the heels can be gradually lowered with time to return to a normal hoof angle by 2 to 3 months.

PROGNOSIS

Early diagnosis and treatment are critical in the treatment and salvage of horses for athletic activity. When the septic process is allowed to become chronic, the chances of salvage for riding purposes is considerably reduced. Careful consideration of the overall cost and likely poor outcome for horses with chronic sepsis is vital. Resolution of the septic process may take several months, and the lameness can rarely be completely resolved. Restrictive adhesions almost always occur between the tendons and tendon sheath and, combined with an exquisitely sensitive tendon sheath, result in chronic pain with movement.

BIBLIOGRAPHY

McIlwraith CW: Diseases of joints, tendons, ligaments, and related structures, in Stashak TS (ed): *Adams' Lameness in Horses.* Philadelphia, Lea & Febiger, 1987, pp 477–478.

Van Pelt RW: Idiopathic tenosynovitis in foals. *J Am Vet Med Assoc* 1969;155:510–517.

Van Pelt RW, Riley WF: Treatment of bilateral septic tenosynovitis in a foal. *J Am Vet Med Assoc* 1971;159:1032–1034.

89 Tendon Lacerations

Alan J. Nixon

Traumatic division of the flexor or extensor tendons of the lower limb occurs relatively commonly in horses. Division of the superficial flexor tendon and/or the gastrocnemius tendon forming the Achilles apparatus is less common but more debilitating. Trauma is almost always involved, and most injuries result from contact with sharp metal, wire fences, floor boards, or glass objects.

DIAGNOSIS

The flexor tendons between the hock or carpus and fetlock are most prone to laceration. An open skin wound on the flexor surface of the limb generally signals the need for deeper examination to evaluate the tendons. Laceration of only the superficial digital flexor tendon results in moderate lowering of the fetlock. Involvement of both superficial and deep digital flexor tendons allows the toe of the foot to rock up with weight bearing and permits further sinking of the fetlock. Rarely, the deep digital flexor tendon is lacerated without complete disruption of the superficial tendon. In this instance, only the toe rocks upward without appreciable lowering of the fetlock. Deep lacerations to the pastern and heel region of the foot frequently sever part or all of the deep digital flexor tendon. Severe lacerations of the flexor tendons proximal to the fetlock may also disrupt the suspensory ligament and neurovascular structures. When both flexor tendons and suspensory ligament are severed, the fetlock often touches the ground and the toe rocks markedly upward with weight bearing. Hemorrhage is profuse when the common digital artery or its branches are involved.

Disruption of the common or long digital extensor tendons frequently occurs with lacerations over the dorsal metacarpal or metatarsal and fetlock regions. Typically the horse "knuckles" over at the fetlock when attempting to stride forward and place the foot, since the toe and fetlock cannot be adequately advanced to take weight and position for extension. Many horses can flip the limb forward and bear weight normally if not hurried or distracted. Involvement of the lateral digital extensor in the laceration can occur but has little additional clinical effect on the function of the limb. Laceration of the lateral digital extensor alone has no discernible effect, since the intact long or common digital extensor tendons provide the majority of the extensor function to the lower limb.

Laceration of the Achilles apparatus is often a devastating injury with complete loss of weight-bearing capacity. These injuries frequently occur from kicking out at sharp objects, including farm machinery, gates, and fences, and occasionally from entrapment of the limb in walls, doors, and trailer floors. Depending on the level of injury proximal to the hock, the superficial digital flexor or gastrocnemius tendon is more superficial and more readily severed. When both structures are completely disrupted the hock has no support and drops markedly with attempted weight bearing. Rupture of only the gastrocnemius tendon allows the hock to flex and drop, but not to the extent that follows rupture of both tendons. The horse can usually advance the limb and walk with some difficulty. If the gastrocnemius tendon of both hind limbs is severed, the horse assumes a squatting position and is unable to straighten its hind limbs.

SURGERY

Methods of surgical treatment and postoperative support vary according to the tendon involved, associated soft tissue damage, duration since injury, and degree of tendon damage. No one surgical protocol is satisfactory for all tendon lacerations.

EXTENSOR TENDONS

Severed extensor tendons are the easiest to treat and have a better prognosis than lacerations involving the flexor tendons. Fresh lacerations with sharp severance

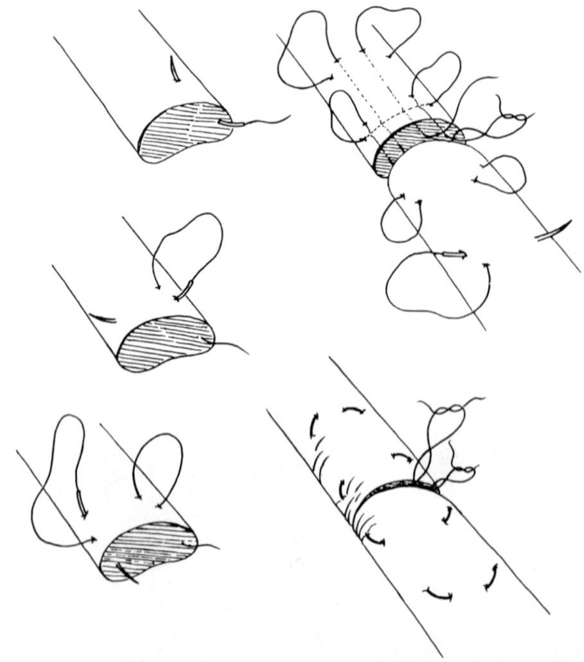

Figure 89–1. Two separate locking loop tendon sutures are used to appose the severed tendon ends. Each suture consists of two axially positioned suture strands spanning between the two tendon ends secured by a loop formed by a transverse penetration that locks on the tendon fibers.

of the extensor tendon can be cleaned and débrided where necessary, and occasionally primary suture of the tendon and skin wounds performed. Apposition of the severed ends of an extensor tendon is often difficult, and where any débridement of damaged tendon is performed the ends can rarely be approximated. Fortunately, extensor tendons heal comparatively well when supported by a cast, or padded bandage and extension splint, for 3 to 4 weeks. The distal portion of the tendon readily attaches to surrounding tissues to prevent knuckling of the fetlock and foot. An extended toe shoe is applied at the time of cast or splint removal to provide a more cranial fulcrum to the lower limb, further preventing knuckling. Restoration of a discrete extensor tendon rarely occurs, but a functional union of the severed ends can provide limited gliding action.

Severely contaminated or infected extensor tendon lacerations should be débrided to remove debris, devitalized and infected tissue (including tendon and paratenon), and irregular skin flaps. The wound is allowed to heal by second intention under a bandage or, if an extensive soft tissue deficit exists, under a cast.

Digital Flexor Tendons

Severed digital flexor tendons are more difficult and time consuming to treat adequately; however, the principles are similar to those for extensor tendons. Fresh, clean lacerations of the flexor tendons can be treated by primary suture repair and postoperative casting. With the horse under general anesthesia, the wound is clipped, shaved, and scrubbed with antibacterial solutions and rinsed with sterile saline or lactated Ringer's solution until all debris has been removed. The skin wound may need to be opened further to débride any devitalized paratenon or tendon tissue. The tendon ends should be trimmed back to healthy tendon. Aseptic technique should be used, including sterile waterproof draping materials.

With the wound clean and with minimal loss of tendon tissue, the severed ends of the tendon may be approximated using a series of locking loop sutures (Fig. 89–1). Two complete and separate locking loops using size 2 monofilament nylon or polypropylene are usually adequate, although the deep digital flexor tendon can accommodate three locking loops. The sutures all need to be placed before any are tightened to ensure correct placement. It is also important that the longitudinal strands of the suture loops are directed deep to the transverse strand, thereby forming a secure loop around a bundle of tendon fibers. In vitro studies in equine superficial digital flexor tendons indicate that the tensile strength of the double locking loop is almost twice that of a single locking loop, and three locking loops have 2.3 times the holding power of a single locking loop. The advantages of locking loops over the Bunnell suture techniques include less interference with tendon blood supply, less tendency for gap formation under load, and minimal exposed suture material. The use of plain or braided wire is not recommended because of the poor relaxation of the suture loops when tension on the anastomosis is relieved with the stride of the horse. A faster suture pattern to apply is the three loop pulley (Fig. 89–2). In equine tendons, this pattern has an in vitro failure strength approximately equal to three locking loops but has less gap at failure and takes only one third the time to apply. The main disadvantage of the three loop pulley is its greater propensity to strangulate the intrinsic tendon blood supply at the sutured ends.

After suture of the tendon ends, the subcutaneous tissue and skin can be closed routinely or, if loss of skin prevents primary closure, the skin wound can be left to heal by second intention. A cast is always applied.

Extensive flexor tendon wounds, especially those of several days' duration, are treated as infected open wounds. Wound cleansing, débridement of all infected tissue (including tendon and paratenon), and casting with slight flexion at the fetlock should be performed. Drains are rarely used under the cast. If wound infection is particularly severe, initial débridement and packing with antibacterial agents may be combined with splinting until the wound begins to granulate. The wound can be further débrided and a cast applied. No attempt to suture the tendon ends is warranted under these conditions.

Tendon lacerations within the digital flexor sheath heal more slowly and often with less satisfactory functional results. Infected tendon and tendon sheath lacerations can be severely crippling, and serious consideration of the economic and personal worth of each horse is warranted (see Chapter 88). Early treatment increases the likelihood of a satisfactory outcome. Open lavage and débridement of the tendon and tendon sheath is warranted when they are heavily contaminated or infected. After thorough cleansing of the

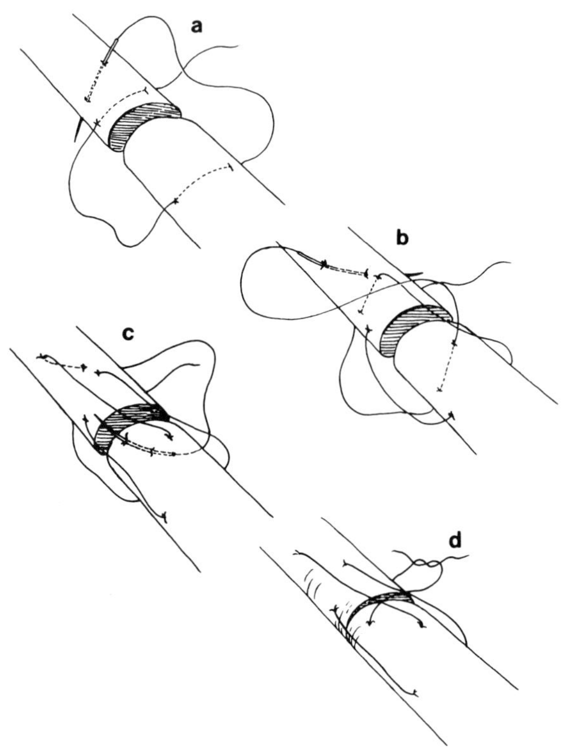

Figure 89–2. The three-loop pulley tendon suture pattern is inserted using a continuous loop applied in three separate longitudinal planes in the tendon. **A.** Horizontal plane placed. Sixty degree insertion commencing. **B.** Sixty degree plane complete. Beginning second sixty degree plane. **C.** Completing second sixty degree plane. **D.** Completed suture with three loops aligned in planes separated sixty degrees to each other.

wound, a decision to suture the tendon can be made based on the tendon deficit and appearance of the wound. In general, tendon lacerations within the tendon sheath result in retraction and atrophy of the tendon ends. Although some function can be regained by adhesion of the distal tendon segment to the tendon sheath, true tendon continuity is rarely established and attempts to rejoin the tendon ends by suturing are generally warranted. Locking loop or loop pulley patterns are satisfactory for use in these tendons. Adhesions of the sheath and surrounding tissues to a tendon repair are unavoidable when there is extensive trauma and contamination. In acute cases where infection can be minimized by lavage, débridement, and antibiotics, closure of the tendon sheath and injection of sodium hyaluronate may decrease adhesion formation and promote tendon healing. Studies of a concentrated sodium hyaluronate gel (Synoflex; Chesapeake Biological Laboratory) injected intrathecally, using an equine tendon adhesion model, revealed a decreased number and strength of adhesions between the deep digital flexor tendon and surrounding structures. Ingress and egress drainage of the tendon sheath is generally not possible with the affected limb immobilized in a cast postoperatively.

Repair of tendon lacerations with carbon fiber may promote the union of the tendon ends with tendon-like tissue containing well-organized type I collagen. Original reports described the carbon fiber acting as an inert scaffold onto which fibroblasts and later collagen attached in an ordered manner. It is now generally considered that such an idealized degradable scaffold does not develop, but rather the carbon incites an increased type III collagen reaction that is somewhat dependent on the quantity of implanted material. One experiment compared monofilament nylon and 20,000 carbon filaments for repair of transected superficial digital flexor tendons and found the carbon repair resulted in a large but significantly weaker tendon than did the repair with nylon. The immature tissue surrounding the carbon bundles was speculated to have weakened the tendon. Further studies with 40,000 and 60,000 carbon filaments showed progressively increasing tendon size. When 60,000 carbon filaments were used, the tendon was stronger than the normal superfical digital flexor tendon from the opposite, nonoperated, forelimb. However, the cosmetic defect at 6 months was considerable. Seemingly, a clean tendon transection does not need carbon implantation for successful healing and the cosmetic appearance may further detract from its use. Where an extensive tendon gap exists as a result of contraction or débridement, carbon filaments may assist by inciting a fibrous bridge for the tendon ends. This may be of particular relevance for repairs of the Achilles tendon, where a massive fibrous response may assist in reestablishing the tendon function before support by casts and braces can no longer be maintained. Carbon fiber implantation is generally contraindicated if contamination or infection is established.

With all digital flexor laceration repairs, a cast is needed to support the sutures or to maintain the tendon ends in reasonable approximation if suturing is not performed. The cast is applied with the fetlock and interphalangeal joints in sufficient flexion to relieve tension on the repair. Despite this, research studies reveal most suture repairs cannot prevent some tendon gap formation, especially in repair of the deep digital flexor tendon within the digital sheath. Casting for 2 weeks is generally sufficient for deep digital flexor tendon lacerations that can be immediately protected by an extended heel shoe. For lacerations of the superficial digital flexor tendon, a fetlock support shoe can allow removal of the cast 2.5 to 3 weeks postoperatively. Correct tension and adequate padding of the support strap of the shoe to give support to the fetlock without creat-

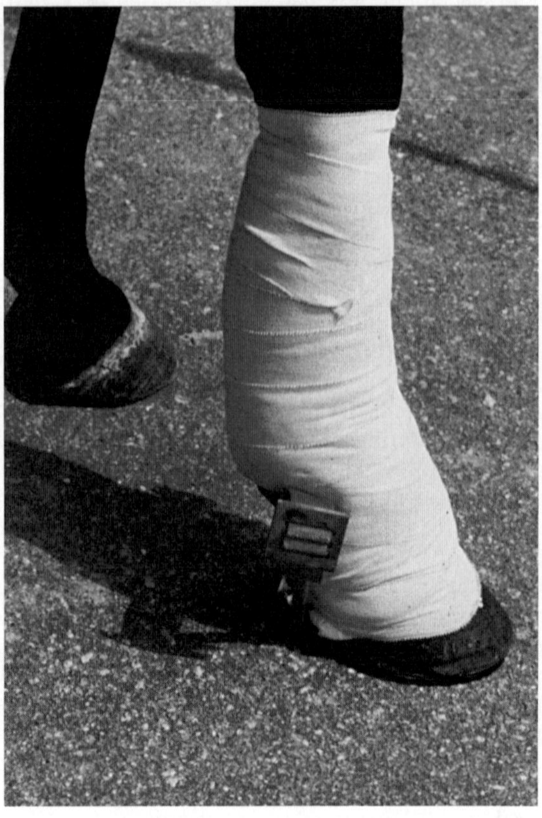

Figure 89–3. A fetlock support shoe with a padded strap preventing sinking of the fetlock during weight bearing.

ing pressure necrosis of the flexor surface of the limb is important (Fig. 89–3).

Achilles Apparatus

Lacerations to the Achilles apparatus are the most serious of tendon transections. Even partial-thickness lacerations need careful attention since these can become complete with normal weight bearing. Inspection and palpation of wounds proximal to the hock over the caudal aspect of the limb are always warranted to evaluate the damage to the superficial digital flexor and gastrocnemius tendons. Complete disruption of these structures results in obvious dropping of the hock; however, substantial partial lacerations without pathognomonic signs may need treatment with a full-length cast and/or a modified Thomas splint or brace to prevent progression to complete separation. Principles of wound and tendon débridement are similar to tendon lacerations at other sites. More extensive attempts at restoration of tendon continuity are vital to a successful repair. Multiple locking loops using size 2 monofilament nylon, size 5 multifilament nonabsorbable suture material (Mersilene; Ethicon Inc), or carbon fiber are acceptable. Lacerations directly adjacent to the calcaneal tuber calcis may need a transverse bone tunnel through the tuber for effective attachment of suture or carbon fiber. For more proximal lacerations, close to the myotendinous junction, a locking weave (Fig. 89–4) or a multiple locked loop pattern (Fig. 89–5) can be used. Both suture patterns are easy to place, resist constriction or purse-stringing muscle and tendon tissues, and resist pulling through the fibers.

Following primary reconstruction of the Achilles mechanism, external support is needed. A fiberglass cast extending as far proximal as the tibial crest will provide considerable support to the sutured tendon. Nevertheless, without the stifle immobilized considerable tension is transmitted to the Achilles tendon. Additional support can be provided for a limited period by a modified Thomas splint; however, pressure necrosis of the medial groin region limits the usefulness of these splints.

POSTOPERATIVE CARE

Preoperative antibiotics are commenced when a decision to treat the tendon laceration is made. Broad-spectrum bactericidal antibiotics such as procaine or crystalline penicillin G and an aminoglycoside are generally selected initially, pending results of cultures of fluid and tissues taken during surgery. An antibiotic specific for anaerobic bacteria, such as metronidazole, may also be used for several days depending on the depth and cause of the wound. Tetanus prophylaxis is necessary. Following surgery, antibiotics can be continued for 4 to 10 days.

Flexor tendon repairs are supported in a cast for varying periods of time as previously described. Daily evaluation of the cast limb is essential, particularly when the normal joint angles are changed to relieve tension on a flexor tendon. Cast pressure abrasions are common, and some horses may need anesthesia and recasting. At the time of final cast removal, a supportive

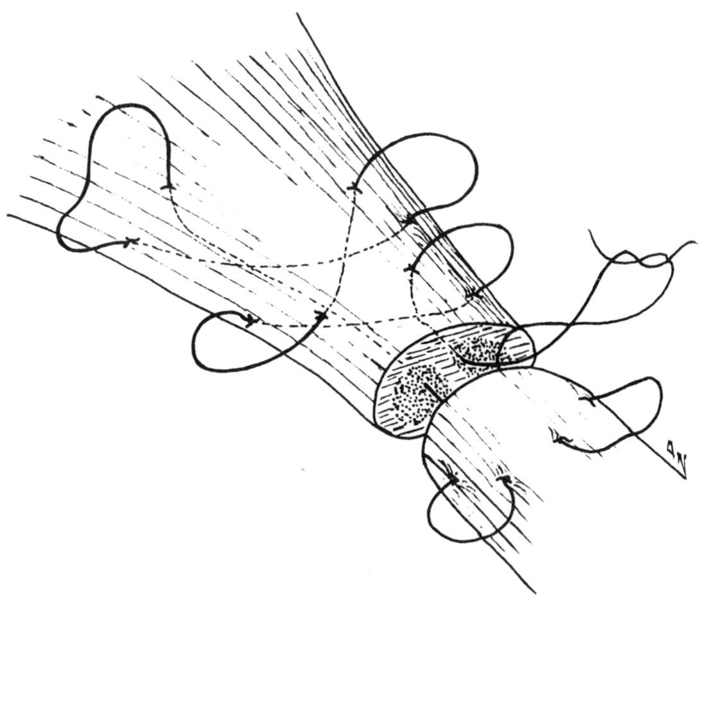

Figure 89–4. The locking weave suture pattern for laceration repair at the myotendinous junction. Multiple loops in different planes of the muscle reduce suture pullout.

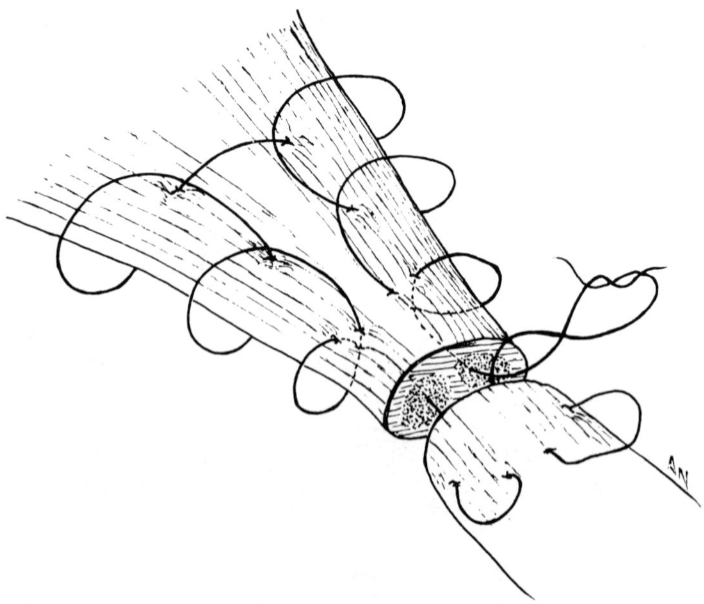

Figure 89–5. The multiple locked locking loop pattern for tendon repair at the myotendinous junction.

therapeutic shoe (extended toe for extensor tendon repair, extended heel for deep digital flexor tendon transection, and extended heel with fetlock support for superficial digital flexor tendon lacerations) needs to be immediately applied. An extended toe shoe may need to be maintained for 2.5 to 3 months. The digital flexor tendon repairs also need support by special shoes for a minimum of 6 to 8 weeks.

Complete stall rest is indicated when the horse has a cast limb. When the support shoes have been fitted, a gradually increasing exercise program of slow controlled walking can commence. At the time of shoe removal, the horse should be able to accommodate 10- to 15-minute walks twice daily. Gradual reduction in the previously elevated heels should also minimize sudden changes in stress on the repaired tendon.

PROGNOSIS

Laceration of the extensor tendons carries the most favorable prognosis. Rarely are, secondary reparative surgeries necessary to establish function of the extensor mechanism. Conversely, transections of the flexor tendons are nearly always serious. Combined superficial and deep digital flexor tendon transections are common but can be repaired to restore a horse to athletic use. One report of eight horses in which both tendons were severed and subsequently repaired indicated seven of the eight horses recovered, five of which were being actively exercised. The eighth horse was lost to follow-up. Deeper lacerations often involve the suspensory ligament or its branches and the neurovascular structures between this ligament and the deep digital flexor tendon. Horses with these injuries are difficult to salvage and a poor prognosis for future use is always warranted (see Chapter 121). Nevertheless, not all horses need necessarily be destroyed, and the literature cites horses successfully repaired and being ridden.

Any involvement of the tendon sheaths is debilitating, and the long-term results are often discouraging. A subacute to chronic tendon laceration through the tendon sheath will frequently become intractably infected, and lameness can be permanent.

Achilles breakdown injuries and lacerations are rarely successfully treated and a significant case series has not been published. Adequately treated horses usually have a permanently thickened Achilles region; however, some of these horses can be ridden and others are successful in breeding activities.

BIBLIOGRAPHY

Aragona J, Parsons JR, Alexander H, Weiss AB: Soft tissue attachment of a filamentous carbon-absorbable polymer tendon and ligament replacement. *Clin Orthop* 1981;160:268–278.

Easley KJ, Stashak TS, Smith FW, Van Slyke G: In vitro comparison of the mechanical properties of four suture patterns for transected equine tendon repair, in *Proceedings of the Veterinary Orthopedic Society meeting*, 1988, p 2.

Krackow KA, Thomas SC, Jones LC: A new stitch for ligament-tendon fixation. *J Bone Joint Surg [Am]* 1986;68:764–766.

McIlwraith CW: Diseases of joints, tendons, ligaments and related structures, in Stashak TS, (ed): *Adams' Lameness in Horses*. Philadelphia, Lea & Febiger, 1987, pp 447–481.

Nixon AJ, Stashak TS, Smith FW, Norrdin RW: Comparison of carbon fiber and nylon suture for repair of transected flexor tendons in the horse. *Equine Vet J* 1984;16:93–102.

Pennington DG: The locking loop tendon suture. *Plast Reconstruct Surg* 1979;63:648–652.

Valdez H, Clark RG, Hanselka DV: Repair of digital flexor tendon lacerations in the horse, using carbon fiber implants. *J Am Vet Med Assoc* 1980;177:427–435.

Valdez H, Coy CH, Swanson T: Flexible carbon fiber for repair of gastrocnemius and superficial digital flexor tendons in a heifer and gastrocnemius tendon in a foal. *J Am Vet Med Assoc* 1982;181:154–157.

Vaughan LC, Edwards GB, Gerring EL: Tendon injuries in horses treated with carbon fiber implants. *Equine Vet J* 1985;17:45–50.

90 Carpal Canal Syndrome

Alan J. Nixon

The carpal canal or carpal tunnel syndrome is an uncommon cause of lameness in horses that results from pressure on the neurovascular structures coursing through the carpal canal. Any trauma to the soft tissue structures within the canal or the development of space-occupying lesions in the canal may cause carpal canal syndrome. Unlike the syndrome in humans, where the diagnosis is supported by wick catheter pressure measurements, the syndrome in horses has not been substantiated to be only a pressure-related phenomenon. On the contrary, many investigators hypothesize that a significant inflammatory tenosynovitis component exists in horses.

The most common cause of carpal canal syndrome in horses is fracture of the accessory carpal bone. Although fracture of this bone may result in an acute syndrome due to the inflammatory swelling and hematoma, more commonly it results in a chronic lameness as the fibrosis and mineralization of the healing fracture compress the contents of the carpal canal, bounded by the indistensible carpal flexor retinaculum. Other known causes of carpal canal syndrome include tendinitis of the superficial or deep digital flexor tendons within the canal and osteochondroma of the distal radius, which can protrude into and chronically irritate the flexor tendon sheath.

Although some evidence of discomfort can be seen in the standing animal, the symptoms are exacerbated by flexion of the carpus, as pressure within the carpal canal causes nerve trauma and vessel claudication, producing distal ischemia and pain. The marked resting pain recorded in humans with acute carpal canal syndrome has not been confirmed in horses, although an appreciation of this would be difficult to establish. Rather, most horses present with a history of moderate, chronic, and occasionally intermittent lameness. Most horses have swelling of the carpal flexor tendon sheath, which protrudes laterally between the lateral digital extensor and the ulnaris lateralis tendons (Fig. 90–1). Moderate swelling can also be evident medially, immediately proximal to the carpus, with the tendon sheath bulging between the tendons of the flexor carpi radialis and flexor carpi ulnaris. The tenosynovitis results from irritation of the tendons within the tendon sheath, external trauma to the sheath and carpal retinaculum, or irritation from a fractured accessory carpal bone or protruding osteochondroma from the distal radius.

Occasionally a horse with carpal canal syndrome will improve with rest, but rapidly becomes lame and the tenosynovitis returns with the resumption of exercise. Tenosynovitis of the flexor tendon sheath within the carpal canal is not necessarily a sign of carpal canal syndrome, because this sheath can be chronically distended without producing marked lameness. This is especially true when the inflammation is due to protruding osteochondromata of the distal radius.

DIAGNOSIS

If there are visible signs of lameness and palpable distention of the flexor tendon sheath within the carpal canal, there is a need for further evaluation. Reduced

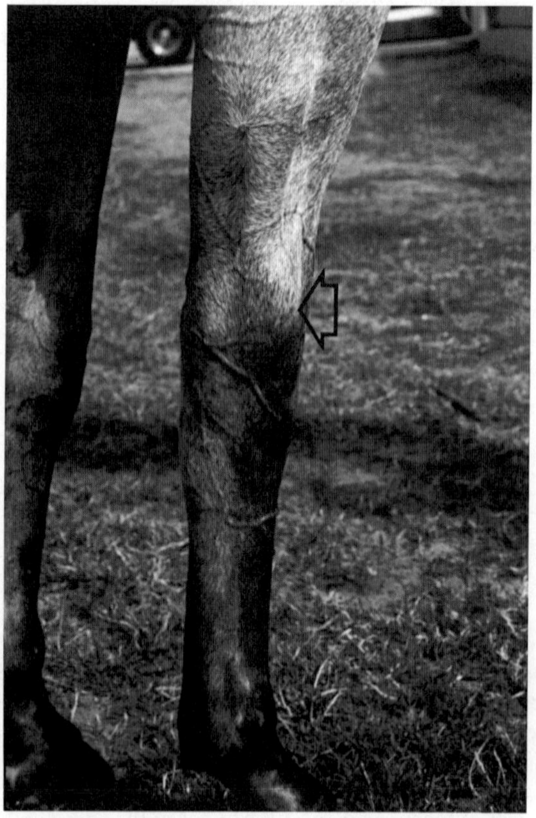

Figure 90–1. Chronic carpal canal syndrome in the right forelimb of a Thoroughbred racehorse. The fluctuant and distended carpal flexor tendon sheath (*arrow*) protrudes between the lateral digital extensor and ulnaris lateralis tendons, proximal to the carpus.

carpal flexion angle and considerable pain on flexion are hallmark signs of carpal canal syndrome. Avoidance behavior, and occasionally attenuation of the peripheral digital pulse, may be elicited by flexion of the carpus. Palpable thickening of the lateral aspects of the accessory carpal bone and excessive lateral-to-medial movement of this bone may signal a chronic fracture. Radiographs are important in evaluating the bony structures forming the boundaries of the carpal canal as well as in identifying osteochondromas of the distal radius, and other intraarticular lesions that may be contributing to the lameness. Not all accessory carpal bone fractures result in the carpal canal syndrome. However, where bony callus and fibrosis markedly reduce the diameter of the canal, a constriction is likely.

The diagnosis of carpal canal syndrome can be confirmed by the intrathecal injection of 5 ml mepivacaine and repetition of the lameness examination, including flexion of the carpus. Differentiation of a true compressive syndrome from direct trauma to the nerves or a painful tenosynovitis may require pressure recordings using catheters placed in the carpal canal. Percutaneous wick catheters can be easily inserted, and a dramatic pressure elevation with limb flexion is diagnostic of the carpal canal syndrome.

Ultrasonography may also be helpful in diagnosing carpal canal syndrome because of the enlargement of the tendons within the canal due to tendinitis.

TREATMENT

Surgical decompression of the carpal canal by sectioning the carpal flexor retinaculum is the only definitive therapy. Medical therapy using corticosteroids injected intrathecally into the carpal canal will usually provide some relief and, when combined with rest, result in improved lameness until exercise is resumed. If a tendon strain has caused the problem, adequate rest to allow for tendon healing can lead to resolution without surgery.

Additional surgical therapy such as repair of a fractured accessory carpal bone or removal of a radial osteochondroma can be combined with division of the constrictive flexor retinaculum. Although a fractured accessory carpal bone may result in significant acute compression of the carpal canal, a more protracted syndrome is far more common. Under the latter circumstances, surgical fixation of the accessory carpal bone is of little value.

SURGICAL TECHNIQUE

The horse is anesthetized and positioned in lateral recumbency with the affected limb down. After sterile skin preparation and draping, a 12-cm skin incision is made on the caudomedial surface of the carpus. The incision is centered over the accessory carpal bone in a craniocaudal dimension and extends 6 cm distal and 5 cm proximal to this bone (Fig. 90–2). Several vessels are covered by or embedded in the carpal flexor retinaculum. The medial palmar vein and radial artery (previously named the medial palmar artery) are just cranial to the correct plane of division in the retinaculum. The lateral palmar nerve, artery, and vein lie caudal to this dissection. These vessels need to be identified and preserved. A thin elliptical strip of flexor retinaculum is excised from between these two groups of neurovascular structures and is discarded. The elliptical incision generally spans the entire length of the flexor retinaculum where it forms an indistensible boundary to the carpal canal. The proximal and distal extremities of the carpal flexor retinaculum are not involved and need not be incised. Fibrous enlargements and adhesions between the flexor retinaculum and the tendon sheath are commonly exposed. These are transected and excised as much as possible.

The flexor tendon sheath within the carpal canal also needs to be incised longitudinally if there are adhesions or fibrous masses within it. The medial palmar artery (previously named the common digital artery) and the medial palmar nerve, both contained within the tendon sheath, must be preserved when freeing the tendons from adhesions and strictures. These neurovascular structures are most vulnerable to the effects of increased pressure within the carpal canal, because they are located deep within the canal. The medial palmar nerve should be carefully freed of fibrous adhesions and examined for intraneural fibrosis, a common cause of failure to regain complete nerve function in humans. Where intraneural fibrosis is suspected, a fine longitudinal incision in the nerve often provides some eventual nerve response. Tendinitis of the superficial or rarely the deep digital flexor tendon within the carpal canal can result in pressure on adjacent structures, and additional decompression can be gained by opening

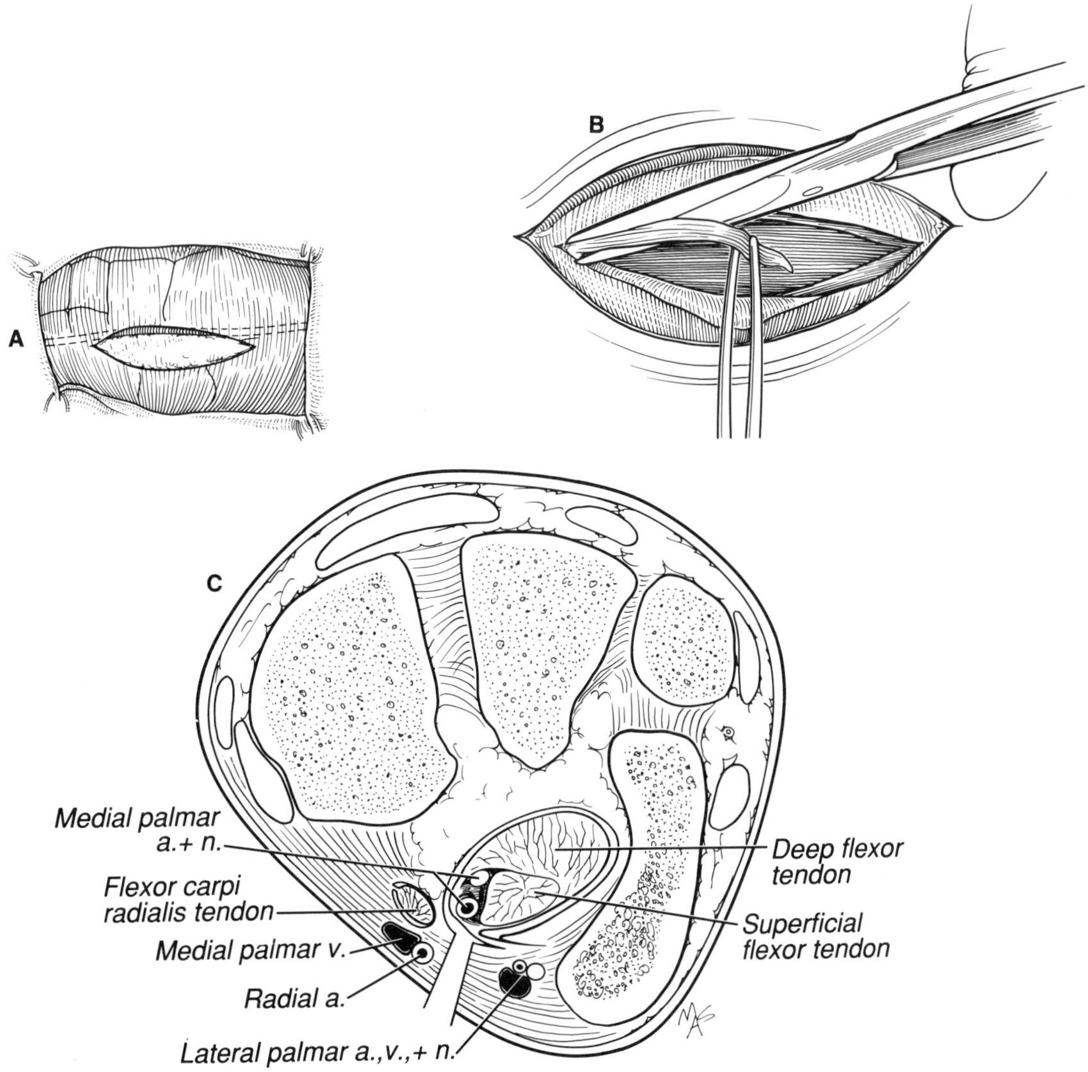

Figure 90–2. Division of the carpal flexor retinaculum forming the carpal canal. **A.** Skin incision on the medial aspect of the carpal canal and centered on the accessory carpal bone. The radial artery is visible in the cranial aspect of the incision. **B.** The carpal flexor retinaculum is incised longitudinally 1 cm caudal to the radial artery and a strip of the retinaculum is excised and discarded. **C.** Cross-section of a right carpus showing the carpal canal and associated structures. (*Figure continues.*)

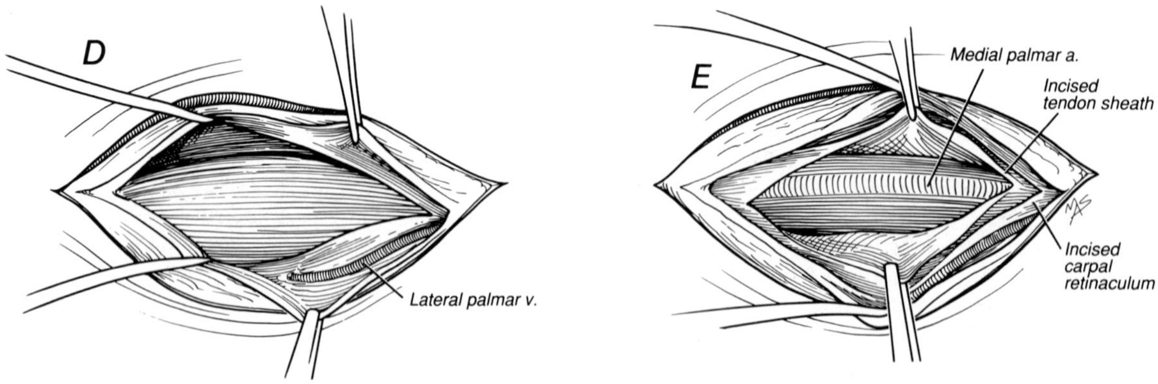

Figure 90–2 (*continued*). **D.** The carpal retinaculum is retracted, exposing the contents of the carpal canal. **E.** The common sheath of the flexor tendons is incised, revealing the medial palmar artery and nerve and the superficial and deep digital flexor tendons.

the surrounding tendon sheath. Most decompression, however, arises from sectioning the carpal flexor retinaculum.

Only the subcutaneous tissues and skin are closed, using 2–0 synthetic absorbable and nonabsorbable suture materials, respectively. The wound is covered with a sterile dressing and a firm cotton bandage is applied.

POSTOPERATIVE CARE

If antibiotics are administered preoperatively, they can be terminated 24 hours after surgery. Anti-inflammatory medication, such as flunixin meglumine or phenylbutazone, is usually administered for 3 to 5 days after surgery. Early institution of walking exercise and pain-limited range of motion exercises are important in reducing fibrosis within the carpal canal and between structures immediately adjacent to the canal. Most horses respond immediately to release of the carpal retinaculum, and this can be regarded as a positive sign for complete recovery. Continued bandaging for 2 to 3 weeks is important to minimize edema at the surgery site and the potential for further pressure on the nerves within the canal. Return to active exercise often depends on the cause of the initial problem, but a protracted recovery may be expected if a fractured accessory carpal exists.

PROGNOSIS

The outlook for horses with chronic carpal tunnel syndrome is fair to good. This response to surgical decompression suggests that intermittent low-grade pressure without extensive fibrous adhesions is most common. Immediate and permanent relief can often follow opening of the carpal canal by transecting the carpal flexor retinaculum. Complications, including poor relief of pain, continued tendon sheath distention, tendon adhesions, and intraneural fibrosis, can lead to unsatisfactory results. Diagnosis and treatment of secondary problems resulting in narrowing of the carpal canal are important.

BIBLIOGRAPHY

Auer J: Diseases of the carpus. *Vet Clin North Am Large Anim Pract* 1980;2:95.

Bauman TD, Gelberman RH, Mubarak SJ, Garfin SR: The acute carpal tunnel syndrome. *Clin Orthop* 1981;156:151–156.

Easley JE, Schneider JE: Evaluation of a surgery for repair of equine accessory carpal bone fracture. *J Am Vet Med Assoc* 1981;178:219–223.

Ford DJ, Ali MS: Acute carpal tunnel syndrome. Complications of delayed decompression. *J Bone Joint Surg [Br]* 1986;68:758–759.

Gelberman RH, Hergenroeder PT, Hargens AR, et al: The carpal tunnel syndrome—a study of carpal canal pressures. *J Bone Joint Surg [Am]* 1981;63:380–383.

Mackay-Smith MP, Cushing LS, Leslie JA: Carpal canal syndrome in horses. *J Am Vet Med Assoc* 1972;160:993–997.

Radue P: Carpal tunnel syndrome due to fracture of the accessory carpal bone. *Equine Pract* 1981;3:8–18.

Turner AS: Carpal canal syndrome in the horse, in Jennings PB (ed): *The Practice of Large Animal Surgery*. Philadelphia, WB Saunders Co, 1984, pp 934–935.

91 Luxation of the Superficial Flexor Tendon at the Calcaneal Tuber

Alan J. Nixon

Luxation or dislocation of the superficial digital flexor tendon from the calcaneal tuber is a relatively rare condition of horses. Several isolated case reports have been described in the literature, and the surgical treatment to reestablish the normal position of the tendon has varied with each. The superficial digital flexor tendon is located superficial to the tendon of insertion of the gastrocnemius muscles at the point of the hock and is maintained in position on the calcaneal tuber by dense fibrous attachments laterally and medially. These attachments represent the tarsal insertions of the tendon. Rupture of the medial attachment, allowing lateral displacement of the tendon, occurs most commonly, although rupture of the lateral attachment has also been described. Trauma, especially impact injuries to the point of the hock, and occasionally severe tension as a result of sudden stopping with the hock partially flexed, are the causes of the displacement.

DIAGNOSIS

An acute onset of lameness is usually accompanied by considerable swelling over the point of the hock. As the lameness declines, some swelling usually persists and the superficial flexor tendon can be identified in a displaced location either laterally or medially on the calcaneal tuber. In the more acute stages of the condition, the prominent swelling is often mistaken for a capped hock. Residual lameness is generally slight and the gait deficit represents a mechanical disability rather than a response to pain. Careful palpation will usually permit identification of the displaced tendon, and in most instances the tendon can be temporarily replaced in its normal location. Further manipulative tests are rarely necessary for a diagnosis; however, radiographs are important to evaluate the bony integrity of the calcaneus. Displaced fractures of the calcaneus can occur concomitantly with complete dislocation of the tendon, both resulting from direct external trauma.

SURGICAL TREATMENT

Because continued mechanical disability and variable discomfort arise from the repeatedly dislocating tendon, surgery is generally recommended to repair the torn tarsal attachment and return the superficial digital flexor tendon to its normal position. Surgical treatment aims to return the tendon to its normal position and to prevent redisplacement. Direct suture of the torn tarsal insertion of the tendon is followed by reinforcement with synthetic mesh or screws or pins inserted into the calcaneus.

The disrupted lateral or medial tarsal insertion of the superficial digital flexor tendon is exposed by a 12-cm curvilinear skin incision, centered over the remnant of the torn attachment. The incision is deepened, exposing the frayed ends of the tendon insertion and the edge of the luxating tendon. The tendon can usually be forced into its normal position over the calcaneal tuber. After débridement of the frayed ends of the tarsal insertion, apposition of these tissues may require partial release of the intact lateral or medial insertion. This can be performed with a scalpel passed through the calcaneal bursa deep to the superficial digital flexor tendon. The tissue to be sutured is often friable, and a near-far–far-near suture pattern using size 2 monofilament nonabsorbable material is indicated for maximum strength of the repair. Nevertheless, supplemental techniques are needed to strengthen the tarsal attachment. The most common method is a reinforcing strip of polypropylene mesh (Marlex Mesh; Davol Inc) secured over the tendon repair using preplaced mattress sutures of heavy monofilament nonabsorbable suture material. Alternatively, bone screws or Steinmann pins can be inserted into the calcaneus alongside the tendon but opposite the ruptured tarsal insertion, thereby preventing displacement of the tendon. Although the screw heads or pin ends block the path of tendon displacement, they provide less support to the suture repair than does a synthetic mesh overlay. Furthermore, these devices eventually need to be removed to prevent irritation of the tendon. Alternative techniques for tension relief on the sutured tendon insertion include a series of deep preplaced mattress sutures penetrating the tendon insertion on the calcaneus and returning to the superficial digital flexor tendon itself. These sutures allow some longitudinal movement of the tendon without allowing subluxation to occur laterally or medially. Nevertheless, the most popular method of suture reinforcement remains the synthetic mesh overlay.

The subcutaneous tissues are apposed using a continuous pattern of size 0 or 1 synthetic absorbable suture. The skin is sutured with monofilament nylon placed in a vertical mattress pattern to provide precise skin edge apposition with some tension relief. After a light dressing has been applied to the sutured wound, the limb is immobilized in extension with a fiberglass cast applied up to the proximal aspect of the tibia.

Complicating injuries to the calcaneus may need surgical treatment in addition to the repair of the disrupted tendon attachment. Scott described the successful bone plate and screw fixation of a comminuted calcaneal fracture before suture repair of the disrupted tendon attachments. Occasionally small calcaneal tuber fractures may accompany a displaced superficial digital flexor tendon, and these fragments are removed or lag screwed into place depending on their size.

POSTOPERATIVE CARE

The affected limb is maintained in a cast for 4 to 6 weeks after surgery. The opposite hind limb is also supported up to the hock with a heavy bandage. Antibiotics are commenced at the time of surgery, especially if a skin wound resulted from the initial traumatic event. Procaine penicillin (22,000 IU/kg intramuscularly) and gentamicin sulfate (2 mg/kg intramuscularly) are suitable choices. Other antibiotics can be substituted as culture results of any open wounds in the region become known. Antibiotics are administered for 3 to 5 days postoperatively. Phenylbutazone is routinely administered prior to surgery (6.6 mg/kg intravenously) and is continued at lower dose rates (4.4 mg/kg by mouth) for 3 to 7 days after surgery. Some horses may need phenylbutazone intermittently for the entire period of cast immobilization and especially for 2 to 4 days after cast removal.

A heavy padded bandage is applied following removal of the cast and maintained for 4 to 5 weeks. Although stall rest is continued after cast removal, several minutes of daily controlled walking exercise can commence within 3 to 7 days, depending on the degree of swelling, pain, extent of the injury, and temperament of the animal. Early mild exercise and forced flexion and extension of the hock and stifle are important in the rehabilitation of the injured limb.

Complicated cases with additional fracture fixation should be evaluated by radiography to determine the earliest possible time for removal of implants since these may interfere with movement of the superficial digital flexor tendon or plantar ligament. It has been proposed that the soft tissue reaction to the implants may be minimized by their early removal and that long-term function of the hock may be improved by early physical therapy.

PROGNOSIS

Displacement of the superficial digital flexor tendon as a result of simple disruption of its lateral or medial tarsal insertion can be effectively treated by suture repair and cast immobilization with good results. The majority of horses return to their former activity, albeit with some reduction in range of hock motion. The injury and resulting tendon displacement are debilitating and surgery is required if an athletic career is anticipated. However, in sedentary horses permanent displacement with fibrosis can result in a pasture-sound animal without the need for surgery.

Chip and comminuted fractures of the calcaneus complicate the healing process with additional fibrosis and callus. Although one horse resumed race training after repair of a comminuted fracture and tendon dislocation, most surgically stabilized comminuted calcaneal fractures preclude such a favorable outcome.

BIBLIOGRAPHY

Fessler JF, Amstutz HE: The musculoskeletal system, in Oehme FW, Prier JE (eds): *The Textbook of Large Animal Surgery.* Baltimore, Williams & Wilkins Co, 1974, p 249.

Meagher DM: Tendon injuries and tendinitis caused by trauma and infection, in *Proceedings of the Annual Conference for Veterinarians.* Fort Collins, Colorado State University, Press, 1981.

Scott EA, Breuhaus B: Surgical repair of dislocated superficial digital flexor tendon in a horse. *J Am Vet Med Assoc* 1982;181:171–172.

Scott EA: Surgical repair of a dislocated superficial digital flexor tendon and fractured fibular tarsal bone in a horse. *J Am Vet Med Assoc* 1983;183:332–333.

Stashak TS: Dislocation of the superficial digital flexor tendon off the calcaneal tuber (luxation of the superficial digital flexor), in Stashak TS (ed): *Adams' Lameness in Horses,* ed 4. Philadelphia, Lea & Febiger, 1987, pp 718–720.

Turner AS: Luxation of the superficial flexor tendon in the hindlimb, in Jennings PB (ed): *The Practice of Large Animal Surgery.* Philadelphia, WB Saunders Co, 1984, pp 936–937.

UNIT VIIIA

Developmental Musculoskeletal Disorders

92
Brachygnathia

Richard M. DeBowes

Brachygnathism is a relatively uncommon condition of young horses that may be associated with serious consequences if left untreated. Although it is considered to be a congenital malformation, foals reportedly have been born clinically normal and have subsequently developed the condition at 3 to 6 months of age. Since this condition minimally affects the young foal's ability to nurse the mare, there are no early signs associated with its presence that would outwardly attract the owner's attention. The abnormality may go unnoticed until an oral examination is performed.

Diagnosis of brachygnathism is made by direct inspection of the dental arcades and identification of imperfect occlusion (Fig. 92–1). In this condition the mandible is shorter than the maxillae. This gives the appearance of an "undershot jaw," with the mandibular incisors positioned caudal to the upper incisors. This deformity is of little immediate consequence because of the liquid nature of the foal's diet. As the affected individual matures, however, the lack of apposition in the dental arcades will become potentially more troublesome. Failure of the premaxillary and mandibular incisors to occlude normally and the development of enamel points on the second upper premolar and the third lower molar teeth on both sides of the arcade may affect the horse's ability to graze and masticate.

SURGICAL TREATMENT

Surgical correction of this condition is possible and involves the placement of temporary wire braces on the upper arcade to retard incisive bone and maxillary bone growth until continued mandibular development has overcome the growth disparity. Surgical treatment should not be pursued until the affected foal has attained 10 weeks of age, by which time the second deciduous upper incisors have erupted. It is desirable to have the second maxillary deciduous incisors present to serve as anchoring points for placement of the incisure tension band devices.

The surgery is performed with the foal anesthetized and positioned in dorsal recumbency. Although either gaseous or intravenous anesthetic agents are effective, the use of gaseous anesthesia administered through a nasotracheal route has been most satisfactory. Preoperative preparation of the patient includes clipping and cleansing of the lateral facial regions and rinsing of the oral cavity with dilute povidone-iodine.

After rinsing the mouth, clipping, and preparing the sides of the facial region, stab incisions are made through the skin and buccal mucosa between the second and third deciduous premolar teeth on both sides of the maxillary arcade. Using a 3.2-mm drill and drill guide to protect the soft tissues, a hole is created in the alveolar bone between the first and second maxillary cheek teeth just below the level of the gingival for the placement of 1.2-mm cerclage wire (Fig. 92–2). The wire is passed through the drill hole and directed cranially with 50% of the wire on the lingual surface of the teeth and 50% on the labial surface. The wire is twisted together for 2 to 3 cm as it traverses the diastema. The wire is then positioned around the deciduous incisors. One strand of the wire is positioned across the midline of the incisors along the labial surface of the incisors and passed through a hole that has been drilled between the central and second deciduous incisors on the opposite side of the premaxillary midline. This wire is then passed back across the midline along the lingual surface of the teeth and passed rostrally through a hole drilled between the central and second deciduous incisors on the side of its maxillary anchorage. The other strand of the wire is directed across the lingual surface of the teeth and passed through a hole drilled between the central deciduous incisors. These two pieces of wire are twisted together over the labial surface of the second deciduous incisor and the ends are cut and folded down between the central and second incisors (Fig. 92–3). The process is then repeated on the opposite side of the upper arcade to complete placement of bilateral tension bands (Fig. 92–4). The buccal stab incisions are closed in two layers with a synthetic absorbable monofilament suture material.

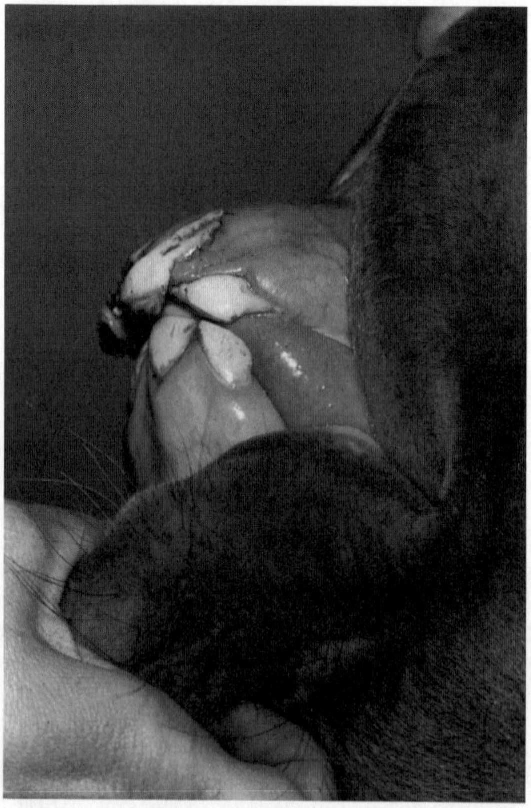

Figure 92–1. The disparity between the upper and lower incisive arcades is generally obvious on physical examination.

POSTOPERATIVE CARE

Broad-spectrum antibiotics should be given during the perioperative period for management of the transient bacteremia that is presumed to occur during surgery of the oral cavity. Gingival, labial, buccal, and lingual soft tissues should be routinely evaluated for evidence of lacerations secondary to the placement of the dental wires. The foal's mouth is rinsed several times daily during the first 3 to 5 postoperative days with a dilute solution of povidone-iodine (<1.0%) to cleanse the braces and remove feed materials that may become impacted in and around the gingival wounds. Foals are observed for evidence of pain while eating or nursing. Occasionally, it is necessary to administer a nonsteroidal anti-inflammatory agent for 72 to 96 hours following surgery to reduce postoperative discomfort in these patients. Although this procedure does not appear to be excessively stressful to the foal, some clinicians recommend the administration of ranitidine (Zantac, 4.4 mg/kg p.o., b.i.d.) to hospitalized foals to reduce the risk of ulcerative gastrointestinal disease. Foals should be evaluated periodically for evidence of wire loosening or breakage.

Several weeks or months may be required for resolution of the mandibular growth disparity. The owners are advised to evaluate the foal's postoperative progress on a weekly basis until normal incisor occlusive symmetry is achieved. Foals that eventually develop a normal degree of incisor occlusion should have the dental wire removed immediately. Wires are readily removed from the standing patient following sedation with xylazine. Failure to remove the implants following the return of a normal degree of incisor occlusion may allow overcorrection of the deformity or prognathism.

PROGNOSIS

In my experience, this procedure may be very effective if performed in patients less than 6 months of age that

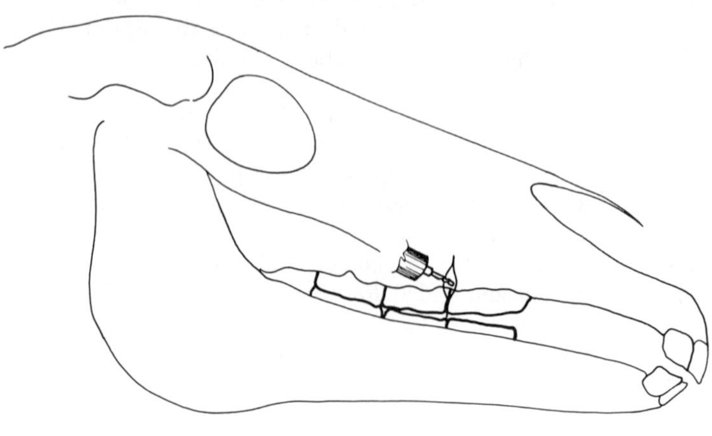

Figure 92–2. A 3.2-mm hole is drilled between the upper cheek teeth for passage of a 1.2-mm wire.

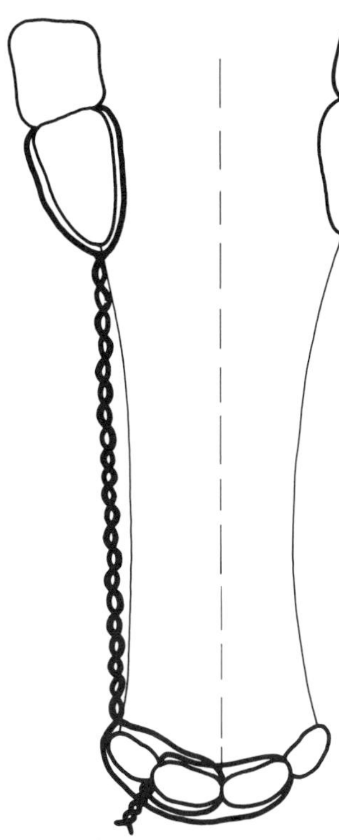

Figure 92–3. Wires are placed around the maxillary teeth and directed toward the incisors, around which they are twisted and secured on the labial surface of the teeth.

are affected with a minimal or moderate deformity. Minimal deformity is one in which the mandibular incisor remains in contact with the maxillary incisior. Moderate deformities are those in which the disparity is less than or equal to the width of one incisor tooth. Horses with extreme incisor malocclusion that suffer a disparity of alignment greater than two incisor widths have not been successfully managed with this surgical technique unless they have been operated at an age of less than 6 months. Horses in excess of 1 year of age do not have adequate compensatory mandibular growth to permit resolution of moderate to severe deformities. Rarely an affected horse that has undergone a successful surgical correction will subsequently reacquire the brachygnathic condition during a period of rapid musculoskeletal growth. While such cases are unusual in my experience, clients should be cautioned as to this possibility. Although I have not observed cases of overcorrection, it is conceivable that this could occur if the braces are not removed when the mandibular and maxillary arcades are realigned.

The ethical question of providing a cosmetic and functional therapy for a condition that may be transmitted genetically has been debated. Although most investigations have suggested that the condition is genetically transmitted in cattle, there are no definitive studies confirming the heritable nature of this condition in the horse. At the present time, I am cautioning the owners of affected animals presented for surgery of the possibility of a familial tendency to develop this condition. Owners are encouraged to neuter or eliminate affected individuals from intended use as breeding stock.

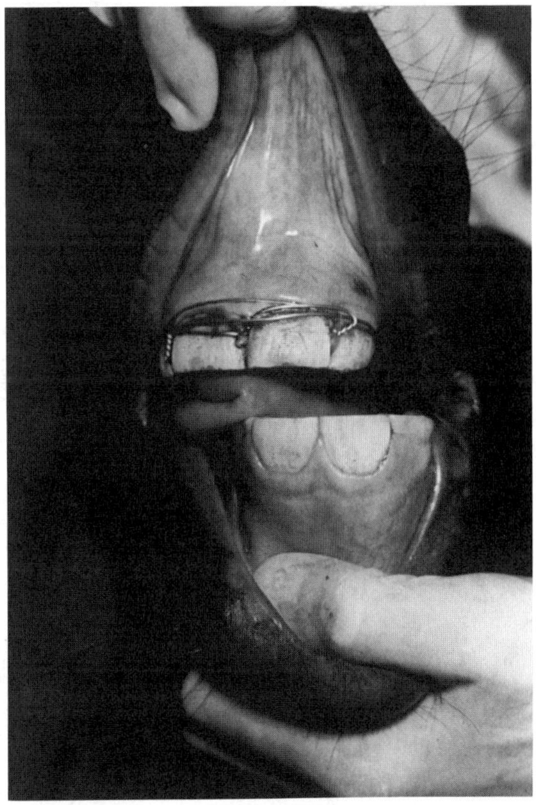

Figure 92–4. Bilateral applications of tension band wires have been made to this maxillary arcade. The wire ends are twisted together and positioned between the incisors.

BIBLIOGRAPHY

Bunton TE: Spontaneous craniofacial malformations and central nervous system defects in an aborted equine fetus. *J Comp Pathol* 1985;95:131–135.

Crowe MW, Swerczek TW: Equine congenital defects. *Am J Vet Res* 1985;46:353–358.
Heidari M, Vogt DW, Nelson SL: Brachygnathism in a herd of Angus cattle. *Am J Vet Res* 1985;46:708–710.
McIllwraith CW: Brachygnathia, in Jennings PD (ed): *The Practice of Large Animal Surgery*. Philadelphia, WB Saunders Co, 1984, pp 558–560.

93 Flexural Deformity of the Distal Interphalangeal Joint (Contracture of the Deep Digital Flexor Tendon)

Pamela C. Wagner

Flexural deformity of the distal interphalangeal joint has also been referred to as contracture of the deep digital flexor tendon, flexural deformity of the coronopedal joint, and "club foot." The condition is usually an acquired condition of the rapidly growing foal between the ages of 2 and 8 months. In some cases the owner is unaware of the condition until the chronic appearance of the deformity becomes more noticeable. Rarely, the condition occurs in the newborn foal. When it does, it is usually associated with deformity of joints other than just the distal interphalangeal joint, suggesting multiple defects.

DIAGNOSIS

Most affected foals are rapidly growing and on a high plane of nutrition when the deformity is noted. Typically, the condition occurs bilaterally in the forelimbs, although one leg is usually more affected than the other. In cases in which the foal is still nursing, the mare may be a very heavy milk producer, and nutritional excess is difficult to control. Curtailing of exercise in young horses being fed and conditioned for show increases the incidence.

In most cases the owner notices the steepness of the hoof when the foal is between 2 and 4 months of age. He or she often reports lengthening of the heel and cracking of the toe. The owner's early complaint often is not lameness, because the foal appears to ambulate well on the affected limbs, but rather the cosmetic appearance of the distal limb. Another common complaint is prominence of the coronary band.

There are several different physical presentations of this condition. The clinical appearance has been divided into stages I and II to indicate the degree of flexural deformity. Stage I deformities are those in which the dorsum of the hoof has not passed the vertical line from the coronary band to the ground, whereas stage II deformities are those in which the dorsal aspect of the hoof has passed vertical and the horse walks on a portion of the dorsum of the hoof (Fig. 93–1). Stage I deformities may have different appearances depending on the duration of the condition. Acute cases present with an elongated heel or a heel that will not touch the ground. Effusion in the distal interphalangeal joint makes the coronary band appear prominent. In stage I deformities that have existed for a longer period of time, especially when attempts have been made to keep the heel on the ground by trimming or shoeing, there is a concave appearance to the front of the hoof wall. As the pull of the deep digital flexor tendon on the distal phalanx continues, there is some separation of the distal phalanx from the hoof wall and the concavity is accentuated (Fig. 93–2). In stage I deformities that are chronic and untreated, a box-shaped hoof is seen in the older horse. Stage II deformities may vary in severity, but in all cases the horse stands on the toe with no sole or frog touching the ground.

Although clinical appearance is often enough to make a diagnosis of flexural deformity, palpation of the soft tissues of the limb and radiographs of the digit should be performed prior to the rendering of a prognosis and prescribing of a treatment. Palpation of the flexor tendons in the elevated, standing, and hyperextended positions should be performed. Hyperextension is achieved by placing the toe on a board to tighten the flexor tendons. In stage I contractures, the deep digital flexor tendon will be tight in the flat and hyperextended positions. In stage II contractures, the deep digi-

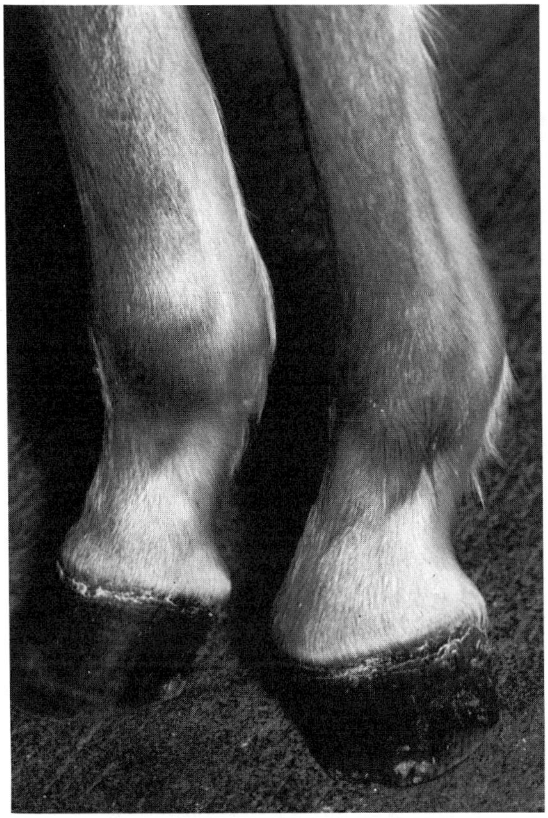

Figure 93–1. Acute onset of flexural deformity of the distal interphalangeal joint, which has already advanced to stage II. The foal walks on the toe and the heel often will not touch the ground.

tal flexor tendon may feel slack until hyperextension is achieved. Lateral and dorsopalmar radiographs of the digit should be made to evaluate the degree of flexion in the distal interphalangeal joint, the degree of separation of the distal phalanx from the hoof wall, the amount of osseous change (if any) in the joint, and the remodeling changes in the distal phalanx and the navicular bone. In cases in which these changes are absent or minimal, the prognosis for future soundness is good with appropriate therapy.

SURGERY

Mild cases of flexural deformity of the distal interphalangeal joint may not require surgery. Conservative therapy consists of diet management, increased exercise, and application of an extended toe shoe with reduction of the heel length starting as soon as the condition is diagnosed. Diet changes should include reduction of total caloric intake and balancing of trace minerals. If prompt response to therapy is not seen, if the clinical signs worsen, or if the deformity is moderate to severe when first seen, corrective surgery is indicated. Stage I and some stage II deformities respond to distal check desmotomy. In severe stage II deformities and all deformities that recur after distal check desmotomy, salvage may be possible with a tenotomy of the deep digital flexor tendon.

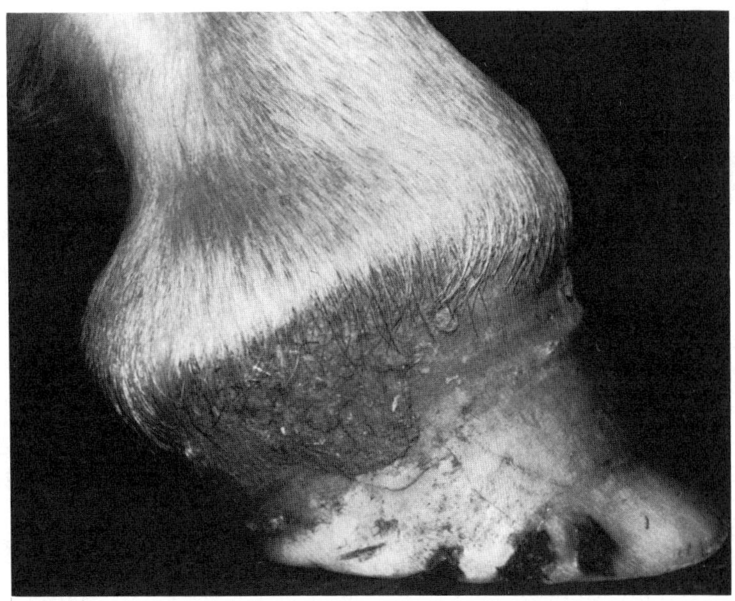

Figure 93–2. Chronic distal interphalangeal joint flexural deformity may present as a "dished" hoof in those horses treated with corrective trimming (stage I).

Distal Check Desmotomy

Distal check desmotomy was first described in 1969. Since then it has been reported to be efficacious in returning the distal limb to correct alignment and the horse to functional performance. The distal check ligament originates at the palmar carpal ligament and inserts on the deep digital flexor tendon in the proximal portion of the metacarpus. The check ligament provides support for the digit through the deep flexor tendon and prevents overstretching or strain of the digital flexor muscle bellies during extension of the digit. As the digit extends, the flexor muscle bellies stretch until the check ligament tenses. When the muscle-tendinous unit is functionally too short, as in flexural deformity of the distal interphalangeal joint, severance of the distal check ligament allows lengthening of the unit and proper axial realignment of the bones of the digit.

Transection or resection of a portion of the distal check ligament can be done from either the medial or lateral side of the limb (Fig. 93–3). The approach is somewhat more difficult from the medial side because of the neurovascular structures to be avoided. A tourniquet is placed above the carpus and after surgical preparation of the limb an incision is made beginning 2 cm below the carpus just dorsal to the flexor tendons. A deep incision through the carpal flexor retinaculum is made to reveal the underlying tendons and check ligament. The division between the deep digital flexor tendon and the distal check ligament is located, and the check ligament is elevated and severed. Care is taken to cut all fibers of this structure. Extension of the foot allows the surgeon to ascertain that the ligament is completely transected. In some cases, escape of synovial fluid indicates the carpal sheath has been entered; however, this does not present a problem. Closure of the flexor retinaculum, subcutaneous tissue, and skin are sufficient to prevent synovial leakage. Pressure wraps are applied and maintained for at least 2 weeks to prevent swelling and ensure cosmetic healing.

Corrective shoeing is done either immediately before or after surgery to hold the foot in the correct position during healing. Several types of shoes may be applied depending on the severity of the deformity. In mild cases an elevated toe plate with open heels is used. The open heels allow the periodic rasping of the rear portion of the foot to keep the correct alignment. More severe cases require a toe extension to force the heels down and prolong breakover. Placing this shoe prior to surgery avoids working with the limb immediately after surgery. Recently, a "mushroom"-shaped shoe has been used to provide support for the hoof wall–third phalanx interface while forcing the heel to the ground. In the young horse, shoes are often difficult to keep in place. Casting material placed over the nails or wires used to hold the shoes in place may be helpful. Recently, glue-on plastic shoes with toe extensions (Glu-Strider; Mustad Inc) have been used with success.

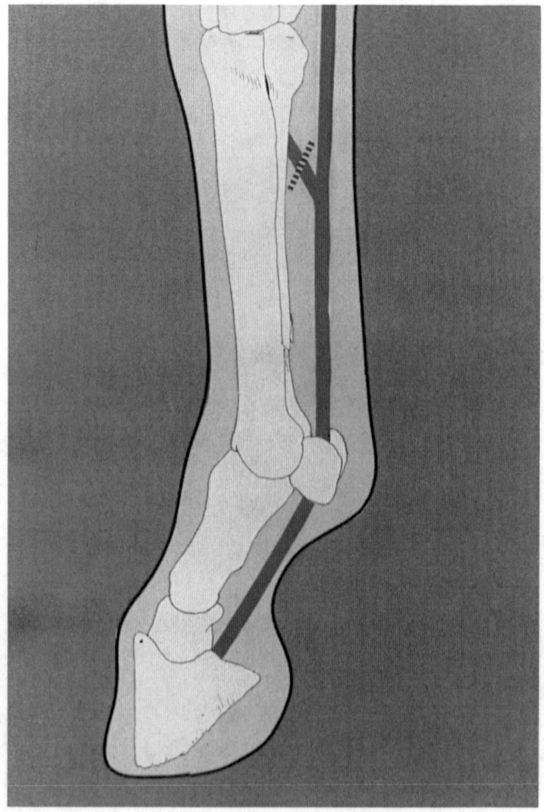

Figure 93–3. The distal check ligament can be approached from either the medial or the lateral side.

Postoperative care includes maintenance of leg wraps and controlled exercise. Over the course of 3 months, the severed ends of the check ligament are reunited by fibrous scar tissue. It is important, therefore, to hold the foot in proper alignment during this time with corrective shoes. Twelve to 18 weeks of corrective shoeing is sufficient to allow healing of the now-lengthened check ligament. After this time, corrective shoeing may be discontinued. The hoof deformity will grow out and be replaced by normal-appearing hoof wall in 4 to 6 months.

Complications of this surgery are few unless contamination occurs. Infection in this area has serious consequences but is avoided by careful aseptic technique. Minimizing tissue dissection and excessive use of suture material minimizes scarring. Generally scarring is most evident in older horses (over 2 years of age). Recurrence of the deformity can occur if corrective trimming and shoeing are not used or if the horse is not exercised after surgery. If the check ligament heals prior to achieving proper foot angulation, the deformity can recur. The majority of cases, however, are successful, as shown in a follow-up study where the outcome was favorable in 87% of 40 horses treated as judged by the ability of the horses to become athletes following surgery.

Deep Digital Flexor Tenotomy

In severe cases of stage II deformities or in those cases of stage I deformity that do not respond permanently to distal check desmotomy, transection of the deep digital flexor tendon at the palmar aspect of the middle phalanx may be considered.

A skin incision is made on the midline of the affected limb at the level of the pastern. When skin and subcutaneous fascia are divided, the tendon sheath of the deep digital flexor tendon is encountered. The sheath is opened and the tendon is transected. Extension of the foot confirms that the entire tendon has been severed. The subcutaneous and cutaneous tissues are closed and the leg bandaged.

After surgery realignment of the digit is variable. In some cases the process is rapid and overcorrection can occur. When this happens the toe elevates and subluxation of the distal interphalangeal joint can occur. Corrective shoeing in the form of a shoe with heel extension is needed. In some horses overextension may be permanent. In other horses, the deformity corrects slowly and proper alignment is eventually achieved. With the variable results associated with this technique, it is recommended for salvage of the horse used for breeding or for a pasture-sound horse, although some horses can go on to athletic activity.

POSTOPERATIVE CARE

Controlled but forced exercise is recommended to maintain normal foot angulation and eventual normal hoof regrowth. Corrective shoeing and trimming is necessary to achieve good results, and surgery should not be undertaken unless follow-up hoof care is ensured.

PROGNOSIS

Stage I deformities treated by distal check desmotomy have a good prognosis for return to function. In long-term studies, over 80% of the treated animals eventually fulfilled their owner's expectations for use. Since many affected animals are intended for show, the cosmetic appearance of the limb was important. In horses less than 1 year of age at the time of surgery, most have minimal scarring. The procedure can correct a chronic condition seen in the aged horse. However, older horses are usually left with a blemish at the surgery site.

When the deformity is so severe that tenotomy of the deep digital flexor must be performed, the prognosis for athletic pursuits is poor but the animal may be salvaged for breeding.

BIBLIOGRAPHY

Fackelman GE, Auer JA, Orsini J, von Salis B: Surgical treatment of severe flexural deformity of the distal interphalangeal joint in young horses. *J Am Vet Med Assoc* 1983;182:949–952.

Flecker RH, Wagner PC: Therapy and corrective shoeing for equine tendon disorders. *Compend Cont Educ Pract Vet* 1986;8:970–976.

Hintz H: Nutrition and its role in angular deformities, in *Proceedings of the Horsemans Short Course.* Yakima, WA, Washington Horse Breeders Assoc, 1979, pp 129–140.

Lewis LD: The role of nutrition in musculoskeletal development and disease, in Stashak TS (ed): *Adams' Lameness in Horses.* Philadelphia, Lea & Febiger, 1987, p 277.

Lysholt B, Sonnichsen HV: Senestylfefod hos fol og plage. *Nord Vet Med* 1969;21:601.

McIlwraith CW: Diseases of joints, tendons, ligaments and related structures, in Stashak TS (ed): *Adams' Lameness in Horses.* Philadelphia, Lea & Febiger, 1987, p 458.

McIlwraith CW, Fessler JF: Evaluation of inferior check ligament desmotomy for treatment of acquired flexor tendon contracture in the horse. *J Am Vet Med Assoc* 1978;172:293–298.

Owen JM: Abnormal flexion of the corono-pedal joint or "contracted tendons" in the unweaned foal. *Equine Vet J* 1975;7:40–45.

Shively MJ: Functional and clinical significance of the check ligaments. *Equine Pract* 1983;5:37–42.

Wagner PC, Grant BD, Kaneps AJ, Watrous BJ: Long-term results of desmotomy of the accessory ligament of the deep digital flexor tendon (distal check ligament) in horses. *J Am Vet Med Assoc* 1985;187:1351–1352.

94
Flexural Deformity of the Metacarpophalangeal Joint (Contracture of the Superficial Digital Flexor Tendon)

Pamela C. Wagner

Abnormal flexion of the fetlock in the horse has been termed "contracture" of the superficial digital flexor tendon, "posty" legs, and flexural deformity of the fetlock or metacarpophalangeal joint. It can occur congenitally or may be acquired in horses between 8 and 18 months of age. The condition has been considered a consequence of unequal lengthening of the muscle-tendon unit of the superficial digital flexor muscle and the osseous structures of the limb, but recent clinical studies suggest that the deep digital flexor tendon and the suspensory ligament are involved in at least some cases.

CONGENITAL DEFORMITY OF THE METACARPOPHALANGEAL JOINT

Diagnosis

The diagnosis is obvious when the foal stands or attempts to stand. In mild cases the foal stands very upright (Fig. 94–1) and in moderate cases the fetlock buckles forward. In severe cases the foal may be unable to stand (Fig. 94–2). The foal is usually full term and well developed. The condition is most commonly seen in the forelimbs or in all four legs. In cases of severe contracture other skeletal abnormalities may be present, especially prognathism.

The joints should be checked for manual extendibility. If the joint can be manually placed in correct alignment, the prognosis for resolution is good with treatment. If the joint cannot be extended, radiographs of the area should be made to rule out osseous abnormalities prior to undertaking therapy. If no radiographic abnormalities are seen, the prognosis for resolution is fair to good. Rupture of the common digital extensor tendon should be suspected in all cases because it can present with a similar conformation.

Surgery

Surgery for correction of congenital flexural deformity is reserved for severe cases or cases unresponsive to conservative therapy. Mild congenital flexural deformities of the metacarpophalangeal joint usually resolve uneventfully as the foal stands and walks. Resolution typically takes 2 to 5 days. Bandaging with light-weight wraps may speed the relaxation of the tight structures. Moderate to severe deformities require splints or casts to obtain correction. Casting achieves greater relaxation but the disadvantages of casting young horses should be weighed against the need to correct the deformity. In general, if the deformity can be reduced easily by manipulation, the use of splints over thick bandages will result in correction. If the deformity is so severe that the foal's leg cannot be kept straight by use of a splint, a light-weight cast can be applied. If both forelimbs must be cast, the foal will require periodic assistance in standing to assure adequate frequency of nursing. If the deformity is so severe that it cannot be manually straightened, a distal check desmotomy will usually allow straightening. If this is not helpful, severing of the superficial digital flexor tendon or the suspensory ligament may allow straightening. If tenotomy or desmotomy is done, support of the limb by splint or cast may be necessary for 10 to 14 days. Long-term care includes reduced activity for several months postoperatively while the structures heal.

Postoperative Care

Casts on young foals must be closely monitored. One should palpate the cast several times daily to check for hot areas indicative of pressure/rub sores. The foal should be kept in a stall to avoid excessive or strenuous exercise with casts that may result in trauma to the limbs. After removal of the casts, the limbs may appear weakened with excessive tendon laxity, but tightening

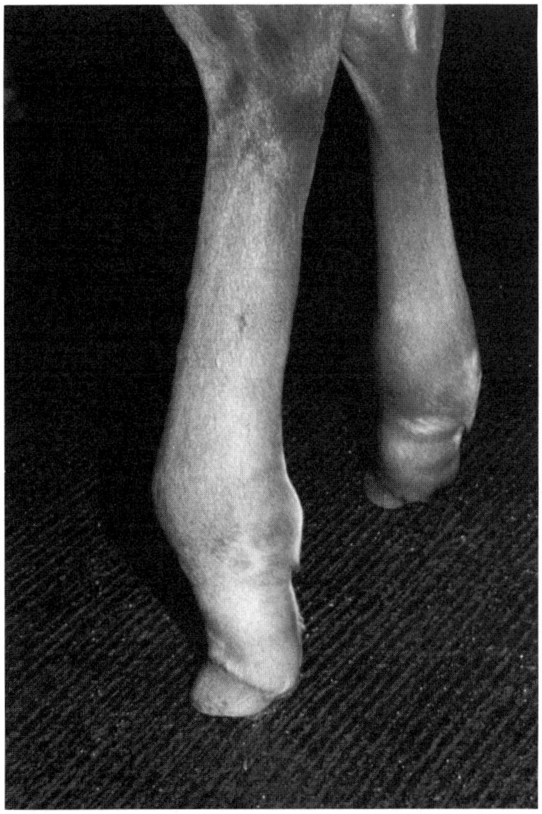

Figure 94–1. Mild congenital flexural deformity of the metatarsophalangeal joint.

of the tendons occurs rapidly. Stall rest with intermittent exercise should be maintained until alignment is near normal. If the limbs are not extended after the casts are removed, the casts must be reapplied. Monitoring the foal for proper maintenance of nutrition and for signs of stress-induced gastric ulcers is important during this therapy.

Prognosis

In general, congenital contractures of the fetlock have a better prognosis than carpal contractures. If the limbs can be manually straightened at birth, the prognosis is good. Nonreducible deformities have a guarded to poor prognosis, although individual cases have responded to radical surgery.

ACQUIRED FETLOCK FLEXURAL DEFORMITIES

Diagnosis

Acquired flexural deformities of the metacarpophalangeal joint usually occur in horses 8 to 18 months of age. Although it is most common on the forelimbs, the hind limbs can be affected. If the condition is bilateral, one limb is usually more severely affected. The onset of signs is gradual, with the leg first becoming upright, then flexed forward at the joint. Horses intended for show, especially halter horses, are most often affected and they appear to be most suseptible during periods of rapid growth.

The normal dorsal angle of the metacarpophalangeal joint is 135 degrees in the weight-bearing stance. Flexural deformity of this joint results in an increase of the angle to 180 degrees in the mild case and to 225 degrees or greater in severe cases. The fetlock joint appears to flex forward and, depending on involvement of other structures, the foot may be in a normal position or have an elevated heel. The horse will be noted to "pop" the fetlocks forward while initially unweighting the limb. As the condition worsens, the fetlock tends to stay in the "knuckled over" or the flexed position (Fig. 94–3).

As with flexural deformity of the distal interphalangeal joint, the etiology of this deformity is probably

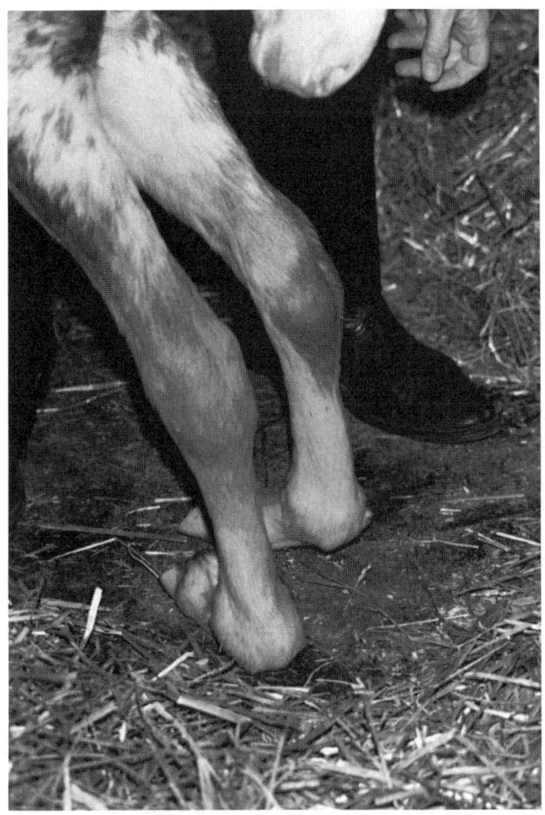

Figure 94–2. With severe congenital fetlock deformities the foal cannot stand unassisted.

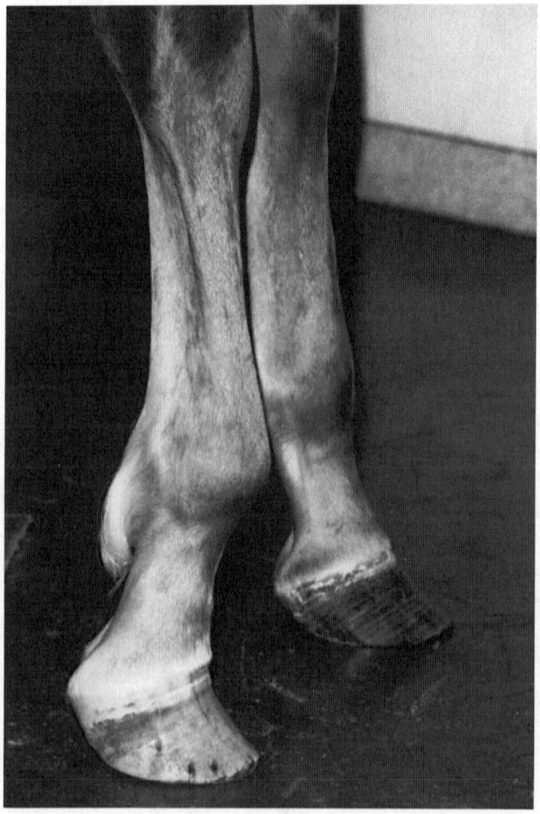

Figure 94–3. Unilateral acquired flexural deformity of the metacarpophalangeal joint.

multifactorial. Most affected horses are rapidly growing and on diets high in energy and/or protein. Pain from physitis at the distal radial growth plate and osteochondrosis of the shoulder and fetlock may be contributory. Pain from hind limb fractures can cause this flexural deformity in the fore, hind, or all four limbs. An unequal growth rate between the osseous structures and the muscle-tendon unit of the superficial digital flexor has been postulated as the pathogenesis. As the tendon unit (stay apparatus) becomes functionally too short, the fetlock flexes forward, shortening the distance between the origin of the superficial flexor tendon, the deep flexor tendon, and the suspensory ligament and their sites of insertion on the proximal, middle, and distal phalanges. Secondarily, the common distal extensor tendon, extensor branches of the suspensory ligament, and dorsal joint capsule stretch, while the palmar joint capsule fails to lengthen. These changes reinforce the flexural deformity of the metacarpophalangeal joint. In severe cases, where manual straightening of the joint is no longer possible, involvement of the suspensory ligament is suspected. In some cases a reflex contracture to pain is also suspected as a cause. Horses with this response will improve with anti-inflammatory drug therapy or resolution of a painful lesion. Trauma to the superficial digital flexor tendon due to tendonitis or lacerations may result in scarring that, as it contracts, also causes an acquired flexural deformity of the joint.

The appearance of the fetlock and foot is usually sufficient to make the diagnosis. Palpation of the tendons both with the limb in the relaxed position and with the toe elevated on a board helps determine if more than one structure is involved. This is important to ascertain because correct treatment depends upon determination of all involved structures. If the superficial digital flexor tendon is most taut with the toe elevated, it is the most involved structure; if the deep digital flexor tendon and suspensory ligament are also taut, the prognosis is poor because all three structures are involved.

Radiographs of the fetlock and digit should be made to determine the degree of osseous change in the metacarpophalangeal and distal interphalangeal joints. In mild cases the articulation between the metacarpus and proximal phalanx is upright and arthritic changes are not present or are only slight. In moderate cases the distal interphalangeal joint may be subluxated with the proximal middle phalanx angled dorsally. These changes increase with severity and duration of the deformity. In very severe cases, changes are seen in the proximal and distal sesamoid bones, the third metacarpal bone, and the distal phalanx. Such changes indicate a grave prognosis with any treatment.

Surgery

Surgery for correction of flexural deformity of the metacarphophalangeal joint is mostly recommended for moderate cases of the condition. Mild cases usually do not require surgery and very severe cases rarely respond to surgery.

In mildly affected horses, the use of a shoe with an elevated heel and toe extension provides adequate correction. Theoretically, the elevated heel unweights the deep digital flexor tendon and preferentially loads the superficial digital flexor tendon and suspensory ligament. This theory is not supported by strain gauge evaluation of tendon and ligaments in response to changes of heel angle. However, clinical response is documented. Dietary changes to reduce the growth rate help to prevent progression of the deformity. Bandaging and/or casting have not been reported to significantly alter the deformity in the acquired form of the condition.

If the condition is moderate, surgical intervention should be considered. The structures contributing to the deformity as determined by palpation will dictate which surgery will be helpful. If only the superficial digital flexor tendon is affected, severance of the accessory ligament of the superficial digital flexor tendon (proximal check ligament) is adequate to restore proper axial alignment of the limb. If both the superficial and deep digital flexor tendons are involved, severance of both the proximal and distal check ligaments is recommended. Moderate cases may respond to severing of either accessory ligament. After surgery, splinting with a polyvinylchloride splint for 5 to 10 days and corrective shoeing help to maintain separation of the ends of the check ligaments.

Proximal check desmotomy is performed from the medial side of the limb, proximal to the radial carpal joint. The skin incision is made dorsal to the cephalic vein and palmar to the radius, approximately 12 cm proximal to the joint. The vein is retracted in a palmar direction and the deep incision is continued through the antebrachial fascia. The flexor carpi radialis is retracted from the radius and the proximal check ligament can be palpated. This ligament has a fan-shaped portion that attaches to the medial side of the radius as well as a thick band that attaches on the palmar surface of the radius (Fig. 94–4). Both should be severed to ensure complete transection of the structure. The thick band is elevated with a heavy Crile hemostat and severed. Heavy Mayo scissors are used to cut the ligament, taking care not to cut vessels of the rete carpi palmares. Closure of the fascia, subcutaneous tissues, and skin completes the surgery. A pressure bandage is placed over the incision, followed by a heavily padded bandage. A polyvinylchloride splint is placed on the limb from elbow to fetlock after recovery to maintain alignment. Corrective shoeing with a toe extension is done to prolong breakover and, thus, increase the time that strain is placed on the superficial digital flexor tendon. The heels may be elevated as an adjunct to the surgery if necessary. Distal check desmotomy is described in Chapter 93.

In severe cases, desmotomy of both check ligaments is inadequate to restore correct angulation to the fetlock. Tenotomy of the superficial digital flexor in the midmetacarpal region may be helpful but is not cos-

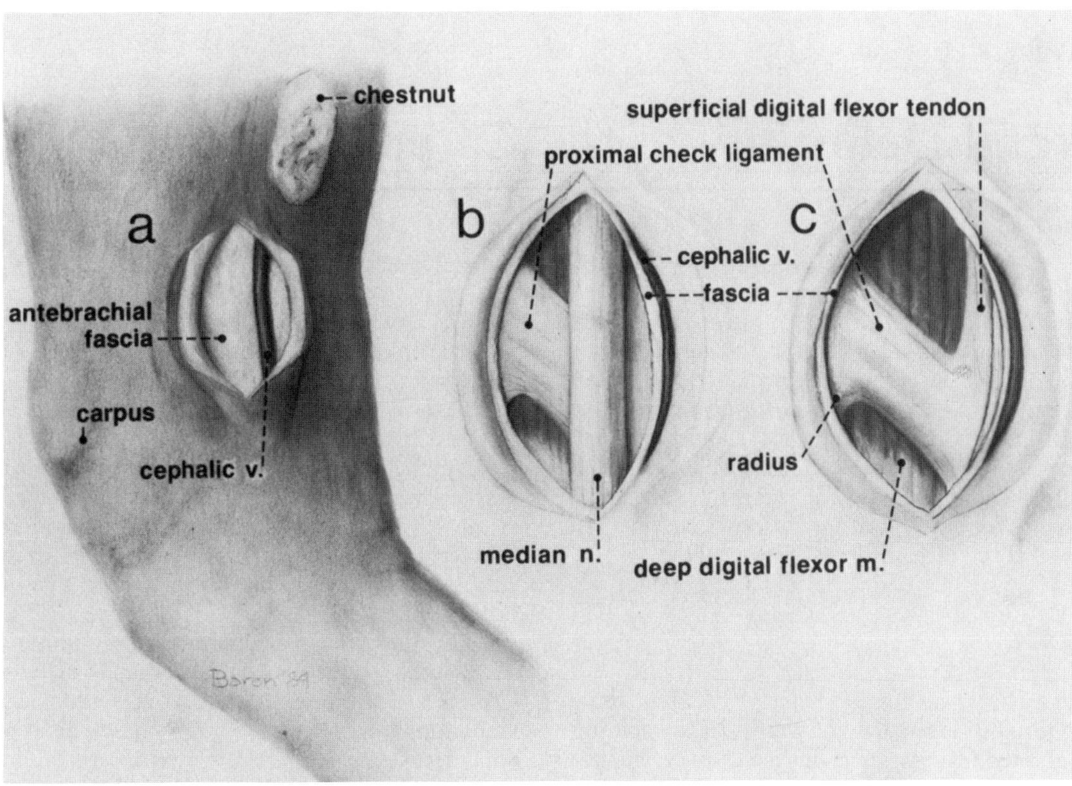

Figure 94–4. The surgical anatomy of the approach to the proximal check ligament. **A.** Skin incision. **B.** Fascial incision. **C.** Check ligament attachment.

metic and can be quite painful. Suspensory desmotomy may also correct the deformity but may result in subluxation of the pastern joint and excessive dropping of the fetlock. Both surgeries should be reserved for the unresponsive case that is to be salvaged for breeding or a pasture-sound pet.

The response of this deformity to surgical therapy is not as consistent as that of deformity of the distal interphalangeal joint. Immediate postoperative improvement is not always apparent, and 4 to 7 days may be required to appreciate improvement. Phenylbutazone therapy is often helpful to establish full weight bearing, which helps maintain the correct conformation after surgery. At 8 to 10 weeks after surgery, the condition may recur. Exercise and corrective shoes will help reduce this complication. In cases in which pain with reflex flexor contracture is suspected as a cause of the deformity, restriction of exercise may be necessary to prevent further contracture. In a study of 15 cases of metacarpophalangeal deformity, severe cases were rarely returned to previous or anticipated levels of performance, whereas mild and moderate cases were responsive to treatment.

BIBLIOGRAPHY

Blackwell RB: Response of acquired flexural deformity of the metacarpophalangeal joint to desmotomy of the inferior check ligament. *Proc Am Assoc Equine Pract* 1982; pp 107–111.

Fackelman GE: Equine flexural deformities of developmental origin. *Proc Am Assoc Equine Pract* 1980; pp 97–105.

Fackelman GE: Flexure deformity of the metacarpophalangeal joints in growing horses. *Compend Cont Educ Pract Vet* 1979;1:51–59.

Jann HW, Beroza GA, Fackelman GE: Surgical anatomy for desmotomy of the accessory ligament of the superficial digital flexor tendon (proximal check ligament) in horses. *Vet Surg* 1986;15:378–382.

Lochner FK, Milne DW, Mills EJ, Groom JJ: In vivo and in vitro measurement of tendon strain in the horse. *Am J Vet Res* 1980;41:129.

Metcalf S, Wagner PC, Balch-Burnett O: Corrective trimming and shoeing in the treatment of tendon disorders of young horses. *Equine Pract* 1982;4:6–15.

Wagner PC, Shires GMH, Watrous BJ, Kaneps AJ, Schmotzer WB, Riebold TW: Management of acquired flexural deformity of the metacarpophalangeal joint in Equidae. *J Am Vet Med Assoc* 1985;187:915–918.

95
Flexural Deformity of the Carpus

Pamela C. Wagner

While the flexural deformities that affect the fetlock and distal interphalangeal joint may be congenital or acquired, those of the carpus are invariably congenital. The deformity may be very slight, resulting in a forward angle of the carpus when the foal stands, or it may be so severe that a normal delivery is impossible. Severely affected animals have been termed "contracted foals," and other skeletal abnormalities have been associated with the carpal flexural deformity.

DIAGNOSIS

The foal with carpal flexural deformity cannot bring the limb into full extension voluntarily. If the deformity is slight, the foal can stand but the carpi are bucked forward (Fig. 95–1). The common digital extensor tendon may appear very taut or may even rupture, giving rise to soft fluctuant masses on the lateral side of the carpus. Severely affected foals cannot stand. Manual pressure on the dorsal surface of the carpus may reduce the flexion partially or not at all (Fig. 95–2). In severe cases all the structures on the palmar aspect of the carpus feel tight. Often there are other congenital defects, including prognathism, scoliosis, kyphosis, flexural deformities in other joints, and in some cases extreme laxity in the lower limb. The more severely affected foals are often premature, but despite their small size they may cause dystocia because of in utero limb flexion.

The causes of carpal contracture are unknown but are assumed to be congenital rather than hereditary. Uterine malpositioning of the fetus is offered as an explanation; however, the deformity has been seen in prenatal fetuses of less than 9 months' gestation when crowding would not be significant. Genetic causes have been postulated but occurrence of contractures from different lines on the same farm has made this

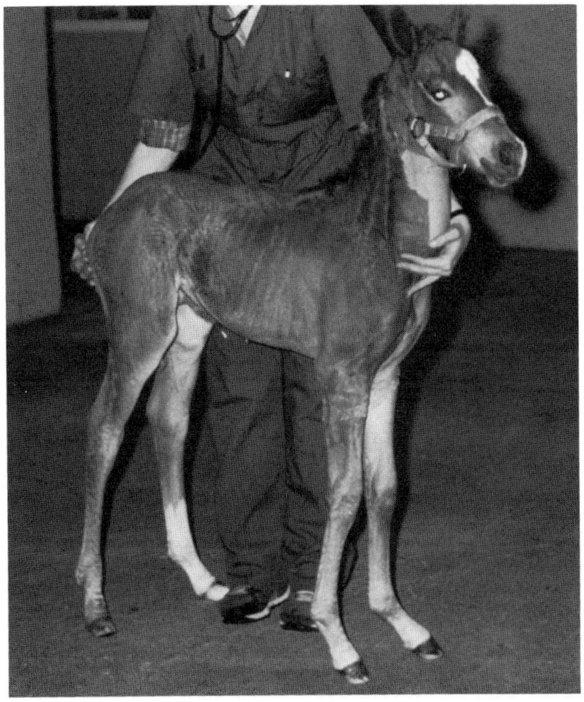

Figure 95–1. Mild flexural deformity of the carpus usually responds to conservative therapy.

unlikely. Proof of a genetic cause is not reported. Teratogenic factors affecting mares in the first 3 months of gestation are the most likely causes, and cases have been documented following ingestion of locoweed or Sudan grass and following influenza outbreaks. One author has suggested the primary defect is in the formation of an abnormal fetal skeleton. Instability of joints leading to the tendency of the soft tissues to contract to stabilize the joint has been suggested and is confirmed by evidence of osseous malformations in some severely contracted foals.

Although the pathogenesis of carpal contractures is unknown, numerous authors have documented that the restricting tissues are the palmar ligaments and palmar joint capsules of the carpus. In necropsy evaluation of severely affected foals, the limbs can only be straightened when these structures are severed.

The foal should be thoroughly examined for accompanying abnormalities before therapy is undertaken. Radiographs should be made of the affected joints to determine whether cuboidal bone malformation or abnormalities are present. The skull and mandible should be inspected for closure defects and malocclusion. Neurologic evaluation may be difficult in the recumbent foal but should be attempted because of the tendency for spinal abnormalities to be present in conjunction with the flexural deformity.

TREATMENT

Mild contractures may improve spontaneously. Those mild cases that do not straighten completely in the first few days of life may be treated by bandaging and splinting the limb from just below the elbow to the fetlock. Heavy bandages should be placed on the limb and the leg should be firmly pulled back to a heavily

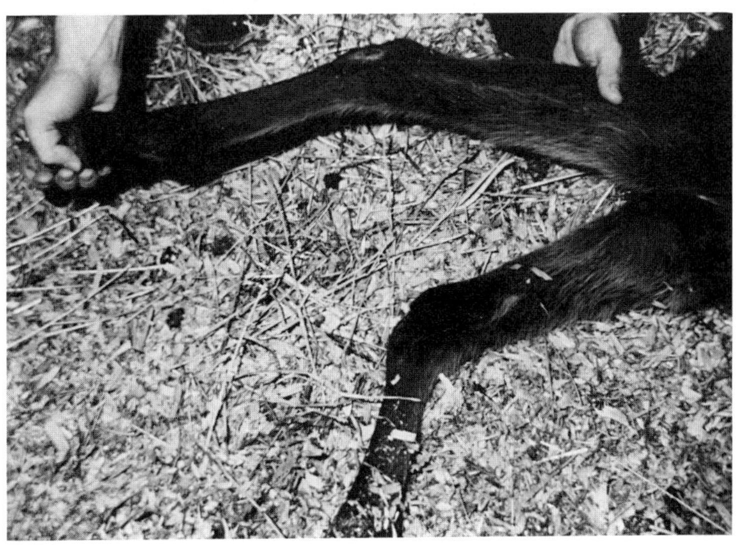

Figure 95–2. Severe carpal flexural deformities cannot be manually reduced.

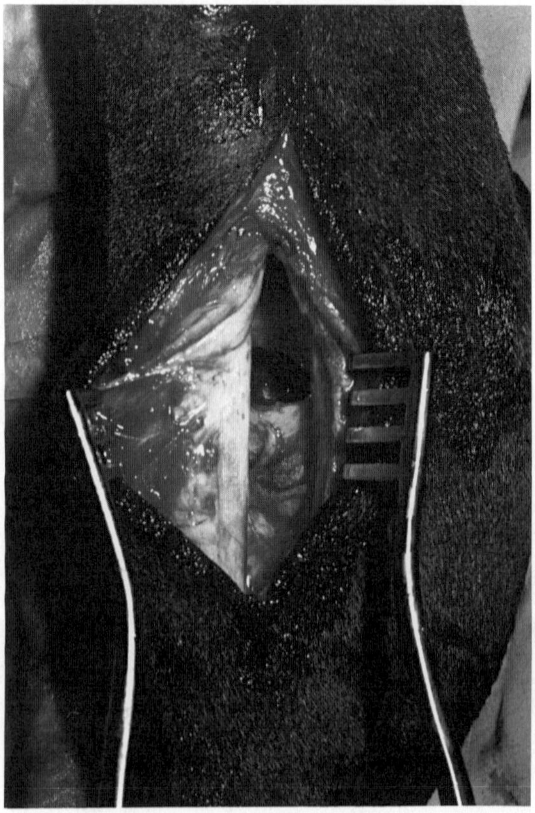

Figure 95–3. Some cases of severe carpal flexural deformity will respond to palmar carpal capsule release.

padded polyvinylchloride splint and taped. Monitoring of splints is important because the splints often rotate and slip, causing pressure sores. Resetting of splints twice daily may be needed. If the foal cannot stand without help after application of the splints, assistance in feeding may be needed. Correction is usually noticeable by 4 to 7 days of age.

Severe cases that do not respond to splinting may benefit from release of the palmar carpal capsule, which may be achieved through a medial approach to the carpal canal (Fig. 95–3). A skin incision is made dorsal to the flexor tendons and continued through the carpal retinaculum. The flexor tendons are retracted and a curved scalpel blade is used to incise the exposed joint capsules of the radiocarpal and middle carpal joints. Pressure is exerted against the dorsal aspect of the carpus and, if straightening can be achieved, the incision in the carpal retinaculum, subcutaneous tissue, and skin is closed. The limb is then splinted in extension. If the limb cannot be straightened at surgery, chances for recovery are poor and humane destruction is advised. Although this procedure has been used only to salvage animals for breeding, some horses recover enough to become functional riding horses.

BIBLIOGRAPHY

Hutt FB: Genetic defects of bones and joints in domestic animals. *Cornell Vet* 1968;58(suppl):104–113.

McIlwraith CW: Diseases of the joints, tendons and ligaments and related structures, in Stashak TS (ed): *Adams' Lameness in Horses.* Philadelphia, Lea & Febiger, 1987, pp 451–454.

McIlwraith CW, James LF: Limb deformities in foals associated with ingestion of locoweed by mares. *J Am Vet Med Assoc* 1982;181:255–258.

Prichard JT, Voss JL: Fetal ankylosis in horses associated with hybrid Sudan pasture. *J Am Vet Med Assoc* 1967;150:871–873.

Rooney JR: Contracted foals. *Cornell Vet* 1966;56:172–187.

Wagner PC: Caudal carpal capsule release as a treatment for severe congenital carpal flexural deformities in foals, in *Proceedings of the 14th Veterinary Orthopedics Society Meeting.* Sun Valley, Idaho, Vet Orthopedic Society, 1987.

96 Appendicular Deviations

Jörg A. Auer

CARPAL DEVIATIONS

Diagnosis

Signalment. Angular limb deformities are seen in horses from 1 day of age up to maturity; however, they are predominantly diagnosed in young foals. No breed or sex predilection has been established.

History. Most foals are born with a certain degree of deviation of the carpi and tarsi. During the ensuing weeks and months, many of these deformities correct on their own. However, a prediction as to whether the deformity will correct spontaneously cannot be made. Spontaneous correction depends, to a certain extent, upon the severity of the deformity. Some foals that are born with straight limbs develop a deviation over the following months. This is primarily seen in the carpal and fetlock regions, and less frequently in the tarsal region. Trauma to the growth plate may also result in deviation. Crushing injuries of the growth plate (Salter-Harris type V fractures) result in deviations of the affected joint because of the development of a local epiphysiodesis that stops the growth on one side of the bone. Physeal fractures, despite rapid and correct treatment, may cause disproportional growth at the level of the physis, resulting in a deviation. Continuous overload of a limb due to a chronic weight-bearing lameness in the contralateral limb has been reported to result in deviation. By placing most of the weight on one limb, the joints and growth plates are loaded excessively. The main weight-bearing limb is displaced toward the sagittal plane of the horse to be closer to the center of gravity. This results in uneven weight bearing of the involved limb along the physis, facilitating development of mainly varus deviations.

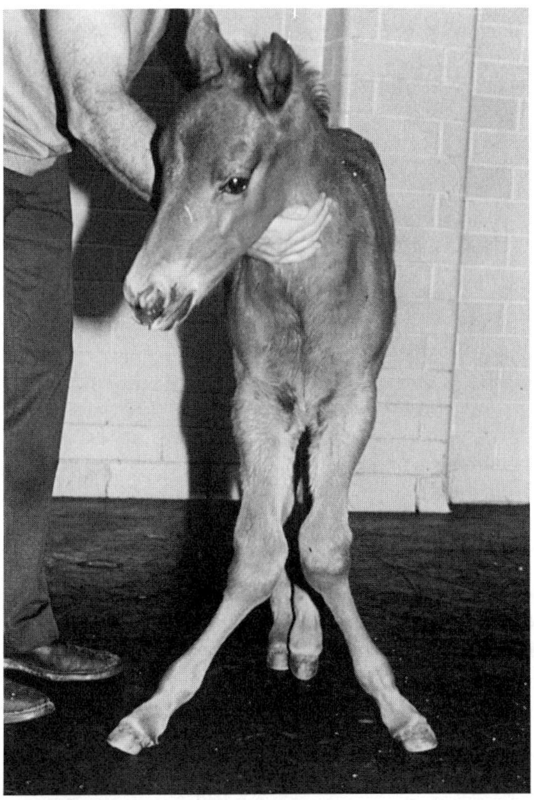

Figure 96–1. Severe carpal valgus deformity in a 2-week-old foal.

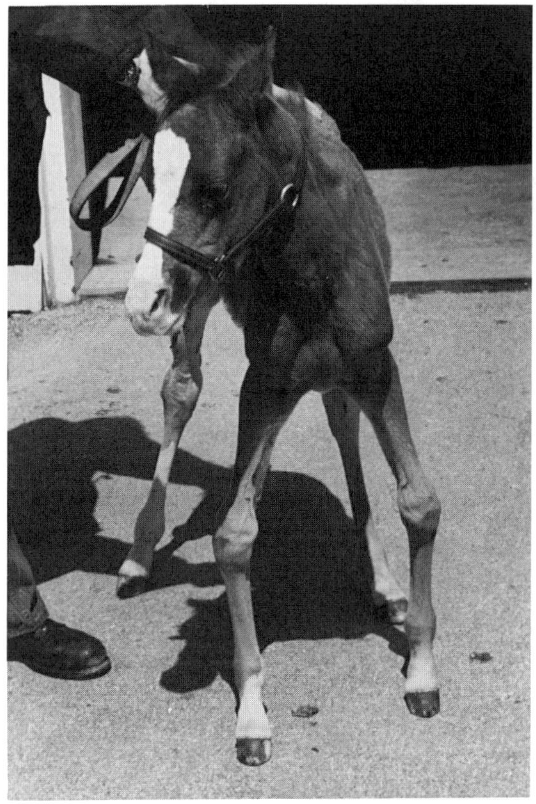

Figure 96–2. Severe carpal varus deformity in a 2-week-old foal.

Presenting Signs. Animals with deviations are presented with a valgus deformity (Fig. 96–1), which by definition is a lateral deviation of the limb distal to the location of the deformity, or a varus deformity (Fig. 96–2), defined as a medial deviation of the limb distal to the location of the problem. Most animals with either type of deviation also have a certain amount of rotational deviation, consisting of an outward rotation (splay footed) in valgus deformities and medial rotation of the feet (pigeon toed) in those foals with varus deformities. This is initially only a postural deviation through rotation of the limbs outward or inward. With time, however, the bone adapts to the abnormal loading according to Wolff's law and a permanent rotational deformity may develop. Rarely is lameness associated with a deformity. When lameness is associated with the deformity, a very grave prognosis for a

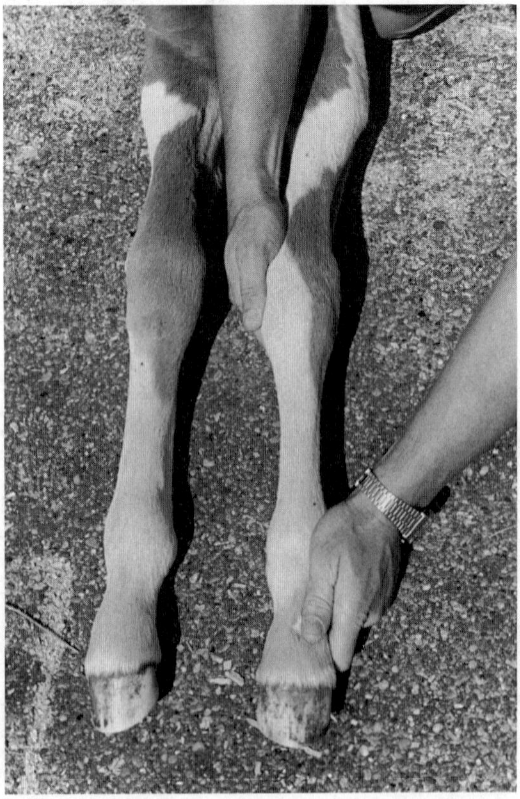

Figure 96–3. By applying manual pressure to the medial aspect of the carpus and counterpressure to the lateral aspect of the phalangeal region, the valgus deformity in the carpus due to joint laxity in a newborn foal can be temporarily corrected.

future athletic career has to be given and the animal should, in most cases, be euthanized.

Confirmatory Tests. The deviations are evaluated by inspection and, in most cases, are easily identified. In carpal and tarsal deviations of newborn foals, applying pressure to the medial aspect of the carpus/tarsus in a lateral direction while simultaneously applying counterpressure to the lateral aspect of the metacarpophalangeal joint in a medial direction may temporarily correct the problem (Fig. 96–3). This test differentiates incomplete ossification or flaccidity of the periarticular supporting structures and developmental deviations due to disproportionate growth at the level of the physis. To establish the exact location and amount of deviation, radiographs are, in most cases, mandatory. This is particularly true for carpal and metacarpal deviations. Lateral and medial deviations in the tarsal region are difficult to diagnose with radiographs because of the anatomic configuration of the tarsus. In this joint the tibia and the tarsus/metatarsus are not located in the same frontal plane.

Care must be taken to direct the radiographic beam vertical to the frontal plane of the bone proximal to the deviation. In the case of the carpus, the radiographic beam is centered perpendicular to the distal radius.

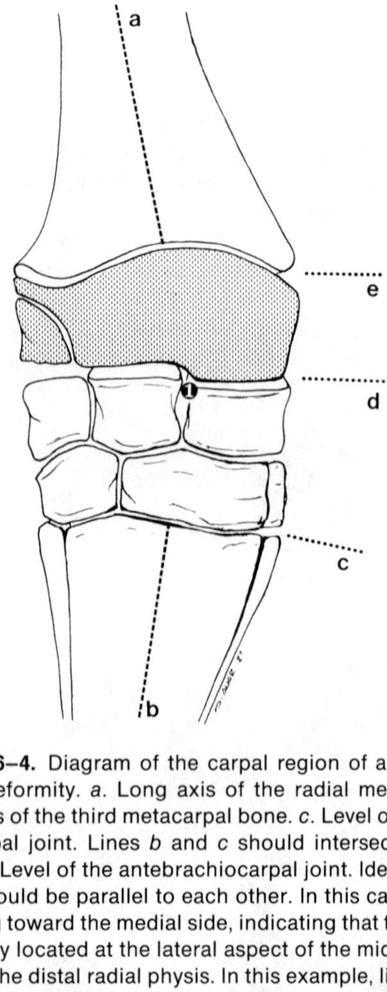

Figure 96–4. Diagram of the carpal region of a foal with a valgus deformity. *a*. Long axis of the radial metaphysis. *b*. Long axis of the third metacarpal bone. *c*. Level of the carpometacarpal joint. Lines *b* and *c* should intersect at a right angle. *d*. Level of the antebrachiocarpal joint. Ideally, lines *c* and *d* should be parallel to each other. In this case, they are diverging toward the medial side, indicating that the problem is partially located at the lateral aspect of the middle joint. *e*, Level of the distal radial physis. In this example, lines *d* and *e* are parallel, as they should be, demonstrating that the epiphysis is evenly developed at the medial and lateral side.

In a straight-legged foal, lines *e* and *a* should intersect at a right angle, which they are not doing in this case, demonstrating that the medial aspect of the metaphysis is longer than the lateral aspect. This suggests that there is disproportional growth at the level of the metaphysis, which could be corrected by means of surgical intervention. The pivot point of the joint (*1*) is derived by the intersection of lines *a* and *b*. Using geometric analysis (lines *a* through *e*) allows a much more precise diagnosis of the angular deformity.

The use of long, narrow radiographic cassettes (7 × 17 in) is strongly encouraged. The exact geometric evaluation of the radiograph is discussed for the carpal region (Fig. 96–4). The long axis of the radius (*a* in Fig. 96–4) and that of the third metacarpal bone (*b* in Fig. 96–4) intersect in the carpal region (*1* in Fig. 96–4 is the pivot point) of a foal with a carpal deviation. In a foal with straight limbs, these two lines should coincide and should be an extension of each other. More precise geometric evaluation of the carpal articulations is aided by lines drawn through the levels of the radiographic joint spaces as well as the physis. Ideally, all four lines are parallel to each other and should be perpendicular to the long axis of the radius and third metacarpal bone. Deviations from the ideal localize the deformity. The total deformity may be a composite of deformities at various sites in the carpal region.

Surgery

Not all deviations have to be corrected surgically, because many of them straighten out spontaneously. Foals with incomplete ossification of the carpal and tarsal bones, as well as those foals with flaxidity of the periarticular supporting structures, are best treated by means of splinting or casting, as described in Chapters 94, 95 and 97. Splinting and casting a limb having disproportionate growth at the level of the physis is contraindicated, however, because the bone cannot adapt easily and pressure sores will develop. This is also true for special braces such as the "Farley brace." The surgical techniques applicable for correction of angular deformities are:

1. Growth acceleration
2. Growth retardation
   a. Staples
   b. Screws and figure eight wires
   c. Small screws and small bone plate
3. Corrective osteotomies
   a. Closing wedge osteotomy
   b. Dome osteotomy
   c. Step osteotomy

The growth acceleration and growth retardation techniques will be described using the carpal region as an example. The corrective osteotomy, will be discussed as it pertains to the fetlock. Subsequently, each location will be discussed as to anatomy, differences in surgical technique, and special considerations.

Growth Acceleration.

Anatomy. The anatomic landmarks for periosteal transection and elevation at the lateral aspect of the distal radius consist of the common digital extensor tendon

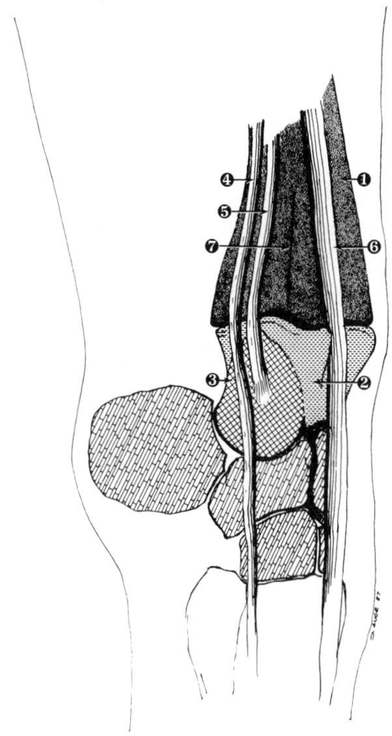

Figure 96–5. Anatomic landmarks of the lateral aspect of the carpal region. *1*, Metaphysis of the distal radius; *2*, epiphysis of the distal radius; *3*, ulnar styloid process; *4*, lateral digital extensor tendon; *5*, rudimentary fibrous ulna; *6*, Common digital extensor tendon; and *7*, straight vertical incision used for periosteal transection surgery.

cranially, lateral digital extensor tendon and rudimentary fibrous ulna caudally, and the physis distally (Fig. 96–5). These landmarks circumscribe the triangular-shaped surgical field used for correction of a valgus deformity. This area is covered only by subcutaneous tissue and skin. Correction of a varus deformity is carried out at the medial aspect of the distal radius just proximal to the physis. There are no other surgical landmarks in the surgical field.

Technique. The skin and subcutaneous tissues are incised over a distance of 2.5 cm, with the distal-most extension of the skin incision located 2 cm proximal to the physis. Care is taken to incise down to, but not through, the periosteum. A curved hemostatic forceps is subsequently advanced cranially perpendicular to the longitudinal incision between the subcutaneous tissues and the periosteum. It is important to stay in close proximity to the periosteum and not to allow subcutaneous tissues, including blood vessels, to lie between the hemostatic forceps and the periosteum during this process. The common digital extensor tendon is undermined and is palpated between the skin and the hemostat forceps. The hemostat is then advanced to a level between the common digital extensor tendon and the extensor carpi radialis tendon. Once in that location, the hemostatic forceps is opened and the subcutaneous tissues are separated from the periosteum. By elevating the soft tissues located between the skin and the hemostat in a cranial direction, a space is created to allow insertion of a no. 12 scalpel blade, placed on its handle, into the correct location at the tip of the hemostatic forceps. The hemostat is subsequently withdrawn and, by applying gentle pressure onto the scalpel blade while withdrawing it slowly, the periosteum is transected in a horizontal direction. The periosteal incision is stopped at the lateralmost aspect of the bone.

The same procedure is repeated on the caudal aspect of the distal radius. The hemostat is advanced to the level of the lateral digital extensor tendon, again separating the subcutaneous tissues from the periosteum. Once the hemostat has passed the rudimentary ulna, its direction is altered into a frontal plane and the fascia is crossed through using a sharp stabbing motion.

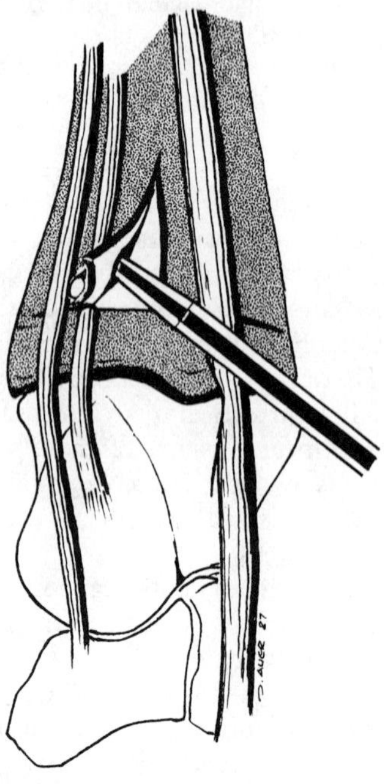

Figure 96–6. Diagram of the periosteal stripping technique. The inverted *T* incision has been carried out through the periosteum. The rudimentary ulna is transected and the two periosteal flaps are elevated.

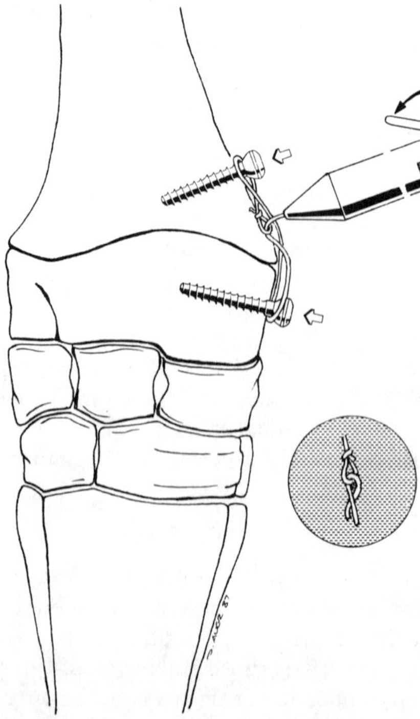

Figure 96–7. Application of screws and cerclage wire growth retardation technique to the distal radius in a case of a valgus deformity.

Once positioned behind the radius, the hemostat is opened, allowing separation of the soft tissues from the periosteum and easy positioning of the scalpel blade to the caudal aspect of the distal radius. The scalpel blade is withdrawn in a fashion similar to that described previously and the periosteum and rudimentary fibrous ulna are transected. Care is taken to connect the two horizontal incisions at the lateral-most aspect of the radius. In about 20% of foals the rudimentary ulna is partially ossified. In those instances, a 1-cm piece of ulna is removed using rongeurs. After the horizontal incision is performed, the inverted *T* incision is completed by making a vertical incision started 2 cm proximad at the lateral-most aspect and advanced to the horizontal incision (Fig. 96–6). This allows subsequent atraumatic elevation of the two triangular periosteal flaps by a periosteal elevator, which is introduced at a 45-degree angle at the distal corner of the flaps. After elevation of the periosteum, a 0.5-cm gap should be evident between the ends of the periosteum. The flaps are carefully laid back onto the bone. Particular attention is given to prevent folding over the edges of the periosteum, because this would result in periosteal new bone formation. The subcutaneous tissues are sutured using a 2–0 monofilament absorbable suture material (PDS; Ethicon Inc) with a simple continuous suture pattern. An intradermal suture line is placed to appose the skin edges, again using the same suture material and suture pattern. The knots of the intradermal suture are buried. No skin sutures are used.

Postoperative Considerations. A bandage is applied over the surgery site consisting of a nonadhesive dressing (Telfa pad, The Kendall Corp) covered by unfolded 4 × 4 sponges and an elastic tape (Elasticon; Johnson & Johnson) that overlaps the sponges by 2 cm proximally and distally. Care is taken not to apply too much pressure and thus to inadvertently compromise the blood flow through the limb and cause pressure sores of the fragile skin underneath the bandage.

Growth Retardation.

Anatomy. In contrast to techniques to promote growth acceleration, growth retardation surgery is carried out at the convex aspect of the bone. The implants used for the various techniques temporarily bridge the physis. The anatomic landmarks for growth retardation procedures performed to correct a valgus deformity include the medial aspect of the distal radius, the physis, the antebrachial carpal joint, and the metaphyseal bone, being covered only by skin, subcutaneous tissue, and periosteum.

Staples Titanium or stainless steel staples are still used in equine practice. However, this technique is very well described in the literature and will not be discussed here.

Screws and Wires This technique is presently the most frequently used growth retardation technique (Fig. 96–7). A slightly curved skin incision of about 8 cm in length is made starting at the level of the antebrachiocarpal joint and extending to about 5 cm proximal to the physis. The incision is centered over the distal radial physis with the curve pointing toward the caudal aspect of the limb. The subcutaneous tissue is transected down to the periosteum in a linear fashion over the medial-most aspect of the distal radius (Fig. 96–7). The level of the physis is easily identified as the most prominent part of the distal radius and there is no need to place a needle into the physis for identification. The collateral ligament is vertically incised parallel to the direction of its fibers about 1.5 cm distal to the level of the physis. A 3.2-mm diameter hole is drilled to an approximate depth of 34 mm with the drill bit protected by a drill guide. Using the 4.5-mm tap through the tap sleeve, threads are cut into the epiphyseal bone. A cortical bone screw of about 30 mm length is subsequently inserted into the prepared hole. An additional hole is prepared in an identical fashion 2 to 3 cm proximal to the physis. Both screws are not completely inserted to allow easy application of a 1.1-mm diameter cerclage wire in figure eight fashion around the two screwheads. Using either a Richards (Richards Co) or ASIF (Synthes Inc) wire tightener, the figure eight wire is tightened snugly (Fig. 96–7). A second wire is applied over the screwheads in similar fashion. The ends of the twisted and tightened wire are carefully bent in a distal direction. Subsequently both screws are fully inserted and tightened, which tightens the wires and thereby applies additional pressure across the physis. The subcutaneous tissues and the skin are closed as described for the periosteal transection procedure.

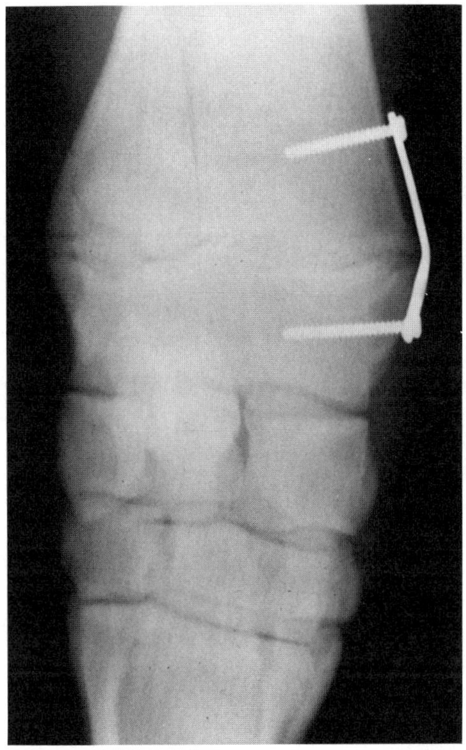

Figure 96–8. Dorsopalmar radiograph of the carpal region of a foal in which a 2.7-cm bone plate was applied over the medial aspect of the distal radial physis and connected to the epiphysis and metaphysis by means of 3.5-mm bone screws. This type of growth retardation gives excellent cosmetic results.

Screws and Small Bone Plate This is the growth retardation technique I prefer (Fig. 96–8). The surgical approach to the bone is identical to that described for the screw and wire technique. A 3.5-mm cortical bone screw of 26 mm length is inserted through the distal-most hole of a 2.7-mm fingerplate into the previously

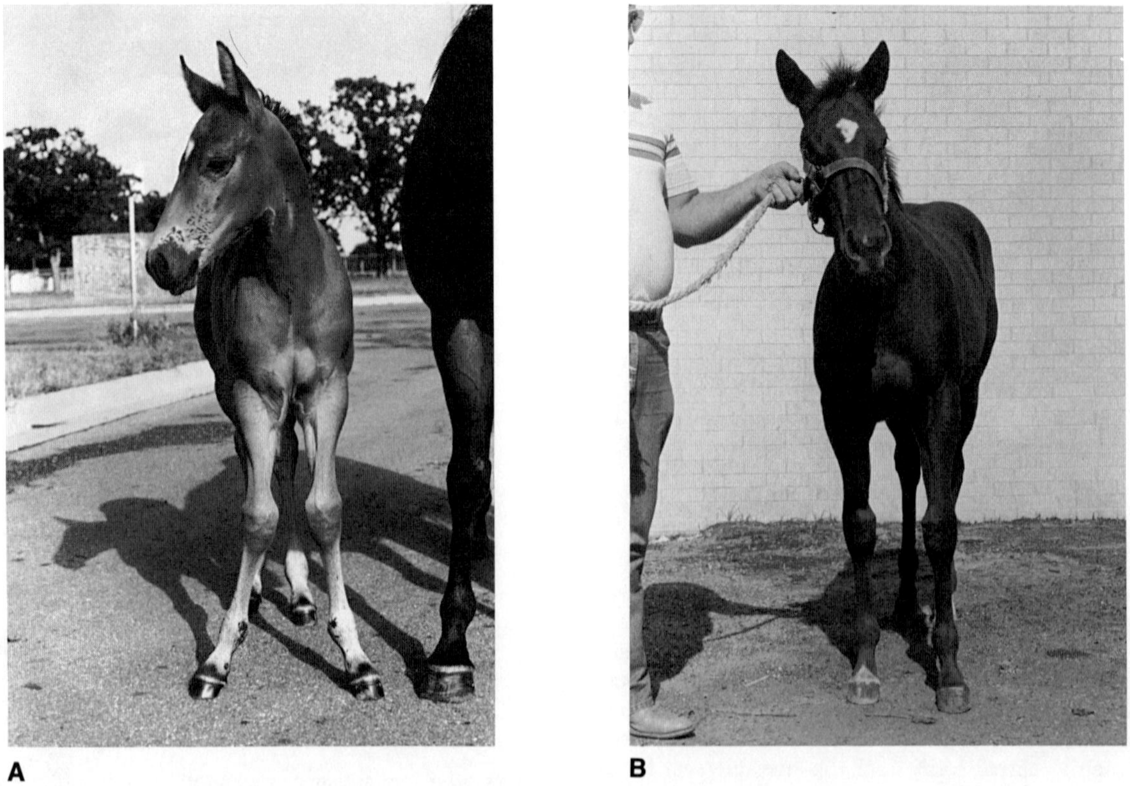

Figure 96–9. A. A 1-month-old foal with marked bilateral carpal valgus deformity. B. The same foal 4 months after periosteal transection and stripping. Note the excellent correction and cosmetic appearance for both carpi.

prepared 3.5-mm diameter hole in the epiphysis. The plate can be bent manually to match the contour of the bone. The location for the proximal hole is marked. By drilling the second hole 1 mm further proximal than the most proximal hole of the plate, a certain amount of compression can be applied once the screw is inserted. The screw hole is tapped, and the screw inserted and tightened. The soft tissues over the 3.5-mm screws and the 2.7-mm seven-hole bone plate are closed as described previously.

Growth retardation procedures may be carried out on horses up to 2 years of age, as long as there is still potential growth left in the physis. However, growth is slow, particularly after 1 year of age.

Postoperative Care

The bandage applied at the end of the surgery is changed 3 days after surgery and a second bandage is left in place for an additional 5 to 6 days. At that point, the bandage can be removed and no additional bandage is needed. Because the skin incision was closed intradermally, no sutures have to be removed. To aid in the correction, it is advisable to slightly lower the outside of the foot for a valgus deformity or the inside of the foot for a varus deformity. In the young foal, this is done at biweekly intervals by simply rasping the desired area of the foot. In an older foal, it is possible to apply a shoe to the previously trimmed foot. Stall rest is advised for 3 weeks, followed by pasture exercise.

It is important to evaluate the straightening of the limb carefully. In the very young foal, straightening may occur within 1 month. The rapidity of straightening is obviously dependent upon the severity of the deformity and the age of the foal at the time of surgery (Fig. 96–9). The older the foal the slower the rate of correction. If the deformity has not corrected adequately 2 months after periosteal transection and stripping, the procedure can be repeated to obtain additional correction. The growth retardation implants, however, stay in place until the deviation is corrected. When implants are used, it is very important to evaluate each limb separately and to remove the implants as soon as the limb is straight. This might entail two separate surgeries in a foal with different degrees of deviations in both forelimbs. One should not wait until both limbs are straight, because at that point the first limb might already be overcorrected, resulting in a new deformity.

Prognosis

The prognosis for complete correction and future ability to enter an athletic career are excellent in foals that are treated at a young age (1 or 2 months). The longer the animal runs on deformed legs, however, the more damage may occur to the cartilage and the more readily degenerative changes may occur during future life. The treatment of choice in very young foals is the growth acceleration technique, which has produced excellent

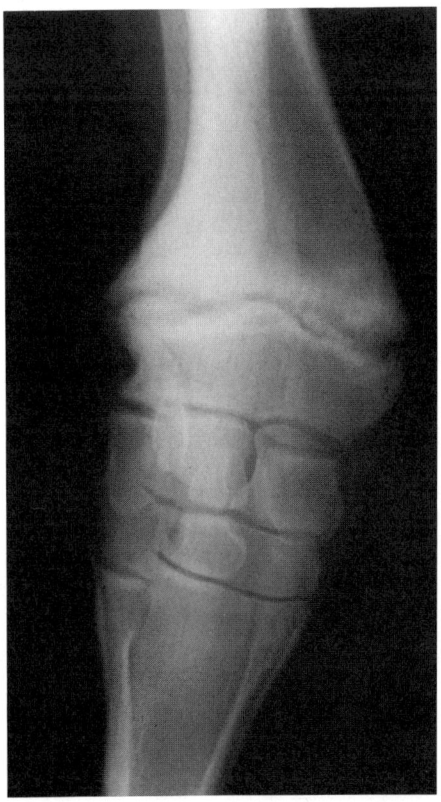

Figure 96–10. Dorsopalmar radiograph of the carpal region of a 7-month-old foal. All three joint spaces are parallel and the bones are developed normally. The distal radial epiphysis, however is narrowed at the lateral aspect and has an abnormal shape. The physis is abnormally shaped and the medial aspect of the radial metaphysis is longer than the lateral aspect.

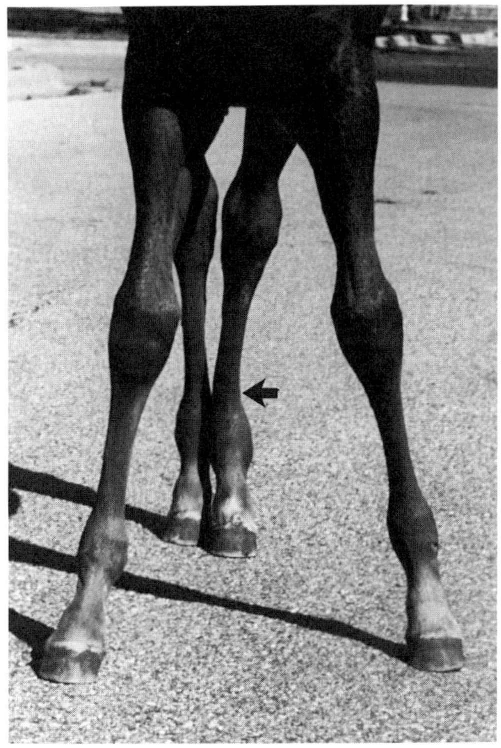

Figure 96–11. A 2-week-old foal with a valgus deviation in the left third metatarsal bone (*arrow*).

results. In severe cases (Fig. 96–10), the growth acceleration technique may be combined with one of the growth retardation techniques to produce more rapid and more complete correction of the deformity. Thus, the goal in treatment of such deviations is to initiate therapy as early and as rapidly as possible.

METACARPAL/METATARSAL DEVIATIONS

Diagnosis

Signalment. Valgus (Fig. 96–11) and varus deformities may occur in the third metacarpal (MCIII)/third metatarsal (MTIII). It has been reported previously that such deformities can be corrected by means of closing wedge osteotomies.

History. These deformities are more and more frequently diagnosed in the very young foal. In most cases, the animals are born with a deformity and do not develop it.

Presenting Signs. These animals show either a varus or valgus deformity.

Confirmatory Tests. Manually these deformities cannot be straightened, and radiographically the exact location as well as degree of deviation can be identified in the metaphysis or diaphysis of MCIII/MTIII.

Surgery

Growth Acceleration. Periosteal transection in a vertical and horizontal fashion (Fig. 96–12) has been carried out to correct these deformities. The surgery is performed over the metaphyses and the diaphysis of the bone at its concave aspect. A vertical skin incision is made from the most proximal aspect of MCIII/MTIII to the distal physis of the bone. The periosteum is transected in the same line. At the proximal- and distal-most aspects of the vertical incision, horizontal skin incisions are made. The two periosteal flaps are elevated from the bone, and the subcutaneous tissues as well as the skin are closed and the leg bandaged as described previously.

A bench-kneed conformation in a young foal can be corrected by combining the above technique on the medial aspect of MCIII with a periosteal transection at the lateral aspect of the distal radius.

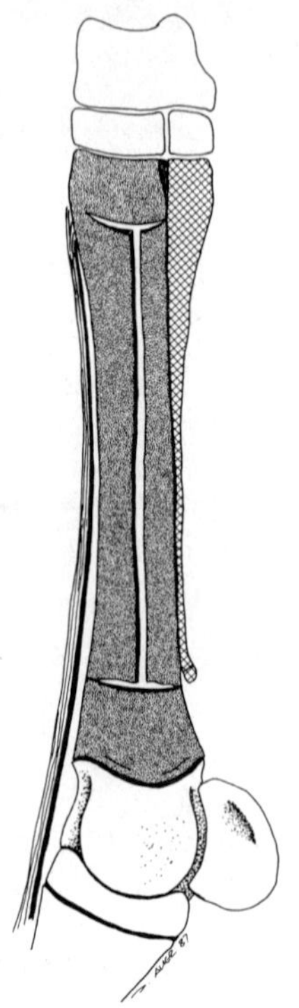

Figure 96–12. Diagram of the location of the periosteal incision and periosteal elevation for growth acceleration of the metaphysis and diaphysis of the third metacarpal/metatarsal bone. An *I*-type incision is performed and the two flaps are elevated over the total length of the incision.

Growth Retardation. Growth retardation is not applicable in these types of deformities.

Corrective Osteotomies. As mentioned above, corrective osteotomies have been described as treatment of such deformities. However, this is only a last resort when the growth acceleration surgery is not successful (see "Metacarpophalangeal Metatarsophalangeal Deviations", below).

POSTOPERATIVE CARE

The postoperative care is identical to that described for carpal deviations.

Prognosis

If periosteal transection is carried out within the first month of life, a good prognosis for complete correction can be given (Fig. 96–13). Corrective osteotomies contain an increased risk of failure as a result of the complexity of the surgery and the risk of postoperative complications.

METACARPOPHALANGEAL/ METATARSOPHALANGEAL DEVIATIONS

Diagnosis

Diagnosis of deviations of the fetlock region is identical to that described for the carpal region. The owner often complains that the foal is toeing out from the fetlocks. However, closer inspection of the deformity verifies that the rotation is secondary to a problem located in the carpal region. In such cases it would obviously be contraindicated to try to correct the deformity in the fetlock region.

It may be beneficial to elevate the forelimb at the carpus and let the distal limb hang down. Such manipulation arranges MCIII and the phalanges in the same frontal plane and facilitates radiography.

Special Considerations. Because most of the growth of MCIII/MTIII occurs during the first 3 months of life, it is important to perform any type of corrective surgery, other than the osteotomy, before the foal is 3

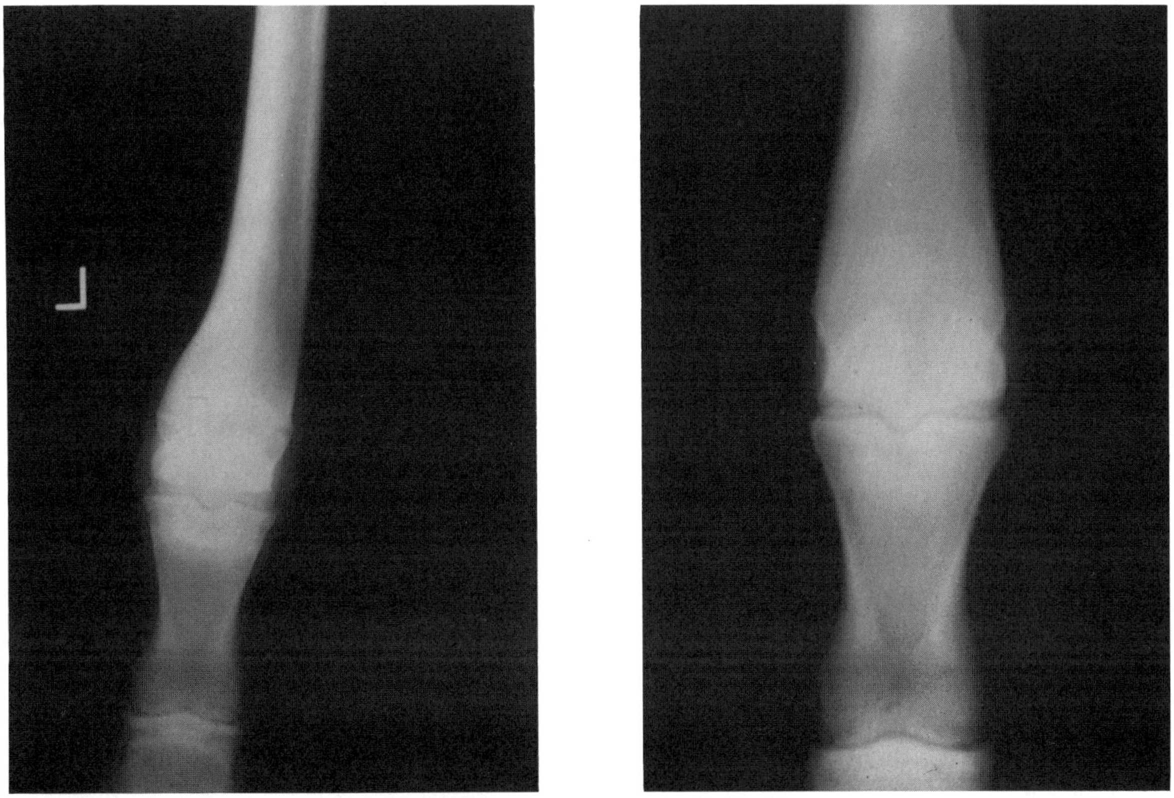

A B

Figure 96–13. A. Dorsopalmar radiograph of the distal metacarpal region of a 6-month-old foal with a severe metaphyseal angular limb deformity. **B.** Dorsopalmar radiograph of the distal metacarpal region 5 months after periosteal stripping of the lateral metaphysis and diaphysis.

months old. Otherwise, only partial correction can be expected. Whenever a deviation is noted in the fetlock region, the distal MCIII/MTIII and the proximal phalanx should be evaluated (Fig. 96–14). It has been reported that compensatory deformities may develop in the proximal phalanx, which may mask a more severe deviation at the distal MCIII (Fig. 96–15).

Surgery

Growth Acceleration.

Anatomy. The surgical landmarks for performing growth acceleration surgery for correction of a varus deformity at the distal MCIII include the distal-most aspect of the second metacarpal bone (MCII) and the medial aspect of the distal metaphysis of MCIII (Fig. 96–16). Surgical landmarks for performing growth acceleration surgery at the proximal phalanx include: the level of the proximal physis of the proximal phalanx, the concave aspect of the metaphysis of the proximal phalanx, and the medial or lateral extensor branch of the suspensory ligament.

Technique. A straight surgical incision of 2.5 cm length is performed to, but not through, the periosteum. Curved hemostat forceps are inserted perpendicular to the incision to separate the subcutaneous tissue from the periosteum in a horizontal fashion at the level of the distal MCII. Periosteal transection is subsequently performed as described for carpal deviation. It is interesting to note that the periosteum covering MCIII/MTIII is much thinner than at the distal radius or tibia. The periosteum is elevated and the surgical incision closed as previously described.

Should a deviation be noted in the proximal phalanx during the first 3 months of life (Fig. 96–17), growth acceleration surgery can be carried out. Again, the pro-

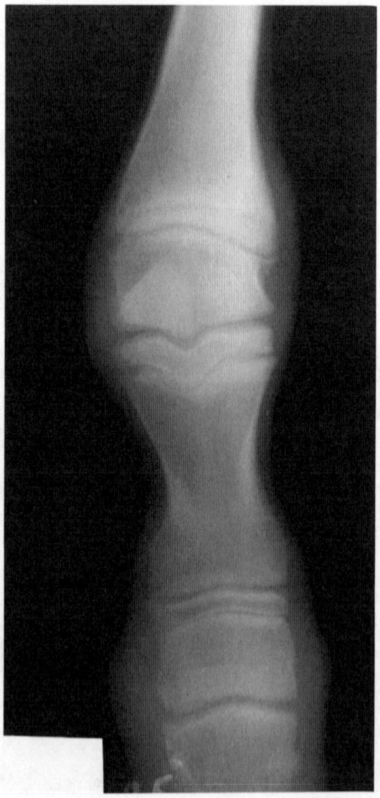

Figure 96–14. Dorsopalmar radiograph of the fetlock region of a 2-month-old foal with a severe varus deformity. Note the wedging of the distal epiphysis of the third metacarpal bone. (From Auer JA: Periosteal transection of the proximal phalanx in foals with angular limb deformities of the metacarpo/metatarsophalangeal area. *J Am Vet Med Assoc* 1985;187:496–499.)

cedure is performed on the concave aspect of the bone. Thus, the surgical site will be the medial aspect of the bone in case of a varus deformity (Fig. 96–16). A vertical skin incision of 2 cm in length is centered over the medial extensor branch of the suspensory apparatus at the medial side of the proximal phalanx. The subcutaneous tissues are separated and the periosteum identified. Using the same dissection technique as previously described, the subcutaneous tissues are separated from the periosteum in both the dorsal and palmaro/plantar directions. The periosteum is transected between the extensor branch of the suspensory apparatus and the proximal physis of the proximal phalanx. At that level, some fibers of the medial oblique distal sesmoidean ligament are transected at their point of insertion; however, this is not of any consequence (Fig. 96–18). The vertical incision is created from the horizontal periosteal incision distally over a length of 1 to 2 cm. The branch of the suspensory ligament must be undermined and not inadvertently transected. The two flaps are elevated and the skin incision is closed as previously described.

Growth Retardation. Using the technique described for the distal radius, screws and wires or small screws and a bone plate are inserted at the convex aspect of the bone. The landmarks consist of the physis and the lateral aspect of the bone in case of a varus deformity. All the previously described steps are followed.

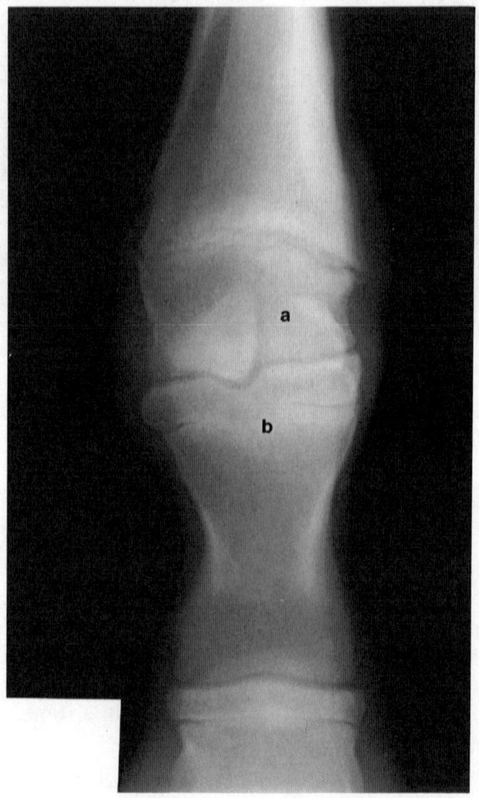

Figure 96–15. Dorsopalmar radiograph of the fetlock region of the foal in Figure 96–14 4 months later. There is still wedging of the distal third metacarpal epiphysis (*a*). In addition to that, an opposing deformity is located in the proximal aspect of the proximal phalanx (*b*). These two deformities result in a straight axis of the limb with the metacarpophalangeal joint not being loaded perpendicular to the ground but at an angle. (From Auer JA: Periosteal transection of the proximal phalanx in foals with angular limb deformities of the metacarpo/metatarsophalangeal area. *J Am Vet Med Assoc* 1985;187:496–499.)

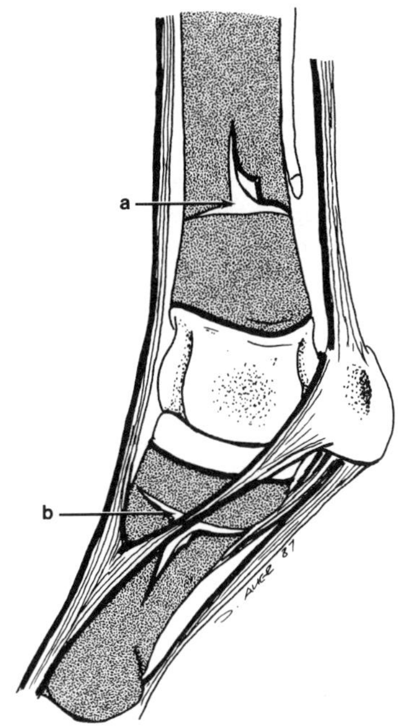

Figure 96–16. Diagram of the locations where periosteal transection may be performed: (*a*) at the distal third metacarpal bone and (*b*) at the the proximal aspect of the proximal phalanx.

Corrective Osteotomy. Corrective osteotomies provide the only surgical solution for foals with a closed physis in the presence of a valgus or varus deformity. These surgical procedures are very demanding and need to be planned in detail. These surgeries should be carried out by a specialist in orthopedic surgery.

The *closing wedge osteotomy* (Fig. 96–19) has been repeatedly described in the literature and the technique will not be discussed in further detail here. The reader is encouraged to study the literature for details on the surgical technique.

The *dome osteotomy* has been used in humans and in one equine case (Fig. 96–20). The technique is described in the literature and will not be described here.

The *step osteotomy* (L.R. Bramlage, personal communication) can be carried out in two different configurations: in the sagittal plane (removal of a bone wedge) (Fig. 96–21) and in the frontal plane without bone removal (Fig. 96–22). The step osteotomy in the sagittal plane will be described in detail as representative of corrective osteotomies for a varus deformity of the distal MCIII. It is important to clip and prepare the limb from the foot to the distal radius. Applying a sterile adhesive drape over that region allows intraoperative evaluation of the adequacy of the correction achieved.

Technique. A skin incision is made over the lateral digital extensor tendon from the proximal aspect of MCIII to the distal physis of MCIII and, from that point, is continued laterally toward the metacarpophalangeal joint. The lateral digital extensor tendon and the periosteum are split longitudinally. Subsequently, subperiosteal dissection is performed around the bone.

Prior to surgery, the pivot point for the deviation is determined by drawing bisecting lines through MCIII and the phalanges (Fig. 96–23). The intersection of these two lines is called the pivot point. These lines were drawn on an acetate foil and laid over the radiograph. By comparing the anatomic landmarks, the pivot point for the deviation is marked on the bone. A 3.2-mm hole is drilled across the bone perpendicular to

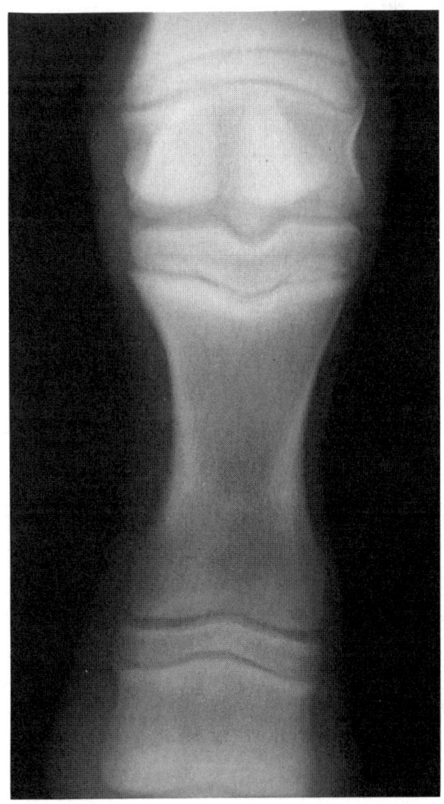

Figure 96–17. Dorsopalmar radiograph of the proximal phalanx in a 1-month-old foal with a deviation. Note the uneven length of the medial and lateral sides of the bone. (From Auer JA: Periosteal transection of the proximal phalanx in foals with angular limb deformities of the metacarpo/metatarsophalangeal area. *J Am Vet Med Assoc* 1985;187:496–499.)

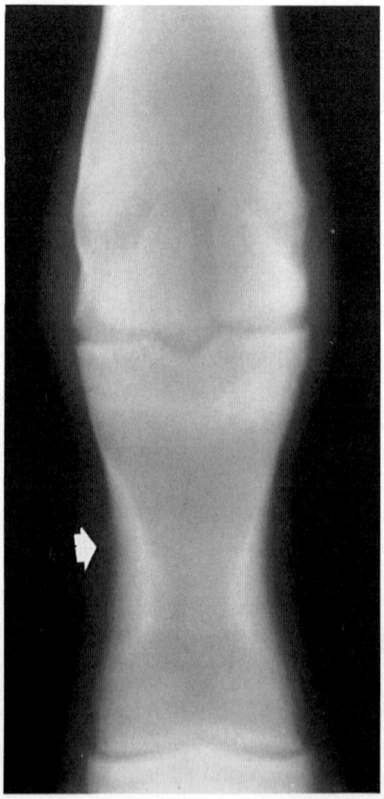

Figure 96–18. Dorsopalmar follow-up radiograph of foal in Figure 96–17 5 months postoperatively. Note the correction of the deformity and the minimal new bone formation at the surgery site (*arrow*). (From Auer JA: Periosteal transection of the proximal phalanx in foals with angular limb deformities of the metacarpo/metatarsophalangeal area. *J Am Vet Med Assoc* 1985;187:496–499.)

the frontal plane. An additional 3.2-mm hole is drilled 3 to 4 cm proximad on the axis of the bone. Using the oscillating saw, a saw cut is performed across the bone between the two 3.2-mm holes. Subsequently, an aluminum template outlining the angle of the wedge, which was previously prepared and sterilized, is laid onto the bone with one side parallel to the first saw cut. The second cut is carried out in the same plane as the first saw cut, (perpendicular to the frontal plane), along the other side of the aluminum wedge. The *Z*-plasty of the bone is completed by a horizontal cut at the lateral and proximal aspect, as well as at the distal and medial aspect of the bone. The bone wedge is subsequently removed and the two bone portions rotated to close the gap created by the removed bone wedge. In doing so, the deformity is corrected. An eventual rotating deviation may be corrected at the same time by removing an additional bone wedge from the dorsal or palmar/plantar cortex.

The adequacy of the correction is evaluated and any necessary adjustments are made. Lag screws may be inserted across the vertical portion of the saw cut and the correction is again evaluated. A bone plate is contoured to the medial aspect of the bone and secured with 4.5- or 5.5-mm diameter cortical bone screws (Fig. 96–24). Care is taken to use the bone screws in lag fashion across the vertical saw cut. The gap created at the distal medial aspect of the bone is filled with bone from the removed wedge. The incision is subsequently closed. The lateral digital extensor tendon is the first layer to be sutured, followed by subcutaneous and subcuticular layers. In selected cases, skin sutures are used. The limb is bandaged and placed in a splint for recovery.

Special Considerations. The holes drilled at the proximal and distal end of the vertical cut reduce stress concentration at these locations and prevent postoperative breakdown at that level. The advantage of the step osteotomy over the closing wedge osteotomy includes better bone-to-bone apposition and prevention of the development of a rotational deformity. Also, the fixation is moved further proximad, away from the pivot point, which allows placement of additional implants across the distal fragment. The achievement of adequate fixation is a major problem in the closing wedge osteotomy when carried out at the pivot point, which is, in most cases, located close to the joint. Rotational deformities can easily be corrected with the step osteotomy, as mentioned before, and still allow good stable fixation and interfragmentary compression across the osteotomy cut. Bone length is maintained, which is an advantage over the closing wedge osteotomy, in which bone length is reduced. The step osteotomy is presently the best technique available to correct deformities in the presence of a closed growth plate. This gives the horse a chance to be used for pleasure riding and, in selected cases, as an athlete (Fig. 96–25). The number of foals treated with this technique is presently too small to allow a more precise prognosis. Nevertheless, the prognosis for being a pasture-sound animal is excellent and better than with either the closing wedge or the dome osteotomy.

Postoperative Care

The postoperative care for growth acceleration and growth retardation procedures is identical to that described for carpal deviations. This includes removal of the implants in the growth retardation procedures, as well as hoof care.

Figure 96–19. Diagram of a deformity in the distal third metacarpal bone and its possible correction by means of a closing wedge osteotomy. The osteotomy is performed at the level of the pivot point. The bone fragment is shown on the right side of the diagram. The axis is corrected.

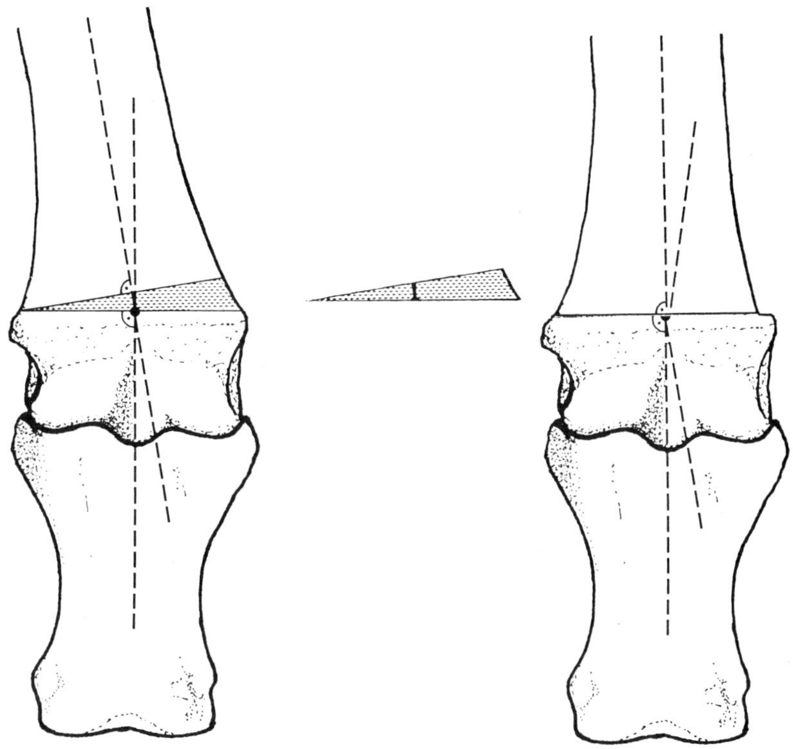

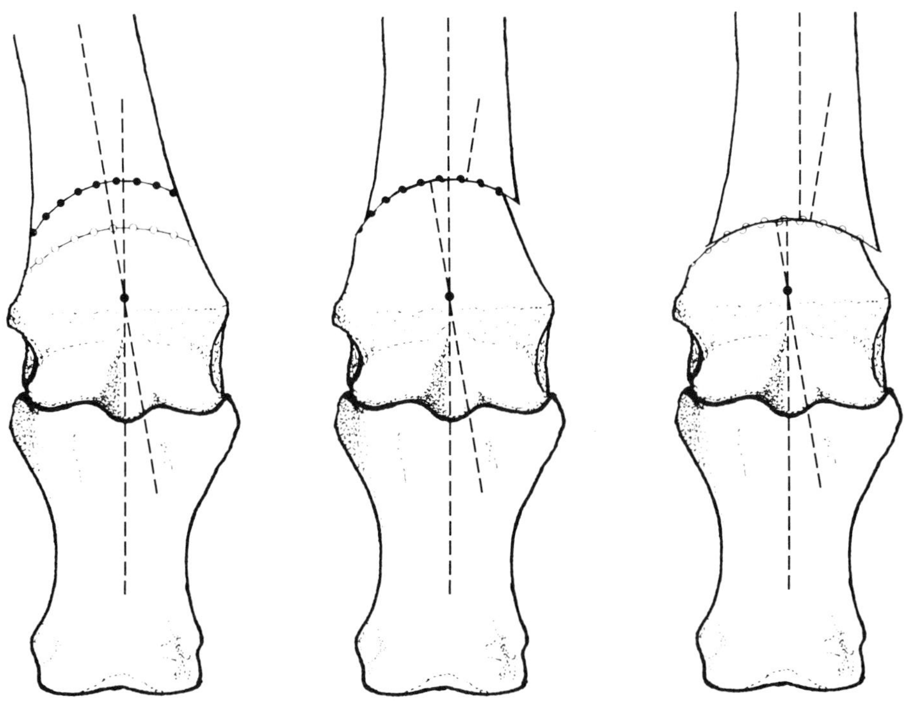

Figure 96–20. A diagram of a deviation of the distal third metacarpal bone and its potential correction through a dome osteotomy. **Left.** Two arches are drawn. The *black dots* represent an arch with a radius whose center is the pivot point. The *open dots* represent an arch closer to the pivot point and whose radius is larger than that of the black dot arch. The dots represent the 2-mm drill holes that are drilled across the bone. **Middle.** The correction when the osteotomy is performed through the black dots. **Right.** The correction through the open dots. It can be seen that the bone axis is aligned; however, the axes are parallel to each other and offset (4 mm).

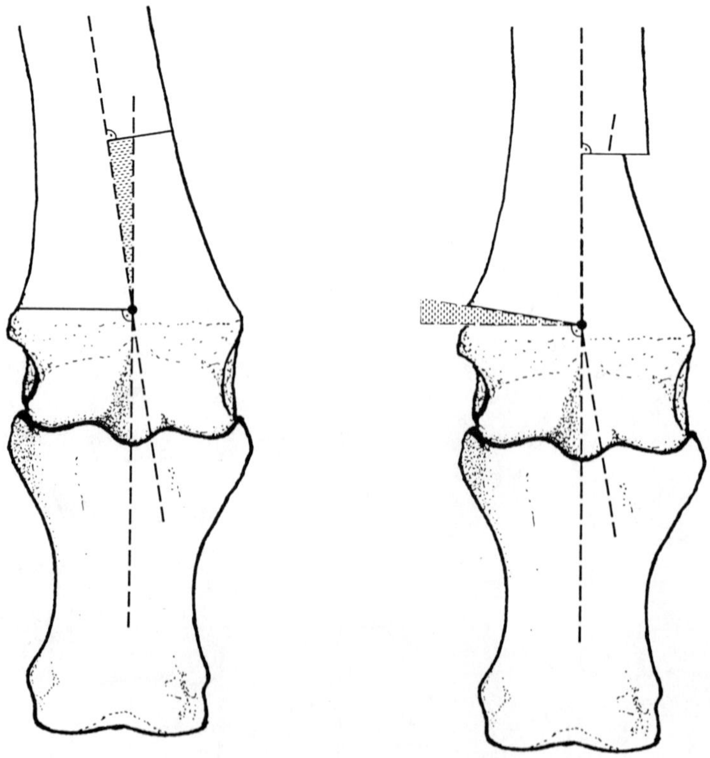

Figure 96–21. A diagram of a deformity of the distal third metacarpal bone and its potential correction through a step osteotomy in the sagittal plane. The triangle of bone that is removed from the metaphysis is inserted into the gap that developed from rotating the proximal portion of the bone into alignment with the distal portion. The plate is placed over that gap in buttress fashion.

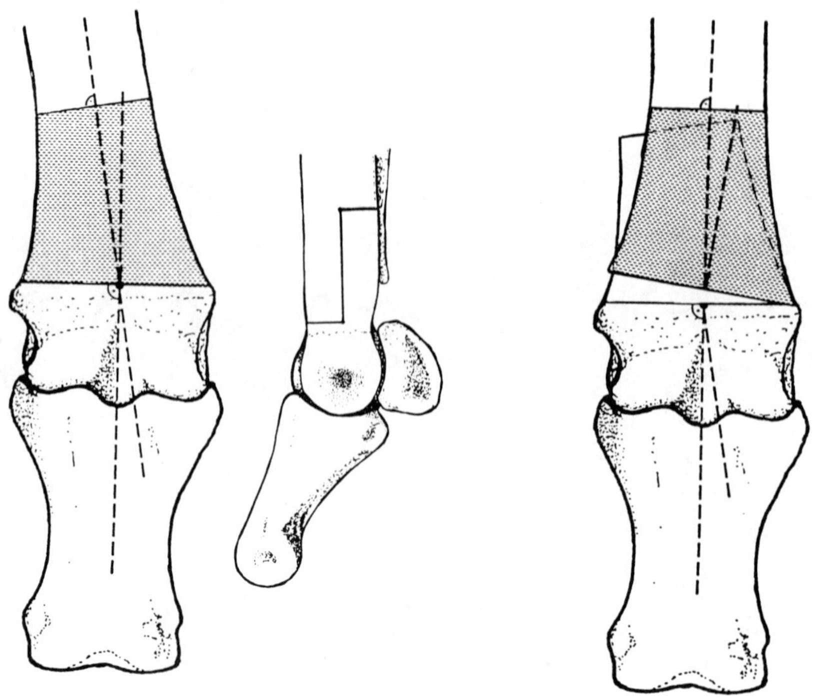

Figure 96–22. A diagram of a step osteotomy in the frontal plane. In this type of osteotomy no bone wedge is removed. The two bone pieces are rotated into alignment relative to each other.

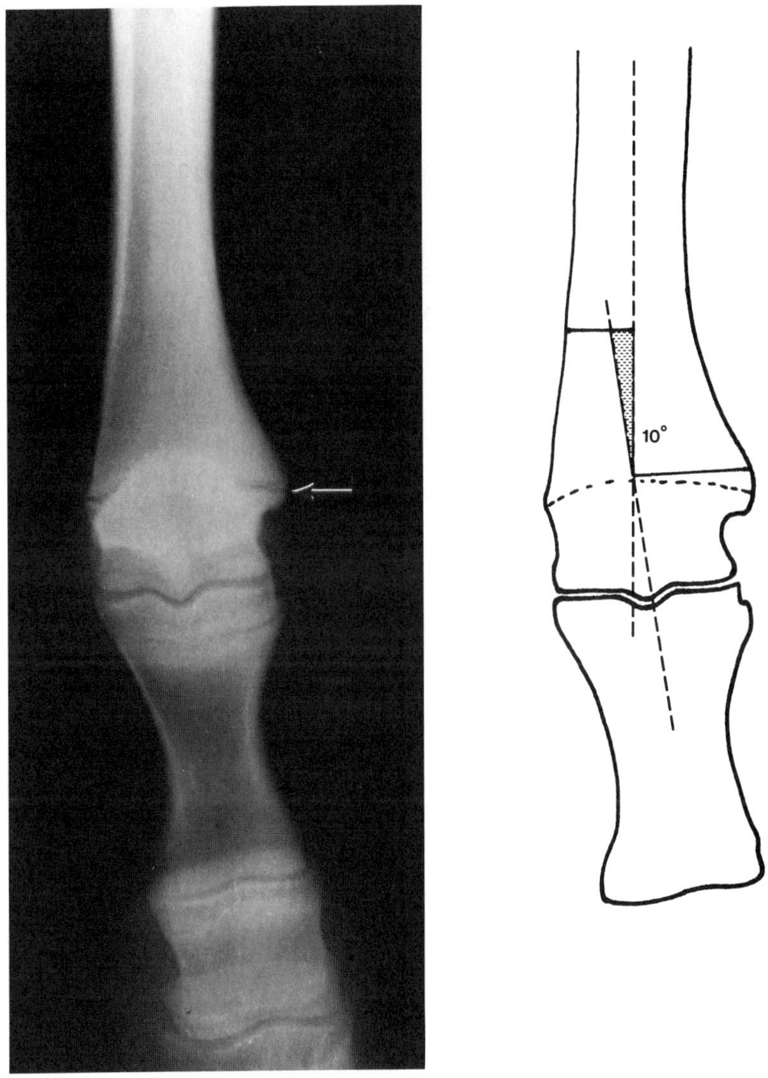

Figure 96–23. A varus deformity of the right limb and a diagram of the possible correction through a sagittal step osteotomy. The growth plate is still visible; however, it is bridged at the medial aspect (*arrow*).

Postoperative care for corrective osteotomies involves maintenance of the splint or cast for 2 to 3 weeks. The bandage should be changed every 3 to 4 days. After removal of the splint or cast, a bandage should be maintained for an additional 2 weeks. Stall rest is required for a total of 2 months, or until there is radiographic evidence of bone healing.

Prognosis

If the growth acceleration and/or growth retardation surgeries are carried out early, a good prognosis for a future athletic career can be given. Because an exostosis may develop at the surgery site in selected cases (Fig. 96–26), careful tissue handling is advised. Foals that have undergone a corrective osteotomy have a good prognosis as breeding animals.

TARSAL DEVIATIONS

Diagnosis

Valgus deviations of the tarsus are the most frequent types of deviations treated in this location. The diagnostic procedures are identical to the ones previously described. Radiographs are not very useful in determining valgus or varus deformities in the tarsal region because the third metatarsal bone and tibia are not arranged in the same frontal plane. Therefore, minimal

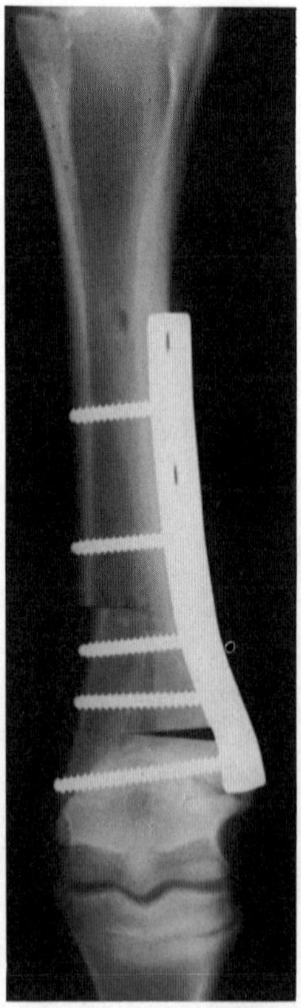

Figure 96–24. Intraoperative radiograph of the step osteotomy performed on the limb described in Figure 96–23. The gap between the two distal screws was subsequently filled with the wedge of bone. The remaining two cortical bone screws were inserted. Good correction was maintained.

deviations from the perpendicular beam angle in relation to the frontal plane of MTIII may demonstrate deformities that are not present in life and vice versa.

Surgery

Growth Acceleration.

Anatomy. The surgical landmarks for correction of valgus deformities in this region include the lateral digital extensor tendon and the lateral aspect of the physis (Fig. 96–27).

Technique. The vertical skin incision may be made cranially or caudally to the lateral digital extensor tendon. The subsequent steps of the surgical procedure are identical to the ones described for the distal radius. It is interesting to note that the periosteum may be up to 2 mm thick in this region. These procedures should be carried out before the foal reaches 3 months of age.

Growth Retardation. *Anatomy.* The anatomic landmarks for correction of a valgus deformity consist of the medial physis of the distal tibia, the collateral ligament, and the tarsocrural joint. Because of the geometric appearance of the tarsocrural joint, the distal implant must be positioned carefully. The screws and wire as well as the screw and bone plate techniques may be applied in this region. The stapling technique is discouraged because of the ease with which the tarsocrural joint may be penetrated with such implants.

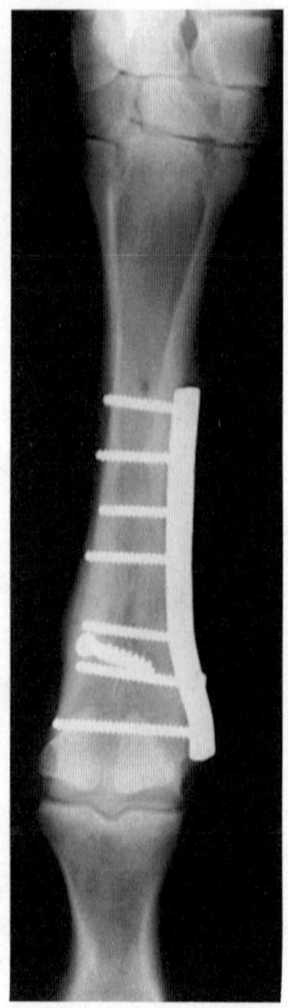

Figure 96–25. Five-month follow-up radiograph of the same limb as in Figure 96–23. Note the healing of the osteotomy site and the callus formation around it. Good correction of the deformity was maintained. The plate could be removed at that point of time.

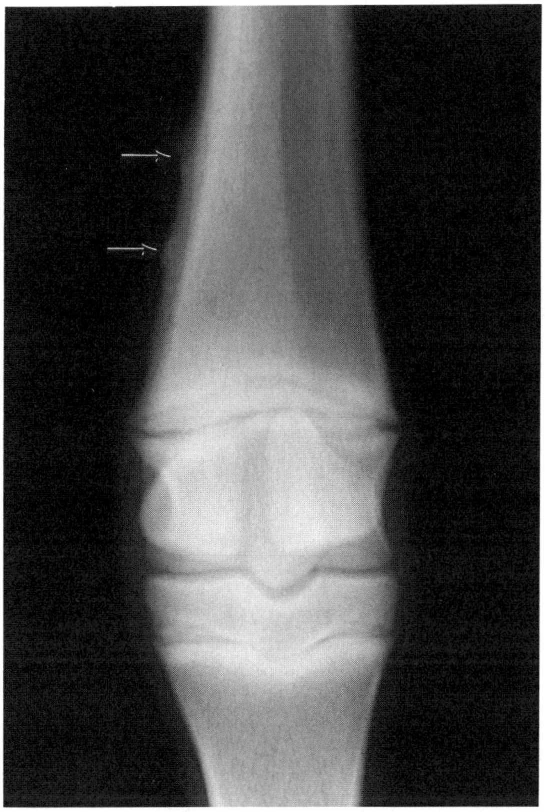

Figure 96–26. Periosteal new bone formation is demonstrated at the previous surgery site, where a periosteal transection technique was performed at the distal third metacarpal bone (*arrows*).

Technique. After performing the skin incision, the fibers of the collateral ligament over the medial malleolus of the distal tibia are separated longitudinally and a screw is inserted from a medial-distal to a lateral-proximal direction (Fig. 96–28). In doing so, penetration of the tarsocrural joint is avoided. The screw hole is prepared for 20 to 25 mm depth, and a 20-mm screw is used. The reason such a short screw may be used is the favorable angle by which tension will be applied by the wire or bone plate. If a longer screw is used the growth plate may be entered and possibly transfixed to the metaphysis, resulting in growth problems in the future. The site for the screw hole proximal to the physis is dependent upon the technique used. This hole is positioned 1 mm proximal to the most proximal hole of the small bone plate, or 2 to 3 cm proximal to the physis when the screws and wire technique is used. Figure eight wires (Fig. 96–28) or the bone plate are inserted according to the specific technique used. Closure of the incision is routine.

Corrective Osteotomy. In selected cases, corrective osteotomies may be performed in this region. However, this is a very difficult surgery in this location.

Postoperative Management

Bandaging techniques and postoperative care are identical to that described for the surgeries involving the radius.

Prognosis

The prognosis for successful correction of the deformity is good, especially if it is carried out in a young animal. Growth retardation in foals older than 5 months of age may not be adequate to correct a severe

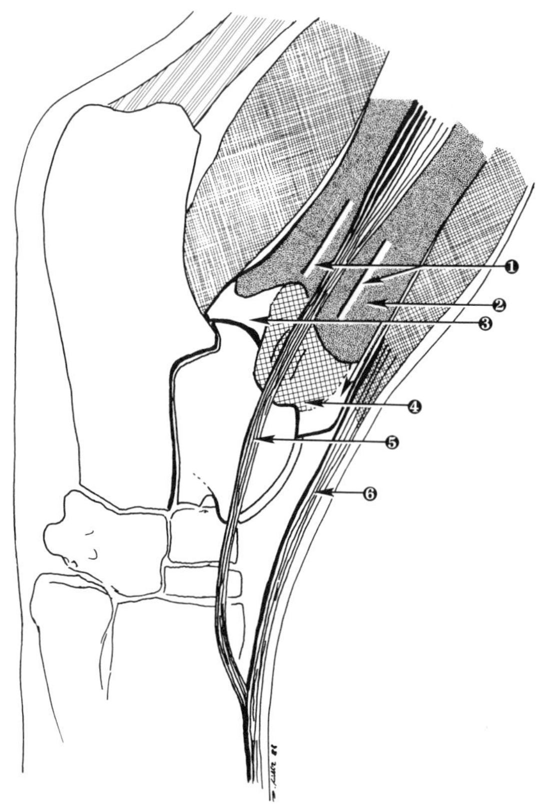

Figure 96–27. Diagram of the lateral aspect of the tarsal region. *1*, Sites for the skin incision to perform periosteal transection surgery; *2*, distal metaphysis of the tibia; *3*, distal epiphysis of the tibia; *4*, lateral malleolus of the distal tibia; *5*, lateral digital extensor tendon; and *6*, long digital extensor tendon. The skin incision may be performed cranial or caudal to the lateral digital extensor tendon.

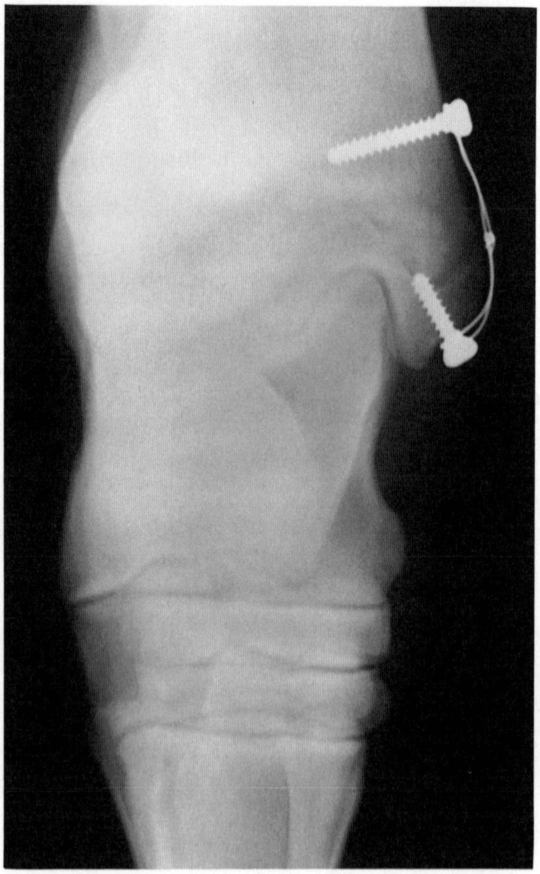

Figure 96–28. Dorsopalmar radiograph of the tarsal region of a foal. A growth retardation procedure was carried out in this foal consisting of two bone screws connected with a figure eight wire. Note the angle of the distal screw relative to the joint surface. Insertion of this screw in a horizontal direction would have resulted in penetration of the joint. Because of the complicated anatomy in this region, staples are very difficult to use and their application is discouraged.

deformity. As with all angular limb deformities, one has to remember that the animal has to *grow* in order to correct the deformity. This is especially important in miniature horses, in which the tendency is to breed smaller and smaller horses.

BIBLIOGRAPHY

Auer JA: Periosteal transection of the proximal phalanx in foals with angular limb deformities of the metacarpo/metatarsophalangeal area. *J Am Vet Med Assoc* 1985;187:496–499.

Auer JA, Martens RJ, Morris EL: Angular limb deformities in foals Part I Congenital factors. *Compend Cont Educ Pract Vet* 1982;4:330–339.

Auer JA, Martens RJ, Morris EL: Angular limb deformities in foals Part II Developmental factors. *Compend Cont Educ Pract Vet* 1983;5:29–35.

Auer JA, Martens RJ, Williams EH: Periosteal transection and periosteal stripping for correction of angular limb deformities in foals. *J Am Vet Med Assoc* 1982;181:459–466.

Bertone AL, Turner AS, Park RD: Further observations of the use of periosteal transection and stripping for treatment of angular limb deformities in foals. *J Am Vet Med Assoc* 1985;187:145–152.

Fackelman GE: Deformities of the appendicular skeleton, in Jennings PB (ed): *The Practice of Large Animal Surgery.* Philadelphia, WB Saunders Co, 1984, pp 950–982.

Fretz PB: Angular limb deformities in foals. *Vet Clin North Am Large Anim Pract* 1980;2:125–150.

Fretz PB, Cyubaluk NF, Pharr JW: Quantitive analysis of longbone growth in the horse. *Am J Vet Res* 1984;45:1602–1609.

Fretz PB, McIlwraith CW: Wedge osteotomy as a treatment for angular limb deformities of the fetlock in horses. *J Am Vet Med Assoc* 1983;182:245–250.

LaMont RL, Prasad B: Experiences with dome shaped osteotomy of upper tibia for multiplane correction. *Clin Orthop Rel Res* 1973;91:152–157.

White KK: Diaphyseal angular limb deformities in three foals. *J Am Vet Med Assoc* 1983;182:272–279.

97
Carpal and Tarsal Cuboidal Bone Anomalies

Richard M. DeBowes

DIAGNOSIS

The medical history attending the clinical presentation of horses affected by cuboidal bone abnormalities is principally concerned with the evaluation of an angular deviation of a limb from its normal longitudinal axis. This deviation may be either unilateral or bilateral and is generally observed within a few days following birth. The deformity usually involves the carpus and is commonly a valgus deformity. The tarsus may also be affected, but with less frequency than the carpus. Typically, the deformity may be reduced by manipulation during physical examination. The presence of a reducible deformity suggests a variety of possible diagnoses, including periarticular laxity of the soft tissues, agenesis of the cuboidal bones, cuboidal bone hypoplasia, or incomplete ossification of the cuboidal bones.

The diagnosis is confirmed by radiographic examination of the clinically affected articulations. Geometric evaluation of the radial or tibial axis compared to the metacarpal or metatarsal axis will identify the specific location of the angular deformity within the carpal or tarsal joints, respectively. The absence of any cuboidal bone on a carpal or tarsal radiographic examination of a full-term foal confirms a tentative diagnosis of cuboidal agenesis (Fig. 97–1). The presence of misshapen bones is consistent with a diagnosis of cuboidal hypoplasia or malformation (Fig. 97–2). The observation of thickened articular cartilage or small rounded centers of ossification within the cartilaginous precursors of the cuboidal bones may support a diagnosis of delayed cuboidal ossification (Fig. 97–3). The ulnar, third, and fourth carpal bones are most commonly affected. Laterally the ulnar and fourth carpal bones are misshapen. The third carpal bone may be wedge shaped and narrowed along its lateral aspect. In the hind limb, the central and third tarsal bones are often affected (Fig. 97–4). Occasionally, deformities are of a complex nature and have both cuboidal, epiphyseal, and metaphyseal components.

All foals should be evaluated for radiographic evidence of degenerative joint disease. The presence of degenerative disease in a young foal constitutes a poor prognostic sign and may preclude the possibility of an athletic future for the affected individual. The absence of radiographic evidence of degenerative changes does not necessarily improve the prognosis. The ultimate outcome of any case cannot be readily determined from radiographic examination because the damage to cartilaginous structures cannot be completely appreciated.

PATHOGENESIS

The pathogenesis for these conditions is not completely understood. Several possible explanations have been offered, including uterine malposition, toxic compounds, and nutritional problems. The possibility that relative dysmaturity may play a role in the pathogenesis has been shown. Cuboidal bones are known to undergo ossification late in the gestational period. Thus, premature foals must subject their underdeveloped cuboidal bones to the pressures of weight bearing, a situation that leads to plastic deformation of the cuboidal bones and fissuring of the articular surface. Foals that are born with a suboptimal thyroid status or hyperplastic goiter have been shown to experience a delayed ossification of carpal and tarsal bones. This phenomenon has been most evident in the tarsus, where the third and central tarsal bones have developed pathologic fractures after physical activity. In the carpus, the ulnar carpal bone is the last cuboidal bone to complete the process of ossification. Its cartilaginous template is often subjected to plastic deformation and malformation, a situation that results in the production of a carpal valgus deformity. The thickened cartilage surface may fissure and develop flap lesions similar to those of osteochondritis dissecans. Conformational defects such as rotational defects (toe-in or toe-out posture) and periarticular soft tissue laxities place asymmetric pressures on the articular surfaces and may contribute to the deformation of hypoplastic or incompletely ossified carpal bones.

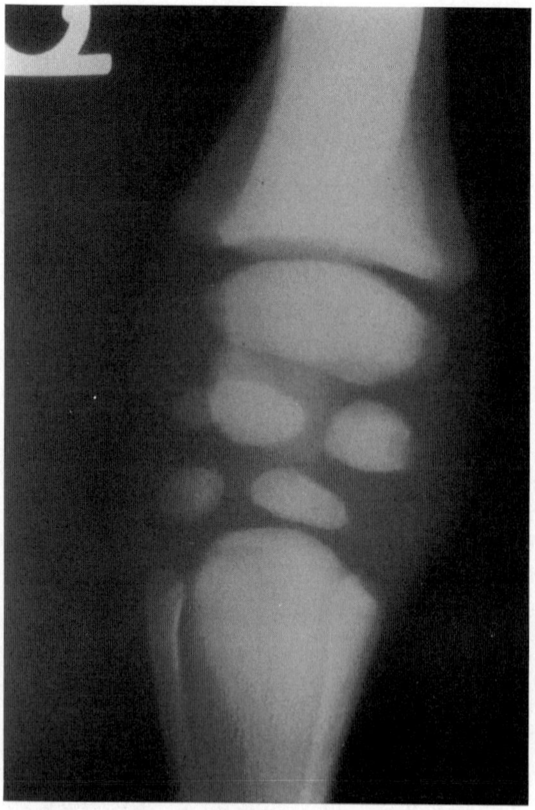

Figure 97–1. Agenesis of the second carpal bone is evident on this radiographic projection.

TREATMENT

Treatment of this condition depends to some extent on the severity of the lesion, and the intended use of the affected individual. Agenesis of the cuboidal bones is difficult to treat by either surgical or medical means. Depending on the specific bone or bones that have failed to develop, it may be impossible to obtain either an orthopedically straight limb or a sound patient following therapy. Although temporary transphyseal bridging and periosteal stripping techniques may be utilized to correct the angular deformity of the limb, these techniques will provide no curative effect for the articular deficits. Some caution should be used in diagnosing carpal or tarsal agenesis. In some cases the cartilagenous model is present but may take several weeks to be identified radiographically.

Cuboidal hypoplasia or incomplete ossification are more readily treatable and may in some cases be managed to obtain both a straight limb and a sound patient. Therapy is directed at the maintenance of a true longitudinal axis of the affected limb so that continued ossification of the cartilaginous cuboidal templates may progress without further distortion of the cartilage model. Failure to achieve the normal longitudinal arrangement of load-bearing bones will lead to the continuation of asymmetric articular loading and compressive remodeling of the cartilaginous cuboidal bone templates. Affected individuals should be confined to stalls and exercised by controlled walking to reduce the amount and intensity of articular trauma. The longitudinal axis may be maintained with either splints or tube casts. Splints that are applied to the limb must be padded at all pressure points to prevent the formation of decubital sores. Sections of polyvinylchloride pipe or cast material molded to the affected limb can serve as splinting material for this purpose. The need to fre-

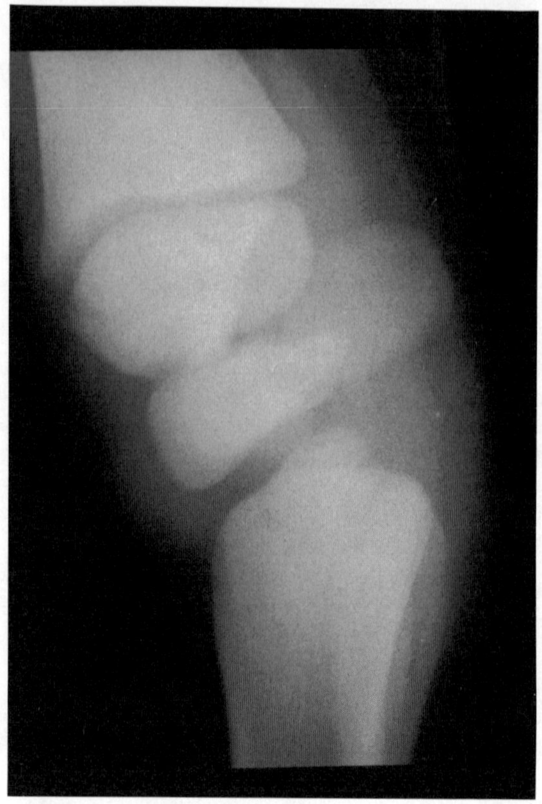

Figure 97–2. Hypoplasia of the third carpal bone is evident on this radiographic projection.

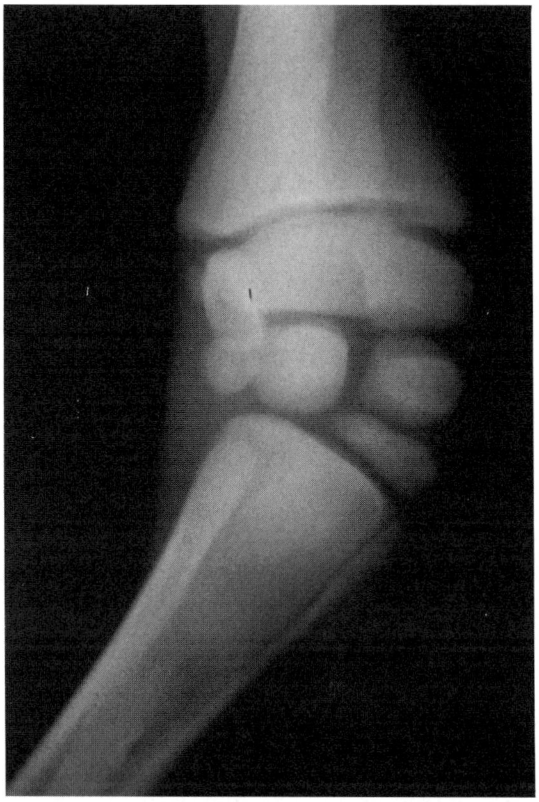

Figure 97–3. Incomplete ossification of the cuboidal bones is evident in this radiographic examination of the carpus.

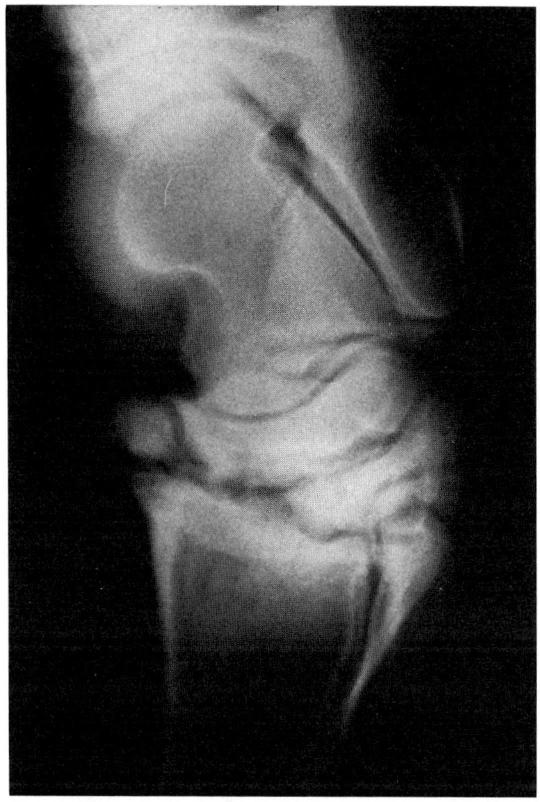

Figure 97–4. Collapse of the third tarsal bone has occurred several months after incomplete ossification of this bone was diagnosed at birth.

quently evaluate the placement of the splints makes them less desirable than tube casts. Tube casts are applied to the affected limbs from the proximal radius/tibia to the distal metacarpus/metatarsus. The casts are well padded at their distal limit and over the distal radial epicondyles and the tibial malleoli to reduce the formation of decubital sores. By avoiding the enclosure of the hoof within the cast, the foal will continue to bear weight in a nearly normal fashion and maintain some degree of tension within the musculotendinous units. Enclosure of the entire distal limb is not recommended because of the tendon laxity and hoof atrophy that may result. Tube casts are generally applied for 14 to 21 days; however, the ossification process should be evaluated by radiographic examination prior to discontinuation of the therapy.

If rotational deformities are concurrently present, corrective trimming of the hooves may help straighten the limb. In most cases the most effective trimming is leveling the hoof and shortening or squaring the toe. Trimming to shorten the hoof wall on one side or the other may be effective, but must be done cautiously to prevent angular deformity of the foot or pastern.

BIBLIOGRAPHY

Auer JA, Martens RJ, Morris EL: Angular limb deformities in foals: Part II Developmental factors. *Compend Cont Educ Pract Vet* 1983;5:S27–S35.

Facklemann GE: Deformities of the appendicular skeleton, in Jennings PB (ed): *The Practice of Large Animal Surgery.* Philadelphia, WB Saunders 1984, vol 2, pp 950–952.

Leitch M: Musculoskeletal disorders in neonatal foals, in Symposium on Neonatal Equine Disease. *Vet Clin North Am Equine* 1985;1(1):189–206.

McIlwraith CW: Angular limb deformities in foals, in Mansmann RA, McAllister ES, Pratt PW (eds): *Equine Medicine and Surgery*, ed 3. Santa Barbara, CA, American Veterinary Publications, 1982, vol 2, pp 1098–1109.

McLaughlin BG, Doige CE: A study of ossification of carpal and tarsal bones in normal and hypothyroid foals. *Can Vet J* 1982;23:164–168.

McLaughlin BG, Doige CE, Fretz PB, Pharr JW: Carpal bone lesions associated with angular limb deformities in foals. *J Am Vet Med Assoc* 1981;178:224–230.

Pharr JW, Fretz PB: Radiographic findings in foals with angular limb deformities. *J Am Vet Med Assoc* 1981;8:812.

98 Rotational Limb Deformities

Melinda K. Krpan

Rotational deformity of the limb (a toe-in or toe-out stance) is a common conformational fault affecting the horse. Outward rotation (a toe-out stance) appears to be most common. Rotational deformity causes a greater amount of stress to be placed on the side of the limb opposite the direction of rotation, affecting soft tissues and bone and wearing the hoof wall excessively on that side. In addition, the foot swings inward abnormally during the advance phase of the stride and may interfere with the opposite limb. Consequently, soft tissue blemishes and periostitis or fracture of the small metacarpal bones may occur. Excessive wear of the hoof wall on one side causes the foot to break over off center. The unbalanced foot that results may further exacerbate the degree of rotation.

Rotational deformities occur in foals of all breeds. The condition may be unilateral or bilateral and may affect forelimbs and hind limbs. There does not appear to be any sex predilection. Rotational deformities may be primary or secondary. Primary rotational deformities are usually congenital and are presumed to be inherited, although this is unproven.

Rotational deformities may occur secondary to angular limb deformities originating in the carpal and tarsal regions. Since they develop subsequent to the angular deformity, secondary rotational deformities are acquired when the foal is a few days to several months old. The etiology of secondary rotational deformities is unknown. In humans, secondary rotational deformities are believed to result from torsional forces applied perpendicular to the axis of physeal growth and parallel to the plane of the physis. Angular deviation of the limb may create these forces. A similar hypothesis has been proposed to explain the association of angular and rotational deformities in the foal. In addition, a relationship exists between the type of angular limb deformity and the direction of rotation. Varus deformity (deviation of the distal limb toward the midline of the body) is associated with inward rotation of the limb and a toe-in stance results. Limbs affected with valgus deformities (deviation of the distal limb away from the midline of the body) exhibit outward rotation and a toe-out stance results.

Primary rotational deformities may arise at any level of the limb or may occur at multiple sites, increasing the overall severity of the deformity. Secondary rotational deformities occur at or below the level of the angular deformity affecting the carpal or tarsal region.

Primary rotational deformities of the equine limb have traditionally been treated by a combination of corrective trimming and shoeing; however, these methods are not without risk. Trimming the unworn side of the hoof wall to level the foot and applying a shoe that raises the worn side are recommended to force breakover at the center of the toe and improve the way the horse travels. Such methods create a foot that is once again unbalanced and, except in the mildest cases, only partially correct the rotational deformity.

Correction of the primary angular limb deformity and corrective hoof trimming have been proposed as means of treating secondary rotational deformities. However, despite early and complete correction of the angular deformity, the rotational deformity often persists and may actually increase in severity. Alternatively, transfixation of the lateral styloid process of the ulna to the distal radial epiphysis has been proposed for simultaneous correction of angular and rotational deformities. The rationale for the surgical technique is based on a theory that the styloid process is unstable in the foal and provides inadequate support for the ulnar carpal bone. The result is a valgus deformity and outward rotation at the level of the carpus. The suggested pathogenesis does not explain rotation in the lower forelimb or the hind limb or the association of varus deformity and inward rotation. For these reasons, the proposed pathogenesis has been criticized and the surgical technique has had limited use.

Failure of the traditional methods to produce complete correction of the rotational deformities indicated a need for more effective methods of treatment. A surgical technique utilizing transphyseal bridges at the involved physis was developed as a direct approach to correction of rotational deformities. The technique was evaluated in 12 foals with rotational deformities created at the distal metacarpal physis. Subsequently, five clinical cases with either primary rotational deformities or outward rotation secondary to valgus deformity were treated with the same technique.

DIAGNOSIS

The diagnosis of rotational deformities and planning for their correction rely on gross visual and radiographic examinations of the affected limbs. With the foal standing squarely and bearing weight equally on all limbs, the humeroradial, carpal, and metacarpophalangeal joints are palpated. The plane dividing each joint into medial and lateral halves is determined and marked on the dorsal surface of the joint with a narrow piece of white adhesive tape. The median plane of the limb is determined by dropping a weighted line from the point of the scapulohumeral joint to the ground. The examiner then stands in front of the foal and observes the alignment of the three pieces of tape with each other and with the weighted line. Alternatively, the examiner may stand caudolateral to the limb being evaluated and view the alignment of the median plane of the limb and the three joints from the point of the scapulohumeral joint distally.

Alignment of the median, humeroradial, and carpal planes, but malalignment with the plane through the metacarpophalangeal joint localizes rotation to the third metacarpal bone (MCIII). When the median and humeroradial planes align but do not coincide with the carpal and metacarpophalangeal planes, rotation exists within the radius. Malalignment of the median and humeroradial planes places the rotational deformity in the humeroradial joint or proximad. When rotational deformity is associated with a moderate to severe angular limb deformity, the site of rotation within the limb can be more difficult to determine. Angular deviation of a joint prevents an exact determination of the bisecting plane and its alignment with the median plane of the limb. In such cases, observing the limb from above the scapulohumeral joint without tape applied to the affected joint has been beneficial.

Radiographic examination of the affected limbs from the proximal aspect of the radius to and including the first phalanx should be performed. Two radiographic projections (dorsopalmar and lateromedial) should be evaluated for abnormalities in osseous structures. When an angular deformity is present, the etiology may be determined and a decision made as to whether correction can be achieved with conservative therapy (splints or sleeve casts) or if surgical intervention is necessary.

SURGERY

Surgical Planning

Use of the oblique transphyseal bridge surgical technique is limited to deformities originating within the radius or distal in the limb. Rotational deformities originating proximal to the radius cannot be corrected with this technique because of poor surgical access to the physes. Deformities of the radius or carpal region are corrected using the distal radial physis, whereas deformities of the metacarpophalangeal region are corrected using the distal physis of MCIII.

No specific age limits have been established for surgical correction of rotational deformities. As a guideline, the age recommendations proposed for correction of angular deformities using the distal radial and metacarpal physes may be followed. Long bone growth studies indicate that growth altering procedures involving the distal radial physis should be performed before 9 months of age. Although long bone growth of the radius continues well beyond this age, the growth rate is slow and the growth potential is considered inadequate to correct moderate to severe deformities. The optimal age for surgical intervention at the distal radial physis is during the first 3 months of life. If the foal is older than 2 months of age, incomplete correction of moderate to severe deformities should be expected.

For primary rotational deformities and secondary rotational deformities distal to the site of angular deviation, a one-stage surgery is planned. Transphyseal bridges are placed on both the medial and lateral sides of the limb. To correct outward rotation, the transphyseal bridges are oriented as shown in Figure 98–1. The distal bone screw of the medial bridge is positioned at the dorsomedial aspect of the epiphysis and the proximal bone screw is positioned at the palmaromedial aspect of the metaphysis. The distal bone screw of the lateral bridge is positioned at the palmarolateral aspect of the epiphysis while the proximal bone screw is positioned in the dorsolateral metaphysis. To correct inward rotation, oblique transphyseal bridges are also placed on the medial and lateral sides of the limb, but the bone screws are positioned in the opposite orientation with respect to the epiphysis and metaphysis.

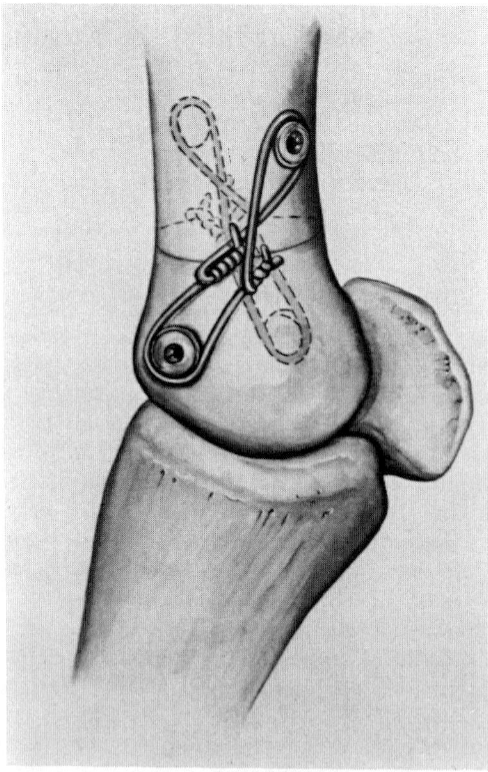

Figure 98–1. Orientation of the medial oblique transphyseal bridge (*solid outline*) and lateral oblique transphyseal bridge (*dashed outline*) for correction of a primary outward rotational deformity or a secondary outward rotational deformity distal to the site of angular deviation at the distal physis of the third metacarpal bone.

To correct rotational deformities secondary to angular deviation originating at the same site, a two-stage surgery is often necessary. During the first surgery, an oblique bridge is placed on only one side of the limb to retard longitudinal growth at the physis asymmetrically, and is oriented to produce derotation. In two clinical cases affected with such deformities, correction of angular deviation preceded complete derotation, requiring a second surgery. In such cases, an oblique transphyseal bridge is added to the opposite side of the limb to correct the remaining rotational deformity and prevent overcorrection of the angular deformity. To correct outward rotation and a valgus deformity, an oblique bridge is placed on the medial side of the limb. The distal bone screw is positioned at the dorsomedial aspect of the epiphysis. The proximal bone screw is positioned at the palmaromedial aspect of the metaphysis (Fig. 98–2). To correct inward rotation and concurrent varus deformity, the bridge is placed on the lateral side of the limb. The distal bone screw is positioned dorsolaterally and the proximal bone screw is positioned in the palmarolateral metaphysis. A second bridge is added if the rotational deformity remains following correction of the angular deformity.

Surgical Technique

With the foal anesthetized and placed in lateral recumbency, the surgical site is aseptically prepared and draped. A 23-gauge, 1-in needle is inserted into the physis. An additional needle is then inserted into the physis on each side of the first needle to define the plane of the physis on the side of the limb. Needle placement within the physis is confirmed with a dorsopalmar radiograph.

A 5-cm curvilinear incision is made, centering over the physis. The incision is started at the proposed posi-

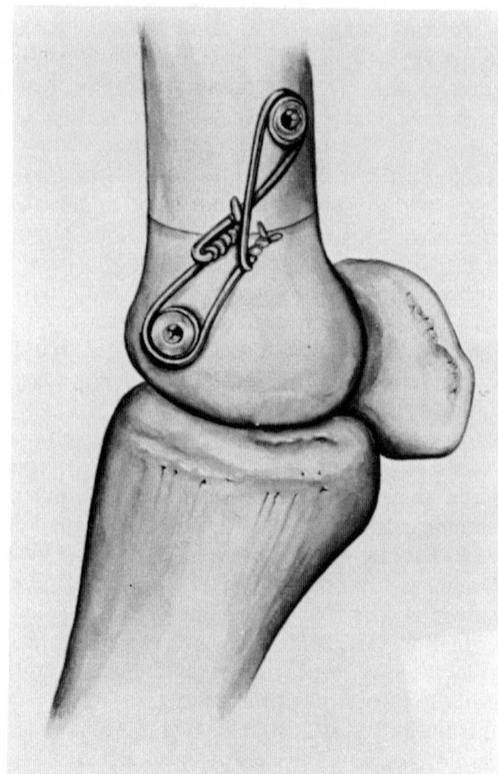

Figure 98–2. Orientation of the oblique transphyseal bridge across the distal third metacarpal physis placed on the medial side of the limb for correction of a valgus angular limb deformity and outward rotation originating at the same site. A lateral bridge is added during a second surgery if rotation persists following correction of the valgus deformity.

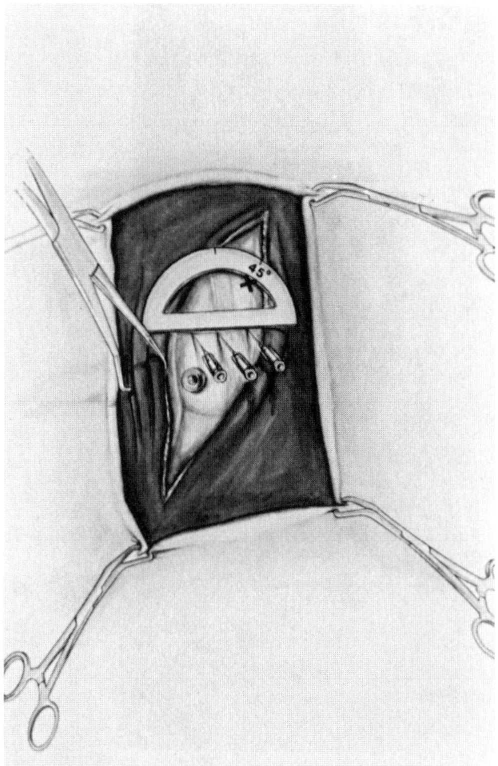

Figure 98–3. A sterile protractor and three needles are used to determine the plane of the physis and the 45-degree angle for placement of an oblique transphyseal bridge. The epiphyseal bone screw has been inserted and the position of the metaphyseal bone screw is marked (*X* below 45° symbol on protractor).

tion of the metaphyseal bone screw and curves toward the anticipated position of the epiphyseal bone screw. The skin flap is dissected free of underlying fascia and reflected toward the base of the incision. During reflection of the skin flap, the physeal needles are removed and reinserted into the exposed physis.

The position for each bone screw is determined using the physeal needles and a protractor placed on the bone surface with its base against the needles (Fig. 98–3). The first bone screw is placed in the epiphysis on a line that bisects the most radial or lateral aspect of the physis and that is at a 45-degree angle to the plane of the physis, midway between the physis and joint space (Fig. 98–3). The metaphyseal bone screw is placed equidistant from the physis on the same bisecting line. A 1-cm stab incision is made through the subcutaneous tissues and periosteum to mark the position of each screw. A 3.2-mm hole is drilled to a depth approximately one half the bone diameter as determined from preoperative radiographs. The drill bit should be aligned to ensure that the screws are parallel to the plane of the physis. The holes are tapped and 4.5-mm cortical bone screws of appropriate length are inserted, leaving two to three threads exposed above the bone surface. The screws are connected by 18- or 20-gauge stainless steel wire in a figure eight pattern. The wire ends are twisted tightly, cut, and bent back toward the bone surface. The screws are then tightened. Subcutaneous tissues are apposed by a simple continous pattern of absorbable suture material. The skin is closed with a simple interrupted pattern using nonabsorbable suture material. If transphyseal bridges must be placed on both sides of the limb for correction of primary rotational deformities, the foal should be repositioned to the opposite side for placement of the second set of screws and wire.

Following placement of the oblique transphyseal bridges, dorsopalmar and lateromedial radiographic projections should be obtained to check the position of each bone screw and rule out the possibility of penetration of the physis or articular cartilage. The skin incisions are covered with sterile nonadherent dressings and full-limb cotton wraps are applied. The hooves are trimmed to ensure medial to lateral foot balance. The foal is then recovered from anesthesia.

Complications

Soft tissue proliferation at the surgical site is a consistent complication associated with placement of oblique transphyseal bridges, similar to reports of transphyseal bridging for correction of angular limb deformities. Subjectively, the size of the soft tissue blemish appears to be greater with the oblique transphyseal bridges.

In the five clinical cases noted above, blemishes resulting from surgery at the distal metacarpal physis were more apparent than those overlying the distal radial physis. Soft tissue proliferation after surgery at the distal metacarpal physis was less in two foals given restricted exercise for the first 30 days following surgery. Removal of the transphyseal bridges following correction of the rotational deformity was associated with a decrease in the size of the blemish. However, lengthening and circumferential growth of each foal's limbs during the 2-year follow-up period did not significantly affect blemish size. As a result, a less than satisfactory cosmetic appearance was achieved in foals that underwent surgical correction of rotational deformities at the distal metacarpal physis. The owners must be advised of this fact before surgery.

Functionally, the limbs were unaffected by the soft tissue proliferation. A decrease in range of motion of

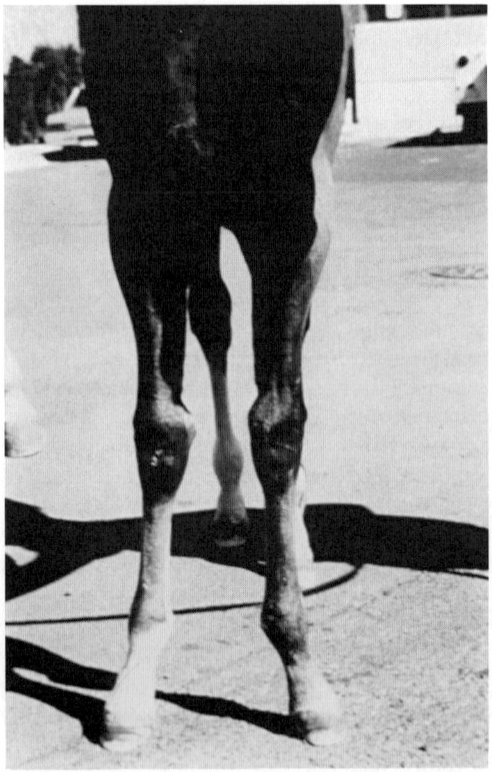

Figure 98–4. A 55-day-old female Appaloosa foal before surgery. Primary outward rotation was localized to two levels in both forelimbs: proximal to the radius and at the third metacarpal bone. Oblique transphyseal bridges were placed on both sides of each forelimb at the distal metacarpal physis to correct the rotational deformity of the third metacarpal bone.

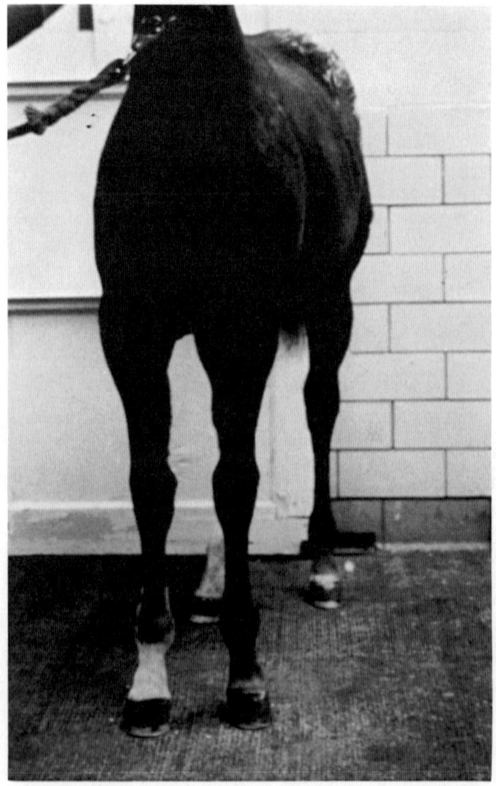

Figure 98–5. The same foal as in Figure 98.4 at 1 year of age, 8 months following removal of the implants. Mild outward rotation remains in both forelimbs as a result of rotation proximal to the radius. Alignment of the carpal and metacarpophalangeal regions is good in both forelimbs. Soft tissue blemishes are evident at the distal metacarpal region.

the joint adjacent to the surgical site was not observed. All foals were sound following surgery and remained sound during the 2-year follow-up period.

POSTOPERATIVE CARE

The foal should be confined to a stall with the mare for 30 days. Controlled exercise in the form of daily controlled walking with the mare can begin 14 days following surgery. The limbs are kept wrapped until suture removal. After 30 days, the mare and foal are allowed free exercise in a small paddock, which is continued until the time of implant removal. The foal's hooves are evaluated at weekly intervals and trimmed as often as needed to maintain medial-to-lateral foot balance.

The owner is instructed to evaluate the affected limbs for correction of the deformity at weekly intervals using the method outlined for diagnosis and localization of rotational deformities. When correction of the deformity is complete, the foal is returned for evaluation and removal of the implants. If more than one limb is affected, it is important to stress that each limb be evaluated independently and the transphyseal bridges be removed as needed to avoid overcorrection.

If the foal has reached the age for closure of the physis, yet correction of the rotational deformity is incomplete, radiographs should be obtained. Closure of the physis would prevent further derotation. In such cases, removal of the bridges is still advised to improve the overall cosmetic appearance of the limb.

PROGNOSIS AND SPECIAL CONSIDERATIONS

Follow-up of the five clinical cases at 1 year of age revealed that complete correction of the rotational deformity was achieved in 3 foals. Incomplete correction, resulting in a very mild rotational deformity, was evident in the two remaining foals. One foal had primary outward rotation originating proximal to the radius and at MCIII of both forelimbs. The mild deformity remaining after removal of the transphyseal bridge from the distal metacarpal region was due to rotation proximal to the radius (Figs. 98–4 and 98–5). The second foal was affected with concomitant angular and rotational deformities of the distal aspect of the radius. Following correction of the angular deformity, the owners were satisfied with the appearance of the limb and the foal did not undergo the second surgery to complete correction of the rotational deformity.

At 2 years of age, three of the horses were available for follow-up. They were considered sound and the alignment of the limbs was acceptable. By 2.5 years of age two horses were being used for pleasure riding and one was in race training. The cosmetic appearance of the limbs at the surgical sites had prevented the two horses used for pleasure riding from starting show careers. It is important, therefore, to consider this postoperative complication and discuss it with the owner before proceeding with the surgery. Generally, the need for a functional limb outweighs the subsequent cosmetic appearance.

The presence of an angular limb deformity at the same level has not been a problem. Simultaneous correction of both deformities occurred in the two animals so affected, although correction of rotation lagged behind correction of the angular deformity, requiring a second surgery. The rotational deformity was corrected after placement of the second oblique transphyseal bridge.

Trimming the hoof wall to produce absolute medial-to-lateral balance of the foot is a necessary adjunct to the surgical treatment of rotational deformities in foals. It should be done at the time of surgery and repeated as often as needed to maintain a balanced foot. Severe rotational deformities may require trimming as frequently as every 7 to 10 days. This will prevent exacerbation of the deformity caused by uneven wear of the hoof wall and minimize asymmetric stresses on the soft tissues and joints of the limb as the deformity is being corrected.

BIBLIOGRAPHY

Fretz PB, Cymbaluk NF, Pharr JW: Quantitative analysis of long-bone growth in the horse. *Am J Vet Res* 1984;45:1602–1609.

Heinze CD: Correction of bone deformities by physeal stapling, in Catcott EJ, Smithcors JF (eds): *Equine Medicine and Surgery*, ed 2. Wheaton, ILL, American Veterinary Publications, 1972, pp 901–905.

Heinze CD: Transfixation of the lateral styloid process. *Proc Am Assoc Equine Pract* 1977; pp 294–300.

McIlwraith CW: Angular limb deformities in foals, in Mansmann RA, McAllister ES, Pratt PW (eds): *Equine Medicine and Surgery*, ed 3. Santa Barbara, CA, American Veterinary Publications, 1982, pp 1098–1109.

Swanson AB, Greene PW, Allis HD: Rotational deformities of the lower extremity in children and their clinical significance. *Clin Orthop* 1963;27:157–175.

99
Osteochondrosis: Current Concepts

Gayle W. Trotter

Osteochondrosis in horses includes a number of clinical conditions that represent developmental disorders of the growing skeleton. These conditions have previously been grouped under the heading of metabolic bone disease. Because cartilage is primarily affected in this disease, a more descriptive term for osteochondrosis might be "dyschondroplasia." However, the term "osteochondrosis" is well established in the veterinary literature and osteochondrosis should be considered one manifestation of developmental orthopedic disease in horses. In osteochondrosis, cartilage of the epiphyseal and metaphyseal physes does not mature properly and the hypertrophied layer persists in areas that normally would ossify. Necrosis subsequently occurs in these areas of thickened cartilage and, depending on the extent of cartilage involvement, one or more of the clinical manifestations of osteochondrosis develops. Osteochondritis dissecans (OCD) and subchondral cystic lesions (involvement of epiphyseal physis) and physitis or epiphysitis (involvement of metaphyseal physis) are considered manifestations of osteochondrosis. Not all subchondral cystic lesions and occurrences of physitis are considered manifestations of osteochondrosis. Trauma may also directly lead to development of some of these lesions. Osteochondrosis may also contribute to some angular and flexural limb deformities, and involvement of cervical vertebrae can result in cervical vertebral malformation and subsequent neurologic signs of wobbler syndrome. Further discussion in this section will concentrate on the clinical entities of OCD and subchondral cystic lesions. Both conditions involve growth cartilage of the epiphysis, and therefore they can affect the final shape of the epiphysis as well as the congruity of the joint surface. If articular surface irregularities or shape changes become excessive, secondary degenerative joint disease often results.

ETIOPATHOGENESIS OF OSTEOCHONDROSIS

Much of the information concerning etiology and development of early changes of osteochondrosis has been extrapolated to the horse from studies done in other species. In recent years, more research has been directed toward study of this disease in horses. This increased interest in osteochondrosis probably reflects the impression of many veterinarians that the incidence of the disease has increased significantly over the past 10 to 15 years.

Early descriptions of osteochonrosis in horses assumed ischemic necrosis of subchondral bone resulted in changes that eventually developed in the overlying cartilage. This theory was extrapolated from what was presumed to occur in osteochondrosis in humans. Recently, evidence of microscopic and submicroscopic vascular changes has been associated with osteochondosis lesions in swine. The role of primary vascular insufficiency in development of osteochondrosis, however, remains to be proven.

In studies done in swine and poultry, the earliest morphologic change of osteochondrosis was focal thickening of epiphyseal cartilage. This thickening was shown microscopically to be due to retention of chondrocytes of the hypertrophied cartilage layer. There is evidence that this also represents the earliest morphologic change of osteochondrosis in horses. Depending on extent of cartilage involvement, and perhaps on local biomechanical forces, necrosis of this cartilage can result in either chondral or osteochondral flap formation, or necrotic cartilage can persist in the subchondral bone, leading to formation of subchondral cystic lesions.

Much research interest is currently directed toward identification of the factors which render cartilage maturation abnormal. There is little doubt that numerous factors may cause and/or predispose an animal to develop osteochondrosis. Overnutrition or malnutrition, trauma, genetics, and endocrine imbalances have all been incriminated as causative factors.

Osteochondrosis has typically been postulated to be due to overfeeding or overnutrition in young, fast-growing animals. Experimental work in swine, cattle, and poultry implicated excessive energy intake leading to rapid growth as the major factor leading to development of osteochondrosis. It is not always clear from these studies whether growth rate is increased or rate of weight gain is increased. In certain studies done in swine, increased rate of weight gain was accompanied by an increased incidence of osteochondrosis; in other studies, disease incidence was unrelated to growth rate and rate of weight gain. Does overfeeding of energy in certain cases induce sufficiently rapid growth that deficiencies of other nutrients are created, or is the problem related directly to certain nutrient excesses that exert an effect independent of growth rate or rate of weight gain? These questions remain to be answered.

The effect of varying levels of protein on growth and calcium metabolism in horses has recently been investigated. It was concluded that excessive protein intake in young horses did not increase growth rate when compared to a diet that provided recommended protein levels. Calcium absorption and retention were also unaffected by high protein intake. In this study, all other nutrients were provided at levels that met National Research Council recommendations. In a separate study where excessive levels of *both* protein and energy were fed to young horses, abnormalities of growth plate cartilage were seen. Epiphyseal and metaphyseal growth plate cartilage had increased cellularity, but decreased cartilage matrix glycosaminoglycan and collagen content. These cartilage matrix changes could adversely affect capillary penetration necessary for normal endochondral ossification. The role of excessive energy and protein in development of these changes is still unclear.

Other nutritional aspects to consider in the pathogenesis of osteochondrosis are calcium, phosphorus, and vitamin D metabolism. In studies done in swine, altering levels of calcium and phosphorus did not consistently result in changes in the incidence of osteochondrosis. However, in dogs fed a high-calcium diet (three times the recommended calcium level, with all other nutrients fed at normal levels), more osteochondral lesions were seen than in dogs fed normal calcium levels. Based on histomorphometric data and levels of circulating parathyroid hormone and calcitonin, it was hypothesized that excessive calcium intake caused relative hypercalcitoninism and relative hypoparathyroidism, resulting in inhibition of osteoclastic bone resorption, retarded cartilage maturation, and an increased incidence of osteochondral lesions. A similar hypothesis has been proposed for osteochondrosis in horses, presumably based on these and other studies done in dogs. How often horses might be subjected to calcium intakes of this level and what effect it might have still remains speculative. Both 1,25-dihydroxycholecalciferol (vitamin D) and its metabolite 24,25-dihydroxycholecalciferol are important to calcium/phosphorus homeostasis and normal development of the immature skeleton. Abnormal vitamin D metabolism also cannot be ruled out as a contributing factor in some cases of osteochondrosis.

Trace mineral nutrition may also play a role in development of osteochondral lesions. Low serum copper levels were found in a number of Thoroughbred foals from two farms where the incidence of osteochondrosis was high. Although serum zinc levels were high in some affected foals, a copper deficiency due to zinc toxicosis could not be proven. In another survey, incidence of developmental orthopedic disease (which included osteochondrosis) on 19 breeding farms was compared to farm scores for feeding practices (types, amounts, and composition of feed available for foals and broodmares) and foal and broodmare management. A relationship was shown to exist between dietary content of calcium, phosphorus, copper, and zinc and the prevalence of developmental orthopedic disease (osteochondrosis, physitis, contracted tendons). In this survey, farms with the highest scores for disease incidence were also those where the lowest protein levels were being fed. Further work by the same group supported dietary copper deficiency as a causative factor in development of osteochondrosis. Broodmares were fed a copper-supplemented or non–copper-supplemented ration and similarly supplemented rations were fed to the foals when they began to consume dry matter. Foals were euthanized and examined for skeletal manifestations of osteochondrosis at 90 or 180 days of age. Incidence of osteochondrosis was three to four times higher in the non–copper-supplemented group. Subsequent studies completed by other research groups have failed to confirm the above findings with low dietary copper levels and it is possible that regional differences may exist regarding relative influence of etiologic factors. Copper deficiency could result in abnormal collagen metabolism due to decreases in the copper-containing enzyme lysyl oxidase.

Popular current feeding practices could contribute to trace mineral imbalances. Alfalfa hay contains higher levels of calcium than does grass hay and, in other species, diets containing higher levels of calcium and phosphorus have been associated with decreased absorption of copper and zinc. Soybean meal, a common protein supplement used in diets for young horses, contains phytic acid, which can form insoluble complexes with zinc and other minerals rendering them less available. It would seem that ration quality may be as or more important a factor to regulate than ration quantity. A nutrionally balanced diet should be provided, and the assistance of an animal nutritionist should be sought where dietary imbalances are suspected or confirmed.

Trauma and mechanical stress have also been considered causative factors in development of osteochondrosis because lesions occur more commonly in some anatomic sites than others. The seemingly increased incidence of osteochondrosis in fast-growing animals is also compatible with increased weight per unit area of growth cartilage. Conversely, osteochondrosis has been seen in a 3-day-old foal, suggesting trauma is not always a contributing factor.

In a study where cystic lesions in the medial femoral condyle of horses were evaluated, subchondral bone plate microfractures and fragments of nonvital bone within the cystic cavity were identified microscopically. It was suggested that trauma to subchondral bone was of primary etiologic significance in development of these lesions. In a further study, subchondral cystic lesions were induced in ponies by surgically creating linear full-thickness incisions in the weight-bearing articular cartilage of the medial femoral condyle. No subchondral lesion developed, however, when a full-thickness elliptical piece of articular cartilage was excised. Subchondral cystic lesions could therefore develop subsequent to trauma that caused a full-thickness cartilage injury. It is possible that trauma is the initiating insult in development of some osteochondral lesions, but the presence of lesions in the very young is more compatible with abnormal cartilage maturation from causes other than direct trauma. Trauma may be more important in development of some subchondral cystic lesions, and as a triggering factor in rendering some osteochondral lesions clinically significant. The sudden onset of clinical signs in some cases of OCD is compatible with traumatic loosening or dislodgement of a chondral/osteochondral fragment.

A genetic predisposition to developing osteochondrosis lesions may exist. In other domestic animals, certain breeds, families within breeds, or offspring from certain matings seem predisposed to developing osteochondrosis. Inherited predisposition for osteochondrosis was also shown in a study on Standardbred and Warmblood horses in Sweden. One stallion in each breed had a significantly higher frequency of osteochondrosis in his progeny compared to progeny groups of other stallions. The pattern of inheritance could not be determined because of small sample size. Body size of the stallion did not seem to be a major determining factor.

Endocrine imbalances have also been suggested as causative factors in osteochondrosis, and some supportive evidence exists. Chronic administration of the glucocorticoid dexamethasone to pony and horse foals was associated with development of osteochondral lesions. Thyroxine is necessary for normal chondrocyte maturation and for normal bony replacement of epiphyseal and metaphyseal growth cartilage. Abnormal endochondral ossification has been seen in the carpal and tarsal bones of hypothyroid foals. The effect of ingestion of soluble carbohydrates on thyroid hormone and insulin metabolism in young horses was also recently investigated. Carbohydrate-induced dissociation of thyroid hormone and insulin secretion was determined. Because of the influence these hormones have on growth cartilage, it was hypothesized that chronic dissociation might adversely affect skeletal development.

In summary, there seems little doubt that a multifactorial etiology is related to development of osteochondral lesions in horses. Of the many factors involved, diet quantity and quality remain those over which some degree of control may be exerted.

TREATMENT FOR OSTEOCHONDROSIS

Effective treatment of horses affected with osteochondrosis is also of importance to veterinarians. Numerous recent reports describe results of conservative or surgical treatment for osteochondrosis. Treatment differs depending on which joint is involved, and whether the lesion is an OCD lesion or a subchondral cystic lesion. Clinical improvement with conservative mangement has been recognized for a variety of clinical syndromes of osteochondrosis. In 76 horses with osteochondrosis, 47% improved to be competitive athletes using conservative treatment. Conservative treatment included modifying the training schedule relative to the degree of lameness, and using nonsteroidal anti-inflammatory medication as required to improve patient comfort. Success included horses that were able to effectively perform their intended function as well as those that could compete successfully at a vocation other than their intended one (racehorse becoming a successful jumper). Success was recorded for both OCD and subchondral cystic lesions involving various joints. No horse having osteochondrosis of the shoulder successfully improved, but success was recorded for horses with bilateral as well as unilateral osteochondrosis involving other joints. Thoroughbred racehorses had the poorest success rate (38%), whereas pleasure and other show horses had a 50 to 60% success rate.

Results of conservative management are inconsistent, however, and surgical intervention is considered beneficial and indicated in many cases. Case selection is always important and will be considered in more detail under specific joint involvement. A favorable prognosis has been reported for surgical management of OCD of the femoropatellar, tarsocrural, scapulohumeral, and metacarpophalangeal/metatarsophalangeal joints. The specific management and prognosis for each type of lesion will be covered in Chapters 100 through 103.

BIBLIOGRAPHY

Bridges CH, Womack JE, Harris ED, Scrutchfield WL: Considerations of copper metabolism in osteochondrosis of suckling foals. *J Am Vet Med Assoc* 1984;185;173–178.

Glade MJ, Belling TH: Growth plate cartilage metabolism, morphology and biochemical composition in over- and underfed horses. *Growth* 1984;48:473–482.

Glade M, Luba N: Serum triiodothyronine and thyroxine concentrations in weanling horses fed carbohydrate by direct gastric infusion. *Am J Vet Res* 1987;48:578–582.

Goedegebuure SA, Hazewinkel HAW: Morphological findings in young dogs chronically fed a diet containing excess calcium. *Vet Pathol* 1986;23:594–605.

Hoppe F, Philipsson J: A genetic study of osteochondrosis dissecans in Swedish horses. *Equine Pract* 1985;7:7–15.

Jeffcott LB, Kold SE, Melsen F. Aspects of the pathology of stifle bone cysts in the horse. *Equine Vet J* 1983;15:304–311.

Kold SE, Hickman J, Melsen F: An experimental study of the healing process of equine chondral and osteochondral defects. *Equine Vet J* 1986;18:18–24.

Knight DA, Gabel AA, Reed SM, Embertson RM, Tyznik WJ, Bramlage LR: Correlation of dietary mineral to incidence and severity of metabolic bone disease in Ohio and Kentucky. *Proc Am Assoc Equine Pract* 1985; pp 445–461.

McIlwraith CW (ed): *Proceedings of the AQHA Developmental Orthopedic Disease Symposium.* Dallas, American Quarter Horse Association, 1986.

Rose JA, Sande RD, Rose EM: Results of conservative management of osteochondrosis in the horse. *Proc Am Assoc Equine Pract* 1985; pp 617–626.

Schryver HF, Meakim DW, Lowe JE, Williams J, Soderholm LV, Hintz HF: Growth and calcium metabolism in horses fed varying levels of protein. *Equine Vet J* 1987;19:280–287.

Woodward JC, Becker HN, Poulos PW: Articular cartilage blood vessels in swine osteochondrosis. *Vet Pathol* 1987;24:118–123.

100
Osteochondrosis of the Metacarpophalangeal/Metatarsophalangeal Joint

John V. Yovich

Osteochondrosis of the metacarpophalangeal/metatarsophalangeal (fetlock) joint includes osteochondritis dissecans of the sagittal ridge and metacarpal/metatarsal condyles and subchondral cystic lesions of the proximal phalanx or the distal metacarpal/metatarsal condyles. The lesion initially described as osteochondritis dissecans of the palmar aspect of the distal third metacarpus is no longer considered a manifestation of osteochondrosis in horses. These palmar metacarpal lesions are considered to have a biomechanical basis. The initial lesion appears to be one of ischemia and necrosis of subchondral bone. Resorption of the necrotic subchondral bone occurs, but, if the horse continues in work, fracture and collapse of the subchondral bone can occur with depression of the overlying articular cartilage.

OSTEOCHONDRITIS DISSECANS OF THE SAGITTAL RIDGE OF THE THIRD METACARPAL AND METATARSAL BONES

Osteochondritis dissecans (OCD) of the sagittal ridge is usually diagnosed in horses less than 3 years old. Most affected horses are examined because of synovial effusion of one or more fetlock joints. Usually horses are lame, with lameness predominating in one limb. Occasionally horses are not lame or become lame only when athletic training is commenced. Passive flexion of affected fetlock joints often elicits a response indicative of pain and exacerbates lameness in that limb.

Synovial effusion of the fetlock and response to flexion tests are usually marked enough to indicate disease of the fetlock joint. Intrasynovial anesthesia of the fetlock or a palmar nerve block should relieve the lameness and help rule out other causes of lameness.

When OCD of the sagittal ridge is suspected or diagnosed, a radiographic examination of all four fetlock joints should be made. This is because lesions are usually present in two or more fetlock joints and the severity of radiographic changes observed is not always correlated with the amount of synovial effusion. Lateral and dorsopalmar radiographic projections are most useful. Bony lesions observed vary but are most prominent on the dorsal aspect of the sagittal ridge. Mild flattening to extensive subchondral bone deficits and irregularity of the sagittal ridge are also observed. Osteochondral fragments may be present close to the subchondral bone deficit in the sagittal ridge or away from the defect. The extent of radiographic changes does not necessarily correlate with the degree of lameness in the involved limbs.

Although larger follow-up studies are required to define optimal treatment in this disease, some general recommendations can be made. Young horses in which irregularity or flattening of the sagittal ridge is noted as an incidental finding should be treated conservatively (Fig. 100–1). These horses have a guarded to good prognosis for soundness. Follow-up radiography may reveal a decrease in the irregularity of the sagittal ridge. Arthroscopic surgery is recommended for fragment removal and lesion débridement in horses with bony fragments from the sagittal ridge (Fig. 100–2) and in horses without fragmentation if lameness is referable to the fetlock. Sometimes, a cartilaginous flap may be evident at arthroscopy, whereas only flattening of the sagittal ridge was present on the radiographs. If the lesions are not extensive, a favorable prognosis can be given. In some cases dissecting lesions of the articular cartilage may be observed at surgery extending from either side of the sagittal ridge onto the dorsal aspect of the metacarpal/metatarsal condyle. If this change is ex-

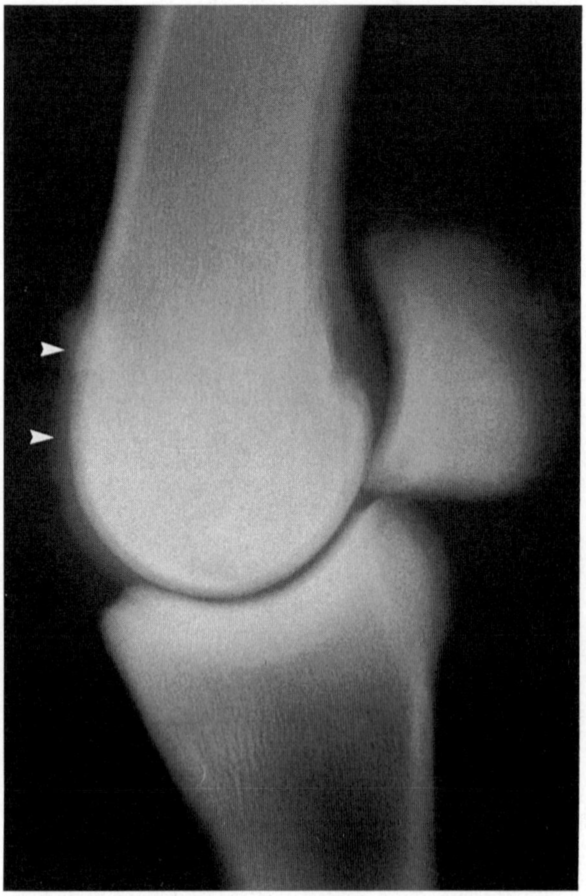

Figure 100–1. Lateromedial radiographic projection of the left hind fetlock of a 2-year-old Quarter Horse filly. Osteochondrosis of the sagittal ridge of the distal metatarsus is present. Note the irregularity of the subchondral bone of the dorsal aspect of the sagittal ridge (*arrows*). (Courtesy of Dr. C. W. McIlwraith.)

tensive, a more guarded prognosis should be given. It is possible to operate all four fetlock joints at one surgery by arthroscopy. Operative technique and postsurgical care are similar to that for osteochondral fractures of the fetlock. With more extensive lesions, a longer postsurgical rest period of approximately 6 months is desirable.

OSTEOCHONDRITIS DISSECANS OF THE THIRD METACARPAL AND METATARSAL CONDYLES

Osteochondritis dissecans of the third metacarpal or metatarsal condyles is an uncommon lesion. This lesion is distinct from OCD lesions of the sagittal ridge and adjacent condyles in that it affects the distal third metacarpal or metatarsal condyles at the distal medial or lateral aspect of the articular surface of the condyle (Fig. 100–3). It is a typical dissecting lesion with flaps of cartilage and attached bone (Fig. 100–4). Affected horses present at a young age with lameness and synovial effusion of the fetlock. On radiographs, irregularity of the subchondral bone is seen, with or without visualization of a dissecting flap depending on the presence of bone in the flap. These lesions are difficult to visualize and remove by any surgical approach. Unless the lesion is small and healing occurs with rest, the prognosis is guarded to poor for soundness. Young horses have been successfully treated by curretage.

Severe lesions of OCD involving the metacarpophalangeal and metatarsophalangeal condyles and the

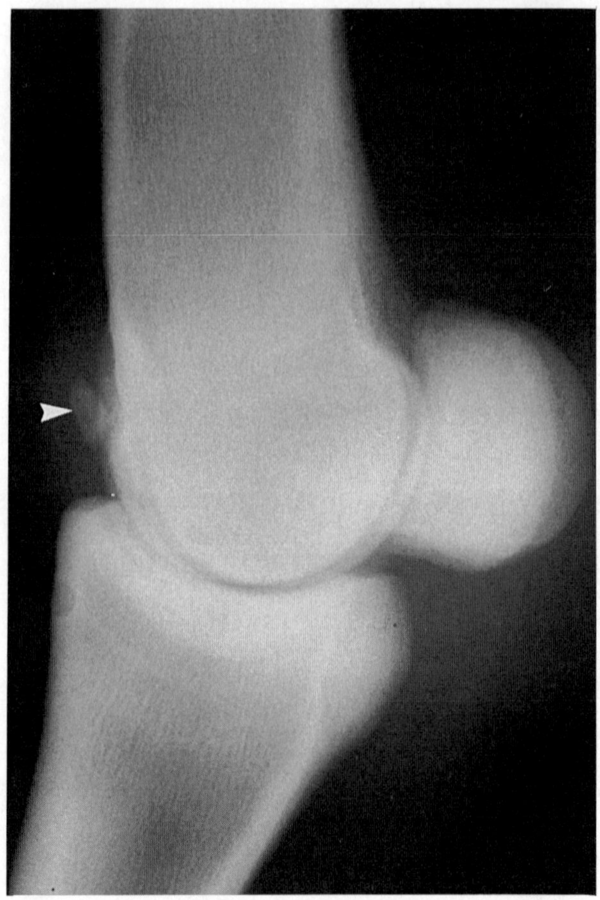

Figure 100–2. Lateromedial radiographic projection of the right front fetlock of a 2-year-old Quarter Horse filly. Osteochondritis dissecans of the sagittal ridge of the distal metacarpus is present. Note the fragment (*arrow*) adjacent to an irregular defect in the subchondral bone.

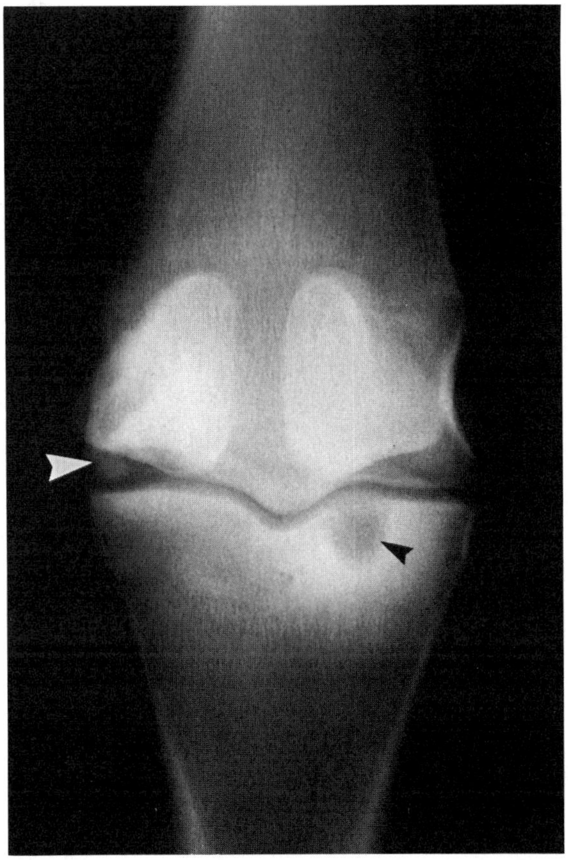

Figure 100–3. Dorsopalmar radiographic projection of the left front fetlock of a yearling Thoroughbred colt. Note the osteochondritis dissecans lesion of the third metacarpal condyle (*white arrow*) and the subchondral cystic lesions of the proximal phalanx (*black arrow*).

proximal surface of the proximal phalanx have been reported as part of a generalized osteochondrosis associated with zinc toxicity or copper deficiency in foals. These generalized lesions are not amenable to treatment.

SUBCHONDRAL CYSTIC LESIONS OF THE FETLOCK JOINT

Subchondral cystic lesions adjacent the fetlock joint are most commonly located in the distal third metacarpal/metatarsal condyle or in the proximal portion of the proximal phalanx (Fig. 100–3). These lesions can occur individually or occur in fetlock joints that also have OCD lesions of the distal metacarpal/metatarsal condyles.

Horses with subchondral cystic lesions of the fetlock joint can become lame as weanlings or yearlings, or not show clinical signs until beginning athletic training. Often there is little synovial effusion to indicate involvement of the fetlock joint. Response to fetlock manipulation is variable, and nerve blocks will be required to localize the problem to the fetlock. Intraarticular anesthesia will not consistently alleviate lameness with subchondral cystic lesions, but a regional palmar nerve block should result in significant improvement.

Subchondral cystic lesions are best seen on lateral-to-medial and dorsal-to-palmar/plantar radiographic projections. Subchondral cysts of the fetlock joint are usually solitary and about 5 to 15 mm in diameter. Cysts have a sclerotic bone margin and a radiolucent center. A small communication with the joint space may or may not be apparent on radiographs.

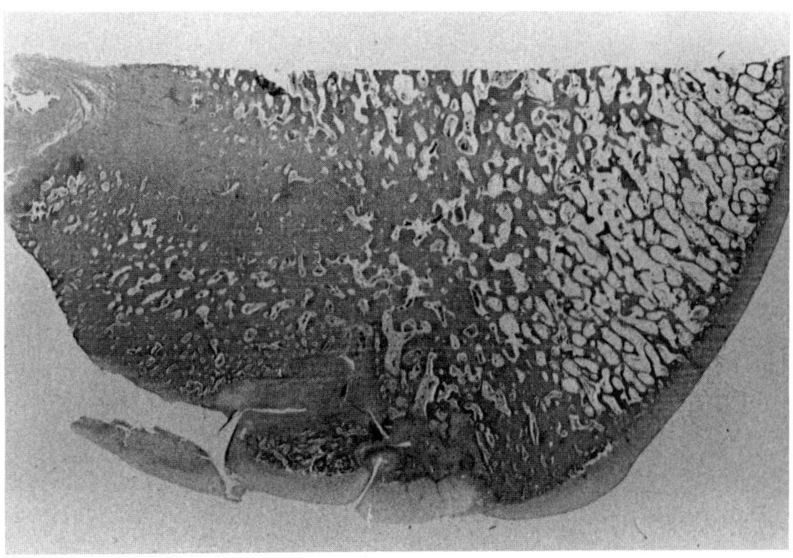

Figure 100–4. Histologic section of the osteochondritis dissecans lesion of the distal third metacarpal bone illustrated radiographically in Figure 100–3. Note the irregular flap of articular cartilage and bone and the surrounding increase in subchondral bone density.

Horses that present with lameness referable to subchondral cystic lesions of the fetlock joint usually have a poor prognosis for soundness with conservative therapy. Filling in of the cyst with bone has been reported to occur over 1 to 2 years. Unfortunately, a series of cases with sufficient follow-up information to allow an accurate prediction to be made is unavailable. Some horses may be sound and a subchondral cyst is noted as an incidental finding. These horses will probably remain sound.

Surgical therapy for subchondral cysts of the fetlock has been performed. Subchondral cysts of the distal metacarpus/metatarsus can be approached by a dorsal arthrotomy of the fetlock. A periarticular approach is used to reach subchondral cysts of the proximal phalanx. The lesions are drilled or curetted and can be packed with cancellous bone. Long-term follow-up is required before the success of surgical treatment is known. Since evidence of concurrent degenerative joint disease is usually minimal in this condition, surgical treatment is worthy of further investigation.

BIBLIOGRAPHY

Hornof WJ, O'Brien TR, Pool RR: Osteochondritis dissecans of the distal metacarpus in the adult racing Thoroughbred horse. *Vet Radiol* 1981;22:98–106.

McIlwraith CW: Osteochondrosis, in Stashak TS (ed): *Adams' Lameness in Horses,* ed 4. Philadelphia, Lea & Febiger, 1987, pp 396–419.

Petterson H, Reiland S: Periarticular subchondral "bone cysts" in horses. *Clin Orthop* 1969;62:95–103.

Yovich JV, McIlwraith CW, Stashak TS: Osteochondritis dissecans of the sagittal ridge of the third metacarpal and metatarsal bones in horses. *J Am Vet Med Assoc* 1985;186:1186–1191.

101 Osteochondrosis of the Shoulder and Elbow

Alan J. Nixon

OSTEOCHONDROSIS OF THE SHOULDER

Diagnosis

Osteochondrosis occurs in the shoulder joint of horses with less frequency than at other sites such as the hock and stifle. Nevertheless, several case studies are reported in the literature, including one retrospective analysis of 38 horses. Osteochondrosis of the shoulder joint usually occurs in young (6- to 12-month-old) horses, but has been reported in horses as old as 3 years. Males are more commonly affected than females. No specific breed predilection has been identified; however, the literature contains a preponderance of affected Quarter Horses and Thoroughbreds. The incidence has also been suggested to be related to body size and rate of skeletal growth, but many affected animals appear normal for breed and age and some even appear smaller and lighter in condition than expected.

Clinical signs of osteochondrosis are often quite insidious but can have a relatively sudden onset. A delay in presentation commonly occurs because of the poorly localized symptoms. At the time of examination, moderate supraspinatus and infraspinatus muscle atrophy has usually developed, the horse is frequently grade 2 to 4 lame (on a scale of 1 to 5) and there is a decreased cranial phase to the stride, with a low foot flight arc. Bilaterally affected animals tend to show a stiff shuffling gait but are generally more obviously lame on one foreleg. Horses with severe disease have a tendency to keep the shoulder joint fixed and partly flexed and extend the forelimb by scapular rotation. This results in a shortened cranial phase to the stride and a tendency to stumble. The stiff gait results in excessive wearing of the toe of the affected foot, and lameness for an extended period of time results in foot contraction.

Manipulative tests of the shoulder are frequently positive. Many horses exhibit a painful response to direct digital pressure cranial or caudal to the infraspinatus tendon directly over the shoulder joint. Joint capsule and periarticular swelling is palpable in only the most severe cases. A painful withdrawal response can often be elicited by extending the limb cranially, which tenses the caudal joint capsule. Additionally, flexion and abduction occasionally result in a painful response, especially in severely affected horses. No manipulative tests are totally specific for the shoulder joint, and in some animals the diagnosis can only be made by systematic regional perineural anesthesia to rule out lower limb lameness and finally intraarticular anesthesia of the shoulder. The diagnosis is then confirmed by radiography. Consistent injection of the shoulder joint requires practice. An 18-gauge 7.5-cm spinal needle is inserted 1 cm cranial to the infraspinatus tendon and 1 cm dorsal to the greater tubercle of the humerus, and directed in a horizontal plane closely following the contour of the proximal humerus to penetrate the cranial cul-de-sac of the shoulder joint. Injection of 12 to 15 mL of local anesthetic usually results in decreased lameness: the response can be quite marked in some horses.

Definitive diagnosis requires radiography of the shoulder. While sufficient detail to make the diagnosis can usually be obtained by radiography in the standing animal, subtle lesions and an accurate assessment of the extent of the lesion will require radiography with the horse anesthetized. The incidence of the various radiographic features of osteochondrosis of the shoulder have been described by Nyack et al. Alterations in the contour of the humeral head and glenoid cavity are the classic changes associated with osteochondritis dissecans (OCD). The majority of cases have involvement of both the humerus and scapula. Secondary changes such as osteosclerosis surrounding the subchondral bone lysis and osteophytes on the cranial and caudal aspects of the glenoid cavity are frequently seen (Fig. 101–1). Osteochondritis dissecans of the horse's shoulder is characterized by the rapid development of degenerative joint disease (DJD), especially when compared to OCD of the hock and stifle. Osteophytes occasionally occur on the caudal humeral head, especially as the disease progresses to advanced DJD. Intraarticular free bodies are a rare feature in the shoulder, but do arise and settle in the voluminous cranial or caudal cul-de-sacs of the joint.

Subchondral cystic lesions are another manifestation of osteochondrosis in horses. Cystic lesions can occur concurrently with OCD lesions in the same shoulder but are more often singular entities. Subchondral cysts

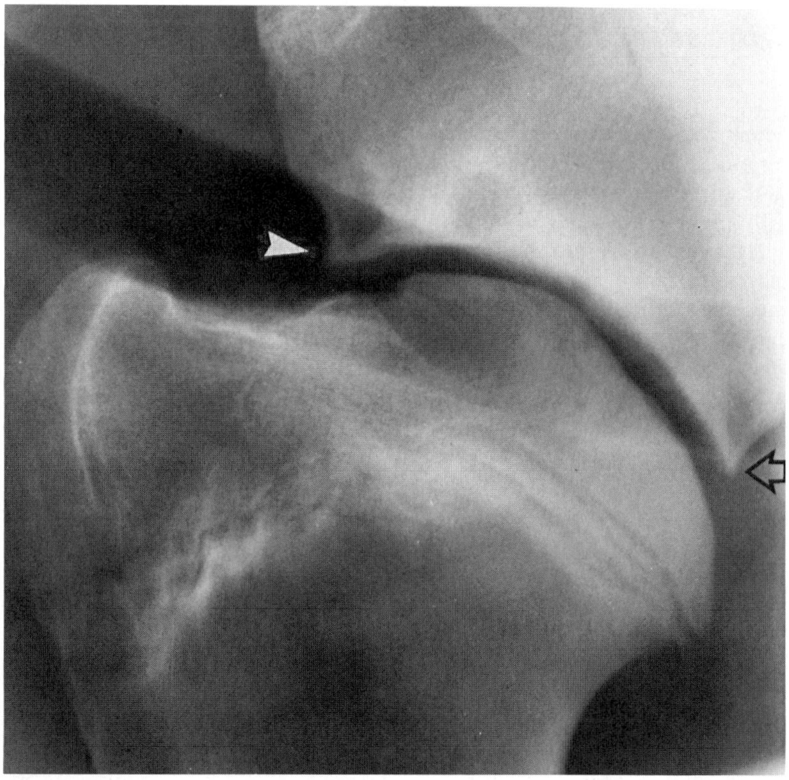

Figure 101–1. Plain radiograph of a horse with OCD of the shoulder. Subchondral lysis of the humeral head and glenoid cavity are prominent. A subchondral cystic defect is also present in the cranial half of the glenoid cavity. Osteophytes on the cranial and caudal aspects of the glenoid cavity (*arrows*) indicate early degenerative joint disease.

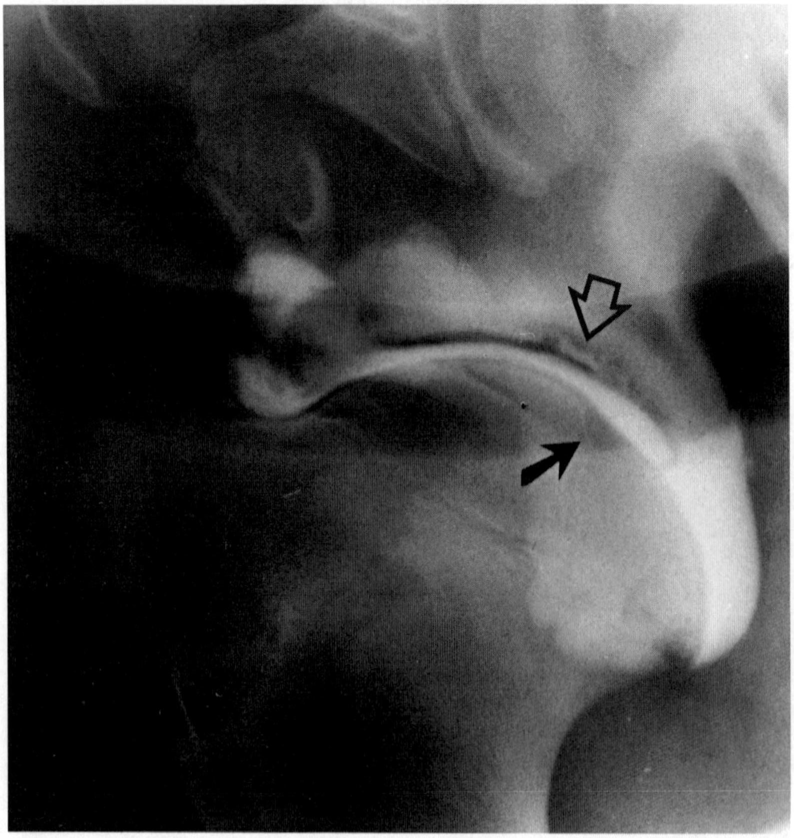

Figure 101–2. Arthrogram of a shoulder joint with an extensively underrun OCD cartilage flap on the glenoid cavity (*open arrow*) and a localized area of cartilage thickening on the humeral head (*arrow*). Surgical débridement of the glenoid lesion is indicated.

occur in the glenoid cavity of the scapula and are quite rare in the humeral head. These lesions are associated with intermittent lameness, and the lameness is more difficult to eliminate by intraarticular anesthesia.

Arthrography is recommended if surgery is contemplated. Contrast delineation allows an accurate assessment of cartilage flap attachments and cyst communication with the joint, thereby providing a more accurate assessment of the need for surgery (Fig. 101–2). Seven to 10 mL of a water-soluble iodinated contrast agent (60%) is sufficient for shoulder arthrography. Enhanced detail can be achieved by adding 30 to 40 mL of air to perform double-contrast arthrography. Smaller areas of subchondral lucency may not represent dissecting cartilage flaps and surgery is not indicated. This is especially important when assessing bilateral lesions, where surgery on both shoulders would result in lengthy operating times.

Synovial fluid analysis is frequently performed but is not specific for OCD of the joint. In most cases an excessive volume of fluid is present with a slightly elevated protein level, and the white blood cell count can be elevated to 1,500 cells/mm^3.

Surgical Treatment

An important feature of shoulder OCD in the horse is the rapid development of secondary DJD. This results in a relatively poor prognosis except in the most mildly affected cases. In a large series of conservatively managed horses with OCD of the shoulder none were able to perform athletically. Another review of 17 cases revealed ten had to be euthanized as a result of substantial and progressive lameness.

Surgical therapy has been reported on 20 cases and there is unpublished data on an additional 13 horses treated by arthrotomy or arthroscopy. Twenty-six of these animals became sound at pasture and 17 of these were known to perform in athletic activities, most commonly racing. Seemingly the prognosis is substantially improved by surgery.

Arthrotomy. Four arthrotomy approaches to the equine shoulder joint appear in the literature. The invasiveness of each varies according to the structures severed in the approach. The muscle-separating techniques appear the least complicated and provide adequate exposure to the lesions.

The integrity of the shoulder joint is largely due to the surrounding tendons. The supraspinatus and infraspinatus tendons of insertion provide major lateral stability, while the biceps and subscapularis tendons and the glenohumeral ligament provide cranial and medial stability. The shoulder joint capsule is extensive and is considerably thickened medially, providing added strength. Most osteochondrosis lesions involve the mid- and caudal portion of the humeral head and glenoid cavity. These areas are readily accessible via a muscle-separating approach in which the infraspinatus muscle is retracted craniad and the deltoideus and teres minor muscles are retracted caudad.

All surgical approaches use lateral recumbency with the affected limb uppermost. After aseptic preparation and draping, a 15-cm curved skin incision is made, centered on the joint and progressing 2.5 cm caudal to the spine of the scapula and infraspinatus tendon of insertion (Fig. 101–3). The brachiocephalicus muscle is exposed and retracted cranially, revealing the deltoideus and infraspinatus muscles. The aponeurotic origin of the deltoideus on the infraspinatus muscle belly is identified and severed, allowing caudal retraction of the deltoid muscle. The exposed teres minor muscle is partially severed at its insertion and retracted caudally, revealing the lateral joint capsule of the shoulder. The joint capsule is opened parallel to the curvature of the glenoid cavity and the joint is explored. Access to the lesion is simple in severe cases because of the remodeling of the humeral head; however, in early and less severely affected cases considerable distraction and abduction are required. Osteochondritis dissecans flaps are readily removed with alligator rongeurs and the subchondral bone curetted to remove fibrosis and expose normal bone. Cystic lesions are more difficult to adequately débride, generally requiring maximal distraction of the joint surfaces and the use of curved rongeurs and curettes. After thorough inspection of the joint for loose fragments, copious saline lavage is used to remove debris and the joint capsule is securely sutured with 2-0 synthetic absorbable suture material. The teres minor insertion, deltoid origin, and brachiocephalicus muscles are reapposed with size 1 synthetic absorbable suture and the subcutaneous tissues closed routinely. The skin can be closed with nonabsorbable suture or stainless steel staples. A stent bandage is sutured over the wound to provide protection. Stall rest for 4 weeks with small amounts of daily walking exercise are routinely recommended. Most horses should not have strenuous activity for 6 months, and there should be a gradual increase in exercise during this recuperative period.

The disadvantages of arthrotomy approaches are the poor access to the caudomedial aspects of the joint, total lack of access to the cranial areas of the joint, severe distraction necessary for adequate débridement of lesions, and the discomfort and cosmetic disfigurement of a large incision.

Arthroscopic Surgery. Two different arthroscopic approaches to the shoulder are reported. Both provide improved access to all areas of the shoulder joint, particularly the cranial portions, without significant dissection, postoperative pain, or cosmetic disfigurement. With a little experience, the débridement of extensive humeral lesions and deep glenoid cystic cavities is more thoroughly accomplished in less time than by arthrotomy.

Arthroscopic techniques differ only in the placement of the arthroscope entry portal either cranial or caudal to the infraspinatus tendon of insertion. For most lesions an insertion caudal to the infraspinatus tendon facilitates complete examination of the joint and lesion curettage. Surgical positioning and preparation are as for arthrotomy. Two 5-mm stab incisions are made, one placed 1 cm cranial to the infraspinatus tendon and a second made 1 to 2 cm caudal to the infraspinatus tendon (Fig. 101–4). An 18-gauge 7.5-cm spinal needle is used to distend the shoulder with 60 mL of lactated Ringer's solution, and the arthroscope sleeve with sharp trocar is inserted directly toward the joint through the caudal skin incision. When the joint surfaces are approximated, the trocar is replaced with an obturator and the arthroscope sleeve is positioned in the lateral joint pouch. The blunt obturator is replaced by the arthroscope and the ingress fluid line and light cable are attached. For most areas a 25-degree oblique forward-viewing 4-mm arthroscope is adequate. A 70-degree arthroscope is helpful to fully examine the caudomedial surfaces of the humeral head and glenoid cavity. If available, a videocamera is attached for remote viewing. Joint distention is maintained by constant infusion of chilled lactated Ringer's solution. An egress cannula is inserted through the cranial stab incision and enters the cranial cul-de-sac of the joint. Examination of the cranial, lateral, medial, and caudolateral aspects of the shoulder joint is readily accomplished by distraction of the joint surfaces to allow the arthroscope to penetrate to the depths of the joint space. Traction on the limb is usually sufficient to distract the joint in horses with OCD. In horses with mild lesions, and especially mature, well-muscled animals, a curved forceps must be placed in the cranial portion of the joint to separate the humeral and glenoid surfaces and allow safe movement of the arthroscope. The forceps enters the joint through the incision cranial to the infraspinatus tendon after removing the egress cannula (Fig. 101–4). A 70-degree arthroscope is

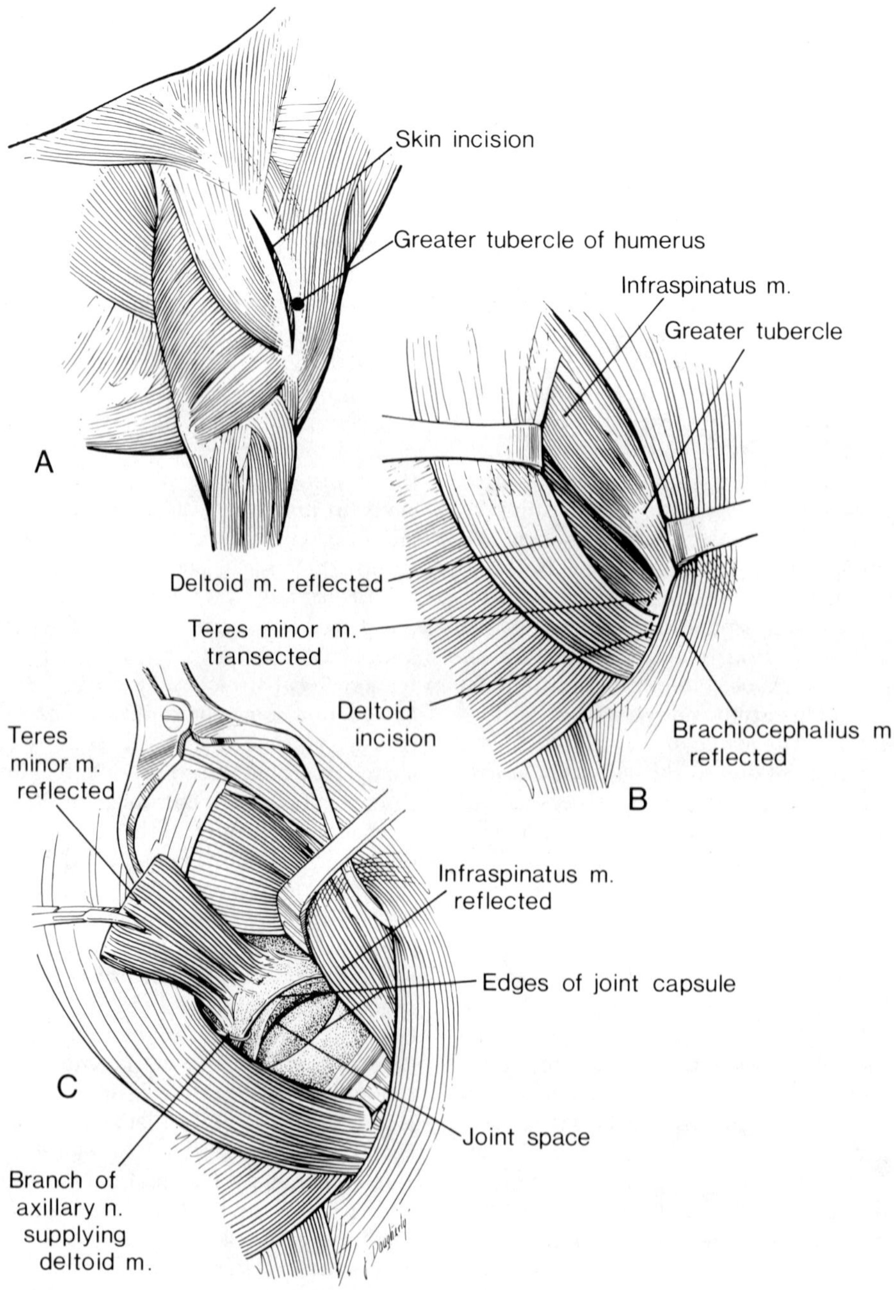

Figure 101–3. A muscle-separating approach to the shoulder joint **(A)** with the infraspinatus tendon retracted craniad and the deltoideus retracted caudad **(B).** The teres muscles are retracted or severed to gain exposure **(C).** (From Nixon AJ, Stashak TS, McIlwraith CW, Aanes WA, Martin GS: A muscle separating approach to the equine shoulder joint for the treatment of osteochondritis dissecans. *Vet Surg* 1984;13:247–256. Reprinted with permission of JB Lippincott Publishing Co.)

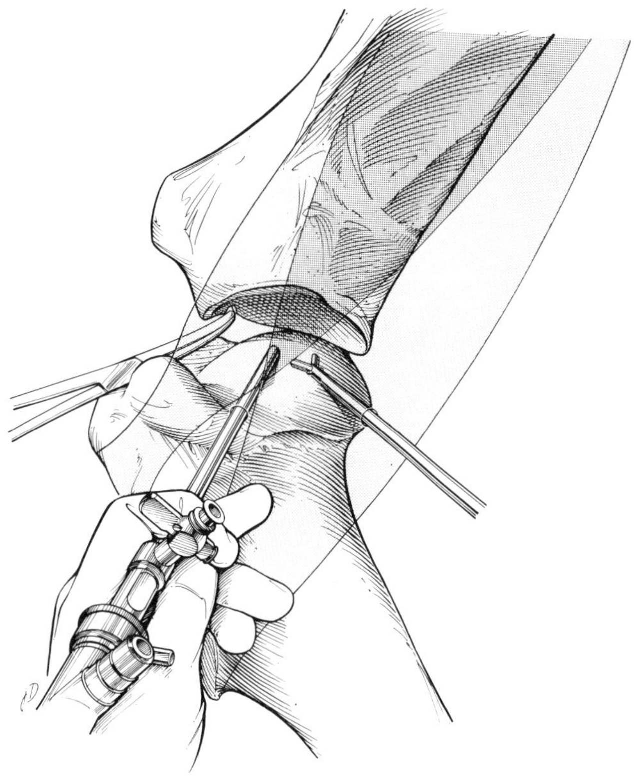

Figure 101–4. Arthroscopic technique used for exploration and surgical débridement of osteochondrosis lesions of the equine shoulder joint. The arthroscope is placed just caudal to the infraspinatus tendon. (From Nixon AJ: Diagnostic and surgical arthroscopy of the equine shoulder joint. *Vet Surg* 1987;16:44–52. Reprinted with permission of JB Lippincott Publishing Co.)

often necessary to adequately evaluate the caudomedial humeral head and glenoid cavity and directly view deep subchondral cystic lesions of the glenoid cavity (Fig. 101–5).

A third 5-mm stab incision 2 to 4 cm caudal to the arthroscope entry portal is used for entry of instruments used to débride OCD lesions by triangulation. Most OCD cartilage flaps of the humeral head and glenoid cavity are readily removed with hand instruments such as rongeurs and curettes. Motorized abraders expedite smoothing of the cartilage edges and subchondral bone, but are not essential. Deeper glenoid lesions, especially subchondral cystic defects, usually require angled rongeurs and frequently are difficult to completely débride. Forage of the sclerotic rim, as commonly performed in subchondral cystic lesions in the distal femur, is not possible with existing equipment.

Following débridement of the lesions, the joint is copiously flushed with lactated Ringer's solution, the excess fluid is expressed from the joint and subcutaneous tissues, and the instruments are removed. The skin incisions are closed with several single interrupted sutures using 2-0 monofilament nonabsorbable material. No bandage is necessary.

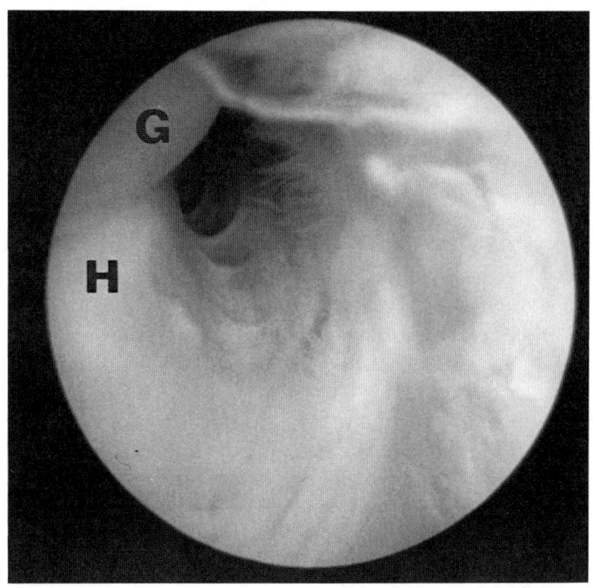

Figure 101–5. View of the caudomedial portions of the humeral head (*H*) and caudal glenoid rim (*G*) using a 70-degree oblique viewing arthroscope.

Postoperative Care

Most clinically affected horses recover from anesthesia without any appreciable increase in lameness; however, severely affected horses with extensive humeral and glenoid lesions can be quite lame postoperatively.

Phenylbutazone is usually administered at a daily dose of 4.4 to 6.6 mg/kg given by mouth in divided doses for 5 to 7 days. Antibiotics are generally not necessary. Polysulfated glycosaminoglycan (Adequan, 250 mg) or sodium hyaluronate (Hylartin V, 20 mg) is generally recommended for an initial intraarticular injection at the time of suture removal. Follow-up weekly injections of polysulfated glycosaminoglycan on four occasions or a second injection of 20 mg sodium hyaluronate 3 weeks after the first are also recommended.

Most horses can be rapidly returned to light exercise following shoulder arthroscopy. Several minutes' walking exercise is commenced 3 to 5 days after surgery. Tolerance range-of-motion exercises are initiated at the same time and the amount of physical therapy is gradually increased. All horses are confined to box stall conditions for 4 to 6 weeks after surgery. The horse may then be moved to a 0.5 to 1 acre pasture for an additional 4 weeks before increasing exercise at pasture. Most weanling- and yearling-age horses are given 4 to 6 months before any attempt is made to break and train the animal.

Follow-up radiographs are recommended at 3 and 6 months after surgery to assess remineralization of the subchondral bone, remodeling of the bone contour of the shoulder, and development of secondary DJD. Many horses have DJD at the time of diagnosis. Most moderately affected horses show minimal further progression of degenerative changes, particularly osteophyte development. Severely affected horses are difficult to salvage for athletic purposes and incapacitating DJD is often a sequel.

Prognosis

The prognosis for all but the mildest forms of OCD of the horse's shoulder is guarded. The shoulder joint is peculiar in its unique tendency for progressive cartilage degeneration and clefting. Degenerative joint disease is commonly present, even at the time of initial diagnosis, and this should be taken into account when deciding on the likelihood of a successful surgery. Two large case series in the literature both present a poor outlook for conservatively managed cases of shoulder OCD. Mildly affected animals can be managed by confinement of exercise and injection of sodium hyaluronate. Severely affected animals with extensive bony remodeling, persistent deep subchondral lysis of the humeral head and glenoid cavity, and advanced secondary DJD usually have a hopeless prognosis for soundness and many are sufficiently lame that elective destruction is warranted. A few can be salvaged by surgery for breeding purposes. Moderate to less severely affected cases generally comprise those selected for surgery with the possibility of return of functional soundness. A fair to good prognosis for athletic soundness exists for those horses with only mild cartilage thickening, not necessarily dissected free from the subchondral bone.

Subchondral cystic lesions of the glenoid cavity are generally considered to be another form of osteochondrosis in the horse. However, the prognosis for conservative therapy is better for these lesions than that cited for OCD lesions in similar areas of the shoulder. Cystic lesions of the glenoid cavity are best treated conservatively for 4 to 6 months. If lameness persists or increases during this time, surgery is warranted. If lameness diminishes, further time usually results in permanent soundness. Conservative therapy usually includes exercise restriction, lowered caloric and protein intakes, increased copper and zinc in the diet, and an injection of the affected joint with 20 mg sodium hyaluronate. If DJD is developing secondary to subchondral cystic lesions, surgical curettage of the cyst is indicated if permanent lameness is to be avoided.

Generally the selection of cases and success of surgery depends upon relatively early recognition of the problem, prompt evaluation (including arthrogram), and rapid surgical débridement of the lesion.

OSTEOCHONDROSIS OF THE ELBOW

Osteochondrosis of the horse's elbow joint is quite uncommon. In three case series involving subchondral cystic lesions in 153 horses, cysts were described at many locations but no mention was made of the distal humerus or proximal radius as possible sites. Two recent reports document subchondral cystic lesions in the elbows of 13 horses. Another three horses are described with OCD flap lesions of the distal humerus.

Diagnosis

Osteochondrosis of the elbow usually occurs in horses 1 to 3 years of age. Seven of the 13 affected animals described in the literature were females and eight of the 13 horses were Quarter Horses.

Clinical signs of elbow osteochondrosis are generally nonspecific. Onset of lameness is often acute, although most improve with time and many are intermittently lame and worsen only with exercise. Lameness is typically grade 2 to 3 and rarely grade 4 (on a scale of 1 to 5).

The affected limb is often normal in appearance, although minor muscle atrophy of the upper limb is common in chronic cases. Horses frequently are observed to straighten the leg with full extension of the carpus early in limb placement rather than as a continuous motion up to weight bearing. Several horses with elbow osteochondrosis were described as maintaining the elbow slightly rotated outward. An obvious tendency to reduce motion of the elbow results in signs similar to, although less marked than, those of a shoulder lameness.

Manipulative tests of the limb rarely result in a localizing response. Several horses described in the literature showed aversion to flexion and extension of the elbow. A flexion test of the elbow has also been positive in some cases, causing an increase in lameness.

Definitive diagnosis is usually made by intraarticular anesthesia of the elbow. Because of the poorly localized signs, most animals have had extensive perineural regional anesthesia and often intraarticular anesthesia of the shoulder before the elbow is finally suspected. The elbow can be injected on the caudolateral aspects, either caudal to the lateral collateral ligament, penetrating the joint between the proximal radius and ulna, or via the voluminous proximal caudal pouch on the lateral aspect between the olecranon process of the ulna and the lateral epicondyle of the humerus. Both techniques require an appreciation of topical anatomic landmarks. The elbow joint cavity is quite spacious and 15 to 20 mL of local anesthetic are required. The response to injection is variable, but most animals improve sufficiently to make a tentative diagnosis of elbow disease.

Confirmation of the type of elbow lesion requires radiography. Good-quality radiographs can be obtained in the standing horse. Five of six cases of osteochondrosis in one report, and four of seven in a second review, involved solitary subchondral bone cysts of the proximal medial aspect of the radius (Fig. 101–6). All other subchondral cysts were in the medial humeral condyle. A third report described OCD flaplike lesions of the lateral humeral condyle, and one other horse had an OCD cartilage flap lesion on the medial humeral condyle. Subchondral cystic lesions of the proximal-medial radius typically are circumscribed, well-defined bony lucencies with an osteosclerotic perimeter and a communicating canal to the elbow joint. The distal medial humeral condyle lesions were less defined, with wider communication with the elbow joint space (Fig. 101–7). OCD lesions have presented as extensive shallow subchondral defects in the contour of the humeral condyle. Secondary DJD is uncommon in cases involving subchondral cystic lesions, even at follow-up several years after the initial diagnosis. Signs of DJD include osteophyte formation on the cranial aspect of the radius, anconeal process of the ulna, and lateral and medial perimeter of the humerus.

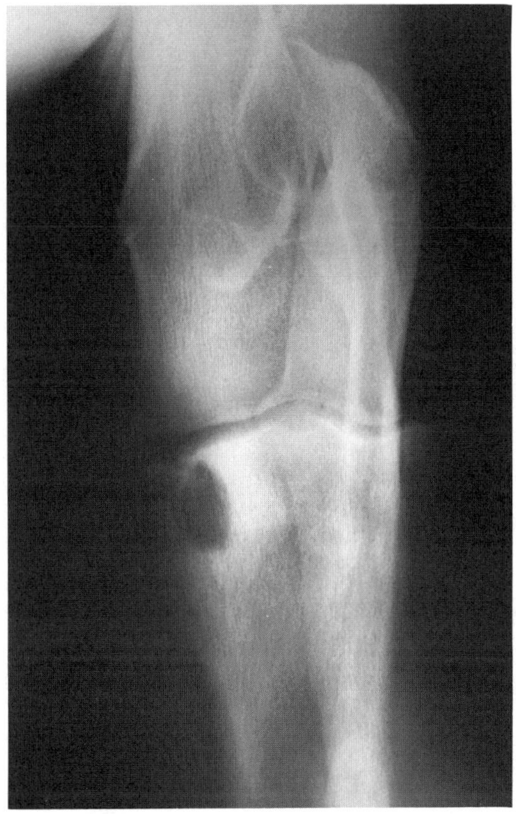

Figure 101–6. Osteochondrosis of the elbow joint. A subchondral cystic lesion of the proximal medial aspect of the radius is present, with an oblique communication with the elbow joint.

Synovial fluid analysis usually reveals increased quantities of fluid with moderately decreased viscosity, normal to slightly elevated white blood cell counts, and normal protein levels.

Treatment

The literature describes ten horses with subchondral cystic lesions of the elbow treated conservatively and three in which an extraarticular transcortical cyst curettage was performed. One report indicated poor results with conservative therapy, with the development of DJD and permanent lameness in three of six horses. Such poor results led to the development of a surgical approach to expose and curette the cyst contents of the latter three horses. A second retrospective analysis of seven horses treated by exercise restriction and injection of sodium hyaluronate or polysulfated glycosaminoglycan indicated five of these horses were sound and entered their intended activity. These ani-

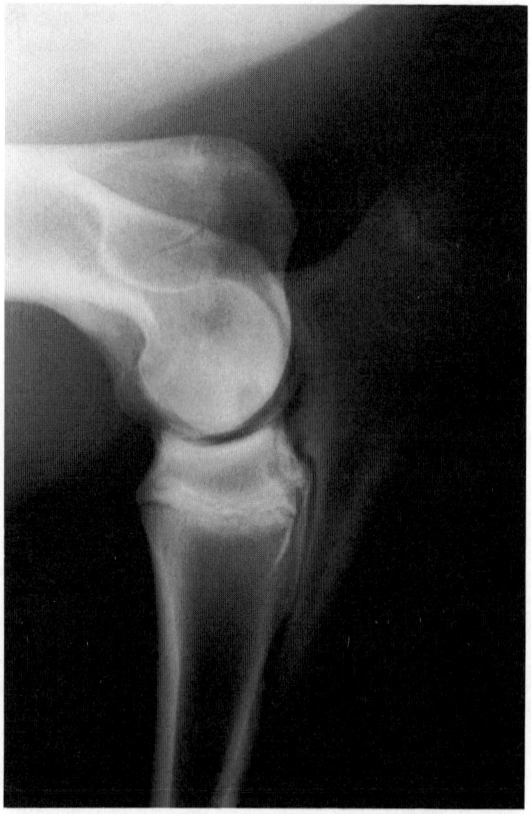

Figure 101–7. Osteochondrosis of the elbow joint. A subchondral cystic lesion is present in the distal articular portion of the medial humeral condyle. A wide communication with the elbow joint is evident.

mals included four horses with subchondral cystic lesions of the proximal radius as well as three with similar lesions of the medial humeral condyle. The two horses remaining lame were 2 and 3 years old at the time of diagnosis and had developed DJD secondary to a lesion in the proximal radius.

Guidelines for selection of animals for surgery are difficult to establish from these two somewhat conflicting reports. Some horses treated conservatively may have had markedly decreased periods of lameness if surgery had been performed. Nevertheless, surgical therapy is not always necessary, and it may be beneficial to reserve surgical curettage for horses in which 3 to 6 months of conservative treatment results in little or no improvement in lameness, or in which early signs of DJD, such as osteophytosis, narrowed joint space, or subchondral sclerosis, are developing. Clearly, an extended delay in surgery may result in irreversible damage to the joint. Repeat examination including radiography is indicated.

Surgical Technique

Two surgical approaches to lesions of the proximal medial radius and distal medial humerus are described.

Extraarticular Enucleation. The elbow joint is a complex, securely interdigitating system of bones, and distraction and exposure to gain access to subchondral cysts of the proximal radius is currently impossible. An extraarticular enucleation approach allowed adequate débridement of the cyst content in the proximal radius of three horses. One of these fractured the radius through the cyst during anesthetic recovery and was destroyed.

Horses are positioned in lateral recumbency with the affected limb down. The medial surface of the affected proximal radius and the adjacent pectoral region are prepared and draped for surgery. A 15-cm skin incision, centered over the radius and flexor carpi radialis muscle, is extended deeper through the muscle fibers of the transverse pectoral muscle. The median neurovascular bundle is identified cranially and preserved, while the flexor carpi radialis muscle is elevated and retracted caudally, exposing the medial radius. The joint space is identified with needles and an approximation of the cyst location is derived from preoperative radiographs. A pilot hole is drilled through the cortex of the radius directly over the expected location of the cyst and parallel to the joint surface. A mediolateral intraoperative radiograph is performed to confirm that the drill has penetrated the cyst cavity. After making corrections as necessary, a 6-mm window is created in the medial cortex of the radius with an osteotome. Curettage of the cyst content can then be accomplished with curettes and rongeurs. Drilling of the sclerotic cyst perimeter must be performed only on the lateral (deeper) portions of the cyst border since fracture of the radius along the path of a distally directed drill hole was described in the original report. The cyst cavity is lavaged to remove fibrous debris and then packed with a cancellous bone graft from the tuber coxa if desired. The benefits of bone grafting after forage are not established.

Closure of the fascia over the flexor carpi radialis and neurovascular structures is avoided since, speculatively, it may induce a compartmental neuropraxia. The pectoral muscle and subcutaneous tissues are closed with absorbable suture material placed in a continuous pattern and the skin is apposed with simple interrupted sutures of 2–0 nylon. A stent bandage is oversewn on the wound to protect it and minimize edema and seroma formation.

Postoperative care includes antibiotics for 2 to 3 days and nonsteroidal antiinflammatory agents for 2 weeks, followed by short but increasing controlled walks for 2 months. Follow-up radiography is recommended to ensure the cyst cavity is filling in before the animal is allowed more active exercise. The two surviving horses of the three animals surgically treated were lame for 1 to 2 months before surgery and were both sound by 2 months postoperatively. Nevertheless, at the final radiographic examination, 2- to 4-mm osteophytes were noted on the proximal aspect of the radius.

None of the horses described in the series of seven cases managed conservatively developed the decreased range of motion, severe osteophytosis, or marked pain on manipulation described in the three horses treated conservatively in the comparative surgery paper. This may reflect different conservative approaches or younger animals in the larger series, or may have been a chance outcome since the total numbers are relatively small.

Arthroscopic Surgery. An arthroscopic approach to the medial aspects of the elbow joint has been developed that provides an intraarticular approach for treatment of subchondral cystic lesions or OCD flaps of the humeral condyles. These lesions generally occur on the caudal portion of the humeral condyles, which are readily accessible to arthroscopic débridement. Patient positioning and preparation are similar to the extraarticular approach to the proximal medial radius. An 18-gauge 7.5-cm spinal needle is inserted into the elbow joint using the medial border of the humeral condyle and medial collateral ligaments as landmarks. The joint is distended with 60 to 80 mL of lactated Ringer's solution. A 5-mm stab incision is made 2 cm distal to the level of the medial humeral condyle, between the palpable muscle bellies of the flexor carpi radialis and flexor carpi ulnaris muscles. The arthroscope sleeve and sharp trocar are inserted and directed proximally until the joint capsule is entered. The sharp trocar is then replaced by the blunt obturator and the arthroscope sleeve is positioned in the caudal joint space of the elbow. The arthroscope is inserted and the light cable and fluid ingress lines are attached.

A complete examination of the caudomedial and caudoproximal areas of the elbow is possible. The voluminous caudoproximal cul-de-sac of the elbow joint enveloping the anconeal process of the ulna can be entered. As the arthroscope is withdrawn, the medial humeral condyle and medial surface of the semilunar notch are examined. Lesions of the medial humeral condyle are readily apparent. The lateral humeral condyle is not as well evaluated; however, lesions on the medial surface of this condyle are accessible for débridement. The proximal surface of the radius is not sufficiently visible for adequate lesion curettage. An instrument entry portal is selected by preplacing a 7.5-cm spinal needle through the skin 2 to 4 cm proximal and caudal to the arthroscope entry point. If the angle of approach to the medial or lateral humeral condyle is adequate, the needle is removed and the skin incised for 5 mm over the needle puncture. An egress cannula is initially inserted for removal of blood and debris, providing a clear view of the articular structures. The instrument entry portal penetrates the muscle belly of the flexor carpi ulnaris. It is important to avoid entering the joint caudal to this muscle belly and proximal to the level of the radiohumeral articulation since the ulnar neurovascular structures are directly vulnerable. Osteochondrosis lesions of the medial humeral condyle are most amenable to arthroscopic visualization and débridement. Further experience may allow lesions of other portions of the joint to be evaluated and treated.

Postoperative treatment following elbow arthroscopy includes phenylbutazone administration for 3 to 5 days and intraarticular injection of sodium hyaluronate or polysulfated glycosaminoglycan 2 to 3 weeks after surgery. Box stall confinement and exercise protocols are similar to those described for shoulder arthroscopy.

Prognosis

Insufficient numbers of horses with elbow osteochondrosis are documented to allow an accurate prognosis or definitive selection of the correct mode of therapy. Present guidelines include the need for surgical curettage of proximal radial or distal humeral subchondral cystic lesions if lameness is unchanged or more severe over a 3- to 6-month period or if serial radiographs document progressive development of DJD. The majority of young animals (less than 2 years) will improve significantly without surgical therapy. The prognosis for return to function of these cases is fair to good. Horses with OCD flap lesions of the humeral condyles carry a guarded prognosis because of progressive cartilage deterioration and development of DJD. Surgery is indicated in all but the mildest forms, and arthroscopic débridement by a medial approach is described for both medial and lateral condyle lesions.

With the low numbers of published cases of elbow osteochondrosis the prognosis described here can only be used as a guideline. Clearly the duration of symptoms and extent of DJD will affect the outcome of any surgical procedure and the attendant prognosis.

BIBLIOGRAPHY

Bertone AL, McIlwraith CW, Powers BE, Stashak TS, Aanes WA, Turner AS: Subchondral osseous cystic lesions of the elbow of horses: Conservative versus surgical treatment. *J Am Vet Med Assoc* 1986;189:540–546.

Bertone AL, McIlwraith CW, Powers BE, Trotter GW, Stashak TS: Arthroscopic surgery for the treatment of osteochondrosis in the equine shoulder joint. *Vet Surg* 1987;16:303–311.

DeBowes RM, Wagner PC, Grant BD: Surgical approach to the equine scapulohumeral joint through a longitudinal infraspinatus tenotomy. *Vet Surg* 1982;11:125–128.

Hopen LA, Turner TA, Colahan PT, Nixon AJ: Subchondral bone cysts in the elbow of horses: Conservative treatment of 7 cases. *J Am Vet Med Assoc* 1989; submitted.

Mason TA, MacLean AA: Osteochondrosis dissecans of the head of the humerus in two foals. *Equine Vet J* 1977;9:189–191.

Nixon AJ: Diagnostic and surgical arthroscopy of the equine shoulder joint. *Vet Surg* 1987;16:44–52.

Nixon AJ, Stashak TS, McIlwraith CW, Aanes WA, Martin GS: A muscle separating approach to the equine shoulder joint for the treatment of osteochondritis dissecans. *Vet Surg* 1984;13:247–256.

Nyack B, Morgan JP, Pool RR, Meagher DM: Osteochondrosis of the shoulder joint of the horse. *Cornell Vet* 1981;71:149–163.

Rose JA, Sande RD, Rose EM: Results of conservative management of osteochondrosis in the horse. *Proc Am Assoc Equine Pract* 1985; pp 617–626.

102 Osteochondrosis of the Tarsocrural Joint

Gayle W. Trotter

Osteochondrosis of the tarsocrural joint includes, in decreasing order of incidence, osteochondritis dissecans (OCD) of the distal intermediate ridge of the tibia, OCD of the lateral trochlear ridge of the talus, and a much lower incidence of OCD of the medial malleolus of the distal tibia and the medial trochlear ridge of the talus.

DIAGNOSIS

Affected horses are usually weanlings or yearlings that are presented because of tarsocrural joint distention (bog spavin). Lameness is uncommon in these horses. The condition is also seen in Standardbred racehorses in training, which may be presented for examination of gait asymmetry that is observed at faster speeds. Young Standardbred and Thoroughbred racehorses may also be presented for examination of bog spavin that appeared with commencement of training.

The most common radiographic lesion is a variably sized, triangular-shaped bony fragment off the distal intermediate ridge of the tibia (Fig. 102–1). Trochlear ridge lesions usually affect the distal aspect of the lateral trochlear ridge. Irregularity of the subchondral bony contour is seen and the presence of one or more mineralized fragments is common at this location (Fig. 102–2). It is uncommon to have a lesion of the talus in conjunction with a lesion of the distal intermediate ridge of the tibia. Medial malleolar lesions can be missed unless radiographs are examined carefully. Radiographically "silent" lesions (normal radiographs but a chondral lesion found at surgery) may also be present. Because lesions are often bilateral, radiographs of the contralateral joint should always be taken, even if current signs of clinical involvement are absent.

TREATMENT

Because lameness is rarely a prominent feature of tarsocrural joint OCD, conservative management has been advocated by some. A favorable outcome was reported in 45% of cases with tarsocrural joint OCD that were treated conservatively; however, it was not reported how many affected horses were racehorses and in what percentage of cases joint effusion resolved. Others recommend that if an athletic career is planned for the horse, surgical removal of fragments is indicated. This was based on retrospective findings of improved performance in racehorses that had OCD fragments surgically removed versus those managed conservatively. It was considered important to remove fragments prior to joint distention becoming well established, because the effusion was considered part of the performance-limiting problem. Where less de-

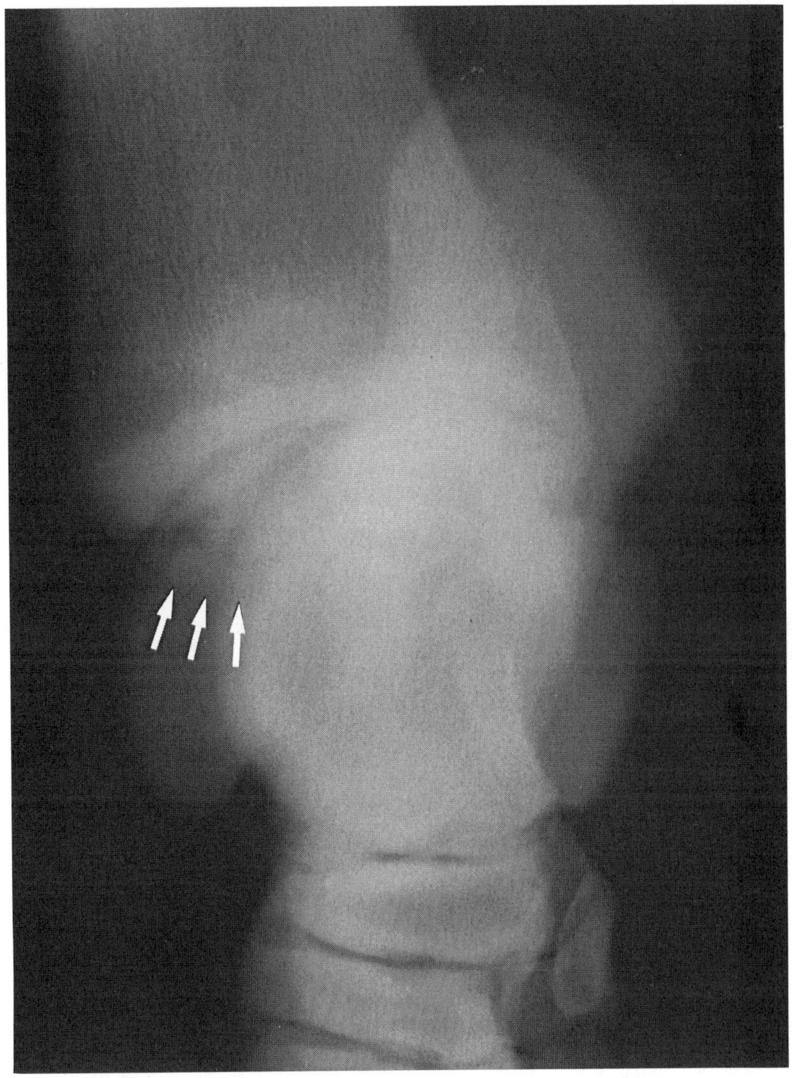

Figure 102–1. *Arrows* outline the distal aspect of an osteochondritis dissecans fragment from the distal intermediate ridge of the tibia.

manding activities are planned, conservative management may suffice.

Dorsolateral tarsocrural joint arthrotomy has been described for surgical treatment of distal intermediate ridge and lateral trochlear ridge OCD lesions. With the patient in either lateral or dorsal recumbency, a surgical approach is made between the long and lateral digital extensor tendons. The incision extends from the lateral malleolus to the middle extensor retinaculum over the tarsus. Good access to lesions at both sites is achieved. If a fragment is free within the joint, it may locate within the dorsomedial outpouching of the joint, requiring a second arthrotomy to retrieve the fragment.

Both intermediate ridge and trochlear ridge lesions are amenable to treatment by tarsocrural joint arthroscopy. A medial arthroscopic portal is used, the entry point being in the middle of the medial joint outpouching and just lateral to the cranial branch of the medial saphenous vein. A small skin incision should be used to allow sufficient visualization of the vein so as to avoid lacerating it during placement of the arthroscope. Fragment removal, and lesion débridement where necessary, are done using a dorsolateral instrument portal. For medial trochlear ridge and medial malleolar lesions, an arthrotomy over the medial outpouching of the joint provides access to the lesion. Both lesions are also amenable to arthroscopic surgery, with

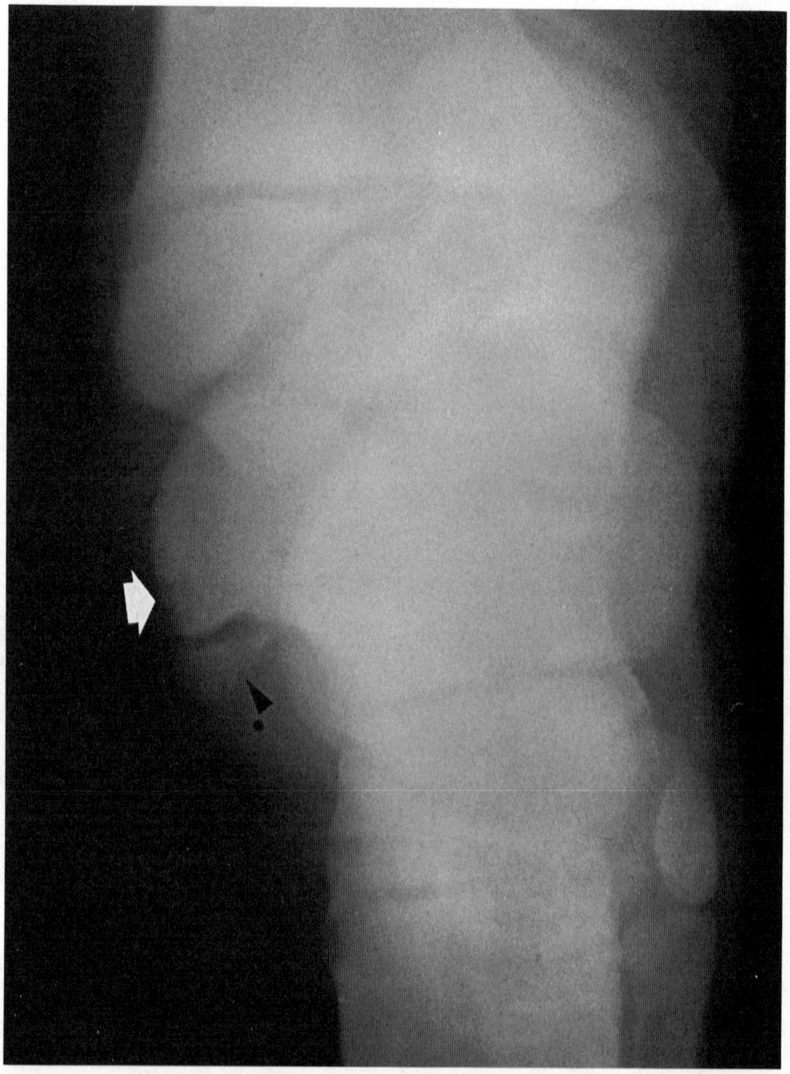

Figure 102–2. An osteochondritis dissecans fragment is seen at the distal aspect of the lateral trochlear ridge of the talus (*black arrow*). A mottled lucent appearance of the trochlear ridge adjacent the fragment is also present (*white arrow*).

the arthroscope and instrument portals both being located medially. Both distal intermediate ridge lesions and malleolar lesions have been diagnosed arthroscopically in horses having tarsocrural joint effusion but lacking radiographic abnormalities.

POSTOPERATIVE MANAGEMENT

With arthrotomy and arthroscopy, the limb is kept bandaged for 2 weeks, after which time controlled walking exercise is started. Exercise is steadily increased over the next 6 weeks. Vigorous training is not recommended for 2 to 4 months, depending on lesion location and extent of involvement.

PROGNOSIS

The prognosis is favorable for full athletic function for distal intermediate ridge lesions and medial malleolar lesions. The prognosis is also favorable for trochlear ridge lesions unless they are extensive. Resolution of joint distention occurs in most cases over 6 to 10 weeks, but resolution may be incomplete where chronic stretching of the joint capsule has occurred before surgery is done.

BIBLIOGRAPHY

Bramlage L: Results of treatment, in *Proceedings of the AQHA Developmental Orthopedic Disease Symposium.*

Dallas, American Quarter Horse Association, 1986, pp 47–48.

McIlwraith CW: Osteochondrosis, in Stashak TS (ed): *Adams' Lameness in Horses.* Philadelphia, Lea & Febiger, 1987, pp 396–419.

McIlwraith CW, Foerner JJ: Diagnostic and surgical arthroscopy of the tarsocrural joint, in *Diagnostic and Surgical Arthroscopy in the Horse.* Edwardsville, Kansas, Vet Med Publishing Company, 1984, pp 103–128.

Romberg B, Rejno S: Osteochondrosis in the horse. I. A clinical and radiologic investigation of osteochondritis dissecans of the knee and hock joint. *Acta Radiol Suppl* 1978; 358:139–152.

Rose JA, Sande RD, Rose EM: Results of conservative management of osteochondrosis in the horse. *Proc Am Assoc Equine Pract* 1985; pp 617–626.

103
Osteochondrosis of the Femoropatellar/Femorotibial Joint

Gayle W. Trotter

Osteochondrosis of the equine stifle includes osteochondritis dissecans (OCD) of the femoropatellar joint and subchondral cystic lesions of the femorotibial joint. In the femoropatellar joint, lesions predominantly involve the lateral trochlear ridge of the distal femur, with lesser involvement of the medial trochlear ridge and the patella. With subchondral cystic lesions, the medial femoral condyle is predominantly affected, with rare involvement of the lateral femoral condyle or the proximal tibial condyles. Both OCD and subchondral cystic lesions are considered to be developmental manifestations of osteochondrosis. However, relative to some recent work on the subchondral lesions, a traumatic etiology or trauma combined with OCD cannot be ruled out for this condition in some horses.

OSTEOCHONDRITIS DISSECANS

Diagnosis

Affected animals are usually presented at 2 years of age or younger, and the most common presenting complaint is distention of the femoropatellar joint. Lameness may be absent at the time joint distention first appears, but most commonly mild lameness is also present. Lameness can be severe in some cases, with some bilaterally affected animals having difficulty rising. In other cases, no overt lameness is seen but the horse has an awkward way of going, with outward rotation of the stifles and prominent-appearing patellae. With severe lateral trochlear ridge involvement, lateral luxation of the patella may occur. Bilateral stifle involvement occurs in approximately 50% of cases.

When lameness is present, it can usually be exacerbated by a hind limb flexion test. Improvement following intraarticular anesthesia is variable. Synovial fluid may have a slight increase in total nucleated cell count, most of which are mononuclear cells. Careful digital palpation between the middle and lateral patellar ligaments may permit identification of some lateral trochlear ridge defects.

The most common radiographic finding is irregularity of subchondral bone contour of the affected trochlear ridge (Fig. 103–1). Mineralized fragments may be present within the trochlear ridge defect or they may be present as detached joint mice. Fragments are more commonly seen in older animals, rather than those 1 year of age or younger. Patellar OCD lesions are reportedly most common at the distal aspect of the patella. Articular defects elsewhere on the patella are usually secondary to trochlear ridge OCD. Remodeling changes and periarticular osteophytes affecting the patella are also occasionally seen. Although contrast arthrography can be used to help delineate undermined flaps of cartilage, it is less valuable than exploring the joint using the arthroscope. Certainly, cartilage defects and free-floating cartilage can be identified at surgery that are not visible on radiographs and that contrast arthrography will not delineate.

Treatment

Both conservative and surgical treatments of femoropatellar joint OCD have been described. Success with

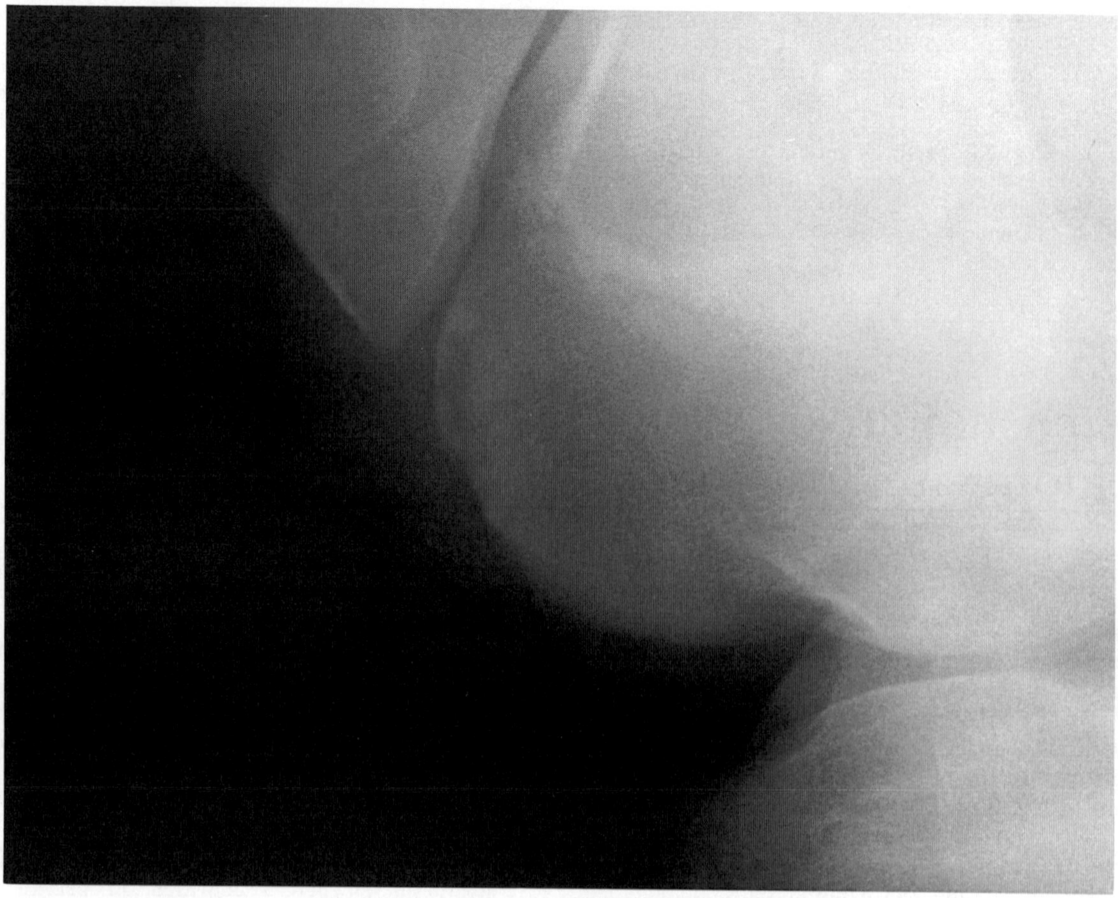

Figure 103–1. An irregular subchondral bone contour is present over an extensive portion of the lateral trochlear ridge. An undermined flap is present at the most proximal aspect of the lesion.

conservative management was reported in approximately 50% of cases with any type of stifle osteochondrosis. However, the degree of clinical and radiographic involvement of affected cases was not reported. Surgical treatment is considered to be indicated in all cases in which lameness and/or mineralized bodies are present. If only mild joint distention and a small subchondral bone irregularity or flattening is seen on radiographs, conservative management may be successful. Conversely, if lameness and joint distention are prominent and extensive articular involvement is seen radiographically, any treatment, including surgery, is unlikely to be beneficial.

Techniques for surgical arthrotomy and lesion débridement of the femoropatellar joint have been described, but arthroscopy has proven to be more useful in evaluation and treatment of affected joints. Arthroscopy also eliminates the problems of seroma formation and incisional dehiscence that accompanied some arthrotomies of the stifle joint. Generally, patients are positioned in dorsal recumbency and the arthroscope is inserted midway between the apex of the patella and the tibial tuberosity and between the lateral and middle patellar ligaments. Depending on lesion location, instrument portals are placed as indicated. A long needle is useful in identifying the optimal instrument portal location. A probe should be used to localize and delineate areas of cartilage that are detached from subchondral bone. Free fragments are grasped and removed, loose fragments in situ are elevated and removed, and abnormal subchondral bone is débrided until bleeding is encountered. A motorized arthroplasty burr is useful in completing lesion débridement.

Postoperative Care

Phenylbutazone is recommended for the perioperative period (2 to 3 days) and the patient is confined to a box stall. Controlled walking is usually started at 2 weeks, and this form of exercise is increased over the next 6 weeks. Access to a larger area can begin 8 weeks after surgery, and, if the animal is of training age, training can begin 3 to 4 months after surgery. The duration of rest after surgery is largely predicated on the severity of the lesion.

Prognosis

Generally, a favorable prognosis for athletic usefulness may be given. Severely affected horses will not be expected to benefit from surgery, but of cases deemed reasonable surgical candidates, 75 to 80% of the horses seem capable of full athletic use. A less favorable prognosis exists if both medial and lateral trochlear ridges are involved, or if degenerative or remodeling changes are present on the patella. Decrease in joint effusion and improvement in lameness reportedly occur early in the postoperative period.

In a limited number of cases in which evaluation of healing of the lesion sites has been possible, fibrous tissue and fibrocartilage have filled the defects. The long-term fate of this reparative tissue is unknown, but in one reported case intact fibrocartilage was present 14 months after surgery. With more focal lesions in younger animals, the radiographic defect may become smaller or even disappear in some cases. More typically, the subchondral bone irregularity on radiographs persists or becomes worse despite dramatic improvement in, or disappearance of, clinical signs.

SUBCHONDRAL CYSTIC LESIONS

Diagnosis

Affected horses are usually 2 years of age or younger and they are presented for examination because of lameness. Some horses are much older before clinical signs of lameness appear. Generally, age at presentation for subchondral cystic lesions is older than for OCD. In younger horses, lameness is usually mild to moderate and either is of sudden onset or becomes apparent at the start of breaking or training. With older horses, mild lameness that is exacerbated by exercise is more common. In this latter group, lameness improves with rest but recurs when heavy work is started. Other less common clinical presentations for horses with subchondral cystic lesions are severe lameness of acute onset or a stiff hind limb action with a shortened anterior phase of the stride.

Usually, specific clinical signs that localize the lameness to the stifle joint are not present. In some cases, femorotibial effusion is palpable, or increased sensitivity to pressure over the medial collateral ligament is present. Hind limb flexion is usually not resisted, and exacerbation of lameness after flexion is quite variable. Although one report states that lameness is always eliminated after intraarticular anesthesia, response to intraarticular anesthesia may be variable. Localization of lameness is based on the presence of specific signs, or by eliminating sources of lameness elsewhere in the limb. Bilateral involvement is seen in approximately 25 to 30% of cases.

The radiographic appearance of the subchondral cystic lesion is that of a circumscribed subchondral lucency with a sclerotic rim (Fig. 103–2). This lucent area is best seen on a caudocranial radiographic projection and it is located in the middle of the femoral condyle. Most lesions open onto the joint surface, either through a wide area of contact or through a narrow channel. Another common radiographic appearance is that of either a flattened or a slightly dome-shaped subchondral bone contour. Rarely, subchondral cystic lesions are seen in the tibial condyles or adjacent to the intercondylar fossa region of the distal femur.

Treatment

Both conservative and surgical treatments have been recommended for treatment of subchondral cystic lesions of the medial femoral condyle. Results of studies in which case follow-up is reported confirm clinical improvement with rest or modified exercise regimens in some cases. In one report, 16 of 25 horses became sound between 4 months and 1 year after diagnosis. Horses 3 years of age or younger with a relatively small lesion had the most favorable prognosis. This improvement was seen despite no change in the radiographic size and density of the lesion over the follow-up period. In a separate report, 14 of 28 horses made a complete recovery at follow-up times ranging between 4 and 33 months. Less favorable results following conservative management have been seen by others, with clinical signs returning with resumption of exercise. This has led some to recommend surgery in any horse in which an athletic career is expected. If lameness is mild and the radiographic lesion is a mild indentation or dome shape to the medial femoral condyle, conservative management with monitoring of progress over 4 to 6 months may be indicated. Where lameness is prominent, or where improvement is not seen with 4 to 6 months of conservative management, surgery is certainly indicated. If radiographic signs of femorotibial joint degenerative joint disease are present, treatment may be unsuccessful.

Most commonly, surgery is done via femorotibial joint arthrotomy. One surgical approach is between the medial collateral ligament and medial patellar ligament, with the horse in lateral recumbency and the affected limb down and in slight flexion. The other approach is between the middle and medial patellar ligaments, with the horse in dorsal recumbency and the limb in full flexion. With both techniques, the crural fascia is incised to expose the fat pad. The fat pad, which is adherent to the underlying joint capsule, is reflected sufficiently to allow a longitudinal incision to be made in the capsule. The limb is then manipulated as necessary to bring the lesion into view.

The typical appearance of the lesion at the articular surface is that of a depressed area of cartilage with a crack or dimple in its center (Fig. 103–3). Cartilage overlying the cystic lesion is sharply excised back to normal margins and debris within the lesion is curetted and removed. Drilling of the sclerotic rim of the lesion (forage) to encourage vascularization that will assist with healing is recommended. Packing the defect with autogenous cancellous bone has also been recommended. The joint capsule, crural fascia, subcutaneous tissues, and skin are closed as separate layers. Tension sutures are placed in the skin, and a stent bandage is sutured over the skin incision. To minimize incisional dehiscence problems, horses can be cross-tied or tied to an overhead wire for 2 weeks after surgery.

Lesions have also been successfully treated using arthroscopic visualization. A curette and motorized burr are used for débridement, and a drill is used for forage. Copious lavage is necessary to flush debris from the joint. Although complications with femorotibial arthrotomy are low, the relatively noninvasive nature of arthroscopy confers advantages here as in other joints.

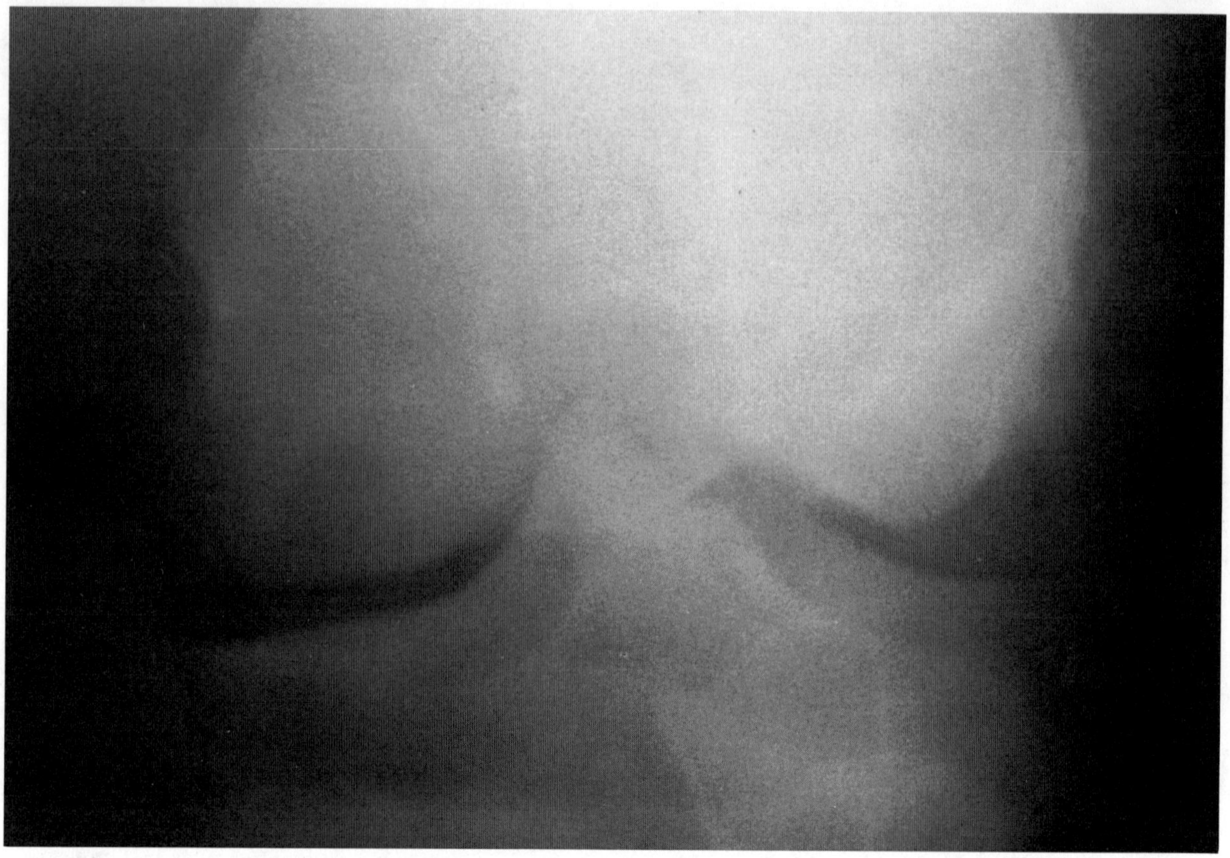

Figure 103–2. A circular-shaped lucent area typical of a subchondral cystic lesion is seen in the middle of the medial femoral condyle.

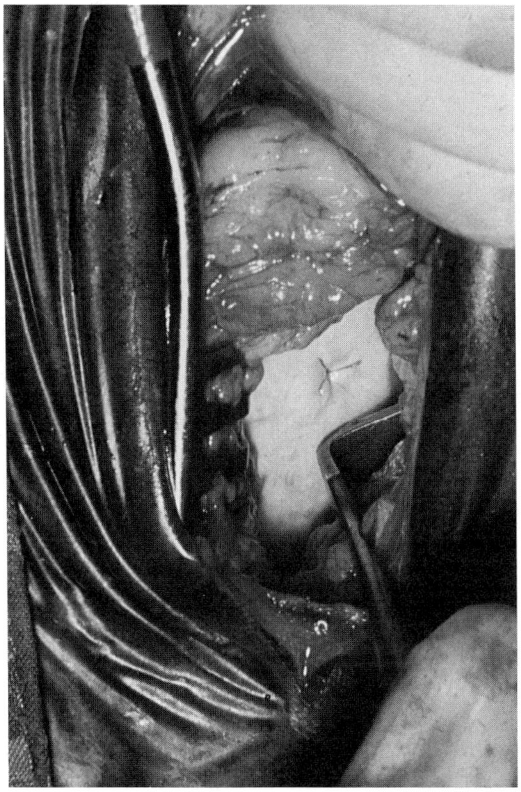

Figure 103–3. Typical wrinkled and indented appearance of the articular surface of a subchondral cystic lesion of the medial femoral condyle.

Postoperative Management

Antibacterial and anti-inflammatory medication is recommended for the perioperative period. Outward signs of discomfort are rarely present and periincisional swelling is minimal. Controlled walking exercise is begun at 2 to 3 weeks after surgery, with the degree of exercise increasing over the next 6 weeks. Paddock rest is maintained until training is started 5 to 6 months after surgery. In cases in which prominent lameness was present before surgery, clinical improvement after surgery may be dramatic and immediate.

Prognosis

Although extensive follow-up data after surgery are unavailable, existing reports document favorable results in 70 to 80% of cases. Some horses still lame 6 months after surgery have been sound by 1 year after surgery. Increased radiodensity of the defect is usually seen if a cancellous bone graft was used, although complete disappearance is rare. Where no graft was used, defects often remain unchanged. There is ample evidence, however, that poor correlation exists betweeen clinical signs and increased radiodensity of the defect. Marked long-term improvement has been reported in many cases in which the radiographic appearance of the defect has remained unchanged.

Incisional complications with arthrotomy (seroma formation, dehiscence) are a low-incidence problem. At incision closure, no attempt should be made to appose successive tissue layers to obliterate dead space because of independent movement of these layers during limb flexion. With arthroscopy, these soft tissue incisional complications are eliminated. Progressive degenerative joint disease of the affected joint is an occasional but uncommon reason for failure to improve. Collapse of the medial femoral condyle has been reported in two horses that did not have surgery but were being exercised as part of their conservative management regimen.

BIBLIOGRAPHY

Kold SE, Hickman J: Results of treatment of subchondral bone cysts in the medial condyle of the equine femur with an autogenous cancellous bone graft. *Equine Vet J* 1984;6:414–418.

Kold SE, Hickman J, Melsen F: An experimental study of the healing process of equine chondral and osteochondral defects. *Equine Vet J* 1986;18:18–24.

Lewis R: A retrospective study of diagnostic and surgical arthroscopy of the equine femotibial joint. *Proc Am Assoc Equine Pract* 1987; pp 887–893.

McIlwraith CW: Subchondral cystic lesions (osteochondrosis) in the horse. *Compend Cont Educ Pract Vet* 1982;4:394–408.

McIlwraith CW, Martin GS: Arthroscopic surgery for the treatment of osteochondritis dissecans in the equine femoropatellar joint. *Vet Surg* 1985;14:105–116.

Pascoe JR, Poole RR, Wheat JD, O'Brien TR: Osteochondral defects of the lateral trochlear ridge of the distal femur of the horse. Clinical, radiographic and pathological examination and results of surgical treatment. *Vet Surg* 1984;13:99–110.

Rose JA, Sande RD, Rose EM: Results of conservative management of osteochondrosis in the horse. *Proc Am Assoc Equine Pract* 1985; pp 617–626.

Stewart B, Reid CF: Osseous cyst-like lesions of the medial femoral condyle in the horse. *J Am Vet Assoc* 1982;180:254–257.

Trotter GW, McIlwraith CW, Norrdin RW: A comparison of two surgical approaches to the equine femoropatellar joint for the treatment of osteochondritis dissecans. *Vet Surg* 1983;12:33–40.

White NA, McIlwraith CW, Allen D. Curettage of subchondral bone cysts in medial femoral condyles of the horse. *Equine Vet J* 1988;Suppl 6:120–124.

104
Physitis

Elwyn C. Firth

Our knowledge of physitis, a disease of young horses, is extremely sparse. The disease is difficult to examine pathoanatomically because, although morbidity is high, there is no threat to life and gross or histologic examination of numerous specimens is thus not possible. Also, the relative ease of clinical diagnosis means that biopsy is not necessary or indicated, and affected tissue is thus very rarely available.

Several names are used for the disease, and correct nomenclature awaits accurate characterization of the disease. The term "physitis" is probably erroneous because it is unlikely that the primary event is inflammation; "epiphysitis" is a term often applied, but also erroneously because the disease involves primarily the physis and metaphysis and not the epiphysis. "Physeal dysplasia" has also been used to refer to the disease. In young horses affected with the articular form of osteochondrosis, obvious lesions in many growth plates were also found, and were characterized as osteochondrosis on the basis of the histomorphologic similarity with the growth plate form of that disease seen in other mammals and birds; the authors indicated that osteochondrosis may be one of the conditions causing "epiphysitis" in young horses. Consequently, appreciation of the known events in the pathogenesis of the disease is more important at this stage of our knowledge than nomenclature. This is especially true because the clinical and radiologic syndromes commonly seen may not be due to the same etiologic factor, or group of factors, in all cases.

ANATOMY AND PHYSIOLOGY OF THE PHYSIS

As in other mammals the equine growth plate consists of resting, proliferative, transitional, and degenerative cell layers. The longitudinal cartilage septa between the chondrocytes are continuous with the primary and secondary spongiosa of the metaphysis. In newborn foals the physis is not yet bound on its epiphyseal side by a subchondral bony plate. This plate forms in the following weeks or months. Until this structure is present, the real physis is apposed on its epiphyseal aspect by unossified epiphyseal cartilage.

As in other species, there are three main blood supplies to the long bone, and each is relevant to growth plate function. First, the terminal branches of the diaphyseal nutrient artery reach the metaphyseal side of the physis, where the capillaries are of central importance in the endochondral ossification process that occurs there. The vascular anatomy at this site is also associated with the predisposition of the mammalian metaphysis to hematogenous bone infection. Second, there are vessels of extraosseous origin that penetrate the metaphysis and nourish the peripheral parts of the growth plate. These vessels, termed epiphyseometaphyseal vessels or metaphyseal vessels, are not prominent in foals more than several weeks of age. Third, there are vessels that enter the epiphysis, and some of these have branches that course toward the metaphyseal growth plate. A number of these branches cross the physis into the metaphysis, where some are morphologically identical to the branches of the terminal nutrient artery and thus appear to nourish the metaphyseal side of the growth plate. The vast majority of vessels cease to cross the metacarpal and distal radial growth plates before the foal is 6 weeks of age. Most epiphyseal vessels enter but do not cross the physis, and penetrate as far as the proliferative layer. As the physis assumes its "mature" thickness and morphology, vessels do not enter the cartilage, and the peglike projections of cartilage projecting into the metaphysis, associated with transphyseal vessels or their remnants, are no longer visible. It is emphasized that the greatest change in these morphologic relationships occurs in the first few months of life, when growth is most rapid.

PATHOGENESIS OF PHYSITIS

Causes of alteration of endochondral ossification in the growing horse include rapid growth, trauma to ossification centers, genetic predisposition, and nutritional imbalances. Knowledge in this area has recently been reviewed by Lewis. Any hypothesis regarding the pathogenesis of physitis must also consider the changing morphology of the equine growth plate, and the documented responses to growth plate injuries in other species. The peak age incidences of physitis are 4 to 8 months and 1 to 2 years, but exact specification of incidence in terms of site, severity, and patient signalment has not been published. It is not known if the structural properties of bone and cartilage and their relationship to the forces placed upon them are exceptional at these times.

Up to certain limits, increased compressive forces experimentally applied across the growth plates of small animals cause an increase in the thickness of the physis. This occurs because proliferation of chondrocytes continues, although conversion into bone does not. This change was also one of the first changes noted on the compression side of ovine bones with angular limb deviation induced by increased weight bearing. Similar changes have also been induced by interruption of the blood supply on the metaphyseal side of the physis of rabbits. Massive compression forces or interruption of the blood supply on the epiphyseal side compromise the germ cell layer, arrest cell division, and cause closure of the growth plate. In horses affected with physitis the most common radiologic finding is irregularity and widening of the physis. Furthermore, histologic descriptions of conditions suggested to be physitis mention an increase in height of physeal cartilage, arrest of ossification, and fissure between metaphyseal cartilage and metaphyseal spongiosa. All of these findings are features indicating an insult to the metaphysis or metaphyseal blood supply and not the epiphysis or epiphyseal blood supply.

It has been suggested, but not proven, that primary spongiosa microfracture precedes cartilage retention in the distal radial growth plate of young foals, but the reverse situation cannot be excluded. Complete closure of the growth plate can occur, as is evident on radiographs of the distal radius of yearlings with physitis and subsequent varus deformity, but it is not clear if this is preceded by physeal thickening, chondronecrosis, and collapse, or if the epiphyseal side of the physis (i.e., the germ cell layer) is insulted primarily by massive compression injury. The cause of physitis in rapidly growing individuals thus may be structural failure of the tissue near the cartilage-bone junction on the metaphyseal side. Presumably the structural integrity of this area may be compromised by imbalances in mineral and trace elements, which have recently been implicated in several diseases including physitis. This could lead to increased predisposition of the metaphysis to normal or abnormal biomechanical influences acting upon it.

DIAGNOSIS

The bones most often involved are the distal metacarpus/metatarsus, radius, and tibia. Rapidly growing, heavily muscled individuals are most often affected. There is occasionally a history of lameness in another limb. The signs are usually bilateral or in all four limbs, and include lameness, stiffness, swelling at the level of the affected physis, and pain on deep palpation. Angular limb deviation may accompany or result from the disease, as may various manifestations of osteochondrosis in other joints. Pathologic fracture of the third metatarsal bone has been recorded. Physitis may be associated with flexural limb deformity of variable severity.

The diagnosis is based on clinical signs and radiologic examination. Involvement of nutritional imbalance or toxicologic factors is determined by examination of the ration and appropriate laboratory examination of body fluids or tissues. Definitive diagnosis can be made by biopsy and histologic examination, but is rarely indicated because the disease is not life threatening, and a strongly tentative diagnosis can be made with clinical and radiologic evidence.

Biopsy for histologic and biochemical examination of physeal cartilage has been described by Belling and Glade. In the sedated, physically restrained horse, local infiltration and perineural analgesia is induced in the area of the distolateral aspect of the radius. A 2.5-cm incision is made through skin, subcutis, and periosteum at the most prominent lateral part of the radius, and the periosteum is reflected cranially and caudally. A 10-mm bone gouge and a hammer are used to remove a piece of bone and physeal cartilage approximately 10 mm in diameter and 8 to 10 mm deep. The wound is closed in three layers using interrupted sutures. The carpal area is bandaged, and antibiotics are administered for several days postoperatively. Recovery from this procedure has been without complications, except that some soreness was evident in the early postoperative period. It is possible that such a large defect could compromise the structural integrity of the metaphysis, with resultant collapse and/or pathologic fracture. Instead of a gouge, a 5- or 8-mm Michele bone biopsy trephine could be used for harvesting the tissue. The sample should immediately be placed in buffered formalin solution, and then decalcified and prepared for routine histology. Sections may show variable involvement, including trabecular microfracture, increased height of the physis, necrosis of cartilage, or retained cartilage in the metaphysis.

TREATMENT

The treatment of physitis is directed toward correcting any management or nutritional errors. Restricted exercise may be allowed, but hard ground should be avoided if possible. Low doses of phenylbutazone may be indicated to encourage free movement and prevent the development of flexural limb deformity. The condition is usually self-limiting and the prognosis is generally good, although it is suspected that a number of affected animals may not race or perform successfully.

Surgical intervention related to this disease concerns growth acceleration or retardation procedures (see Chapter 96).

BIBLIOGRAPHY

Belling TH, Glade MJ: A non-destructive biopsy method allowing the rapid removal of live growth-plate cartilage. *Vet Med* 1984;79:528–531.

Dammrich K: Wachstumstorungen des Skeletts bei jungen pferden. *Pferdeheilkunde* 1985;1:5–13.

Duff SRI: Histopathology of growth plate changes in induced abnormal bone growth in lambs. *J Comp Pathol* 1986;96:15–24.

Firth EC, Poulos PW: Blood vessels in the developing growth plate of the equine distal radius and metacarpus. *Res Vet Sci* 1982;33:159–166.

Firth EC, Poulos PW: Microangiographic studies of metaphyseal vessels in young foals. *Res Vet Sci* 1983;34:231–235.

Firth EC, Poulos PW: Retained cartilage in the distal physis of foals. *Vet Pathol* 1984;21:10–17.

Fretz PB: Angular limb deformities in foals. *Vet Clin North Am* 1980;2:125–150.

Gallina AM: Bone and joint pathology, in Mansmann RA, McAllister ES, Pratt PW (eds): *Equine Medicine and Surgery.* Santa Barbara, CA, American Veterinary Publications, 1982, p 979.

Knight DA, Gabel AA, Reed SM, Embertson RM, Tyznik WJ, Bramlage LR: Correlation of dietary mineral to incidence and severity of metabolic bone disease in Ohio and Kentucky. *Proc AAEP Ann Conven* 1985; pp 445–461.

Lewis LD: The role of nutrition in musculoskeletal development and disease, in Stashak T (ed): *Adams' Lameness in Horses.* Philadelphia, Lea & Febiger, 1987, pp 276–279.

Rejno S, Stromberg B: Osteochondrosis in the horse. II. Pathology. *Acta Radiol (Suppl)* 1978;358:153–178.

Rooney JR: Epiphyseal compression in young horses. *Cornell Vet* 1963;53:567–574.

Sherrod WW: Epiphysitis in foals. Vet Med/Small Anim Clin 1975;70:1443–1448.

Spira E, Farin I: The vascular supply to the epiphyseal plate under normal and pathological conditions. *Acta Orthop Scand* 1967;38:1–22.

Trueta J, Amato VP: The vascular contribution to osteogenesis. III. Changes in the growth cartilage caused by experimentally induced ischaemia. *J Bone J Surg [Br]* 1960;42:571–587.

UNIT VIIIB

Traumatic Musculoskeletal Disorders

105
Articular Cartilage Healing: Current Concepts

Anne Vachon
C. Wayne McIlwraith

STRUCTURE OF ARTICULAR CARTILAGE

Articular cartilage is a highly specialized connective tissue with unique physicochemical properties suited to provide a frictionless bearing surface. Normal articular cartilage has a smooth, glossy appearance. It is avascular, aneural, and without lymphatic vessels. A characteristic feature of the tissue is the paucity of cells interspersed in a highly hydrated extracellular matrix. Mature articular cartilage is composed, by dry weight, of approximately 60% collagen, 30% proteoglycan, and 10% glycoprotein, lipids, and chondrocytes. Water content ranges from 65 to 75%, is freely exchangeable with synovial fluid, and appears to be bound in the form of a proteoglycan-collagen gel. The structure of articular cartilage can be described as a network of type II collagen that forms a system of compartments in which the water-binding proteoglycan complexes are enclosed. Proteoglycans provide the articular cartilage with compressive stiffness. Furthermore, they modulate the degree of pre-stress in the collagen fibers, and hence their stiffness, by controlling the hydration of intrafibrillar and extrafibrillar spaces. The instantaneous deformation of cartilage under load is related to the tensile properties of cartilage and depends primarily on the properties of the collagen network.

Based on the distribution of cells and the orientation of the collagen fibers, four zones have been described: (*a*) a tangential zone in which the cells are elongated with their long axis parallel to the surface, (*b*) a transitional zone in which the cells are rounded and appear randomly distributed, and (*c*) a radial zone in which the cells appear to line up in short, irregular columns. At skeletal maturity, when articular cartilage becomes calcified, the calcified zone (*d*) is separated from the radial zone by the tidemark (a thin, wavy blue line with hematoxylin and eosin staining). The deep surface of the calcified zone merges with the endplate of the underlying subchondral bone.

The concentration of proteoglycans varies inversely with the collagen and water content. This concentration is lower superficially and higher in the deeper zones of uncalcified cartilage. Therefore, tensile strength resides in the collagen-rich tangential layer, whereas compressive strength resides primarily in the proteoglycan-rich transitional layer. Disturbance of this proteoglycan gradient, as occurs in degenerative cartilage or in repair fibrocartilage, will alter the diffusion of solutes to and from the chondrocytes and therefore will affect chondrocyte metabolism and matrix composition, causing biomechanical dysfunction of the tissue. In mature articular cartilage, the role of the surface layer may be of the utmost importance in protecting the tissue from unfavorable mechanical stresses during joint function. Any disruption of the integrity of the surface layer will expose the deeper portion of the tissue to large tensile stresses and strains, which in turn could lead to ultimate loss of articular cartilage.

The biomechanical significance of the tidemark, calcified cartilage layer, and subchondral bone plate have been documented. The tidemark anchors the collagen fibers of the middle and deep zones of noncalcified cartilage to the calcified zone. Its undulating configuration provides resistance against shear stresses that are present at the noncalcified-calcified cartilage interface. Similarly, because the compliance of the calcified cartilage is intermediate to that of noncalcified cartilage and subchondral bone, the calcified zone acts to minimize shear stress concentration at the cartilage-bone interface. The deformation of the subchondral bone plate under load is responsible for shock absorption and joint congruency.

ARTICULAR CARTILAGE RESPONSE TO INJURY AND DISEASE

The skeletal maturity of the patient, the type of the lesion, whether the cause is acute (traumatic) or insidious (degenerative), and the depth of the injury will influence the vascularity and thereby the pattern of the healing process of an injured osteoarticular segment. Other factors, such as the size of the defect and its location within the joint, will also influence the repair and remodeling of the diseased articular surface.

The earliest structural change in the matrix characterizing degenerative joint disease is a decrease in proteoglycan content. This may be due to a release of synovial proteoglycanase caused by a primary synovitis usually traumatic in origin. In addition, the cycle of chondral breakdown and release of proteoglycan, enzymes, and other inflammatory products is believed to induce a vicious cycle of synovitis that promotes further chondral breakdown, either at the site of the original lesion or elsewhere in the joint. The severity of the accompanying synovitis is dependent on the amount of the articular tissue exfoliation. The relative importance of the chondrocytes and synovium as the origin of destructive enzymes is controversial. They are both the source of lysosomal proteoglycanase and collagenase. In addition, the inflamed synovium is a direct source of prostaglandins and an indirect source, via the neutrophils, of superoxide radicals. The prostaglandins may suppress glycosaminoglycan synthesis as well as cause its degradation. Superoxide radicals have the important capability to degrade hyaluronic acid, proteoglycans, and collagen. Recent work has emphasized the potential role of two intercellular messengers (catabolin and interleukin) originating from neutrophils and synovium. These substances are capable of modulating the chondrocyte metabolism to a catabolic state. In other words, while the cartilage plays a major role in matrix breakdown, there appears to be a triggering mechanism from the synovium. The relative contribution of these various pathways in cases of equine degenerative joint disease has yet to be documented.

In response to injury, the chondrocytes increase their mitotic activity and their rate of protein and glycosaminoglycan synthesis up to a certain level. In spite of such attempts, the rate of degradation of proteoglycans always exceeds their rate of synthesis and lower concentration of glycosaminoglycans persists throughout the disease process. The loss of glycosaminoglycans from the transitional zone reduces the viscoelasticity of that zone. It is believed that under loading, forces are concentrated and absorbed in the poorly compressive resistant tangential zone. This would lead to microfracture of the collagen network, and eventually to full-thickness chondral erosion with bone exposure. The morphologic patterns of articular cartilage degeneration vary but the principal and histologic manifestation is that of fibrillation. Arthroscopically, fibrillation appears as "furry" degenerative changes. Microscopically, it is characterized by vertical splitting from the articular surface, extending down into the uncalcified cartilage layers, along the alignment of the matrix collagen framework (Fig. 105–1). Such changes are preceded by a loss of glycosaminoglycans and collagens and an increase in water content. Thin type II collagen fibrils fuse to thicker ones. This disorganization or loosening of the collagen network may allow proteoglycans to bind more water, to swell, or to leak out. This may lead to further collapse of the collagen network.

As fibrillation progresses, erosion of the articular cartilage is evident grossly. Other changes that may be seen on histologic examination include horizontal splitting at the interface between uncalcified and calcified layers of articular cartilage, and fasciculation (vertical fissures in the deeper layers under an intact superficial layer). A partial-thickness injury in mature articular cartilage produces no inflammatory response because of the absence of vessels, nor does the cartilage show more than a minimal attempt at repair. Histologically, the first change occurs in the matrix with the loss of proteoglycans along the margin of the injury.

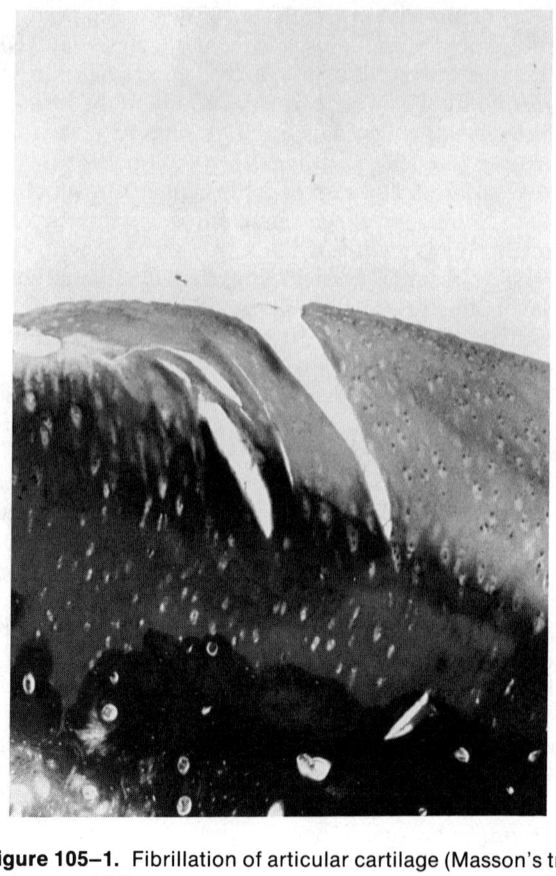

Figure 105–1. Fibrillation of articular cartilage (Masson's trichrome, ×150).

This stimulates an attempt at repair with increased glycosaminoglycan and collagen synthesis. Soon after the injury, cells adjacent to the injured surfaces may show a brief burst of reproductive activity with the appearance of multinuclear chondrones in the defect margins. Despite such attempts at repair, there is no appreciable increase in the bulk of cartilage matrix and the repair process is almost never effective in healing the defects. If the wall of the defect is vertical, inward lipping of the margin of surrounding cartilage, termed "matrix flow," can occur to a limited degree. This response gives a smooth appearance on gross examination. These flow formations are caused by the pressure of weight bearing and shearing forces. Superficial defects are not necessarily progressive and do not necessarily prejudice joint function.

A full-thickness lesion can develop as a result of an acute avulsion of cartilage off intact cortical bone, an osteochondral fracture, or osteochondritis dissecans, or as full-thickness erosion due to degenerative joint disease. The overall response to an injury that extends into the subchondral bone differs from that seen with the superficial lesion. The repair process is dominated by a subchondral angioblastic ingrowth. The response of the articular cartilage itself does not vary much from that following the superficial lesion and provides only limited repair necessary to replace the dead cells and damaged matrix at the margin of the wound. The defects heal by ingrowth of subchondral fibrous tissue that may or may not undergo metaplasia to fibrocartilage. The sequence of events in repair of experimentally induced 5- and 15-mm^2 full-thickness defects of the femoropatellar and carpal joints was recently investigated in the horse. At 1 month, the defects were filled with a poorly organized fibrovascular repair tissue. Changes between 2.5 and 4 months were limited to an increase in the amount and organization of this fibrous tissue. At 5 months, the small lesions were nearly undetectable in the radiocarpal and femoropatellar joints. In contrast, the outline of their 15-mm^2 counterparts was still readily evident. Repair of third carpal bone lesions lagged behind other sites and some of these lesions showed exposed subchondral bone. The presence of fibrocartilage was first documented at 5 months but matrix staining for proteoglycans was still minimal at that time. At 9 months, large defects were filled with fibrocartilage at the level of surrounding articular cartilage. Proteoglycans were increased but still markedly reduced compared to uninjured articular cartilage. In most of the large defects of the third carpal bone, perilesional clefts and undermined flaps of repair fibrocartilaginous tissue were identified.

As with partial-thickness lesions, matrix flow may contribute to the healing of full-thickness lesions. In the horse, matrix flow in induced 5-mm^2 full-thickness defects of the lateral trochlear ridge of the femur reduced the area of the defects by 50 to 90% within the first 2.5 to 4 months. Matrix flow was less obvious in the same size defect induced in the third carpal bone and distal radius.

The subchondral bone defect either heals with bone or fills in with fibrocartilaginous tissue. Duplication of the tidemark and calcified cartilage layer is the exception rather than the rule. Adherence of repair tissue to the surrounding, noninjured cartilage is often incomplete and poor.

Perichondrial and synovial pannus formation may contribute vascular and cellular elements to the repair of cartilaginous defects located adjacent to a bone-synovial junction. Experimentally and clinically in the horse, such lesions repair poorly by fibrovascular ingrowth and are associated with subchondral bone resorption and disruption of perilesional articular cartilage.

Arthroscopic examination of degenerative full-thickness lesions shows areas of exposed, often hemorrhagic subchondral bone covered with interspersed islands of reparative fibrocartilage adjacent to parent, fragmented cartilage. Histologically, the exposed sclerotic subchondral bone is increased in density with thickened trabeculae. The vascularity may increase and penetrate the surface, resulting in focal hemorrhage. Organization of the blood clot results in the formation of fibrous and fibrocartilaginous islands surrounded by necrotic subchondral bone. It is suggested that repair fibrous or fibrocartilaginous tissue does not coalesce unless the necrotic bone is removed by an inflammatory process or surgical débridement.

It is important, whether dealing with osteochondritis dissecans or with traumatic injuries, to consider the possible limitation inherent to the replacement of full-thickness defects imposed by the diameter of the defect. Some have suggested that large osteochondral defects of the human patella or distal femur are unlikely to heal because they lack the support of intact, surrounding cartilage. Previous studies in the horse supported this concept and showed that large, induced osteochondral defects ($>$ 1 cm) in the carpal and femoropatellar joints do not repair as well as smaller ones. Large defects (15 mm^2) had good initial repair but at 5 months perilesional and intralesional subchondral clefts developed. Nonetheless, other surgeons claim that functional healing of large osteochondral defects of the lateral trochlear ridge of the femur occurs in the horse and that restitution of normal subchondral bone contour is not necessary for clinical soundness.

On a cellular basis, the chondrocyte modulates its metabolic activities to modify the biochemical ultrastructures of its surrounding matrix in response to increased functional stress. In accordance with these concepts, Furukawa et al. demonstrated an increased concentration of glycosaminoglycans and type II collagen in weight-bearing areas of the femoral condyle in rabbits. The literature related to the influence of loading on the healing of osteochondral defects is varied and contradictory. Discrepancies of findings may result from the lack of objective biomechanical data in determining the location of the weight-bearing versus non–weight-bearing areas in the various joints studied. This makes comparison of data difficult. Keeping these considerations in mind, Depalma et al. showed that repair of small defects (4 mm) in dogs occurred at a slower and quantitatively inferior rate in the non–weight-bearing area of the distal femoral condyle than in the weight-bearing area. This concept has been experimentally supported in the horse. Small lesions (5 mm^2) in the femoropatellar and carpal joints showed significantly better cellular and matrical indices of cartilage repair in weight-bearing defects, whereas non–weight-bearing defects developed disrupted degenerative fibrous surfaces and ineffective proteoglycan replacement. Fischer et al. contradicted this concept and demonstrated that induced osteochondral defects (6.5 mm) of the non–weight-bearing distal lateral trochlear ridge of the equine talus healed with fibrocartilaginous tissue at a faster rate and more completely as compared to those in the weight-bearing proximal medial trochlear ridge of the talus.

STRUCTURE OF REPARATIVE FIBROCARTILAGE

Reparative fibrocartilage forms following full-thickness injury to hyaline cartilage. It also occurs as a natural repair process in joints with degenerative arthritis. It is grossly whiter and softer on palpation than normal articular cartilage. Both hyaline cartilage and repair fibrocartilage contain proteoglycans, although proteoglycan content as a rule does not reach normal values in the repair fibrocartilage. Repair fibrocartilage is hypercellular but shows cellular characteristics similar to those of hyaline cartilage, with oval cells including eccentric nuclei surrounded by lacunae. This fibrocartilage contains primarily type I collagen as opposed to type II collagen in hyaline cartilage. Comparison between the biochemical properties of repair cartilage and those of normal articular cartilage is advocated to predict its prospect of surviving as a weight-bearing surface. Identification of type II collagen by electrophoresis is considered to be the critical factor that distinguishes hyaline cartilage from repair fibrocartilage.

PHYSICOCHEMICAL PROPERTIES OF REPAIR FIBROCARTILAGE

Repair fibrocartilage does not display normal cellularity or matrix composition nor does it display the characteristic zonal architecture of hyaline articular cartilage. More precisely, fibrocartilage is fibrous and hypercellular. The presence of an abnormal subchondral bone plate and absence of tidemark and calcified cartilage layer creates an increased stiffness gradient and therefore increased shear stresses at the junction of the repaired fibrocartilage and underlying bone. Under loading, the propagation of such shear stresses leads to the degradation of repair fibrocartilage and exposure of the bone. Such mechanical failure of repair tissue has been observed experimentally and clinically in the horse.

Fibrocartilage repair is, therefore, biomechanically unsuitable as a replacement weight-bearing surface and has been shown to undergo mechanical failure with use. One can speculate that the lack of durability is due to faulty biochemical composition of the matrix, to incomplete remodeling of the interface between old and repair cartilage, or to increased stress in the regenerated cartilage due to abnormal remodeling of the subchondral bone plate and calcified cartilage layer.

CARTILAGE HEALING AND CLINICAL RESPONSE

As a general rule, chondral and osteochondral defects have a better potential for healing in immature animals. This is directly related to increased chondrocytic capacity for mitosis, matrix synthesis, and perhaps the presence of an intracartilaginous vascularity. Prognosis for functional healing is good when the amount of articular cartilage damage is small and decreases with more extensive articular damage. Nonetheless, in the equine carpus, up to a certain level (30% of articular surface), articular cartilage damage does not compromise successful return to racing. Loss of 50% of the articular surface or severe loss of subchondral bone is associated with a poor prognosis.

Complete restoration of the ultrastructure and configuration of an osteochondral defect in a hingelike gliding, type joint such as the femoropatellar joint is believed to be unnecessary for clinical soundness. In contrast, an osteochondral defect located in the intercarpal joint is subjected to an unforgiving biomechanical environment and must be given a poorer prognosis.

MODULATION OF HEALING

Even though considerable progress has been made in the field of joint therapy and articular constructive surgery successful management of large chondral and osteochondral defects and of degenerative lesions is still a challenge for the orthopedic surgeon. To provide access to subchondral pluripotential cells, débridement procedures such as partial- or full-thickness chondrectomy combined with subchondral bone drilling and/or spongialization have been advocated to stimulate fibrocartilaginous repair. Breakdown of repair tissue has been observed, and functional healing in high-impact loading joints such as the intercarpal joint of the horse is not achieved.

Partial-Thickness Chondrectomy

Arthroscopic débridement of partial-thickness defects down to relatively healthy chondral tissue (shaving) smooths the fragmented cartilaginous area and may decrease further tissue exfoliation. This procedure may produce, in conjunction with joint lavage, an early remission of the synovitis. Controlled work is necessary to evaluate the usefulness of such débridement. Aggressive scraping of partial-thickness defects down to bone is contraindicated. At no time should solid areas of partial-thickness degenerative hyaline cartilage be removed in an attempt at replacement with repair fibrocartilage.

Full-Thickness Chondrectomy

The extent of the débridement depends on the configuration of the lesion. If the lesion is well defined with perpendicular margins of normal articular cartilage, as occurs in an acute osteochondral fracture, minimal débridement is necessary. If the margins are irregular with undermined flaps, as in the osteoarthritic or osteochondritic case, débridement of the projecting flaps is advocated to promote peripheral attachment of repair fibrocartilaginous tissue. In humans, if a sclerotic lesion is débrided only to the margins of the exposed bone, the result can be an island of repair tissue surrounded by an area of necrotic bone. Débridement in these transition zones must meticulously extend into adjacent tissue to encourage a firm seal from the reparative to the parent tissue.

Subchondral Bone Drilling

Previous studies have evaluated the effects of subchondral bone drilling on the healing of cartilage defects of the third carpal bone in the horse and of the femur in the rabbit, and of chondromalacia of the patella in humans. In the horse, fibrocartilaginous repair tissue found in the drilled defects was interpreted to be superior qualitatively and quantitatively to the fibrous tissue in the nondrilled defects. Absence of osseous bridging of drilled subchondral bone plates and minimal zonal reorganization of repair tissue was observed in humans and in the horse. Conversely, in the rabbit the drill hole filled with hyaline-like cartilage, although the true nature of the reparative tissue was not substantiated by collagen typing. In an osteochondral defect induced in the relatively normal avascular subchondral bone of the third carpal of the horse, intracancellous débridement via drilling offers better potential for fibrocartilaginous repair than superficial cortical débridement via curettage alone. The benefit of subchondral drilling in the treatment of degenerative sclerotic full-thickness lesions needs to be investigated in the horse.

Perichondrial/Periosteal Autografts and Osteochondral Allografts

Perichondrial/periosteal autografts or osteochondral allografts have been advocated when large areas of diseased or denuded joint surfaces are present or when conventional débridement procedures have failed to induce functional healing. The neochondrogenic potential of perichondrium and periosteum has been used experimentally to restore large osteochondral defects in the rabbit, dog, and horse. A few European reports describe the use of these autografts to resurface diseased articular surfaces affected by osteoarthritis, rheumatoid arthritis, and osteochondritis dissecans in humans. Both perichondrium and periosteum possess a chondrogenic layer of undifferentiated mesenchymal cells that, when placed in a synovial environment, can differentiate toward chondroblasts and form hyaline-like cartilaginous tissue. In experimental studies, histopathologic and biochemical similarities between induced neocartilage and articular hyaline cartilage have been documented. There is still controversy regarding which tissue (perichondrium or periosteum) is most chondrogenic and regarding the most effective means of securing the autograft in the recipient osseous bed. Suture techniques usually resulted in poor attachment of the graft, and fixation using synthetic and fibrin adhesives has produced inconsistent results.

Fresh and frozen osteochondral allografts have been used successfully clinically and experimentally to resurface diseased or injured articular surfaces. The biology and immunology of osteochondral grafts have been studied extensively. Chondral allografts evoke a measurable immunologic response but an intact cartilage matrix acts as a filter, restricting ingress and egress of antigens and thereby protecting the chondrocyte. Techniques are now available for storing osteochondral grafts utilizing freezing and cryopreservatives. Although freezing results in death of an appreciable number of chondrocytes, it reduces the immune response directed toward the bony portion of the allograft, the significance of which is controversial. Longevity of an osteochondral allograft depends upon a number of factors, including the age of the donor and recipient, the site of the defect, the size of the graft, the accuracy of fit, and firm incorporation of the transplant into the recipient bed.

The suitability of using periosteal/perichondrial autografts and osteochondral allografts to resurface large osteochondral defects needs to be investigated in the horse.

Motion

There is continuing controversy concerning indications for rest and for motion in the management of traumatic joint injuries. Immobilization has a detrimental effect on the healing of full-thickness cartilage defects. In experimental studies, metaplasia of the healing tissue into hyaline-like cartilage occurs slower and is not as complete with immobilization as with either intermittent active motion or continuous passive motion. Early postoperative weight-bearing ambulation in humans who have sustained a superficial intracortical débridement procedure has been shown to maintain the healing osteochondral defect in a state of hyperemia, which resulted directly or indirectly in delayed chondrification. Although weight bearing in the early stage of healing seems to be detrimental, joint motion in the absence of loading does not maintain normal articular cartilage. In the horse, a fibrovascular response dominates the first 2 months of the natural healing pattern of large osteochondral defects. Thus, restricted activity by stall confinement is likely to be critical during this period.

Electrical Stimulation

Baker et al. showed that an electrical field could enhance the metaplasia of subchondral granulation tissue to hyaline-like cartilage in rabbits. The electrical fields are thought to have an indirect action on the chondrocyte by lowering its local oxygen tension. Lowering of oxygen tension, if it occurs when electrodes are implanted in vivo, would favor both differentiation of cartilage from pluripotential cells and maintenance of preexisting cartilage. This technique has not been tested clinically and cannot yet be recommended for use in the horse.

Intraarticular Therapy

Despite extensive clinical experience, certain aspects of local intraarticular corticosteroid treatment remain controversial (e.g., the potential deleterious effects of their use in treatment of degenerative joint disease). The widespread use of these agents in the athletic horse has proven this therapy, when combined with rest, to be beneficial in reducing synovial inflammation associated with various forms of traumatic and degenerative arthritis. Intraarticular corticosteroids have been shown to inhibit synovial collagenase and prostaglandin release as well as leukocyte superoxide radicals and catabolin production. The corticosteroids also decrease proteoglycan synthesis by chondrocytes (Table 105–1). Whether in some instances this negative effect on proteoglycan synthesis is offset by their beneficial inhibition of enzymatic matrix breakdown is conjectural.

To determine the effect of intraarticular steroids on normal equine articular cartilage, 100 mg of 6-α-

TABLE 105–1. SIGNIFICANT ACTIONS OF INTRAARTICULAR CORTICOSTEROIDS, POLYSULFATED GLYCOSAMINOGLYCAN (PSGAG), AND SODIUM HYALURONATE WITHIN SYNOVIAL JOINTS

Corticosteroids	PSGAG	Sodium Hyaluronate
1. Stabilize lysosomes and inhibit release of: collagenase prostaglandins superoxide radicals catabolin 2. Decrease proteoglycan synthesis in articular cartilage	1. Inhibits proteoglycan and collagen breakdown 2. May also stimulate synthesis of glycocosaminoglycan in articular cartilage 3. Stimulates synthesis of sodium hyaluronate	1. Decreases synovial membrane inflammation 2. Lubricates synovial membrane 3. Permeability control of the synovial membrane and effusion blockade

methylprednisolone was injected three times at 14-day intervals in the intercarpal joints of four horses. A significant decrease in the articular cartilage glycosaminoglycan content was demonstrated. Chondroprotective effects of corticosteroids have been reported in both physical and chemical models of articular cartilage degeneration. Recent studies using a chemically induced arthritis model in the horse did not support these previous findings. Glycosaminoglycan depletion was not prevented when 6-α-methylprednisolone was administered intraarticularly.

Polysulfated glycosaminoglycan inhibits proteoglycan and collagen lysosomal breakdown in osteoarthritic cartilage and also results in high-molecular-weight glycosaminoglycan production by chondrocytes and increased hyaluronate synthesis by synovial cells (Table 105–1). In the horse, the effect of intraarticular polysulfated glycosaminoglycans on repair of chemical and physical articular cartilage injuries was recently evaluated. Polysulfated glycosaminoglycans had chondro-protective properties on chemically induced articular cartilage damage, whereas they had no obvious beneficial effects on healing of induced partial- and full-thickness defects.

The beneficial anti-inflammatory effects of hyaluronate on synovium are well recognized. However, it has been shown that it has no effect on healing of intracartilaginous and osteochondral joint lesions in immobilized and mobile joints.

BIBLIOGRAPHY

Baker B, Becker RO, Spardo J: A study of electrochemical enhancement of articular cartilage repair. *Clin Orthop* 1974;102:251–267.

Bentley G: Articular cartilage changes in chondromalacia patella. *J Bone Joint Surg [Br]* 1985;67:769–774.

DePalma AF, McKeever CD, Subin DK: Process of repair of articular cartilage demonstrated by histology and autoradiography with tritiated thymidine. *Clin Orthop* 1966;48: 229–242.

Dingle ST: The role of cellular interactions in joint erosions. *Clin Orthop* 1983;182:25–29.

Enkvist O, Johansson SH: Perichondrial arthroplasty. A clinical study in twenty-six patients. *Scand J Plant Reconstr Surg* 1980;14:7187.

Fischer AT, Stover SM, Pool RR: Healing of full-thickness articular cartilage defects in the horse: A comparison of weightbearing to non-weightbearing areas (abstr.) *Vet Surg* 1986;15:20.

Furukawa T, Eyre D, Koide S, Glimcher M: Biochemical studies on repair cartilage resurfacing experimental defects in the rabbit knee. *J Bone Joint Surg [Am]* 1980;62:79–89.

Garret JC: Treatment of osteochondral defects of the distal femur with fresh osteochondral allografts. A preliminary report. *J Arthritis Research Surg* 1986;2:222–226.

Hurtig MB, Fretz PB, Doige CE, Schnurr DL: The effect of lesion size and location in equine articular cartilage repair. *Can J Vet Res* 1988;52:137–146.

Johnson LL: *Arthroscopic Surgery Principles and Practice.* St. Louis, CV Mosby Co, 1986, vol 1, pp 500–663.

Mankin HJ: in Bojrab MJ (ed): *Pathophysiology in Small Animal Surgery.* Philadelphia, Lea & Febiger, 1981, pp 557–567.

Maroudas A, Mizrahi J, Wachtel EJ, Soudry M: in Kuettner K (ed): *Articular Cartilage Biochemistry.* New York, Raven Press, 1986, pp 311–320.

McIlwraith CW: Diseases of joints, tendons, ligaments, and related structures in Stashak T (ed): *Adams' Lameness in Horses.* Philadelphia, Lea & Febiger, 1987, pp 339–481.

McIlwraith CW: Arthroscopic surgery for the treatment of osteochondritis dissecans in the equine femoropatellar joint. *Vet Surg* 1985;14:105–116.

McIlwraith CW: Current concepts in equine degenerative joint disease. *J Am Vet Med Assoc* 1980;180:239–250.

McIlwraith CW, Yovich JV, Martin GS: Arthroscopic surgery for the treatment of osteochondral chip fractures in the equine carpus. *J Am Vet Med Assoc* 1987;191:531–540.

Ohlsen L, Widenfalk B: The early development of articular cartilage after perichondrial grafting. *Scand J Plast Reconstr Surg* 1983;17:163–177.

Palmoski MJ, et al: Joint motion in the absence of normal loading does not maintain normal articular cartilage. *Arthritis Rheum* 1980;23:325–334.

Pascoe JR, Pool R, Wheat JD, O'Brien TR: Osteochondral defects of the lateral trochlea ridge of the distal femur of the horse. *Vet Surg* 1984;113:99–110.

Radin EL, Rose RM: Role of subchondral bone in the initiation and progression of cartilage damage. *Clin Orthop* 1986; 213:34–40.

Salter RB, Simmonds DF, Malcolm BW, Rumble EJ, MacMichael D, Clements ND: The biological effect of continuous passive motion on the healing of full-thickness defects in articular cartilage. *J Bone Joint Surg [Am]* 1980;62:1232–1251.

Trotter GW, McIlwraith CW, Yovich JV, Norrdin RW, Wrigley RH: Effect of intra-articular methylprednisolone acetate on equine articular cartilage and synovial membrane. *Am J Vet Res* 1989, submitted.

Trotter GW, McIlwraith CW, Yovich JV, Norrdin RW, Wrigley RH: Effect of intra-articular methylprednisolone acetate on chemically injured equine articular cartilage. *Am J Vet Res* 1989, submitted.

Vachon A, Bramlage L, Gabel A, Weisbrode S: Evaluation of the repair process of cartilage defects of the equine third carpal bone with and without subchondral bone perforation. *Am J Vet Res* 1986;47:2637–2645.

Yovich JV, Trotter GW, McIlwraith CW, Norrdin RW: Effect of polysulfated glycosaminoglycans on chemical and physical defects in equine articular cartilage. *Am J Vet Res* 1987;48:1407–1414.

106
Interphalangeal Degenerative Joint Disease

Gayle W. Trotter

Interphalangeal degenerative joint disease, or ring-bone, refers to degenerative joint disease of the proximal (high ring-bone) or distal (low ring-bone) interphalangeal joints. This condition has also been described as articular versus periarticular ring-bone. With articular ring-bone, radiologic features of degenerative joint disease are present to varying degrees, with or without periarticular new bone growth. With periarticular ring-bone, radiologic features are those of periosteal new bone growth away from the joint margins. This new bone growth can occur at sites of ligament or joint capsule origins or insertions (enthesophytes), or at any other bone site where the periosteum is subjected to external trauma (blunt trauma, wire cut). Periarticular ring-bone can sometimes progress to the point where degenerative joint disease ensues. The following discussion concerns the articular forms of ring-bone.

PROXIMAL INTERPHALANGEAL JOINT DEGENERATIVE JOINT DISEASE (HIGH ARTICULAR RING-BONE)

Diagnosis

High articular ring-bone results from numerous inciting causes. It occurs commonly in horses that make sharp turns and sudden stops, such as polo ponies and Western performance horses. It is also seen as a sequela to intraarticular fractures involving the proximal or more commonly the middle phalanx. Faulty distal limb conformation may result in abnormal joint loading and subsequent articular degeneration. Luxations and subluxations have also been associated with degenerative joint changes. A syndrome has been described in young horses in which lesions of osteochondrosis are seen in conjunction with those of degenerative joint disease.

History and presenting signs vary with the clinical syndrome, and how early in the course of the disease the animal is presented for examination. With high ring-bone in Western working horses, the history is usually one of decreased performance and progressive lameness. Swelling of the pastern usually develops later, although transient swelling that resolves with rest may occur. Eventually, the swelling characteristic of ring-bone persists. Where fractures are involved, a history of sudden-onset lameness is present. With osteochondrosis in young horses, progressive lameness and marked pastern swelling often are present. This condition in young horses seems to involve hind limbs more frequently than forelimbs.

Affected horses may show sensitivity to digital pressure over the pastern region and phalangeal flexion or torsion may exacerbate the lameness. Improvement in the horse's gait will only be partial with a palmar/plantar digital nerve block, but inclusion of dorsal nerve branches (ring block) should greatly improve or eliminate lameness.

Radiographs are necessary for definitive diagnosis. In early cases, radiographic changes may be absent and later reexamination will be required. When radiographic changes are present, they are those of degenerative joint disease and include any or all of the following: partial or complete joint space narrowing, marginal osteophyte formation, subchondral bone sclerosis, and occasionally subchondral bone lysis and periosteal new bone growth. With osteochondrosis in young horses, focal lucencies in the distal proximal phalanx often accompany the other radiographic findings (Fig. 106–1). Phalangeal fractures will be self-evident.

Treatment

Ankylosis of affected joints, either naturally or by surgical intervention, is usually required before pain, lameness, and dysfunction resolve. Although natural ankylosis does occur, the time course may be protracted and periosteal reaction may be excessive. Surgical arthrodesis is associated with the earliest and most predictable joint fusion and subsequent return to function.

Three techniques for surgical fusion of the proximal interphalangeal joint have been described. All involve surgical exposure of the pastern joint and curettage of articular cartilage down to subchondral bone. Stabilization of the proximal phalanx to the middle phalanx is then achieved using:

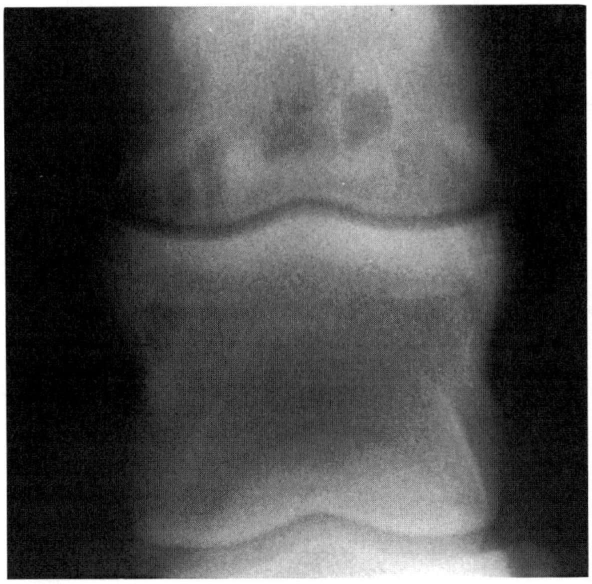

Figure 106–1. Focal lucent areas are present in the distal proximal phalanx of a young horse with bilateral osteochondrosis and high ring-bone affecting both rear pasterns.

1. Three cortical bone screws placed in parallel fashion from the distal dorsal proximal phalanx into the middle phalanx.
2. Two cortical bone screws placed in criss-cross fashion from the distal medial and lateral aspects of the proximal phalanx into the second phalanx.
3. A bone plate (T-plate or dynamic compression plate) placed on the dorsal surface of the phalanges.

In an experimental study in which techniques 1 and 2 were compared, the parallel screw technique resulted in stronger phalangeal union over the first 120 postoperative days. All techniques have been used successfully, however, and technique selection is based largely on personal preference and previous experience.

Horses are positioned in lateral recumbency, with the affected limb uppermost. A pneumatic tourniquet applied just below the carpus/tarsus facilitates surgery. Either an *I*-shaped or *C*-shaped skin incision is made over the pastern area, starting at the middle of the proximal phalanx and ending 0.5 to 1 cm proximal to the coronary band. The skin and subcutaneous fascia are reflected to expose the common/long digital extensor tendon. Using either an inverted *V*-incision or a *Z*-plasty approach, the tendon is incised. The tendon is reflected and the joint capsule is incised. A chisel or osteotome may be required to remove proliferative bone from the dorsal aspect of the joint. Collateral ligaments are incised only enough to allow curettage of articular cartilage from the ends of both phalanges.

When the parallel screw technique is used, a shelf is made with a bone chisel on the distal dorsal proximal phalanx, approximately 2.5 cm proximal to the joint surface. Either two or three (depending on the size of the horse) cortical screws are placed in lag fashion from the proximal phalanx into the middle phalanx, and intraoperative lateral to medial radiographs should be taken after placement of the first screw to ensure that the screw does not protrude beyond the palmar/plantar cortex of the middle phalanx (Fig. 106–2). This is especially important if cortex penetration occurs on the distal middle phalanx, because chronic irritation of the suspensory ligaments of the navicular bone could ensue. With this technique the drill must be positioned closely against the dorsal surface of the fetlock during drilling to achieve correct screw alignment.

When the criss-cross technique is used, the surgical approach and joint surface curettage are performed as previously described. Glide holes are then drilled from the articular surface of the proximal phalanx to exit at or near the eminences for the medial and lateral collateral ligaments on the proximal phalanx. The joint is aligned in extension and pilot holes are drilled into the middle phalanx. An intraoperative radiograph should be taken after screw placement to ensure that the distal interphalangeal joint has not been penetrated.

Both T-plates and dynamic compression plates have been used for arthrodesis of the pastern joint. When the T-plate is used, it is placed in an inverted fashion along the dorsal surface of the phalanges. Bone plates are favored when arthrodesis is performed for middle phalanx fractures. Intraoperative radiographs are taken to ensure that screws do not protrude through the palmar/plantar cortex of the phalanges.

With all techniques, an autogenous cancellous bone graft between the phalanges may be used. This is not a requisite, however, for success with this surgery. The joint capsule and tendon ends are reapposed over the implants and the skin is closed. A cast is applied to the level of the proximal metacarpus/metatarsus.

Postoperative Management

Perioperative antibacterial treatment is optional, but phenylbutazone is given as long as necessary for patient comfort. The patient is kept in a cast for 4 to 8 weeks, depending on postoperative use of the limb and progression of bony ankylosis. When evidence of healing is seen radiographically, the cast is removed standing and a bandage is maintained for a further 1 to 2 weeks to control limb swelling.

Typically, affected horses are lame when the cast is first removed, but lameness improves over the first few

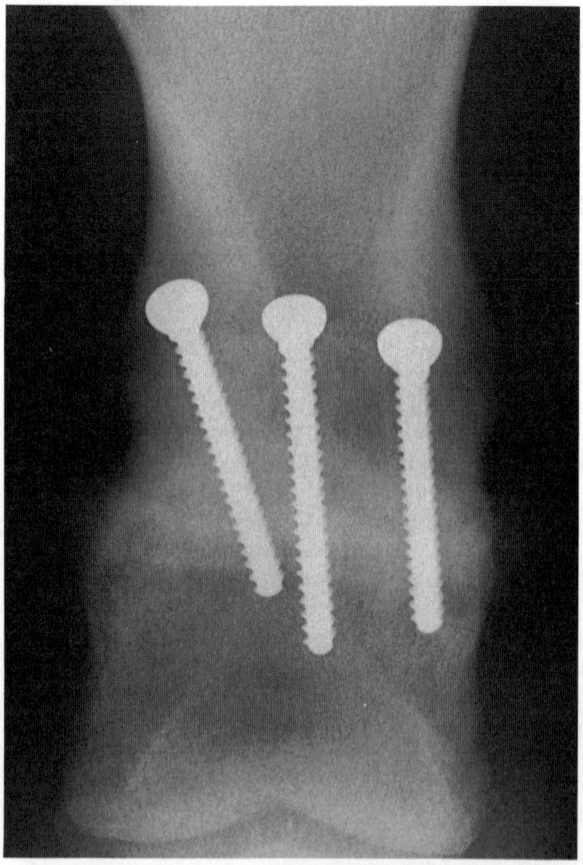

A

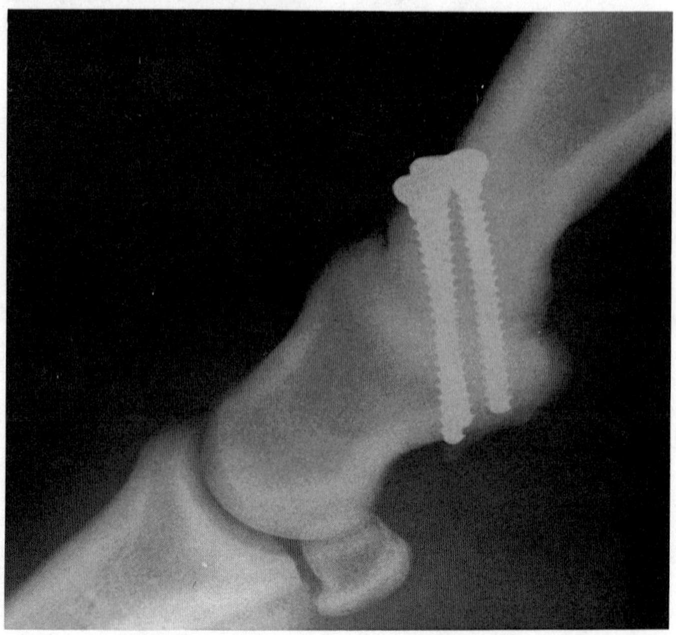

B

Figure 106–2. **A.** Dorsoplantar radiographic projection showing screw placement using the parallel screw technique. Lateral screw was placed obliquely to avoid the fracture plane of a caudal eminence fracture of the middle phalanx. Bony ankylosis is complete. **B.** Lateral-to-medial radiographic projection of same case. All screws should have been oriented more vertically to enter the midarticular surface of the middle phalanx.

weeks. Exercise is initially restricted to walking, the amount of exercise being increased as lameness improves. Radiographs every 2 months will help confirm joint fusion.

Prognosis

Favorable results with all three techniques have been reported for treating lameness due to high ring-bone. Horses have been sound at the trot by 10 to 12 weeks after surgery but return to full athletic usefulness takes from 6 to 12 months. From reported cases, a return to full use can be expected in approximately 75% of surgically treated cases.

One report documents better results for pastern arthrodesis of the hind limb compared to the forelimb. Complications encountered in the forelimb included toe elevation in some horses, as well as a proliferative exostosis on the dorsal surface of the distal phalanx in others. Reasons for these complications could not be explained. Other reported complications using the parallel screw technique are screw breakage, incorrect screw placement in the distal proximal phalanx resulting in phalangeal fracture around the screws, and screw penetration of the palmar/plantar cortex of the distal middle phalanx. Screw penetration of the distal interphalangeal joint has also been reported when using the criss-cross technique. When bone plates are used, plate position must be sufficiently proximal on the middle phalanx to avoid plate infringement on the distal interphalangeal articulation (Fig. 106–3).

Screws and plates do not need to be removed unless lameness associated with the implants persists. It is deemed important to do surgery before bony proliferative changes are so extensive as to affect surrounding soft tissue structures. Successful bilateral pastern arthrodesis has been reported for both the forelimbs and hind limbs.

DISTAL INTERPHALANGEAL JOINT DEGENERATIVE JOINT DISEASE (LOW ARTICULAR RING-BONE)

Diagnosis

Low articular ring-bone is a more confusing clinical entity, because clinical symptomatology is variable and radiographic changes in many cases are absent at the time of initial lameness. It more commonly affects the forelimbs, and affected horses may present for forelimb lameness that clinical examination localizes to the foot. A syndrome of arthrosis involving the distal interphalangeal joint is reportedly common in racing Quarter Horses.

An extreme form of low ring-bone is pyramidal disease, or buttress foot. With this disease, new bone growth occurs at the extensor process of the distal phalanx, and this new bone growth may or may not be accompanied by an extensor process fracture. Where no fracture is involved, it is assumed that new bone growth is due to excessive strain at the insertion of the common/long digital extensor tendon. It has been suggested that horses with animated gaits may be more predisposed to this specific problem. Extensor process fractures also occur most commonly in the forefeet, but they are not always accompanied by excessive bony proliferation. These fractures can contribute, however, to development of distal interphalangeal joint degenerative joint disease.

Clinical signs of low ring-bone vary with the severity of the problem. Some affected horses may point the affected limb(s), and one author claims the gait is characterized by excessive landing on the heel. Digital flexion tests may cause pain and/or exacerbate the lameness. In racing Quarter Horses, bilateral forelimb lameness is seen with the syndrome. Affected horses

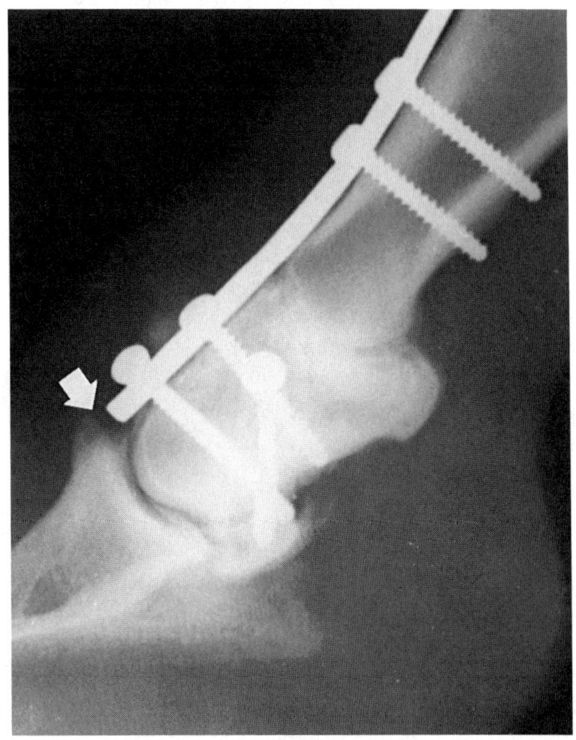

Figure 106–3. Dorsal application of a bone plate for middle phalanx fracture repair and fusion of the proximal interphalangeal joint. Placement of the plate too close to the distal interphalangeal joint can result in low ring-bone (*arrow*). (Courtesy of Nathaniel A White II.)

are short strided and often have an increased digital pulse, with palpable joint effusion along the coronary band. Many of the clinical features resemble those seen with navicular disease syndrome. A complete clarification of this particular clinical syndrome remains to be developed.

With chronicity and further bony proliferation, some horses develop a triangular-shaped foot as a result of a ridge that forms along the dorsal hoof wall (buttress foot). Occasionally, pain to deep digital pressure over the middorsal coronary band will be present. Localization of the site of lameness can be confirmed with a pastern ring block or intrasynovial anesthesia of the distal interphalangeal joint.

Radiographic changes are often absent or minimal (the exception being the radiographic changes seen with pyramidal disease and some extensor process fractures). Osteophyte formation at the extensor process of the distal phalanx may be the only radiographic abnormality.

Treatment

If an extensor process fracture is present, fragment removal, or fragment stabilization through a dorsal midline arthrotomy of the distal interphalangeal joint, may be indicated. Size of the fragment and extent of associated degenerative joint disease must be considered. Some fragments can be removed using arthroscopic techniques. In advanced cases of pyramidal disease, bony proliferation is so extensive that any treatment is likely to be ineffective. There is little information available on response to therapy and prognosis for further athletic use in earlier cases of low articular ringbone. Some horses respond to systemic nonsteroidal anti-inflammatory medication, and shoeing that is designed to minimize joint movement (roller motion shoes). Other horses reportedly respond favorably to intraarticular corticosteroids. For the syndrome seen in racing Quarter Horses, intraarticular corticosteroids plus sodium hyaluronate have proven effective in relieving the lameness. Because many of these horses also have long toes, underrun heels, and a broken pastern axis, corrective measures that address these foot abnormalities are also considered important.

BIBLIOGRAPHY

Ellis DR, Greenwood RES: Six cases of degenerative joint disease of the proximal interphalangeal joint of young horses. *Equine Vet J* 1985;17:66–88.

Genetzky RM, Schneider JE, Butler HC, Guffy MM: Comparison of two surgical procedures for arthrodesis of the proximal interphalangeal joint in horses. *J Am Vet Med Assoc* 1981;179:464–468.

Goodman N: Quarter Horse racetrack practice. *Proc Am Assoc Equine Pract* 1987; pp 835–841.

Hoffman KD, Pool RR, Pascoe JR: Degenerative joint disease of the proximal interphalangeal joints of young horses. *Equine Vet J* 1984;16:138–140.

Martin GS, McIlwraith CW, Turner AS, Nixon AJ, Stashak TS: Long-term results and complications of proximal interphalangeal arthrodesis in horses. *J Am Vet Med Assoc* 1984;184:1136–1141.

Rick MC, Herthel D, Boles C: Surgical management of middle phalangeal fractures and high ring-bone in the horse: a review of 16 cases. *Proc Am Assoc Equine Pract* 1986; pp 315–321.

Schneider JE, Carnine BL, Guffy MM: Arthrodesis of the proximal interphalangeal joint in the horse: a surgical treatment for high ring-bone. *J Am Vet Med Assoc* 1978;173:1364–1369.

Stashak TS: Pyramidal disease (buttress foot) and ring-bone (phalangeal exostosis), in *Adams' Lameness.* Philadelphia, Lea & Febiger, 1987, pp 528–29, 551–558.

Steenhaut M, Verschooten F, DeMoor A: Arthrodesis of the pastern joint in the horse. *Equine Vet J* 1985;17:35–40.

Trotter GW, McIlwraith CW, Norrdin RW, Turner AS: Degenerative joint disease with osteochondrosis of the proximal interphalangeal joint in young horses. *J Am Vet Med Assoc* 1982;180:1312–1318.

107
Fractures of the Metacarpophalangeal/Metatarsophalangeal Joint

John V. Yovich

OSTEOCHONDRAL FRACTURES OF THE DORSAL PROXIMAL ASPECT OF THE PROXIMAL PHALANX

This is the most common type of fracture of the metacarpophalangeal/metatarsophalangeal joint and it occurs almost exclusively in the forelimbs. The medial dorsal proximal aspect of the proximal phalanx is involved more than twice as frequently as the lateral aspect. Both the medial and lateral aspects of the proximal phalanx may be fractured in the same fetlock joint. Fracture is considered to occur during racing or fast training when extreme extension of the joint causes compression of the dorsal proximal aspect of the proximal phalanx against the distal part of the third metacarpal bone. Clinical signs are most prominent during the first few days after injury, with a mild to moderate lameness and usually obvious pain during joint flexion. Later, especially with rest, lameness may be inapparent unless the horse is in race training.

The fracture is most readily identified on dorsopalmar-lateromedial oblique (Fig. 107–1) and mediolateral oblique radiographic projections. Recent fractures are not usually accompanied by radiographic evidence of degenerative joint disease.

Treatment for this fracture type has evolved from conservative management to surgical treatment via arthrotomy and, in recent years, arthroscopic surgery. Surgical removal of the fracture fragment via a dorsal arthrotomy was the treatment of choice for many years. Unfortunately, dorsal arthrotomy sometimes resulted in decreased range of joint motion secondary to fibrosis at the surgical site, joint capsule thickening, and calcification and adhesions of the joint capsule close to the articular edge of the proximal phalanx. In consideration of these complications, a conservative approach was adopted. Although a percentage success rate is not documented, the fracture can potentially heal and horses can return to racing without lameness after 3 to 6 months' rest. If the horse remains lame after rest, or as an initial palliative therapy, intraarticular medication has been used.

Horses in which conservative treatment will be successful are not readily predictable at the time fracture occurs. Not all dorsal proximal phalanx fractures remain undisplaced and not all horses are rested immediately after fracture occurs. In consideration of the variables described above, arthroscopic surgery is recommended for this type of fracture (Fig. 107–2). Results for arthroscopic surgery for fractures of the dorsal proximal phalanx have been documented. Horses treated included those rested after injury and operated on within a few weeks, horses kept in race training after the fracture occurred with or without intraarticular corticosteroid treatment, and horses that had been rested a month or more after injury but had subsequently becoming lame when returned to race training. Arthroscopic surgery resulted in 82.6% of horses returning to athletic performance at least equal to that before injury.

The technique for arthroscopic surgery of the affected joint has several advantages over conservative therapy or arthrotomy. Both medial and lateral aspects of the fetlock and more than one fetlock may be safely operated in one procedure. Aftercare is minimal, with suture removal at about 10 days and lower limb bandaging for about 10 to 14 days. Two months' convalescence is recommended; however, horses have returned to training after convalescence of only 6 weeks.

Arthroscopic surgery does not result in periarticular enlargement or loss of joint motion. Should another injury occur, previous arthroscopic surgery will not adversely influence the ease of further surgical intervention.

DORSAL FRONTAL FRACTURES OF THE PROXIMAL PHALANX

Dorsal frontal fractures are an uncommon proximal phalanx fracture. Dorsal frontal fractures commence at

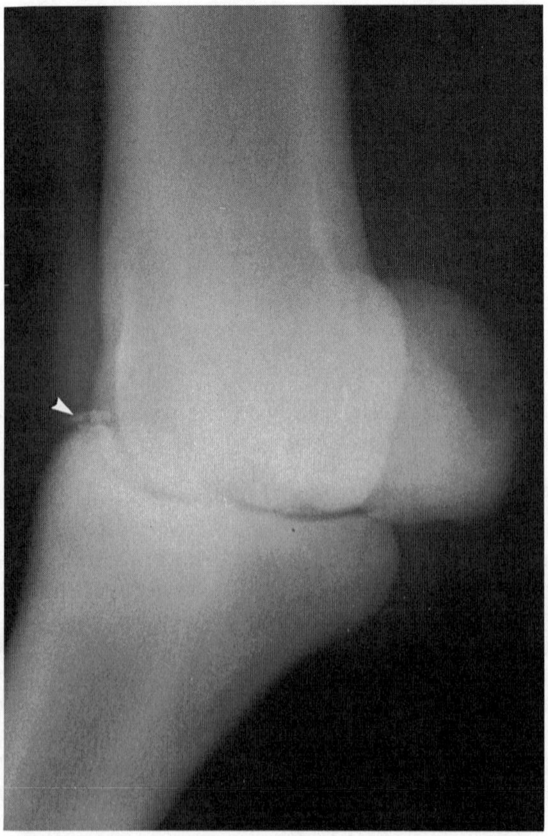

Figure 107–1. Medial oblique radiographic projection of the left front fetlock of a 2-year-old Thoroughbred. Note the osteochondral fracture of the medial aspect of the dorsal proximal aspect of the proximal phalanx (*arrow*).

the proximal dorsal articular surface of the proximal phalanx, extend in the frontal plane and, if complete, continue through the dorsal cortical surface. The fracture usually occurs during fast work. In one report, all dorsal frontal fractures occurred in the hind limb; however, this fracture type has been seen in the forelimbs. It is usually unilateral, but bilateral fractures are reported. In a series of nine cases, eight horses were Thoroughbreds and one was a Standardbred. Dorsal frontal fractures produce only a mild lameness with minimal synovial effusion. The lateromedial radiographic projection provides the best visualization of this fracture (see Chapter 118).

Therapy for this fracture depends on whether the fracture is complete and displaced or incomplete and nondisplaced. Complete and displaced dorsal frontal fractures should be treated surgically by lag screw fixation. A dorsal arthrotomy of the fetlock joint should be made to débride the fracture bed and allow fracture reduction. This can usually be completed with the arthroscope as well. The midportion of the fragment is approached via a stab incision in the long digital extensor tendon. The fragment is compressed to the parent bone with a 3.5-mm cortical bone screw inserted using the lag technique. Postoperatively the limb is kept in a support wrap and the horse is confined for 6 to 8 weeks. Bony healing of the fracture should be radiographically evident by 3 months following surgery, and horses can return to training at this time with a good prognosis for soundness.

Incomplete, nondisplaced dorsal frontal fractures may be managed conservatively. Bony healing of the fracture will be evident after 4 to 6 months of stall rest with a support wrap on the limb. Prognosis for soundness is excellent.

FRACTURES OF THE PROXIMAL PALMAR/PLANTAR PROCESS OF THE PROXIMAL PHALANX

Fractures of the palmar/plantar process of the proximal phalanx may be nonarticular or articular. Local swelling may be observed in the fracture area. Both nonarticular and articular fractures result in mild lameness at a trot. Flexion of the joint will exacerbate the lame-

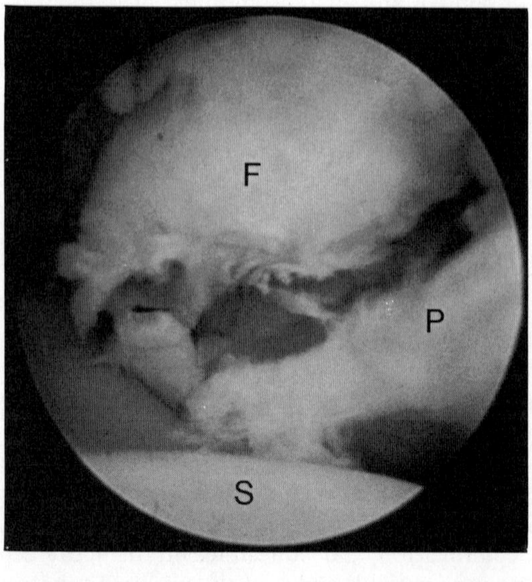

Figure 107–2. Osteochondral fracture of the dorsal proximal aspect of the proximal phalanx as viewed during arthroscopic surgery. *F*, osteochondral fragment; *P*, proximal articular margin of the proximal phalanx; *S*, midsagittal ridge of the distal third metacarpus. (Courtesy of Dr. C. W. McIlwraith.)

ness, particularly if the fracture is articular. Synovial effusion is more likely with an articular fracture. After a recent fracture, xanthrochromic synovial fluid may be obtained upon arthrocentesis in the case of an articular fracture. Intrasynovial anesthesia should relieve the lameness with an articular palmar/plantar process fracture. A palmar/ plantar nerve block will be required to resolve the lameness with a nonarticular fracture. Finally, radiographs are examined to determine if the fracture is articular. Consideration of clinical findings and the result of local anesthesia are important in cases in which the radiographs do not allow a definitive decision as to fracture location. The lateral plantar process is most commonly fractured.

Nonarticular palmar/plantar process fractures tend to occur in younger horses, often yearlings at pasture. Because this fracture type may also be an incidental finding, conservative treatment is recommended. Horses should be stall rested for approximately 1 month, followed by controlled walking or pasture exercise for 2 to 3 months. The prognosis for soundness is good to excellent, with a mean time to return to soundness being 3 months. Bony union of the fracture may occur, but a fibrous union is more common.

Articular palmar/plantar process fractures occur most frequently in horses about 3 years of age in race training. The most common presentation is a plantar process fracture in a Standardbred horse. Rest alone does not usually result in a permanent reduction in lameness after this fracture. Surgical removal of the fracture fragment is recommended.

To remove an articular palmar/plantar process fracture, the horse should be positioned in lateral recumbency with the fracture site uppermost. A vertical incision is made on the abaxial surface of the affected joint dorsal to the palmar/plantar neurovascular structures at the level of the proximal portion of the proximal phalanx. The distal portion of the annular ligament of the fetlock is incised and then the joint capsule is incised immediately distal to the collateral sesamoidean ligament and proximal to the proximal surface of the proximal phalanx. Exposure of the fracture fragment is achieved by flexion of the joint and retraction of the joint capsule. The fragment can then be dissected free. Occasionally, the fracture fragment will be large enough to repair by internal fixation using one or two cortical screws inserted in a lag fashion. Closure is routine and the annular ligament of the joint should be sutured in this procedure. After surgery, the limb should be kept in a support wrap for 2 weeks. One to 2 months' stall rest is recommended before pasture exercise is permitted. In one series, nine racehorses with this type of fracture were treated by fragment removal (eight cases) or internal fixation (one case). All horses became sound at a mean of 5 months after surgery. Linear abrasions on the articular surface of the distal third metacarpal/metatarsal bone were observed in seven of these horses at surgery. Apparently, this observation should not deter giving a favorable prognosis for return to athletic performance after surgery.

FRACTURES OF THE PROXIMAL PALMAR/PLANTAR ARTICULAR MARGIN OF THE PROXIMAL PHALANX

Although palmar/plantar articular process fractures can involve the articular margin of the proximal phalanx, this group of fractures is discussed separately for clarity. This section deals with osteochondral fractures from the palmar/plantar aspect of the proximal phalanx that arise axial to the processes and medial or lateral to the sagittal groove of the proximal phalanx.

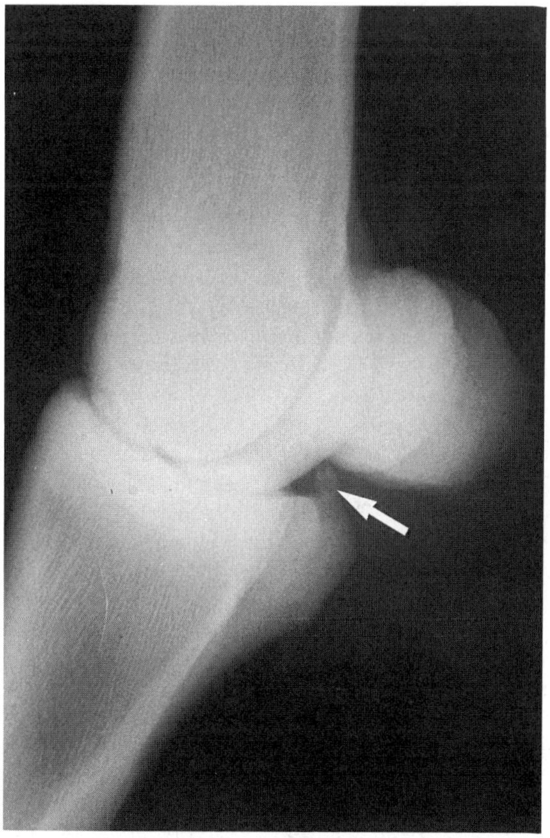

Figure 107–3. Oblique radiographic projection of the right hind fetlock of a 7-year-old Thoroughbred. Note the fracture from the plantar articular margin of the proximal phalanx (*arrow*). (Courtesy of Dr. C. W. McIlwraith.)

This fracture type has been observed in young horses prior to training, indicating the possibility of osteochondrosis as well as trauma as an etiology. Standardbreds are the most common breed affected. Lameness is first noticed when fast training is begun. Synovial effusion is variable, with some cases having marked distention while others have none. Flexion of the joint usually does not exacerbate the lameness. In the case of fracture in the hind limb, careful differentiation of lameness originating in the hock is necessary. Tarsal flexion may increase the lameness because of concurrent flexion of the metatarsophalangeal joint. Intrasynovial or regional anesthesia of the metatarsophalangeal joint will relieve the lameness and the exacerbation of lameness by hind limb flexion tests. In the forelimb, flexion tests and intrasynovial or regional anesthesia should localize the lameness to the metacarpophalangeal joint.

On initial radiographic examination the fracture fragments will be detected on the lateral-to-medial projection and sometimes the dorsopalmar(plantar) view. Oblique radiographic projections will highlight the fragments and confirm the side of the joint involved if the dorsopalmar (plantar) view is inadequate (Fig. 107–3). An oblique projection with the x-ray beam projected 15 degrees down from horizontal is useful to identify some fragments. Because this lesion type can occur bilaterally, the contralateral joint should be radiographed when a palmar/plantar proximal phalanx fracture is diagnosed. The medial plantar aspect of the proximal phalanx is the most common location for this fracture.

Conservative therapy and intrasynovial medication are generally not successful in maintaining or returning horses to optimal athletic performance with this type of fracture. Surgical removal of osteochondral fragments via arthrotomy or arthroscopy is recommended if the fragments are causing lameness. In either case, the horse is positioned in lateral recumbency with the side of the fracture uppermost. For removal by arthrotomy, a vertical incision is made through the palmar/plantar reflection of the joint capsule. Flexion of the joint improves exposure of the fracture; however, it may be necessary to extend the incision distally through the collateral sesamoidean ligament to permit removal of the fragment. Alternatively, the fracture fragment can be approached by an arthrotomy made at the level of the proximal surface of the proximal phalanx where it meets the distal metacarpal/metatarsal condyle and the base of the proximal sesamoid bone. This approach will also transect a portion of the collateral sesamoidean ligament. The fracture fragment is freed by sharp transection of its soft tissue attachments. Closure of the arthrotomy includes suture layers in the collateral sesamoidean ligament, subcutaneous tissue, and skin.

Fracture fragment removal by arthroscopy is less traumatic to the soft tissue than arthrotomy and is recommended. The arthroscope is inserted through the palmar/plantar joint capsule reflection between the suspensory ligament and the metacarpus/metatarsus. The joint must be flexed to allow passage of the arthroscope between the distal metacarpus/metatarsus and proximal sesamoid bones. A needle is used to locate an appropriate instrument portal, which is usually 4 to 5 cm distal to the arthroscope, passing through the collateral sesamoidean ligament. The joint capsule at the articular margin is probed to locate the fracture fragment. Once located, the fracture fragment is cut free using a sharp-ended elevator, a double-bladed tendon-splitting knife, or a Beaver blade. After separating the fragment, it is removed using rongeurs.

Postoperatively, bandaging of the limb is recommended for 7 to 14 days. Stall rest with controlled walking for about 1 month is suggested, with a return to training in 4 months after arthrotomy or 2 to 3 months after arthroscopic surgery. The prognosis for return to athletic soundness after treatment of this fracture is good to excellent.

BIBLIOGRAPHY

Barclay WP, Foerner JJ, Phillips TN: Lameness attributable to osteochondral fragmentation of the plantar aspect of the proximal phalanx in horses: 19 cases (1981–1985). *J Am Vet Med Assoc* 1987;191:855–857.

Bukowiecke CF, Bramlage LR, Gabel AA: Palmar/plantar process fractures of the proximal phalanx in 15 horses. *Vet Surg* 1986;15:383–388.

Copelan RW, Bramlage LR: Surgery of the fetlock joint. *Vet Clin North Am Large Anim Pract* 1983;5:221–231.

Haynes PF: Diseases of the metacarpophalangeal joint. *Vet Clin North Am Large Anim Pract* 1980;2:37–49.

Markel MD, Martin BB, Richardson DW: Dorsal frontal fractures of the first phalanx in the horse. *Vet Surg* 1985;14:36–40.

McIlwraith CW (ed): *Diagnostic and Surgical Arthroscopy in the Horse.* Edwardsville, KS, VM Publishing Inc, 1984.

Raker CW: Calcification of the equine metacarpophalangeal joint following removal of chip fractures. *Arch Am Coll Vet Surg* 1975;4:66–68.

Yovich JV, McIlwraith CW: Arthroscopic surgery for osteochondral fractures of the proximal phalanx of the metacarpophalangeal and metatarsophalangeal (fetlock) joints in horses. *J Am Vet Med Assoc* 1986;188:273–279.

108
Synovial Pad Proliferation in the Metacarpophalangeal Joint

Nathaniel A. White II

ANATOMY AND PATHOLOGY

The metacarpophalangeal joint has a synovial pad or plica at the dorsal joint recess. This pad covers the transition zone between the condylar cartilage and the attachment of the joint capsule of the third metacarpal bone, which is also the site of contact of the proximal rim of the proximal phalanx during full fetlock extension. The pad has a fibrous structure with a linear arrangement of fibrous connective tissue containing a small number of blood vessels. The pad normally tapers to a thin edge at the top of the metacarpal condyles. Although its function is unknown, its position and structure suggest that the pad acts as a cushioning surface or contact interface between the proximal phalanx and the third metacarpal bone where these are in contact during full extension of the joint.

The pad can become thickened and has been reported to form large nodules that are associated with lameness, effusion of the metacarpophalangeal joint, and

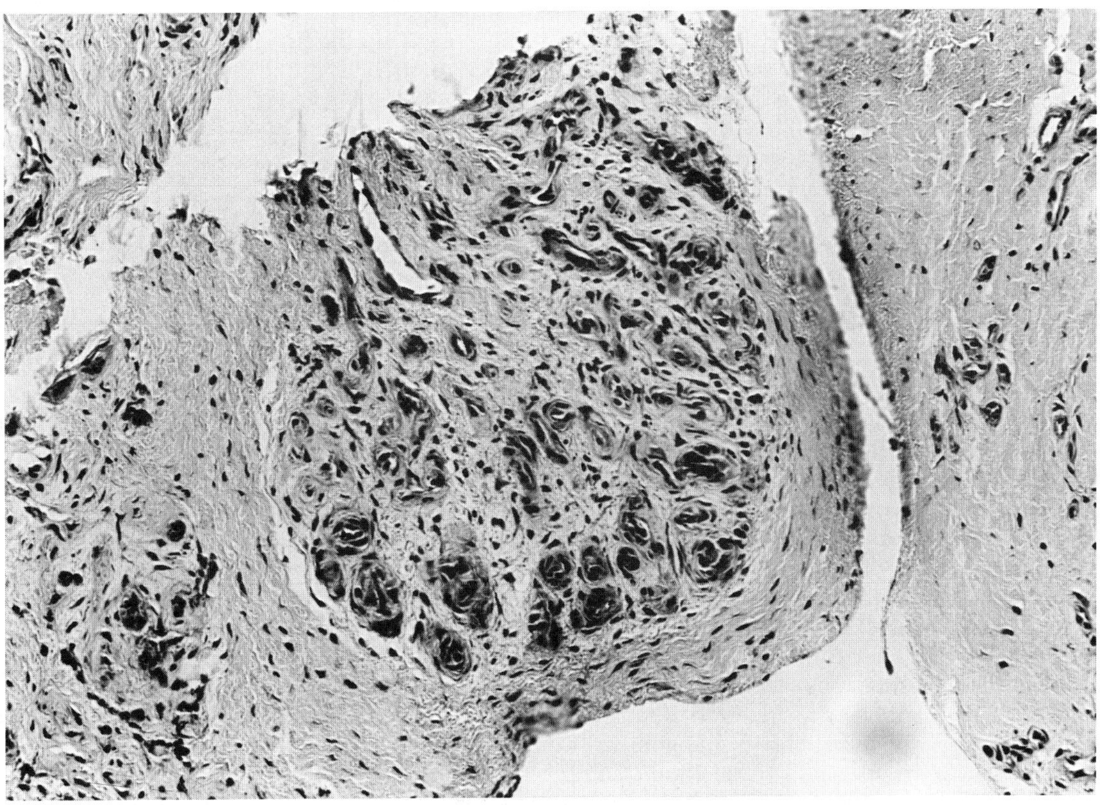

Figure 108–1. Nodules in the pad are rounded areas of fibroblastic and vascular proliferation. There are rarely any inflammatory cells within the tissue. The normal metacarpophalangeal synovial pad is composed of relatively acellular linear connective tissue similar to tendon or meniscus. The pad tapers to a thin border at its distal edge and is covered with a single layer of synovial mesothelium.

remodeling of the dorsal surface of the third metacarpal bone. This condition has been referred to as villonodular synovitis and may occur on either side of the sagittal ridge of the third metacarpal bone. The thickening may be swelling of the entire pad, which eliminates the normal tapered contour of the pad. Other changes that are seen include rounding of the edge of the pad and nodule formation within the body of the pad.

The nodules have two histologic features. One is fibrous proliferation along the edge of the pad and the other is nodule formation within the normal fibrous connective tissue. The nodules consist of fibrous tissue proliferation with increased vascularity, and an abundance of fibroblasts (Fig. 108–1). Centers of collagen necrosis within nodules have also been observed. These areas are characterized by loss of fibrocytes with no apparent fibrous or vascular reaction and a complete absence of an inflammatory response. Chondroid metaplasia and some dystrophic calcification occur in rare instances.

DIAGNOSIS

The fibrous proliferation with nodule formation is diagnosed most often in racing Thoroughbreds in association with proximal dorsal phalangeal fractures. Horses with synovial pad proliferation have chronic joint effusion and a history of poor performance or lameness. Horses often respond temporarily to intraarticular injection of corticosteroids or sodium hyaluronate when combined with rest. The relief is temporary because recurrence of joint effusion and lameness is common upon resumption of training or racing. Enlargement of the synovial pad is normally not visible on the dorsal surface of the metacarpophalangeal joint except in severe cases in which the nodule can be palpated or seen protruding from the dorsal surface of the joint. The swelling and nodule can be visualized during arthroscopic exploration of the dorsal surface of the metacarpal condyles.

Fibrous proliferation of the synovial pad and nodule formation can occur without concurrent chip fractures, although in these cases there is usually some cartilage erosion along the opposing rim of the proximal phalanx. The synovitis that normally occurs with the pad proliferation causes palpable fluid swelling of the palmar pouches and pain on fetlock flexion. Joint fluid analysis will often only reveal a nonspecific joint effusion.

Radiographically the pad cannot be seen without a contrast arthrogram. Occasionally the dorsal surface of the third metacarpal bone at the junction of the shaft of the bone and the condyles will be concave. This is not present in all cases and large nodules can be present without this finding. Although the condition may be suspected from plain radiographs, a definitive diagnosis can be made by contrast arthrography or ultrasound examination. The arthrogram utilizes a intraarticular injection of radiopaque contrast medium (Renographin; Solvay Veterinary, Inc). This will outline a thickened soft tissue mass or nodule that is otherwise not visible radiographically.

Ultrasound is less invasive and can also provide definitive information about synovial pad size and density and the character of the underlying bone surface. A real-time or linear ultrasound scan can be used. The real-time scan can image both a transverse and a sagittal view (Fig. 108–2). The normal pad has a thin, tapered edge and is less than 4 mm in thickness on the sagittal view (Fig. 108–3). The nodular shape of the pad

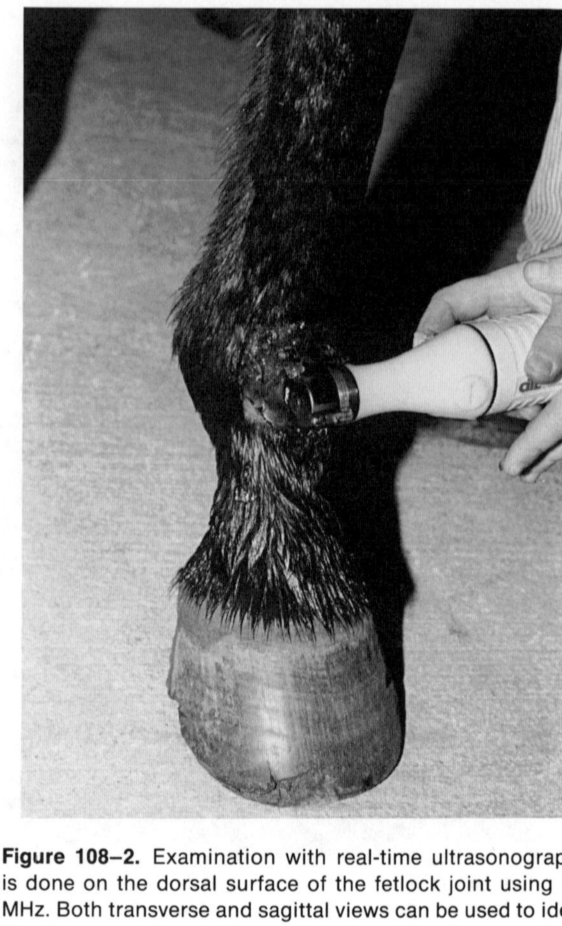

Figure 108–2. Examination with real-time ultrasonography is done on the dorsal surface of the fetlock joint using 7.5 MHz. Both transverse and sagittal views can be used to identify the synovial pad. The nodule formation is normally to either side of the sagittal ridge of the third metacarpal bone.

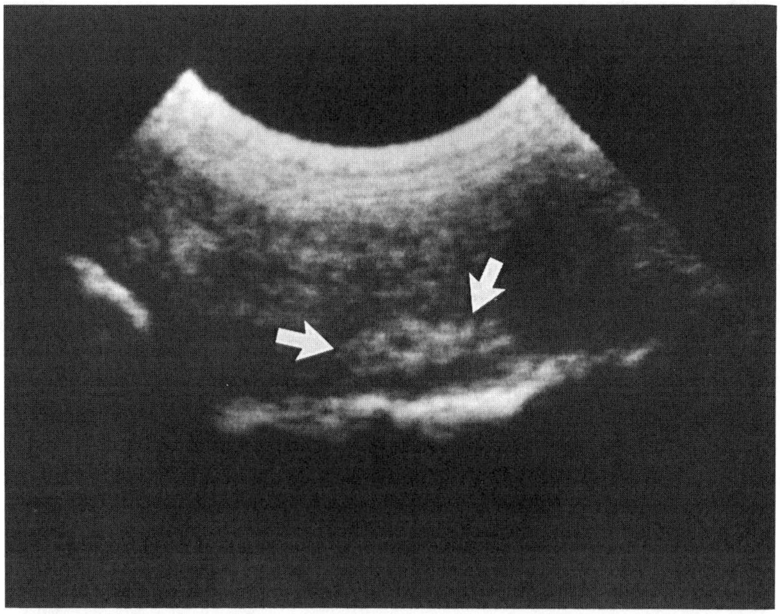

Figure 108–3. A normal sagittal ultrasonic view of the synovial pad (*arrows*). The pad tapers at its distal edge and has a uniform density except for a small hypoechoic region in the center of the pad.

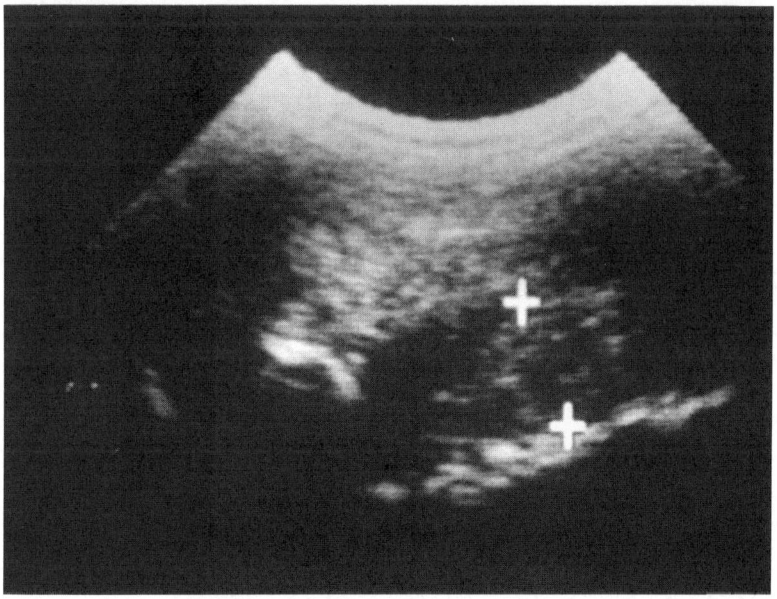

Figure 108–4. A sagittal view of an enlarged synovial pad (mass between the *crosses*) that is identified by increased thickness, rounding of the distal edge, and a hypoechoic region in the center of the enlarged mass.

can be outlined ultrasonically using a sagittal view (Fig. 108–4). Occasional hypoechoic areas seen within the pad are thought to be areas of new disorganized fibrous proliferation (Fig. 108–4). The region beneath the pad can also be visualized with ultrasound to identify the concurrent concave crater and roughening of the underlying third metacarpal bone.

Whenever chip fractures of the proximal rim of the proximal phalanx are diagnosed, acute inflammation or nodular enlargement of the synovial pad should be suspected. Synovial pad changes should also be suspected in horses with nonresponsive synovitis of the joint. There may be no radiographic evidence of joint disease in these cases.

TREATMENT

Removal of the affected portion of the synovial pad proliferation is the best treatment to assure a satisfactory response. The decision for surgical removal is usually made during removal of chip fractures. If no fracture is present and nodule formation is suspected, surgery is usually performed after failure of intraarticular anti-inflammatory therapy.

Although arthrotomy has been reported, the procedure should be done by arthroscopic removal to avoid formation of fibrotic scar tissue at the surgery site. The synovial pad is probed to determine the extent of thickening and the presence of a nodule. Generalized thickening of the synovial pad that remains elastic and resilient does not indicate removal. Fibrous proliferation, when probed, will be firm and inelastic. This may include the entire pad, a portion of the pad, or a focal nodule.

Removal of focal lesions can be done with a pituitary or laminectomy rongeur, leaving the unaffected portion of the pad intact. To remove the entire paid or a segment, two instrument portals may be needed, one for grasping the nodule and a second positioned dorsad to the first to insert a scissors or blade to cut along the attachment of the pad. In this way the entire pad can be removed. The bone beneath the pad is often soft and frayed. This bone should be removed by curettage to expose normal subchondral bone. There is evidence that the synovial pad does not regenerate. However, regrowth after two years has been seen in one case.

Medical treatment is symptomatic and can be used for temporary relief. Several horses I have managed surgically had not responded permanently to intraarticular therapy of sodium hyaluronate or corticosteroids but did respond to surgical removal. Once the nodular area was removed, joint effusion decreased or disappeared and horses returned to training and racing without soreness. Some horses continue to have some joint effusion but do not have lameness while training or racing.

The diagnosis of nodular proliferation can be associated with generalized joint degeneration. The horse should be carefully examined for other signs of joint disease before concluding that the synovial pad is the only reason for the soreness and effusion in the fetlock joint. In racing horses the synovial pad should be evaluated ultrasonically to determine if fibrous synovial pad proliferation is present.

BIBLIOGRAPHY

Jann HW, Fackelman GE, Koblik PD, Perdue BD: Electrosurgical arthrotomy and excision of soft tissue masses in the metacarpophalangeal joint of the horse. *Vet Surg* 1986;15:429–434.

McIlwraith CW: *Diagnostic and Surgical Arthroscopy in the Horse.* Edwardsville, KS, Veterinary Medicine Publishing Co, 1984, pp 74–77.

Modransky PD, Rantanen NW, Hauser ML, Grant BD: Diagnostic ultrasound examination of the dorsal aspect of the equine metacarpophalangeal joint. *Equine Vet Sci* 1983;3:56–58.

Nickels FA, Grant BD, Lincoln SD: Villonodular synovitis of the equine metacarpophalangeal joint. *J Am Vet Med Assoc* 1976;168:1043–1046.

Turner AS: Large animal orthopedics, in Jennings P (ed): *The Practice of Large Animal Surgery.* Philadelphia, WB Saunders, 1984, pp 832–833.

Van Veenendaal JC, Moffatt RE: Soft tissue masses in the fetlock joint of horses. *Aust Vet J* 1980;56:533.

White NA, Sullins KE, Spurlock SL, Parker GA: Diagnosis and treatment of metacarpophalangeal synovial pad proliferation in the horse (abstr). *Vet Surg* 1988;17:46.

109
Fractures of the Proximal Sesamoid Bones

Albert A. Gabel

The proximal sesamoid bones are an important part of the suspensory apparatus. They are bony bearings intercalated between the elastic suspensory ligament and the relatively inelastic distal sesamoidian ligaments (Fig. 109–1). The sesamoids articulate with the distal end of the third metacarpal/metatarsal bone when the foot is hyperextended (dorsiflexed) during weight bearing.

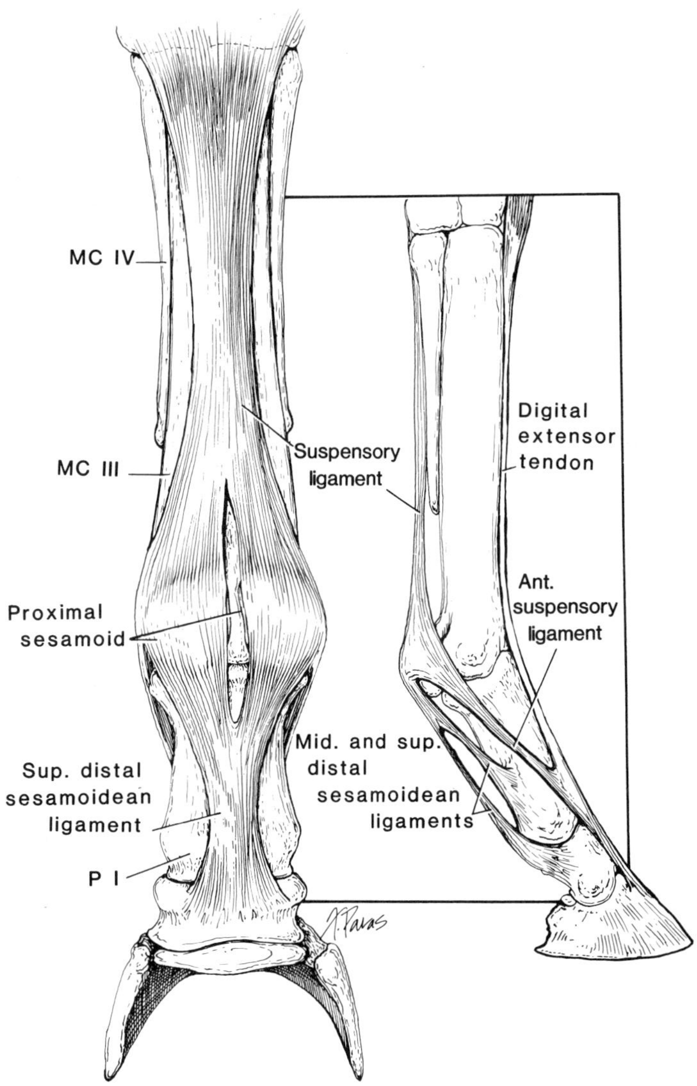

Figure 109–1. Drawing of the suspensory apparatus, including the suspensory ligament, the proximal sesamoid bones, and the distal sesamoidean ligaments.

Injury to any part of the suspensory apparatus can occur, depending on the breed, use, and degree of fitness of the horse, as follows:

1. Avulsion of part of the origin of the suspensory ligament, which occasionally occurs in young Standardbreds when they first race.
2. Sprain of the origin of the suspensory ligament, which occurs most commonly in horses used over fences and Standardbreds.
3. Midsuspensory ligament sprain, which occurs commonly in Standardbreds.
4. Sprain of a branch of the suspensory ligament, which is the most common lameness problem in Standardbreds except for sore feet.
5. Sesamoiditis, which occurs most commonly in toed-in or toed-out horses. It is not common, but is very serious. Even if the horse is rested for a long period, sesamoiditis often recurs when the horse is trained near race speed again.
6. Fractures of sesamoids.
7. Distal sesamoidean ligament sprains, which are not very common. They are seen mostly in racing Thoroughbreds and horses used over fences.

TESTING THE SUSPENSORY APPARATUS TO FAILURE

To test the strength of the suspensory apparatus, Standardbred and Thoroughbred limbs were placed in a weight-bearing position in a testing machine and tension was applied until fracture. The tension required to cause failure in the suspensory apparatus from horses in training was significantly higher than those from six horses not in training. In the horses not in training, 22 out of 24 limbs had either acute rupture of the suspensory ligament or insidious stretching of the ligament allowing the fetlock to sink to the ground with no specific area of ligament rupture. However, horses in training had 17 apical fractures, 2 basilar fractures, and 1 midbody fracture of the sesamoid when tension was applied to failure. Thus, exercise strengthens the suspensory ligament, allowing failure at the proximal sesamoids. However, my observations indicate that an exercise program in Standardbreds that includes much long slow work (jogging) followed by a cautious, gradual increase in speed work results in fewer sesamoid fractures in horses being trained for the first time.

SIGNALMENT

Generally the sesamoid bones fracture during fast work. In Standardbreds, the lateral rear sesamoids are most commonly affected, with a high incidence in horses training near race speed or in their early races. Trainers often want to believe that the horse kicked the stall wall at an angle to cause the fracture, but this is unlikely. If a horse suffers a fractured sesamoid before it does fast work, it is likely to be inherently unsound and unlikely to be a successful racehorse. There are significant fractures of sesamoids in the front legs of both Thoroughbreds and Standardbreds of all ages. Twisting of the leg on placement or uneven track surface may be a factor in these injuries.

HISTORY

The horse is usually lame after a workout or race, and is more lame by the next day. The area of the sesamoid may be swollen, and the proximal pouch of the fetlock is usually distended by the day after the fracture occurs. The branch of the suspensory ligament above insertion on the sesamoid is often swollen. Prognosis is better if the suspensory ligament is not injured. If a pressure bandage is kept on the limb, as soon as the injury is suspected, it is easier to palpate to determine if the suspensory ligament is damaged. Ultrasound examination of the suspensory ligament is also useful in determining the severity of the injury and the prognosis. Rarely, horses with small nondisplaced apical fractures, especially of the rear sesamoids, will show only mild lameness and no swelling will be evident. Except for these rare instances, it is easy to localize the injury.

Diagnosis is made by radiography. A dorsopalmar/plantar, lateral, and 45-degree oblique view in each direction should be taken to accurately assess the fracture (Fig. 109–2)

APICAL FRACTURE

Since the sesamoid bone heals poorly because of lack of periosteal and endosteal activity, all affected horses should have surgery. The fracture fragment heals to the parent bone very slowly with a weak fibrous union. After removal of the fragment the fibers of the associated branch of the suspensory ligament scar and reattach to the fractured surface of the bone. Therefore, a long period of rest or controlled exercise is required to increase the strength of this attachement if the horse is to stay sound with fast work.

The branch of the suspensory apparatus attaches to the proximal palmar/plantar and abaxial part of the sesamoid, at a point about halfway down the vertical dimension of the bone (Fig. 109–1). The larger the apical fractures the poorer the prognosis, since more of the fibers of the branch of the suspensory ligament must be cut from the fragment. It is unwise to remove the fragment if it is larger than one third of the vertical dimension of the sesamoid (i.e., approximately one fourth the mass of the bone).

SURGERY

General anesthesia and aseptic technique are required. An incision is made through the skin, fascia, and joint capsule from the apex of the proximal pouch to the attachment of the collateral sesamoidean ligament, which is at the level of the middle of the sesamoid bone. The incision should be in the middle of the pouch so neither the suspensory ligament nor the small vessels on the third metacarpal/metatarsal bone are damaged. When making the incision on the lateral pouch of the hind leg, great care should be taken not to cut the distal end of the great metatarsal artery at the proximal end of the incision. If it is accidently cut, the laceration should be sutured with continuous fine suture material.

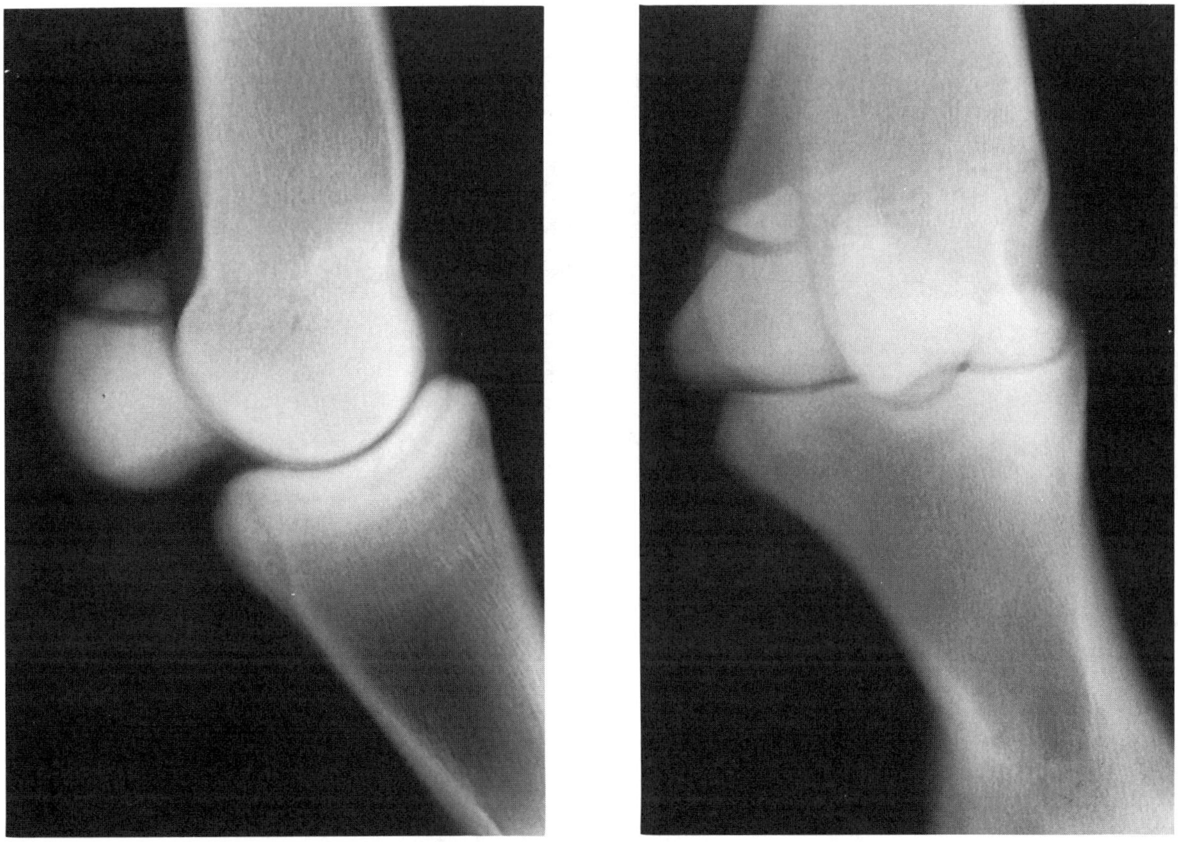

A B

Figure 109–2. An apical sesamoid fracture depicted in two views (**A,** 45-degree oblique; **B,** lateral). This is the most common fracture and is the most amenable to surgical treatment. Four well-marked radiographic views should be taken so any other fracture can be detected and so it is certain if the lateral or medial sesamoid is fractured.

Retraction of the incision by an assistant with a thyroid retractor on the sesamoid side and a knee retractor on the third metacarpal/metatarsal bone side is most satisfactory. Best exposure is obtained by partial flexion of the fetlock. This is best controlled by the surgeon using his/her abdomen against the foot, which is double draped with impervious material (sterile gloves). The fragment is removed using a no. 15 blade, a right-angle Beaver blade, and a meniscus knife (Fig. 109–3). When the fragment is nearly loose, a periosteal elevator can be used to pry it away so it can be completely cut free. The goal is to do as little damage as possible to the fibers of the suspensory ligament. The articular edge of the fracture of the parent bone should be curetted very conservatively and the joint lavaged thoroughly. The joint capsule is closed with 2-0 synthetic absorbable simple interrupted sutures that are preplaced, then tied. The subcutaneous tissue is sutured with a continuous 3-0 synthetic absorbable suture.

Postoperative Care

A pressure bandage should be used for about 3 weeks with bandage changes every 5 days, or sooner if the bandage becomes wet, dirty, or loosened. It would be best if the horses could start slow, gradually increasing exercise about 6 weeks after surgery to encourage reattachment (scarring) of the fibers of the suspensory ligament to the proximal fracture surface of the sesamoid. Since this can seldom be done safely, we recommend that the horse be kept in a stall and be walked daily for the first 3 months, then turned out until 6 months after surgery, at which time the horse can be put back in training. Racing should not be resumed until 11

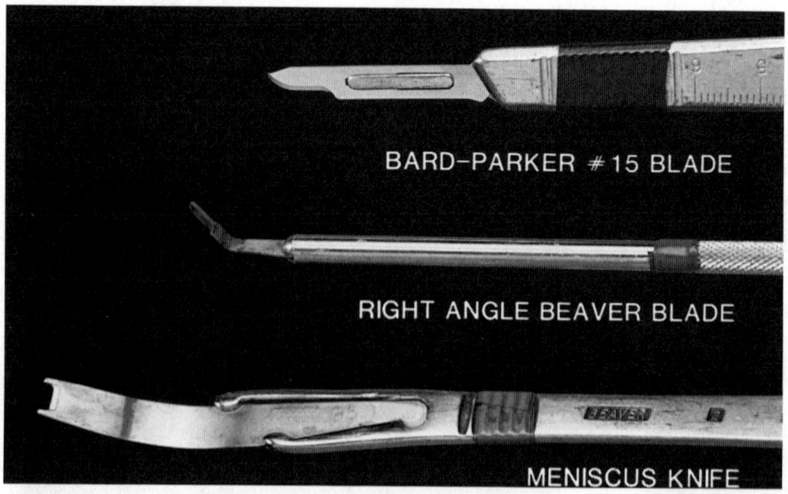

Figure 109–3. Instruments useful for sharp dissection of the apical fragment away from the suspensory ligament.

months after surgery. Follow-up radiographs are of little value in determining prognosis as the horse recovers, but should be taken if complications or slow return to soundness occur.

Prognosis

In a series of 80 Standardbreds in which apical fractures were removed, 45% had raced prior to the injury and 50% raced after the surgery. Sixty-four percent of the horses that raced before surgery raced again after surgery. Of the horses that had raced or trained near race speed, had no suspensory ligament damage, had not been jogged or trained after the injury, and had been operated on within 30 days of injury, 70% raced as well as before surgery or as well as would be predicted by the average of the population. Only 36% of horses with palpable suspensory ligament damage above the fracture site raced after the surgery.

Twenty-nine horses with apical fractures were treated nonsurgically. Sixty-nine percent had raced before injury, and 37% raced after injury. The performances of the horses that raced after injury was significantly poorer than their preinjury performance. However, there was bias in selecting patients for nonsurgical treatment.

It appears that the prognosis for horses with apical fractures of the front legs is poorer than for those with apical fractures of the rear legs. It is obvious that horses with apical fractures can be used for breeding without surgery if no major injury has occurred.

MIDBODY FRACTURES

Midbody fractures of both sesamoids are often involved in breakdown injuries of racing Thoroughbreds (Fig. 109–4). The treatment of such injuries is not addressed in this chapter (see Chapter 121).

Unilateral midbody fractures are much less common than apical fractures. The proximal fragment cannot be

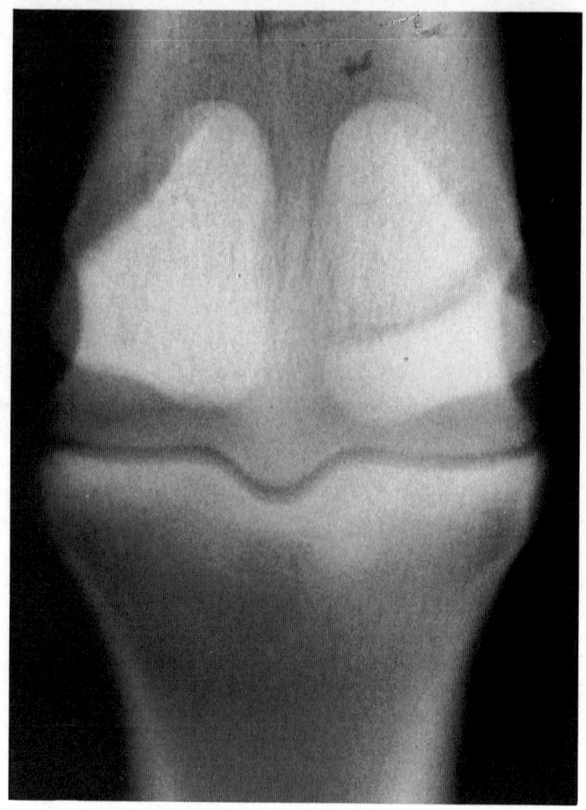

Figure 109–4. Midbody sesamoid fracture.

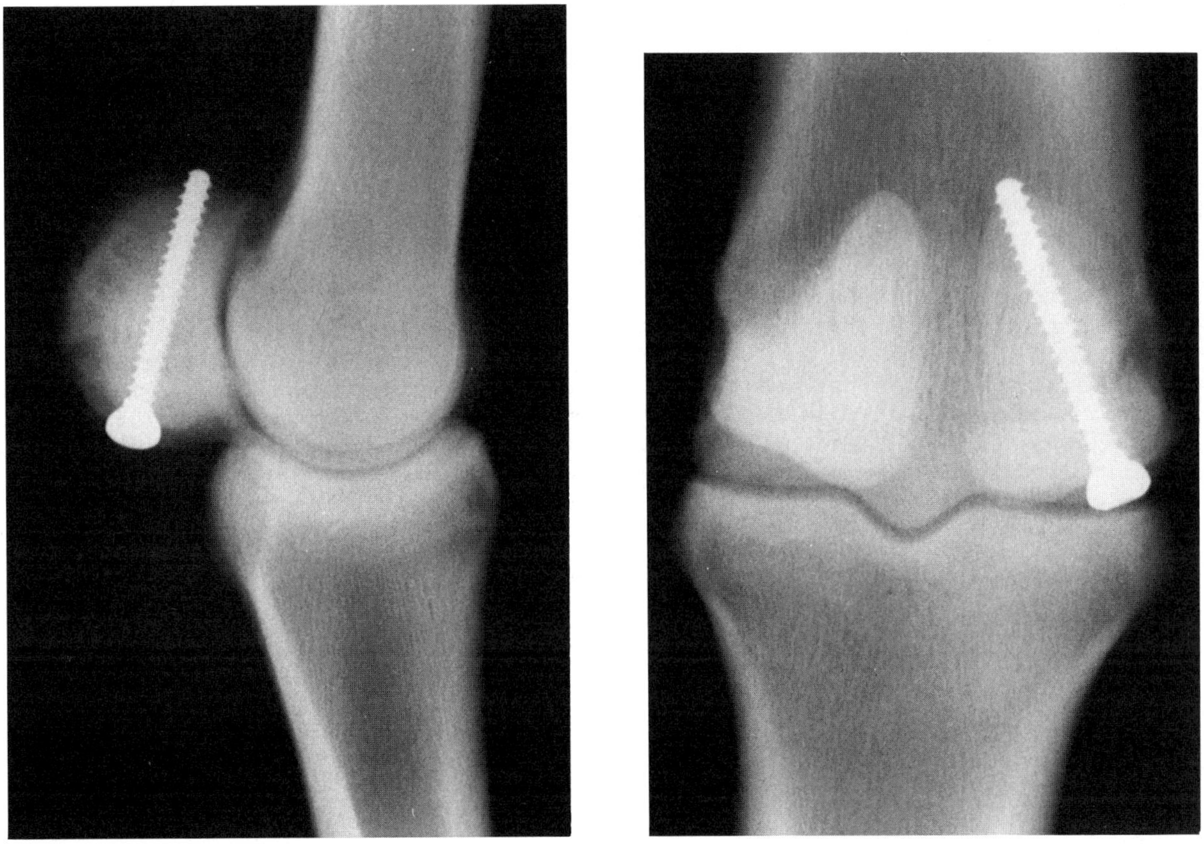

A B

Figure 109–5. Midbody sesamoid fracture after cancellous bone graft and application of a compression screw. **A.** Forty-five–degree oblique view. **B.** Dorsopalmar view.

removed successfully because it interrupts all or nearly all of the fibers of the associated branch of the suspensory ligament. Even with long periods of stall rest, the healing is by fibrous union, which cannot withstand the tension of the suspensory apparatus when the horse does fast work. Compression screws applied from either the distal or proximal aspect of the bone have been used to fix the two fragments together, but these techniques have not been very successful in getting horses to race profitably unless bone grafts are also used. Some success has resulted from using bone grafts alone with a caudal approach.

Surgery

The most successful surgical treatment of midbody fractures has been to place a bone graft between the fragments through an arthrotomy in the proximal pouch of the fetlock (Churchill approach) and to apply a compression screw from distal to proximal (Fig. 109–5). The incision used for removal of apical sesamoid fractures is made. This is a great help in accurately placing the screw whether or not the ASIF sesamoid clamp is used. Next, a second incision is made distal and abaxial to the fractured sesamoid, retracting the digital vessels and nerve caudally. The dissection is continued between the straight and cruciate ligaments of the sesamoid.

Methods of Placing the Screw. I prefer free-hand drilling using a 2-mm marker drill bit centered in the distal fragment. This drill bit is positioned 90 degrees to the fracture plane and aimed at the apex of the bone, which is palpated through the proximal incision. Dorsopalmar and lateral radiographs are taken and must be precise in all directions to prevent distortion. If it is not in the way, the marker drill is left in place while the 4.5-mm drill bit is used to make the glide hole in the distal fragment. There is difficulty in most cases in getting the drill axial and cranial enough to get the correct angle because of the bulb of the heel. Although it is usually best to severely extend the foot, in some cases severe flexion will solve this problem. The drill used should have a very small chuck to minimize interference with the heel. Long drill bits can also be used to prevent this interference. The distance from the end of the tissue protector guide to the chuck is measured when starting to drill to determine when the thickness of the distal fracture fragment has been penetrated. If this cannot be determined by the feel of the drill, a second set of radiographs are taken when the thickness of the distal fracture has nearly been penetrated. Since the position of this hole is somewhat deep in the tissue, a long Kirschner wire or 2-mm drill bit is placed in the hole when the 4.5-mm drill bit is removed. This makes it easier to place the 3.2-mm inside/4.5-mm outside diameter sleeve in the hole by rotating it over the Kischner wire or small drill bit. If there is distraction of the fragments, the fetlock is flexed or maneuvered to reduce the fracture. The 3.2-mm drill bit is then drilled through the sleeve through the apex of the sesamoid, the hole tapped, and the screw positioned in the glide hole. The countersink instrument is not used. Through the proximal incision, as much cancellous bone graft as possible is placed in the fracture gap using flat dental instruments, small periosteal elevators, or small retractors. It is easiest to take the graft from the medial side of the tibial plateau of the down leg, making a 4.5-mm drill hole and using a curette to scoop out the graft material.

If the ASIF sesamoid clamp is used, it is placed in the position of entrance and exit of the screw hole, using the same incision described above. After placing the clamp, it is essential that accurate dorsopalmar and lateral radiographs are taken to verify the location. There are drill sleeves for both the 4.5-mm and 3.2-mm drill bits in the clamp. Because they are shaped to fit only one side of the leg, a pair of these instruments should be purchased. Although they work satisfactorily, I find I do better with the free-hand method.

Dorsopalmar and lateral radiographs are taken to check screw length (usually 36 to 38 mm) and reduction of the fracture before closing the incisions. In some cases surgeons elect to recover horses from anesthesia with the leg in a cast up to the carpus or hock following repair, to prevent fracture of the repaired bone. Although a safety precaution, this is not necessary if the bone is well reduced and fixed.

Postoperative Care

The limb should be bandaged for 3 weeks after surgery. Stall rest and controlled walking should be the only activity for at least 3 months, and the horse should be sound when trotted on a lead shank before it is put in a small paddock alone. The horse should not be put back in training until at least 8 months after surgery, and should be given gradually increasing work so it races no sooner than 14 months after surgery. Follow-up radiographs are of some value in determining progress and prognosis, but the appearance of nonarticular mineralization should not be cause for alarm if the horse is sound on a sensible schedule of rehabilitation.

Prognosis

If screw compression repair is done without bone grafting, the prognosis is poor. If bone grafting is included, it appears that nearly 70% of the horses will race again, provided cases are selected in which severe distraction of the proximal fragment has not occurred, and the surgery is done within a few weeks of the injury. Hind limb fractures have a better prognosis.

The only alternative management of these cases is a long period of stall rest, which results in a fibrous union that usually results in a horse satisfactory for breeding. Horses with "breakdown injuries" that include fractured sesamoid(s) should be treated by arthrodesis of the fetlock joint.

BASILAR SESAMOID FRACTURES

Basilar sesamoid bone fractures are most commonly seen in the front limb of racing Thoroughbreds and usually cause severe lameness (Fig. 109–6). Surgical treatment appears to improve the prognosis little compared to a long period of rest. Horses often race again but become unsound after racing. Horses with very small distal fragments that appear to be nonarticular can often race satisfactorily after a period of rest to allow the associated ligaments to heal. Horses with larger *T*-shaped fractures have very little chance of returning to racing. The distal sesamoidean ligaments heal poorly and tend to become painful when strenuous exercise is resumed. The prognosis for basilar fractures probably depends on the degree of damage to the distal sesamoidean ligaments regardless of method of treatment.

Surgical Techniques

Removal of Fragment. The surgical approach for removal of basilar sesamoid fracture fragments is similar to that for apical sesamoid fractures. The incision should be continued distally through the collateral ligament of the sesamoid. Sharp dissection during flexion of the limb permits removal of the fragment through the joint. Alternatively, the fragments can be dissected

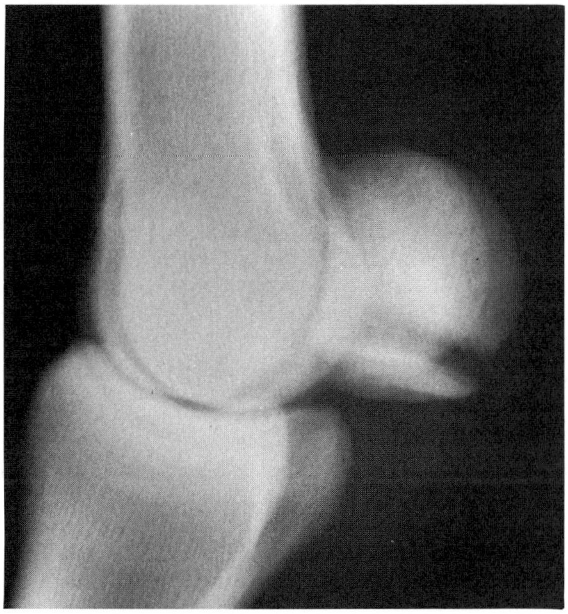

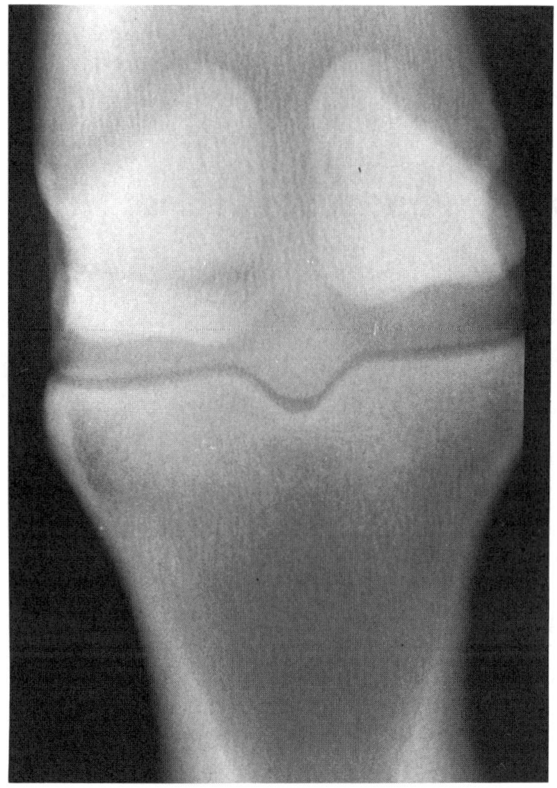

Figure 109–6. Basilar sesamoid fracture. **A.** Forty-five–degree oblique view. **B.** Dorsopalmar view.

free from the distal sesamoidean ligaments by a distal approach similar to that used for screw placement in midbody fractures. A method to remove the basilar fragment by approaching the fractured proximal sesamoid bone on the abaxial aspect of the fetlock and severing the collateral ligaments has been advocated as being less traumatic than the palmar or plantar approach.

Bone Grafting. The use of cancellous bone grafts to stimulate healing of these fractures and substantially improve the prognosis has been reported. A vertical incision should be made through the skin only, directly over the digital vein over the fractured sesamoid, and continued through the fascia a few millimeters palmar/plantar and axial to the digital vein, artery, and nerve. These structures should be retracted dorsally. Needles can be used to locate the fracture line and, if necessary, to outline the sesamoid bone. Radiographs may be taken if necessary. An incision then should be made through the fibrous tissue to the fracture line and a small periosteal elevator inserted into the fracture line horizontally, then rotated 90 degrees vertically to distract the fracture. Cancellous bone is packed in the fracture site. The fibrous layer should be sutured meticulously with strong nonabsorbable suture and the fascia and skin sutured routinely and bandaged.

Postoperative Care

Regardless of how basilar sesamoid fractures are treated, the return of the horse to exercise should be very conservative. Horses should be turned into a small paddock alone after 3 months or more of rest only if they are sound when trotted on firm ground.

ABAXIAL SESAMOID FRACTURES

Many abaxial sesamoid fractures are nonarticular and best managed conservatively with stall rest until the lameness subsides. Articular abaxial fractures that do not involve a large part of the insertion of the suspensory ligament branch should be removed. Some large articular abaxial sesamoid fractures can be repaired by screw fixation. Small articular fragments may be removed by arthroscopic visualization through the palmar/plantar joint pouch.

SAGITTAL SESAMOID FRACTURES

Sagittal sesamoid fractures usually occur with condylar fractures and have a poor prognosis for future athletic performance. Some can be repaired by screw fixation.

CONCLUSION

A proximal sesamoid bone injury must be considered as an injury to the suspensory apparatus rather than only an injury to the bone. Treatment must be aimed at normalizing the suspensory apparatus. In injuries of the sesamoid bones, fibrous repair is unacceptable since the horses will become unsound when they race. The aim of any surgical treatment must be to obtain functional reconstruction of strength of the suspensory apparatus without further sacrificing any normal structures.

BIBLIOGRAPHY

Barclay WB, Foerner JJ, Phillips TN: Axial sesamoid injuries associated with lateral condylar fractures in horses. *J Am Vet Med Assoc* 1985;186:278–279.

Bramlage LR: Autologous cancellous bone grafting in the horse. *Proc Am Assoc Equine Pract* 1981;27:243–247.

Bramlage LR, Gabel AA, Hackett RP: Avulsion fractures of the origin of the suspensory ligament in the horse. *J Am Vet Med Assoc* 1980;176:1004–1010.

Bukowiecki CF: A comparison of three different methods of the repair process of midbody sesamoid fractures in the horse. Read before the 20th Annu Meeting of the ACVS, Feb, 1985.

Bukowiecki CF, Bramlage LR, Gabel AA: *In vitro* strength of the suspensory apparatus in training and resting horses. *Vet Surg* 1987;16:126–130.

Churchill EA: Surgical removal of fracture fragments of the proximal sesamoid bone. *J Am Vet Med Assoc* 1956;128:581–582.

Copelan RW, Bramlage LR: Surgery of the fetlock joint. *Vet Clin North Am Large Anim Pract* 1983;5:221–233.

Fackelman GE: Compression screw fixation of proximal sesamoid fractures. *J Equine Med Surg* 1978;2:32–39.

Fackelman GE, Nunamaker DM: *Manual of Internal Fixation in the Horse*. New York, Springer-Verlag, 1982, pp 53–55.

McKibbin LS, Armstrong KN: Bone screws as a method of immobilizing sesamoid fractures. *Proc Am Assoc Equine Pract* 1970; pp 203.

Medina LF, Wheat JD, Morgan JP, Pool R: Treatment of basal fractures of the sesamoid bone in horses using an autogenous bone graft. *Proc Am Assoc Equine Pract* 1980; pp 345–380.

Sevelius F, Tufvesson G: Treatment for fracture of the sesamoid bones in horses. *J Am Vet Med Assoc* 1963;142:981–988.

Spurlock GH, Gabel AA: Apical fractures of the proximal sesamoid bones in 109 Standardbred horses. *J Am Vet Med Assoc* 1983;183:76–79.

Wheat JD, Rhode EA: Surgical treatment of fractures of the proximal sesamoid bones in the horse. *J Am Vet Med Assoc* 1958;132:378–382.

110
Carpal Bone Fractures

Dean W. Richardson

Carpal chip and slab fractures are almost exclusively an injury of the racehorse. Most occur in younger horses and there are very distinct sites of predilection. In Thoroughbreds and Ouarter Horses, the distal radial carpal bone (Fig. 110–1), distal lateral radius (Fig. 110–2), and proximal intermediate carpal and proximal third carpal bones (Fig. 110–3) are the most common sites of fracture. In Standardbreds, lesions are almost uniformly restricted to the distal radial carpal bone and proximal third carpal bone. Steeplechasers and other jumpers have a higher prevalence than other athletic horses of fractures involving the accessory carpal bone or other bones on the palmar aspect of the carpus. Comminuted fractures can occur as accidents at pasture in horses not used for racing. Other types of carpal fractures are uncommon in these horses.

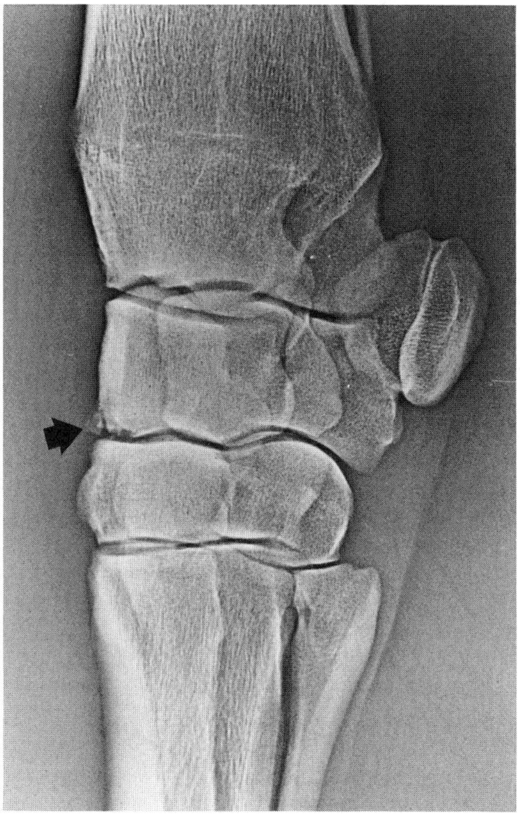

Figure 110–1. Xeroradiograph of a displaced distal radial carpal chip fracture (*arrow*). This is the most common fracture found in Thoroughbred and Quarter Horse racehorses.

DIAGNOSIS

The history and presenting clinical signs associated with carpal fractures are widely variable depending on the specific type of fracture. A horse with a small distal radius chip might cool down from a race and be mildly lame with a slight effusion. This horse may be sound enough to train in a day or two. A horse with a more serious fracture, such as a displaced slab fracture of the third carpal bone, will be much more lame and remain so for a longer time. Horses with comminuted fractures are usually non–weight bearing. A misleading history that is frequently associated with chronic carpal fractures is that the horse has "big knees" because of banging them on the stall wall. Such activity is an unlikely cause of carpal chip fractures.

Clinical signs include lameness, effusion, and pain upon flexion in most cases, but occasionally the primary complaint will only be decreased performance, a widened shuffling gait, or a tendency to lug in or bear out away from the affected side. Diagnosis in horses with obvious localizing pain and swelling is made with radiographs. In more subtle cases, intraarticular anesthesia is necessary to localize the cause of the lameness prior to taking radiographs. A complete series of high-quality radiographs is essential. In most cases, standing and flexed lateral-to-medial views, both oblique projections and a flexed tangential view ("skyline"), of the distal carpal row are recommended. Occasionally, dorsopalmar views or tangential projections of the proximal joint are needed to identify a fracture. Finally, arthroscopy can be used to confirm the presence, extent, or degree of displacement of a fracture and associated cartilage damage.

SURGERY

The anatomy of the dorsal aspect of the carpus is quite straightforward and easy to master using either arthrotomy and arthroscopy. The broad extensor carpi ra-

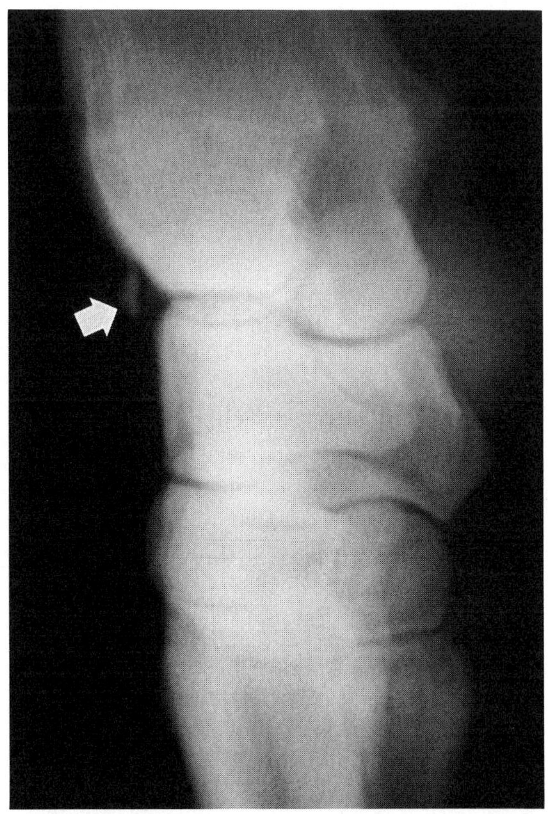

Figure 110–2. Typical displaced chip fracture (*arrow*) of the distal dorsal lateral aspect of the radius.

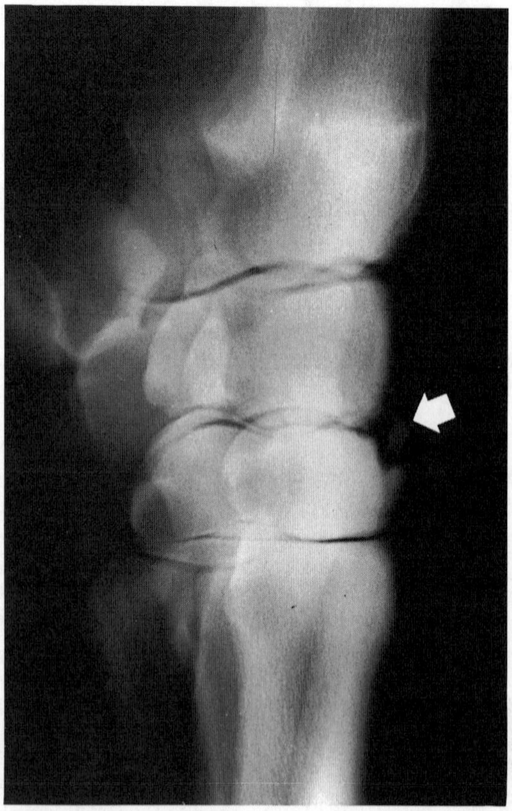

Figure 110–3. Wedge-shaped fracture (*arrow*) of the proximal dorsal medial aspect of the third carpal bone. Such fractures are most common in Standardbreds.

dialis tendon with its synovial sheath covers the middorsal aspect of the joint, and the common digital extensor tendon with its smaller sheath is parallel and a few centimeters lateral to it. The two most common sites of entry to the carpus are either side of the extensor carpi radialis tendon. Less frequently used are the spaces lateral to the common digital extensor tendon and an outpouching proximal to the head of the fourth metacarpal bone. The anatomy of the palmar aspect of the carpus is more complex and fortunately is seldom approached. If necessary, most structures on the palmar aspect of the carpus can be approached by dissecting through the carpal canal.

Arthroscopy has replaced arthrotomy as the preferred technique for all routine carpal surgeries. Major reconstruction of large fragments remains the primary exception to this rule. Arthroscopy offers the advantages of superior evaluation of both hard and soft intraarticular tissues, decreased tissue trauma, the ability to easily operate multiple joints, decreased chance of infection or wound problems, more rapid return to function, better cosmetic appearance, and (with practice) shorter surgical times.

Chip Fractures

Because a general principle of arthroscopy is not to insert the arthroscope close to the lesion, the horse should be positioned either in dorsal recumbency or in lateral recumbency with the suspect site away from the surgeon. For a routine distal radial carpal chip, the arthroscope portal is made midway between the two extensor tendons and the instrument portal is 10 to 12 mm medial to the edge of the extensor carpi radialis tendon. With the carpus slightly flexed, sterile saline or polyionic fluid is infused through a 20-gauge needle until the joint is firmly distended. A 5- to 6-mm skin incision is then made for the arthroscope portal and the cannula with its sharp trocar is used to penetrate the joint capsule. The sharp trocar is replaced by the blunt obturator and the cannula is positioned further across the joint. The arthroscope is then inserted and a complete visual inspection of the joint is performed. The visual examination is easiest at that time because joint distention is maximal and hemorrhage is minimal before the instrument portal is made.

A no. 11 scalpel is used to make the instrument portal. The location of the instrument portal is selected by observing the interior wall of the joint while externally palpating or by placing a small-gauge needle into the joint prior to making the incision. In addition, it is helpful to pass the scope medially and transilluminate the joint from the interior so that larger blood vessels can be avoided. The incision should be *V* shaped, widest at the skin and quite small through the capsule. Grasping forceps (Schlesinger Intervertebral Disc Rongeurs, 5-in shaft, serrated jaws, 3 × 10-mm bite; Scanlan Surgical Instruments Inc) or rongeurs (Ferris Smith Rongeurs, 7-in shaft, 4 × 10-mm bite; Scanlan Surgical Instruments Inc) are used to remove any loose fragments of bone and cartilage. A curette or motorized burr is used to cut back undermined or focally degenerate cartilage to healthy margins. Extensive débridement or motorized abrasion arthroplasty of large areas of the carpal bones is generally not performed unless the cartilage is very seriously damaged or poorly attached to the subchondral bone. If a narrow rim of normal cartilage along the dorsal surface of the bone (particularly the third carpal bone) remains after débridement, it also is removed since subsequent stress concentration and fracture may occur there. The joint is thoroughly lavaged to remove any floating fragments and the skin is sutured.

Surgery of the intercarpal joint is easier than that of the radiocarpal joint because there are fewer and smaller blood vessels, a more capacious joint capsule, and a relative flat surface along the proximal surface of the distal row of carpal bones. Most lesions are well predicted from the radiographs, but osteophytes and fractures from the dorsal lateral corner of the radial carpal bone and dorsal medial corner of the intermediate carpal bone are frequently found as "surprises." So-called incomplete slab fractures that are seen only on the tangential view (Fig. 110–4) usually are found to be linear, ovoid, or even circular areas of degenerate cartilage with crumbling subchondral bone. Débridement of the loose bone and cartilage can result in dramatic improvement postsurgically. Screw fixation is not indicated since no evidence of a complete fracture line is seen. A normal fibrous band exists that extends from the second carpal bone and medial joint capsule to the juxtaarticular surface of the distal dorsal radial carpal bone. It varies slightly in prominence and position between horses but should not be mistaken for a pathologic adhesion.

The radiocarpal joint is generally operated with the limb more extended because the rim of the distal radius, where chips frequently occur, may be obscured during flexion. "Kissing" lesions of the proximal intermediate or radial carpal bones are extremely common and may be almost entirely cartilaginous, and hence not evident on the preoperative radiographs.

Slab Fractures

Slab fractures of the third carpal bone occur in three forms: fractures in a frontal or nearly frontal plane (Fig. 110–5), fractures of the lateral corner of the third carpal bone (Fig. 110–6), and sagittal or near-sagittal fractures (Fig. 110–7). The frontal fractures always involve the radial facet, but larger fragments can extend across the intermediate facet. The larger the slab fragment is, the more likely it is that there are other fractures, particularly off the distal palmar radial carpal bone. Treatment options include rest, internal fixation, and fragment removal. Rest as the sole therapy is indicated only in nondisplaced fractures, and even in those instances some decrease in healing time and improvement of articular healing may be obtained with lag screw fixation. Usually a minimum of 6 months' rest is necessary, and frequently it is a year or more before the horse is able to race again.

Lag screw fixation of third carpal slab fractures can be done under arthroscopic visualization or directly via arthrotomy. Bone screws 3.5 mm in diameter (3.5-mm cortex screw with fine thread, catalog no. 204; Synthes Ltd) are preferred to the 4.5-mm screws because: (*a*) the screw head is smaller and rarely requires countersinking, (*b*) it is easier to place two or more screws when indicated, (*c*) the smaller screw is less likely to split thin fragments, and (*d*) satisfactory strength of fixation can be achieved in most cases. The 4.5-mm screws are used when fragments are extremely large or unstable because of comminution along the fracture line. Lag screw fixation under arthroscopic control involves defining the limits of the fracture with needles. A 3.5-in spinal needle is positioned to bisect the proximal articular surface of the fracture and to align the drill in the correct dorsal-to-palmar angle. The drill is centered in the proximodistal aspect between this needle and another small needle placed in the carpometacarpal joint just distal to it. The drill is kept perpendicular to the axis of the metacarpus and parallel with the directing needle. When centering the needle, the magnification of the structures close to the end of the arthroscope may create the illusion that the structures visualized

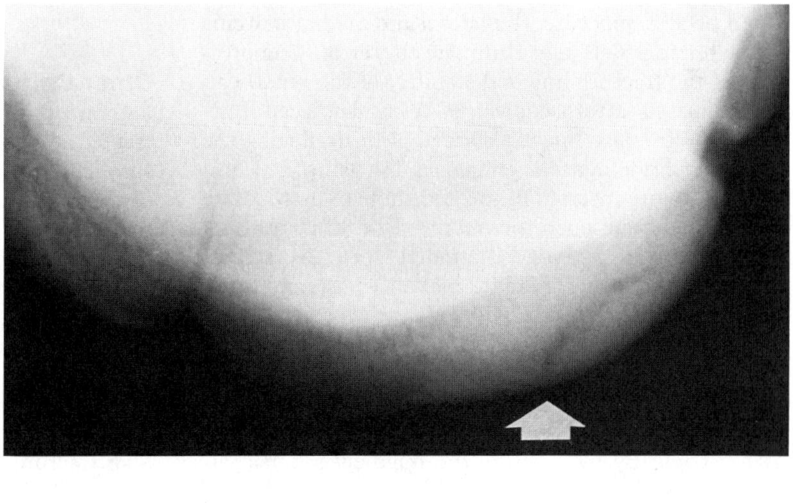

Figure 110–4. Radiolucent line seen on the tangential projection of the third carpal bone may be found at the time of arthroscopic examination to be a fracture involving only the proximal articular surface.

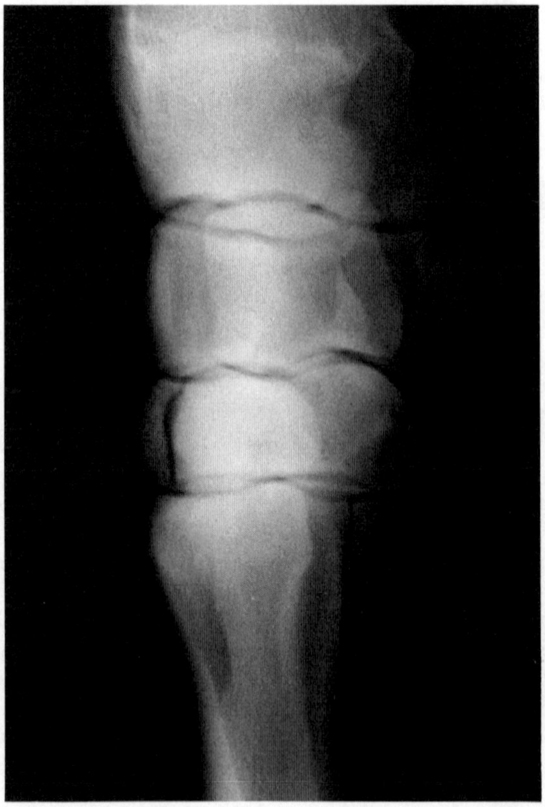

A

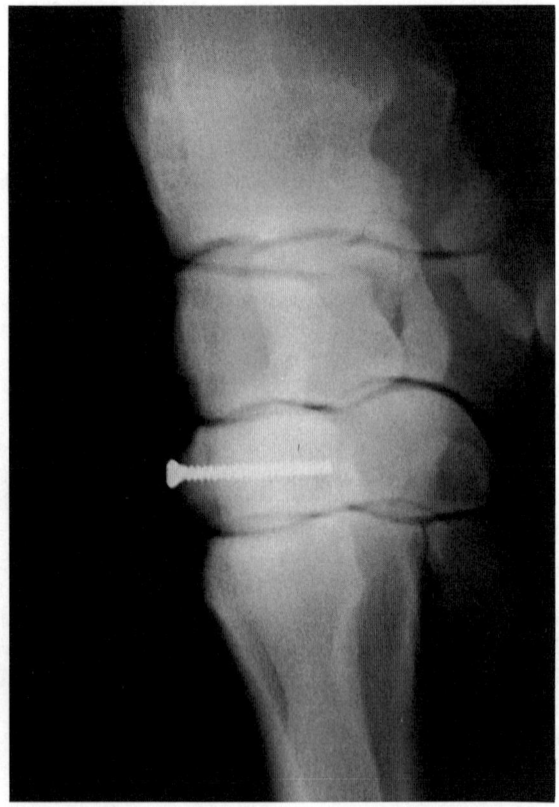

B

Figure 110–5. A. Dorsolateral-palmaromedial oblique projection demonstrating a typical slab fracture of the radial facet of the third carpal bone. **B.** Repair of a small frontal slab fracture with a single 3.5-mm cortical lag screw. Larger slab fractures require additional screws.

are farther away than they really are, causing the tendency to place the screw too close to that side. Two small needles placed at the lateral and medial margins of the fracture will help eliminate this error. Compression of the fracture line and stability of the repair can be evaluated arthroscopically. With displaced fractures, the fracture line is débrided prior to placing the screw. Debridement is enhanced by using a 3-mm Kirschner wire inserted in the glide hole to manipulate the fragment and open the fracture line. In larger fractures that extend beyond the radial facet, two screws are recommended for additional strength and rotational stability.

Removal of slab fracture fragments should be considered when the fragment is particularly thin or lytic (Fig. 110–8), comminuted, or otherwise unsuited for internal fixation. Slab fragments can be removed arthroscopically by severing the fragment's dorsal attachments, but the surgery is more easily performed through an arthrotomy.

Other Carpal Bone Fractures

Lateral corner fractures of the third carpal bone are treated similarly to slab fractures. They are usually smaller, rarely requiring more than one screw. Because of the size of the fragment and the screw head's proximity to the fourth carpal bone, the 3.5-mm screws should be used. Sagittal fractures are often nondisplaced and rest is frequently the selected therapy. Fractures that are truly sagittal propagate toward the articulation between the second and third carpal bones and can be repaired with a lag screw. Many fractures tend to parallel this articulation, which makes it impossible to place a lag screw perpendicular to the fracture line. Slab fractures of the fourth, radial, and intermediate

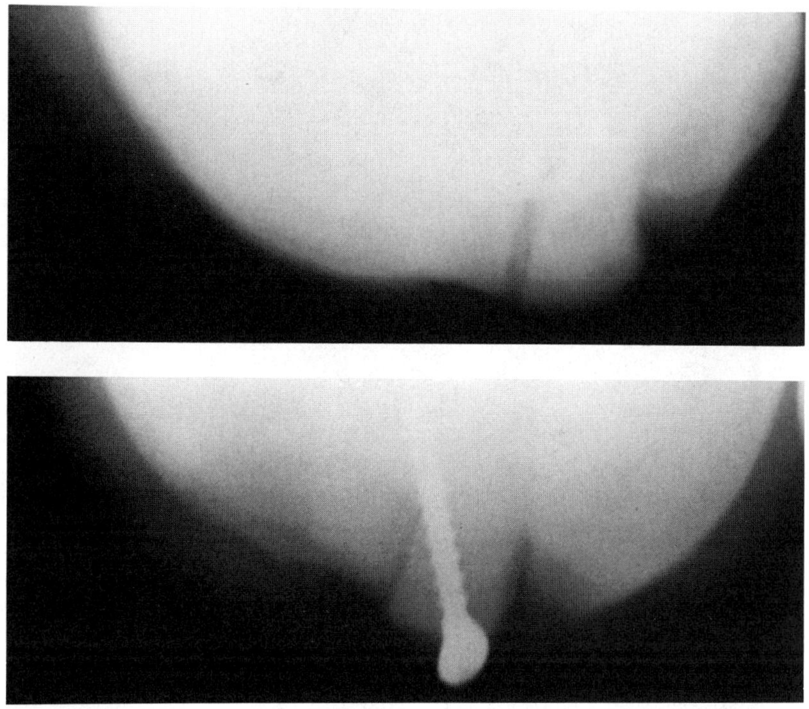

Figure 110–6. A. Lateral corner slab fracture of the third carpal bone. **B.** Repair with a single 3.5-mm lag screw.

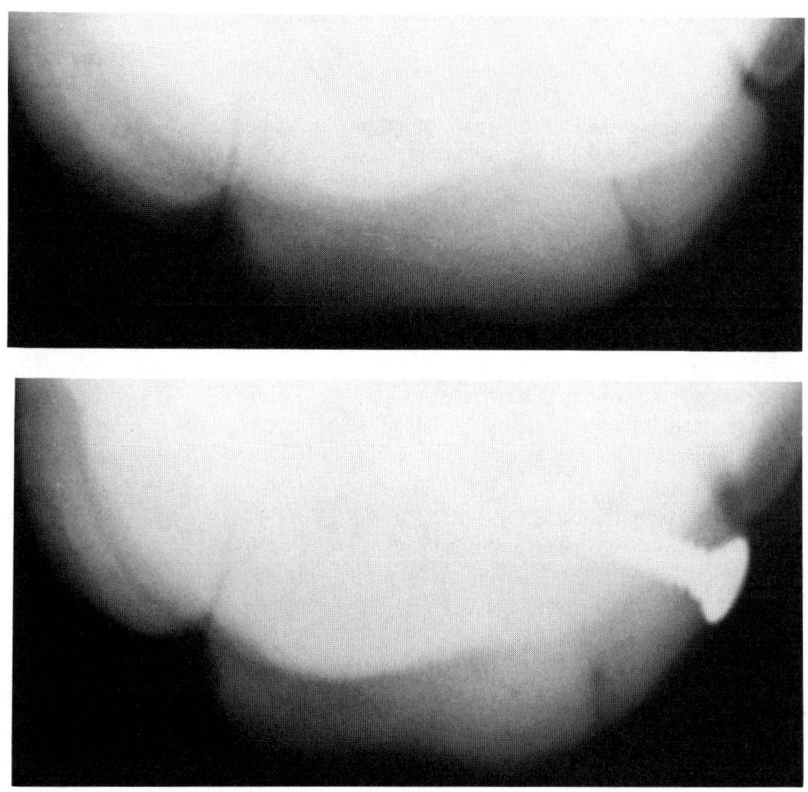

Figure 110–7. A. Tangential view of the third carpal bone demonstrating a near-sagittal fracture of the medial aspect of the third carpal bone. **B.** When such fractures are displaced, repair with a carefully placed lag screw is recommended.

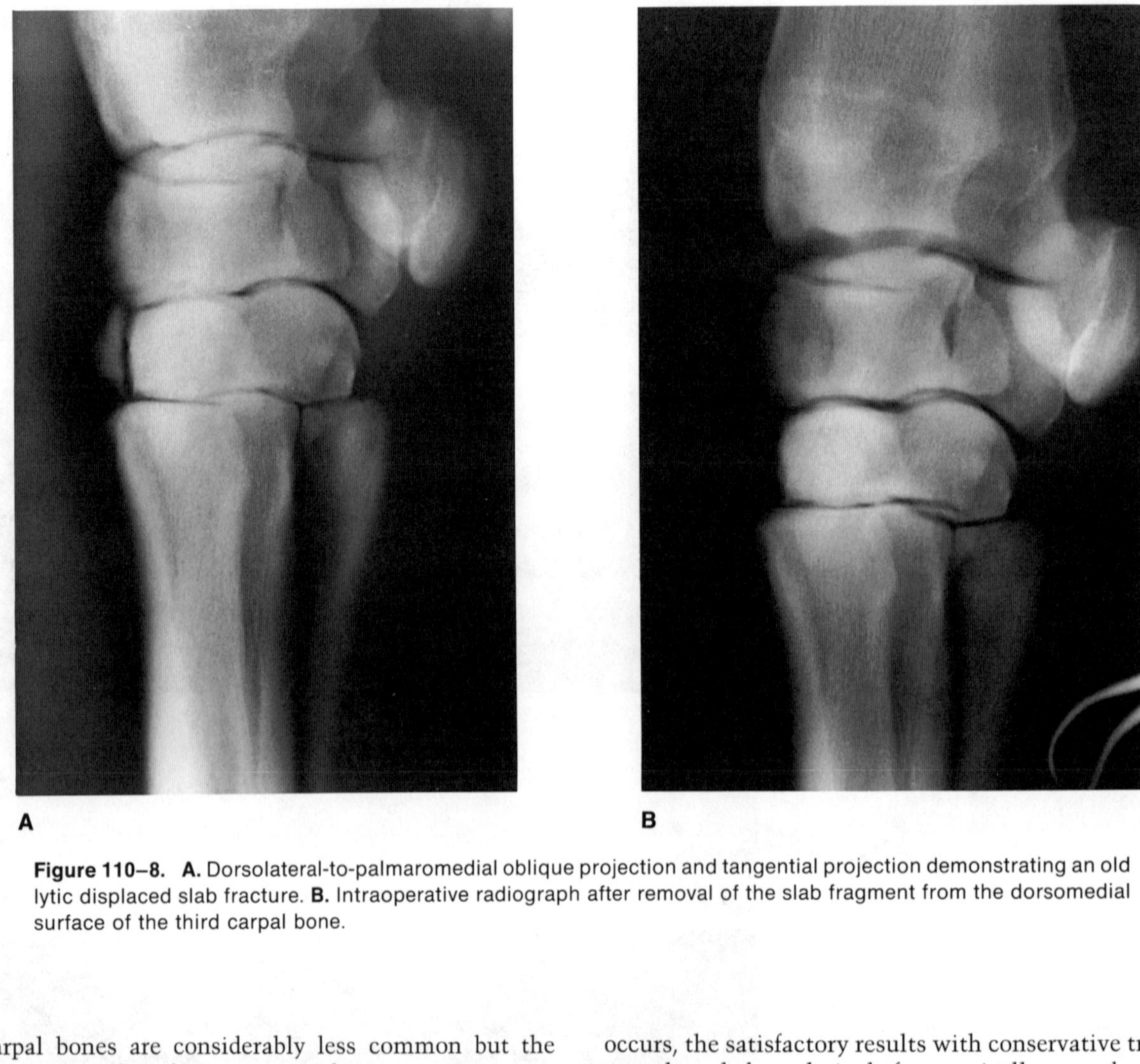

A B

Figure 110–8. **A.** Dorsolateral-to-palmaromedial oblique projection and tangential projection demonstrating an old lytic displaced slab fracture. **B.** Intraoperative radiograph after removal of the slab fragment from the dorsomedial surface of the third carpal bone.

carpal bones are considerably less common but the same principles of treatment apply.

Accessory Carpal Bone Fractures

Accessory carpal bone fractures are usually nonarticular and occur in a vertical and frontal plane. Comminution, especially at the proximal edge of the fracture line, is common. Horses usually have pronounced lameness immediately after injury but the lameness is reduced rapidly. Flexion may exacerbate the lameness and an effusion of the carpal flexor sheath may be present. A prolonged period of rest (usually about 1 year) will result in most horses becoming serviceably sound. There has been a technique described for internal fixation of these fractures with two lag screws using a specially designed C-clamp. Although theoretically there should be an advantage to internal fixation of these fractures since a fibrous nonunion generally occurs, the satisfactory results with conservative treatment have led to relatively few surgically treated cases.

Comminuted Carpal Fractures

Comminuted carpal fractures are life-threatening injuries and treatment is for salvage purposes only. If the fragments are large enough, stability of the carpus can be improved by lag screw reconstruction of the individual bones. If comminution is too severe, a pancarpal (radius to metacarpus) or intercarpal/carpometacarpal arthrodesis with plates and screws should be considered. If at all possible, the radiocarpal joint should not be fused since the functional result will be superior if the horse still has some flexion of the carpus. Simple external coaptation with bandages, splints, or casts is occasionally successful, but the extreme instability of these injuries frequently leads to severe rub sores, skin loss, infection, and nonunion. Even if the carpus fuses with this treatment, a severe carpus varus deformity often develops. With any selected treatment, laminitis of the contralateral foot is a common complication.

POSTOPERATIVE CARE

Postoperative care of horses with chip fractures treated arthroscopically depends upon the degree of articular damage. In simple, clean distal radial chips, the horse can begin walking or swimming 2 weeks after surgery and be returned to training 6 to 8 weeks postoperatively. More extensively damaged joints appear to benefit from additional time, but more than 4 to 6 months rest is rarely indicated following any chip fracture surgery. With arthroscopy, prolonged bandaging of the limb is not necessary because the swelling associated with the surgery resolves within a week in most cases. Phenylbutazone is given for a day or two following surgery to lessen pain and swelling. Antibiotics are not necessary in an otherwise healthy horse if aseptic technique is used.

Sodium hyaluronate (20 to 40 mg) is often administered intraarticularly a week or two following surgery. In horses with evidence of diffuse early cartilage damage, a series of three to five intraarticular injections of 250 mg polysulfated glycosaminoglycan (Adequan) is recommended. If multiple joints are involved or if the horse has had an adverse reaction to intraarticular drugs, three to five weekly or biweekly intramuscular injections of 500 mg polysulfated glycosaminoglycan are recommended.

In most horses, the postoperative morbidity is so low that a progressive swimming or walking program can begin 2 weeks or so following surgery. If there is extensive damage or postoperative pain, however, return to a complete range of motion can be achieved by daily passive flexion of the carpus.

Although postoperative radiographs should always be taken for medicolegal reasons, follow-up films before returning to training are not always useful. It is surprisingly difficult to predict success or failure by these films and, in most cases, the horse will be trained regardless. Horses with slab fractures, on the other hand, should be evaluated at about 2-month intervals since a reasonable estimate of healing can be made radiographically.

PROGNOSIS

All horses undergoing carpal surgery are at risk for a drop in level of performance or, if they have not previously raced, not reaching their previously predicted potential. The great majority of horses undergoing carpal surgery will return to race, although a significant proportion will drop in class. There is considerable room for doubt about the "true" prognosis associated with individual fractures. Some studies have shown no relationship between the location of the fracture and the outcome. Other reports and our own experience suggest that there is such a relationship. In particular, horses with small chips in the radiocarpal joint have a better prognosis (70 to 80% chance of performing successfully) than those with chips in the intercarpal joint (50 to 60%). In particular it appears that, of the common chip fractures, those involving the third carpal bone have the poorest prognosis.

In a recent retrospective study of 150 slab fractures in Thoroughbreds and Standardbreds, a definite correlation of various fracture characteristics with outcome was not found, although it appears that deep slab fractures (i.e., those with a wide dorsopalmar thickness) have a particularly poor prognosis. The presence of existing degenerative change in a joint with a third carpal slab or chip fracture does not preclude a successful outcome. It appears that the horse's racing ability proven prior to injury is the greatest predictor of success, irrespective of the method of treatment or fracture characteristics. A surprising result in this study was the relatively high success rate following slab fragment removal. In general, however, although a majority of horses will return to racing, a drop in class can be expected following a slab fracture repair.

BIBLIOGRAPHY

Easley KJ, Schneider JE: Evaluation of a surgical technique for repair of equine accessory carpal bone fractures. *J Am Vet Med Assoc* 1981;178:219–223.

Fackelman GE, Nunamaker DM: *Manual of Internal Fixation in the Horse.* New York, Springer-Verlag, 1982, pp 37–40.

Gabel AA: Selection of cases for carpal surgery and results, in *Proceedings of the 5th Annual Bain Fallon Memorial Meeting.* Sydney, Australian Equine Veterinary Medical Association, 1983, pp 134–139.

Lindsay WA, Horney FD: Equine carpal surgery: A review of 89 cases and evaluation of return to function. *J Am Vet Med Assoc* 1981;179:682–685.

McIlwraith WGC Yovich JV, Martin GS: Arthroscopic surgery for the treatment of osteochondral chip fractures in the equine carpus. *J Am Vet Med Assoc* 1987;191:531–540.

Palmer SE: Prevalence of carpal fractures in Thoroughbred and Standardbred racehorses. *J Am Vet Med Assoc* 1986;188:1171–1173.

Park RD, Morgan JP, O'Brien T: Chip fractures in the carpus of the horse: A radiographic study of their incidence and location. *J Am Vet Med Assoc* 1970;157:1305–1312.

Pendergast K: An analysis of the racing performance of horses following carpal fractures. *Aust Vet Pract* 1979;9:179–182.

Richardson DW: Technique for arthroscopic repair of third carpal bone slab fractures in horses. *J Am Vet Med Assoc* 1986;188:288–291.

Speirs VC, Anderson GA, Bourke JM: Assessment of prognosis for racing after carpal surgery in 210 Thoroughbreds. *Equine Vet J* 1986;18:187–192.

Stephens PM, Richardson DW: Slab fractures of the 3rd carpal bone in Standardbreds and Thoroughbreds: 155 cases (1977–1984). *J Am Vet Med Assoc* 1988;193:353–358.

Thrall DE, Lebel JL, O'Brien T: A five-year survey of the incidence and location of equine carpal chip fractures. *J Am Vet Med Assoc* 1971;158:1366–1368.

Wyburn RS, Goulden BE: Fractures of the equine carpus: A report on 57 cases. *NZ Vet J* 1974;22:133–142.

Unit VIIIC

Septic Musculoskeletal Disorders

111
Infectious Arthritis in Foals

Elwyn C. Firth

Infectious arthritis in the foal is almost always hematogenous, and should not be considered alone because (*a*) the disease is usually part of an infectious disease process affecting other body systems, and (*b*) the majority of bacterial arthritis cases are associated with accompanying infection in adjacent bone tissue. The joint and bone lesions have been classified as synovial, epiphyseal, physeal, or tarsal. More than one type can be present at one time in a given foal. A synovial lesion means that only synovitis is present, and that bone infection is not. An epiphyseal lesion implies the presence of infectious arthritis accompanied by osteomyelitis of the epiphysis or the adjacent bone. A physeal lesion implies osteomyelitis is present near the physis, usually in the metaphysis; arthritis may be present in these cases. A tarsal lesion refers to osteomyelitis in the small tarsal bones.

DIAGNOSIS

Signalment

Polyarthritis/polyosteomyelitis occurs in foals up to the age of 4 months, and most patients are less than 6 weeks old. Most foals with only polysynovitis (synovial) are less than 2 weeks old, and those with concurrent bone infection are from several days to 4 months of age. Tarsal osteomyelitis has been recorded in foals aged less than 30 days of age. Most affected foals in the upper age range have single physeal lesions. Despite these general trends, the age range for each lesion type is too broad to allow accurate prediction of lesion type based simply on the foal's age. No breed predisposition has been described, excluding the general susceptibility of those breeds with a high incidence of congenital immunodeficiency.

History

Abnormalities at or shortly after birth are almost always demonstrable. The mare may have lost colostrum before birth, or may have had a genital tract infection. The foals often are underweight at birth, are born early, are born after dystocia, have not stood or sucked promptly, or have been sick soon after birth. Furthermore, these problems may have been treated with apparent success. Foals with synovial lesions are thus often presented with a history of signs of foal septicemia (weakness, dehydration, prostration, multilimb lameness). Other foals may present with milder or no signs of systemic disease, but with joint swelling and lameness of variable duration, severity, and speed of onset.

Presenting Signs

Increased rectal temperature and other cardinal signs of infectious disease may not be present. The foal may be recumbent because of the systemic consequences of infection or because of multilimb lameness. Lameness can be isolated to a single limb, and is usually severe. The nature of the swelling in and around joints is important in differentiating the lesion type. Foals with synovial lesions have many swollen warm joints. Epiphyseal lesions are associated with joint effusion. By contrast, physeal lesions are initially associated with subtle swelling at the level of the affected physis. Joint effusion may be undetectable or very slight until generalized periarticular edema supervenes and masks these changes. Physeal lesions that have extended via the joint capsule or epiphysis into the joint cavity cause more obvious effusion. Chronic physeal lesions may rupture into periosseous tissues and produce fluctuant subcutaneous or fistulating swelling at, and just ventral to, the level of the metaphysis. Foals with tarsal osteomyelitis may present with one or more of the following signs: moderate to severe lameness, localized swelling at the level of the small tarsal articulations, cranial angulation of the tarsus, and effusion of the tibiotarsal joint.

Arthrocentesis of involved joints yields synovial fluid with a macroscopic appearance that varies widely. The fluid may resemble pure pus in some synovial lesions or be of relatively normal color and clarity in physeal lesions. Turbidity is almost always present.

Confirmatory Tests

The synovial fluid has an increased leukocyte count and clear neutrophil predominance. It has been suggested that in infectious arthritis the leukocyte count must be greater than a certain level (e.g., 50,000 cells/μL), but this may not be true of cases that are early, very chronic, treated with anti-inflammatory drugs, or caused by a relatively avirulent bacterium. Neutrophil predominance, however, is almost always present. Changes in protein, mucin precipitation, erythrocyte count, and enzyme levels consistent with inflammation are evident.

Definitive etiologic diagnosis is dependent on the demonstration of microorganisms from affected synovial fluid, synovial tissue, or bone by culture or staining techniques. These are often negative because of poor collection, storage, and laboratory technique, prior administration of antibiotics, or partial success of the foal's immune system in containing the infection. It is recommended that arthrocentesis be performed before treatment of any kind is begun, that a blood culture medium be inoculated immediately, that a Gram's stain of the aspirate be performed, and that culture for anaerobes be included. Microbiologic examination will often be negative, at least in the first instance, so if macroscopic characteristics and cytologic findings of the synovial fluid suggest infection, ASSUME bacterial arthritis and osteomyelitis are present until disproven, and treat accordingly.

The diagnosis of osteomyelitis is supported by radiologic demonstration of bone lesions. Good-quality radiographs are needed because there may be only slight osteolysis in early lesions. Accurate interpretation of the radiographic findings demands knowledge of lesion site predisposition and of radiographic anatomy of the developing skeleton. If bone lesions are not visible on first examination, radiographs should be repeated after 7 days, although in some cases osteolysis may appear earlier than this. Clinical, laboratory, and radiologic findings must be considered together. Bone lesions cannot be demonstrated without radiology, and osteolytic lesions can be wrongly interpreted without consideration of synovial findings. This is particularly true when osteochondrosis and infectious synovitis are present in the same joint.

There are further tests that can confirm the etiologic agent (chromatography), the presence and localization of inflammation (technetium bone scanning, scanning after iridium labeling of the foal's own leukocytes), and the presence of bone lesions (intraosseous phlebography, ultrasound). However, these are not widely available or applicable in practice, or are not yet well tested. Further invasive (operative) diagnostic techniques are presented below.

TREATMENT

Systemic antibiotic administration is the most important aspect of treatment, but antibiotic administration combined with aspiration of abnormal synovial fluid using regular-sized needles is associated with poor results. If such conservative treatment does not result in clinical improvement within 1 to 2 days, more aggressive therapy is indicated.

Joint Lavage

The technique of joint lavage is described in Chapter 112. Joint flushing can be conveniently done at the time of diagnostic arthroscopy. If this is not performed, the joint should be lavaged using 4- to 5-mm bore needles or cannulas; the fact that even an arthroscope sleeve sometimes becomes obstructed by fibrin clots indicates that using smaller gauge needles has little chance of removing all debris. Flushing can be repeated several times at intervals of about 2 days if clear improvement is not evident. Lavage is not as simple in foals as in adults, because there are usually several joints involved.

Arthrotomy

The technique of arthrotomy in cases of infectious arthritis is described in Chapter 112. The openings made in the joint are kept open by latex Penrose drains or orthopedic drains; sterility is maintained by sterile wraps, which must be changed regularly. This is not possible for some joints (e.g., the stifle), and although arthrotomy may be indicated in cases in which lavage has failed, the management of polyarthritis cases so treated is daunting.

Arthroscopy

Arthroscopy may be either diagnostic or operative. Diagnostic synovial biopsy under arthroscopic visualization is possible but may be superfluous if collection and culture techniques for synovia are correct and exhaustive. The proliferation and inflamed appearance of the synovial membrane, and the presence of fibrin in cases of arthritis, help support the diagnosis but also impede examination of the joint. Diagnostic arthroscopy to determine the presence of epiphyseal osteomyelitis lesions is feasible, because the sites of the lesions are reasonably constant. There are some limitations, however, because some lesions occur in sites that are not accessible, or accessible only with difficulty, and the only lesions detectable are those that have extended so far into cartilage that they can be directly visualized or found by probing. This means that negative findings have no meaning, and lesions that are evident are far advanced.

Operative arthroscopy is appropriate for removal of necrotic cartilage and bone of epiphyseal lesions that have nearly penetrated into the joint. One case of angular deformity following bone and cartilage removal in the lateral styloid process of the radius has been described, but disruption of the growth plate in other sites may not be deleterious to function (e.g., distal talar condyle).

Osteotomy

The purpose of osteotomy is either diagnostic or therapeutic. There may be a place for diagnostic drilling of the metaphysis in cases of suspected metaphysitis that are radiographically negative, although it is not easy to determine the precise site of maximum pain and swelling. If this procedure is to be performed a 6- to 7-mm incision is made onto bone just on the metaphyseal side of the metaphyseal growth plate (under radiographic or fluoroscopic guidance if necessary). Care is taken to avoid vessels and the joint capsule. The metaphysis is drilled with a 5-mm bit and the material removed in the drill is saved for microbiologic and histologic examination. One should not expect to see pus well up in the osteotomy site, as occurs in humans and cattle. In some cases, the metaphysis can be penetrated by a blunt instrument after probing of the area accessible through the skin incision.

Therapeutically, osteotomy is said to be effective in limiting extension and progression of early bone lesions by relieving tissue pressure in the enclosed space of the bone, and by allowing drainage. Although not proven, this may be true in the horse. The wound should be kept open with a drain, flushed daily, and kept under a sterile bandage. The removal of radiographically demonstrable bone lesions through osteotomy has also been suggested, and is simpler than the above method because the operative site can be identified by radiography. The lesion is approached by drilling, curetted carefully, flushed, and kept open with a drain. In physeal lesions, the curette should be directed toward the diaphysis so that if the physis is still intact, its blood supply will not be damaged. In epiphyseal lesions, the defect is approached by entry through the epiphysis. The articular cartilage must not be penetrated. It is clear that the use of osteotomy is limited by the site and morphology of some bone ends.

Abscess Removal in the Umbilical Area

Infectious processes in the navel area include abscessation of the umbilical arteries, umbilical vein, and urachus. Extraabdominal umbilical abscessation may also occur, but usually without systemic consequences. Septic omphalophlebitis may not be evident externally, where only a normal dry navel may be palpable. Consequences of abscessation include involvement of the abdominal wall, uroperitoneum after bladder wall necrosis, or peritonitis with subsequent bacteremia and infectious arthritis. Diagnosis of the presence of such abscesses can be difficult, and ultrasound examination is indicated. Incrimination of an abscess as the source of bacteremia is also difficult, and strict guidelines for removal of umbilical abscesses in cases of arthritis/osteomyelitis are lacking (see Chapter 146).

If resection is elected, the foal is operated under general anesthesia and in dorsal recumbency. Prior microbiologic examination of material issuing from a fistula will have specified the choice of perioperative antibiotic therapy. If a fistula is present, one should determine its direction by the use of a probe, and then close the opening with skin sutures. The abdominal cavity should be approached through a 4-cm incision at a site where there is least likelihood of encountering the abscess or associated adhesions. Although this will often be cranial to the navel, involvement of the umbilical vein should also be suspected and care taken to avoid this structure. Digital exploration of the abdominal cavity will reveal the site and extent of abnormal masses in the unbilical area. The abdominal incision is then lengthened around the mass, so that it can be elevated out of the abdominal cavity, draped off, and resected after appropriate clamping. The umbilical vessels should be ligated and the stumps covered with adjacent connective tissue. One must ensure that the resection surface is viable, and the bladder wall should be closed with a double layer of 2-0 absorbable suture material if the bladder was entered. Body wall closure is routine.

POSTOPERATIVE CARE

Whether or not surgical intervention has been part of the treatment of infectious arthritis/osteomyelitis, specific antibiotic therapy should be continued long after clinical signs have abated. Nonsteroidal anti-inflammatory drugs may have a place in the therapy of infectious arthritis to reduce the acute and chronic effects of infection on articular cartilage. The effect of these drugs on the leukocytic response of an immunocompromised patient may be more than is presently appreciated. Furthermore, the risk of gastrointestinal toxicity induced by these agents in foals is well known. Consequently, one should not exceed recommended dose rates and durations.

The provision of rest for the affected tissues is more dependent on the consequences of inflammation on articular cartilage than on the effects of the surgical procedures, which if correctly performed are of a minor and innocuous nature. All patients should be confined for several weeks after an incident of infectious arthritis, because the proteoglycan matrix of the cartilage may be depleted, and the collagen framework in which it is enmeshed may be disrupted. These effects of infectious arthritis mean the cartilage will be less resistant to the compression associated with locomotion, and secondary degenerative joint disease can result several months later. The amount of rest necessary to ensure that the articular cartilage of the rapidly growing foal can withstand physiologic stresses will depend on the duration and virulence of the joint infection. Unless the infection has been recognized and treated successfully within 2 to 3 days, one should assume that matrix depletion has occurred and, therefore, should not allow free exercise for at least several weeks. If arthritis has continued for longer than 5 to 6 days, one should assume that collagen damage has also occurred and prolong the period of rest. These are only guidelines based on other species, because no species-specific work in the horse is reported. The period of rest after osteotomy should also include consideration of the healing of the osteotomy itself, which weakens the bone. If the defect is small, and the guidelines for treatment of joint cartilage are followed, there is probably little danger of fracture. If the created defects are large, immobilization may be indicated.

It should be noted that no treatment, or combination of treatments, of infectious arthritis in foals has been prospectively evaluated and published. Follow-up clinical and radiologic examination of the foal is thus mandatory, preferably at around 6 months after discharge.

PROGNOSIS AND SPECIAL CONSIDERATIONS

The prognosis for infectious arthritis and osteomyelitis remains guarded to grave. There is some evidence that prognosis is dependent on the number of joints involved, the number and extent of bone lesions, the time since disease onset, and the promptness of the response to treatment. The number of animals achieving adulthood and athletic function is low. The need for prompt diagnosis and immediate instigation of antibiotic therapy, followed by joint lavage, cannot be overemphasized.

112 Infectious Arthritis in Adult Horses

Alicia L. Bertone

Infectious arthritis in adult horses is usually a sequela to traumatic joint puncture, an extension of cellulitis through the joint capsule, or secondary to iatrogenic bacterial inoculation. Hematogenous origin of infectious arthritis is less common in the adult horse than in foals. Infectious arthritis is a devastating equine joint disease because articular destruction occurs rapidly, the agent can be difficult to eradicate, and the byproducts of infection (i.e., fibrin, neutrophils) worsen the articular destruction, leading to degenerative joint disease. The immunologic response of the host to the bacterial and cartilage degradation products compounds the joint inflammation and articular destruction. The major goals of therapy, therefore, are rapid intervention to eliminate the infectious agent, removal of the by-products of infection, control of inflammatory events, and provision of the appropriate articular environment during convalescence for maximal cartilage and synovial repair.

PATHOGENESIS

The reaction of the synovial membrane to the infectious agent is the initiator of the articular cartilage destruction and, in in vitro studies, also appears to be the initiator of chondrocyte metabolism changes that impede replacement of the lost cartilage matrix. The amount of reactive inflammation in the synovial membrane depends on the virulence of the bacteria and the immune response of the host. The bacteria act as antigens and promote the rapid accumulation of neutrophils in the synovial membrane and fluid. Growth factors are released by synovial cells and inflammatory cells that promote the in situ proliferation of mononuclear cells. Enzymes are released from many cell types that rapidly (<48 hours) degrade the articular cartilage glycosaminoglycan, which is part of the proteoglycan aggregate matrix. The proteoglycan–hyaluronic acid aggregates are responsible for the compressive stiffness of the articular cartilage and help protect the collagen and chondrocytes from mechanical damage. The degree of collagen loss depends on the organism and the release of collagenase, but can occur as early as 9 days after inoculation. Alterations in synovial fluid (i.e., fibrin accumulation, loss of viscosity) can impede nutrition of chondrocytes, further thwarting the anabolic state needed for matrix repair.

The loss of the cartilage matrix (proteoglycans, hyaluronic acid, and collagen) leaves the chondrocytes unprotected and necrosis can occur. The metabolism of the remaining chondrocytes is slow relative to other tissues, and repair is frequently incomplete and overcome by mechanical stresses. Ensuing osteoarthrosis often results in permanent lameness.

DIAGNOSIS

Infectious arthritis must be considered a major diagnostic rule-out in any horse that develops a severe or non–weight-bearing lameness, particularly if a history of a periarticular wound or intraarticular injection exists. Fresh open joint injuries that are contaminated but not yet infected may not be associated with severe lameness. At least one half of open joint injuries will develop infectious arthritis, and therefore aggressive diagnostics to document joint involvement should be performed.

Any horse is susceptible to infectious arthritis if adequate bacterial numbers are inoculated into the joint. With some bacteria, such as *Staphylococcus aureus*, this may occur with as few as 100 organisms. Compromise of the host immune response from either systemic disease or local inflammation or ischemia to the joint (such as open joint injuries) may allow established infection with even fewer numbers of bacteria. The lower limb may be more frequently involved in infection in the adult horse, since wounds and open joint injuries are more common at that site (see Chapter 20).

The most prominent clinical sign of infectious arthritis is severe lameness with pain on manipulation of the joint; however, all the cardinal signs of inflammation are present, including heat and effusion. Joint effusion may be difficult to detect if periarticular swelling (edema and cellulitis) is also present. Synovial hypertrophy can be palpated in some joints, such as the carpus. Systemic signs including depression, hypophagia, fever, and alterations in the complete blood count values are common in the acute phases of infection (Fig 112–1). Typically by the third day after infection the peripheral packed cell volume will fall and fibrinogen will rise. By the tenth day, the total protein concentration in plasma, peripheral white blood cell count, and neutrophil count will rise.

Confirmatory tests for infectious arthritis include synovial fluid analysis, culture, and joint radiology. Synovial fluid should at least be analyzed for color, clarity, white blood cell count and differential, total protein, viscosity, and mucin clot–forming ability, and a Gram's stain should be performed. Infected synovial fluid is usually amber or dark yellow, turbid, and of poor viscosity and mucin-clot–forming ability. The synovial white blood cell count is elevated from less than 800 to greater than 30,000 cell/μL and more commonly to 100,000 to 200,000 cells/μl. Most cells are neutrophils (>95%) even after infection is of several weeks' duration, and the synovial membrane contains equal numbers of mononuclear and polymorphonuclear cells. As much synovial fluid as possible should be inoculated into a brain-heart infusion broth blood culture bottle containing PABA, 0.1% agar, vitamin K, hemin, CO_2, and sodium polyanetholesulfonate for aerobic and anaerobic culture (BBL Microbiology Systems). The advantages of using a large volume of inoculum and medium are that very low numbers of bacteria can be detected and growth inhibitors are diluted. Incubation of cultures should be for a minimum of 1 week, with subculturing employed as necessary. With aggressive culture techniques, isolation of organisms is as successful from synovial fluid as from synovial membrane. Antibiotic susceptibility testing should be per-

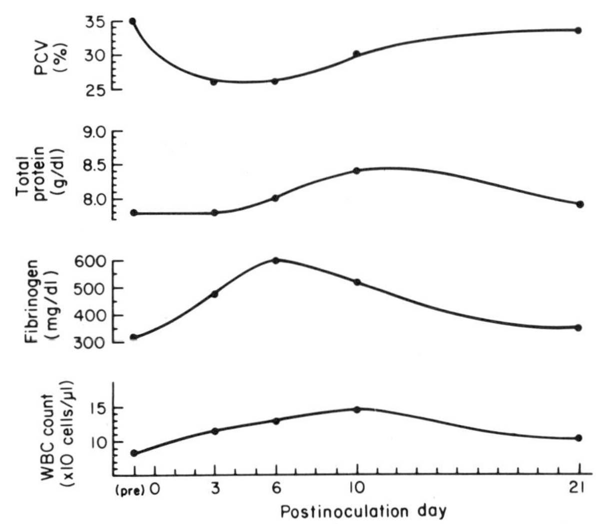

Figure 112–1. Hemogram changes with time in horses with experimental infectious arthritis of the tarsocrural joint. (From Bertone AL, McIlwraith CW, Norrdin RW, Jones RL, Radin JM: Comparison of treatments for experimentally-induced equine infectious arthritis. *Am J Vet Res* 1987;48:524.)

formed on all isolates. *Streptococcus, Staphylococcus,* and *Mycoplasma* are more commonly isolated from adult horses, whereas, the common pathogens for foal joints are *Salmonella* or *Escherichia coli*. Establishing the pathogen and its antibiotic susceptibility may be the most important component of patient care, since appropriate antibiotic therapy may provide the largest contribution to success.

Radiography of infected joints not associated with an open joint injury has not been of much benefit in the diagnosis of acute joint infection, but has been significantly helpful (along with contrast radiography) in the diagnosis of joint involvement with periarticular wounds. This procedure also is of value in identifying the presence of concomitant osteomyelitis. Since these findings may alter the course of therapy and/or prognosis, radiography is still recommended as a diagnostic procedure in infectious arthritis or any open joint injury.

TREATMENT

Antibiotics

Aggressive systemic antibiotic therapy is the most critical part of the treatment for infectious arthritis. Early antibiotic therapy can alleviate the signs associated with septicemia and, at high levels of administration, significantly help eliminate the joint infection. Most antibiotics will reach concentrations in the synovial fluid equivalent to plasma levels. In infected synovial fluid that has more protein and a lower pH (normal pH 7.35, infected synovial fluid pH 7.1 to 7.25), the antibiotic concentration varies depending on drug solubility, pK_a, and many other factors associated with the inflammatory state of the infection. In infected synovial fluid in horses, a trimethoprim-sulfadiazine combination (Tribrissen) administered orally at 60 mg/kg divided into two daily doses reached therapeutic concentrations for both trimethoprim and sulfadiazine against *S. aureus* for the entire interdosing period. Ampicillin may attain higher concentrations in inflamed equine joints than in the serum. Most antibiotics adequately penetrate infected synovial membrane in experimental models of infectious arthritis in rabbits. Some antibiotics, such as cephadrine and flucloxicillin, have not been able to adequately penetrate infected synovial membrane in humans.

To attain maximal tissue concentrations of the antibiotic, the first dose should be administered intravenously and subsequent doses continued intravenously or by other parenteral routes. Intraarticular administration of antibiotics is currently not recommended because of the ensuing synovitis and rapid distribution of the drug to the systemic circulation. This method, however, may achieve higher levels of antibiotic within the joint and overcome in vivo deterrents to antibiotic activity while simultaneously avoiding systemic toxicity. This is commonly practiced and is currently being investigated.

Antibiotic administration should continue for at least 3 weeks beyond clinical improvement. In horses with tarsocrural infectious arthritis, 42% of the joints still contained bacteria after 3 weeks of antibiotic therapy and marked clinical improvement, confirming this premise.

Joint Drainage

Joint drainage provides relief of joint pressure and removal of protein, fibrin, bacteria, cellular enzymes, and inflammatory cells. Some form of drainage is considered mandatory in the treatment of infectious arthritis. In horses, articular cartilage glycosaminoglycan content was significantly higher 3 weeks after inoculation with *S. aureus* when a drainage procedure and high level of antibiotic were used than when no drainage procedure and a lower level of antibiotic were used. The method of joint drainage did not affect the bacterial isolation rates. Bacterial isolation was most affected by antibiotic level.

Currently, the three most commonly recommended joint drainage techniques in the horse include through-and-through lavage, arthrotomy with lavage, and arthroscopy with lavage. Each of these techniques provides good dispersion of a large volume of irrigation solution.

Through-and-through lavage is the most commonly performed joint irrigation technique (Fig. 112–2). Soft-tipped catheters should be used to avoid damage to or inoculation of the articular cartilage with bacteria. Disadvantages of through-and-through lavage include inability to perform joint débridement or synovectomy, to obtain synovial membrane for histology or culture, or to inspect articular cartilage. Fibrin cannot be removed from the joint with this technique and this may provide a barrier to adequate lavage (Fig. 112–3). Based on bacterial isolation from the synovial fluid, synovial membrane histology, or articular cartilage histochemistry in horses with infectious arthritis, no advantage was detectable whether through-and-through lavage was performed once, twice, or three times. Through-and-through lavage is simple and practical and can be performed in the tractable animal without general anesthesia.

Arthrotomy with joint débridement and lavage allows direct inspection of articular cartilage, and provides exposure to synovial membrane and access to fibrin. Additionally, if the arthrotomy is allowed to

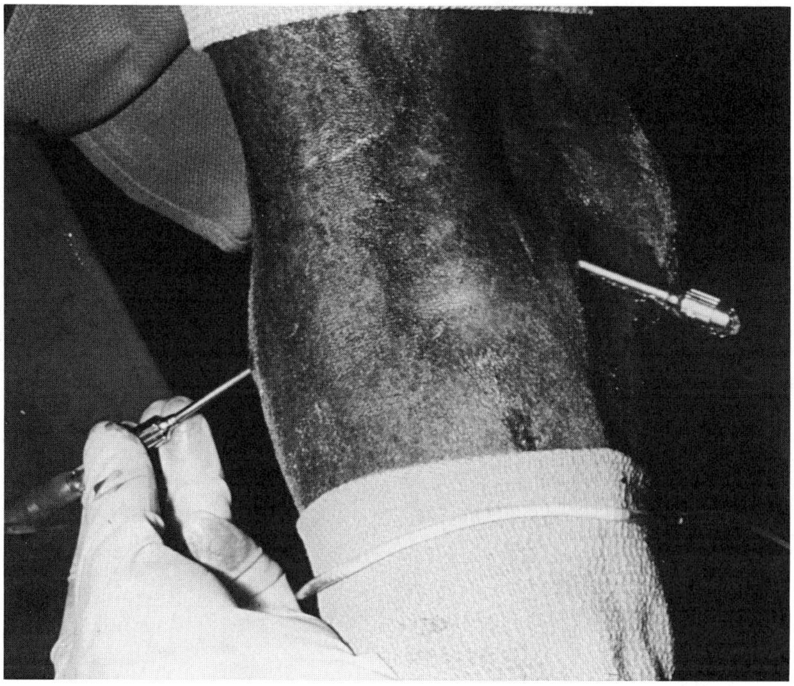

Figure 112–2. Through-and-through lavage of the tarsocrural joint. Several liters of fluid can be rapidly flushed through the joint from the dorsomedial pouch out the plantarlateral pouch. (From Bertone AL, McIlwraith CW, Powers BE, Radin JM: Effect of four antimicrobial lavage solutions on the tarsocrural jonts of horses. *Vet Surg* 1986;15:307.)

heal by second intention, continual drainage is established and synovial fluid production can act as a constant internal lavage system. Indwelling lavage systems such as orthopedic drains can be inserted for additional lavage during the acute phases. Drains are not without problems, however, because they can induce pain, mechanical pressure, and damage to articular cartilage and they can break off in the joint. Visualization of the joint is limited with arthrotomy, and healing of the incision is delayed as a result of the infection and drainage. Production of exuberant granulation tissue complicates healing, and peri-incisional fibrosis may limit range of joint motion. The long-term disturbances of joint function associated with arthrotomy need to be investigated and may be dependent on the joint involved and the arthrotomy location. In horses with infected joints, arthrotomy did produce significantly less synovial inflammation and fibrin accumulation than through-and-through lavage, although cartilage histochemistry was similar.

Arthroscopy can provide more complete visualization of the joint and access to synovial membrane than arthrotomy, and initial reports on its use in human cases of infectious arthritis are encouraging. Portal incisions can be left unsutured to provide some temporary drainage. Indwelling lavage systems can be inserted under arthroscopic guidance. Arthroscopy may provide the advantages of arthrotomy (decreased synovial membrane inflammation) without the disadvantages (delayed and complicated incisional healing).

Irrigation Solution. Joint lavage with an isotonic balanced electrolyte solution produces a mild, transient synovitis and undetectable articular cartilage damage in the horse. Joint lavage with dilute povidone-iodine solution [1% Betadine, 1:100 dilution (1.0% Betadine contains 0.1% povidone-iodine and 0.01% available iodine); Purdue Frederick Co] produces a similar response. More concentrated solutions of povidone-iodine produce additional inflammation and some loss of articular cartilage glycosaminoglycans. Higher concentrations are not necessary since dilute povidone-iodine (0.1%) is as bactericidal or more than the higher concentrations. Dilute chlorhexidine solution (Nolvasan solution, 2% chlorhexidine w/v; Fort Dodge Laboratories) induces severe pain and synovitis in the horse and should not be used for joint lavage.

In horses with infectious arthritis, the use of 0.1% povidone-iodine solution for through-and-through lavage was of no benefit over a balanced electrolyte solution in eliminating the infection or in reducing synovial inflammation or the loss of articular cartilage glycosaminoglycan content, despite its bactericidal activity. Mechanical removal of joint debris may be the most important effect of lavage.

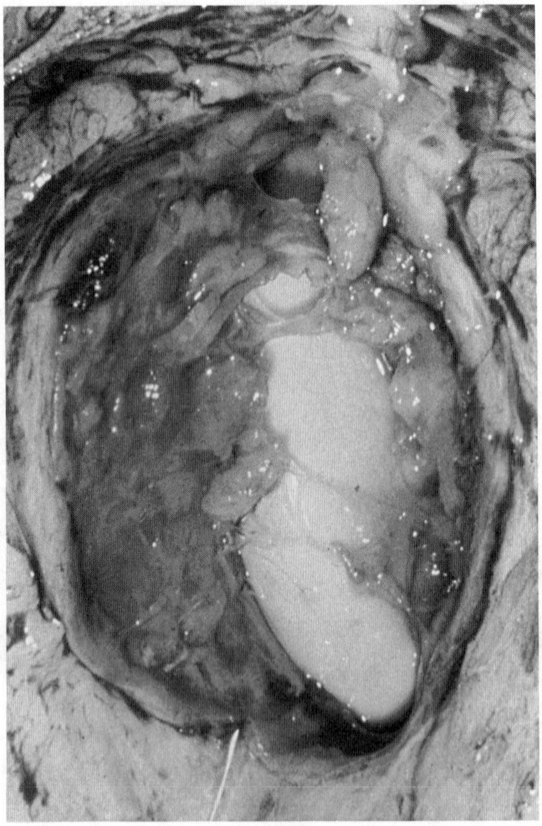

Figure 112–3. Fibrin accumulation in a joint 3 weeks after *S. aureus* inoculation and repeated through-and-through lavage. The fibrin could not be removed by this method of joint drainage. (From Bertone AJ, McIlwraith CW, Norrdin RW, Jones RL, Radin JM: Comparison of treatments for experimentally-induced equine infectious arthritis. *Am J Vet Res* 1987;48:526.)

POSTOPERATIVE CARE

General postoperative care consists of close monitoring, continued systemic antibiotic administration, repeated synovial cultures and aseptic cleaning and bandaging of incisions and arthrocentesis portals. Special considerations for infectious arthritis include joint motion and anti-inflammatory treatment.

Joint Motion

During the early acute phases of inflammation, joint rest is indicated to minimize joint injury and decrease pain. In the horse, this usually means intermittent active motion such as that afforded by stall rest. Fortunately, weight bearing is often minimal because of pain. Passive range of motion exercises (swimming and physiotherapy) should be initiated as soon as joint heat and swelling are reduced (usually in less than 7 days). Movement of the joint helps regain soft tissue flexibility that is lost through immobilization and fibrosis of the joint capsule and may also minimize synovial adhesions to cartilage. These soft tissue structures are the major shock absorbers of the joint and therefore are important for maximal long-term joint function.

Anti-inflammatory Treatment

Anti-inflammatory medication is an important component to treatment of infectious arthritis. The inflammatory cascade within the joint is the main contributor to articular cartilage damage. Prostaglandins are released in large quantities by synovial cells during inflammation and are known to increase proteoglycan degradation and inhibit its synthesis.

Nonsteroidal anti-inflammatory agents have repeatedly been shown to be beneficial in reducing joint destruction in arthritis models in other species. Nonsteroidal anti-inflammatory medication should be administered for both the anti-inflammatory and analgesic effects.

Corticosteroids are a potent anti-inflammatory agent, but are contraindicated in the treatment of infectious arthritis. Intraarticular corticosteroids suppress microbial killing and reduce the number of bacteria necessary to establish infection. In the horse, intraarticular steroids delayed but did not suppress the inflammatory response to bacterial joint inoculation.

Sodium hyaluronate has been shown by experiment to reduce joint swelling, lameness, and synovial fluid white blood cell count and produce less synovial lining damage than occurred in untreated infected joints. Its use is recommended, although the number of times it should be used is still questioned.

Many other substances and procedures are of potential benefit in the postoperative treatment of infectious arthritis, such as intraarticular administration of polysulfated glycosaminoglycans, dimethylsulfoxide, orgotein, and hyperimmune serum and the application of pulsating electromagnetic fields. Further research is needed to investigate the possible benefits of these treatments.

PROGNOSIS AND SPECIAL CONSIDERATIONS

The prognosis for infectious arthritis is dependent on the pathogenicity of the causative organism, the duration of infection prior to treatment, and the physiologic state of the joint and animal. Although the prognosis has been generally stated as poor, it is not hopeless. In horses, specific reports of prognosis are limited, but in open joint injuries, 39% of horses that developed infectious arthritis survived for a useful function. The controlled study of more treatments and adjunctive drug and physical therapy will likely improve the outcome in the future.

It has repeatedly been shown that early diagnosis and treatment (<24 hours) is important in controlling infection and outcome. The suspicion of an infected joint should be treated as a diagnostic emergency. An infected or contaminated joint should be treated as a surgical emergency.

BIBLIOGRAPHY

Bertone AJ, Jones RL, McIlwraith CW: Serum and synovial fluid steady-state concentrations of trimethoprim and sulfadiazine in horses with experimentally induced infectious arthritis. *Am J Vet Res* 1988;49;1681–1687.

Bertone AJ, McIlwraith CW, Jones RL, Norrdin RW, Radin JM: Povidone-iodine lavage treatment of experimental equine infectious arthritis. *Am J Vet Res* 1987;48:712–715.

Bertone AL, McIlwraith CW, Norrdin RW, Jones RL, Radin JM: Comparison of treatments for experimentally-induced equine infectious arthritis. *Am J Vet Res* 1987;48:519–529.

Bertone AL, McIlwraith CW, Powers BE, Radin JM: Effect of four antimicrobial lavage solutions on the tarsocrural joints of horses. *Vet Surg* 1986;15:305–315.

Firth EC, Klein WR, Nouws JFM, Wensing TH: Effect of induced synovial inflammation on pharmacokinetics and synovial concentration of sodium ampicillin and kanamycin sulfate after systemic administration in ponies. *J Vet Pharmacol Therap* 1988;11:56–62.

Gibson KT, McIlwraith CW, Turner AS, Stashak TS, Aanes WA, Trotter GW: Open joint injuries in horses: 58 cases (1980–1986). *J Am Vet Med Assoc* 1989;194:398–404.

Goldenberg DL, Reed JI: Bacterial arthritis. *N Engl J Med* 1985;312:764–771.

McIlwraith CW: Antibiotic use in musculoskeletal disease. *Proc AAEP Ann Conven* 1986;pp:241–249.

Salter RB, Bell RS, Keeley FW: The protective effect of continuous passive motion on living articular cartilage in acute septic arthritis. *Clin Orthop* 1981;159:223–247.

Schurman DJ, Hirshman HP, Nagel DA: Antibiotic penetration of synovial fluid in infected and normal knee joints. *Clin Orthop Rel Res* 1978;136:304–310.

Stover SM, Pool RR: Effect of intraarticular gentamicin sulfate on normal equine synovial membrane. *Am J Vet Res* 1985;45:2485–2491.

Tulamo RM, Bramlage LR, Gabel AA: The influence of corticosteroids on sequential clinical and synovial fluid parameters in joints with acute infectious arthritis. *Equine Vet J* 1989;21:332–337.

Von Essen R, Holtta A: Improved method of isolating bacteria from joint fluids by the use of blood culture bottles. *Ann Rheum Dis* 1986;45:454–457.

UNIT IX

Fractures

113 Mandibular Fractures

Robert K. Schneider

Mandibular fractures can be classified into 4 groups based on the anatomic location of the fracture within the mandible: incisive fractures, interdental space fractures, fractures involving the cheek teeth, and fractures of the vertical ramus of the mandible. Fractures of the incisive area and those involving the interdental space are the more common types. Fractures of the vertical ramus of the mandible are rare, usually unilateral, and normally are not repaired.

DIAGNOSIS

Mandibular fractures result from the horse entrapping its lower incisors under an immovable device (i.e., a stall door latch) and suddenly jerking backward, fracturing the mandible through the incisors or through the interdental space. These fractures can also result from a kick to the rostral part of the lower jaw. Mandibular fractures are more common in foals and young horses because of their inquisitive nature; they frequently bite or play with objects in their environment by grasping with incisor teeth, or put their nose where it doesn't belong and receive a kick from another horse.

Horses with incisive fractures may have few external signs of a problem; some salivation or dysphagia may be observed. Oral examination reveals displacement of the involved incisors, which is diagnostic for a fracture. Fractures through the interdental space usually involve both rami of the mandible and are unstable. These animals are uncomfortable, have difficulty eating, salivate excessively, and may have swelling around the lower jaw. Oral examination reveals malalignment of the upper and lower incisors; this is easily observed when the mouth is closed and the lips are separated to demonstrate the malocclusion. Instability can be detected by manipulating the cranial mandible. Fractures through the cheek teeth are infrequent because the mandible is wider and reinforced by the roots of the teeth in this location. These fractures are usually unilateral and result from trauma to the lower, lateral jaw. A large force is required to fracture the mandible in this location and the overlying skin and soft tissues are frequently damaged and/or opened by the injury. Dysphagia, excess salivation, swelling, and malalignment of the incisors are seen with these fractures. Displacement of the cheek teeth in the lower arcade also may be observed on examination of the oral cavity.

Mandibular fractures are the primary differential diagnosis to consider in horses with dysphagia, excess salivation, and swelling around the lower jaw. Radiographs of the mandible will confirm the presence of a fracture. Radiography is not always necessary in horses with fractures through the incisive area because they can be adequately evaluated by examination and palpation of the displaced incisors. However, radiographs of the incisive area will demonstrate the extent of the fracture; this area of the mandible is best evaluated on a ventrodorsal projection taken with the casette in the horse's mouth. Fractures of the interdental space and cheek teeth are best evaluated on lateral and oblique projections of the mandible.

SURGICAL REPAIR

Fractures of the Incisive Area

Fractures in this location usually involve the corner incisors and a small piece of the surrounding bone (Fig. 113–1). Stabilization of the fracture is accomplished using overlapping wires placed around the incisor teeth. The fracture line is débrided and flushed to remove debris and feed material. A curette is helpful to scrape away debris and necrotic bone. A 14-gauge needle is placed through the mucous membrane at the base of the incisors as a guide for the 18-gauge wire. The end of the wire is directed into the sharp end of the needle, the needle is removed, and the wire is left in place between the teeth. Two overlapping loops are used to maximize stability and to maintain the fixation should one of the wires break. The loops of wire are preplaced and then tightened by twisting the wire until the fracture is reduced and stable. The wire that passes to the outside of the corner incisor may slip off the tooth. To avoid this complication, the mucous membrane and mandible are cut or grooved, creating a notch to support the wire when it is tightened. When the fracture involves the corner of the mandible and ex-

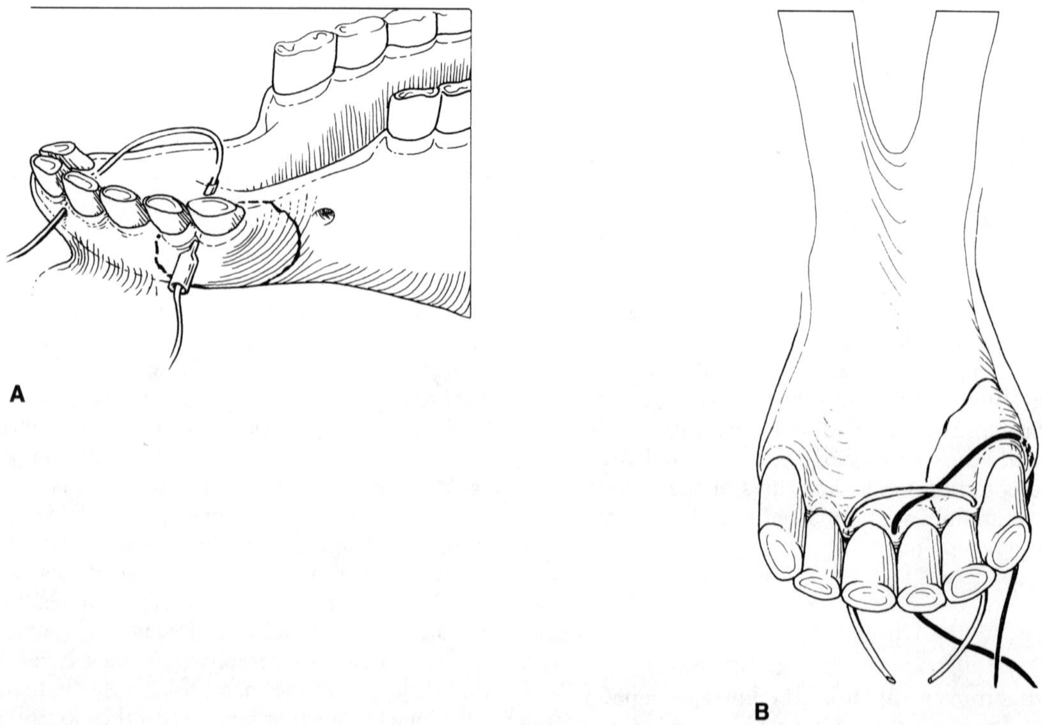

Figure 113–1. Overlapping wire repair of a fracture through the incisive area of the mandible. **A.** A 14-gauge needle is placed through the gums between teeth as a guide for the 18-gauge wire. **B.** The wires are preplaced around the teeth before twist-tightening them to stabilize the fracture.

tends into the interdental area, an oral acrylic splint may be necessary to achieve stability. An acrylic splint may also be indicated if one or two of the incisor teeth are missing. The splint is secured to the other incisors with wire and if necessary to the ramus of the mandible caudal to the symphysis (see Fig. 113–3). The twisted ends of the tightened wire are cut and bent over into the mucous membrane to prevent lacerations to the buccal surface of the lips.

The prognosis for incisive fractures is good. In tractable horses, the wires can be placed and tightened with the horse sedated and standing, but frequently general anesthesia is necessary. The wires are removed in 8 weeks, after the fracture has healed.

Fractures in the Interdental Space

Fractures in the interdental space are usually unstable and bilateral, involving both horizontal rami of the mandible. The fractures are not often comminuted. Several techniques have been employed to stabilize these fractures. A tension band wire between the incisors and the cheek teeth or an intraoral acrylic splint are preferred because of their ease of application and low incidence of complications. General anesthesia is necessary because reduction and repair are accomplished working inside the horse's mouth. Nasal intubation with the endotracheal tube will allow more room in the mouth, which facilitates placement of the wires.

The tension surface of the unstable mandible is on the oral side of the bone; contact between the upper and lower incisors causes dorsoventral bending of the mandible and distraction of the fracture along the oral surface. Wiring the incisors to the cheek teeth stabilizes the fracture and prevents distraction. The horse is anesthetized and positioned in dorsal recumbency. The skin over the left and right cheeks is prepared for aseptic surgery. The space between the first and second left lower cheek teeth is located and a small stab incision is made in the skin overlying this space at the gum line. Using blunt dissection with curved Kelly forceps, the buccal tissues are separated until only the thin mucous membrane is left. This prevents excessive hemorrhage, which frequently occurs when a full-thickness stab incision is made through the cheek with a scalpel. The oral mucous membrane is then incised. A 3.2-mm drill bit is placed through the incision into the space between the first two cheek teeth just ventral to the gum line. While protecting the soft tissues of the cheek, a hole is drilled between the two teeth. The same approach and drill hole are made over the right lower dental arcade. The stab incisions in the cheek facilitate passage of the wire around the first cheek tooth. The end of the wire is passed into the mouth along the buccal surface of the cheek and out through the stab incision; the wire is then passed back through the incision into the 3.2-mm drill hole. This allows the wire to be passed directly from lateral to medial through the drill hole, since the restricted space in the mouth makes it extremely difficult to pass the wire into the hole without these incisions. An 18-gauge wire is placed around the incisor teeth at their base using a 14-gauge needle through the mucous membrane as a guide (Fig. 113–2). A piece of wire approximately 40 cm in length is bent in the middle and the two ends are passed between the first and second incisors on the right and left side of the mandible from the buccal to the lingual side of the teeth. The end of the wire on the right is passed back around the remaining right incisor teeth, directed caudally around the right first cheek tooth as previously described, and returned to the incisors. The wire is passed back to the midline space between the two first incisors by weaving it around the base of the three incisors. The end of the wire on the left is placed around the left incisors and the first cheek tooth in a similar fashion. The weave of the wire around the incisors will end with the wire passing out the midline space between the first pair of incisors. The ends of the wire are twist-tightened over the wire and the ends are cut and bent over into the gingiva. The two wires along the interdental space are then toggled together using a curved mosquito forceps

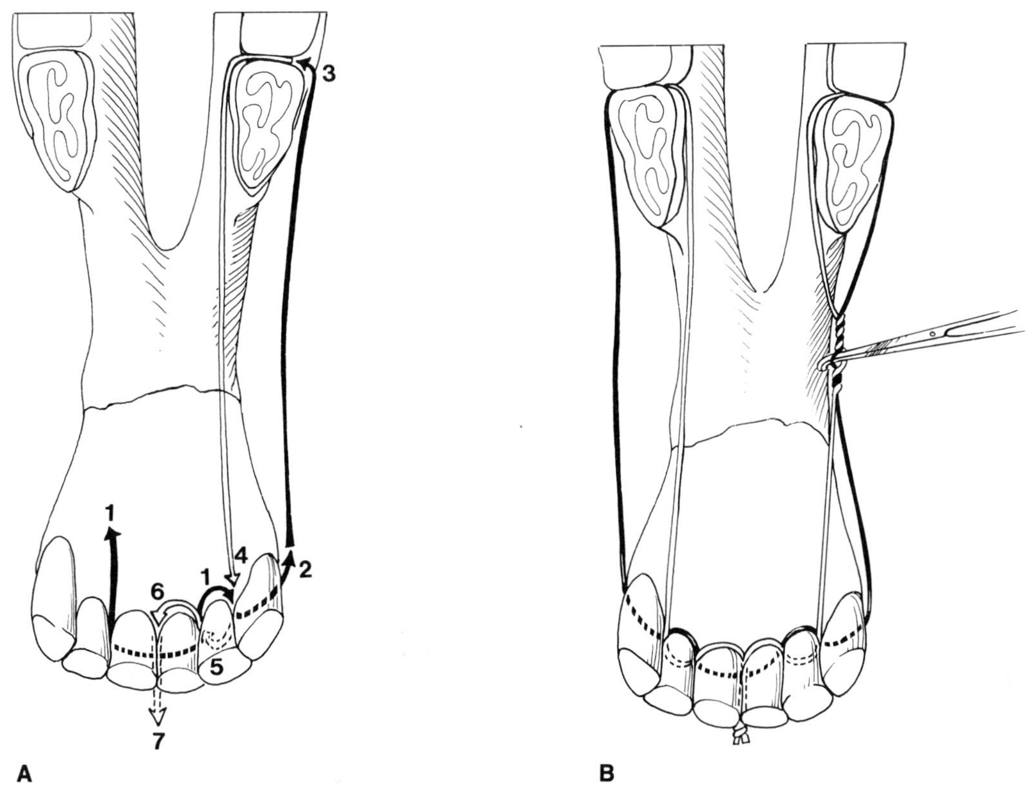

Figure 113–2. Tension band wire placement for repair of a fracture in the interdental space of the mandible. **A.** A piece of large-gauge wire is woven around the lower incisors, passed caudally around the first cheek tooth, and back around the lower incisors again. The numbers refer to the order in which the wire is passed around the teeth. Once both ends of the wire are placed around the teeth on both sides of the mouth, the ends of the wire will end up in the space between the two first incisors. **B.** The ends of the wire are twist-tightened over the middle of the wire. The two wires in the interdental space are then toggled together until the wires are tight. The wire functions as a tension band on the oral side of the fracture.

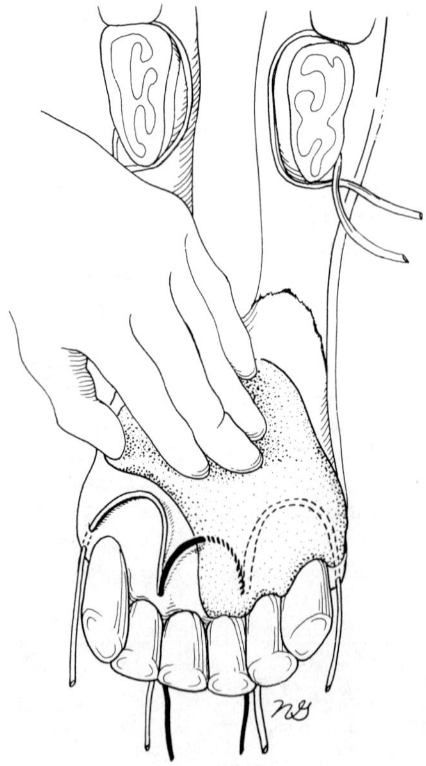

A

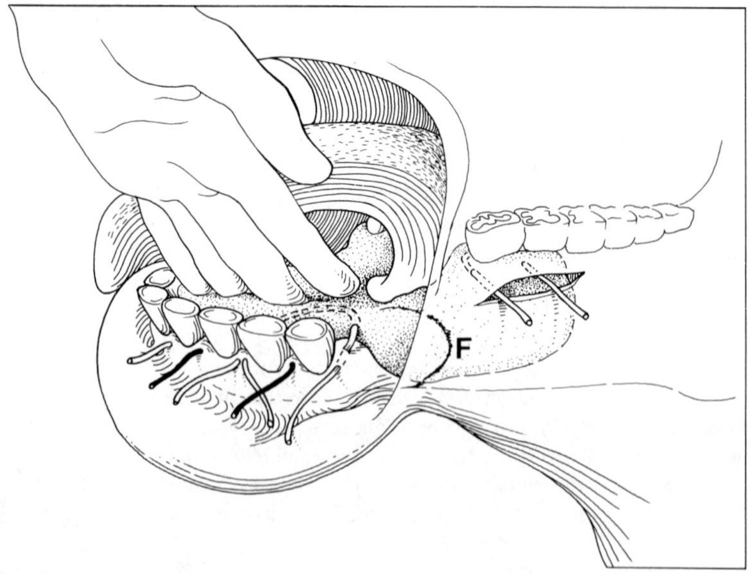

B

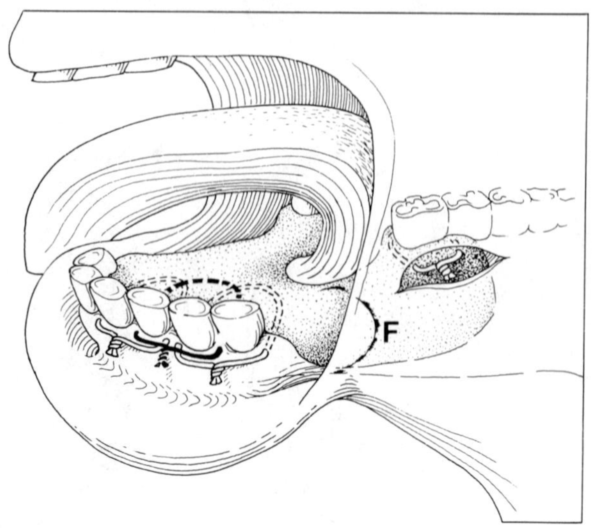

C

Figure 113–3. Intraoral acrylic splint repair of a fracture through the interdental space of the mandible. **A.** The wires are preplaced around the teeth using a 14-gauge needle as a guide. The loops are left loose and extend into the oral cavity for a short distance. Methylmethacrylate is mixed and molded to the oral side of the incisors, incorporating the wires into the acrylic. **B.** The acrylic is placed along the mandible caudally to the first cheek teeth. **C.** In a few minutes the acrylic becomes hard. Then the wires are twist-tightened, securing the splint to the incisors and first cheek teeth. *F* shows the location of the fracture line.

to wrap one wire over the other, twisting them together until the wire is tight (Fig. 113–2). This is done on both sides of the mandible until the fracture is reduced and stable. The two stab incisions through each cheek are left open to heal by second intention.

Intraoral splints made from cold-setting methylmethacrylate acrylic (Howmedica, Inc) can also be used to fix fractures through the interdental space of the mandible. Individual wires are preplaced around the incisors using a 14-gauge needle as a guide through the gum; the wires are not tightened (Fig. 113–3). Individual wires are also preplaced around each of the first cheek teeth through stab incisions in the cheeks. Once the wires are in place the fracture is reduced, and the methylmethacrylate is mixed and, when clay-like in consistency, is molded to the mandible within the mouth. The methylmethacrylate extends caudally from the incisors along the horizontal ramus of each mandible to the lingual and buccal side of each of the first cheek teeth. The preplaced loops of wires are incorporated into the soft methylmethacrylate on the lingual side of the teeth. The methylmethacrylate splint sets up in a few minutes. Once hard, the wires are tightened, stabilizing the mandible to the acrylic splint (Fig. 113–3). Further fixation of the mandible to the splint can be achieved by passing wire loops submucosally around the ramus of the mandible and over the acrylic splint. This is rarely necessary and is indicated only in young foals that may have just two erupted incisors or in foals with comminuted fractures. Once the acrylic hardens, the wires are twist-tightened and the ends are bent over and embedded in the gingiva.

Fractures through the Cheek Teeth

Fractures through the cheek teeth are usually unilateral and some stability is provided by the intact opposite ramus of the mandible. They can be repaired using a dynamic compression plate placed along the lateral surface of the mandible or by external fixation with transfixation pins incorporated in an external acrylic brace.

Internal fixation of mandibular fractures is accomplished through a ventrolateral approach. The skin is incised along the ventrolateral edge of the mandible. Part of the attachment of the masseter muscle must be elevated off the caudal mandible. The transverse facial artery, vein, and parotid salivary duct should be preserved where they cross the mandible at the rostral edge of the masseter muscle. The fracture is reduced and a broad dynamic compression plate is applied to the lateral surface of the mandible (Fig 113–4A). It is not necessary to avoid the roots of the cheek teeth when placing the screws. A special cement drill bit (Masonry Drill Bit; Black and Decker) can be used to drill through the hard teeth roots. Even in infected, open fractures screw placement directly into the tooth roots has not always resulted in infection and loss of the tooth. The plate holds the fracture stable until it is healed; the implants are then removed because these fractures are open and frequently infected.

External fixation is accomplished by driving large intramedullary pins through the fractured ramus of the mandible into the ramus on the opposite side (Fig. 113–4B). This is accomplished through small stab incisions. Once the intramedullary pins are in place, they are cut off leaving about 4 cm lateral to the skin. A cardboard paper towel roll or piece of rubber hose is placed over the ends of the pins and filled with acrylic. (Technovite; Jorgensen Labs). The acrylic is mixed in liquid form and poured into the tube before it hardens. Once the acrylic hardens it forms an external brace that stabilizes the fracture.

POSTOPERATIVE CARE

Fractures repaired with wire fixation or intraoral acrylic splints require minimal postoperative care. The mouth is flushed daily with water to keep feed material from accumulating around the wires or splint or in the fracture site. Once the fracture is stabilized, there is minimal postoperative pain. Phenylbutazone may be given for the first few days following surgery but is usually not continued over the long term. A soft diet of soaked alfalfa pellets may be given to minimize chewing. Fractures of the incisors, once stabilized, rarely require the horse to have a special diet. Careful attention to bending the wires and smoothing the edges of the acrylic splint will prevent lacerations and minimize discomfort from intraoral fixation. In contaminated or open fractures systemic antibiotics may be indicated; their use should be based on the needs of the individual case. Open skin wounds are cleaned and flushed daily with a dilute povidone-iodine solution.

Once the mandibular fractures are stabilized, most of the aftercare can be accomplished by the owner. The owner also can monitor the fixation by parting the horse's lips and checking the position and occlusion of the upper and lower incisors. Therefore, these patients do not require postoperative care in the hospital beyond a few days. Open fractures of the cheek teeth area can be an exception and may require more complex care after fixation. By 8 to 12 weeks the fracture is healed and the wires and acrylic splints can be removed, usually with the horse standing while sedated. Transfixation pins and the external acrylic splint may loosen in 6 to 8 weeks and should be removed or new pins placed in new holes if the fracture is not yet healed.

PROGNOSIS

The prognosis for fractures of the mandible is good, especially for the more common types involving the

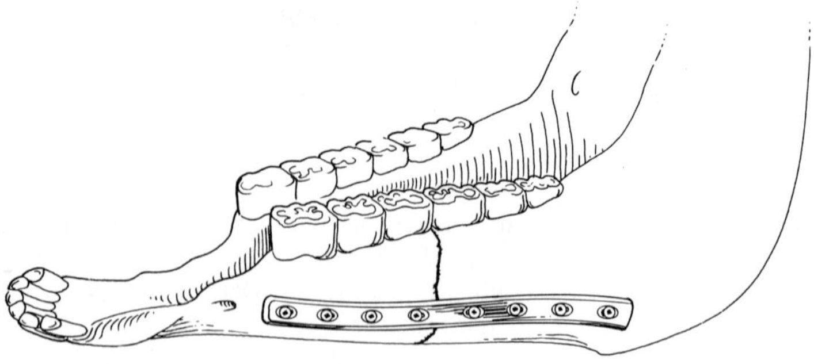

A

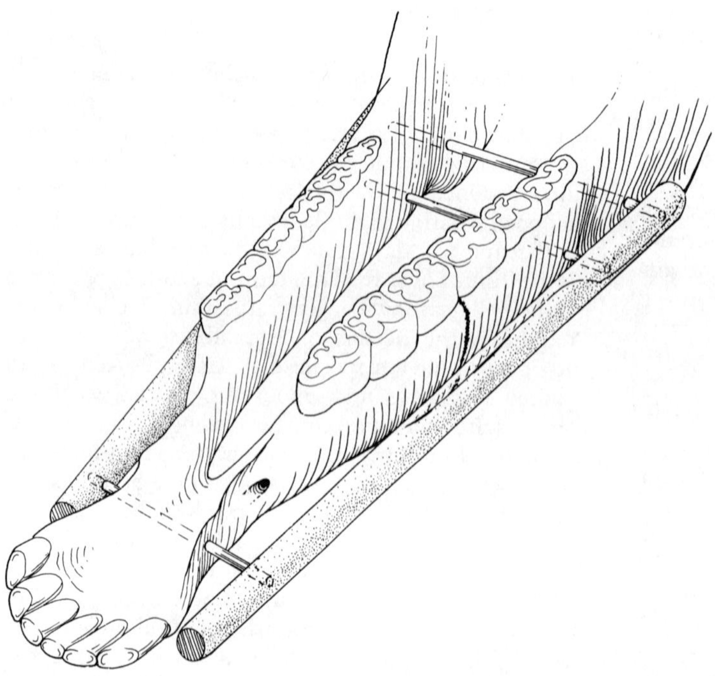

B

Figure 113–4. Two methods of repair for fractures through the cheek teeth of the mandible. **A.** A broad plate and screws are placed on the ventral lateral horizontal ramus of the mandible. **B.** Transfixation pins and an external acrylic splint can also be used to stabilize these fractures.

incisors and interdental space. The rich vascular supply to the mandible and surrounding tissues allows rapid fracture healing, and even open, contaminated fractures heal with few complications. Both tension band wires and acrylic splints are effective in stabilizing mandibular fractures cranial to the cheek teeth. Oral acrylic splints have advantages; they can function as a tension band to resist dorsoventral bending forces, but they also stabilize the jaw against movement caused by forces acting against the cranial mandible (such as the foal bumping the lower jaw against a feeder). The acrylic splint also has an advantage in foals with only one set of incisors, in comminuted fractures, or in fractures involving the incisors and a small amount of bone. It is difficult to stabilize these fractures with just a tension band wire around the teeth, and more fixation to the splint can be obtained by wiring around the ramus of the mandible over the splint.

Fractures through the cheek teeth are frequently open into the oral cavity and to the outside as well. Repair with transfixation pins and an external acrylic splint is preferred to a dynamic compression plate because it involves less tissue dissection and minimizes the risk of disseminating the infection. However, loosening of the pins limits the length of time that fixation can be maintained. Plate fixation is more stable but has greater risk of complications.

BIBLIOGRAPHY

Colahan PT, Pascoe JR: Stabilization of equine and bovine mandibular and maxillary fractures, using an acrylic splint. *J Am Vet Med Assoc* 1983;182:1117–1119.

Monin T: Tension band repair of equine mandibular fractures. *J Equine Med Surg* 1977;1:325–329.

Turner AS: Large animal orthopedics, in Jennings P (ed): *The Practice of Large Animal Surgery*. Philadelphia, WB Saunders Co, 1984, pp 893–897.

114 Facial Bone Fractures

Jeffrey P. Watkins

Fractures of the facial bones are usually the result of striking immovable objects or receiving kicks from other horses. The frontal, nasal, lacrimal, zygomatic, and maxillary bones are commonly affected. In addition, fractures in this area may concurrently affect the paranasal sinuses, nasal cavity, nasal septum, teeth, and globe.

Individuals frequently affected include young horses, horses that are easily startled, and horses that tend to be aggressive toward other horses. Often the history indicates the horse became startled during restraint and violently threw its head. The injury results either from striking a nearby object, such as a restraining stanchion, or from the force applied by a halter with a securely tied lead rope. Horses may also strike their head by attempting to run through a fence or gate. This may result in severe facial trauma, especially in areas where welded pipe fencing is commonly used. Aggressive behavior is frequently implicated in facial fractures in horses that have been kicked. The use of padded restraint stocks, care in securing lead ropes, the use of fences with less potential for causing injury, removing excessively aggressive horses from the herd, and behavior modification of "head shy" horses may help reduce the incidence of these injuries.

DIAGNOSIS

Horses with facial fractures are usually presented with a history of blunt trauma, deformity of facial contour, and occasionally an open wound. In some cases facial deformity may not be evident. This is the result of soft tissue swelling and hematoma filling in the depressed area of the fracture and obscuring the abnormal facial contour. With resolution of the hematoma and soft tissue swelling, the deformity usually becomes obvious. Immediately after the injury, crepitation, instability, and pain on palpation are frequently present. However, these abnormalities become less evident as the injury becomes chronic and fibrosis occurs. When the fracture enters the nasal cavity or paranasal sinuses, epistaxsis will be an additional physical finding. The degree of hemorrhage is usually not severe and in most cases the hemorrhage has stopped by the time a veterinarian is consulted. However, epistaxsis implies that the mucosa of the upper respiratory tract has been penetrated and, although a skin wound may not be present, indicates that an open fracture exists.

The diagnosis of a facial fracture requires a thorough history, physical examination, and radiographic evaluation, with primary emphasis placed on the previously described physical findings. The identification of fracture fragments and crepitation may require deep palpation because of soft tissue swelling and hematoma formation. However, the examination must be done carefully so as not to cause further injury. In chronic injuries with advanced fibrosis, it may not be possible to find palpable evidence that a fracture exists.

To confirm fracture location, establish the degree of displacement, and identify nondisplaced fracture lines, radiographic evaluation is required. Radiographic views tangential to the suspected fracture fragments are most diagnostic (Fig. 114–1). Nondisplaced fracture lines or changes in contour that are not oriented tangential to the x-ray beam are not well visualized or may not be evident. Radiographs also aid in determining if other structures, such as a cheek tooth alveolus, are involved with the fracture. The presence of a fluid line secondary to hemorrhage into a paranasal sinus indicates that the fracture has penetrated the mucosal lining of the sinus.

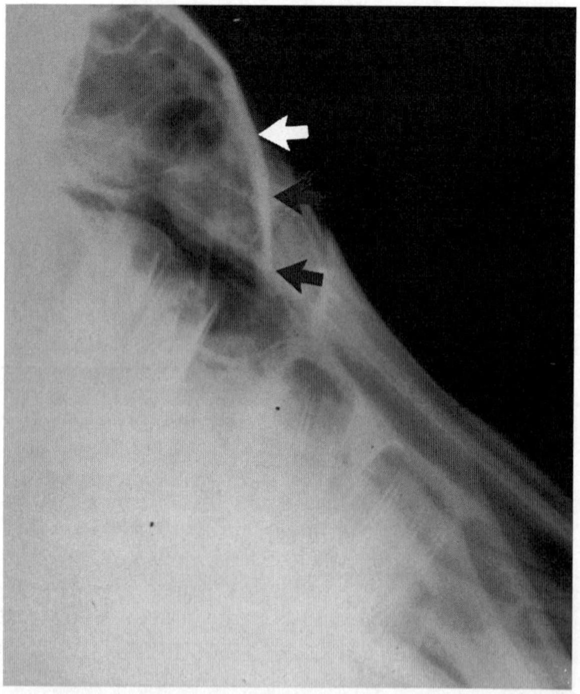

Figure 114–1. Radiograph taken tangential to a depression fracture of the nasal bone (*arrows*).

TREATMENT

When fracture fragments are minimally displaced and if vital structures and functions are not impaired, conservative management may be considered. Protective bandages to minimize swelling and prevent the accumulation of subcutaneous emphysema are recommended for fractures that enter the upper respiratory tract. Antimicrobial drugs are indicated when the fracture involves the nasal cavity or paranasal sinus but will not always prevent infection from developing at the fracture site. The potential to develop sinusitis and bone sequestra from these fractures exist. Fortunately, sequestration is not common following facial fractures because there is an excellent blood supply to the region.

Horse with significant facial deformity or impairment of vital functions should have reconstructive surgery. In many instances the degree of facial deformity may be underestimated because of soft tissue swelling and the presence of a fracture hematoma. There may be a tendency in these cases to elect conservative treatment; however, an unsightly deformity may subsequently develop, the degree of which depends on the amount of fibrosis and callus formation. When conservative therapy is under consideration, the ultimate facial contour is best predicted by radiographs taken tangential to the fracture. Although reconstruction can be undertaken after soft tissue swelling has resolved and fibrosis has occurred, a better cosmetic effect is obtained by primary open reduction when the fracture is less than 72 hours old.

Fracture Reduction Technique

Reconstructive surgery should be performed on an elective basis as soon after the fracture as possible. Delays of over 72 hours may be associated with the inability to anatomically reduce fracture fragments. Recommendations for exposure of the fracture are to utilize generous curvilinear incisions extending beyond the fracture lines. Using this approach, the incision does not lie directly over fracture lines or implants. Optimal exposure of healthy adjacent bone, which may be required for reduction and stabilization as well as providing a better soft tissue seal over the fracture site, is achieved if these principles are followed. Once the fracture is exposed, the hematoma should be carefully removed to preserve the periosteal attachments to the fracture fragments. The risk of infection can be minimized with fractures associated with skin wounds or wounds into the respiratory tract by careful cleansing and débridement. Small fragments devoid of periosteum should be discarded if their removal will not compromise stability.

A number of methods have been used successfully for reduction. One technique is to position holes in healthy bone adjacent to the fracture through which instruments can be introduced and used to elevate the fragments into place from beneath without disturbing the edges of the fracture. Holes may also be drilled into the bone fragments and a bone hook introduced to elevate the fragments into proper position. Alternatively, periosteal elevators or thin osteotomes can be placed into the fracture line and used to pry the displaced fragment into a normal position. Many of these fractures are stable once they have been reduced because of and interdigitating nature of the fragments. Occasionally internal fixation is required and in these cases 18- or 20-gauge stainless steel wire is used to attach the fragments to normal bone. Horses with facial fractures open into the upper respiratory tract or associated with a skin wound are candidates for perioperative antimicobial drug administration. During recovery from anesthesia, the head should be protected with a padded helmet to reduce the potential for additional trauma to the fracture region. Postoperatively, head bandages are indicated to protect the wound from environmental contamination. In addition, bandages provide pressure for obliteration of dead space and aid in preventing the accumulation of subcutaneous emphysema and wound fluids. Bandaging is accomplished by taping or by using large stockinette to make a form-fitting bandage for the entire head.

Sinus and Nasal Cavity Fractures

Severe injuries associated with a significant loss of skin and bone may predispose to formation of a mucocutaneous fistula into the affected sinus or nasal cavity. Reconstruction of these defects is accomplished either by creation of periosteal flaps and skin mobilization or by muscle flap closure combined with skin mobilization or grafting techniques. Complications related to infection include sequestration and sinusitis. Removal of small fragments devoid of soft tissue attachments combined with thorough débridement and pressure lavage will minimize sequestra formation. Lavage tubes should be positioned to provide for postoperative sinus lavage in cases with a high risk for developing sinusitis, especially in fractures entering a sinus that are associated with a heavily contaminated skin wound. Upper respiratory obstruction may develop as a result of thickening and deformation of the nasal septum when it is involved with the fracture. Nasal septum resection may be required in these cases as airway compromise becomes evident. Residual facial deformity may occur from an inability to completely reduce the fracture fragments, often due to a delay in surgical therapy. Implantation of a fluorocarbon polymer (Proplast; Dow Corning Corp) has been utilized to restore normal facial contour associated with this complication.

Periorbital Fractures

Periorbital fractures are usually depression fractures that may result in permanent damage to the eye if the fragment is putting pressure on the globe. Periorbital fractures most commonly affect the zygomatic process of the frontal bone (Fig. 114–2). Clinical signs include soft tissue swelling, chemosis, proptosis, and occasionally trauma to the globe. In addition to the previously described signs, periorbital fractures that occur at the medial canthus involve the osseous lacrimal canal and maxillary sinus. Displacement of bone fragments into the retrobulbar area may occur with periorbital fractures and cause entrapment of the eye, exophthalmos, and pain. In some cases the periorbital injury causes severe trauma to the globe and the eye cannot be salvaged.

The management of periorbital fractures is similar to that for other depression fractures of the facial bones. The goals of treatment are to reduce displaced fragments and restore vital functions.

Zygomatic Process Fractures

Zygomatic process fractures can usually be reduced by a noninvasive technique. A bone hook can be carefully passed into the conjunctival fornix and positioned beneath the fracture fragments, which are then elevated as needed to achieve reduction. Reduction of the fragments often results in adequate stability because of the interdigitating nature of the fragments. If the desired results cannot be obtained by the noninvasive technique, open reduction for depression fractures is indicated. When reducing fractures adjacent to the medial canthus, care must be taken to avoid injury to the lacrimal canal. Orthopedic wires are used for stabilization if wedging the bone fragments into position does not provide adequate stability. Retrobulbar fragments that may cause entrapment of the eye may be identified by careful palpation through the conjunctival fornix and

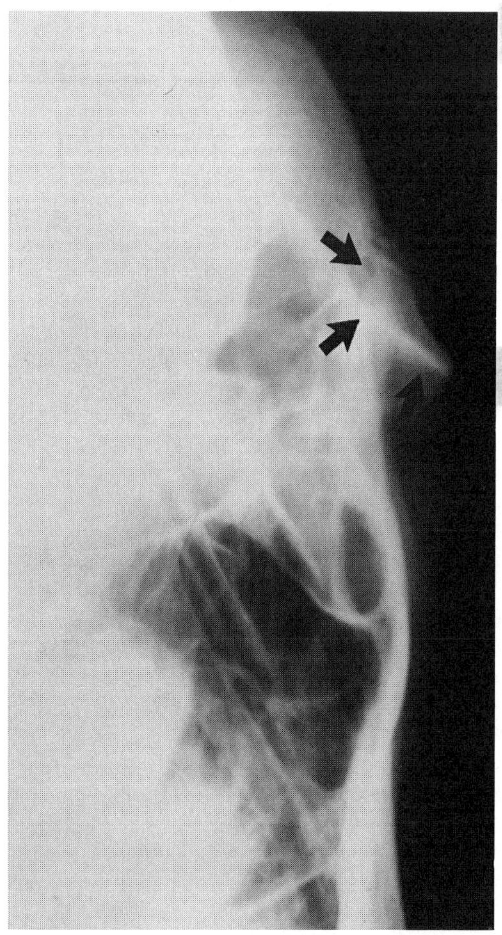

Figure 114–2. Oblique view demonstrating fracture of the zygomatic process of the frontal bone (*arrows*).

should be removed to prevent complications associated with ocular entrapment.

Other Considerations

Perioperative considerations in addition to those described for facial bone fractures include prevention of infection associated with placement of the bone hook through the conjunctiva and ophthalmic therapy for coexisting lesions.

BIBLIOGRAPHY

Blackford JT, Hanselka DV, Heitmann JM, Boyd CL: Noninvasive technique for reduction of zygomatic process fractures in the horse. *Vet Surg* 1985;14:21–26.

Campbell ML, Peyton LC: Muscle flap closure of a frontocutaneous fistula in a horse. *Vet Surg* 1984;13:185–188.

Caron JP, Barber SM, Bailey JV, Fretz PB, Pharr JW: Periorbital skull fractures in five horses. *J Am Vet Med Assoc* 1986;188:280–284.

Schumacher J, Auer JA, Shamis L: Repair of facial defects with periosteal flaps in two horses. *Vet Surg* 1985;14:235–239.

Tulleners EP, Raker CW: Nasal septum resection in the horse. *Vet Surg* 1985;12:41–47.

Turner AS: Surgical management of depression fractures of the equine skull. *Vet Surg* 1979;8:29–33.

Valdez H, Rook JS: Use of fluorocarbon polymer and carbon fiber for restoration of facial contour in a horse. *J Am Vet Med Assoc* 1981;178:249–252.

115
Fractures of the Distal Phalanx

Mark C. Rick

Fractures of the distal phalanx occur most commonly in racehorses, with the highest incidence in the Standardbred. The forelimb is most frequently involved and trauma is the primary cause for the fracture. Racing on hard or frozen racetracks partially accounts for the increased occurrence in Standardbreds. Foals have the second highest prevalence as a population group. A combination of rough terrain in the pastures, soft feet, and their tendency to run and play all have some role in these fractures in young horses.

DIAGNOSIS

Affected horses usually have a moderate to severe weight-bearing lameness on the fractured limb. Trotting on a hard surface markedly accentuates the degree of lameness, as does circling the horse. An increased digital pulse, sensitivity to hoof testers over the sole, painful withdrawal of the foot after sharp percussion, and fluid swelling around the coronary band may all be noted. Some horses with fractures of the distal phalanx show marked improvement with palmar digital nerve anesthesia, but many require that the entire foot be desensitized by perineural anesthesia of the digital nerves at the abaxial surface of the proximal sesamoids before substantial improvement in gait is seen. Arthrocentesis of the distal interphalangeal joint yields a blood-tinged synovial fluid if the acute fracture has an articular component. Once the clinical exam has isolated a foot-related problem, confirmation of a fracture requires a high-quality radiographic examination.

The radiographic examination necessitates that several views of the distal phalanx be obtained. Often, to best identify the fracture, several stand-down oblique views are required to position the primary x-ray beam directly over the fracture. The four routine radiographic views include the 60-degree dorsoproximal-palmarodistal (stand-down) with the horse standing on the cassette, lateral-medial with the foot elevated on a block, 60-degree stand-down taken 45 degrees lateral to medial oblique, and a 60-degree stand-down taken 45 degrees medial to lateral oblique. If there is still doubt about the existence or extent of a particular fracture, additional oblique radiographs may be taken. This is especially true for some fractures involving the alar portions of the distal phalanx when a question exists about possible joint involvement (Fig. 115–1). Because airspace trapped in the frog sulci can sometimes be confused with fracture lines, careful packing and positioning of the foot are paramount. Vascular channels can also sometimes mimic fracture lines. If the clinical signs indicate a possible fracture of the distal phalanx but the initial radiographs are negative, resting the horse for 2 weeks and subsequent radiographic exam will sometimes delineate small fractures that have

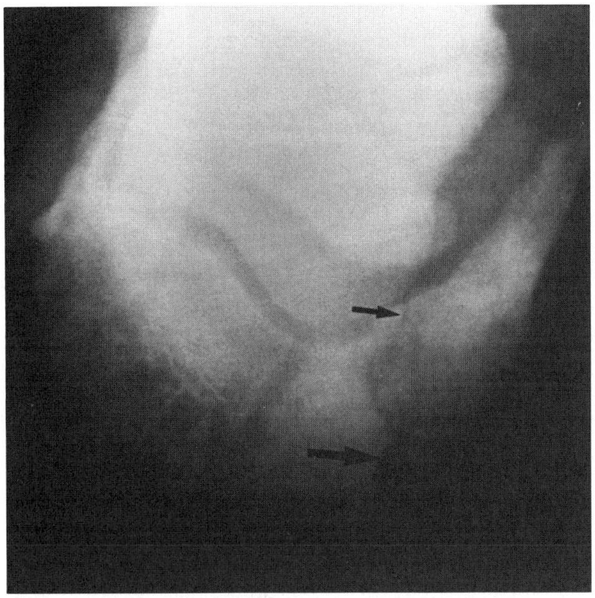

Figure 115–1. Sixty-degree stand-down radiographic view taken 45 degrees lateral to medial oblique to demonstrate an articular alar fracture. *Arrow* points to fracture and minimal, yet very important, involvement of the distal interphalangeal joint.

opened slightly or demineralized along the fracture line.

CLASSIFICATION

Fractures of the distal phalanx have been classified by their configuration (Fig 115–2). The involvement of the distal interphalangeal joint heavily influences the future outcome of the fracture and soundness of the patient. Fractures that involve the articular surface usually account for more lameness, increased length of convalescence, greater necessity of surgical repair, and a poorer prognosis for return to serviceability. Conversely, nonarticular alar fractures and solar marginal fractures carry a much better prognosis. Table 115–1 lists the classifications of distal phalangeal fractures, their preferred treatments, and the subsequent prognosis.

TREATMENT AND PROGNOSIS

Provided the diagnosis is made rapidly and appropriate therapy is instituted, most distal phalangeal fractures in horses 1 year of age or less heal with resolution of the lameness. Older horses may be able to return to their former use but they seldom achieve a bony union and will need to be managed accordingly with therapeutic shoeing to allow for function and to prevent recurrence.

Therapeutic shoeing generally consists of a bar shoe with heavy quarter clips or a full-rim shoe to prevent expansion of the hoof wall. Most horses will improve, some with marked improvement, a short time after application of the bar shoe. This initial improvement may encourage too early a return to full use, which in turn may result in inadequate healing. Preferably the horse should receive 3 to 9 months of stall rest and maintenance of the foot in therapeutic shoes.

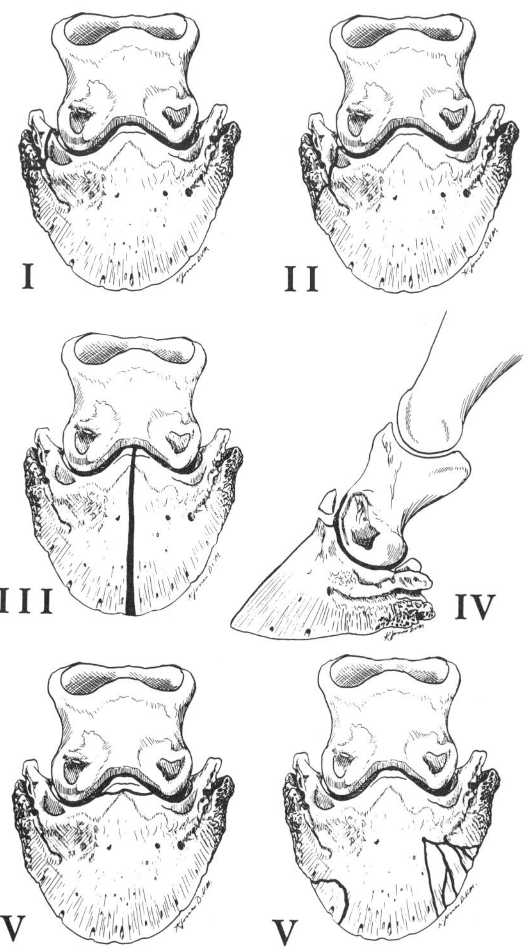

Figure 115–2. Five different types of fractures of the distal phalanx. **I.** Nonarticular wing. **II.** Articular wing. **III.** Midsagittal. **IV.** Extensor process avulsion. **V.** Marginal and miscellaneous fractures.

TABLE 115–1. FRACTURES TYPES, METHODS OF TREATMENT, AND PROGNOSIS

Fracture Type	Treatment	Prognosis
I	Stall rest 3–6 months Therapeutic shoeing Possible neurectomy	Good
II	Stall rest 6–12 months Therapeutic shoeing for life of horse Possible neurectomy Possible internal fixation	Guarded; good for young horses
III	Stall rest 6–12 months Therapeutic shoeing for life of horse Internal fixation	Guarded; good for young horses
IV	Surgical removal (small) Internal fixation (large) Stall rest (small)	Guarded to poor depending on size of fracture and duration
V	Correct the primary problem Therapeutic shoeing	Good to guarded depending on inciting cause

Healing of distal phalangeal fractures is determined by sequential radiographs. Complete osseous union requires at least 6 to 12 months and may lag behind the disappearance of lameness. Lack of osseous union with continued radiographic evidence of a fracture gap indicates a fibrous union.

Type I Fractures

Nonarticular alar fractures (Type I) carry a good prognosis. With 3 to 6 months of stall rest and therapeutic shoeing, most of these horses can be expected to return to their former use. Occasionally these horses may benefit from an ipsilateral palmar digital neurectomy to resolve any residual lameness.

Type II Fractures

Articular alar fractures (Type II), the most prevalent distal phalangeal fracture, carry a guarded to poor prognosis and often leave the horse with some pain even after extended periods of rest. Palmar digital neurectomies have been performed, but because of the involvement of the distal intephalangeal joint and the dorsal position of the fracture, there usually is incomplete or transient resolution of the lameness following neurectomy. Older horses with larger articular alar fractures should be considered candidates for internal fixation. If completed, eventual removal of the lag screw may be necessary to totally resolve the lameness after fracture healing.

Type III Fractures

Sagittal fractures of the distal phalanx (Type III) rarely occur but can be very discouraging to treat because of their prolonged healing and the likelihood of degenerative joint disease. Internal fixation should be considered for all horses 3 years and older. Prior to surgery, the foot is carefully cleaned and gently rasped and an iodine-soaked bandage applied. Lead pellet markers, washers, or wire mesh can be taped to the foot and the correct site for screw placement etched in the hoof wall before anesthetizing the horse. If an image intensifier is available, the marking can be done once the horse is on the surgery table.

The correct site for screw insertion is midway between the articular surface and the center of the semilunar canal and parallel to the dorsal surface of the bone. At this point the width of the foot is measured with sterile calipers and an 8-mm (3/8-in) diameter hole is trephined through the horny wall. The thickness of the hoof wall is then measured and this measurement doubled and subtracted from the original hoof width measurement to arrive at the width of the distal phalanx at this location, which equals the proper screw length. A 4.5-mm glide hole is then drilled through the near fragment with radiographic confirmation that the drill does go all the way to the fracture line. A 3.2-mm drill guide is inserted and the far fragment is then drilled and tapped. The hole can be gently countersunk and the cortical screw of predetermined length is inserted and tightened. Correct screw length should be checked with intraoperative radiographs because a screw that is too long will impinge on the sensitive laminae and probably cause lameness.

The hoof wall defect is packed with an antibacterial ointment and covered with sterile wraps and elastic tape. Preferably, a therapeutic shoe is applied immediately following the surgery or as soon as possible. Alternatively, the foot may be encompassed in a fiberglass cast for the immediate postoperative period before application of the therapetic shoe. Systemic antibiotics are recommended perioperatively and for 3 to 5 days. Within 3 to 4 weeks, the hoof wall will have grown past the screw head and the defect can be covered with an acrylic material or left open to cornify. Strict stall rest is prescribed for 8 weeks. Controlled walking may then be resumed, and follow-up radiographs should indicate fracture healing within 3 to 6 months. If lysis around the screw head or other signs of infection should appear, the screw should be removed. In young horses the midsagittal fracture will heal if treated with stall confinement and restriction of the hoof wall movement. The prognosis is excellent if the fracture is not displaced.

Type IV Fractures

Extensor process fractures (Type IV) are very rare and may occur unilaterally or bilaterally. Excessive tension on the common digital extensor tendon is thought to give rise to these fractures. When these "fractures" are present in both front feet, separate centers of ossification must be considered. The degree and duration of lameness are variable. If the condition has been present for several months, there generally tends to be a triangular shape to the hoof, which is called a buttress foot. Pain may be elicited with pressure over the center of the coronary band, and local anesthesia at the level the abaxial surface of the proximal sesamoids is necessary to eliminate the soreness. Radiographic confirmation is based on a lateral-medial view, which would demonstrate the avulsed fragment and the presence or absence of degenerative joint disease.

Small fragments can be removed surgically via a midline incision located over the center of the common digital extensor tendon and just proximal to the coronary band. If necessary, the incision can be extended into the coronary band. The incision will subsequently heal without ill effects on either the growth or the integrity of the hoof wall. A large fragment should be considered a candidate for internal fixation. The approach is similar to that for fragment removal. The ASIF navicular screw has been recommended because of its smaller head and ability to compress without overdrilling of the fragment. The 3.5-mm ASIF screw also has excellent applicability to this size of fracture fragment. Overtightening of the screw is to be avoided, especially in the young horse or in a fracture of longstanding duration, because the screw can pull through the fragment or lead to dehiscence. If the fragment should dehisce during the attempted repair, it would be most advisable to remove the screw and fragments. Following surgical repair, the foot is placed in a cast up to the carpus or tarsus for 1 month, followed by an additional month of stall confinement after cast removal. The horse should have 6 months of rest to allow for adequate fracture healing and to minimize joint movement before the articular surfaces have healed. Only the larger fragments should be considered for surgical repair, and case selection should entail careful examination of the radiographs for evidence of secondary degenerative joint disease so that accurate predictions can be made for eventual resolution of lameness.

Type V Fractures

Fractures that occur at the tip of the distal phalanx (Type V) are commonly secondary to pedal osteitis, chronic laminitis, or osteomyelitis, which may all represent a type of avascular necrosis (Fig. 115–3). In such cases the solar margin of the bone is weakened, demineralized, and prone to pathologic fracture. As a rule, these solar marginal fractures are not of primary concern themselves, but rather an indication of another underlying condition. Horses with pedal osteitis and marginal fractures may benefit from shoeing with

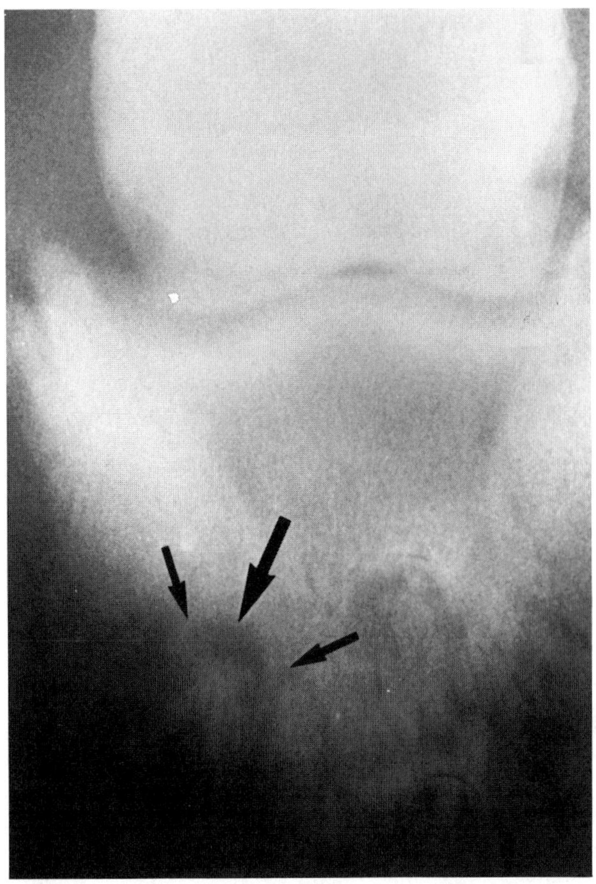

Figure 115–3. Radiograph taken at 60 degrees dorsoproximal-palmarodistal of hind limb of 1-year-old horse with osteomyelitis of the distal phalanx and pathologic fracture and sequestration involving the solar margin.

thick neoprene pads or aluminum, rigid plastic, or steel sole plates. Smaller marginal fractures will be resorbed and not be evident on the radiographs after 2 to 3 months.

BIBLIOGRAPHY

Duncan DB, Dingwall JS: Surgical removal of avulsed portions of the extensor process of the third phalanx in the horse. *J Am Vet Med Assoc* 1971;159:201–203.

Fackelman CE: Sagittal fractures of the third phalanx in horses. *Vet Med/Small Anim Clin* 1974;69:1317–1324.

Gabel AA, Bukowiecki CF: Fractures of the phalanges. *Vet Clin North Am Large Anim Pract* 1982;00:183–191.

Haynes PF, Adams OR: Internal fixation of fractured extensor process of the third phalanx in a horse. *J Am Vet Med Assoc* 1974;164:61–63.

Pettersson H: Conservative and surgical treatment of fractures of the third phalanx. *Proc AAEP Ann Conven* 1972; pp 183–191.

Scott EA, McDole M, Shires MH: A review of third phalanx fractures in the horse: Sixty-five cases. *J Am Vet Med Assoc* 1979;174:1337–1343.

Stashak TS (ed): *Adams' Lameness in Horses,* ed 4. Philadelphia, Lea & Febiger, 1987, pp 521–528.

Yovich JV, Stashak TS, DeBowes RM, Ducharme NG: Fractures of the distal phalanx of the forelimb in eight foals. *J Am Vet Med Assoc* 1986;189:550–554.

116
Navicular Bone Fractures

Mark C. Rick

Fractures of the navicular bone are an infrequent cause of lameness in the horse. Simple (transverse or oblique) fractures, avulsion or chip fractures, and comminuted fractures comprise the three types of navicular bone fractures previously described (Fig. 116–1).

The forelimb is more commonly involved and racehorses have a higher incidence than horses used for pleasure riding. Those patients with hind limb navicular bone fractures invariably have a history of kicking a wall, the back of a horse trailer, or some other solid object. Pathologic fractures can occur following sepsis from a puncture wound into the navicular bursa and the development of osteomyelitis.

AVULSION FRACTURES

The avulsion or chip fracture is detected most commonly in horses that have moderate to severe degeneration of the navicular bone. These fractures involve the distal border (margo distalis) of the navicular bone, range from 2 to 12 mm in size, and are rectangular in shape (Fig. 116–2). With improved radiographic techniques and higher resolution film-screen combinations, more avulsion fractures are being detected. On some occasions a lucent fracture bed can be seen from which the chip fracture has originated. Other apparent fragments may represent dystrophic calcification within the distal navicular (impar) ligament and are not true fractures. As such, they would be classified as a pathologic lesion associated with navicular disease but do not, by themselves, influence the clinical signs or the prognosis.

SIMPLE FRACTURES

Diagnosis

The horse with a simple transverse or oblique navicular bone fracture commonly presents acutely lame and demonstrates unwillingness to set the heel down firmly. There is increased sensitivity to hoof testers placed over the heel and central frog regions. After several days of stall rest, the pain subsides and the horse shows mild to moderate lameness of the affected limb at a walk. Light work accentuates the lameness and circling the horse significantly increases the degree of lameness. If this horse had prior navicular bone degeneration, the anamnesis may be slightly misleading. In these instances, the horse may have previously demonstrated signs of lameness of a lesser degree, on either the affected limb or both front limbs. Palmar digital nerve anesthesia ameliorates the lameness. If lameness of the opposing front limb is then evident, there may be an ongoing degenerative process involving both navicular bones and the fracture may have occurred secondar-

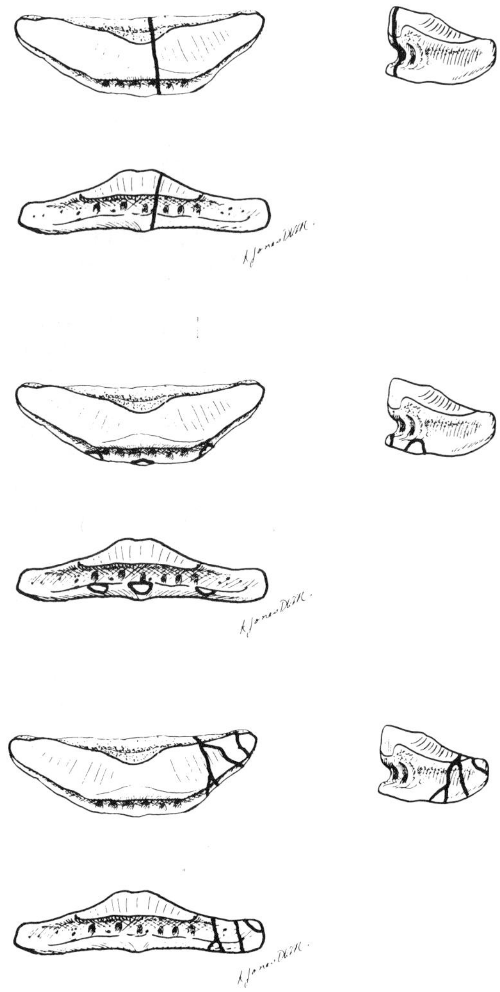

Figure 116–1. Three types of navicular bone fractures: *top*, simple (transverse or oblique); *middle*, avulsion or chip; and *bottom*, comminuted.

ily to the increased porosity of the bone. Enlarged foramina and osteoporosis of the bone can weaken it and increase the likelihood of fracture occurrence. These fractures can also occur in normal navicular bones, especially if the horse's foot lands on a solid object.

Radiography confirms the diagnosis of a navicular fracture. It is very important to carefully trim and clean the foot before taking the radiographs to eliminate all artifacts. Packing the frog sulci with a claylike material or standing the horse in a specially designed water tank will lessen the chances of radiolucent air shadows being mistaken for fracture lines. Routine radiographic views taken to outline the navicular bone should include a 60-degree dorsoproximal-palmarodistal view, often referred to as the stand-down or high coronary projection, a 45-degree stand-down view, a lateral-medial view, and a palmaroproximal-palmarodistal or flexor tangential view (Fig 116–3).

Radiographic evidence of healing of navicular fractures is not always associated with the degree of lameness. Even after extended periods of rest, fractured navicular bones will usually develop only a fibrous union between the fragments. Because of fracture instability and the likelihood for adhesions to the deep flexor tendon to develop, the prognosis for eventual resolution of the lameness is guarded to poor. Fracture fixation has been performed to provide compression and promote healing; however, if there is concomitant navicular bone degeneration associated with the fracture itself, lameness may persist following the healing process. Therefore, both resolution of lameness and healing of the fracture need to be carefully evaluated on the basis of the clinical exam as well as radiographic findings.

Treatment

Corrective Shoeing With or Without Neurectomy. A conservative means of handling the horse with a simple navicular bone fracture entails shoeing with a bar shoe and heavy quarter clips, and a minimum of 6 weeks of strict stall rest. This allows for development of the initial fibrous union without endangering the deep flexor tendon as it passes over the fracture fragments. If additional time off is allowed, 4 to 6 months of stall rest or confinement in a small paddock with the bar shoe and clips will be helpful in stabilizing the fibrous union. A small percentage of horses handled in this fashion will return to serviceability with only a slight degree of lameness. For light pleasure horses or brood mares, this may be acceptable. Analgesic therapy may help lessen any residual lameness. Continuation of shoeing with a bar shoe may lessen the movement of the ununited fragments and decrease damage to the flexor tendon. Contracture of the heels is an expected sequela.

When an extended rest is not acceptable and/or the horse will be expected to perform at higher levels of competition, the horse should be reevaluated after the initial 6- to 8-week rest for a possible palmar digital neurectomy. Improvement or elimination of the lameness following local anesthesia of the palmar digital nerves validates a neurectomy procedure. The standard approach to the palmar digital nerves is utilized (see Chapter 26). Epineural capping, cryoneurectomy, electrocoagulation, simple transection, or combinations of the above are all methods currently in use. Complica-

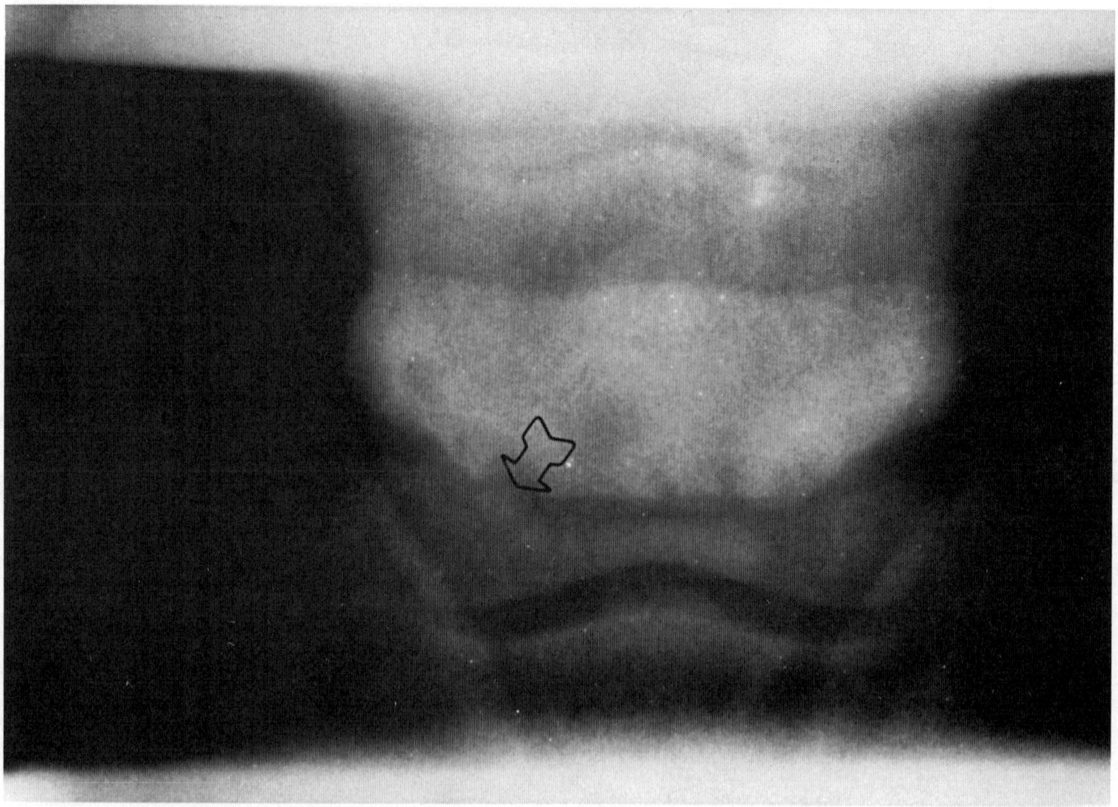

Figure 116–2. Radiograph of avulsion or chip fracture with associated fracture bed from the distal border of the navicular bone as visualized on 60-degree stand-down projection.

tions include the development of painful neuromas, incomplete amelioration of the lameness, or overuse of the limb and further damage to the deep digital flexor tendon from the fracture fragments. Close physical examination and diagnostic ultrasonography may provide early diagnosis of distal deep flexor tendonitis and forewarn of tendon fraying and possible tendon rupture. Excessive effusion within the deep digital flexor sheath at the palmar aspect of the pastern region can be seen, felt, and demonstrated on an ultrasound examination of this region. If tendon damage or fraying does occur, the prognosis for continuation of the horse's career is poor. If the deep digital tendon does rupture, the prognosis for salvage is guarded because of the lost support of the distal phalanx. Various forms of long-term stabilization, such as casts, sustained flexion splints, and special shoes, can be used to provide support for the weakened or missing tendon (see Chapter 83). Eventually fibrous tissue will bridge the gap and provide support, but the horse will most likely only be salvaged for pasture exercise.

Fracture Fixation. If continuation of the career of a horse with a simple transverse navicular bone fracture is of utmost importance, the animal should be considered as a candidate for fracture fixation. Fracture stabilization should lessen chances for future tendinous disruption at upper levels of competition. Concurrent neurectomy should be performed when there is radiographic or clinical suggestion of navicular bone degeneration.

One technique aimed at surgical stabilization and compression of the fragments offers a reasonable prognosis for those patients that suffered from an acute transverse navicular bone fracture. Implantation of a screw, in lag fashion, has resulted in adequate compression to ensure healing within as short a time span as 6 weeks when evaluated by radiographic disappearance of the fracture line. The technique does require very precise radiographic monitoring, or preferably fluoroscopic image intensification equipment in the surgery suite. Also, a specially developed apparatus that allows for precise positioning of the screw is mandatory.

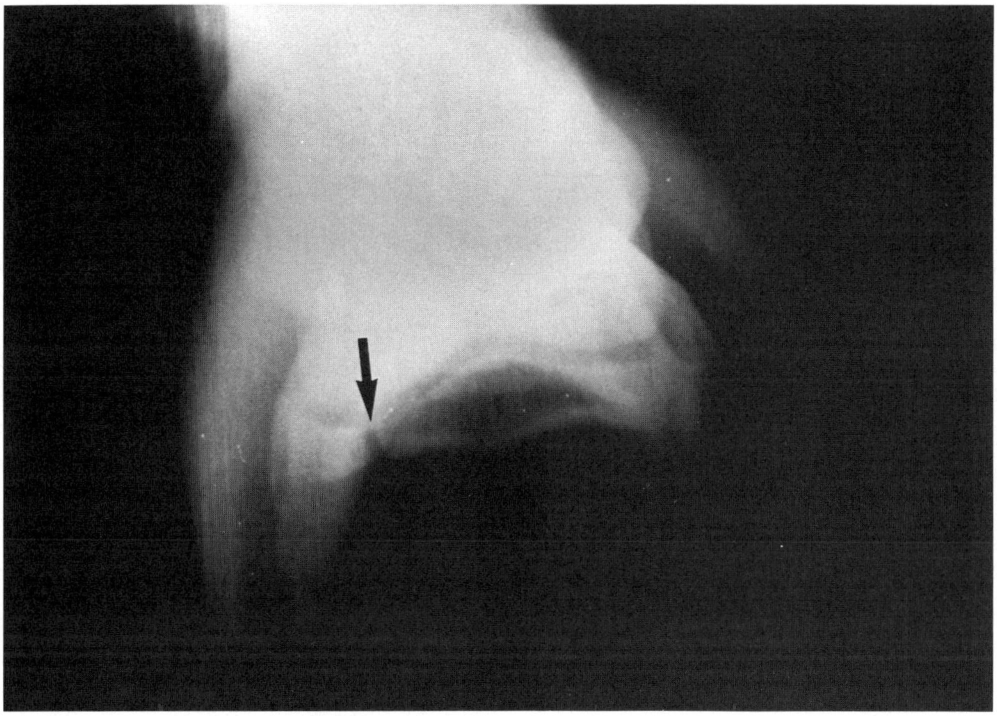

Figure 116–3. Radiograph of simple transverse navicular bone fracture (*arrow*) as seen on flexor tangential view.

Prior to surgery adequate hoof preparation includes cleaning, rasping, and soaking the foot in iodine for 24 to 48 hours. Systemic antibiotics are begun preoperatively. The horse is anesthetized in lateral recumbency with the affected limb uppermost. By utilization of fluoroscopic visualization or several radiographs and placement of needles for markers in the hoof, the ends of the navicular bone are identified. Again, after fluoroscopic or radiographic confirmation, the threaded drill guides attached to a special hoof clamp are positioned over the ends of the navicular bone, being certain to maintain absolute alignment along the transverse axis of the bone. A 3.5-mm drill hole is then drilled through the hoof wall, sensitive laminae, lateral cartilage, alar of the distal phalanx, and through the end of the navicular bone up to the fracture line. Then a 2-mm drill hole is made through the far fragment. Additional tissue and bone are removed up to the near fragment to allow for passage of the screw head and screwdriver. The far fragment is tapped and a 3.5-mm cortical screw of proper length is inserted. The size and shape of the navicular bone dictates that the first drill hole be accurate. For those horses with navicular bone degeneration, the feasibility of fracture repair must be questioned. Even with a healed fracture, the patient may still be lame as a result of bone degeneration, tendon-to-bone adhesions, bursitis and distal interphalangeal degenerative joint disease.

BIBLIOGRAPHY

Hauser ML, Rantanen NW, Modransky PD: Ultrasound examination of distal interphalangeal joint, navicular bursa, navicular bone and deep digital tendon. *J Equine Vet Sci* 1982;2:95–97.

Johnson JH: The foot, in Mansmann RA, McAllistor ES, Pratt PW (eds): *Equine Medicine and Surgery,* ed 3. Santa Barbara, CA, American Vet Publications, Inc. 1982, p 1104.

Morgan JP: *Radiology in Veterinary Orthopedics.* Philadelphia, Lea & Febiger, 1972, pp 26–27.

Nemeth F, Dik KJ: Lag screw fixation of sagittal navicular bone fractures in five horses. *Equine Vet J* 1985;17:137–139.

Stashak TS: *Adams' Lameness in Horses,* ed 4. Philadelphia, Lea & Febiger, 1987, pp 514–515.

Toal RL: *Textbook of Veterinary Diagnositic Radiology.* Philadelphia, WB Saunders Co, 1986, pp 206–209.

Turner TA: Dystrophic calcification of the deep digital flexor tendons resulting from navicular disease. *Vet Med/Small Anim Clin* 1982;77:571–573.

Turner TA, Fessler JF: The anatomic, pathologic, and radiographic aspects of navicular disease. *Compend Cont Educ Pract Vet* 1982;8:350–355.

117
Fractures of the Middle Phalanx

Mark C. Rick

Middle phalangeal fractures usually occur as acute injuries. Sudden stops and sharp turns, maneuvers required of Western event horses and polo ponies, are commonly incriminated in the pathogenesis of these fractures. Shoeing these horses with heel caulks and rim shoes provides additional traction but also anchors the foot on the ground and thereby increases torsional stress transferred to the middle phalanx. Middle phalangeal fractures may also occur during unrestrained paddock or arena exercise.

DIAGNOSIS

Those middle phalangeal fractures that occur during strenuous exercise are often felt by the rider. The horse will become suddenly very lame, often non–weight-bearing on the affected limb, and be highly resentful of lower limb manipulation. Swelling will be evident in the pastern area and crepitation may be felt upon manipulation. Highly comminuted fractures demonstrate abnormal angulation of the pastern as a result of total loss of bony support and concomitant collateral ligament damage. Horses with fractures involving the proximal corner eminence may not initially have severe lameness, and the crepitation may not be evident; however, the painful response upon torsion or flexion of the pastern area will aid in the presumptive diagnosis.

Extensive lameness examinations requiring local anesthesia are only necessary for patients with relatively small and minimally displaced proximal corner eminence or proximal midsagittal fractures. Otherwise, the horse presents with such obvious lower limb pain that it is best diagnosed with radiography only. The configurations of fractures of the middle phalanx can be variable (Fig. 117–1).

The four radiographic views necessary to fully characterize the extent of the fracture(s) are the dorsopalmar, lateral-medial, dorsopalmar lateral to medial oblique, and dorsopalmar medial to lateral oblique. The foot should be elevated on a block to provide adequate visualization of the distal interphalangeal joint.

FRACTURE MANAGEMENT

The majority of middle phalanx fractures have, until relatively recently, been dealt with primarily on a conservative nonsurgical basis. Despite available surgical techniques, the overall prognosis was not considered to be significantly better with internal fixation in combination with casting than with casting alone. Even though up to 100 days in casts is sometimes necessary for comminuted middle phalanx fractures to heal and despite costs of several general anesthesias and several casts, many times the conservative approach has been chosen and the results accepted (Fig. 117–2).

Recently, several surgeons have advocated various surgical approaches to repair these fractures as a means of offering a better prognosis and shorter convalescence. Because of the accessibility of most of the dorsal aspect of the middle phalanx, allowing for some interfragmentary compression and arthrodesis of the proximal interphalangeal joint, several means of surgical repair have been completed with return of a serviceably sound horse. The basic tenets of fracture fixation apply to the middle phalanx. Compression of fragments, establishment of normal bone alignment, use of an autogenous cancellous bone graft, and arthrodesis of the proximal intephalangeal joint have enabled a larger population of horses to return to former use or more quickly become pasture-sound breeding animals than without surgery.

Middle phalanx fractures involving only one proximal corner eminence are amenable to fixation with a bone screw. A linear skin incision, located over the apex of the avulsed fragment, is made. Utilizing meticulous radiographic assistance a single 4.5-mm cortical bone screw can be inserted, in lag fashion, to reattach the fragment to the parent bone and preserve joint congruence.

Comminuted middle phalanx fractures, encountered four times more frequently than the single avulsions, require evaluation of many factors, such as involvement of the distal interphalangeal joint, expected use for the horse, and expense, before the decision for surgery versus conservative management is made. If the

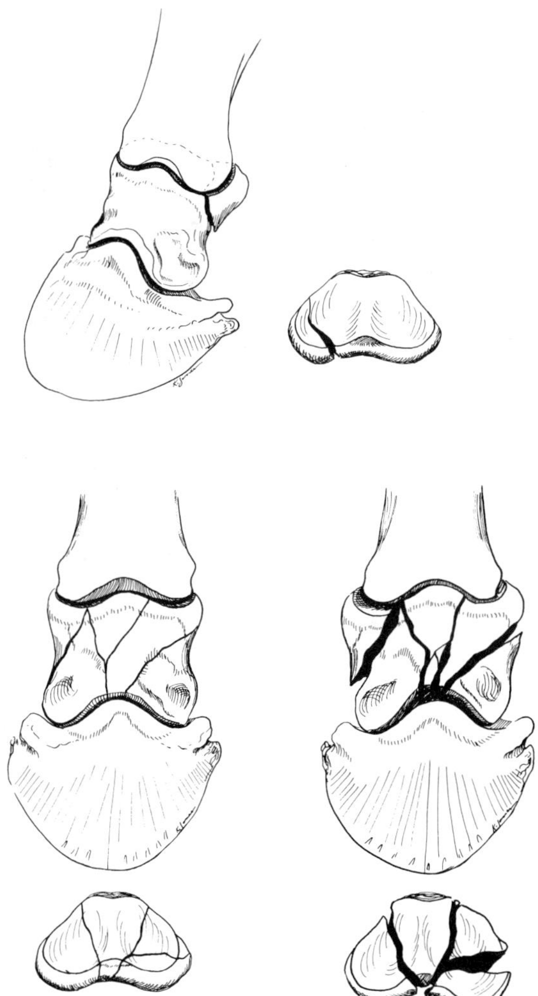

Figure 117–1. Diagrammatic representations of four different types of middle phalangeal fractures.

distal interphalangeal joint is not involved, or is only minimally so, then pastern arthrodesis and fracture repair is an option. The technique for repair will vary somewhat depending on the fracture configuration. A T-plate, ASIF compression plate(s), two criss-cross screws, and three parallel screws have all been used successfully. Use of the T-plate or compression plate has the inherent advantage of reestablishing a bony strut of support, preventing the proximal phalanx from further displacing the fracture fragments (Fig. 117–2A), and, by placement of screws into the proximal palmar aspect of the middle phalanx, reestablishing the tension of the straight distal sesamoidean ligament.

Surgical Technique

For surgery the horse is positioned in lateral recumbency with the affected leg uppermost. An Esmarch bandage and pneumatic tourniquet are utilized and routine aseptic preparation of the leg from the coronary band to midmetacarpal region is performed. An *I*- or *C*-shaped skin incision is made and a *Z*-plasty or inverted *V* incision is made through the long/common digital extensor tendon. Removing all the articular cartilage off the distal proximal phalanx and proximal middle phalanx allows for bone-to-bone contact. Lag screws can be placed separately or screws can be placed in lag fashion through the plate to achieve compression of the larger bone fragments (Fig. 117–3). Care must be taken to ensure that none of the screws penetrates too far palmar/plantar because several important structures lie just palmar to the middle phalanx (the navicular bone, its suspensory ligaments and surrounding

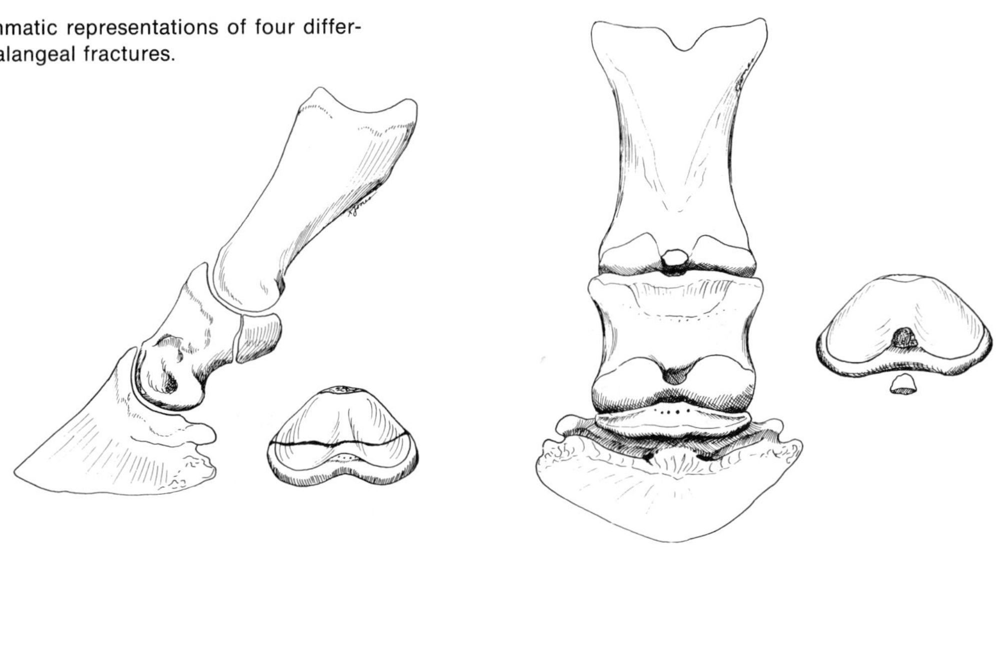

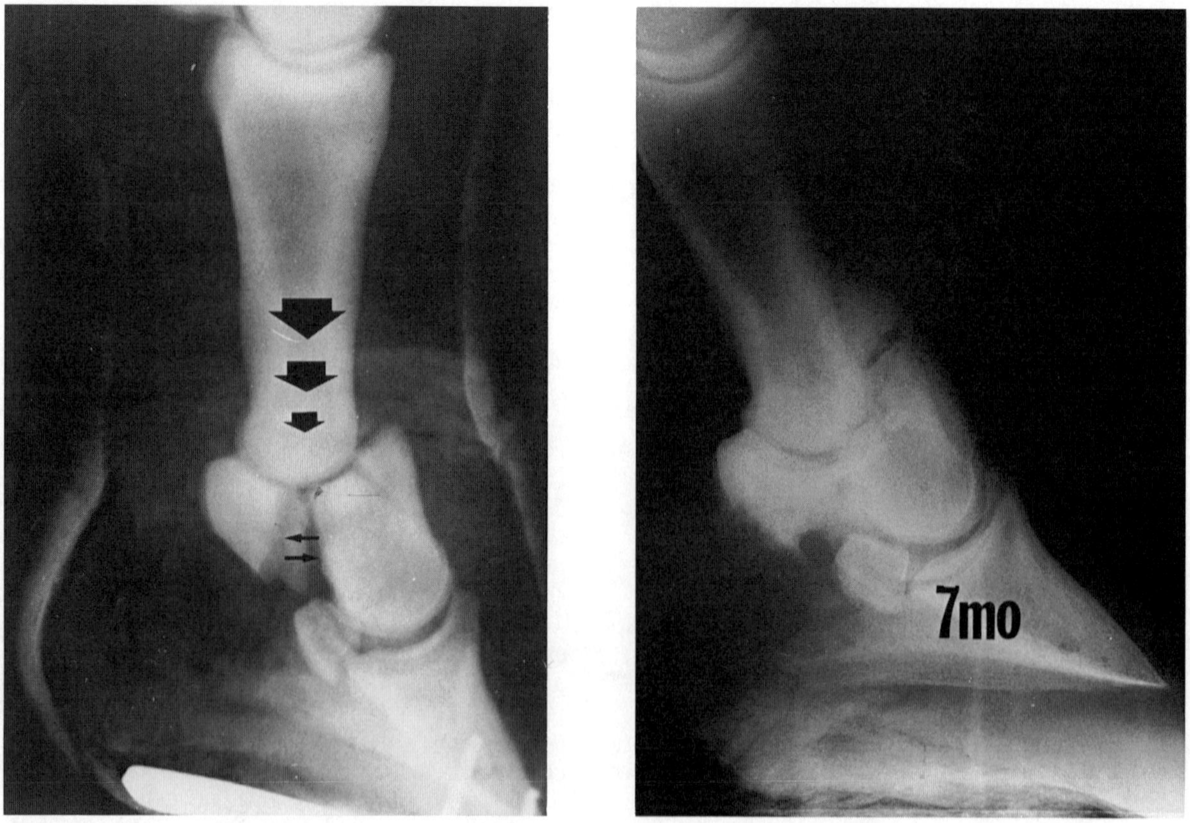

A B

Figure 117–2. **A.** Radiographic demonstration of the proximal phalanx wedging down into (*vertical arrows*) and separating (*horizontal arrows*) middle phalanx fracture fragments. **B.** The fracture was treated by casting alone for 3 months. Note excessive exostosis and abnormal pastern angle after remodeling of the callus at 7 months.

bursa, and the deep digital flexor tendon). Intraoperative radiographs assist in proper screw placement. The proximal interphalangeal joint itself is immobilized utilizing the plate under compression or by lagging screws from the proximal phalanx into the middle phalanx.

Perioperative antibiotics are considered important because of the proximity of the hoof wall to the surgical incision, the difficulty in adequate preoperative surgical preparation because most patients are in a cast, and the intraoperative time required with use of internal fixation. Autogenous cancellous bone grafting aids the stabilization and shortens the convalescence by increasing bony accretion. The tuber coxa or sternum may be utilized as a source for the cancellous bone graft.

Total surgery time for a well-coordinated middle phalanx fracture repair, pastern arthrodesis including bone graft, and cast application is approximately 3 hours. Because many of these horses will be well-muscled Quarter Horses, minimizing surgery time is very important to decrease the likelihood of recumbency or anesthetic-related myopathy.

POSTOPERATIVE CARE

Recovery should include a cast encompassing the foot to the carpus or tarsus that the horse will wear for at least 4 weeks. The need for a second cast will be determined by the radiographic signs of early healing, the adequacy of the fracture repair, and the temperament of the patient. Stall confinement during the initial cast period and for an additional 30 days after cast removal is advised. Following cast removal a heavy wrap should be applied to control swelling and provide support to

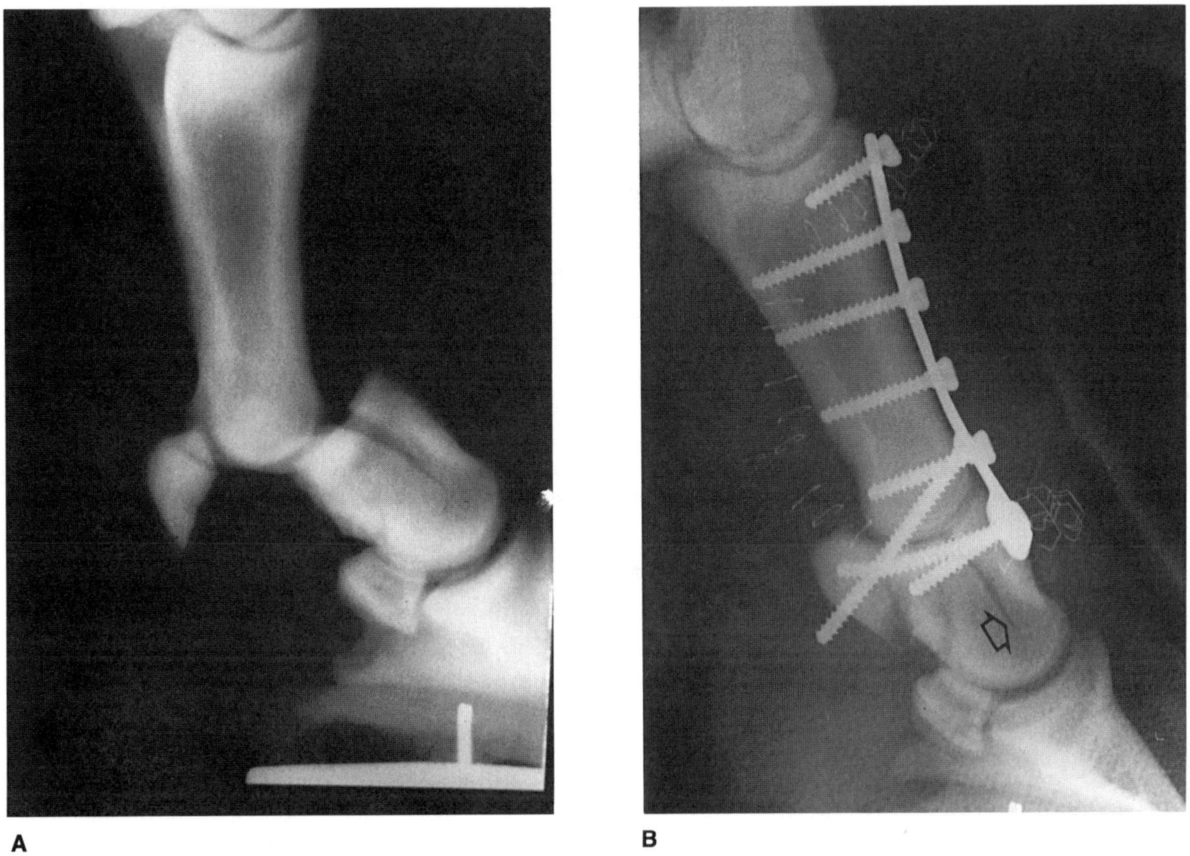

Figure 117–3. Severely displaced and comminuted middle phalanx fracture (**A**) and subsequent repair with T-plate and one separate cortical bone screw (**B**). Note how the fracture can be compressed at the distal interphalangeal joint (*arrow* in **B**). The separate cortical bone screw was too long and should have been replaced with a proper-length screw. Metallic skin staples were utilized in the closure.

the lower limb. Seventy-five to 90 days postoperatively the radiographs should demonstrate progression of bony union and loss of the proximal interphalangeal joint space. At this time the horse may have access to a small paddock and begin limited walking exercise. Monthly reexaminations should be performed and increasing amounts of exercise prescribed depending upon clinical and radiographic progress. Usually light exercise can commence 4 to 6 months following surgery. Possible reasons for residual lameness past the sixth month would include screw penetration into a navicular bone suspensory ligament, excessive periosteal response, degenerative joint disease of the distal interphalangeal joint, or failure of the pastern arthrodesis. Nine months to 1 year should be allowed before ultimate success or failure of the repair is determined relative to the soundness of the patient.

PROGNOSIS

Almost all horses with middle phalanx fractures can be saved unless, in the extremely rare exception, the fracture should be compound. With external coaptation alone, the majority of these fractures would heal in 3 to 5 months. Excessive exostosis, abnormal lower limb angulation, degenerative changes within the distal interphalangeal joint, and tendinous restrictions are all inherent complications when conservative techniques are utilized alone (Fig. 117–2B). Horses with comminuted middle phalanx fractures have about a 1:10 chance for return to athletic function without surgery.

With surgical intervention the chance for return to athletic soundness can be increased to over 50%. Surgical repair seems best suited for hind limb fractures that do not involve two articulations. The corner eminence fractures, although occasionally lagged back into place by screw fixation, are more commonly dealt with via pastern arthrodesis. Comminuted middle phalanx fractures, with excessive wedging apart of fragments, would best be handled by internal fixation, rather than casting alone, to prevent migration of fragments through the skin, ensure normal bone alignment, and lessen convalescence (Fig. 117–3).

BIBLIOGRAPHY

Colahan PT, Wheat JD, Meagher DM: Treatment of middle phalangeal fractures in the horse. *J Am Vet Med Assoc* 1981;178:1182–1185.

Doran RE, White NA, Allen D: Use of a bone plate for treatment of middle phalangeal fractures in horses: Seven cases (1979–1984). *J Am Vet Med Assoc* 1987;191:575–578.

Fackelman GE, Nunamaker DM: *Manual of Internal Fixation in the Horse.* New York, Springer-Verlag, 1982, pp 74–79.

Genetzky RM, Schneider EJ, Butler HC, Guffy MM: Comparison of two surgical procedures for arthrodesis of the proximal interphalangeal joint in horses. *J Am Vet Med Assoc* 1981;179:464–468.

Martin GS, McIlwraith CW, Turner AS, Nixon AJ, Stashak TS: Long-term results and complications of proximal interphalangeal arthrodesis in horses. *J Am Vet Med Assoc* 1984;184:1136–1140.

Modransky PD, Grant BD, Rantanen NW, Corey DG: Surgical treatment of a palmar midsagittal fracture of the proximal second phalanx in a horse. *Vet Surg* 1982;11:129–131.

Rick MC, Herthel DJ, Boles C: Surgical management of middle phalangeal fractures and high ringbone in the horse: A review of 16 cases. *Proc AAEP Ann Conven* 1986, pp 315–321.

Schneider JE, Carnine BL, Guffy MM: Arthrodesis of the proximal interphalangeal joint in the horse: A surgical treatment for high ringbone. *J Am Vet Med Assoc* 1978;173:1364–1369.

Turner AS, Gabel AA: Lag screw fixation of avulsion fractures of the second phalanx in the horse. *J Am Vet Med Assoc* 1975;167:306–309.

118
Fractures of the Proximal Phalanx

Mark D. Markel

DIAGNOSIS

Fractures of the proximal phalanx occur frequently in the horse. The most common major fracture of the proximal phalanx is the midsagittal type. The majority of proximal phalanx fractures occur in 2- to 6-year-old Standardbred and Thoroughbred racehorses of either sex. The degree of lameness after the injury depends on the type and severity of the fracture. Most horses are moderately to severely lame with fetlock joint effusion, increased digital pulse, and pain on forced flexion or rotation of the joint. Diagnostic regional anesthesia usually is not necessary to confirm the cause of the lameness, but palmar nerve anesthesia at the level of the sesamoid bones often improves the horse's gait. The clinician should use diagnostic regional anesthesia with great caution on horses with severe lameness because of the possibility of causing the fracture to become complete or displaced when the horse increases weight bearing.

Radiographic examination of the proximal phalanx is necessary for a definitive diagnosis. Proximal phalanx fractures can be classified as noncomminuted or comminuted. Noncomminuted fractures have been divided into six types.

1. *Midsagittal fractures* (Fig. 118–1). Midsagittal fractures exist primarily in the sagittal plane. This fracture classification is divided into three subgroups:
   a. Short, incomplete midsagittal fractures. These fractures arise from the proximal articular surface of the proximal phalanx and are less than 30 mm long.
   b. Long, incomplete midsagittal fractures. These fractures are longer than 30 mm.
   c. Complete midsaggital fractures.
2. *Dorsal frontal fractures* (Fig. 118–2). These fractures start at the metatarso- or metacarpophalangeal joint in the frontal plane and extend toward the dorsal aspect of the proximal phalanx.

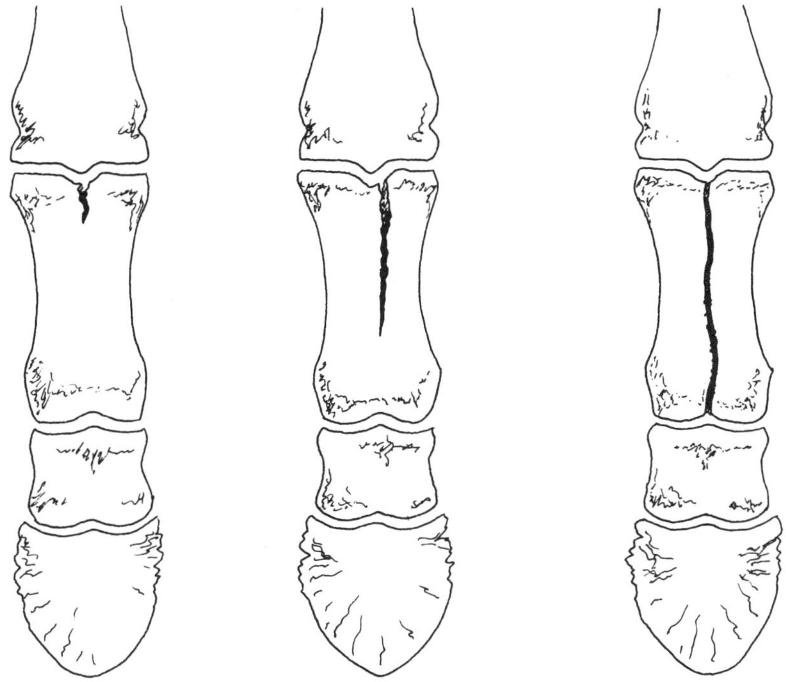

Figure 118–1. Three stages of midsagittal fractures of the proximal phalanx.

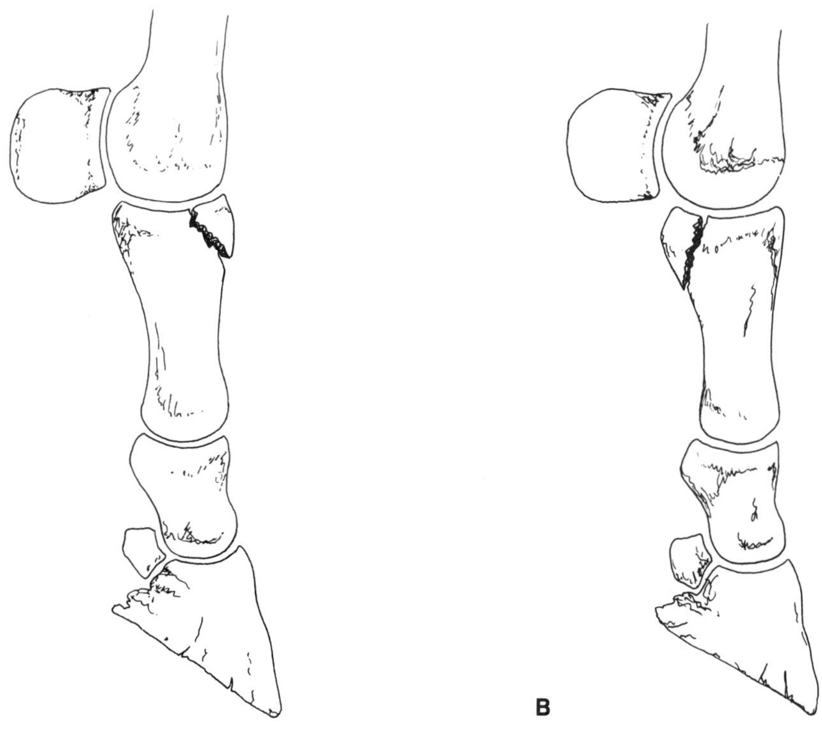

A B

Figure 118–2. **A.** Dorsal frontal fracture of the proximal phalanx. **B.** Palmar/plantar process fracture of the proximal phalanx.

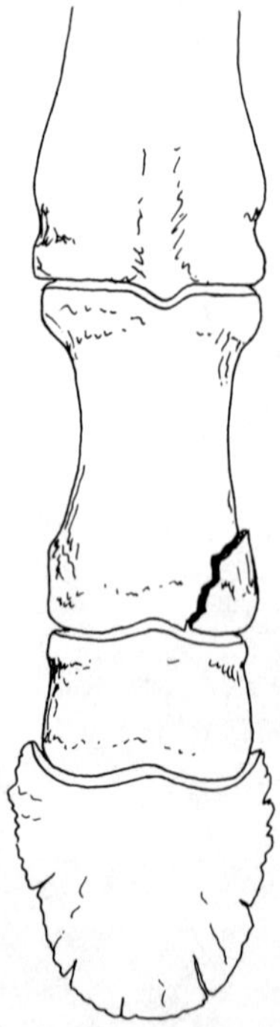

Figure 118–3. Distal joint fracture of the proximal phalanx.

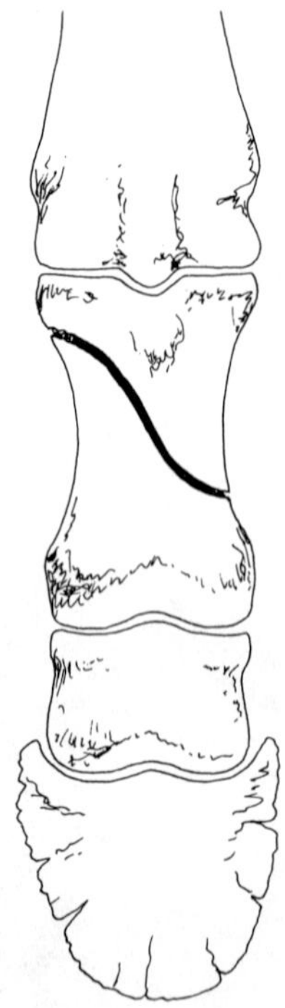

Figure 118–5. Oblique fracture of the proximal phalanx.

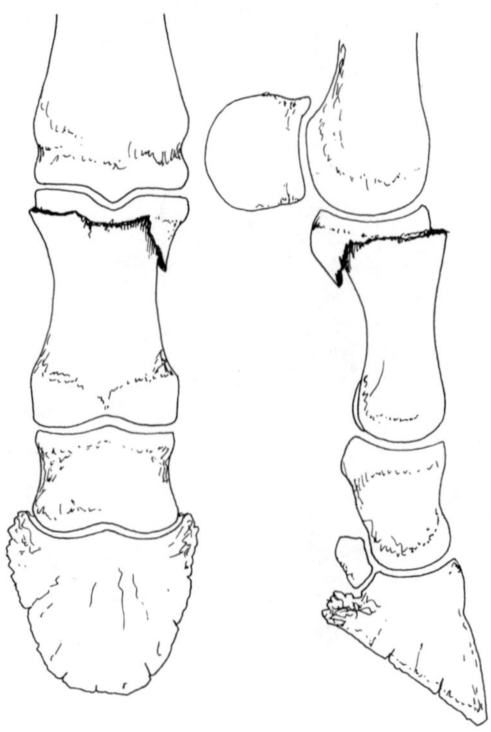

Figure 118–4. Salter-Harris type II fracture of the proximal phalanx.

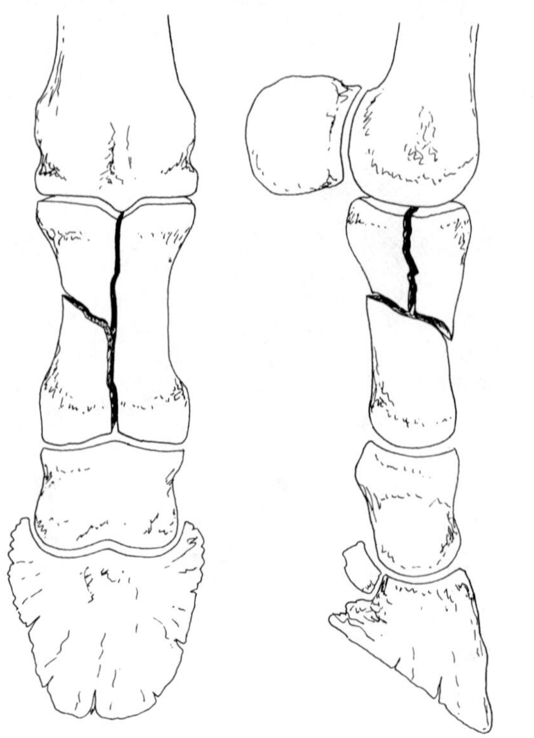

Figure 118–6. Comminuted fracture of the proximal phalanx with an intact cortex (strut) of bone from the proximal to the distal joint.

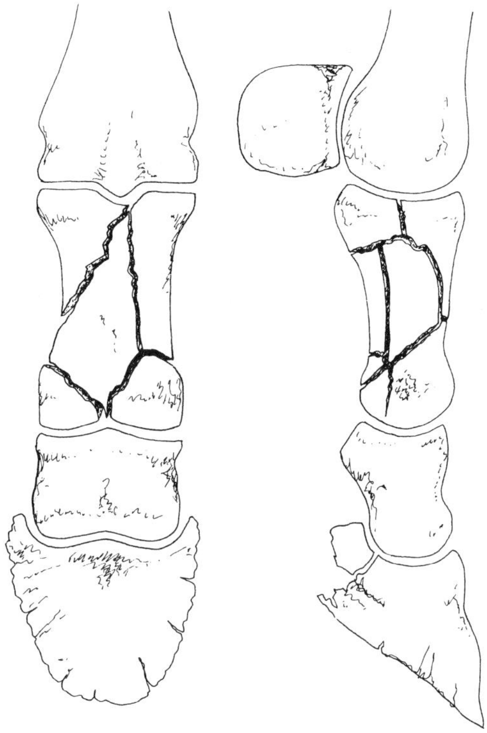

Figure 118–7. Comminuted fracture of the proximal phalanx without an intact cortex (strut) of bone from the proximal to the distal joint.

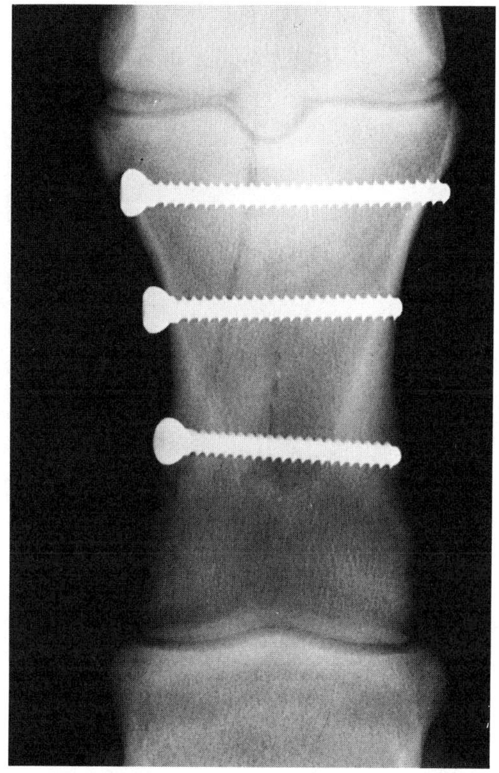

Figure 118–8. Incomplete midsagittal fracture repaired with three 4.5-mm cortical bone screws.

3. *Distal joint fractures* (Fig. 118–3). These fractures communicate with the proximal interphalangeal joint only.
4. *Palmar or plantar process fractures* (Fig. 118–2). These fractures are proximal articular fractures.
5. *Physeal fractures* (Fig. 118–4). These fractures usually are Salter-Harris type II fractures.
6. *Oblique or transverse diaphyseal fractures* (Fig. 118–5). These fractures do not affect the physis or either articular surface of the bone.

Comminuted fractures (three or more major fragments) can be divided into two types: fractures with an intact cortex (strut) of the proximal phalanx extending from the proximal to the distal joint (Fig. 118–6) and fractures lacking a strut (Fig. 118–7). Fractures that have only two major pieces and other smaller fragments can be repaired as if the smaller fragments are not present.

FRACTURE MANAGEMENT

The method selected for repair of proximal phalanx fractures depends on the fracture type and severity, and the horse's age and projected use. Midsagittal fractures are repaired using lag screw fixation with 4.5- or 5.5-mm cortical bone screws (Synthes, Ltd.) (Fig. 118–8). Incomplete fractures can be repaired by placing the screws through stab incisions using radiographic or fluoroscopic control. For complete, displaced midsagittal fractures, the metacarpophalangeal joint should be entered through a dorsal longitudinal incision to permit accurate reconstruction of the proximal articular surface of the proximal phalanx.

Dorsal frontal fractures can be treated either surgically or conservatively, depending on whether the fracture is complete or incomplete. Complete fractures should be repaired surgically to reestablish articular congruity (Fig. 118–9). The fragment is compressed to the parent bone with a 3.5-mm cortical bone screw applied in lag fashion in a dorsoplantar direction. Incomplete dorsal frontal fractures can be managed by placing the horse in a stall for 6 to 8 weeks with a firm support wrap on the affected limb or by the surgical method described for complete fractures. Distal joint fractures can be managed either surgically or conservatively. Displaced fractures should be reduced and stabilized with 4.5- or 5.5-mm cortical bone screws applied

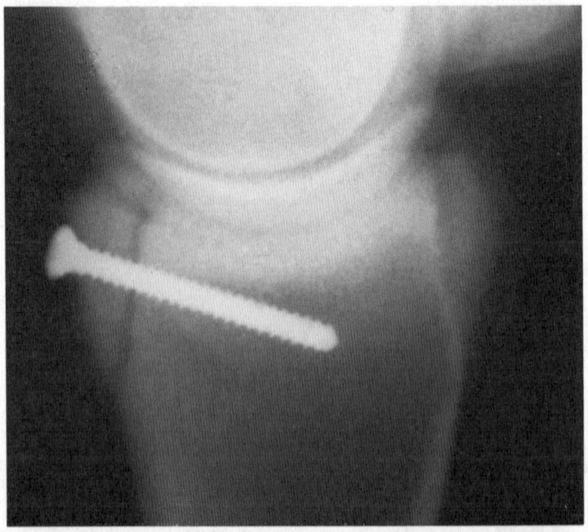

Figure 118–9. Complete dorsal frontal fracture repaired with one 3.5-mm cortical bone screw.

in lag fashion. Horses with nondisplaced fractures can be managed conservatively by placing the affected limb in a cast for 6 to 12 weeks.

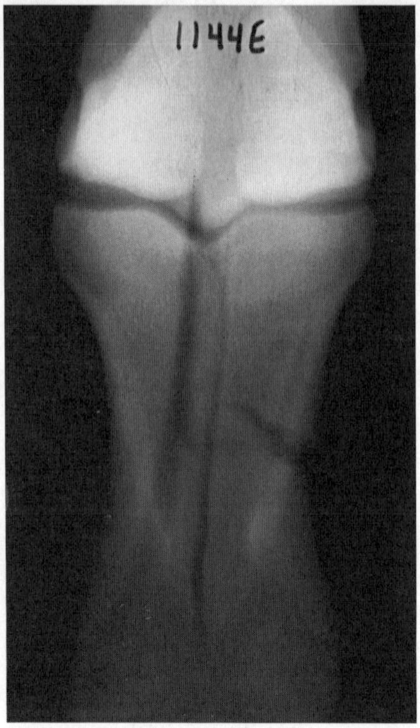

Figure 118–10. Comminuted fracture of the proximal phalanx with an intact cortex (strut) of bone from the proximal to the distal joint.

Plantar process fractures can be managed surgically or conservatively. Surgical therapy is best reserved for horses with acute fractures; large fragments are stabilized with one or two 3.5-mm cortical bone screws, and small fragments are removed. The radiographic appearance of some plantar process fractures is consistent with a chronic nonunion of the fracture. One explanation for this appearance is the possibility of the fracture having occurred early in the horse's life. There is a variable degree of lameness associated with this lesion, and the nonunion fracture may be an incidental finding in some horses.

Physeal fractures should be managed with stall rest and external coaptation of the fracture with a cast for 3 to 4 weeks. Fractures may heal with a moderate degree of malunion, but the bone will develop a more normal appearance as it remodels. In young foals reduction of the metaphyseal fragment by bone pin fixation or small screws helps maintain axial alignment.

Oblique fractures can be managed surgically or conservatively, depending on the configuration of the frac-

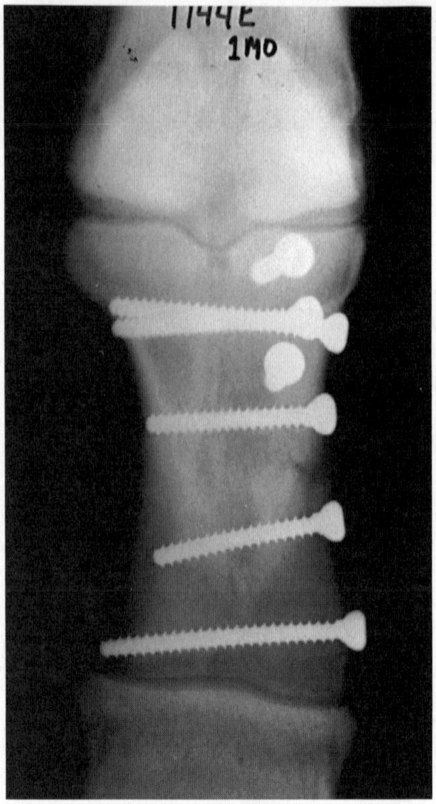

Figure 118–11. Radiographic examination of horse in Fig. 118–10 1 month after lag screw fixation of proximal phalanx with 4.5-mm cortical bone screws.

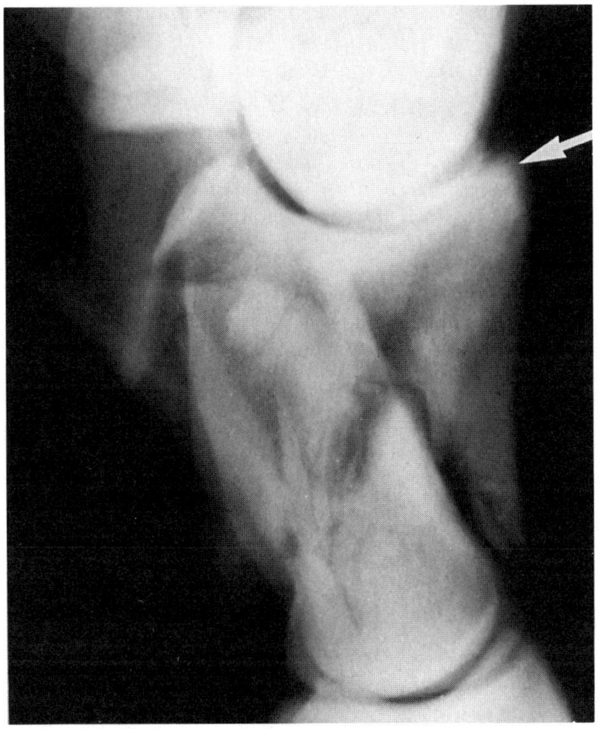

Figure 118–12. Comminuted fracture of the proximal phalanx without an intact cortex of bone from the proximal to the distal joint. The dorsal aspect of the proximal phalanx is displaced dorsally, potentially forcing the fragment through the fetlock joint (*arrow*).

ture. If the fracture is a long oblique fracture, the fragments can be compressed using lag screw fixation with cortical bone screws. Horses with minimally oblique fractures or transverse fractures of the proximal phalanx can be managed using a narrow 4.5-mm dynamic compression plate applied on either the lateral, medial, or both lateral and medial surfaces of the proximal phalanx.

Comminuted fractures with an intact strut of bone should be managed surgically. The bone is usually approached from the side opposite the intact strut of bone (which is usually medial) (Figs. 118–10 and 118–11). The skin incision is curvilinear, and starts at the distal lateral aspect of the third metacarpal or third metatarsal bone and crosses the dorsal aspect of the fetlock joint, extending distally toward the lateral aspect of the proximal interphalangeal joint. The collateral ligament is incised and the fetlock joint is luxated to expose the proximal articular surface. The fracture fragments are reduced to rebuild the proximal articular surface of the proximal phalanx. The fragments are stabilized by lag screw fixation with cortical bone screws. After reduction and stabilization of the fracture fragments, the collateral ligament and joint capsule are reapposed with simple interrupted sutures. Following closure of the skin, the limb is placed in a cast for 6 to 12 weeks.

Comminuted fractures lacking an intact column of bone are very difficult to manage. The severe comminution usually precludes surgical reconstruction of these fractures. Some horses can be managed by placing the limb in a cast, but the cast must be diligently monitored for pressure sores. The third metacarpus or third metatarsus often displaces distally, forcing fragments of the proximal phalanx through the dorsal aspect of the fetlock joint (Fig. 118–12). Horses with comminuted fractures without an intact cortex of bone can also be managed using external skeletal fixation with transfixation pins (Fig. 118–13) (see Chapter 121). This fixation device allows immobilization of the first phalanx for healing. There is risk of third metacarpal/metatarsal fracture at the transfixation pin holes after the device is removed, which must be considered when choosing this method of treatment.

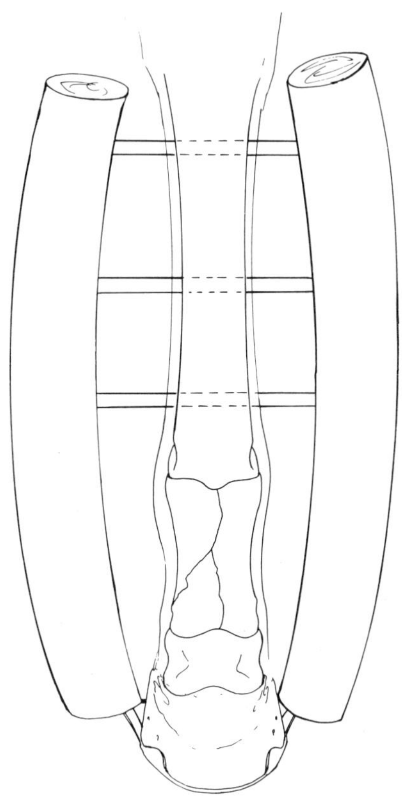

Figure 118–13. Comminuted fracture of the proximal phalanx managed with external skeletal fixation.

POSTOPERATIVE CARE

Horses that are managed with open reduction and lag screw fixation or horses with comminuted proximal phalanx fractures should have broad-spectrum antimicrobial agents administered perioperatively. Antimicrobial agents should be continued for 24 to 48 hours after surgery unless there is significant vascular compromise at the surgical site, in which case the antimicrobial agents should be continued for 10 to 14 days. Horses should be given phenylbutazone to minimize pain and to protect the contralateral limb from excessive weight bearing and possible laminitis.

Most repaired fractures should be stabilized with a cast while the horse recovers from anesthesia. The majority of horses with noncomminuted fractures do not require a cast after recovery, so the cast can be removed immediately. A firm support wrap should be applied to the limb for 8 to 12 weeks.

Comminuted fractures with an intact strut of bone that have been managed surgically by incising the collateral ligament to reduce and stabilize the fracture fragments should be kept in a cast for 6 to 12 weeks. Horses with comminuted proximal phalanx fractures without an intact strut of bone should be managed in a cast or external skeletal fixator until there is radiographic evidence of bony union.

All fractures should be monitored every 4 to 6 weeks with radiographs to evaluate fracture healing. After bony union of the fracture, horses are turned out to pasture for a 4- to 6-month convalescent period. Passive flexion of the metacarpophalangeal and proximal interphalangeal joints during fracture healing may minimize fibrosis and loss of range of motion of these joints.

PROGNOSIS AND SPECIAL CONSIDERATIONS

Horses with noncomminuted proximal phalanx fractures have an excellent prognosis for survival. A retrospective study of 63 horses with noncomminuted proximal phalanx fractures revealed that four horses were euthanized because of persistent lameness on the fractured limb. Of the 59 remaining horses, 34 returned to racing, 7 were used as show or pleasure-riding animals, 8 were used for breeding, and 10 were lost to follow-up.

In the same study, more Standardbreds with noncomminuted proximal phalanx fractures returned to racing than did Thoroughbreds. Of 30 Standardbreds that raced or trained before the fracture, 23 returned to racing: 8 to their previous level of performance, 11 to a lower level of performance, and 4 to an unknown level of performance. The Standardbreds that returned to racing were horses with physeal fractures (2/2); long, incomplete midsagittal fractures (4/4); complete midsagittal fractures (11/16); short, incomplete midsagittal fractures (4/7); distal joint fractures (1/2); and plantar process fractures (1/2). Of 21 Thoroughbreds that raced or trained before the injury, 11 returned to racing: 7 to their previous level of performance, and 4 to a lower level of performance. The Thoroughbreds that returned to racing were horses with distal joint fractures (1/1); dorsal frontal fractures (4/5); long, incomplete midsagittal fractures (2/3); plantar process fractures (1/2); and complete midsagittal fractures (3/11).

A recent review by Ellis et al of 119 horses with fractures of the proximal phalanx revealed that horses with short (60 horses) or long (17 horses) incomplete fractures had a good prognosis for return to performance following conservative treatment. Forty-seven of 77 horses with these fractures raced again. Of 13 horses with midsagittal fractures that required internal fixation, 6 raced after the injury, and 5 were retired to stud.

Horses with comminuted fractures of the proximal phalanx with an intact cortex of bone have a fair prognosis for survival. Of seven horses treated with this type of fracture, four (57%) were alive more than 1 year after treatment. Two were mildly lame on the affected limb and one was moderately lame on the limb. Horses with comminuted proximal phalanx fractures without an intact strut of bone have a poor prognosis for survival. Of 13 horses treated with these fractures, 3 were alive more than 1 year after treatment. The most common reason for euthanasia in these horses was infection secondary to attempts at surgical stabilization of this fracture. Strong consideration should be given to the use of transfixation pins to prevent collapse of severely comminuted proximal phalanx fractures.

BIBLIOGRAPHY

Barclay WP, Foerner JJ, Phillips TN: Lameness attributable to osteochondral fragmentation of the plantar aspect of the proximal phalanx in horses: 19 cases (1981–1985). *J Am Vet Med Assoc* 1987;191:855–857.

Bowman KF, Fackelman GE: Management of comminuted fractures in the horse. *Compend Cont Educ Pract Vet* 1980;11:98–103.

Bukowiecki CF, Bramlage LR, Gabel AA: Palmar/plantar process fractures of the proximal phalanx in 15 horses. *Vet Surg* 1986;15:383–388.

Ellis DR, Simpson DJ, Greenwood RES, Crowhurst JS: Observations and management of fractures of the proximal phalanx in young Thoroughbreds. *Equine Vet J* 1987;19:43–49.

Fackelman GE: Sagittal fractures of the first phalanx in the horse. *Vet Med/Small Anim Clin* 1973;68:622–636.

Gable AA, Bukowiecki CF: Fractures of the phalanges. *Vet Clin North Am Large Anim Pract* 1983;2:233–260.

Markel MD, Richardson DW: Noncomminuted fractures of the proximal phalanx in 69 horses. *J Am Vet Med Assoc* 1985;186:573–579.

Markel MD, Richardson DW, Nunamaker DM: Comminuted first phalanx fractures in 30 horses: Surgical vs. nonsurgical treatments. *Vet Surg* 1985;14:135–140.

Nunamaker DM, Richardson DW, Butterweck DM, et al: A new external skeletal fixation device that allows immediate full weightbearing; Application in the horse. *Vet Surg* 1986;15:345–355.

Schneider RK: Incidence and location of fractures of the proximal sesamoids and proximal extremity of the first phalanx. *Proc AAEP Ann Conven* 1979, pp 157–158.

119 Third Metacarpal/Metatarsal Condylar Fractures

Dean W. Richardson

Vertical fractures involving the distal extremity of the third metacarpal or third metatarsal bone are among the most common major fractures that occur in racehorses. A typical condylar fracture is usually only seen following vigorous training or racing activity and is quite rare in nonracing breeds. Two- to 4-year-old Thoroughbreds, are the most commonly affected horses, but the fracture is prevalent over a broader age range in Standardbreds.

DIAGNOSIS

Most horses have a history of acute, severe lameness following hard training or a race. Usually there is no specific inciting cause, but occasionally a collision or stumble by the horse will be reported. Affected horses have marked joint effusion and pain on manipulation of the fetlock. It is notable that there is a poor correlation of the degree of lameness with size or displacement of the fracture. The third metacarpal bone is affected approximately twice as often as the third metatarsal bone in the Thoroughbred, whereas, the Standardbred has a more nearly equal distribution between the two sites.

A dorsopalmar(plantar) radiograph is diagnostic (Fig. 119–1A). Lateral and oblique views are used to further characterize the fracture and a 125-degree dorsopalmar projection (a horizontal beam view with the fetlock in partial palmar flexion) is useful to evaluate the distal palmar metacarpal surface for comminution or subchondral erosion (Fig. 119–2). A well-exposed dorsopalmar (plantar) view is also needed to identify the occasional axial sesamoid fracture that may occur in conjunction with the condylar fracture. With any incomplete fracture, a full complement of radiographs of the length of the bone is recommended. This is imperative in any fracture involving the medial condyle since either an upward spiraling or middiaphyseal *Y* configuration is usually present.

FRACTURE MANAGEMENT

The primary anatomic concern in treatment of all condylar fractures is perfect reconstruction of the articular surface. The fetlock is a very unforgiving joint and minor incongruities can cause very poor results in athletes. The specific technique of lag screw fixation (Fig. 119–1B) is recommended in all complete displaced fractures and in incomplete fractures in athletes. True "hairline" cracks without displacement can be managed conservatively with success in most cases. The advantages of lag screw repair are important, however, and include improved articular surface healing, prevention of fracture propagation, a more rapid return to complete weight bearing, and probably a shorter overall convalescence. The disadvantages are the need for and risks of general anesthesia, risk of infection, additional expense, and the possibility of needing a second surgery for screw removal.

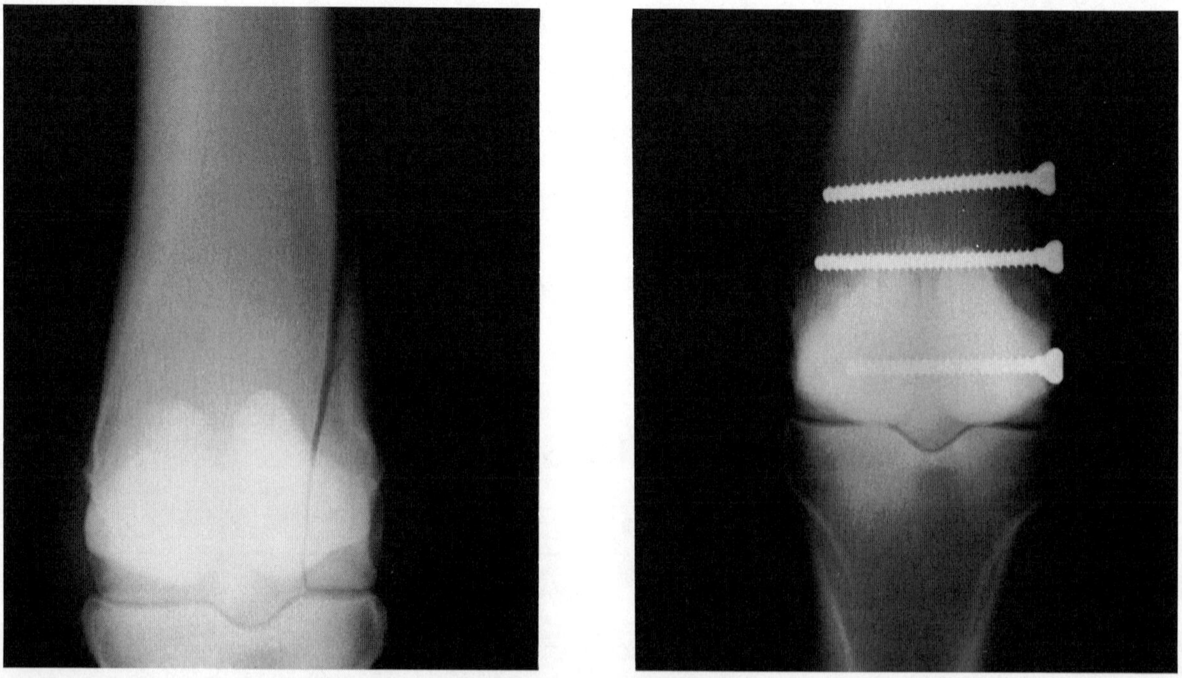

A B

Figure 119–1. A. Complete displaced lateral condylar fracture. **B.** Typical repair with three 4.5-mm lag screws.

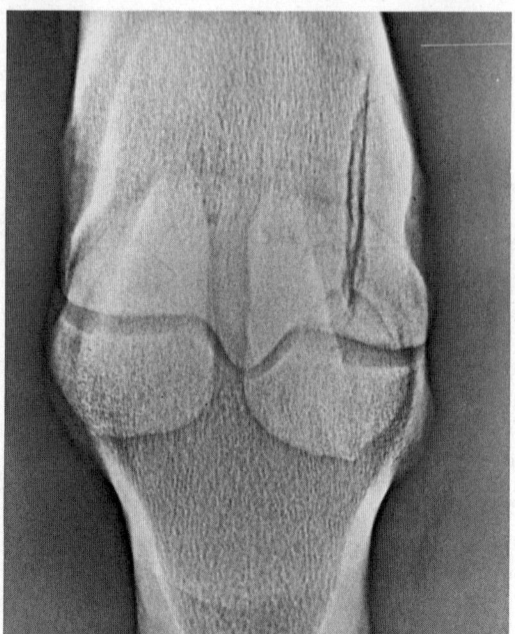

Figure 119–2. A 125-degree dorsopalmar xeroradiographic projection of the fetlock that silhouettes the distal palmar aspect of the bone. This is useful to identify focal areas of comminution or subchondral lysis.

Incomplete Condylar Fractures

Incomplete condylar fractures are repaired with lag screws placed through stab incisions since reduction of the fracture is not a problem. The distal screw is positioned at the deepest point of the condylar fossa through a longitudinal stab in the collateral ligament. It is considered that the disadvantage of irritation to the ligament is outweighed by the advantage of maximizing compression at the joint surface. Accurate central placement and transverse direction of this screw are essential to avoid having the screw too close to the articular surface, since subchondral stiffening may enhance cartilage deterioration. Use of 4.5-mm screws is recommended over 5.5-mm screws since the thinner screws have been shown by experience to be strong enough for this repair and their lower stiffness may cause fewer cases of exercise-associated, screw-related lameness. The smaller screw is also much less expensive.

The basic technique of lag screw placement is well described in various texts. In this particular application the far cortex should not be penetrated when placing the distal screw in order to avoid trauma to that collateral ligament. A relatively short (48-mm) screw will generate more than enough compressive force since the condylar bone is so dense. When working through stab incisions to place lag screws, a small Kirschner wire should be placed in the hole while changing instruments to avoid "losing" the hole. One or more screws, depending on the length of the fracture, are placed proximal and parallel to the initially placed distal screw. Screws are positioned at about 2-cm intervals. The proximal screws should never be placed less than 10 to 15 mm from the proximal end of the fracture since the fractures are often quite narrow near their apex. The more proximal screws are usually placed by drilling completely across the bone and are countersunk slightly to avoid bending of the screw head. Intraoperative radiographs are essential to assure correct screw position and length, especially when working through stab incisions.

Displaced Condylar Fractures

Displaced fractures should always be at least partially opened to assure anatomic reconstruction. Fresh, minimally displaced fractures can be checked for a perfect interdigitating fit at their proximal end through a short incision. Older fractures with less definite interdigitation must be checked for reduction at the articular surface. The simplest approach is to identify the fracture line with needles and make a straight incision through the skin and subcutaneous tissue into the fracture line.

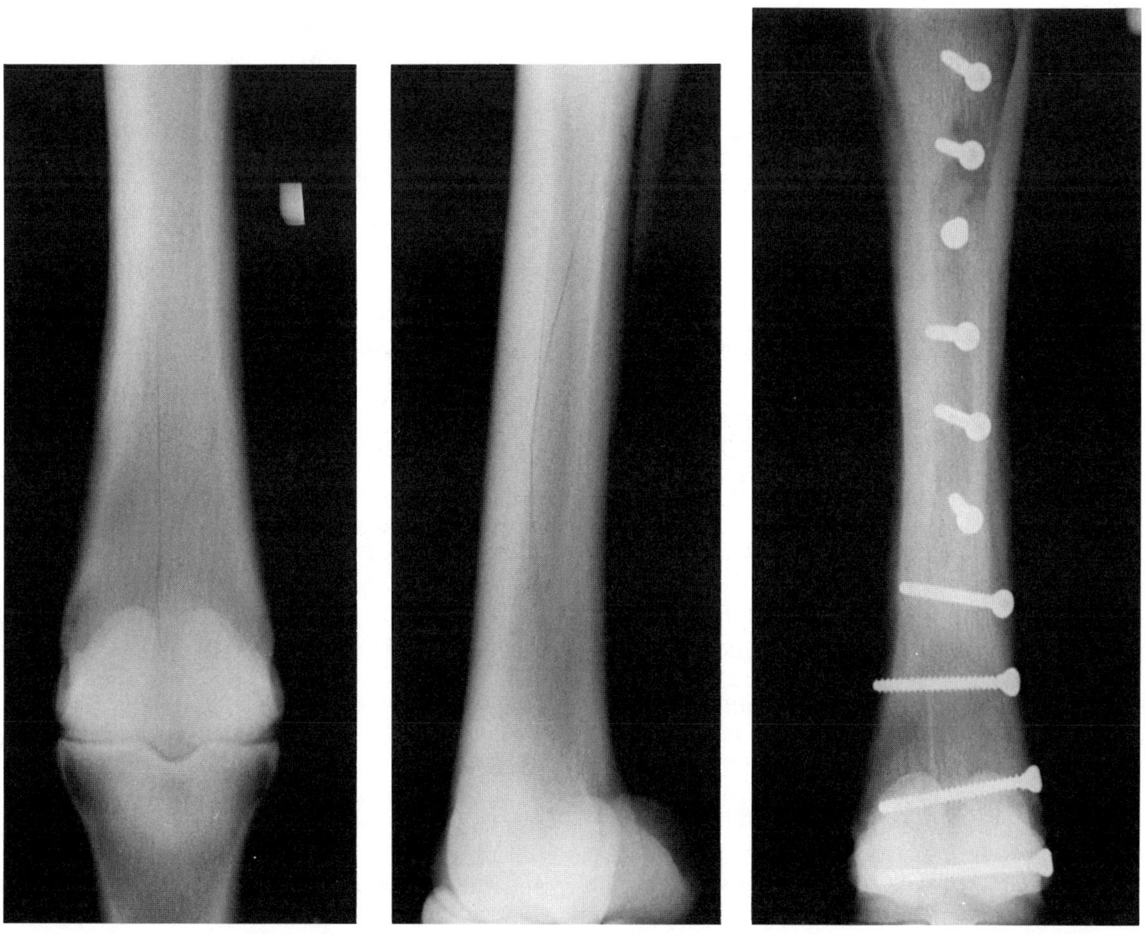

A B C

Figure 119–3. A. and **B.** Spiraling of a medial condylar fracture can only be seen with a complete series of radiographs. The extent of the fracture is seen by using both the dorsopalmar (**A**) and oblique (**B**) views of the third metacarpus. **C.** Repairs are performed with multiple lag screws placed through an open exposure or under careful intraoperative radiographic control.

This allows complete débridement of the fracture, easy visualization of the reduction, and an easy wound closure. An alternative approach that allows retrieval of fragments, which are usually found on the palmar surface of the condyle, is to make a gently curved incision originating at the apex of the fracture extending over the palmar pouch. The deep incision follows the fracture line down to and through the collateral sesamoidean ligament. This incision does cause more hemorrhage unless a tourniquet is used, but affords excellent visualization of the articular surface. In addition, the palmar approach allows evaluation of the articular surface of the sesamoid, and with displaced condylar fractures there is a very high incidence of significant articular damage to the sesamoid directly behind the fracture edge.

With both approaches, the distal screw is still placed through a stab incision but the skin and subcutaneous tissue are easily retracted for insertion of the more proximal screws. The surgeon must always be prepared to expose the joint enough to confirm accurate reduction. Similarly, if comminution is known to exist on the distal palmar surface, loose fragments should be removed by widely spreading the fracture and grasping through the fracture line or by using a palmar approach and a sharp curved hook to help extract the fragment.

Medial Condylar Fractures

Medial condylar fractures must be carefully evaluated with radiographs before deciding on a surgical approach. If a spiral component can be identified, lag screws are inserted perpendicular to the fracture plane over the length of the identifiable fracture (Fig. 119–3). Usually six to ten screws are required. Although one can usually estimate the configuration of the spiral fracture well enough to place screws through stab incisions, it is safe, reliable, and easy to expose the entire dorsal diaphysis of the third metacarpal/metatarsal bone through a dorsomedial incision made adjacent to the extensor tendon. After the periosteum is elevated, the fracture lines are easily identified, allowing accurate placement of the screws. Technically, it is easier and faster to place the screws with the bone exposed and it is easier to avoid inadvertent injury to the suspensory ligament or splint bones.

Medial condylar fractures of the third metatarsal bone that cannot be shown to spiral must be treated with extreme caution because they are prone to complete oblique middiaphyseal fracture (Fig. 119–4). Horses with hairline cracks can be treated by absolute stall rest, but fractures with the slightest degree of displacement are probably best treated surgically. Routine lag screw repair is used for the visible portion of the fracture and the horse is recovered from anesthesia as carefully as possible. Judicious tranquilization during emergence from anesthesia, manual assistance by lifting the tail of the horse, and the use of a special recovery system such as deep foam mats are all recommended. The application of a full-leg cast for anesthetic recovery or as a primary treatment merits consideration, but the cast itself holds significant risk of injury. A half-leg cast does not prevent middiaphyseal failure and may even be contraindicated. "Prophylactic" plating of a typical medial condylar fracture is a possible consideration in a breeding animal but is probably not necessary in the majority of cases and is definitely not recommended in the athlete unless the "Y" fracture is evident.

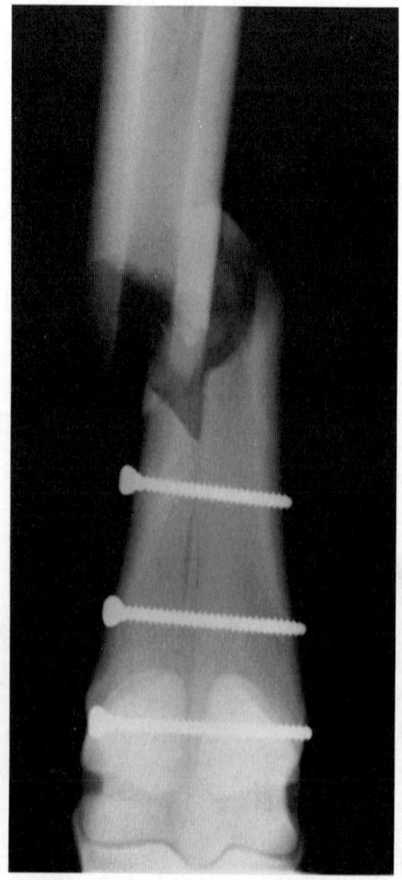

Figure 119–4. Complete middiaphyseal fracture of medial condylar fractures can occur both while awaiting surgery or during transportation, or even following repair of the distal aspect of the fracture.

Lateral Condylar Fractures

Lateral condylar fractures of the third metacarpal bone are at relatively low risk during recovery from anesthesia so routine bandaging and recovery procedures are used. Because of the torsional forces the horse places on the hind leg during recovery, all third metatarsal fractures are considered to be at risk and handled accordingly. With hind leg fractures, a heavily padded, full-leg bandage is useful to prevent the horse from lying with the affected limb down. Cross-tying the horse with a high-risk fracture would be a consideration but is not done routinely with metatarsal fractures.

POSTOPERATIVE CARE

All horses with condylar fractures are given 4 months' stall rest before considering a return to training or screw removal. As much passive flexion as is feasible is recommended with all fractures, and carefully controlled walking is permitted as soon as the horse is comfortable enough. Most horses with condylar fractures will not require screw removal, but removal is advocated if more than three screws are involved (i.e., the screws involve the diaphysis) or if the shaft of the distal screw is less than 10 mm from the articular surface. If the horse has a specific race or series of races that is considered essential, then screw removal is recommended whenever possible to avoid training the horse up to its important races only to have to remove the screws at that time. The horse is walked or lightly jogged for 8 weeks following screw removal before returning to regular race training.

PROGNOSIS

The prognosis for all incomplete minimally displaced fractures is excellent for return to racing function, with probably 80% or more of horses returning to racing

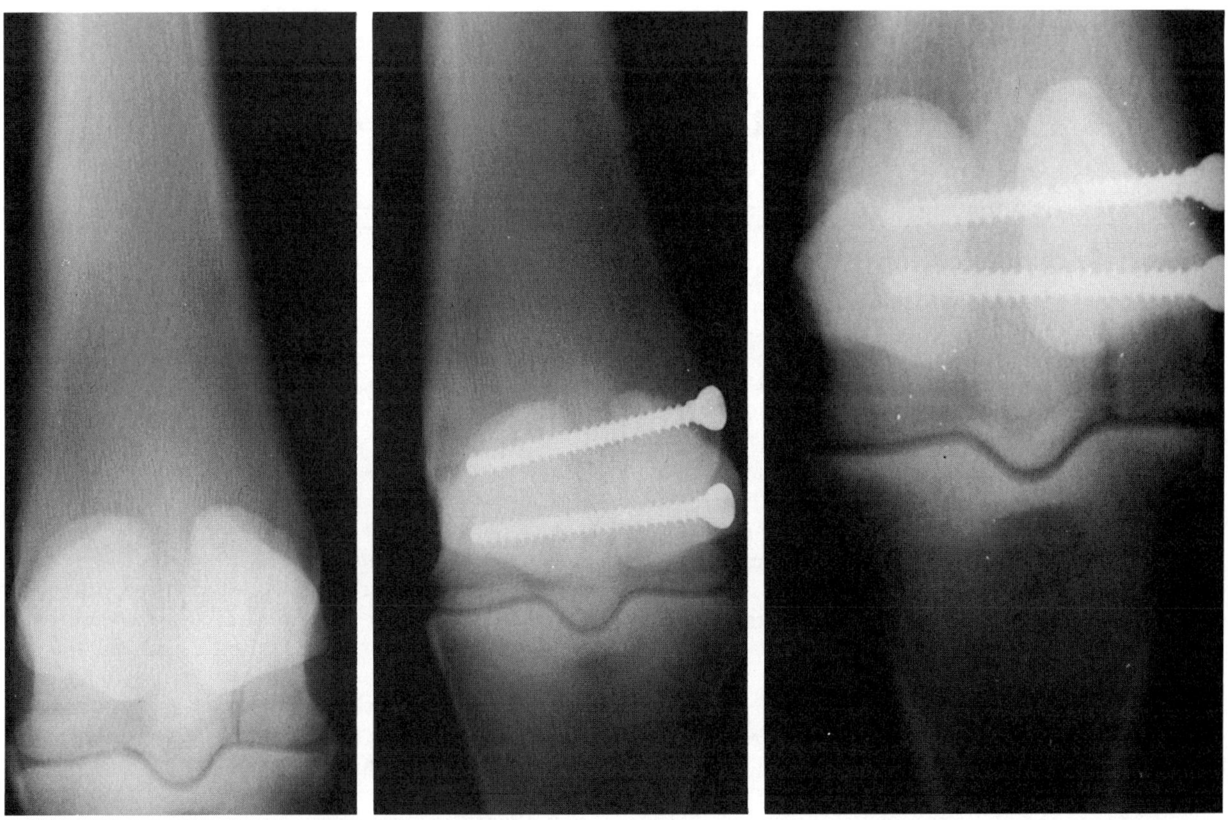

A B C

Figure 119–5. Incomplete, nondisplaced lateral condylar fracture, **(A)** was repaired with two lag screws that appeared to adequately reduce the fracture **(B)**. A postoperative radiograph taken after 10 weeks demonstrates lysis along the distal margin of the fracture **(C)**. This may be due to some unsuspected comminution at the time of the original injury or inadequate compression with the distal screw.

soundness if there was not extensive degenerative joint disease present at the time of repair. Although a complete obliteration of the fracture line should ideally occur before returning the horse to work, a faint remnant of the fracture near the articular surface will often persist and may even be evident after the horse has successfully returned to racing. This occurs more frequently with incomplete débridement of the fracture line or less than optimal compression at the joint surface by the distal screw (Fig. 119–5). Horses with displaced fractures have a much less favorable prognosis even with adequate repair since there is usually more damage to the articular surface and joint capsule. Even a small amount of lysis or comminution along the distal palmar condyle is associated with a poor prognosis for racing soundness, so accurate evaluation of this site is essential. All horses with condylar fractures have a good prognosis for breeding soundness or pasture comfort if properly handled.

BIBLIOGRAPHY

Adams SB, Turner TA, Blevins WE, Shamis LD: Surgical repair of metacarpal condylar fractures with palmar comminution in two Thoroughbred horses. *Vet Surg* 1985;14:32–35.

Barclay WP, Foerner JJ, Phillips TN: Axial sesamoid injuries associated with lateral condylar fractures in horses. *J Am Vet Med Assoc* 1985;186:278–279.

Hornof WJ, O'Brien TR: Radiographic evaluation of the palmar aspect of the equine metacarpal condyles: A new projection. *Vet Radiol* 1980;21:161–167.

Richardson DW: Medial condylar fractures of the third metatarsal bone in horses. *J Am Vet Med Assoc* 1984;185:761–765.

Rick MC, O'Brien TR, Pool RR, Meagher D: Condylar fractures of the third metacarpal bone and third metatarsal bone in 75 horses: Radiographic features, treatments, and outcome. *J Am Vet Med Assoc* 1983;183:287–296.

Turner AS: Surgical repair of fractures of the third metatarsal bones in a Standardbred gelding. *J Am Vet Med Assoc* 1977;171:655–658.

120
Stress Fractures of the Third Metacarpal Bone

David M. Nunamaker

Stress fractures of the third metacarpal bone represent one expression of a complex series of events that occur in the dorsal cortex of the third metacarpal bone during vigorous training for racing. The condition results from an interaction of the biologic aspects of bone modeling and remodeling combined with the mechanical aspects of fatigue and creep in bone associated with high-speed work. Although the Thoroughbred appears to be at greatest risk for this condition, it also occurs in the racing Quarter Horse and, to a limited extent, in the Standardbred racehorse.

PATHOGENESIS AND PATHOMECHANICS

A partial understanding of the pathogenesis and pathomechanics of the condition is necessary before one can either assess the condition in an individual patient and arrive at a rational treatment, or design a regimen for prevention. Because our present understanding of the pathogenesis is incomplete, some review and speculation will be necessary. Stress fractures of the third metacarpal bone seem linked to the bucked shin syndrome, so any discussion must include this condition as well.

Pathomechanics

Bone Modeling. The average Thoroughbred racehorse is broken to be ridden at the end of its yearling year. Subsequently, 2-year-olds start training on a racing surface a month or more before their 2-year-old year begins. The superimposition of race training on growth and development of the equine skeleton appears to play an important part in the development of bucked shins. Initially a middiaphyseal cross-section of a yearling Thoroughbred's third metacarpus would be relatively round, with the medullary cavity being large and centrally located. As the animal matures, however, both the area of the bone and the area of the medullary cavity enlarge. The shape that this bone takes is related to the exercise patterns that the horse experiences. Training for racing will superimpose strains (deformations) on the bone that ordinary pasture activity would not. The bone responds to these strains by bone modeling.

Bone modeling represents the change in the shape of the bone that occurs during growth and development by the apposition of new bone on the surfaces of the bone, and appears to be related to the strain history of the bone. Thus, as a result of these strains, the bone modifies its shape. Because the deformations on the bone presumably involve bending of the bone in a dorsopalmar direction, most of the new lamellar bone is formed on the dorsal or dorsomedial surface where these strains are compressive. As the bone changes its shape, the inertial properties of the bone also change, making it stronger in bending in that direction. The end result is that the bone undergoes a reduction of strain during that exercise period. Therefore, a young 2-year-old in training may suffer deformations of its third metacarpus of 0.5%, whereas the modified bone of an older horse (4-year-old) would undergo strains of only about 0.3% when running at speed (Fig. 120–1). This change of 0.2% deformation in the bone may account for the fact that older horses do not develop the periosteal new bone formation that occurs with bucked shins, since these older horses would have presumably already changed the shape of their bone to reduce bone strain.

Bucked Shins. When bone models it may add bone to increase its diameter by appositional rates of approximately 1 μm/day. When modeling occurs on the bone's surface, the internal remodeling that is responsible for the reconstitution of the cortex is inhibited. This process allows the bone to accumulate cyclic deformations that induce fatigue and/or creep damage. As fatigue in bone progresses, the bone loses its stiffness, thereby increasing the deformations that occur at the bone's surface at a given load. This in turn causes the bone to continue its efforts to add new bone (modeling) to increase the inertial properties. Once the bone surpasses its limits for normal lamellar bone formation, the formation of fibrous bone begins. The appearance of this periosteal new bone formation is the first radiographic appearance of bucked shins. Although clinicians consider this periosteal new bone to be abnormal, it is important to remember that this is a normal response of the bone to a loading history that exceeds the ability of the bone to form normal lamellar bone. The timing and duration of these events appear to be related to the number of strides (cycles) that the horse galloped and the surface over which the animal trained.

The onset of bucked shins is related to the onset of training and not the chronologic age of the horse. Although most horses buck their shins as 2-year-olds, horses that start training in their third or fourth year will also be at risk for the condition since their bones have not modeled for training and racing.

Stress Fractures. Stress fracture of the third metacarpal bone seems to represent a sequela to bucked shins. Most horses that develop these stress fractures have a history of "shin problems." Generally, the stress fractures follow the bucked shin episode by a few months

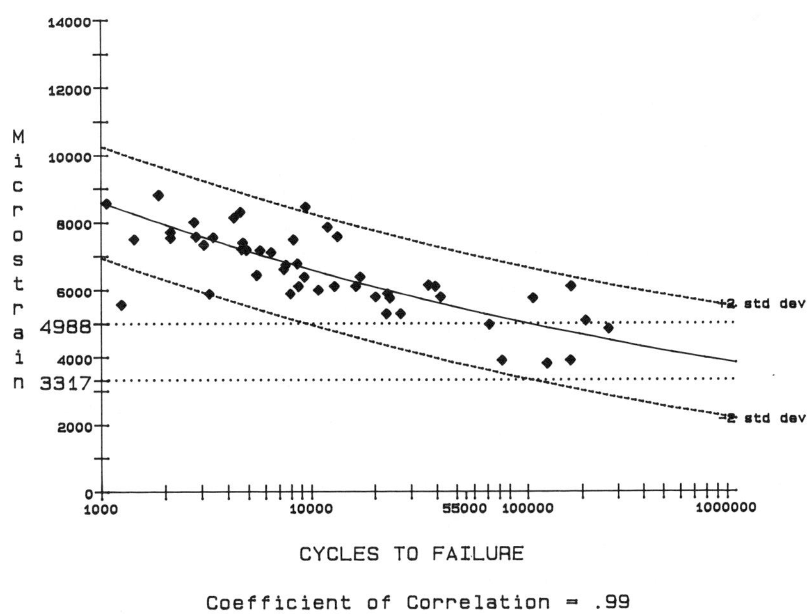

Figure 120–1. Relationships of strain versus number of cycles to failure that was achieved in in vitro studies on equine third metacarpal bone. The dotted line originating at 4988 μm on the y axis shows the strain levels achieved by 2-year-olds in training at racing speeds. The dotted line originating at 3317 μm on the y axis shows the strain on the third metacarpal bone of an older horse. Note the intersection of these two dotted lines (3317 and 4988 μm) with the fatigue data. Young horses produce high strains while running and therefore are at risk for fatigue failure long before older animals. In fact, the older animals would have time to remodel their bone before fatigue would occur.

to a year and occur in 3- or 4-year-old horses. However, if the horse started training after its 2-year-old year, the fractures will occur later.

The radiographic lesion will usually be on the dorsal or dorsolateral aspect of the third metacarpal bone and can be identified as an oblique radiolucent line that progresses to the middle of the dorsolateral cortex (Fig. 120–2). The lesion may occur anywhere along the length of the bone, and multiple lesions on the same bone are common. The fracture lines usually start distally on the cortical surface and progress proximally, but occasionally may start proximally and progress distally. Sometimes the fracture may be truly saucer-shaped and have a cortical connection both proximally and distally (Fig. 120–3). Computerized axial tomography scans may show a radiolucency that progresses into the marrow cavity as well. The occult continuation of the fracture into the medullary cavity may also be manifested by an endosteal callus (personal communication, Dr. Howard Seeherman, Tufts University School of Veterinary Medicine, June, 1987).

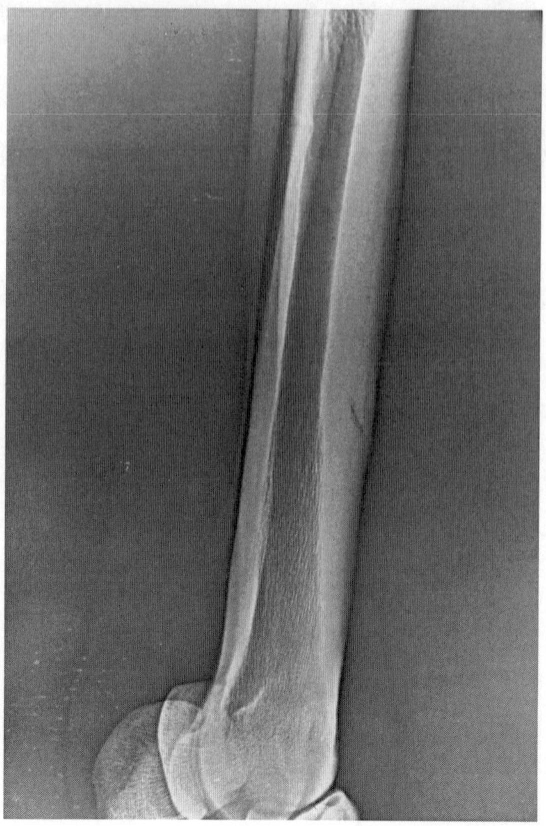

Figure 120–2. Xeroradiograph depicting a middiaphyseal lesion that is typical of a stress fracture.

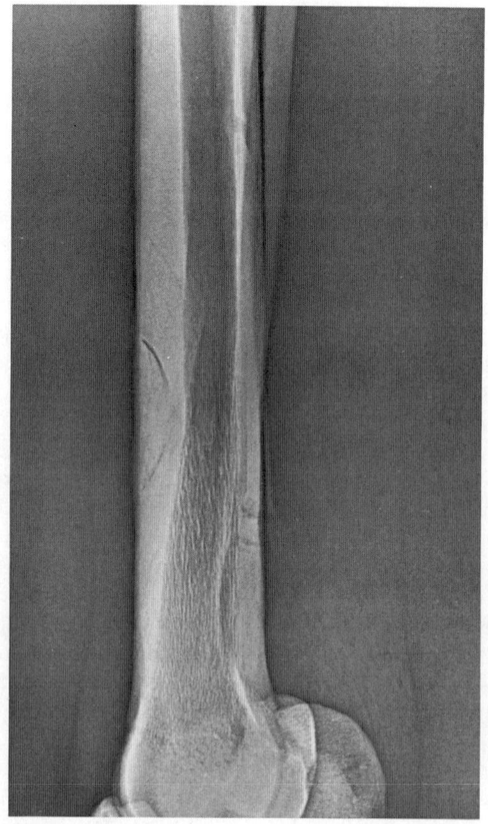

Figure 120–3. The fracture lines evident on this xeroradiograph have progressed to a complete "saucer fracture."

Pathogenesis

The limited information available on the histologic picture of this condition indicates that it is an area of intense remodeling. Radiographically, the lesion is a fracture, and the clinical picture of sudden lameness certainly implies that a fracture exists. Specimens for histologic examination are not easily obtained, however, so the pathogenesis of stress fractures remains incompletely understood.

Speculation about the pathogenesis of the condition relies heavily on the coincidence of bucked shins with the subsequent occurrence of stress fractures. If, during the progression of bucked shins, bone remodeling is inhibited for the entire time that the periosteal new bone is being laid down and modeled on the outer surface, the cortical bone would be accumulating cyclic fatigue. The dorsolateral cortex, having less periosteal new bone formation than the dorsomedial cortex, may experience equally high strains while the animal is running, and high-strain cyclic fatigue of bone may produce these stress fractures. Histologic evidence seems to indicate that this portion of the cortex does not undergo remodeling, at least during the period when bucked shins occur, thereby allowing the accumulation of cyclic fatigue.

After the decrease in cortical modeling associated with inertial property changes that occur secondary to the vigorous exercise involved in race training, the bone may then enter a period of increased activation of cortical remodeling. If this is true, then the bone may be more porous than normal, subjecting this structure to high-stress cyclic fatigue.

CLINICAL SIGNS AND TREATMENT

Bucked Shin Complex

The usual history of an animal with bucked shins involves a period of training with clinical signs developing at or near the onset of fast work. Some people believe that the use of the starting gate is an important etiologic event. The animal may develop clinical signs ranging from minimal pain to severe lameness. Pain usually precedes radiographic evidence of periosteal new bone formation.

Treatment is usually directed at reducing pain and lameness. Rest and analgesics (phenylbutazone) play an important role, but the training regimen may be most important. Many horses that are rested through their painful episode will have an exacerbation of the condition following the resumption of training. Careful evaluation of the training program may be the key to successful treatment.

Experimental studies in racehorses using strain gauges attached to the third metacarpal bone have shown that peak strains diminish as the animal grows older. These studies also show that the principle directions of the peak strains change considerably as the animal's speed increases. Since it is thought that the bone remodels in relation to the strains and their principle directions, it becomes evident that many Thoroughbred racehorses remodel their bone for training and not for racing. Thus, the onset of fast work places demands on the bone that the modeling-remodeling process has not satisfied. Consequently, these horses are the ones most at risk to develop bucked shins. In the treatment of this condition the physiology of the bone must be understood relative to the mechanical history. It would appear that short periods of high-speed work would be necessary to turn on the proper modeling-remodeling sequence. Long work at high speed may cause injury and long work at slow speeds will not affect the bone in a positive manner.

Stress Fractures

The clinical signs of stress fractures are similar to those of bucked shins. The condition is usually seen acutely after training and is diagnosed radiographically. Serial radiographs may demonstrate the lesion if initial films are negative.

Treatment of this condition has changed dramatically over the years but even today some horses are resistant to therapy. Conservative treatment involves rest until the area is not painful. Controlled walking can be performed during this period. Controlled exercise programs progress through ponying, jogging on the track in a clockwise direction, slow galloping, and eventually the resumption of training. Radiographic assessment continues at monthly intervals and training resumes as the fracture line begins to fade radiographically. The possibility of a catastrophic fracture through this stress fracture exists, making the decision to resume training and racing a difficult one. Although this regimen works in many cases, it is obvious from the above discussion that a complete understanding of the pathophysiology does not exist for this condition. When following the "healing" of this condition, the normal time constants of bone activation, resorption, and formation that occur in bone remodeling must be considered. This process cannot be hurried.

Surgical treatment of stress fractures consists of single cortical lag screw fixation through the lesion or perforation drilling of the lesion with or without the use of a cancellous bone graft. The techniques may be used together, but recently there seems to be less use of the screw technique. Clearly, the older technique of double cortical lag screw fixation through the dorsal and palmar cortex has been discontinued. In part this may be explained by the necessity of screw removal and the possibility of refracture through the area. It should be remembered that removal of any screw will create a stress concentration in the bone that will take at least 8 weeks to be dissipated. Resumption of training earlier than this could leave the bone at risk for a complete disruptive type of fracture.

BIBLIOGRAPHY

Carter DR, Caler WE, A cumulative damage model for bone fracture. *J Orthop Res* 1985;3:84–90.

Copelan RW: Incidence, location and principles of treatment of stress fractures of the third metacarpal bone. *Proc AAEP Ann Conven* 1972; pp:159.

Fackelman GE, Nunamaker DM: *Manual of Internal Fixation in the Horse.* New York, Springer-Verlag, 1982.

Frost HM: *Intermediary Organization of the Skeleton.* Boca Raton, FL, CRC Press, 1986.

Norwood GL: The bucked shin complex in Thoroughbreds. *Proc AAEP Ann Conven* 1978; pp:319–336.
Nunamaker DM, Butterweck DM, Black J: Fatigue failure of equine third metacarpal bone: An in vitro comparison of the thoroughbred and standard racehorse. *AJVR* 1989 (in press).
Nunamaker DM, Butterweck DM, Black J: Fatigue fractures in Thoroughbred racehorses: Relationships with age, peak bone strain and training. Submitted to J Orthop Res, 1987.
Nunamaker DM, Butterweck DM, Provost MT: Some geometric properties of the third metacarpal bone: A comparison between the Standardbred and Thoroughbred racehorse. J Biomech 1989;22:129–134.

121 Metacarpophalangeal/Metatarsophalangeal Breakdown Injuries

Jack R. Snyder

Traumatic disruption of the suspensory apparatus most often occurs in the Thoroughbred racehorse. The injury usually involves a single forelimb and affects both right or left limbs with equal frequency. In a normal stride, the suspensory apparatus functions to transfer forces across the tension surface of the fetlock as the limb becomes weight bearing. During maximum stride effort, as occurs during racing, the fetlock undergoes hyperextension, placing maximal strain on the suspensory apparatus, and making it vulnerable to injury.

The suspensory apparatus becomes disrupted by three mechanisms: fractures of both the medial and lateral sesamoid bones, avulsion of the distal sesamoidean ligaments, and rupture of the suspensory ligament or the extensor branches (Fig. 121–1). These injuries, alone or in combination, result in loss of mechanical support to the fetlock. Recently, in a review of 25 cases with fetlock breakdown injuries, the majority ($n = 15$) were caused by fractures of the medial and lateral sesamoid bones. Presently there are no factors reported to predispose to these injuries.

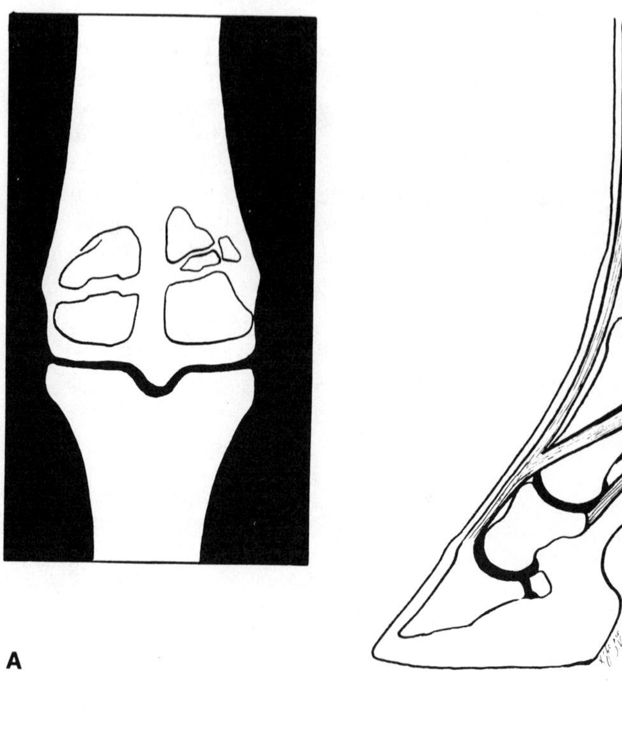

A

Figure 121–1. Drawings of traumatic disruption of the suspensory apparatus, caused by fractures of both the medial and lateral sesamoid bones **(A)**, avulsion of the distal sesamoidean ligaments **(B)**, and rupture of the suspensory ligament **(C)** or extensor branches of the suspensory ligaments **(D)**. These injuries either alone or in combination result in loss of the suspensory apparatus and fetlock support. (*Figure continues.*)

Figure 121–1. (*continued*)

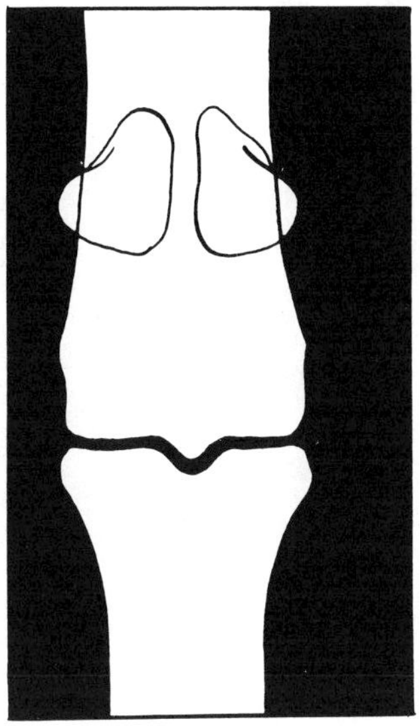

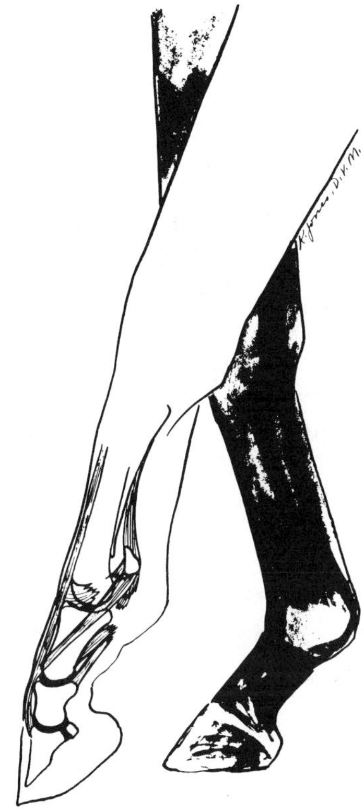

B

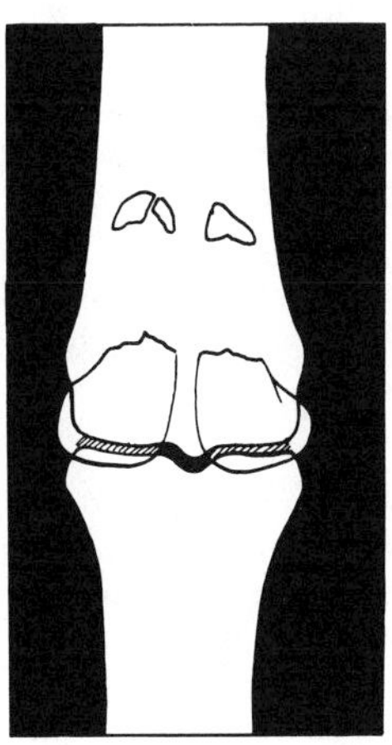

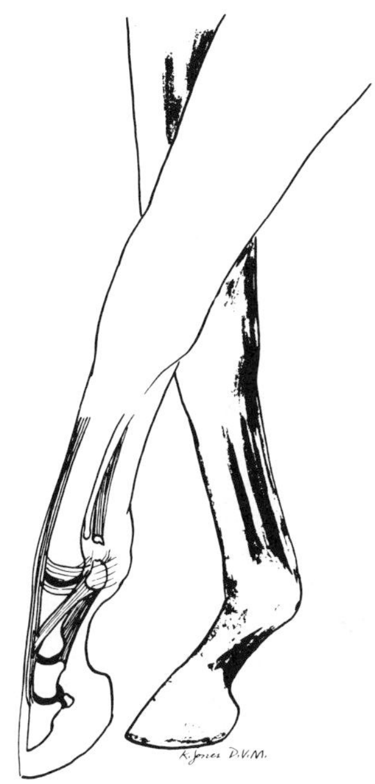

C

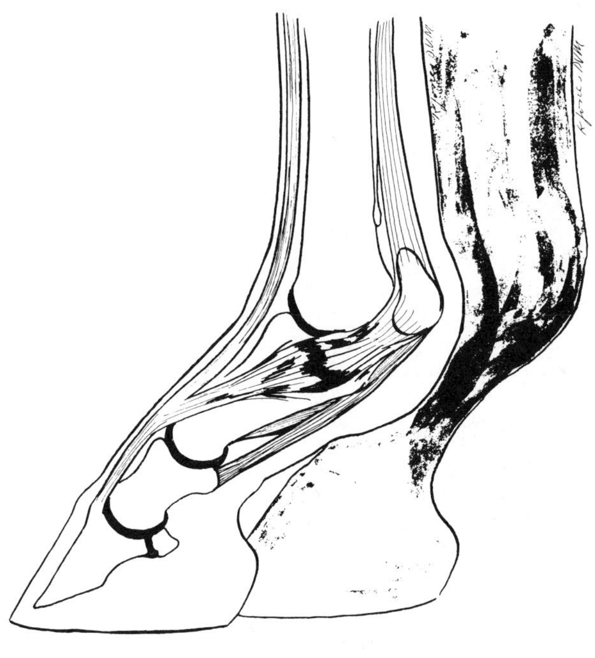

D

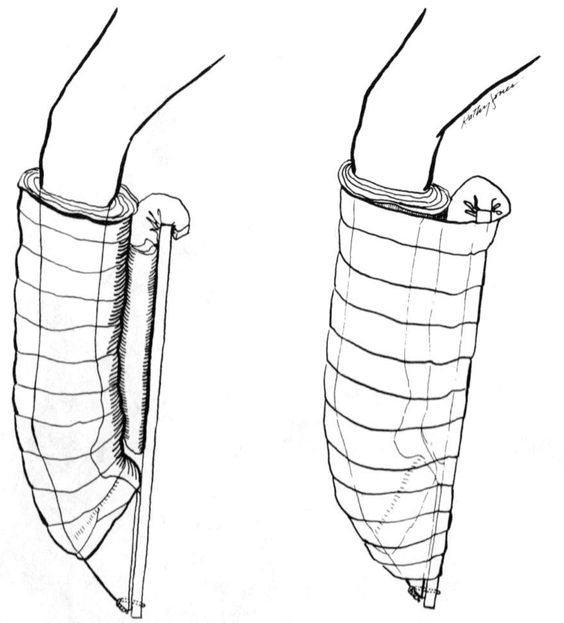

Figure 121–2 Application of the board splint. Using 9-gauge wire the board splint is secured to the hoof through predrilled holes. The limb is padded with bandage material before the board is positioned onto the caudal aspect of the third metacarpal bone, placing the fetlock in hyperflexion.

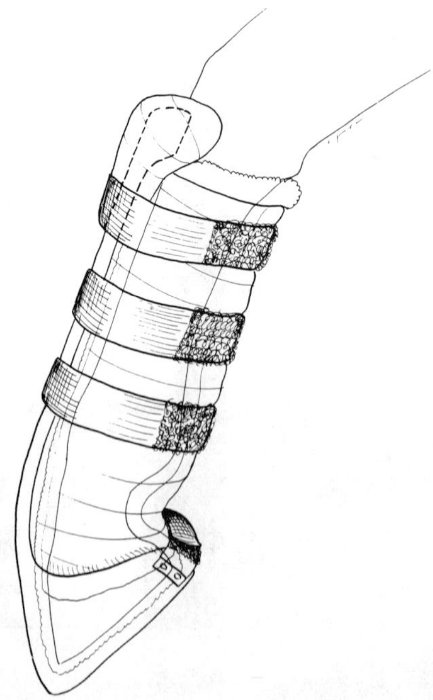

Figure 121–3 Application of the metal splint. The splint is placed on the dorsal aspect of the limb and secured to the limb using Velcro straps. As with the board splint the limb must be padded with bandage material before application of the device. The metal splint places the fetlock in hyperflexion.

Immediately after injury, the horse is incapable of placing weight on the affected limb without causing hyperextension of the fetlock. Because of the violent forces involved in this injury, extensive soft tissue damage frequently occurs. In many cases, the high-speed ground contact at the time of injury results in an open, contaminated skin wound. Frequently the vascular supply to the foot becomes compromised either by direct trauma or by stretching of the digital vessels from the joint instability. To prevent further tissue and vascular damage, the horse should not be moved or transported without adequate fetlock support. Stabilization of the fetlock immediately after injury can be accomplished by using either a board or a metal splint. Before either splint is applied, the limb should be generously padded with bandage material. The wood splint (2 × 12 × 45 cm) is placed on the palmar aspect of the limb and secured to the foot by a length of 9-gauge wire drilled through the hoof at the toe. The board is secured to the limb with additional bandage material, thus placing the fetlock in hyperflexion (Fig. 121–2). Alternatively, a commercially available metal splint (Kimzey, Inc) can be positioned on the dorsal aspect of the limb and secured over padding by straps (Fig. 121–3).

FRACTURE MANAGEMENT

Various therapeutic methods have been attempted, including surgical arthrodesis and conservative approaches using external support. Techniques for surgical arthrodesis include internal and external skeletal fixation. Initially, it may be beneficial to leave the limb in the external support splint for 24 to 48 hours prior to surgical intervention, allowing evaluation of vascular integrity and débridement of debris or necrotic tissue in those cases in which wounds are present.

Surgical Arthrodesis

Internal Skeletal Fixation. Internal fixation utilizes principles of bone plating and tension band wiring. The horse is positioned in lateral recumbency with the affected limb up. If there is no evidence of vascular damage, an Esmarch's bandage is used and a tourniquet positioned on the proximal aspect of the metacarpus. The skin incision is made on the dorsal aspect from the proximal aspect of the metacarpus to just above the coronary band. The deep incision is continued longitudinally through the center of the extensor tendon and periosteum for the length of the plate. The joint capsule is incised over the fetlock. Using subperiosteal dissection, the periosteum and the fetlock joint capsule are lifted from the bone, allowing for direct plate-to-bone contact.

A broad dynamic compression plate with sufficient length to span the entire length of the proximal phalanx and the distal two thirds of the third metacarpal bone is used. The plate is contoured on the dorsal aspect of the proximal phalanx and third metacarpal bone by dorsiflexing the fetlock 10 degrees, which because of the normal tapering of the proximal phalanx creates an overall fetlock angle of 30 degrees to the long axis of the limb. Two tension band wires are positioned on the caudal aspect of the fetlock joint in a figure-eight pattern. Holes are drilled from medial to lateral in the proximal phalanx and distal one third of the third metacarpal bone in a frontal plane for wire placement. A wire-passing instrument can be used to aid the placement of the wires dorsal to the sesamoid bones. The wires are then crossed immediately caudal to the joint space. Care is taken to assure that the wires are flat against the osseous structures. However, the wires are not tightened at this point in the procedure.

In attempting surgical arthrodesis, an important step is removal of the articular cartilage, which is facilitated by creating a condylar fracture with an oscillating bone saw after plate selection and contouring. A 3.2-mm hole is predrilled to ensure anatomic reduction for repair. The fragment should be wide enough to allow lag screw compression without risk of comminution. The condylar fragment is elevated and retracted caudally, while the joint is luxated, exposing the articular surface. All articular cartilage is removed either by hand curetting or chiseling or with motorized equipment. The subchondral bone from the distal metacarpal bone and the proximal phalanx is drilled with a 2-mm drill bit at 1-cm intervals, allowing access to the vascular supply and mobilization of osteogenic cells.

The fetlock joint is reduced and the condylar fracture repaired using a lag screw through the predrilled hole. An alternative technique to creating a condylar fracture is the transection of the medial collateral ligament, which also allows joint luxation. The collateral ligament is repaired with absorbable suture material. The caudal tension band wires are tightened until the joint is in slight ventriflexion. The plate is positioned on the dorsal surface and initially secured to the phalanx. As an option, compression is applied across the joint using the removable compression device at the proximal end of the plate to aid in maintaining plate position while the remaining screws are positioned and tightened. The screws on either side of the joint are applied across the articular space using lag principles (Fig. 121–4).

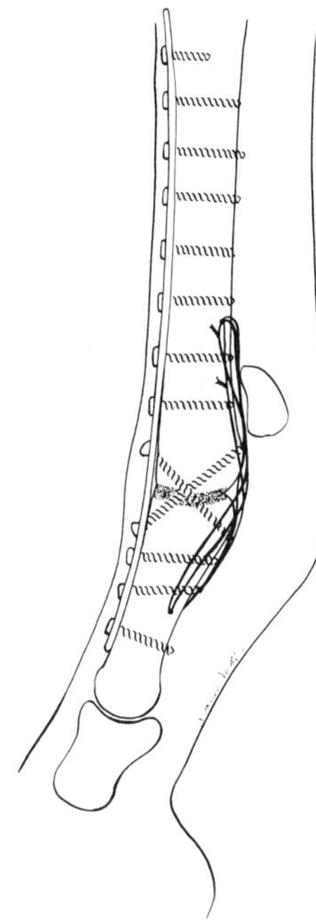

Figure 121–4. Drawing of a fetlock arthrodesis using a dorsally applied plate, two tension wires on the caudal aspect of the joint, and transection of the medial collateral ligament for exposure of the fetlock joint surfaces.

The soft tissue and skin are closed over the plate. A fiberglass cast should be applied that encloses the foot and extends to the proximal third metacarpal bone. The cast may be changed or removed in 2 to 3 weeks, at which time the skin sutures are removed.

An alternative to plate fixation is the use of stainless steel baskets packed with cancellous bone inserted in holes drilled into the dorsal surface of the metacarpophalangeal joint. This technique requires cast application and has not been tested in clinical cases.

External Skeletal Fixation. In patients with extensive soft tissue damage, the use of internal fixation may increase the risk of infection and further vascular damage. In these patients the use of external skeletal fixation is an alternative technique for arthrodesis of the fetlock joint. The technique involves an external frame connecting a foot plate to transfixation pins placed through the third metacarpal bone.

Three stab incisions are made laterally over the third metacarpal bone for the transfixation pins. The first incision is made in the middle of the bone and the other two are positioned approximately 6 to 7 cm proximal and distal to the first incision. Initially, a 4.5-mm hole is drilled transversely through the bone at each of the three sites. These holes are widened with an 8.73-mm drill bit. Three stainless steel self-tapping pins (9.6 mm outside diameter, 8.6 mm inside diameter) are positioned across the bone. As the pins exit out the medial side of the bone, 1-cm incisions are made in the skin.

The articular cartilage and a portion of the subchondral bone is removed using a drill through a 4- to 7-cm incision made over the dorsal aspect of the fetlock joint. The incision is made through the skin, common digital extensor tendon, and joint capsule. Following curettage, the articular space is carefully packed with a previously harvested cancellous bone graft. The tendon and skin are closed over the joint.

The transfixation pins are fixed to a frame consisting of a foot support with ascending vertical bars. The frame is constructed from 1.27-cm diameter tubular steel fitted to a cast aluminum foot plate. The foot plate is secured to a tapped steel bar shoe that is placed on the foot using standard techniques. The plate is designed to elevate the heel approximately 25 degrees, aligning the fetlock joint with the limb.

The vertical bars are secured to the transfixation pins using a commercial polyurethane material (Sigma Chemical Co). The liquid material is poured into a mold made of foam rubber tubing used for pipe insulation, incorporating the ascending bars and transfixation pins. Care must be taken to properly align the frame when pouring the material, because of the rapid polymerization of the material. Sterile bandages are placed at the skin-pin interface.

The horse should be confined to a box stall and phenylbutazone administered as needed to control pain. Bony fusion is monitored radiographically and the external device removed once fusion has occurred, which usually takes 6 to 7 weeks. After removal of the pins, a sterile bandage should be maintained over the exit sites of the pins until granulation tissue has filled the holes. Exercise is restricted after pin removal for 6 to 8 weeks. Third metacarpal bone fracture through the pin holes has occurred after use of this fixation method.

Conservative Splintage

An alternative method to surgical intervention is the long-term use of an external board or metal splint. The splint is used until fetlock stabilization is achieved by fibrosis. If a wood splint is to be used, it is advisable to secure the splint with two bolts welded to the shoe surface, preventing the complication associated with wire breakage. The external splint is removed every 1 to 3 days for bandage changes, evaluation of joint stability, and evaluation/treatment of pressure sores.

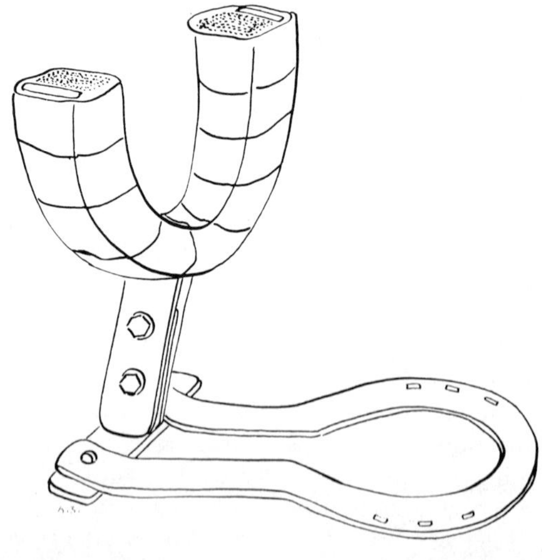

Figure 121–5. Fetlock support shoe with adjustable padded brace. The support to the fetlock can be adjusted by the center post, allowing the fetlock to slowly return to a normal angle after removal from the external splint.

Once the joint is judged to be stable by palpation, which usually takes 4 to 7 weeks, a support shoe is applied (Fig. 121–5). The affected joint is initially placed in the hyperflexed position and the adjustable support on the shoe is gradually lowered over the following 1 to 3 weeks until a normal fetlock angle is reached. During this convalescent period the horse is confined to a stall and phenylbutazone is administered as needed. After removal of the fetlock support shoe, an elevated heel shoe is used for an additional 4 to 6 weeks while slowly increasing the amount of exercise.

COMPLICATIONS

Complications using the methods described for treatment of suspensory disruption are numerous. Postoperative infection following internal fixation requires vigorous therapy. Laminitis may develop in the contralateral foot, especially if the affected limb is non–weight bearing. Sequestra formation may develop from comminuted sesamoid bone fractures. Fragments should be removed surgically at the time of repair or under local anesthesia if sequestration occurs during the convalescent period. With conservative methods the possibility of reinjury exists, because stability is dependent on fibrosis. Although uncommon, if instability occurs the injury can be managed again with the external splint. The development of pressure sores when using the external splints will vary in location depending on which splint is used. Pressure sores usually occur on the palmar aspect of the pastern region with the board splint, whereas with the metal splint sores usually occur at the proximal end of the splint on the dorsal surface of the third metacarpal/metatarsal bone.

PROGNOSIS

Management of this type of injury by any method carries a guarded prognosis. At best, the horse may return to unrestricted pasture exercise with a mechanical lameness of the affected limb as a result of the loss of fetlock mobility. Ideally, internal fixation results in rigid joint fusion and is the treatment of choice for surgical arthrodesis, resulting in greater than 50% of horses having a successful outcome. However, in some patients, because of the extensive soft tissue damage and contamination, internal fixation may be unacceptable and the use of external skeletal fixation is recommended.

Conservative management is a viable alternative, avoiding general anesthesia and the complications associated with surgical intervention. In a report of 17 horses managed by conservative methods, 11 (64%) returned to unrestricted pasture exercise.

At present, the methods described for treatment of disruption of the suspensory apparatus are elected as salvage procedures and are usually employed only in valuable breeding animals. In selected cases in which the fractures are minimally comminuted and vascularity is good, primary repair of both medial and lateral sesamoid fractures has been attempted. This allows some continued function of the fetlock. Screws, screws plus wires, and tension band wires alone have been used in combination with external coaptation.

BIBLIOGRAPHY

Bramlage LR: An initial report on a surgical technique for arthrodesis of the metacarpophalangeal joint in the horse. *Proc AAEP Ann Conven* 1981; pp 257–261.

Crawly GR, Grant BD, White KK, Barbee DD, Gallina AM, Ratzlaff MH: A modified Cloward's technique for arthrodesis of normal metacarpophalangeal joint in the horse. *Vet Surg* 1988;17:117–127.

Richardson DW, Nunamaker DM, Sigafoos RD: Use of an external skeletal fixation device and bone graft for arthrodesis of the metacarpophalangeal joint in horses. *J Am Vet Med Assoc* 1987;191:316–321.

Snyder JR, Wheat JD, Bleifer D: Conservative management of metacarpophalangeal joint instability. *Proc AAEP Ann Conven* 1986; pp 357–364.

122 Transverse and Comminuted Fractures of the Third Metacarpus/Metatarsus

Robert K. Schneider

Transverse or comminuted fractures of the third metacarpal or metarsal bones are readily recognized from the horse's stance and its inability to use the affected limb. Horses with this type of fracture cannot support weight on the unstable leg; attempts to bear weight result in abnormal bending between the fetlock and carpus or tarsus. Third metacarpal/metatarsal fractures are frequently open because there is little overlying soft tissue to protect the bone from external trauma or to prevent sharp ends of the fractured bone from penetrating the skin when the horse attempts to use the leg. If the horse is acutely non–weight bearing, it is advisable to palpate and examine the leg prior to assessing the animal's gait. This precaution may help avoid opening the skin when the horse moves. Pain, crepitation, and lateral-to-medial instability are detected upon manipulation of the lower leg. Severe swelling may not be present. Frequently the proximal, distal, or midshaft location of the fracture within the bone can be determined by palpation. Radiographs are required to assess the configuration of the fracture and the degree of comminution.

Third metacarpal/metatarsal fractures in adult horses are usually open and severely comminuted because of the high energy required to break the dense cortical bone. This fact makes successful treatment of these fractures difficult. Transverse fractures occur more commonly in young foals that have been kicked by other foals or horses. Bandaging and splinting closed fractures is critical to successful treatment. For metacarpal fractures, one splint should be placed over the palmar surface of the leg and a second one over the lateral side of the leg; these two splints at 90 degrees to each other restrict abnormal bending of the leg when the horse moves. The splints should extend over the entire length of the leg to immobilize both the fetlock and the carpus. For metatarsal fractures the plantar splint is extended proximal to the point of the hock and the lateral splint extends proximally over the lateral surface of the hock. This configuration restricts bending of the limb distal to the hock. Once a fracture of the third metacarpus or metatarsus is diagnosed, bandages and splints should be placed on the leg to avoid further insult to the limb and opening of the skin over a closed fracture. Radiographs can be taken through the splint once the animal has been stabilized.

FRACTURE MANAGEMENT

Closed fractures of the third metacarpus/metatarsus can be managed with internal fixation, a full-leg cast, transfixation pins incorporated in a full-leg cast, or external fixation devices. The method used depends on the configuration of the fracture, degree of comminution, location of the fracture within the bone, and size of the horse. Internal fixation with one or two plates provides the most stability in fractures that are amenable to plate fixation; sufficient bone proximal and distal to the fracture must be present. Transverse fractures and fractures with minimal comminution that can be reconstructed to achieve cortical contact between the proximal and distal fragments are candidates for plate fixation.

Open fractures, even in small foals, are poor candidates for internal fixation because the plates frequently cannot maintain stability long enough for the fracture to heal in the presence of infection. Open reduction and internal fixation may still be a consideration for open fractures accompanied by a small break in the skin and minimal contamination (Fig. 122–1). If there is gross contamination, surgical repair will only disseminate the infection throughout the bone. Infected or severely contaminated fractures can be managed with transfixation pins placed in the proximal fragment and/or in the distal radius and incorporated in a full-leg cast. Local wound lavage, débridement, and leaving the wound open to drain will minimize the spread of infection. Interfragmentary compression may be obtained by placing one or two screws across the fracture with minimal surgical dissection. Cancellous bone can be grafted to the fracture site to promote new bone production and fracture healing. Repeated grafts may be necessary. The transfixation pins transfer some of the load normally carried by the bones to the cast and therefore decrease the weight that must be supported by the fracture and lower limb. However, these pins have a limited life span because infection along the pin and weight-bearing forces in the bone act to loosen the pins. For this reason, this technique has limitations in the management of complicated open fractures.

Severely comminuted fractures of the metacarpus/metatarsus are not good candidates for internal fixation because sufficient bone is not available for placement of screws or bone plates (Fig. 122–2). These fractures are best managed with a cast or transfixation pins incorporated in a cast. Shattered third metacarpal bones can sometimes heal in a full-leg cast. If the fracture is closed, the prognosis for healing of a severely comminuted fracture and obtaining a pasture-sound or breeding animal is fair.

SURGICAL TECHNIQUE

Bone plates should be placed on the tension surface of the bone to maximize stability and resist bending forces at the fracture site. The third metacarpus of the horse does not have a strong tension surface since all sides of the bone are compressed during axial loading. Therefore, the plate can be placed on any side of the bone except on the palmar surface because of the suspensory ligament and other important soft tissue structures. Bone plate location around the dorsal half of the bone is determined by the fracture configuration and, to a lesser degree, the presence of open skin wounds. When using a single plate, it is usually located dorsal or dorsolateral. If two plates are used, one is placed on the dorsal surface and the second is located on the medial or the lateral side of the bone depending on fracture configuration. With third metatarsal fractures, the plate is usually placed on the dorsolateral surface, which is the tension side of this bone.

The surgical approach to the dorsal and medial cortices of the third metacarpal bone is through a curvilinear skin incision extending from the carpometacarpal joint distally along the medial aspect of the metacarpus to the fetlock. The incision is curved at its proximal and distal ends so that the flap of skin can be reflected off the dorsal surface of the bone. The incision is continued through the subcutaneous tissues and the subcutaneous tissue is reflected with the skin flap. The periosteum is incised and elevated to expose the frac-

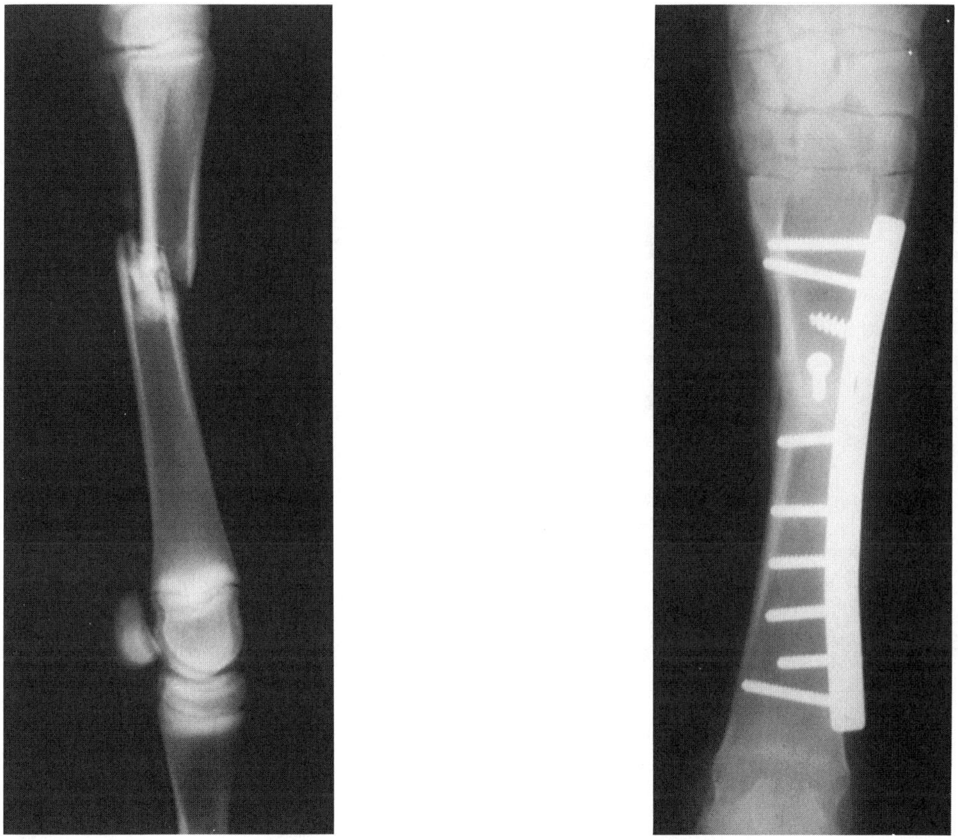

A B

Figure 122–1. **A.** Lateral radiograph showing a transverse, mildly comminuted fracture of the third metacarpus in a 3-month-old Quarter Horse foal. Although there was a small skin laceration over the lateral side of the leg, healing occurred following stabilization of the fracture with a ten-hole broad dynamic compression plate as seen in a dorsopalmar radiograph of the third metacarpus 4.5 months after surgery **(B)**. Internal fixation is the treatment of choice in closed fractures where enough bone is available proximal and distal to the fracture.

ture and bone for bone plate application. The dorsolateral surface is approached through an identical incision on the lateral side of the leg. Access to the dorsolateral cortex of the bone can then be obtained by splitting the common digital extensor tendon and the underlying periosteum. Subperiosteal elevation exposes the dorsal and lateral cortex.

Reduction of the fracture is usually accomplished by having an assistant apply traction on the distal limb while externally or internally rotating the leg as the surgeon manipulates the ends of the bones to align the fracture. Alternatively, the two ends of the fractured bone are lifted upward out of the incision, the far cortex of each end is engaged, and a downward pressure is applied to reduce the fracture. Comminuted fractures are made into two-piece fractures with lag screw fixation of butterfly fragments to the proximal or distal piece. If the fracture is oblique, reduction can be maintained with one lag screw from the proximal to the distal piece. Occasionally plate application is used to obtain axial alignment by first securing the plate to the proximal (or distal) fragment and using self-centering bone-holding forceps to clamp the plate to the distal (or proximal) fragment.

A broad dynamic compression plate that extends over the length of the bone is selected and contoured to the cortical surface of the bone. If circumferential cortical contact is obtained with reduction, the four screws closest to the fracture can be placed in the load position to achieve maximal compression. If there is a cortical defect, loading the screws to compress the fracture may not be indicated. The bone plate in these

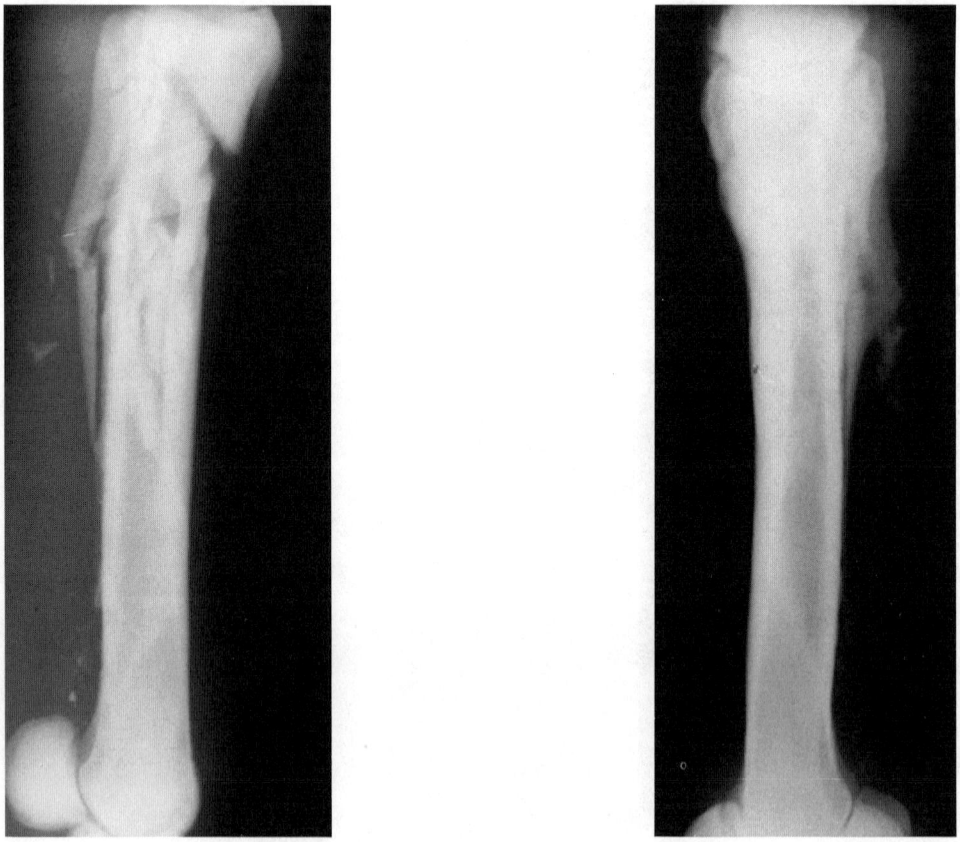

A B

Figure 122–2. A. Radiograph of a 4-year-old Standardbred mare with a closed, severely comminuted fracture of the third metacarpus. This fracture was stabilized in a full-leg cast for 12 weeks. **B.** Six-month follow-up radiograph shows a healed fracture.

cases may be placed over the defect as a neutralization plate to maintain cortical alignment opposite to the defect. In foals large 5.5-mm screws are used in the proximal and distal metaphysis. In adults the 5.5-mm screws are used in all holes in the dorsal plate because of their increased strength and greater holding power in equine bone. A second plate is used to maximize the strength of the fixation. The first bone plate is placed on the dorsal cortex and spans the length of the bone. The second plate is shorter and is placed on the medial or lateral cortex as a neutralization plate. With metatarsal fractures, the second plate should be placed on the lateral cortex because the tension side of this bone is dorsolateral. Screws that can be angled to cross the fracture line should be placed as lag screws to increase interfragmentary compression. The second plate is positioned on the bone such that the screw holes in this plate are between the screw holes in the dorsal plate. Following screw fixation of both plates, luting with methylmethacrylate is recommended to protect the screws against fatigue failure and to increase the ability of the fixation to resist cyclic loading (see Chapter 134).

Cancellous bone grafts are used in many third metacarpal/metatarsal bone fractures repaired with internal fixation because there is usually a cortical defect or the fracture is open. Bone grafts may not be necessary in closed fractures in young horses in which the cortex can be completely reconstructed. On the other hand, grafting cancellous bone into a fractured metacarpus/metatarsus has not been associated with any negative effects.

Suction drains are frequently used to remove blood and serum from the surgery site in the immediate postoperative period. Their use in treatment of third metacarpal/metatarsal bone fractures is at the surgeon's discretion. Drains can be a potential source of infection if they are not managed appropriately and in these fractures, where relatively little space exists for hematoma formation, the risks may outweigh the benefits.

Once both plates are tightly screwed to the bone, the skin is closed. Skin closure is an important step because there are no other soft tissues to cover the plates. Partial dehiscence of the skin postoperatively will expose the implant and fracture, increasing the risk of infection. In horses with fractures that are repaired with two broad plates considerable tension is placed on the skin closure. Thus, subcutaneous closure is used when possible. Several large vertical mattress sutures are placed in the skin with size 2 nylon to relieve tension from the primary sutures. The vertical mattress sutures draw the skin edges together. Size 0 prolene is then placed in a vertical mattress pattern, splitting the thickness of the skin on the superficial portion of the suture pattern. This suture pattern apposes the skin edges and provides a stronger closure than a simple interrupted pattern.

Perioperative antibiotics are recommended because of the duration of tissue exposure during fracture fixation. Antibiotics selected should have a broad spectrum, achieve effective concentrations in bone, and be given intravenously just before surgery. During fracture repair, the surgical field is periodically lavaged with sterile normal saline containing antibiotics.

Recovery and Postoperative Care

Postoperative management of horses with fractures of the metacarpus/metatarsus is not substantially different from horses with other long bone fractures (see Chapter 125).

Following surgical repair, the leg is placed in a full-leg cast or a large Robert Jones bandage. The decision is based on whether the fracture is open and the size of the horse. A full-leg cast will stabilize the limb and further support the internal fixation, and is recommended in closed fractures in full-sized horses. Since open fractures are more difficult to manage under a cast a bandage may be used in smaller horses and foals to improve drainage and wound management. The strength of the repair usually determines whether a cast, is necessary; the added stability obtained by immobilizing the limb is necessary to achieve healing in some fractures repaired with internal fixation.

OTHER MANAGEMENT METHODS

Full-leg casts can be used to treat horses with third metacarpal/metatarsal bone fractures. In horses with closed, severely comminuted metacarpal fractures, they are the treatment of choice and offer a chance for successful healing of the fracture. Proper application of the cast in these horses requires general anesthesia; it is impossible to apply the cast with the horse standing because the horse will not bear weight on the leg. A wire is placed through holes drilled in the heel of the foot and a flat board or twich handle is wired to the bottom of the foot. The handle is used to apply traction, to support the limb, and to position the foot during cast application (see Chapter 25). The cast is applied from the foot to the elbow. The cast will usually need to be changed every 3 to 4 weeks until the fracture heals. Full-leg casts can also be used on the rear limbs and should incorpororate the foot and extend proximally to the tibial crest. Ten to 12 weeks of cast fixation will be required to achieve bony union provided healing is not delayed by infection. Although the prognosis for open fractures is poor, they can also be managed with a full-leg fiberglass cast. The fiberglass cast allows wound fluids to drain through the cast. Drainage can be promoted by soaking the cast in Epsom salts and dilute Betadine.

Transfixation pins can be placed in the distal radius/tibia or proximal third metacarpal/metatarsal bone and

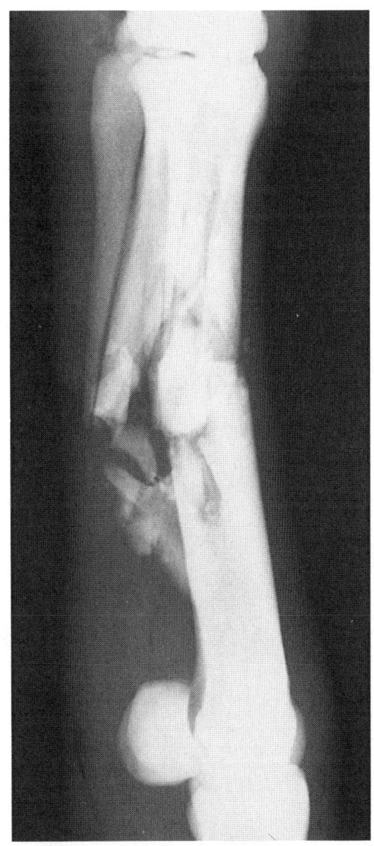

Figure 122–3. Lateral radiograph of severe comminution that frequently occurs with fractures of the metacarpus in full-sized horses. Unlike the case in Figure 122–2, this fracture was open. Successful repair of an open third metacarpal/metatarsal bone fracture is extremely difficult with methods currently available.

incorporated into a full-leg cast, or metal or acrylic splints. The transfixation pin transfers weight from the bony column to the cast during weight-bearing, decreasing the load that must be supported by the fractured bone. The pin and cast also stabilize the bone against torsional forces. Pins are placed through small stab incisions in the skin into drill holes smaller than the outer diameter of the pin. Threaded pins placed in pretapped holes are better than smooth pins. The pins are cut off with enough pin protruding to be incorporated into the cast. The cast is applied and any space around the pin in the cast is filled with Technovite hoof acrylic. The smooth pins will loosen between 4 and 8 weeks as a result of infection entering the bone along the pin and normal weight-bearing forces causing bone resorption at the bone-pin interface. Threaded pins remain tight for a longer period. A combination of transfixation pins and cast followed by pin removal and immobilization in a cast may be required to maintain stability long enough to allow the fracture to heal.

PROGNOSIS

Fractures of the equine metacarpus/metatarsus still challenge the available methods of treatment. There is not a good method for stabilizing and healing open fractures; unfortunately many of these fractures are open (Fig. 122–3). Infection and compromise of the periosteal blood supply frequently results in sequestration of part of the cortical bone and/or a nonunion. Injury to the main source of blood supply through the nutrient artery severly reduces the chance for fracture healing and increases the risk of infection and nonunion. Rigid stabilization, regardless of the technique employed, is difficult to maintain beyond 8 weeks in infected fractures subjected to normal weight-bearing forces, even in small foals. Furthermore, treatment of these fractures is expensive. Therefore, at this time it may be best to consider humane destruction of horses with open, contaminated third metacarpal/metatarsal bone fractures. Closed fractures that can be stabilized with internal fixation carry a better prognosis, especially in smaller horses and foals. Even severely comminuted fractures can be managed in a full-leg cast with a reasonable chance for successful fracture healing. Better success in treating these fractures in the future relies on the development of improved methods of fixation, better ways of combating infection, and new techniques to promote vascularization and healing of the fractured bone.

BIBLIOGRAPHY

Bramlage LR: Long bone fractures. *Vet Clin North Am Large Anim Pract* 1983;5(2):285–310.

Bramlage LR: Current concepts of emergency first aid treatment and transportation of equine fracture patients. *Compend Cont Educ Pract Vet* 1983;5:564–573.

Nunamaker DM, Bowman KF, Richardson DW, et al: Plate luting: A preliminary report of its use in the horse. *Vet Surg* 1986;15:289–293.

Nunamaker DM, Richardson DW, Butterweck DM: A new external skeletal fixation device that allows immediate full weight bearing: Application in the horse. *Vet Surg* 1986;15:345–355.

Turner AS, Mills EJ, Gabel AA: In vivo measurement of bone strain in the horse. *Am J Vet Res* 1975;36:1573–1579.

Yovich JV, Turner AS, Smith FW: Holding power of orthopedic screws in equine third metacarpal and metatarsal bones: Part I Foal bone. Part II Adult horse bone. *Vet Surg* 1985;14:221–234.

123 Fractures of the Small Metacarpal and Metatarsal Bones

Dean W. Richardson

DIAGNOSIS

"Splint" bone fractures occur in all age horses as a consequence of direct external trauma and in racehorses as a consequence of an acute overload. The history varies with the type of fracture. The typical distal splint fracture in which the extremity of the bone is fractured is seen in young racehorses as an acute injury with moderate focal pain, swelling, and an overt lameness. In some older horses, especially Standardbreds, the fracture appears to be a sequela to suspensory desmitis and may have a more insidious onset of clinical signs. Fractures of the upper half of the small metacarpal or metatarsal bones nearly always are caused by direct trauma, such as an interference, a kick, or a fall. The most commonly affected bone is the fourth metatarsal, since horses back up to kick one another when they fight. Proximal second metacarpal fractures in racehorses, especially proximal articular fractures, can occur as racing accidents while leaving the starting gate or in a collision with another horse. Proximal splint fractures usually have marked soft tissue swelling and articular fractures will cause effusion of the intercarpal joint.

A special case of fractured splint is often seen when the original traumatic incident resulted in a skin wound. The pain and swelling are frequently ascribed to the visible soft tissue injury and radiographs are not taken. The wound usually heals initially only to open and drain days or weeks later. Radiographs then reveal the fracture, which is frequently a septic nonunion since the drainage extends directly into the fracture line (Fig. 123–1). There may or may not be sequestrum and involucrum formation.

Diagnosis of all splint fractures is by localizing heat, pain, and swelling and confirmatory radiographs. Oblique, lateral, and dorsopalmar projections are always recommended to identify all fracture lines, any sequestra, and any concurrent injury of the third metacarpal/metatarsal bone.

SURGICAL ANATOMY

The surgical anatomy of the splint bones is very straightforward, with the only critical vascular structure being the great metatarsal artery (dorsal third metatarsal artery) adjacent to the dorsal margin of the fourth metatarsal bone. The metacarpal or metatarsal arteries on the axial aspects of the bones are relatively small and easily avoided by remaining close to the axial surface during dissection. The weight-supporting function and importance of articular congruity of the proximal extremities of the bone should not be underestimated, especially when considering treatment of proximal fractures. Finally, the insertion of the medial collateral ligament and flexor carpi radialis and extensor carpi obliquus muscles on the proximal second metacarpus produce significant tensile forces that can result in failure of some fixation techniques not allowing for these forces. Similarly, the lateral collateral ligament and ulnaris lateralis insertion tend to abduct the proximal fourth metacarpus. In the hind limb, the proximal small metatarsal bones serve for the insertion of collateral ligaments.

SURGICAL TECHNIQUE

Distal Fractures

The surgical technique for removal of the distal extremity of the splint bone has been previously described in numerous textbooks. All that is required is a linear incision over the affected portion of the bone, dissection of the fragment and any callus from the adjacent bone, and a beveled transection proximal to the fracture. It is doubtful that any functional difference is found between removing or leaving the splint periosteum. There may be an improvement in cosmetic appearance and less chance of new bone production if a surrounding portion of the metacarpal periosteum is excised. Wound closure and postoperative bandaging are routine and complications are very rare.

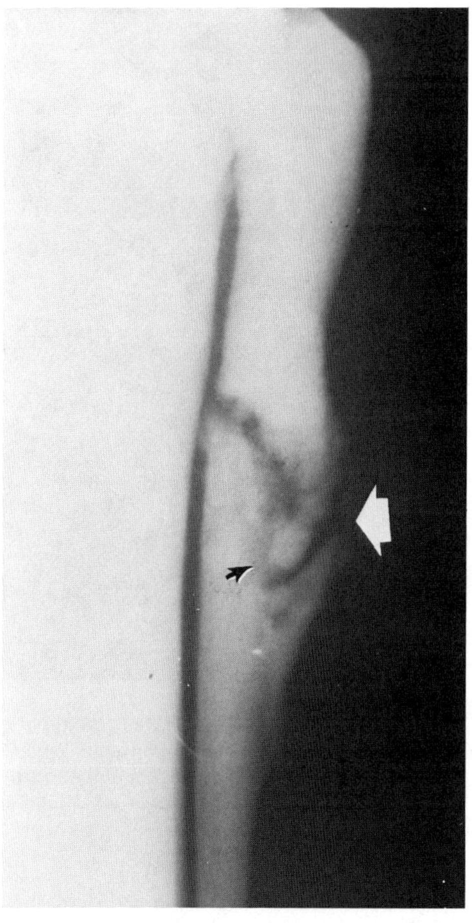

Figure 123–1. Septic nonunion of the proximal fourth metatarsal bond. There is a sequestrum (*black arrow*) and early involucrum formation (*white arrow*).

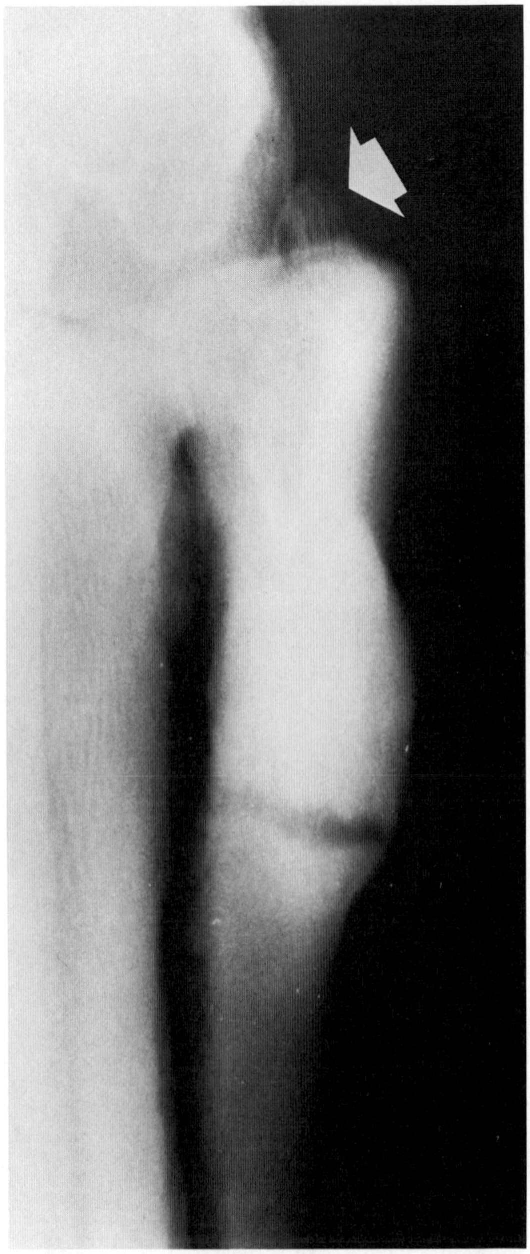

Figure 123–2. A conservatively treated proximal fourth metatarsal fracture 3 months after the original injury. An enthesiophyte involving the proximal aspect of the fourth metatarsal has developed (*arrow*). The horse was lame and responsive to distal intertarsal injection.

It is generally accepted that no more than the distal two thirds of the splint should be removed to avoid loss of axial support. It probably is advisable, where possible, to repair any fracture involving the proximal half of a splint bone, especially the second metacarpus, which is heavily loaded. Closed fractures of the proximal splint may be articular or nonarticular. Nonarticular fractures may be treated conservatively with good results unless there is significant displacement of the proximal fragment, which can affect joint alignment (Fig. 123–2). Stall-rested horses should be reradiographed at 4- to 6-week intervals or with any change in degree of lameness. Displacement can occur as a late event and requires surgical intervention.

Proximal Fractures

Displaced proximal splint fractures and especially articular fractures should optimally be treated with open reduction and internal fixation. Although some success has been seen with lag screw repairs, plate fixation is strongly recommended because of the need to overcome the tensile forces distracting the abaxial surface of the proximal fragment and to avoid the fixation of the splint bone to the third metacarpal/metatarsal bone with transverse screws. The latter technique frequently results in either overt failure of the screw(s) or lysis and pain around the screw(s) as a result of the marked difference in elastic modulus between stainless steel and bone.

The recommended approach is a slightly curved incision dorsal to the anticipated site of plate placement so that the incision is not directly over the implants. Subperiosteal dissection is carried out to expose the fracture line, which is débrided as needed. A 3.5-mm dynamic compression plate or reconstruction plate is placed with standard technique (Fig. 123–3). Whenever possible, the screws engage only the splint bone so as to maintain the normal amount of relative motion between the bones. With articular fractures, the joint surface can be exposed to assure perfect reduction. The subperiosteal plane of dissection must be extended proximally, elevating the tendinous and ligamentous insertions to place the proximal part of the plate closely against the bone. Most proximal splint fractures are oblique enough to permit the use of at least one lag screw in the repair. Additional lag screws adjacent to the plate can be used to augment the repair if the fracture configuration allows.

Open Fractures

Acute open fractures that are displaced are also best treated with internal fixation following meticulous débridement. Even if infection ensues, stability is usually adequate to assure healing and the infection can be resolved by later plate removal. Chronic infected fractures a few centimeters distal to the articulation are very common, however, and usually a decision must be made whether to risk internal fixation in the presence

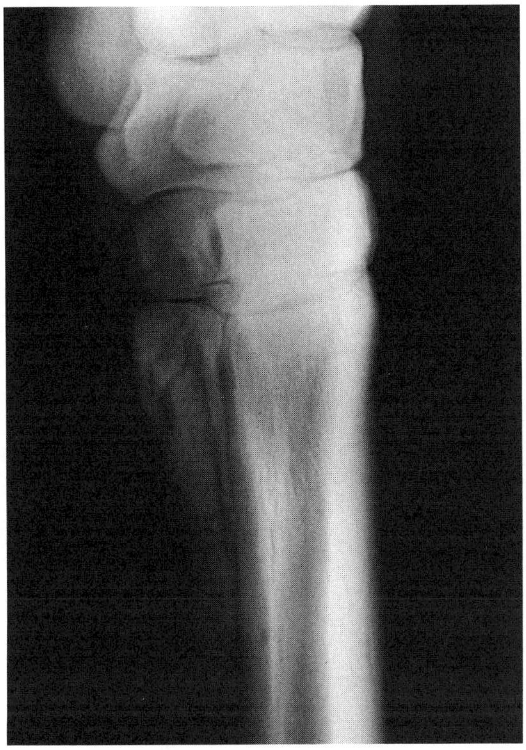

A

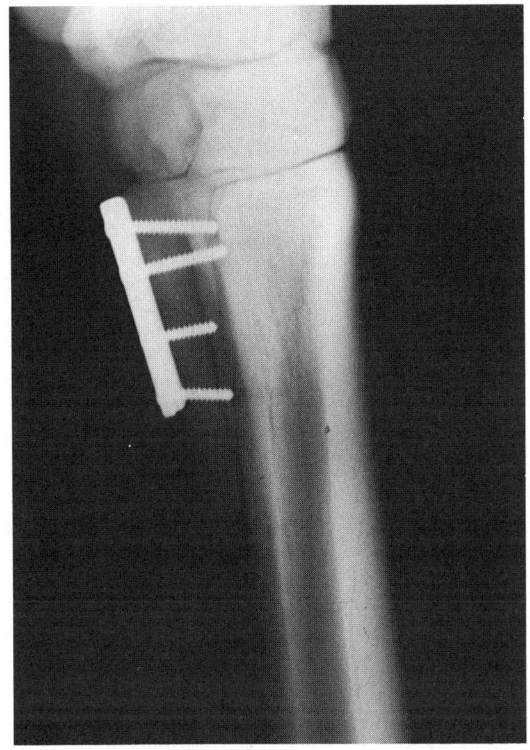

B

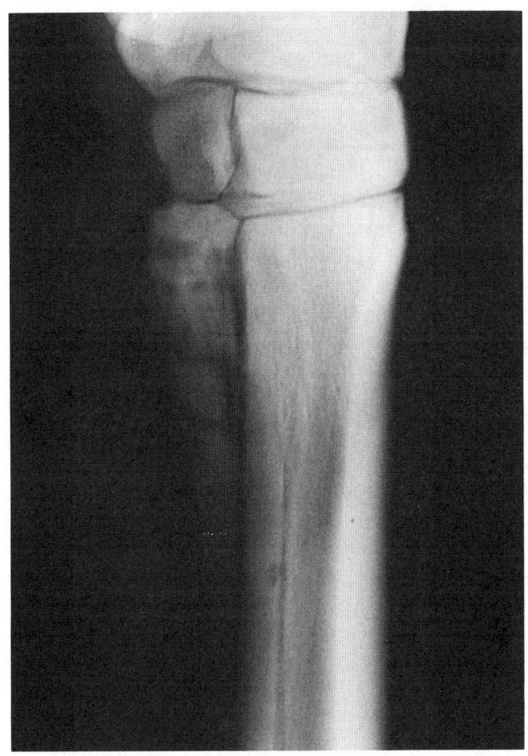

C

Figure 123–3. **A.** displaced articular fracture of the proximal second metacarpal in a Thoroughbred racehorse. **B.** Repair of the fracture with a four-hole 3.5-mm dynamic compression plate. **C.** Plate removal at 4 months following surgery. The horse returned to stakes-winning form.

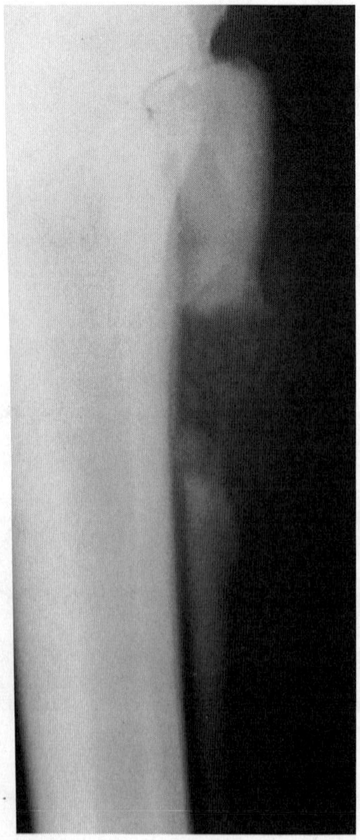

Figure 123–4. En bloc excision of the septic nonunion seen in Figure 123–1. The defect is filled with an autologous cancellous bone graft.

of the established infection. An alternative method of handling such fractures is an en bloc excision of the infected area and replacement of the removed splint with an autologous cancellous bone graft that is placed in a tapered form to simulate the shape of the removed bone (Fig. 123–4).

Multiple Fractures or Sequestration

In cases in which multiple splint bone fractures or sequestration with excessive callus are present, total excision of the fracture and the distal portion of the splint bone may provide the best cosmetic and functional outcome. In these cases, the periosteum is removed with the splint bone or the callus and is similarly removed around the attachment of the third metacarpal/metatarsal bone to the small metacarpal or metatarsal bones. This helps the proximal portion of the fractured bone heal to the third metacarpal/metatarsal. Similarly, old fractures that have already healed with attachment of the small metacarpal or metatarsal bones to the third metacarpal or metatarsal should not be disturbed other than to remove the excessive callus and the distal portion of the bone. Although this would seem to interfere with the normal movement between the two bones during weight bearing, this technique is usually successful with no complicating lameness in fractures involving the distal 60 to 75% of the bone. In cases in which there is sequestration with contamination or infection, thorough débridement and total removal of all inflamed tissue allow primary closure with first-intention healing.

POSTOPERATIVE CARE

Well-padded, firmly wrapped compression bandages are used following all splint surgeries. A roll of gauze can be placed over the incision and under the bandage padding to help keep focal pressure and minimize swelling. This may be important in the end cosmetic result, especially following excision of a large fragment of distal splint bone. Casts are not indicated, even for complicated fractures. Postoperative management of uncomplicated distal splint fractures involves a very short period (3 to 6 weeks) of rest *unless*, as is often the case, concomitant suspensory desmitis requires a longer convalescence. Horses with plated fractures are usually not allowed free exercise for about 3 months and plates may be removed at about 4 months (Fig. 123–3C). Plate removal is recommended if any of the screws engage the third metacarpal/metatarsal bone or if there is any apparent loosening of the implants or infection. An additional 2 months of gradually increasing exercise is recommended before returning the horse to hard training. Horses with infected fractures treated with en bloc excision and grafting are given about 4 months of stall rest and controlled walking before returning to work.

PROGNOSIS

Complications following distal splint fractures are extremely rare, but implant failure and infection are occasional problems in proximal fractures, especially open fractures. The prognosis for distal splint fractures as a solitary lesion is excellent, but the surgeon must be aware of other more serious lesions seen with the fracture, such as suspensory desmitis or sesamoiditis.

The prognosis for proximal splint fractures, even articular fractures, is good with proper repair. Even open fractures generally have a satisfactory outcome. The results with "simple" lag screw repairs using the third metacarpal/metatarsal bone as the transcortex have been disappointing, and plating or grafting techniques are strongly recommended.

BIBLIOGRAPHY

Allen D, White NA: Management of fractures and exostosis of the metacarpals and metatarsals II and IV in 25 horses. *Equine Vet J* 1987;19:326–330.

Bowman KF, Fackelman GE: Surgical treatment of complicated fractures of the splint bones in the horse. *Vet Surg* 1982;11:121–124.

Caron JP, Barber SM, Doige CE, Pharr JW: The radiographic and histologic appearance of controlled surgical manipulation of the equine periosteum. *Vet Surg* 1987;16: 13–20.

Jones RD, Fessler JF: Observations on small metacarpal and metatarsal fractures with or without associated suspensory desmitis in Standardbred horses. *Can Vet J* 1977;18: 29–32.

Peterson PR, Pascoe JR, Wheat JD: Surgical management of proximal splint bone fractures in the horse. *Vet Surg* 1987;16:367–372.

Verschooten F, Gasthuys F, DeMoor A: Distal splint bone fractures in the horse: An experimental and clinical study. *Equine Vet J* 1984;16:532–536.

124 Ulnar Fractures

Dean W. Richardson

DIAGNOSIS

Ulnar fractures are relatively common fractures in all age horses. External trauma from a blow or fall is the most common history, although missteps made by a horse running at speed can also be a cause. In most cases, the horse is acutely and severely lame, but some horses, particularly foals, with nondisplaced, incomplete fractures will be more subtly lame. Swelling directly over the fracture site is generally palpable, although markedly displaced proximal olecranon fractures may occasionally be initially misdiagnosed as humeral injuries. Both the medial and lateral aspects of the ulna should be palpated for swelling and crepitus. The horse's appearance is characteristic; the elbow is "dropped" as a result of loss of triceps support and concomitant carpal flexion. Pain is evident with virtually any manipulation of the limb. Radiographs are confirmatory for the diagnosis. Nearly all ulnar fractures can be identified on lateral-to-medial radiographs alone, although a craniocaudal view may reveal comminution. This view is also necessary to define the specific configuration of the fracture. In young foals, a flexed (stressed) view of the elbow may be needed to identify a Salter-Harris type I fracture of the olecranon process. Concomitant injury to the radius with an ulnar fracture is quite common in young horses, and the proximal radial physis should be examined (Fig. 124–1).

FRACTURE MANAGEMENT

The functional anatomy of the equine ulna is simple, with the olecranon process serving as the triceps-powered lever arm that extends the elbow. The ulna forms a major part of the elbow articulation and is the origin of several flexor muscles. Fractures of the ulna have been classified according to their location and degree of comminution.

Nondisplaced and minimally displaced fractures of the olecranon can be successfully treated conservatively. Healing of these fractures may be complicated, however, because displacement may occur as a result of the powerful pull of the triceps. Nonsurgical management is best reserved for fractures at or below the proximal radioulnar articulation. If the animal is very lame, the limb should be splinted from the ground to the proximal forearm to prevent carpal flexion and eventual contracture.

Surgical management is indicated in nearly all displaced and most proximal ulnar fractures. The primary exception is the severely comminuted fracture in which internal fixation is technically not feasible. Otherwise, surgical treatment is rewarding because of the mechanical factors involved. The action of the triceps affords a well-defined tension surface along the caudal ulna, and the absence of axial weight bearing minimizes torsional and variably directed bending forces.

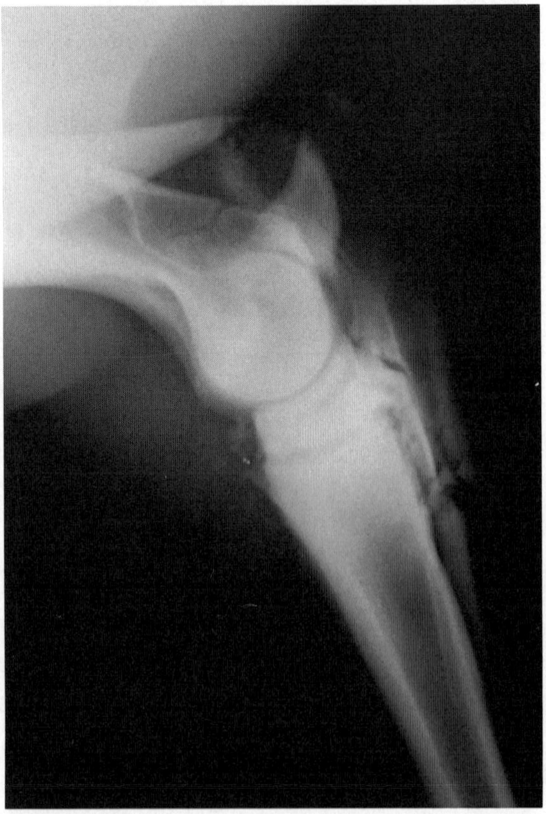

Figure 124–1. A comminuted ulnar shaft fracture with a crushing injury of the proximal radial physis. The prognosis for normal limb length and function is poor in a foal less than 6 months old.

Surgical management of ulnar fractures is dependent both on the configuration of the fracture and the experience, equipment, and preference of the surgeon. All surgical techniques employ the tension band principle.

Surgical Technique

The surgical approach is direct and uncomplicated, varying only in the length of the incision as it is made over the ulnar shaft between the ulnaris lateralis and the ulnar head of the deep digital flexor tendon. This incision is continued proximally in the same line until the proximal aspect of the olecranon is near the end of the incision. To avoid placing an incision near the vulnerable caudal aspect of the olecranon, the incision is curved craniolaterally as a small flap if it needs to be extended. Deep dissection should always be subperiosteal; a very sharp elevator or a scalpel is needed to fully expose the proximal olecranon since a portion of the triceps insertion extends distally on the bone. The only special concerns with surgery of the ulna are excessive dissection and elevation of the triceps attachment or injury to the interosseous vessels between the ulna and radius. These vessels are very difficult to identify and ligate.

Wires alone can be used very successfully to treat ulnar shaft fractures in foals or even yearlings (Fig. 124–2). Because of other supporting elements, medial to lateral bending is negligible distal to the articulation, so only the caudal tensile forces need to be negated. The advantages of the technique are the minimal instrumentation and cost, minimal incision required, and lack of need for implant removal even in a very young foal. A 1.2- or 1.5-mm diameter wire may be used in both figure-eight and simple loop patterns. A 2.5- or 3.2-mm drill bit is used to make two or more transverse holes 2 to 4 cm above and below the fracture line. Although two or three wires are adequate for a 100-kg foal, four or five wires are recommended in larger patients. A definite weight limitation for this technique is not known, but in larger animals (>200 kg) a bone plate is probably safer except in the simplest nondisplaced fracture.

A pins and wire tension band technique can be used to repair virtually all very proximal olecranon fractures and is the recommended technique for foals with proximal fractures. The proximal olecranon is approached as described above and the fracture reduced by extending the elbow. A single pin is placed normograde through or just cranial to the ossific nucleus of the epiphysis. The pin is directed distally down the shaft of the ulna until the tip is engaged. The distal cortex should not be fully penetrated in order to avoid distal pin migration. Figure-eight tension band wires are then passed cranial to the proximal end of the pin and passed transversely through a hole drilled in the ulna distal to the fracture. The wire should be passed close to the bone *under* the triceps attachment; use of a long needle as a cannula or a tunneling instrument facilitates this maneuver. An additional one or two pins and two or more wires are positioned to complete the fixation.

In large horses with very proximal fractures, pin placement is very difficult because of the thickness and density of the bone. Consequently, long 5.5-mm cortical screws are used after drilling and tapping the path of the screw in the same direction described for a pin (Fig. 124–3). At least two screws and five wires are recommended in a 450-kg horse. Articular reconstruction can be performed simultaneously with this technique using accurately directed lag screws from the caudal cortex. Uncrossed wires tightened as a suture laterally, in addition to the figure-eight wires, will help prevent some medial-to-lateral instability.

Bone plating is the most versatile and widely used technique for repair of ulnar fractures, especially in older horses (Fig. 124–4). Because of the mechanical forces, this is one location where a single plate is adequate for even very large individuals. The plate should be applied subperiosteally using standard ASIF technique to compress the fracture line. A 4.5-mm narrow plate can be used in animals up to about 400 kg. Heavier animals usually need a fitted broad plate. Three major mistakes in placing ulnar bone plates should be avoided: (*a*) the screws should not breach any articular surface, (*b*) the screws should not engage the proximal radius in foals less than 6 months old (Fig. 124–5), and (*c*) the plate should be *carefully* aligned straight along the caudal aspect of the ulna. The surgeon may encounter difficulty securing the extremities of the plate if the plate is positioned diagonally. Ideal plate fixation of an ulnar fracture entails at the very least three screws above and three below the fracture.

POSTOPERATIVE CARE

As with most equine long bone fractures, these horses are at risk for disruption of the fixation during the anesthetic recovery phase. Smaller animals should always be manually assisted to their feet. Larger horses should

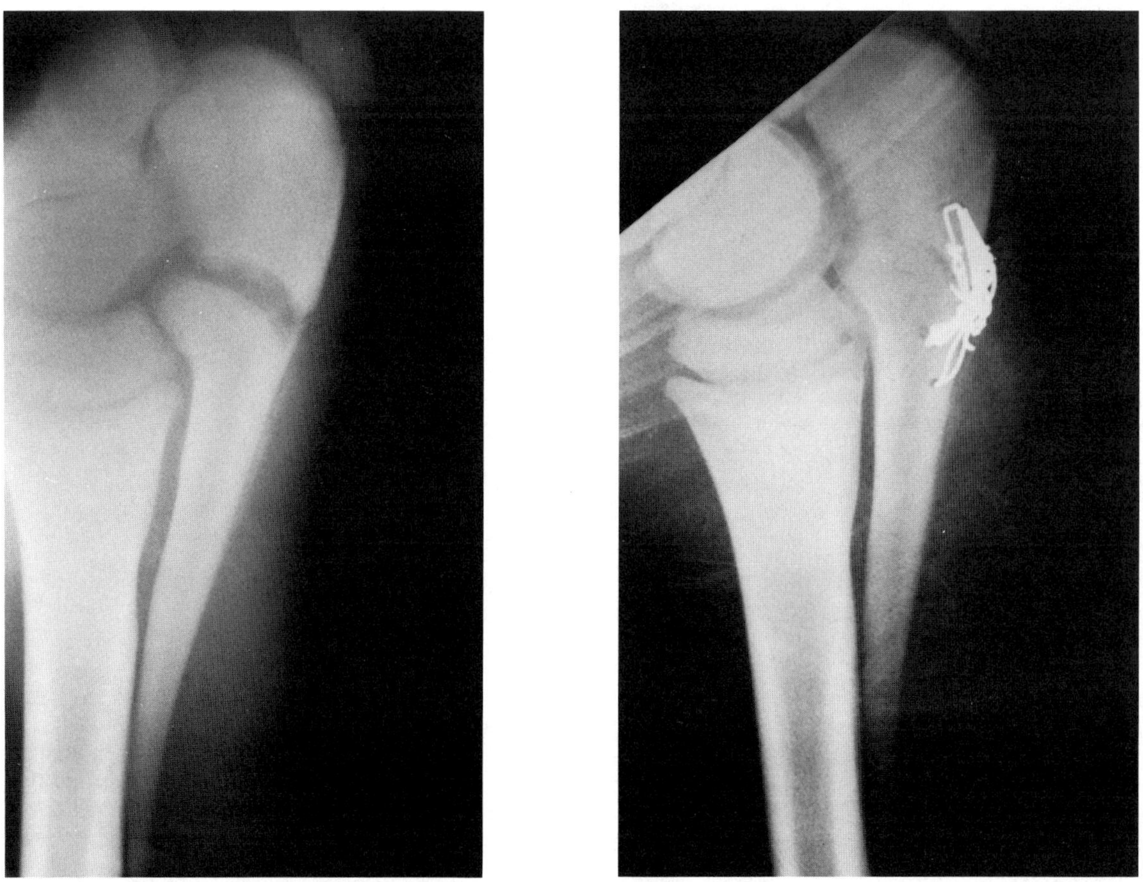

A B

Figure 124–2. A. Displaced olecranon fracture in a 3-month-old foal. **B.** A tension band wire repair of this fracture can be performed through a minimal incision with minimal expense.

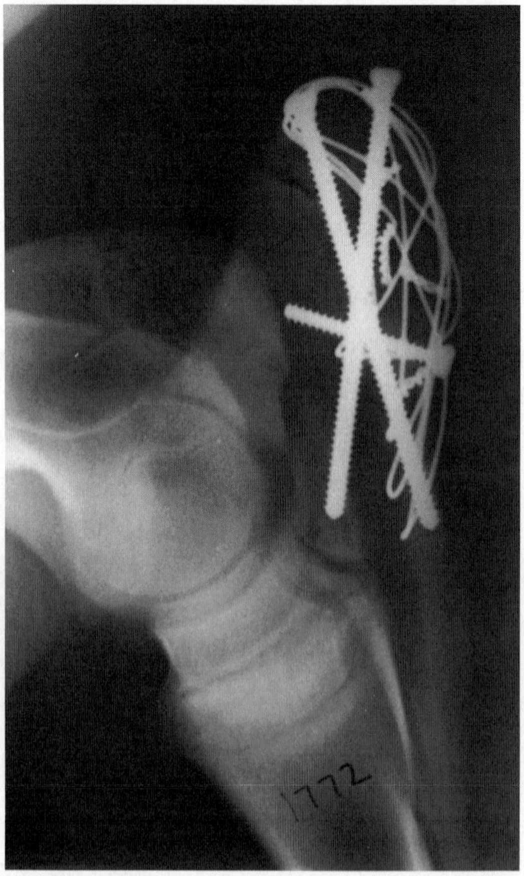

Figure 124–3. A 400-kg yearling with a markedly displaced proximal olecranon fracture that has been repaired by a tension band with two 5.5-mm screws and multiple wires. A single 4.5-mm lag screw was used to reduce the articular surface.

be managed with a deep mat or other special recovery system, if possible. The avoidance of emergence delirium by the judicious use of xylazine or opioids in the recovery phase is important.

Postoperative care of these patients is usually not difficult since they are almost always immediately comfortable on the affected limb. The distal limb is bandaged to eliminate edema and the incision is covered for a few days with an adhesive elastic bandage to prevent contamination from the bedding. Drains are rarely necessary in ulnar fractures unless there is extensive soft tissue trauma associated with the original injury. Unless a drain is present, prophylactic antibiotics are discontinued 24 hours following surgery.

Young foals heal quickly and usually need stall confinement for only 6 to 8 weeks. Adult horses are usually given a minimum of 4 months' rest before allowing vigorous exercise. Foals less than a few months old in which a pin and wire tension band technique was used usually have the implants removed to help prevent long-term complications of premature physeal closure of the olecranon. Although complications with this technique have not been seen to date, it would appear prudent to perform the second surgery in very young horses. In any case, with wires alone, the implants are left in place. The bone plates do not always have to be removed, even in the athletic horse, but pain associated with the plates during vigorous exercise may necessitate their removal. In a breeding animal, implant removal would only be necessary if there was sepsis associated with the implants. In foals, the plate should be removed as soon as healing occurs if any of the screws engage the radius.

PROGNOSIS

The prognosis for soundness is excellent for all simple ulnar fractures that are properly handled. Significant comminution of the proximal fragment definitely lessens the prognosis for athletic soundness, but most horses can still be salvaged for breeding purposes. Badly contaminated, open fractures or postsurgical infection are serious complications since the fractures often involve the elbow joint. In open fractures with mild to moderate contamination, successful management is still possible because of the excellent stability that can be achieved. Local infection along the metallic implant may necessitate its later removal, but as long as stability is present, healing can occur.

BIBLIOGRAPHY

Brown MP, Norrie RD: Surgical repair of olecranon fractures in young horses. *J Equine Med Surg* 1978;2:545–550.

Colahan PT, Meagher DM: Repair of comminuted fractures of the proximal ulna and olecranon in young horses using tension band plating. *Vet Surg* 1979;8:105–111.

Denny HR, Barr ARS, Waterman A: Surgical treatment of fractures of the olecranon in the horse: A comparative review of 25 cases. *Equine Vet J* 1987;19:319–325.

Donecker JM, Bramlage LR, Gabel AA: Retrospective analysis of 29 fractures of the olecranon process of the equine ulna. *J Am Vet Med Assoc* 1984;185:183–189.

Easley KJ, Schneider JE, Guffy MM, et al: Equine ulnar fractures: A review of twenty five clinical cases. *Equine Vet Sci* 1983;3:5–12.

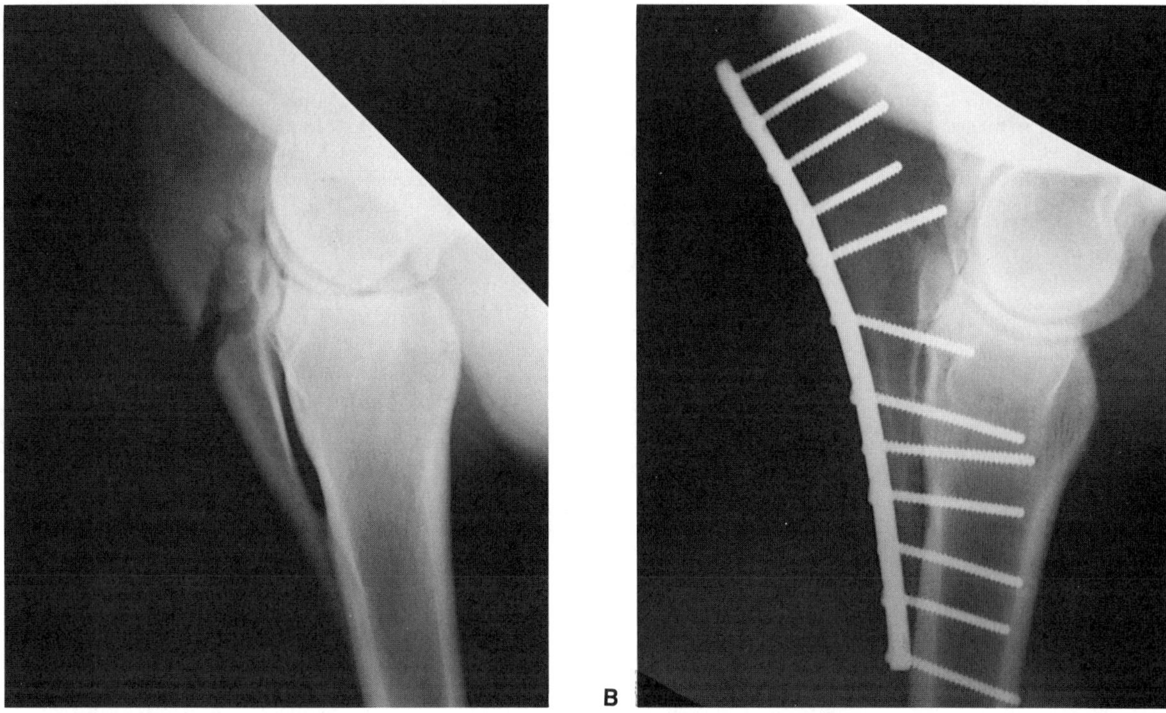

A B

Figure 124–4. Typical ulnar fracture **(A)** and plate repair **(B)** in an aged mare. In a skeletally mature horse, the radius is included in the fixation. Prognosis for this type of fracture is excellent.

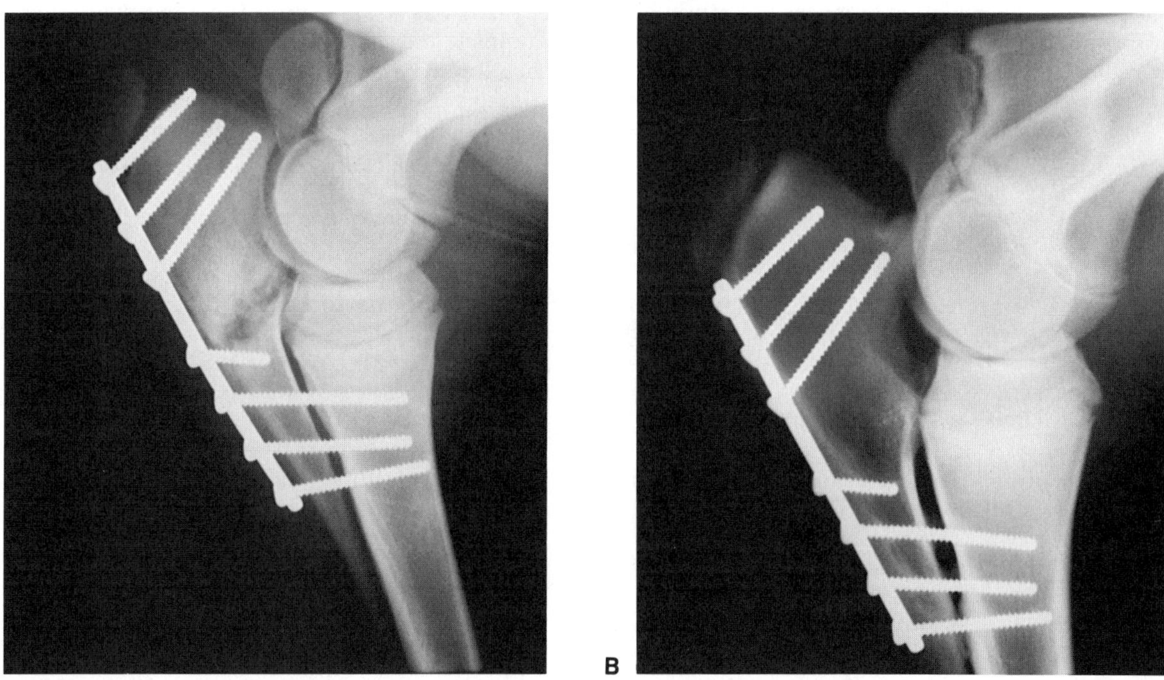

A B

Figure 124–5. A. Inappropriate repair of an ulnar fracture in a 3-month-old foal. The distal screws should not engage the radius. **B.** Six months following the repair, the continued growth of the proximal radial physis has resulted in marked subluxation of the radioulnar articulation.

Fretz PB: Case report: Fractured ulna in the horse. *Can Vet J* 1973;14:50–53.
Levine SB, Meagher DM: Repair of an ulnar fracture with radial luxation in a horse. *Vet Surg* 1980;9:58–60.
McGill CA, Hilbert BJ, Jacobs KV: Internal fixation of fractures of the ulna in the horse. *Aust Vet J* 1982;58:101–104.
Monin T: Repair of physeal fractures of the tuber olecranon in the horse, using a tension band method. *J Am Vet Med Assoc* 1978;172:287–290.
Stover SM, Rick MC: Ulnar subluxation following repair of a fractured radius in a foal. *Vet Surg* 1985;14:27–31.
Wilson DG, Riedesel E: Nonsurgical management of ulnar fractures in the horse: A retrospective study of 43 cases. *Vet Surg* 1985;14:283–286.

125
Fractures of the Radius

Robert K. Schneider

DIAGNOSIS

Complete fractures of the shaft of the radius are not difficult to diagnose. The horse is not able to support weight on the affected limb because of pain and instability. The leg hangs or is carried at the animal's side. Swelling in the forearm is usually present and crepitation and/or instability can be palpated between the elbow and carpus when the distal leg is abducted. Careful palpation and manipulation of the leg frequently allow the examiner to locate the site of the fracture within the radius. Radiographs are necessary to confirm the anatomic location of the fracture within the bone and to assess the degree of comminution. It is important to adequately evaluate the fracture with radiographs to determine the chances for successful repair of the fracture before a decision to destroy the horse is made. This is particularly true when the fracture occurs in a young foal.

Incomplete fractures of the radius offer more of a diagnostic challenge. Horses with these fractures are very lame, but will bear some weight on the leg. Instability is not present on manipulation and swelling may be minimal. This fracture occurs in adults, and affected horses usually are sensitive to direct pressure on the bone or to a firm tap on the medial side of the radius where there is little overlying soft tissue. Incomplete shaft fractures of the radius spiral up and down the long axis of the bone. They should be suspected in horses that have severe occult front limb lameness, especially in those with a history of blunt trauma to the upper forelimb. Radiographs confirm the diagnosis. A large x-ray unit and high-detail films may be necessary to demonstrate the presence of the fracture. Several views, including oblique projections, may be needed because the fissure spirals around the bone.

FRACTURE MANAGEMENT

Incomplete fractures of the radius are not common. However, when they occur there is potential for a disastrous end result if they are not recognized and handled with extreme caution. These horses should be confined and moved as little as possible to avoid complete fracture of the shaft of the radius. Horses with incomplete fractures may develop a complete fracture of the radius while confined to a box stall. Therefore, minimal movement is recommended. The horse should be confined to a tie stall or tied on an overhead wire to prevent it from lying down. The attitude of the horse is also an important consideration; calm, docile animals may do very well in a box stall, but excitable, overactive horses will require more restraint. Daily tranquilization with oral promazine granules (Fort Dodge Laboratories) is a viable consideration in horses that cannot adapt to this degree of restraint. These fractures are not easy to repair with internal fixation because of the difficulty in defining the limits and location of the fracture lines. Without accurate identification of the fracture, it is possible for screws to be placed inadvertently in a fracture line, which will tend to open the fracture further. Screws may also act as stress concentrators, weakening the bone and increasing the likelihood of complete fracture. Therefore, limiting the horse's movement for 8 to 12 weeks is the treatment of choice. The prognosis for soundness is good if complete fracture does not occur. Clients should be forewarned of the inherent risks in managing these cases.

Horses with complete fractures of the radius frequently have a history of being kicked or have experienced blunt trauma to the upper forelimb. In foals less than 1 year of age proximal oblique or transverse midshaft fractures are more common, whereas in adults comminuted shaft fractures are more frequently seen. Cortical bone in adult horses is dense and brittle and a large force is required to initiate the fracture; the high-energy blow leads to comminution when the bone fails. Options for treatment are limited to internal fixation with bone plates and screws, external fixation with a ful-leg cast, or euthanasia. The decision to treat a horse with a fractured radius is based on whether the fracture is open or closed, the economic value of the horse, and the size of the animal. Treatment with a full-leg cast is usually unsuccessful because the cast cannot immobilize the elbow joint proximal to the fracture, and this reduces the stability that can be attained at the fracture site. The final decision is made by weighing the chance for successful treatment with internal fixation against the costs of this type of surgery.

Surgery—Internal Fixation

Aseptic technique is an absolute necessity for internal fixation of equine radius fractures. The chances of healing the fracture are dramatically reduced once infection develops; even in small foals the bone plates may not maintain enough stability to allow fracture healing in the presence of infection. Therefore, every precaution should be taken to prevent infection and every technique employed to maximize stability in the repair.

In bones that undergo strong bending forces during dynamic loading, the plate should be placed on the tension surface of the bone to achieve optimal fixation. The tension surface of the equine radius is slightly to the lateral side of cranial. In addition, the soft tissues on the lateral surface of the bone afford more protection for the implants. In small foals when only one plate is used, the plate should be placed on the cranial or craniolateral surface of the bone. In large foals and adults, two plates are used; one as a tension band on the cranial surface and a second as a neutralization plate 90 degrees lateral to the first plate. The configuration of the fracture and location of cortical defects may necessitate altering the position of the plates; however, the radius is bent so strongly cranial to caudal when loaded that this should only be considered when large cortical defects alter the direction of the bending forces.

The surgical approach is made through a skin incision over the lateral surface of the leg between the muscles of the extensor carpi radialis dorsally and the common digital extensor laterally. The intermuscular septum between these muscles is sharply incised and blunt dissection is used to expose the radius. The extensor carpi radialis is retracted cranially and the common digital extensor caudally. Periosteal elevation minimizes soft tissue dissection and exposes the fractured bone.

Reduction can normally be accomplished using manual traction on the distal limb while manipulating the fragments with bone reduction forceps and/or Hohman retractors. Tenting the proximal and distal pieces upward out of the incision, engaging the fragments along the medial cortex, and replacing the fragment into the surgical field will reduce some fractures. Internal or external rotation of the distal limb may also help to align the fracture fragments during reduction. Comminuted fractures of the radius are reduced by attaching the butterfly fragments to the proximal or distal piece with lag screws, creating a two-fragment fracture, which can then be reduced by manipulation.

Once the fracture is reduced, a broad dynamic compression plate (Synthes, Ltd) is contoured and placed on the cranial surface of the radius. The plate is prestressed over the fracture and should span the length of the bone from the proximal to the distal metaphysis. In foals, the physes are not bridged unless, because of fracture location, this is necessary to gain stability in a proximal or distal fragment. Also in young foals, screws are not placed into the ulna on the palmar surface of the proximal radius; fusion of the radius to the ulna prevents the normal differential growth between these two bones and may lead to elbow dysplasia and arthritis. In adults, a 16- or 18-hole plate is frequently required to span the length of the radius. The four screws closest to the fracture line in the dorsal plate are loaded to maximally compress the fracture. All other screws are placed using the neutral guide. Screws that can be angled to cross the fracture are placed as lag screws by overdrilling the near cortex directly under the plate. In foals the large 5.5-mm cortical screws (Synthes, Ltd.) are used in the proximal and distal metaphysis. In adults, 5.5-mm screws are used in all holes in the dorsal plate. In adult horses and in foals with open fractures a second plate is contoured to the bone and placed as a neutralization plate on the lateral surface. A shorter plate is used to avoid the stress-concentrating effect of ending both plates at the same location on the metaphyses. All of the screws in the second plate are placed in the neutral position; those that can be angled to cross the fracture are placed as lag screws. In adult horses 5.5-mm screws are recommended. The second plate is positioned on the bone so that the screw holes are not superimposed over the screw holes in the initial plate. In closed fractures in neonatal foals a second plate is not always necessary; adequate stabilization can be achieved with one plate.

Plate luting is recommended for all fractures of the radius except those in small, young foals. Once both plates are in place on the bone, the screws in the dorsal plate are loosened and methylmethacrylate is mixed to achieve a claylike consistency and used to fill the space between the plate and bone. The screws are then retightened. The acrylic fills the bone-plate interface as well as the holes in the plate around the heads of the screws. The lateral neutralization plate is loosened and also luted with methylmethacrylate. Luting the plate increases the strength of the fixation by protecting the screws against fatigue failure from cyclic loading.

Cancellous bone grafts are beneficial in treating fractures of the radius to decrease the time required for fracture healing. Long bone fracture healing in the horse is frequently a race between the time required for healing of the bone and the length of time that the implants can hold the bone stable before they loosen or fail. Cancellous bone is rapidly revascularized and promotes osteogenesis at the fracture site, decreasing the time to bony union. It may not be necessary to graft radius fractures in young foals because they heal rapidly. Radius fractures repaired with internal fixation in all other horses should be grafted, especially if the fracture is comminuted and cortical defects are present.

Because of the length of time that the skin is open during double bone plating of the radius, perioperative antibiotics should be given. Antibiotics selected should have a broad spectrum, achieve effective concentrations in bone, and be given intravenously prior to surgery. During the surgical repair, the surgical field is periodically lavaged with sterile normal saline containing antibiotics.

Suction drains are used to remove blood and serum from the surgery site in the immediate postoperative period. A 0.25-in polyethylene tube with multiple holes is placed along the bone plates; the end is brought through the skin distal to the incision and attached to a suction device. The wound is closed over the drain. The intermuscular fascia between the extensor carpi radialis and common digital extensor is closed using interrupted absorable sutures. The subcutaneous tissue is closed with a continuous absorbable suture and the skin is closed in an interrupted pattern with monofilament nonabsorable suture. During skin closure, several large vertical mattress sutures are placed to counteract tension from postoperative swelling. The leg is wrapped in a large Robert Jones bandage. Full-leg casts are not used on equine radius fractures repaired with bone plates because they reverse the normal dorsal-to-palmar bending of the radius during walking. The palmar surface of the bone becomes the tension surface and the dorsal plate is then located opposite the tension surface of the bone. In this location the bone plate is submitted to cyclic compression loads and the fixation is weakened.

Recovery

The greatest stress on the fixation in the 3-month period after surgery will occur during anesthetic recovery. The largest strains recorded from the equine radius occurred during induction and recovery from anesthesia. Quiet, controlled recovery minimizes the number and magnitude of forces acting on the fracture fixation. Difficult, stormy recoveries cause large abnormal forces on the repaired bone and acute failure of the fixation can result. For this reason some surgeons have advocated recovery on a tilt table or in a swimming pool. Both of these systems recover the horse standing so that it does not have to rise to its feet from a recumbent position. Stormy or bad recoveries can still occur with these techniques. However, if the fracture repair is so tenuous that the horse is capable of breaking it while standing up during recovery, the fixation would not be likely to hold the bone in alignment for the 10 to 12 weeks required for fracture healing to occur. Usually the method of recovery does not determine the ultimate outcome, but it is important to protect against a rough recovery. Small doses of xylazine (Rompun, 50 to 100 mg intravenously) administered during the recovery period may quiet the animal and smooth the recovery. In animals that do recover from lateral to standing under their own power, ropes attached to the head and tail through rings high on the recovery stall wall help to stabilize the horse and reduce staggering and misplaced steps with the fractured limb. Unassisted recoveries are unacceptable for equine patients with a fractured radius.

Postoperative Care

Antibiotics are continued during the postoperative period. The decision to halt antibiotic treatment is based on clinical assessment of the surgery site. Antibiotic therapy is usually maintained until the suction drain has been removed and soft tissue swelling is resolving. Antibiotics are continued beyond 3 to 5 days only in those animals showing clinical signs of infection including fever, excessive heat and edema around the incision, or decreased weight bearing on the leg. In horses with postoperative infection, establishing drainage for septic wound fluid is important in controlling and limiting the infection. A ventral-draining fistula to the outside should be established, cultures should be taken from the draining tract, and antibiotic therapy administered based on culture results. Infection is a serious complication that greatly worsens the prognosis, but its presence does not mean fracture treatment will fail in every case.

Phenylbutazone is given for anti-inflammatory and analgesic effect during the first few days following surgery. The antipyretic effects of this drug will not usually mask a fever from local wound infection and the analgesic effect will not mask decreased weight bearing from fixation failure.

Monitoring use of the limb is important in evaluating the state of the fracture repair. Rigid fixation of radius fractures normally allows the horse to put considerable weight on the leg. A sudden change in use of the fractured leg is cause for concern; radiographs of the fracture and careful examination for any signs of infection should be performed.

Progression of fracture healing can be monitored radiographically at 4-week intervals. However, careful evaluation of the horse's clinical status and radiographs of the fracture only when a problem develops is a logical approach for following these cases for the 3 to 4 months required for healing to occur. Infection will prolong the time required for fracture healing. Once the fracture is healed, a decision must be made regarding removal of the plates. Removal of the implants is necessary in infected fixations to resolve the infection. Plate removal is also recommended in horses that are to be used as athletes because of the large forces acting on the radius during active exercise. Removal of the implants should be staged to minimize weakening of the bone due to the stress-concentrating effect of the empty screw holes. Taking out both plates at once

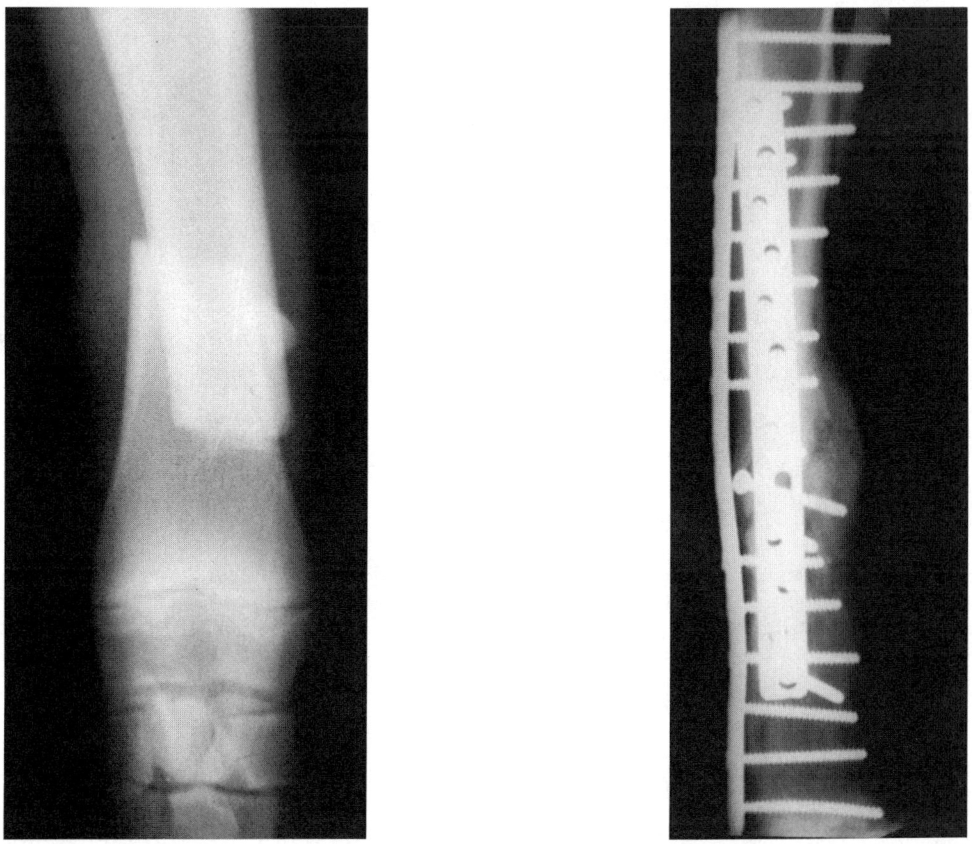

A B

Figure 125–1. Successful repair of a fractured radius in an 800-lb Arabian yearling colt. **A.** A closed, simple transverse fracture was repaired with two bone plates. **B.** The dorsal plate was prestressed and loaded with dynamic compression to function as a tension band, and the second plate was placed as a neutralization plate on the medial cortex. Although this fracture healed, use of 5.5-mm screws instead of 4.5-mm screws is recommended for fracture repair in adult-sized horses.

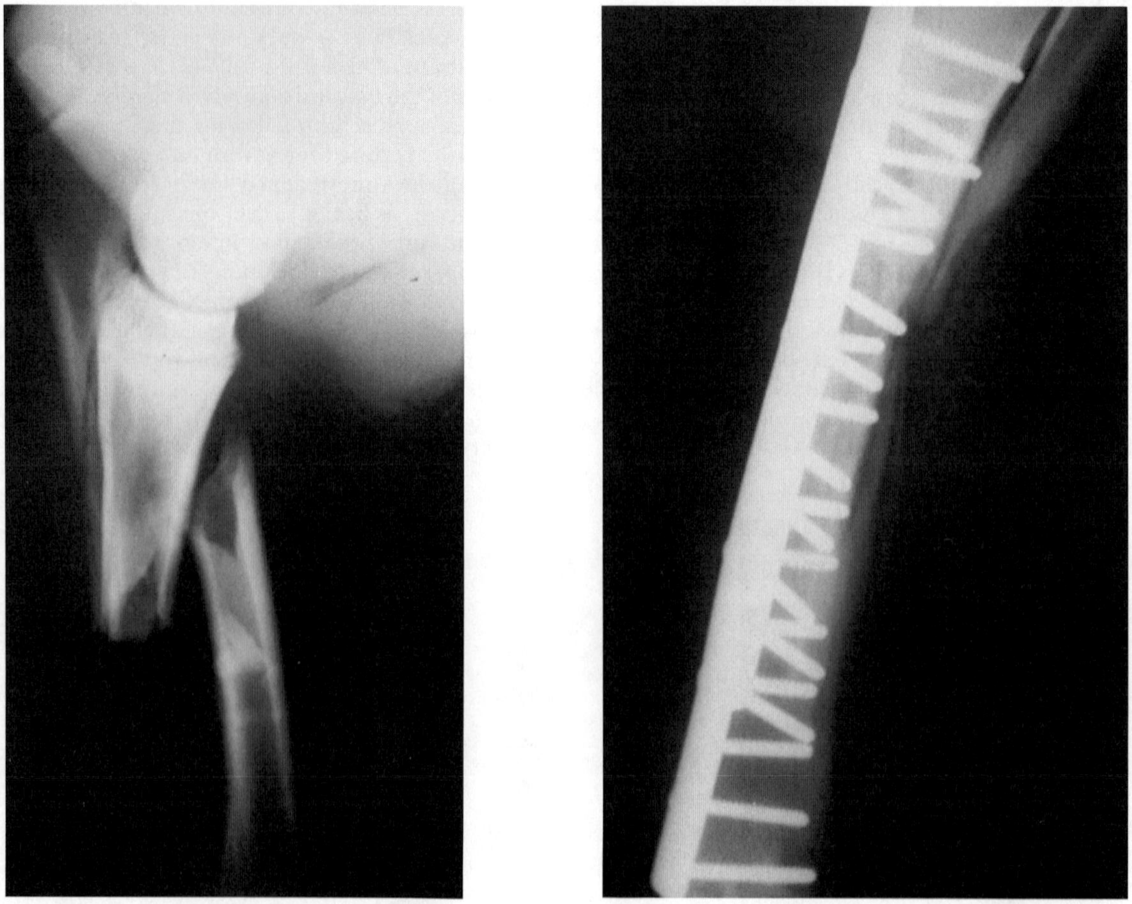

A B

Figure 125–2. Unsuccessful repair of a fractured radius in a 300-lb Arabian foal. **A.** An open transverse fracture was repaired with two bone plates. Despite anatomic reduction and a smaller sized patient than the horse in Figure 125–1, the infected fracture did not heal, continued to drain, and became unstable 8 weeks after surgery. **B.** Radiographs taken 6 weeks after surgery show lysis at the fracture site and absence of any bridging callus. This repair would have been strengthened by using 5.5-mm screws and luting both plates; however, with infection present it is unlikely that it would have altered the outcome. Infection delays or stops fracture healing and eventually screws loosen and the fixation fails.

greatly decreases strength in the healed radius and predisposes the horse to a catastrophic fracture following plate removal. Some plates can be removed standing under sedation with xylazine and butorphanol (Torbugesic, Bristol Labs) and local anesthesia. This is especially true for implants in infected fractures that are walled off from surrounding soft tissues, making dissection and isolation of the plate relatively easy. Following plate removal, exercise should be severely restricted to minimize stress until bone remodeling can occur. At least 60 days should be allowed between removal of the first and second plates; during this time bone remodeling will have removed the stress-concentrating effects of the screw holes. Radiographically the screw holes will still be present because they are filled with woven bone, which is less dense than the surrounding cortical bone.

OTHER MANAGEMENT METHODS

There are currently not many other options for managing radius fractures in the horse. Casts have limitations because they cannot immobilize the elbow, but they have been used successfully in rare instances to treat horses with fractures of the radius. Transfixation pins placed through the radius proximal to the fracture and incorporated in the cast may be useful in horses with distal radius fractures. The pins help support some of the horse's weight and also stabilize the fracture against torsional forces. These treatments should be considered only in open, contaminated fractures when the chances of successful plate fixation are poor because of infection.

PROGNOSIS

The prognosis for horses with a fracture of the radius depends on the size of the horse and whether or not the fracture is open. Closed, transverse diaphyseal radius fractures in young foals under 400 lb have a good prognosis with internal fixation. Over 400 lb, the larger the horse the poorer the prognosis for successful fracture healing. A few adult radius fractures have been successfully treated (Fig. 125–1). Open, contaminated fractures of the radius have a poor prognosis even in small

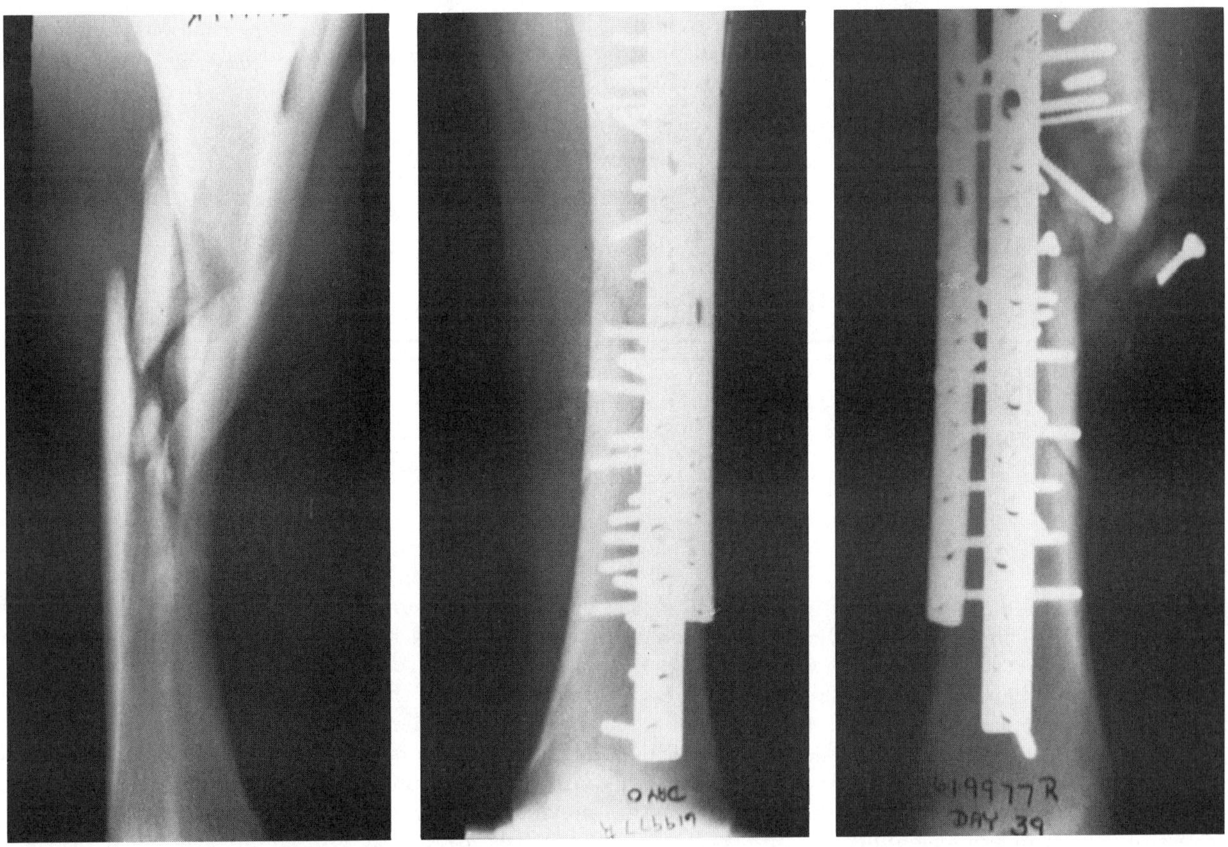

A B C

Figure 125–3 Unsuccessful repair of a fractured radius in a 900-lb Arabian mare. **A.** A closed, comminuted fracture of the radius was repaired with two bone plates. **B.** Anatomic alignment and reduction with full cortical contact was obtained. This mare walked almost sound following surgery. The skin and soft tissues healed without signs of infection. **C.** On postoperative day 39 the mare became acutely lame with swelling at the surgery site. Radiographs revealed breakdown of the internal fixation devices. Plate luting and 5.5-mm screws may have made a difference in this case by increasing the stability of the repair enough to withstand cyclic loading of the screws.

foals because the risk of infection is high and internal fixation cannot hold a 300-lb foal's fractured radius rigid long enough for healing to occur in the presence of infection (Fig. 125–2). Therefore, open fractures of the radius warrant a poor prognosis. Comminuted fractures of the radius also have a poor prognosis, even in fractures that can be completely reconstructed, because of the limited ability of plates and screws to hold the fracture stable until healing can occur (Fig. 125–3). The prognosis is poorer for older horses with radial fractures since they heal more slowly than younger horses and the fractures are usually more comminuted.

New techniques such as plate luting and stronger implants like the 5.5-mm cortical screws have improved our ability to stabilize equine radius fractures. The new Dynamiic Condylar Plate (Synthes, Ltd) is larger and stronger than the largest standard plates available and may allow repair of previously irreparable injuries. This plate may be particularly useful in metaphyseal fractures in the proximal or distal radius where gaining adequate purchase of the epiphysis is difficult.

BIBLIOGRAPHY

Auer JA, Watkins JP: Treatment of radial fractures in adult horses: An analysis of 15 clinical cases. *Equine Vet J* 1987;19:103–110.

Milne DW, Turner AS: Approaches to the radius, in *An Atlas of Surgical Approaches to the Bones of the Horse.* Philadelphia, WB Saunders Co, 1979, pp 98–107.

Nunamaker DM, Bowman KF, Richardson DW, et al: Plate luting: A preliminary report of its use in horses. *Vet Surg* 1986;15:289–293.

Sanders-Shamis M, Bramlage LR, Gabel AA: Radius fractures in the horse: A retrospective study of 47 cases. *Equine Vet J* 1986;18:432–4327.

Schneider RK, Milne DW, Gabel AA, et al: Multidirectional in vivo strain analysis of the equine radius and tibia during dynamic loading with and without a cast. *Am J Vet Res* 1982;43;1541–1550.

126 Fractures of the Humerus

Mark D. Markel

DIAGNOSIS

Fractures of the humerus can occur in horses of any age, breed, or sex, but most often affect foals under 1 year of age, racing or race training Thoroughbreds, and horses used for jumping or steeplechase events. Stress fractures of the humerus occur most frequently in 2- and 3-year-old Thoroughbreds. Lameness is of sudden onset and occurs when the horse is at racing or training speeds rather than during slow work. The lameness ranges from mild to non-weight bearing, and is exacerbated by manipulation of the elbow or shoulder. Diagnosis of stress fractures can be made by radiography or nuclear scintigraphy. Often, radiographs taken at the time of injury do not reveal abnormalities, but within 2 to 3 weeks periosteal proliferation develops at the site of the fracture. Stress fractures of the humerus have two typical locations: the proximal caudal lateral cortex and the distal cranial medial cortex (Fig. 126–1).

Complete fractures of the equine humerus are relatively uncommon because of the bone's short, thick configuration and surrounding musculature. These fractures usually involve the middle one third of the humerus and have two common histories. The first is direct trauma to the humerus in jumping horses when they fall, or in foals from a fall or a kick. The second common history is the occurrence of the injury during racing or race training. Some of these horses have a previous history of intermittent lameness that may have been associated with an undiagnosed stress fracture of the humerus.

Horses with complete humeral fractures invariably have an immediate severe lameness on the affected limb with soft tissue swelling centered over the humerus. The limb presents with the elbow dropped and with the carpus in flexion. Radiographic examination of the limb confirms the diagnosis (Fig. 126–2). Often, massive swelling of the humeral region accompanied

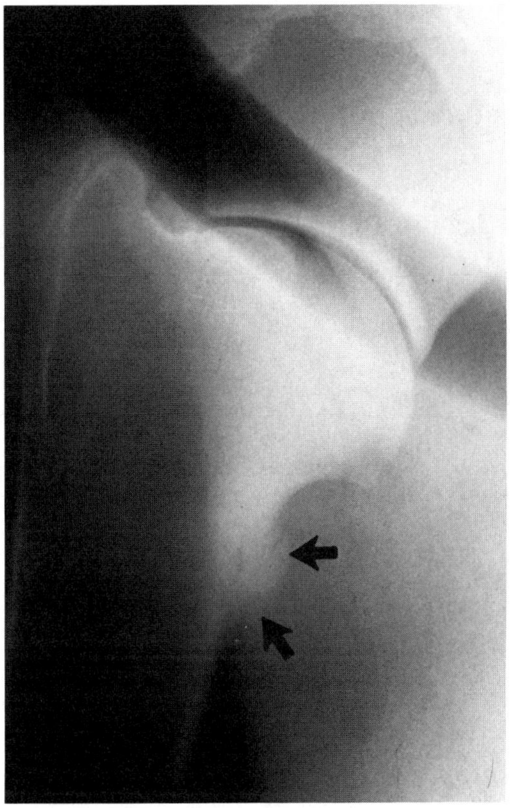

Figure 126–1. Periosteal response secondary to a stress fracture of the caudal proximal aspect of the humerus (*arrows*).

by pain upon manipulation of the limb make accurate radiographic diagnosis of the fracture's configuration difficult. In these cases, radiographic examination of the region with the horse under general anesthesia may be required. Complete fractures of the humerus usually are oblique or spiral, and course from the bone's caudal surface proximally to its cranial surface distally (Fig. 126–3). Humeral fractures in adults frequently are comminuted, complicating their repair.

Other fractures that are seen less frequently are fractures of the deltoid tuberosity and fractures of the greater tubercle. These fractures are secondary to direct trauma such as a kick. Physeal fractures of the humeral head or of the distal humeral condyle may also occur in young animals (Fig. 126–4A).

FRACTURE MANAGEMENT

Horses with stress fracture's are best managed conservatively with stall rest until the lameness resolves. If the horse is severely lame, it should be tied up in a standing stall or on a tie line to minimize the chances of completely fracturing the humerus when the horse gets up or down. After 8 to 12 weeks, the fracture should be reevaluated with radiographs, and if adequate callus has developed the horse can then be turned out to pasture for an additional 3 to 4 months. The humerus should be reevaluated with radiographs before allowing the horse to return to training.

The treatment of horses with complete fractures of the humerus is based on the type of fracture, the age of the horse, and the horse's intended use. Foals less than 6 months of age have been managed in a variety of ways. Conservative therapy with stall rest may allow the fracture to heal in foals with fractures that are minimally displaced (Fig. 126–4B). The limb should be splinted with a polyvinyl chloride (PVC) splint on its caudal aspect to prevent carpal contracture and maintain a straight limb for support. The contralateral limb should be supported with a heavy bandage to prevent breakdown of the flexor tendons. Conservative therapy in foals frequently results in healing of the fracture, but with varying degrees of malunion. Often a residual lameness may persist as a result of shortening of the limb. Breakdown of the contralateral limb occasionally occurs despite support bandaging.

Fracture Stabilization in Foals

Many surgical procedures have been described to stabilize complete fractures in foals less than 6 months of age. These techniques include intermedullary pinning, ASIF nailing, and dynamic compression plating. The technique for intramedullary pinning is similar to that used in small animals, but is much more difficult because of poor surgical exposure, difficult reduction, comminution, and overriding of the fracture. To repair fractures by intramedullary pinning, the humerus should be exposed through a lateral approach. The fracture should be reduced, and an attempt made to minimize overriding of the fracture fragments using traction. With a 1.2-cm auger drill bit, a hole should be placed just medial to the greater tubercle centered between the cranial and caudal aspects of the tubercle. Intramedullary pins (6.4-mm, or 0.25-in, diameter; 30.5-cm length) are directed from the greater tubercle normograde into the medial condyle of the humerus. Care must be taken not to exit the medial cortex of the distal fragment when placing the pins. Multiple intramedullary pins achieve stabilization of the fracture by fixation in the proximal distal metaphysis/epiphysis and by filling the medullary cavity with enough implants to create frictional forces between the pins and the intracortical surfaces that will prevent or minimize motion. Therefore, it is important to fill the medullary

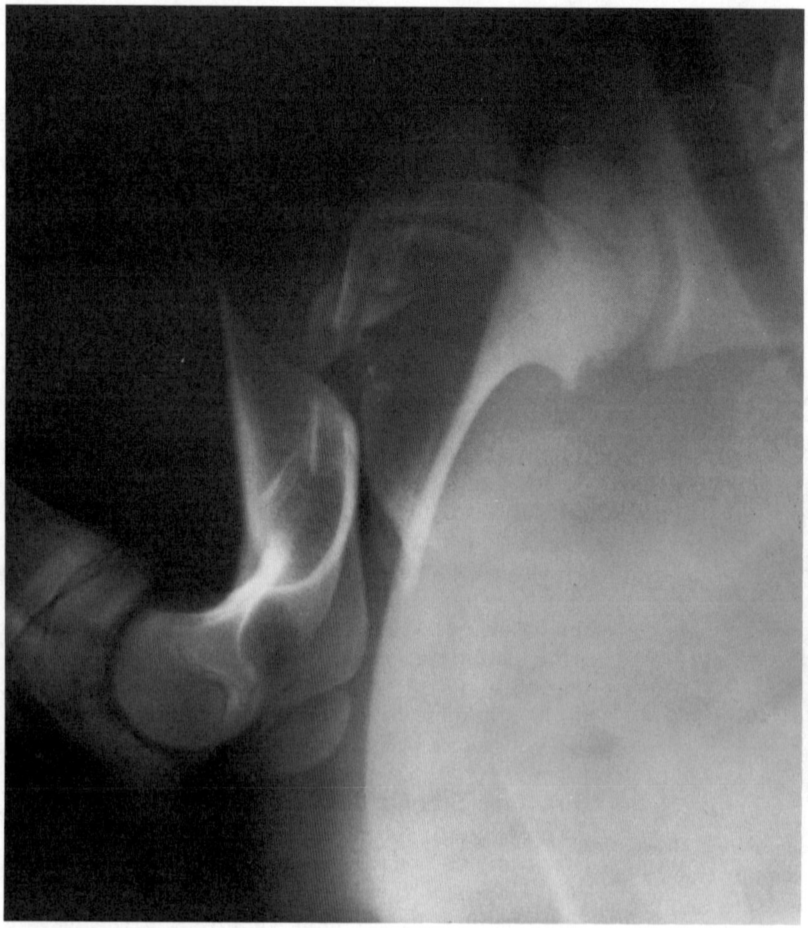

Figure 126–2. Complete fracture of the humerus in a 2-week-old foal.

cavity, but not to such an extent that the pins create further fractures of the humeral cortex. The humerus of foals less than 6 months of age will usually take two to three intramedullary pins (6.4-mm diameter), but smaller pins may have to be used in conjunction with the larger pins to achieve stability. The pins are cut proximally, leaving 2 to 3 cm protruding from the greater tubercle.

ASIF tibial nails (Synthes, Ltd) have been used successfully in foals up to 4 months of age. The medullary cavity must be reamed prior to application of the nail. The nail is placed in the same manner as the intramedullary pins.

Bone plates have been used to repair humeral fractures in foals and yearlings. The plates are placed on the lateral surface of the humerus, requiring elevation of the brachialis muscle and preservation of the radial nerve. The technique is very difficult because of poor exposure and the large deltoid tuberosity of the humerus. Cranial approach to the humerus between the biceps brachii and the brachialis muscles may be used for cranial plate application.

All of these techniques may result in a successful outcome, but complications such as radial nerve paresis or implant failure in the fractured limb, and laminitis or flexor tendon failure of the opposite limb are common.

Fracture Stabilization in Adults

Adult horses with complete fractures have been managed conservatively by being placed in slings, although laminitis of the contralateral limb 3 to 6 weeks after the injury frequently develops. Stabilization of the fracture with either dynamic compression plates or multiple intramedullary pins is currently impractical. Even if the technical difficulties of plate application can be overcome, single compression plating has resulted in implant failure in foals and would appear to lack sufficient strength to achieve stability in adult horses. Double plating of the humerus in adult horses is not feasible because of the bone's configuration. Multiple intramedullary pining alone probably would not achieve sufficient stability to prevent the development of nonunion in adult horses. The frequent comminution of complete fractures in adult horses combined with the distraction and overriding of these fractures minimize this technique's usefulness.

Deltoid Tuberosity Fractures

Deltoid tuberosity fractures can be repaired using lag screw fixation or a combination of tension band wires and lag screw fixation. The deltoid tuberosity is compressed to the parent bone using two 4.5-mm cortical bone screws applied in lag fashion. Lag screw fixation alone probably is adequate for foals and ponies, but in adult horses the technique should be combined with tension band wiring. The wires course from the deltoid tuberosity to a screw or screws in the cranial cortex of the humerus. Fractures of the deltoid tuberosity that are small can be removed rather than reattached to the parent bone.

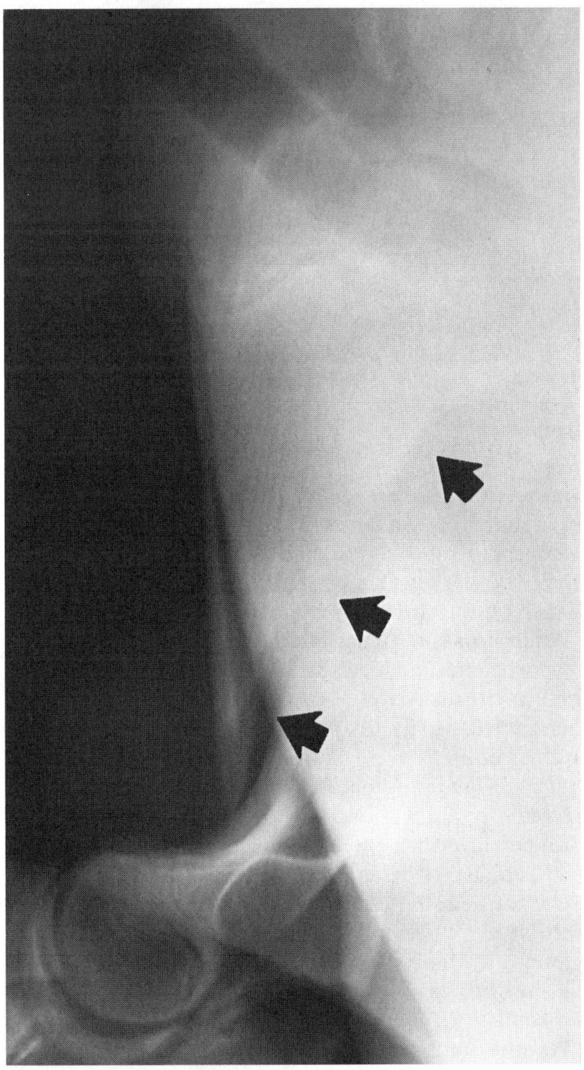

Figure 126–3. Long, oblique fracture of the humerus in a yearling (*arrows*).

Greater Tubercle Fractures

Fractures of the greater tubercle have been managed surgically and conservatively with successful results. Small, nonarticular fractures are managed conservatively with stall rest, and large fractures or articular fractures are removed.

Physeal Fractures

Physeal fractures in foals are best managed conservatively unless displacement is noted. If there is minimal displacement of the fracture, the foal should be managed with a PVC splint from the elbow to the foot. The splint should be applied to the caudal aspect of the affected limb and a support wrap should be placed on the contralateral limb.

POSTOPERATIVE CARE

Foals with complete fractures that are managed conservatively should be stall confined with no exercise until there is radiographic evidence of bony healing of the fracture. Healing usually occurs within 6 to 12 weeks of the injury. The foal typically will be non–weight-bearing lame at the time of injury and over the course of 3 to 6 weeks will gradually begin to bear weight on the affected limb. The opposite limb should be bandaged for support and the affected limb may need to be splinted. The PVC splint, which is applied on the caudal aspect of the limb from the ground to the elbow, should be monitored closely and reapplied every 3 to 4 days until the foal no longer holds the limb in flexion.

Foals with humeral fractures that have been stabilized surgically should be given perioperative broad-spectrum antimicrobial therapy. If drains are placed at surgery, the antimicrobial therapy is continued until removal of the drains.

Migration of the pins proximally should be anticipated if a fracture has been repaired with multiple intramedullary pins. As the pins migrate, they should be cut off so as not to protrude through the skin. After the fracture has healed, the pins should be removed unless growth has incorporated them into the bone.

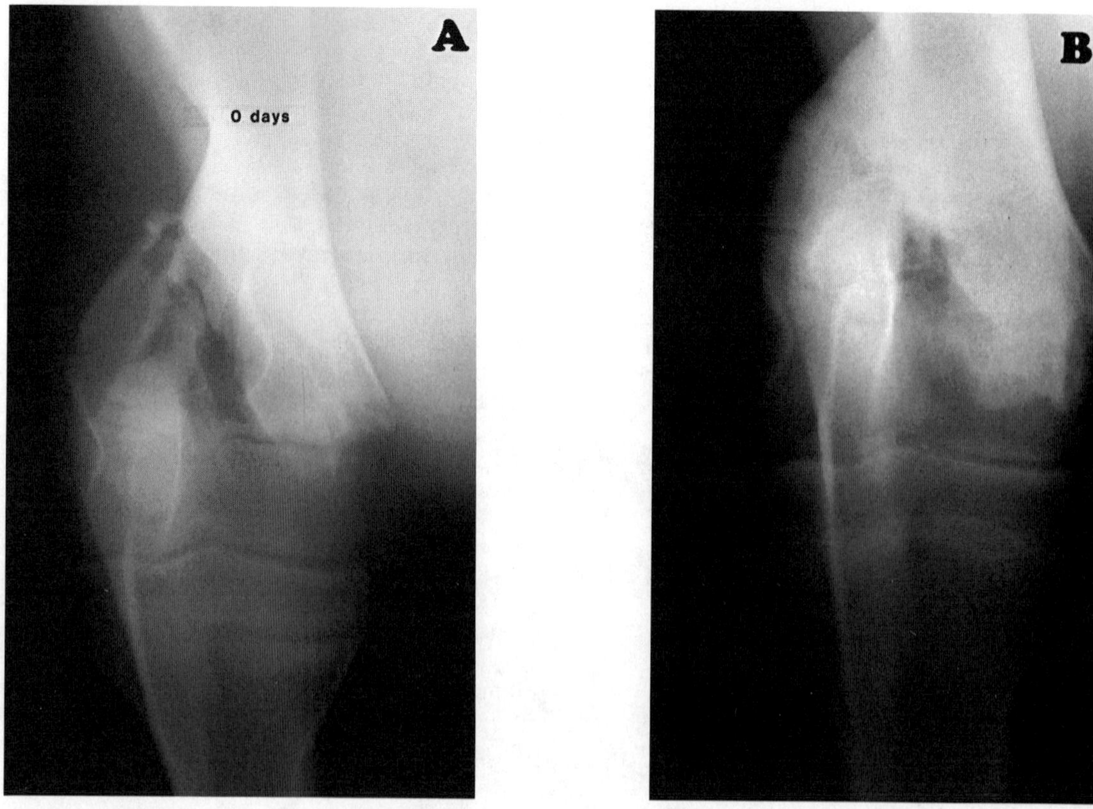

Figure 126–4. **A.** Salter-Harris type II fracture of the humerus in a 4-month-old foal. **B.** Follow-up radiograph of the fracture 100 days after the injury, which was managed conservatively.

Adult horses with complete humeral fractures that are being managed with a sling need intensive nursing care. The sling should be well padded with fleece pads, and the stall deeply bedded and well ventilated to help prevent excessive sweating and secondary pressure sores. The application of a heart bar shoe to the foot of the weight-bearing limb may help prevent rotation of the distal phalanx. Despite these considerations, adult horses with humeral fractures frequently develop laminitis. Flotation tanks have been used to manage horses with debilitating lamenesses. Water allows the horse to float or stand with minimal forces exerted on the painful limb or limbs. Although flotation tanks have many advantages, they are expensive to build and maintain, require intensive and constant care of the patient in the tank, and are not widely available.

PROGNOSIS AND SPECIAL CONSIDERATIONS

Adult horses with stress fractures have an excellent prognosis for soundness and return to performance with conservative therapy. Animals must be monitored judiciously and reevaluated regularly with radiographs during their convalescent period. Owners should be warned that the stress fracture may become a complete fracture if the horse is not rested.

Adult horses with complete humeral fractures have a poor prognosis for survival. Successful surgical repair of these fractures has not been reported and conservative therapy frequently results in nonunion of the fracture and/or laminitis of the contralateral limb, requiring euthanasia. Two methods of repair currently being investigated are multiple intramedullary pinning combined with cerclage fixation, and locked intramedullary nailing. Cerclage fixation enhanced the stiffness of multiple intramedullary pinning, but the two techniques were still significantly weaker than intact bone. The strength of the fixation could be improved by increasing the stiffness of the pins and the tensile strength of the bands.

Another technique that merits investigation is the interlocking intramedullary nail. This technique maintains axial and torsional reduction of the fragments. Conventional interlocking femoral nails accommodate fully threaded proximal screws applied in an oblique position in relation to the long axis of the nail. The technique requires reaming of the medullary cavity after reduction of the fracture. The nail is placed within the humerus and screws are applied either obliquely or transversely in the frontal plane through both the humerus and predrilled holes in the nail. Screw placement requires either a jig and/or intraoperative fluoroscopy or radiography. To the author's knowledge, this technique has yet to be used successfully in an adult horse.

In foals, the chances for survival are much better because of their enhanced fracture healing. In foals treated conservatively, shortening of the affected limb and flexor contracture are common, as are angular deformities and flexor tendon failure of the contralateral limb. Internal fixation of suitable fractures in foals can help minimize these complications, although failure of the repair, pin migration, and osteomyelitis can occur.

BIBLIOGRAPHY

Alexander JT, Rooney JR: The biomechanics, surgery and prognosis of equine fractures. *AAEP Ann Conven* 1972; pp 219–236.

Allen D, White NA II: Chip fracture of the greater tubercle of a horse. *Compend Cont Educ Pract Vet* 1984;6:S39-S41.

Bramlage LR: Long bone fractures. *Vet Clin North Am Large Anim Pract* 1983;5:285–310.

Dyson SJ, Greet TRC: Repair of a fracture of the deltoid tuberosity of the humerus in a pony. *Equine Vet J* 1986;18:230–232.

Fessler JF, Amstutz HE: Fracture repair, in Oehme FW, Prier JE (eds): *Textbook of Large Animal Surgery*. Baltimore, Williams & Wilkins, 1974, pp 314–316.

Kelman DA: Surgical repair of a spiral fracture of a humerus in a foal—a case report. *Aust Vet Pract* 1980;10:257–259.

Mackey VS, Trout DR, Meagher DM, Hornof WJ: Stress fractures of the humerus, radius, and tibia in horses. *Vet Radiol* 1987;28:26–31.

Markel MD, Nunamaker DM, Wheat JD, Sams AE: *In vitro* comparison of three fixation methods for humeral fracture repair in adult horses. *Am J Vet Res* 1988;49:586–593.

Smith GK: Biomechanics pertinent to fracture etiology, reduction and fixation, in Newton DC, Nunamaker DM (eds): *Textbook of Small Animal Orthopaedics*. Philadelphia, JB Lippincott Co, 1985, pp 195–230.

Stashak TS: The humerus, in Stashak TS (ed): *Adams' Lameness in Horses*, ed 4. Philadelphia, Lea & Febiger, 1987, pp 675–678.

Turner SA: Fractures of the humerus, in Jennings PB (ed): *The Practice of Large Animal Surgery*. Philadelphia, WB Saunders Co, 1984, vol 2, pp 798–800.

Valdez H, Morris DL, Auer JA: Compression plating of long bone fractures in foals. *J Vet Orthop* 1979;1:10–18.

Vaughn LC: Limb injuries in foals. *Equine Vet J* 1968;1:4–8.

Yovich JV: Fracture of the greater tubercle of the humerus in a filly. *J Am Vet Med Assoc* 1985;187:74–75.

127
Fractures of the Scapula

Mark D. Markel

DIAGNOSIS

Fractures of the scapula are uncommon and affect horses of any breed or sex. These fractures occur most often in horses less than 2 years of age, and frequently involve the supraglenoid tubercle (Fig. 127–1). The other common sites for scapular fractures are the scapular neck with or without involvement of the articular surface, and the body of the scapula (Fig. 127–2). Scapular fractures usually are secondary to direct trauma. Horses with supraglenoid tubercle fractures have a shortened cranial phase of the stride and lameness upon manipulation of the shoulder. If the fracture is chronic, there will be muscle atrophy over the affected shoulder. Horses with complete neck or body fractures are moderately to severely lame and resist manipulation of the shoulder. Auscultation of the region may reveal crepitance. Soft tissue swelling over the region is often present and radiographic examination of the scapula is required for the diagnosis. Lateral radiographic examination of the scapula reveals the majority of scapular fractures, but body or scapular spine fractures may be best appreciated using a caudal to cranial projection.

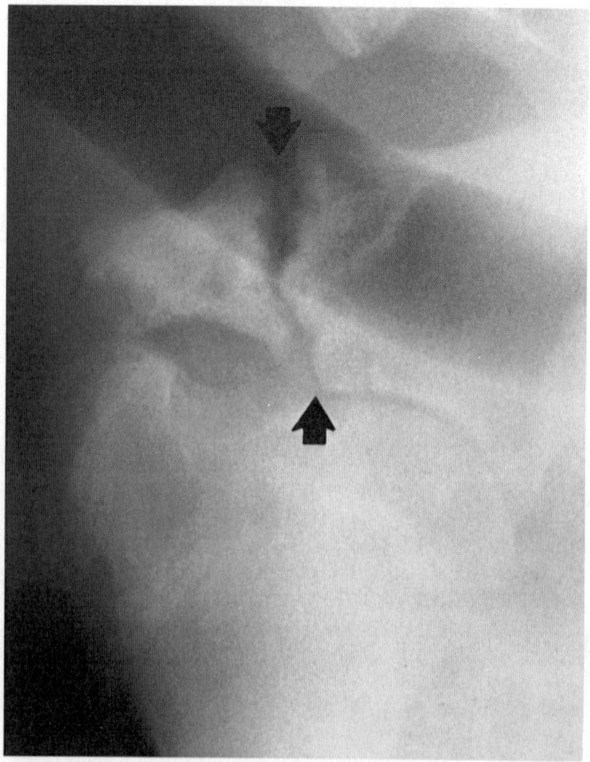

Figure 127–1. Chronic supraglenoid tubercle fracture of the humerus (*arrows*).

ANATOMY

The most cranial prominence of the scapula is the supraglenoid tubercle, which forms the point of the shoulder. The supraglenoid tubercle serves as the origin of the biceps brachii muscle and the two glenohumeral ligaments, which support the scapulohumeral joint. The coracoid process is the medial projection of the supraglenoid tubercle and is the origin of the coracobrachialis muscle. The suprascapular nerve courses along the cranial surface of the scapular neck and may be traumatized when the scapular neck is fractured.

FRACTURE MANAGEMENT

Repair of scapular fractures depends upon the type of fracture, the age of the horse, and the presence of an articular component. Fractures of the supraglenoid tubercle can be managed either surgically or conservatively. Conservative therapy in the form of stall rest for 3 to 4 months and turnout to pasture for an additional 6 to 9 months usually results in improvement of the horse's stride, but there is often a residual lameness and degenerative joint disease as a result of nonunion. Two methods of surgical management of supraglenoid tubercle fractures have been reported: either removal of

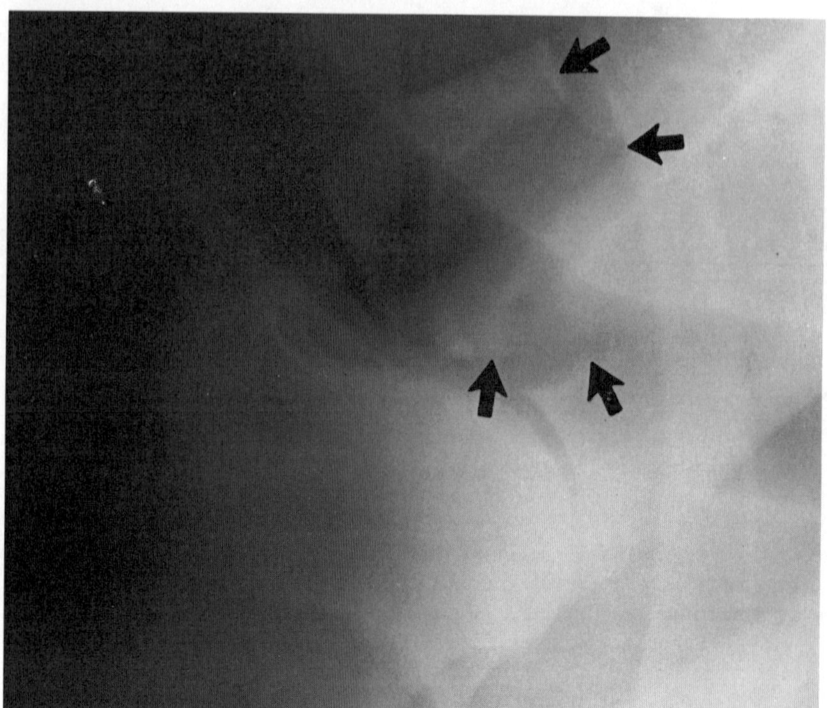

Figure 127–2. A comminuted, articular neck fracture of the humerus with luxation of the scapulohumeral joint. *Arrows* point to the fracture margins.

the fracture fragment or internal fixation of the fragment to the parent bone. In one case review, internal fixation of three fractures resulted in one clinically sound horse and two horses with no improvement. The repair of a supraglenoid tubercle fracture with tension band wires and lag screws has been reported. The horse had no residual lameness on the limb 4 years after repair.

Internal fixation of supraglenoid tubercle fractures is performed through a skin incision centered over the point of the shoulder. After exposing the fracture, fracture hematoma and/or callus are removed to achieve accurate reduction of the fragment. The origin of the biceps brachii tendon is partially severed to lessen the tensile and shear forces on the fixation. Internal fixation is achieved using a combination of lag screw fixation and tension band wiring.

Previous reports indicate successful treatment by rest and by surgical removal of the fragment in supraglenoid tubercle fractures. To remove the supraglenoid tubercle, the horse is anesthetized and placed in lateral recumbency. A skin incision is centered over the supraglenoid tubercle of the scapula and the greater tubercle of the humerus. The brachiocephalicus is incised over the region of the supraglenoid tubercle in the direction of its muscle fibers. The supraspinatus then is divided along its muscle fiber length over the supraglenoid tubercle. Beneath the supraspinatus, the supraglenoid tubercle with its attachment to the biceps tendon will be present. The fragment is sharply dissected from the biceps tendon. On the medial aspect of the fragment the coracobrachialis muscle is attached to the coracoid process. The fragment should be grasped with bone-holding forceps in order to manipulate it into a position that allows incision of the soft tissues away from their attachments. A Cobb periosteal elevator is helpful for much of the tissue separation. Once the attachments of these strcutures are removed, the fracture fragment is removed.

Fractures of the scapular body can be repaired using bone plates. The fracture will often override, requiring distraction to achieve compression. Distraction of the fracture can be performed using an ASIF fracture distractor. (Synthes, Ltd) Two 3.5-mm dynamic compression plates (Synthes, Ltd) are then applied on either side of the scapular spine. Because of the thinness of the scapula, the plates should be applied immediately adjacent to the scapular spine, and may require cancellous bone screws rather than cortical bone screws to achieve purchase in the bone. During the repair of body fractures of the scapula, the surgeon should evaluate the integrity of the suprascapular nerve as it courses over the cranial aspect of the neck of the scapula.

Fractures of the neck that involve the articular surface of the scapula or comminuted neck or body fractures usually are not amenable to surgical fixation because of the configuration of the scapula.

POSTOPERATIVE CARE

Horses that have had surgical repair of scapular fractures should have perioperative administration of broad-spectrum antibacterial agents and nonsteroidal anti-inflammatory agents. In two studies, two of eight horses treated surgically were euthanized because of osteomyelitis. Horses should be stall rested for 8 to 12 weeks, and reevaluated with radiographs before being turned out to pasture. Follow-up radiographs should be taken every 2 to 3 months until bony union is achieved.

Horses managed conservatively should have stall rest for 3 to 4 months and then turned out to pasture. The horse may need to be rested up to 1 year before being returned to work to allow for bone union and muscle regeneration.

PROGNOSIS AND SPECIAL CONSIDERATIONS

Horses with fractures of the scapula should be given a guarded prognosis for return to soundness. Horses with nonarticular supraglenoid tubercle fractures appear to have the best prognosis, because removal of the supraglenoid tubercle usually results in athletic soundness. Care must be taken to minimize dead space when removing these fractures. The grid approach minimizes the potential for seroma formation by requiring only one incision in the supraspinatus muscle. This approach provides minimal intraoperative exposure of the suprascapular vein, artery, and nerve, and the surgeon must carefully locate and preserve these structures prior to removal of the fragment. Removal of the supraglenoid tubercle in chronic fractures is difficult and traumatic. The prognosis for life in horses with supraglenoid tubercle fractures is excellent.

If surgical removal of the supraglenoid tubercle is to be successful, it is important to perform the procedure before degenerative arthritis of the scapulohumeral joint develops. Therefore, early diagnosis is important to maximize the success of surgical therapy.

There has been one reported case of plate fixation of a scapular body fracture. At 1 year after surgery, the horse was clinically normal and showed no lameness or functional disability. Neck, body, comminuted, or articular fractures are very difficult to repair, and horses with these fractures should be given a grave prognosis for future soundness.

BIBLIOGRAPHY

Adams SB: Surgical repair of a supraglenoid tubercle fracture in a horse. *J Am Vet Med Assoc* 1987;191:332–334.

Dyson S: Sixteen fractures of the shoulder region in the horse. *Equine Vet J* 1985;17:104–110.

Goble A, Brinker W: Internal fixation of the equine scapula: A case report. *J Equine Med Surg* 1977;1:341–343.

Leitch MA: A review of treatment of tuber scapulae fractures in the horse. *J Equine Med Surg* 1977;1:234–240.

Pankowski RL, Grant BD, Sande R, Nickels FA: Fracture of the supraglenoid tubercle: Treatment and results in five horses. *Vet Surg* 1986;15:33–39.

Wagner PC, Watrous BJ, Shires GM, Reibold TW: Resection of the supraglenoid tubercle of the scapula in a colt. *Compend Cont Educ Pract Vet* 1985;7:S36-S41.

128 Fractures of the Tibia

Dean W. Richardson

There are several typical fractures of the tibia that are seen in foals and adult horses. In foals, the most common fractures are Salter-Harris type II injuries of the proximal tibia and middiaphyseal fractures. Distal physeal fractures also occur but less frequently. In adults, the most common tibial fractures are catastrophic diaphyseal fractures or subtle incomplete or nondisplaced fractures of the diaphysis.

PROXIMAL PHYSEAL FRACTURES

Foals with proximal physeal fractures range in age from a few days old up to nearly a year old. These fractures are more common during the first few months of life. They usually are a result of trauma, such as a kick to the stifle region while the limb is bearing weight, or some other cause of forceful abduction of the limb distal to the stifle. The mechanics are apparently similar in all cases since the fracture configuration is always similar. Clinically there is swelling of the proximal tibia that is more pronounced medially. The limb is usually held partially flexed and weight bearing is absent or minimal. Motion and/or crepitus can be felt in the proximal medial tibia when the limb is abducted, although the foal objects to the pain from this manipulation.

Radiographically, minimal displacement of the fragments may be apparent on the lateral projection, but is quite evident on the caudal-to-cranial view (Fig. 128–1). The metaphyseal component of the Salter-Harris II fracture is always lateral but its triangular outline varies in size. Overriding of the fracture occurs on the lateral side.

Anatomic considerations of importance are that the extensors of the digit and flexors of the hock are craniolateral and tend to further distract the fracture and that young foals always tend to stand with their limbs spread, which also tends to distract the fracture. Surgical exposure of the lateral aspect of the fracture is more difficult because of the presence of the extensor muscles. Surgical exposure medially is very easy, but soft tissue coverage of implants is difficult.

Conservative treatment of these fractures is not desirable since most foals remain very lame and rapidly develop problems in the contralateral hind limb. Another consequence of conservative treatment is a residual deformity of the tibia due to gapping of the fracture medially and lateral overriding.

Surgical treatment of these fractures is generally quite rewarding. A number of techniques have been described, including transfixation devices and internal fixation with lag screws alone or cross-pins. The latter techniques certainly have marginal strength in larger foals so a medial bone plating technique is preferred. The foal is anesthetized and positioned in lateral recumbency with the affected leg down. A slightly curved incision is made cranial to the medial collateral ligament extending from 1 cm proximal to the tibial plateau distally 7 to 10 cm depending on the length of plate used. After the skin and subcutaneous tissue are incised, a large fracture hematoma is removed from the physeal fracture line. The best reduction possible is achieved by manipulation of the limb and leverage with a Hohman retractor. A five-hole T-plate (Synthes,

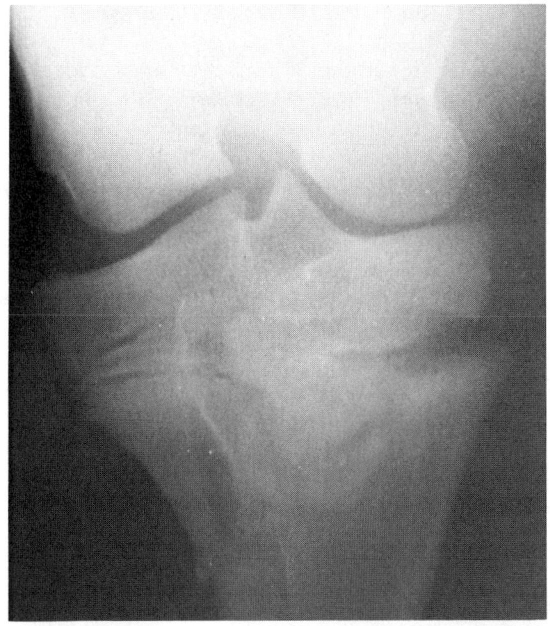

Figure 128–1. Salter-Harris type II fractures of the proximal tibia are quite common and are always similar in appearance. The metaphyseal component is always lateral. Displacement of the distal fragment is always lateral. This results in a consistent tension surface on the medial aspect of the fracture line.

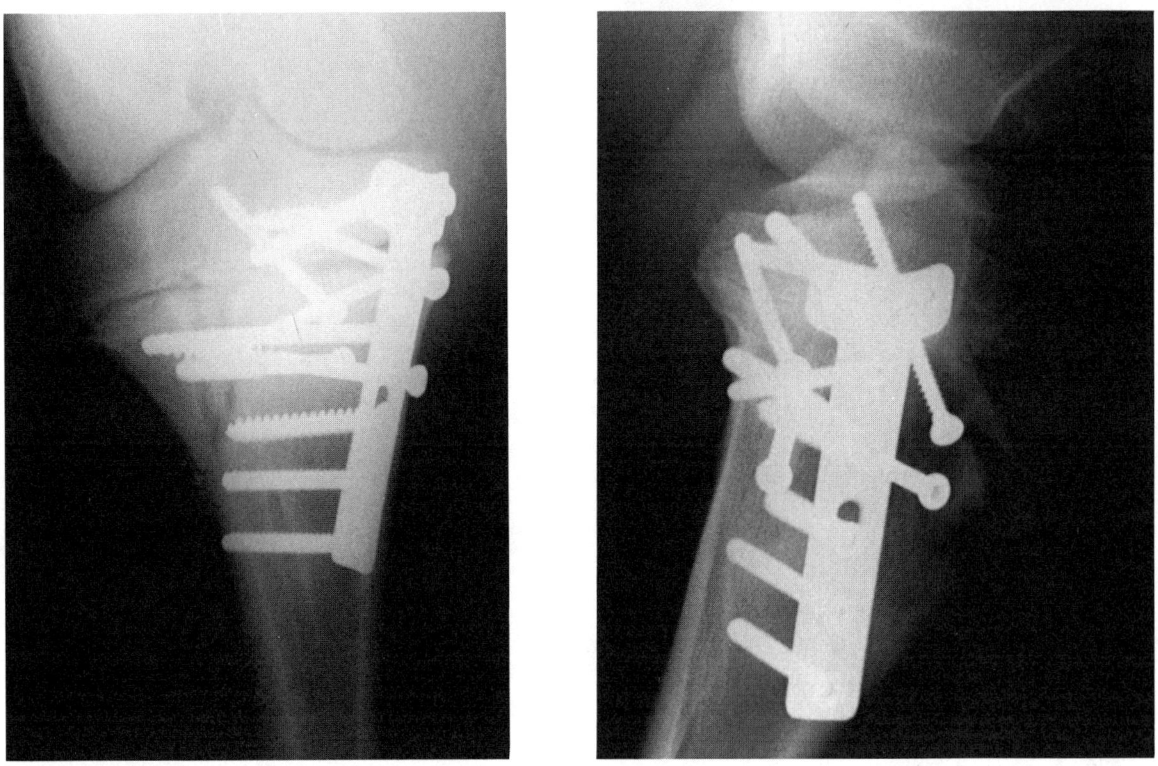

A B

Figure 128–2. Repair of the proximal physeal fracture is easily performed with a T-plate that allows placement of two screws in the epiphysis. Additional lag screws may be added to augment the fixation, especially in larger foals.

Ltd) is used in small foals (Fig. 128–2), but two side-by-side narrow dynamic compression plates (Synthes, Ltd) are recommended in much heavier (>300-kg) foals because of the much larger cross-section of the plate. Size 5.5-mm cortical screws (Synthes, Ltd) are used in the epiphysis. An effort should be made to place the screws nearly parallel with the proximal articular surface to avoid injuring the cartilage and to maximize the usable thread length of this screw. The distal screws are placed in the plate so as to compress the fracture medially. Additional lag screws may be added across the fracture line to enhance stability.

Closure of the wound over the bone plate(s) must be meticulous because of the minimal soft tissue coverage. Vertical mattress tension sutures may be necessary in the skin. An adhesive elastic bandage and gauze bandage are used to avoid direct contamination of the wound. If this technique is used in young foals (<3 months), removal of the implants as soon as healing is evident (6 to 10 weeks) is recommended to avoid permanent physeal bridging and development of an angular deformity. Lag screws across the fracture must be removed or limb shortening may result from compression of the physis. In older foals the implants are left in

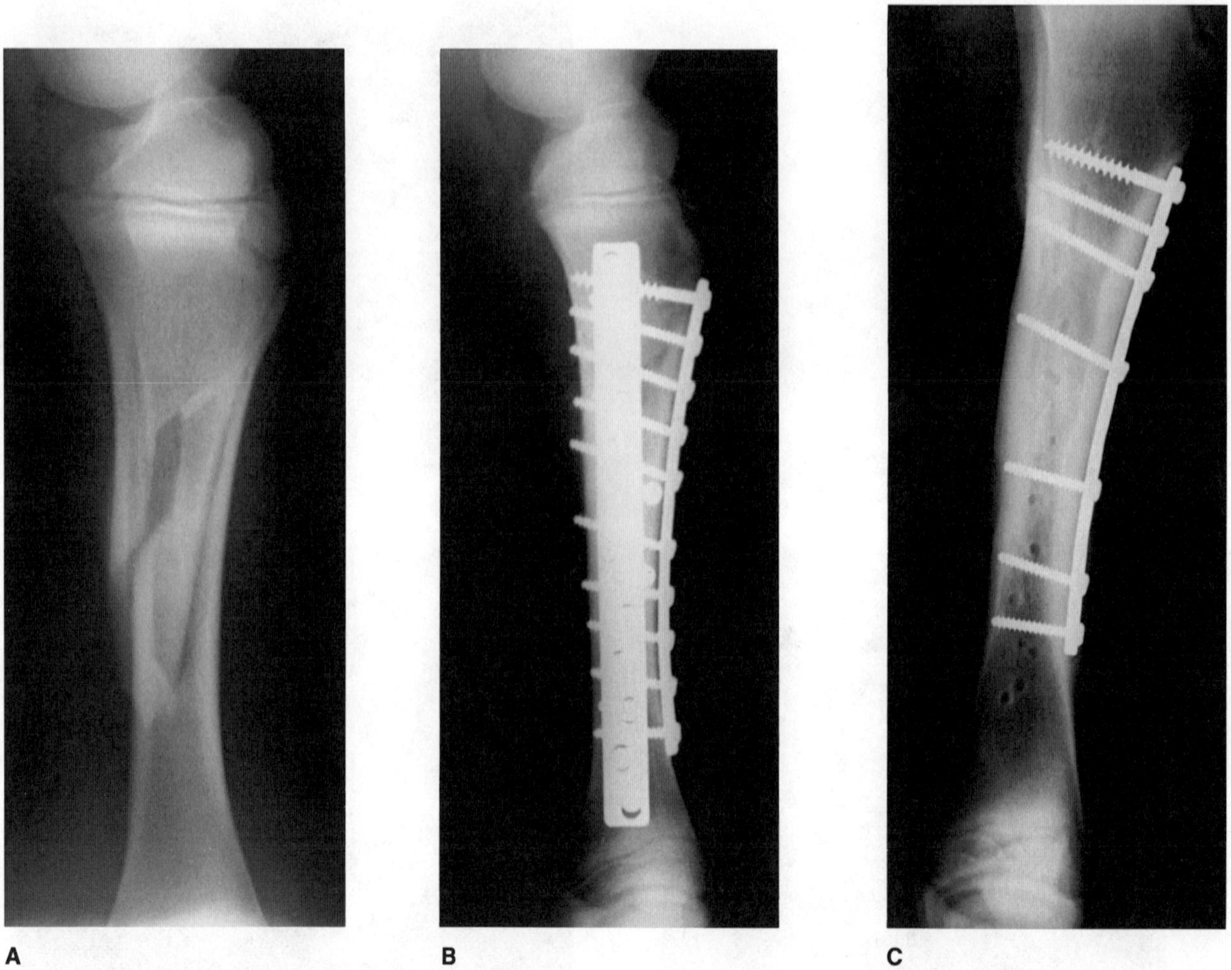

A B C

Figure 128–3. A. Spiral middiaphyseal fracture of the tibia in a 3-month-old foal. Such a configuration is ideal for repair since several lag screws through the plates can be used for interfragmentary compression. **B.** Repair with a cranially positioned narrow plate and a medial broad plate. The medial positioning in this case allowed more interfragmentary lag screws to be used. Note that two separate lag screws were used to maintain the initial reduction while the plates were applied. **C.** Four months postoperatively, the medial plate was removed. There is minimal callus formation. In this case, only some of the screws were removed from the second plate at the second surgery. Simultaneous removal of both plates is currently recommended.

place, especially if the fracture was incompletely reduced. The prognosis for fracture healing and functional soundness is good with these injuries, but the long-term outcome in athletes is still not reported.

Complete Diaphyseal Fractures

Complete diaphyseal fractures occur in any age horse, but in older horses the likelihood of an open fracture is much greater and the prognosis is poor. Most fractures occur as unwitnessed trauma, but direct blows or missteps while galloping are sometimes identifiable causes. Clinical signs are non–weight-bearing lameness, obvious swelling, and instability. Radiographs are confirmatory (Fig. 128–3A).

The surgical approach recommended is cranial and the incision is made over the tibialis cranialis muscle. The configuratiom of the fracture and preference of the surgeon determine the exact position of the incision. If the affected limb is in lateral decubitus, the incision is curved medially to allow application of a longer plate craniomedially. If the longer plate is to be placed craniolaterally, the incision is curved laterally with the leg uppermost. The latter approach has the advantage of placing the longer plate on the tension surface of the bone, but a long medial plate is easier to conform to the proximal tibia and can be placed somewhat more proximally than a lateral plate. Subperiosteal dissection and plate placement are advisable, and leveraged elevation of the tibialis cranialis with Hohman retractors is essential for adequate exposure.

Double plating is mandatory because of the complex forces acting on the tibia (Fig. 128–3B). Whenever possible, two broad dynamic compression plates are used, although a combination of a broad and a narrow plate may be necessary in some foals. Size 5.5-mm screws are recommended in larger individuals, but the surgeon must keep in mind that the plates must be "staggered" to avoid interference of one plate's screws with those of the other plate. This staggering process is more difficult to achieve with 5.5-mm screws. Most diaphyseal fractures of the tibia are oblique so lag screws can be used for compression of the fracture line and to improve stability. Luting beneath the plates is recommended. This involves loosening all the screws in the plate, placing polymethylmethacrylate (Simplex P; Howmedica) under the plate while it is in its doughy stage, and tightening the screws. This results in improved contact between the plate and bone, provides additional support for the screw heads within the elliptical holes of the dynamic compression plate, and prolongs the effective stability of the implant.

Closed suction drainage is optional; it has the advantage of evacuating the inevitable accumulation of serum around the implants but the disadvantage of providing a potential route of contamination. We prefer not to use drains in most cases and rely on meticulous closure and compression bandages.

Foals are strictly confined for 3 to 4 months, at which time implant removal is considered (Fig. 128–3C). Plates are removed in all animals that are destined to be athletes, although their removal in breeding animals or pleasure horses is probably unwarranted.

Adult horses with complete diaphyseal fractures are *much* more difficult to treat, especially because many of these fractures are open and contaminated medially where soft tissue coverage is minimal. Many of these fractures result from severe external trauma or a fall, but severely comminuted fractures can occur as a consequence of a single misstep. Double plating or triple plating with broad plates and 5.5-mm screws is recommended. The same surgical approach as described for foals is used. Special care is needed during recovery since horses tend to experience large torsional stresses in the tibia as they stand up, and refracture is very possible. Repair of tibial fractures in adult horses is still considered a salvage procedure for breeding or other nonathletic purposes.

Incomplete Fractures

Incomplete fractures of the tibia are characteristically seen in young (2 to 4 years) Thoroughbreds with a history of acute severe lameness that sometimes dissipates or disappears within a few days. Although not present in all cases, focal pain can often be elicited with digital pressure over the proximal medial or distal medial tibia. Painful, pitting edema may be noted over the medial gaskin where muscle coverage is minimal. Most limb manipulations will exacerbate the lameness. Occasionally, localizing physical findings are absent and the lesion may only be identified serendipitously on hock or stifle films. Radiographs usually reveal a well-defined linear lucency shortly after the fracture, with periosteal proliferative changes noted after 2 to 3 weeks (Fig. 128–4A,B). The configuration of the majority of incomplete fractures of the tibia appears to be spiral, with the fracture exiting from the distal craniomedial cortex and proximal lateral cortex. A true spiral fracture by definition has a longitudinal component, so the fracture may appear as a vertical line in the diaphysis. In subtle cases, high-detail radiographs with a large x-ray unit and grid cassettes may be necessary. Radionuclide imaging techniques also can be helpful in identifying otherwise occult tibial fractures and may be useful in separating the incomplete spiral fracture from a focal "stress" or fatigue fracture.

Therapy of incomplete spiral fractures is problematic. Stall rest alone has a distinct risk of the horse completing the fracture (Fig. 128–4C). The risk appears

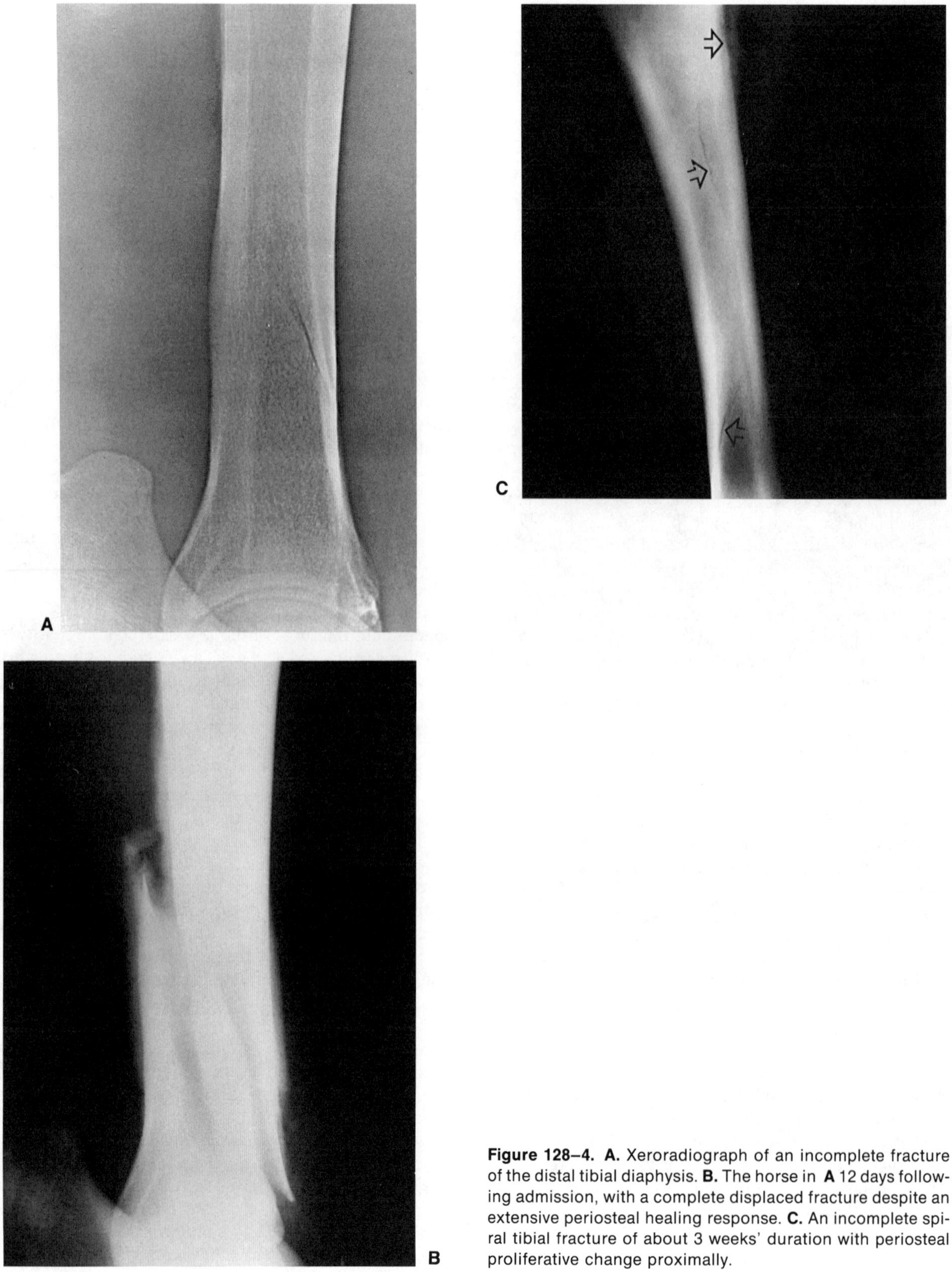

Figure 128–4. A. Xeroradiograph of an incomplete fracture of the distal tibial diaphysis. **B.** The horse in **A** 12 days following admission, with a complete displaced fracture despite an extensive periosteal healing response. **C.** An incomplete spiral tibial fracture of about 3 weeks' duration with periosteal proliferative change proximally.

to be greatest 2 to 3 weeks following the injury. Since the exacerbation of the fracture is believed to be associated with arising from recumbency, stall rest can be augmented by tying the horse's head in cross-ties or to a sliding overhead wire to prevent the horse from lying down. Some horses tolerate this remarkably well, whereas others will simply collapse despite the head tie.

Nondisplaced Fractures

Internal fixation would appear to be a reasonable option for nondisplaced fractures if one could predict with assurance that a given fracture was going to displace. Most affected horses, however, are racehorses and aggressive internal fixation by itself places the horse's career at risk and is additionally quite expensive. End-to-end plating with lag screws through the plate would be the indicated method of repair if this decision were made.

We continue to treat these fractures conservatively since the prevalence of complete dehiscence appears to be less than 50%. Casts or splints are not recommended since the stifle joint cannot be satisfactorily immobilized and there is evidence that they provide insignificant protection. If the horse's temperament allows, cross-tying or other head restraint is recommended along with stall rest. Radiographs are taken at about monthly intervals; usually 4 months are allowed before returning to exercise. The first 3 to 4 weeks appear to be critical; complete failure of the fracture becomes progressively less likely thereafter. If healing is uneventful, the prognosis for soundness is excellent since articular surfaces are not involved and muscle or neurovascular involvement is very unlikely.

BIBLIOGRAPHY

Bramlage LR, Hanes GE: Internal fixation of a tibial fracture in an adult horse. *J Am Vet Med Assoc* 1982;180:1090–1094.

Hayes PF, Watters JW, McClure JR, et al: Incomplete tibial fractures in three horses. *J Am Vet Med Assoc* 1980;177:1143–1145.

Johnson PJ, Allhands RV, Baker GJ, Boero MJ, et al: Incomplete linear tibial fracture in two horses. *J Am Vet Med Assoc* 1988;192:522–524.

Wagner PC, DeBowes RM, Grant BD, et al: Cancellous bone screws for repair of proximal growth plate fractures of the tibia in foals. *J Am Vet Med Assoc* 1984;184:688–691.

Watkins JP, Auer JA, Taylor TS: Crosspin fixation of fractures of the proximal tibia in three foals. *Vet Surg* 1985;14:153–159.

White NA, Blackwell RB, Hoffman PE: Use of a bone plate for repair of proximal physeal fractures of the tibia in two foals. *J Am Vet Med Assoc* 1982;181:252–254.

Young D, Richardson DW, Nunamaker DM, Ross MW, Tulleners EP: Use of dynamic compression plating for treatment of diaphyseal tibia fractures in foals: 9 cases (1980–1987). *J Am Vet Med Assoc* 1989;194:1755–1760.

129
Femoral and Patellar Fractures

Jeffrey P. Watkins

FRACTURES OF THE FEMUR

Femoral fractures commonly result from severe external trauma. In foals this trauma is frequently associated with halter-breaking accidents, falling down with the limb in adduction, or being kicked by another horse. Adult horses with femur fractures usually have a history of suffering a fall or external blow.

Diagnosis

Most fractures of the femoral diaphysis are accompanied by massive soft tissue swelling secondary to hematoma formation. The limb proximal to the stifle will appear two to three times the circumference of the opposite limb when viewed from the caudal aspect. This degree of swelling in conjunction with severe lameness is highly suggestive of a fracture of the femoral shaft. Patients with femoral fractures are generally non-weight bearing in the affected limb, especially those animals with displaced diaphyseal fractures. However, foals with fractures of the proximal femoral physis may be capable of partial weight bearing. Another sign suggestive of a femoral fracture is a relative discrepancy in limb length. With a significant degree of displacement and overriding by the fracture fragments, the hock of the affected limb will be proximal and straight relative to the hock of the normal hind limb. This makes the affected limb appear to be shorter.

Manipulation of the limb usually reveals the presence of crepitation and elicits pain. The large muscle mass overlying the area may make it difficult to detect crepitus; however palpation over the greater trochanter and distal femoral metaphysis, or auscultation over the area, may aid in identifying crepitation. Fractures of the proximal femoral physis may not present with obvious crepitus. The integrity of the vascular supply to the distal limb should also be assessed during physical examination. One case has been reported in which vascular damage was severe enough to result in ischemic necrosis of the distal limb and warranted euthanasia in a foal.

Radiographs are required to confirm the presence of a fracture, and determine its location and severity. The entire femur should be examined to ensure that all fracture lines are identified. Techniques used for stifle radiography are acceptable for fractures of the distal femur but seldom allow acceptable visualization of the entire femur. Radiography of the proximal femur and diaphysis requires general anesthesia and the use of high-capacity radiographic equipment except in small foals. The femur is best viewed with a medial-to-lateral projection using a grid technique. The patient is positioned in lateral recumbency with the affected limb down. The cassette and grid are placed beneath the femoral area and the uppermost hind limb abducted. Two separate medial-to-lateral projections taken at different exposures may be required to fully evaluate the bone since the soft tissue thickness varies from the proximal to the distal femur. After ensuring that the medial-to-lateral projections are acceptable, the patient is repositioned, placing the affected limb uppermost, and a caudal-to-cranial projection is taken. The film cassette is positioned cranial to the femoral area with the limb extended and partially abducted. Although some degree of distortion results, this view allows definition of the fracture in a plane approaching a right angle to the medial-to-lateral projection, thereby providing a better evaluation of the severity and degree of overriding of the bone ends. The proximal femoral physis is best visualized with a ventral-to-dorsal projec-

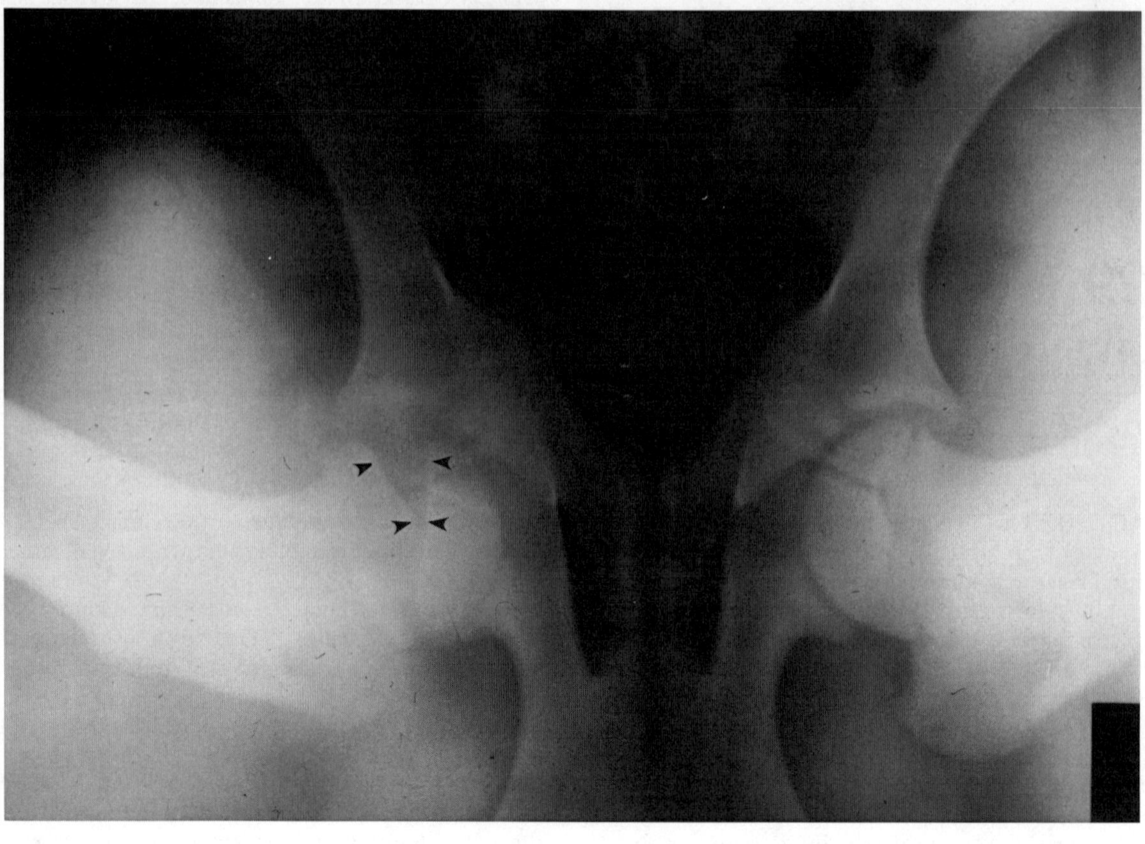

Figure 129–1. Ventral-to-dorsal radiograph of a foal with a Salter-Harris type I fracture of the proximal femoral physis (*arrows*).

tion. The patient is positioned in dorsal recumbency as for pelvic radiographs with the hind limbs in the frog leg (flexed) position and the film cassette positioned beneath the coxofemoral area in question.

Fracture Management

Numerous factors should be taken into consideration when deciding whether or not to pursue treatment of a femoral fracture. Size of the patient is very important. Euthanasia is recommended for horses over 200 kg with displaced fractures of the femoral diaphysis since repair is usually not possible, and prognosis is poor. In many Quarter Horse foals, the size limitations may be more stringent because of the heavy muscling that is characteristic of this breed. Other factors to consider include the intended use and temperament of the patient as well as potential economic constraints. Fracture location, configuration, and accompanying soft tissue damage are also important with regard to the potential for a successful repair. It should be noted, however, that if the fracture can be stabilized and infection does not occur, healing can occur because of the femur's excellent blood supply and soft tissue cover.

Proximal Femoral Fractures. Salter-Harris type I or II injuries are most common at the proximal femoral physis (Fig. 129–1). These fractures are frequently associated with the foal flipping over backward and landing on the greater trochanter. A shear force is propagated through the physis that results in a physeal fracture. With secondary muscle contraction and attempts to use the limb, the femoral shaft often displaces cranial and dorsal. Conservative therapy (box stall rest) has not resulted in acceptable recovery rates in most cases. Ischemic necrosis of the femoral head, degenerative changes in the coxofemoral joint, and permanent disability have been the end result in most foals treated conservatively. Better results have been obtained by open reduction and internal fixation. Either a craniolateral approach as described in dogs or a trochanteric osteotomy is used to expose the coxofemoral joint and proximal femur. The fracture is then stabilized by directing multiple intramedullary pins from the lateral diaphysis through the femoral neck to engage the head of the femur. Because the femoral head is dome shaped, care must be taken to ensure adequate purchase by the implants in the epiphysis, yet avoid entering the coxofemoral joint. Placement of pins in as many directions as possible to engage all parts of the femoral head is recommended.

Distal Femoral Fractures. Fractures of the distal femoral physis are usually Salter-Harris type II or IV injuries (Fig. 129–2). The metaphyseal bone fragment characteristic of type II injuries is most often located either cranially or caudally. Type II fractures with the metaphyseal fragment located caudally usually result from severe external trauma and are characterized by marked displacement of the epiphysis caudally and proximally. Reduction of these fractures can be extremely difficult and may not be possible in some instances.

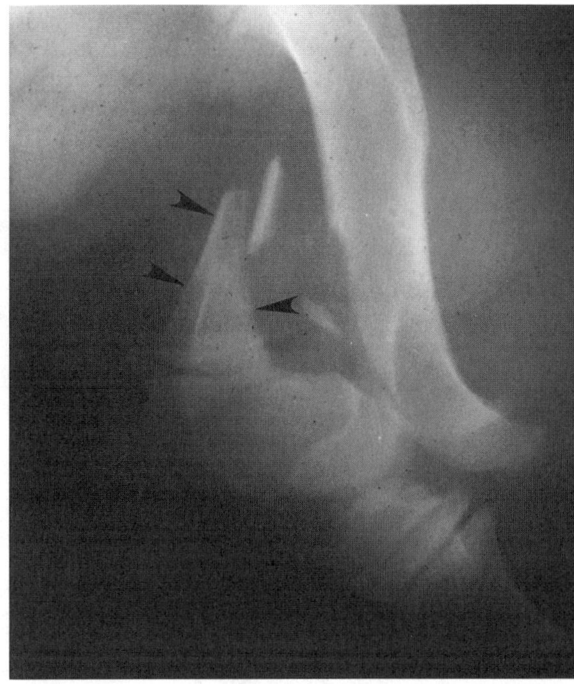

Figure 129–2. Medial-to-lateral radiograph of a foal with a Salter-Harris type II fracture of the distal femoral physis. The metaphyseal bone fragment is located cranially (*arrows*).

Internal fixation of type II fractures of the distal femur should employ implants designed to increase the degree of purchase in the distal epiphysis. These include the angle blade plate, condylar plate, and DCS implant system (Synthes, Ltd). Richardson (personal communication, 1987) has had success in two foals with type II fractures of the distal femur using the condylar plate. In many instances, however, economic constraints and the poor prognosis accompanying this injury influence owners to have affected foals euthanized.

DeBowes et al reported on the successful treatment of a type IV physeal fracture of the distal femur. The fracture extended through the caudal aspect of the physis and entered the femoropatellar joint cranially. Fixation across the fracture was accomplished with multiple cancellous bone screws placed through the articular

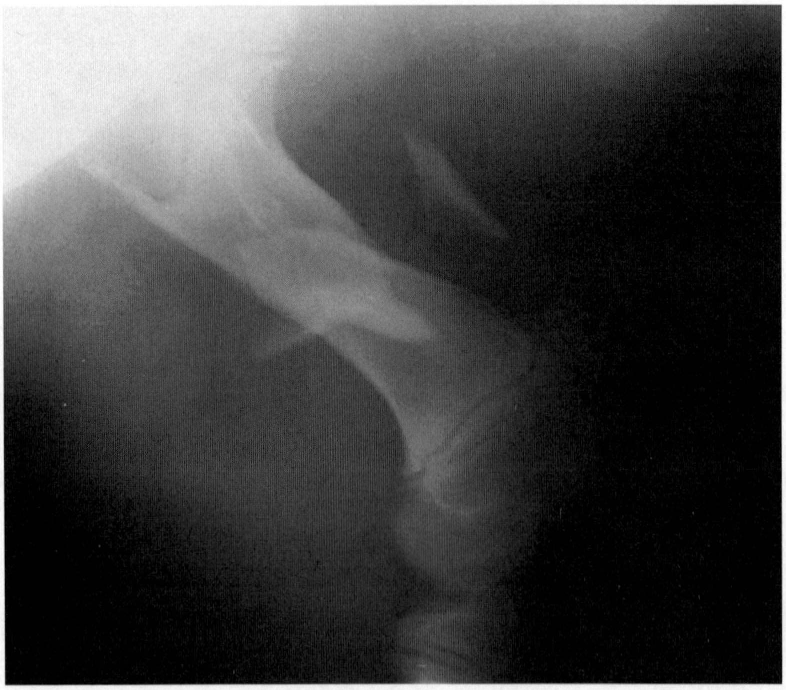

Figure 129–3. Medial-to-lateral radiograph of a foal with a comminuted fracture of the femoral diaphysis.

surface of the femoral trochlea. The screws were recessed into the subchondral bone to prevent subsequent damage to the patella.

Diaphyseal Femoral Fractures. The most commonly encountered fractures of the femur are diaphyseal. They usually occur subsequent to a severe fall, often with the leg in adduction, resulting in oblique or spiral fractures of the mid- to distal diaphysis. The fracture fragments are typically overriding as a result of contraction of the musculature in the area. Occasionally the fracture is comminuted, in which case the prognosis for recovery is greatly reduced, especially if the comminution is in the caudal cortex (Fig. 129–3). There is usually severe soft tissue trauma secondary to the bone ends gouging the adjacent musculature during attempts at weight bearing. In addition, if the popliteal artery is damaged, the distal limb may be predisposed to ischemic necrosis.

Foals of small stature with a simple oblique mid-diaphyseal fracture are good candidates for internal fixation. Two bone plates are recommended for internal fixation of these fractures, one placed laterally and one placed cranially. Plate fixation may not be satisfactory in neonatal foals, as in calves, because the cortical bone may not hold the screws. Intramedullary pin(s) should be considered as an alternative for fixation in these cases.

The fracture is approached between the biceps femoris and the vastus lateralis muscles. Fractures of the distal diaphysis may necessitate extending the exposure distally by transection of the attachment of the biceps femoris to the lateral patellar ligament and opening the lateral aspect of the femoropatellar joint. Once exposed, the fracture hematoma is removed and the fragments are brought into reduction. Reduction can be very difficult because of the problem of overcoming contraction of the powerful musculature in the area. By tenting the bone ends into the incision and using bone-holding forceps to move the bones, the fracture can usually be reduced. Traction on the distal limb is generally of minimal benefit in aiding reduction of the fracture. Once reduced, the fracture is stabilized for plating with one or two lag screws or a bone-holding forceps. Care must be taken when using lag screws not to interfere with placement of the plates. The lateral plate should be applied first and positioned cranial to the third trochanter proximally and supracondylar fossa distally. If the fracture is comminuted or involves the distal diaphysis, additional purchase in the distal epiphysis should be obtained with one of the previously mentioned implants on the lateral aspect of the femur (Fig. 129–4). Plate luting may be used if deemed necessary to increase bone-plate contact and screw support. The cranial plate is then applied extending proximally from the trochlea. Because the deep muscular investment impairs exposure of the proximal femur, difficulty can be expected when placing the proximal screws in the cranial plate.

Prior to wound closure, one or two suction drains are placed beside the plates to evacuate wound fluids and prevent the development of a hematoma at the surgical site. Care should be taken to accurately reconstruct the soft tissues, particulary when the incision is extended distally into the lateral femoropatellar joint. This should include tension-relieving sutures in the fascial attachments of the patella. A stent bandage is recommended to protect the skin incision postoperatively.

Postoperative Care

Prophylactic use of systemic, broad-spectrum, bactericidal antibiotics is indicated beginning immediately prior to surgery and intraoperatively when the surgical procedure is over 3 hours in duration. Antibiotics should be administered postoperatively for 24 hours after removal of the drains. As long as significant fluid is recovered from the surgical site, the suction drains should be maintained in position. Nonsteroidal anti-inflammatory drugs should be used sparingly to relieve postoperative pain. The foal should be encouraged to stand and to nurse regularly after surgery. Most foals will lay with the affected femur uppermost and are able to rise unassisted. However, these foals occasionally need some assistance during attempts at standing in the early postoperative period. The foal is kept confined in a stall until fracture healing has occurred.

Complications

Complications can be numerous when attempting repair of femoral fractures. Problems with reduction and fixation have been addressed. Failure of fixation can occur subsequent to a violent recovery from the often prolonged anesthetic period. In these instances providing assistance during recovery may reduce the chances for an acute failure of the bone-implant system. Fixation failure may also occur when plate stabilization is attempted in newborn foals in which the bone is unable to hold the screws. However, instability with accompanying osteomyelitis is the most common cause of fixation failure. With infection, as bone lysis progresses minor instability worsens and the implants subsequently become detached within 6 to 8 weeks. It appears that when infection develops, the proximal end of the distal fragment may become a sequestrum subsequent to disruption of the nutrient vessels and the endosteal blood supply of the distal fragment.

Complications may occur subsequent to any severe lameness of chronic duration in foals. These complications include fetlock hyperextension and angular limb deformity in the unaffected limb and flexural deformity in the fractured limb. The high propensity for these conditions to result in disability emphasizes the importance of an early return to weight bearing in the fractured limb.

If fistula formation has not occurred, implant removal after the fracture has healed is not recommended. Horses that had successfully treated femur

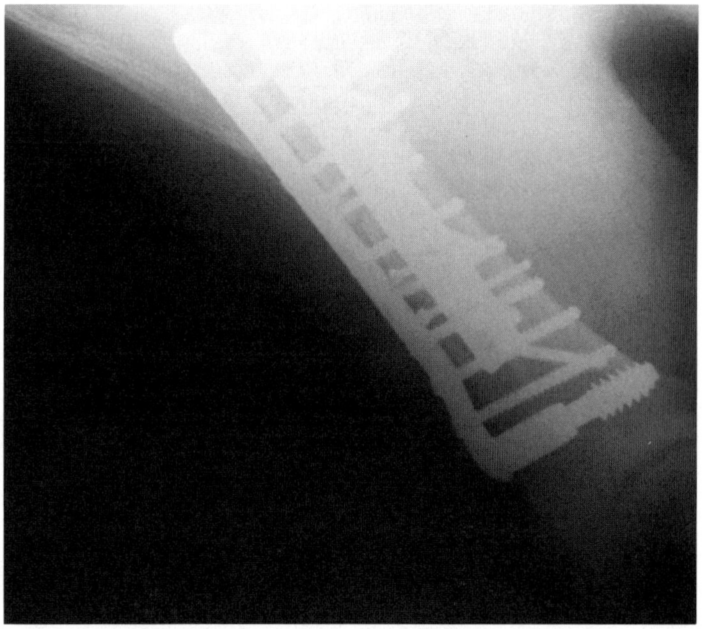

Figure 129–4. Caudal-to-cranial radiograph demonstrating use of the dynamic condylar screw and plate positioned laterally in fixation of a comminuted diaphyseal femur fracture in a foal.

fractures as foals have been able to train successfully with the implants still in place.

FRACTURES OF THE PATELLA

Patellar fractures have been reported both as a rare condition in horses and as occurring more frequently than expected. In my experience, fractures of the patella are infrequent and usually are the result of a direct blow to the patella either from an injury inflicted by another horse or from striking an immovable object. In areas where horses compete over solid fences, patella fractures may be more common because of the tendency for these horses to hit their stifles on the fence at high speeds (D.W. Richardson, personal communication, 1987).

Configuration of the fracture is variable, with longitudinal, transverse, and comminuted fractures occurring. Fractures that are transverse in nature may be severely distracted secondary to contraction of the quadriceps mechanism. Occasionally patellar fractures are open and accompanied by contamination of the stifle joint. Transverse fractures and small avulsion fractures originating from the medial patellar angle at the attachment of the medial patellar ligament and accessory fibrocartilage of the patella have been reported to occur secondary to intense contraction of the quadriceps group.

Diagnosis

Horses with fractures of the patella present with acute onset of severe lameness. There is frequently soft tissue swelling in the region of the patella and crepitation may be noted upon palpation. Effusion in the femoropatellar joint is usually present. Definitive diagnosis requires radiographic examination. Lateral-to-medial and skyline projections are required for a complete examination. If the patient will tolerate flexion of the stifle, the skyline view can be accomplished with the horse standing. With the stifle flexed, the film cassette is positioned horizontally distal to the patella and the beam is directed downward to project the patella away from the trochlear groove (Fig. 129–5). If the patient will not tolerate flexion of the stifle, the skyline projection will require general anesthesia with the patient in dorsal recumbency. The film cassette is positioned proximal to the patella with the limb flexed, and the beam is direct proximally. The skyline view is necessary for delineating avulsion fractures of the medial patellar angle, since these fractures are not visible on the lateral projection.

Fracture Management

Patellar fractures that disrupt the articular surface or disable the quadriceps mechanism are likely to result in disability if treated conservatively. The potential for salvaging an athlete is best if a congruent joint surface and the quadriceps mechanism are restored. Open reduction and internal fixation of major fragments with lag screws has been successful. Augmentation of the lag screw fixation with tension band wiring may be indicated in transverse patellar fractures to offset the distractive forces of the quadriceps mechanism. Small fragments that are articular and cannot be stabilized are best removed. This can be accomplished in some instances utilizing arthroscopic techniques to identify the fragments and strategically located stab incisions to gain access to the joint and remove the fracture fragments. Simple avulsion fractures of the medial patellar angle have been reported to heal satisfactorily with stall confinement and do not require surgical intervention in most cases.

Surgery may be complicated by the presence of severe soft tissue swelling, difficulty in overcoming the quadriceps mechanism to achieve reduction (especially in transverse fractures), and the risk of sepsis involving the stifle joint. As with any surgery in the stifle area, the surgical wound is prone to dehiscence. Controlled recovery from anesthesia is mandatory and, once re-

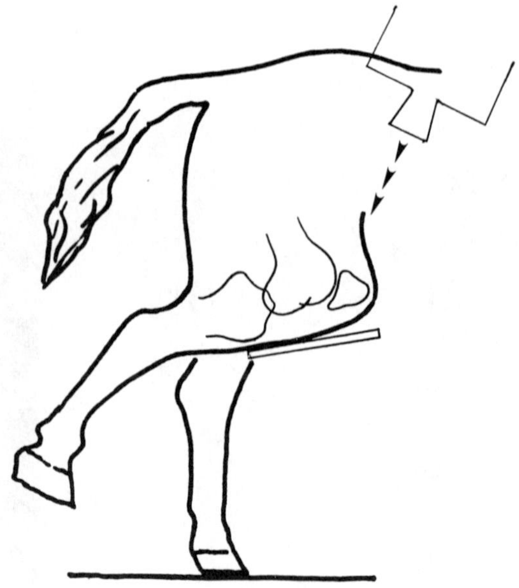

Figure 129–5. Positioning of the x-ray tube and the film plate relative to the patella for a skyline projection of the patella in the standing horse.

covered, the horse should be tied to maintain a standing position for up to 6 weeks postoperatively.

Prognosis

With anatomic reconstruction of the articular surface and restoration of the quadriceps mechanism, the prognosis for a pain-free limb is good. However, because of the nature of most patellar fractures and the potential complications, including degenerative joint disease, a guarded prognosis should be given to the owners prior to surgery.

BIBLIOGRAPHY

Aldrete AV, Meagher DM: Lag screw fixation of a patella fracture in a horse. *Vet Surg* 1981;10:143–148.

Bramlage LR: Long bone fractures. *Vet Clin North Am Large Anim Pract* 1983;5:285–310.

DeBowes RM, Grant BD, Chalman JA, Rantanen NW: Fractured patella in a horse. *Equine Pract* 1980;2:49–53.

DeBowes RM, Grant BD, Modransky PD: Lag screw stabilization of Salter type IV femoral fracture in a young horse. *J Am Vet Med Assoc* 1983;182:1123–1125.

Dik KJ, Nemeth F: Traumatic patella fractures in the horse. *Equine Vet J* 1983;15:244–247.

Milne DW, Turner AS: *An Atlas of Surgical Approaches to the Bones of the Horse.* Philadelphia, WB Saunders Co, 1979, pp 154-167.

Nunamaker DM, Bowman KF, Richardson DW, Herring M: Plate luting: A preliminary report of its use in horses. *Vet Surg* 1986;15:289–293.

Pankowski RL, White KK: Fractures of the patella in horses. *Compend Cont Educ Pract Vet* 1985;7:S566-S573.

Rose PL, Watkins JP, Auer JA: Femoral fracture repair complicated by vascular injury in a foal. *J Am Vet Med Assoc* 1984;185:795–797.

Stashak TS: Fracture of the patella, in Stashak TS (ed): *Adams' Lameness in Horses,* ed 4. Philadelphia Lea & Febiger, 1987, pp 743.

Stick JA, Derksen FJ: Intramedullary pinning of a fractured femur in a foal. *J Am Vet Med Asso* 1980;176:-627–629.

Turner AS, Milne DW, Hohn RB, Rouse GP: Surgical repair of fractured capital femoral epiphysis in three foals. *J Am Vet Med Assoc* 1979;175:1198–1202.

130
Pelvic Fractures

Dean W. Richardson

Pelvic fractures occur in all age horses but appear to have a higher prevalence in younger horses. In a recent retrospective study of 100 cases by Rutkowski and Richardson, 60% of affected horses were less than 2 years old and 76% were under 4 years. In this hospital series, there were more female than male horses affected, but this was probably a consequence of referral decisions. Many horses suffer the fracture as a result of unobserved trauma, but an observed fall is by far the most common known cause of a pelvic fracture. A smaller number of horses develop the fracture during strenuous exercise.

DIAGNOSIS

The important presenting sign is acute lameness. Usually the lameness is severe, although horses with minimally displaced or nondisplaced fractures can have more subtle signs. The characteristic posture of the horse with a pelvic or proximal femoral injury is to stand with the limb slightly cranial to its normal position and with marked external rotation along its entire length. This externally rotated posture is particularly prominent during the anterior phase of the stride. Displacement of the fracture results in pelvic asymmetry that may be grossly visible. Asymmetry may be directly assessed by measuring the distances between pelvic landmarks on the left versus the right; this may be difficult in the extremely lame horse, however, since accurate measurements require a square stance. Internal symmetry of the pelvic canal is assessed by rectal palpation. Acute swelling may be noted in either the cranial gluteal and tuber coxae area or over the thigh and lateral stifle. Internal swelling palpated rectally is probably more common. Crepitus may be palpable externally by placing the hand over the greater trochanter and tuber coxae while rocking weight on and

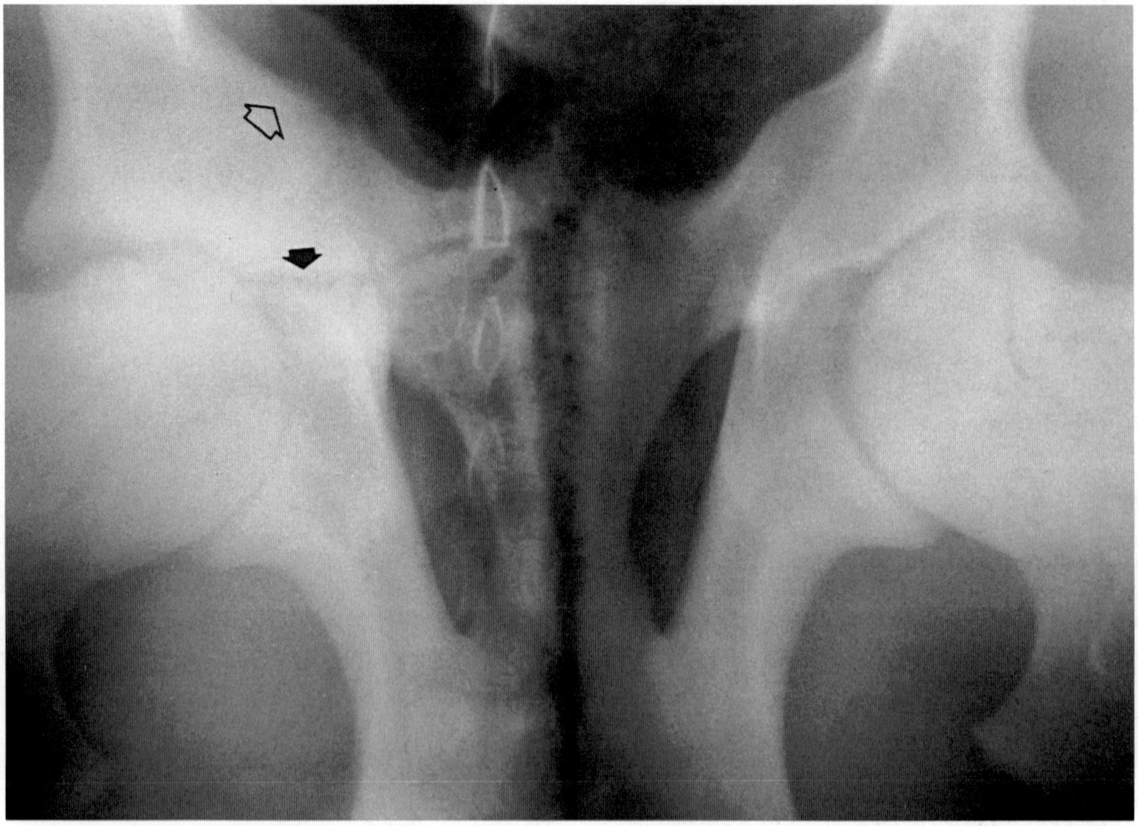

Figure 130–1. Minimally displaced comminuted fracture involving the acetabulum (*black arrow*). There is some callus already present (*open arrow*). Despite the comminution and joint involvement, stall rest affords a good prognosis for breeding soundness.

off the limb. Crepitus palpated rectally is also usually noted by intermittent weight bearing or by walking the horse a few steps during the rectal examination. In horses with fractures of 1 to 2 weeks' duration, there may be visible muscle atrophy on the affected side primarily involving the gluteal muscle.

Although very young, tractable foals may be held in recumbency under sedation for ventrodorsal radiographs, definitive diagnosis in adults requires general anesthesia and an X-ray machine capable of large exposures. Exposures of 90 to 100 kVp and 800 mAs are used with a high-ratio (12 : 1) grid and a 400 film-screen speed to obtain good quality radiographs. Generally a ventrodorsal view is the sole projection, but lateral oblique projections can be helpful in delineating the degree of displacement or even identifying otherwise invisible fracture lines. Without radiographs the diagnosis of pelvic fracture is made on the above-mentioned clinical signs, with pelvic asymmetry and crepitus being the most specific indications of a pelvic fracture. Femoral head or neck fractures must be considered among differential diagnoses.

FRACTURE MANAGEMENT

Successful surgical repair of an equine pelvic fracture has yet to be reported. The mass of muscle overlying the fracture makes for immense difficulties in exposure and reduction. Surgical repairs would be feasible in a very young foal with a suitable fracture, but considerable deliberation would be needed before undertaking the procedure. The results with rest for all minimally displaced fractures have been surprisingly favorable so surgical intervention at this time should probably only be considered in a small foal with a relatively simple displaced articular fracture.

Confinement in a stall with good footing and generous bedding is the currently accepted treatment for virtually all pelvic fractures. Box stall rest for a minimum of 3 to 4 months is recommended, and nonsteroidal anti-inflammatory drugs should be used, especially in the early stages of the rest period to help relieve pain. Radiographs are useful in formulating a prognosis and in making a decision to use stall confinement. A racehorse gelding with a comminuted displaced articular fracture will probably not be sound as an athlete whereas a valuable filly with a minimally to moderately displaced acetabular fracture has a favorable prognosis for breeding soundness (Fig. 130–1). Horses with nonarticular fractures can return to athletic performance, as can those with minimally displaced articular fractures. In our reported series of cases, 18% of all horses with acetabular fractures returned to athletic performance and an additional 23% became successful broodmares. Thirty-four percent were euthanized at the time of diagnosis, frequently for economic reasons. In horses allowed to survive, there was no difference in outcome between those with acetabular and nonacetabular fractures. However, this partially reflects the choice of euthanasia for the horses with the most severe articular fractures. Seventy-seven percent of horses with pelvic fracture were salvaged for breeding or performance purposes. It is important to remember that even though a horse may be extremely lame initially with a pelvic fracture, considerable improvement is often evident within a few weeks. Our results and those of others suggest that conservative therapy is very worthy of consideration in any potential breeding animal.

COMPLICATIONS

Complications of pelvic fractures include those specific for the fracture, such as severe hemorrhage and narrowing of the birth canal, as well as more general complications of serious fractures, such as contralateral laminitis and supporting limb deformity. Laminitis is fortunately a relatively uncommon complication in pelvic fractures. The angular deformities in the contralateral limb, usually tarsus varus, tend to be most severe in young horses. Serious, even fatal, hemorrhage can occur with displaced acetabular fractures that lacerate the iliac or obturator arteries. Dystocia as a consequence of pelvic canal narrowing is a consideration, but appears to be a relatively uncommon complication. A mare with a severely displaced fracture that resulted in obvious pelvic narrowing would be an obvious candidate for elective cesarean section.

Complications associated with the general anesthetic procedure needed for radiographs are uncommon. In instances in which a more accurate prognosis is needed, radiology would appear to be worth the risk.

BIBLIOGRAPHY

Heinze CD, Lewis, RE: Radiographic examination of the equine pelvis: Case reports. *J Am Vet Med Assoc* 1971;159:1328–1334.

Jeffcott LB: Radiographic appearance of equine lumbosacral and pelvic abnormalities by linear tomography. *Vet. Radiol* 1983;24:201–213.

Jeffcott LB: Technique of linear tomography for the pelvic region of the horse. *Vet Radiol* 1983;24:194–200.

Little C, Hilbert B: Pelvic fractures in horses: 19 cases (1974–1984). *J Am. Vet Med Assoc* 1987;190:1203–1206.

Rutkowski JA, Richardson DW: A retrospective study of 100 pelvic fractures in horses. *Eq Vet J* 1989;21(4):256–259.

Stashak TS: in Stashak TS (ed): *Adams' Lameness in Horses,* ed 4. Philadelphia, Lea & Febiger, 1987, pp 752–753.

131
Current Concepts in Bone Grafting

Svend E. Kold

THEORETICAL CONSIDERATIONS

Bone grafts have been used since the 19th century to fuse joints and repair skeletal defects. The basis for the success of bone grafts is the vascularization of devitalized bone and the replacement of the old bone by deposition of new bone on the trabecular framework of the implanted bone. Most surgeons would agree that an autograft, when available in sufficient quantity, is the best graft material because it will not induce adverse immunologic reactions by the host tissue. Fortunately availability and harvesting of graft material is usually not a problem in the horse. However, the collection of an autograft may incur additional surgery time, a higher risk of contamination, and increased discomfort.

Whereas immunologic rejection may prevent the successful use of a fresh allograft and particularly a fresh xenograft, the proven existence of an inductive bone morphogenetic protein within bone matrix may provide enough benefit to consider using preserved allogeneic graft bone when autogenous graft bone fails to meet the demands in terms of quality and availability.

The biologic value of a bone graft is determined by its osteogenic capacity and by the quality and rate of revascularization and graft reorganization. Both cancellous and cortical bone provide these qualities, although in different amounts. The installation of a fresh cancellous bone graft provides undifferentiated mesenchymal cells, an osteoconductive framework, and an osteoinductive stimulus via a bone morphogenetic protein. Further refinement of this bone morphogenetic protein may increase the use of freeze-dried allograft bone in combination with bone morphogenetic protein.

The object of using an autogenous cancellous bone graft is not to transplant viable morsels of bone, but rather is two-fold: (*a*) to seed the recipient site with viable pluripotential cells that will multiply and produce new bone, and (*b*) to provide a strong bone induction potential with transformation of osteoprogenitor cells to osteoblasts. The earliest evidence of osteogenesis within the graft takes place at the interface between graft and host tissues, with bone formation taking place within a porous graft by the accretion of new bone upon old, dead, and disintegrating trabeculae. Internal remodeling of the bone graft is similar to the remodeling of the remaining skeleton, but occurs in a much more exaggerated manner. This process is initiated after approximately 30 days and is almost complete after 90 days.

Selection of the type of autogenous bone graft depends on the purpose for which it is required. As an example, cancellous bone possesses a large surface area and strong osteoinductive and osteoconductive potential, but possesses little mechanical strength. Thus, cancellous bone is of minimal use for replacing complete segments of bone or bone under compression unless another means of structural support can be used during bone healing. Cancellous grafts are therefore used primarily to fill small defects, whereas segments of cortical bone are used primarily to provide support. A corticocancellous bone graft may give some initial support and at the same time provide some callus induction potential and more rapid revascularization. Cancellous and cortical autografts differ histologically in at least two aspects:

1. Cancellous grafts are revascularized more rapidly and more completely than cortical grafts.
2. "Creeping substitution" of cancellous bone involves an initial phase of oppositional bone formation, followed by a resorption phase, whereas cortical grafts remain a mixture of necrotic and viable bone.

The use of bone substitutes, in particular calcium phosphate ceramics such as hydroxyapatite and tricalcium phosphate, has received wide attention. Their chemical properties resemble those of bone minerals, but they have a relatively low mechanical strength and their clinical application is therefore limited to non–weight-bearing areas or bone cavities.

BONE GRAFTS IN EQUINE ORTHOPEDIC SURGERY

There are few reports in the literature on the use of bone transplant techniques in equine orthopedics. However, the benefit of autogenous cancellous bone grafting as an adjunct to the treatment of certain orthopedic problems has been recognized, especially the use of bone grafting in the treatment of open compound fractures with cortical defects.

Fackelman et al. investigated the formation of new bone in decalcified, allogeneic grafts implanted heterotopically and noted that it took between 7 and 9 weeks. Similarly, Jones et al. used frozen segmental cortical allografts for skeletal reconstruction and found that it took 6 months for complete replacement with no signs of rejection. Experimental studies examining the incorporation of an autogenous equine cancellous bone graft found that the graft was infiltrated by an intricate network of blood vessels 10 weeks after grafting and that almost all the cancellous graft bone had been replaced by 20 weeks. The amount of bone replacement during this process was found to be underestimated if judged from conventional radiographs.

Investigations with an equine third metacarpal bone model found that equine bone reacts to autogenous cancellous bone grafts in a manner similar to that in other mammals, with all installed graft trabeculae showing signs of nonvitality and gradually disintegrating. Two processes of new bone formation occur. First, immature projections of new trabeculae originate from the graft-host interfaces, and second, a gradual accretion of osteoid and woven bone upon disintegrating graft trabeculae occurs uniformly throughout the graft. The graft adapted to the structure of the host bone by corticalization and trabecularization in each respective area (Fig. 131–1).

The use of cortical grafts is rare in clinical cases. Harvesting and banking of the bone is required, and successful replacement of entire segments of bone re-

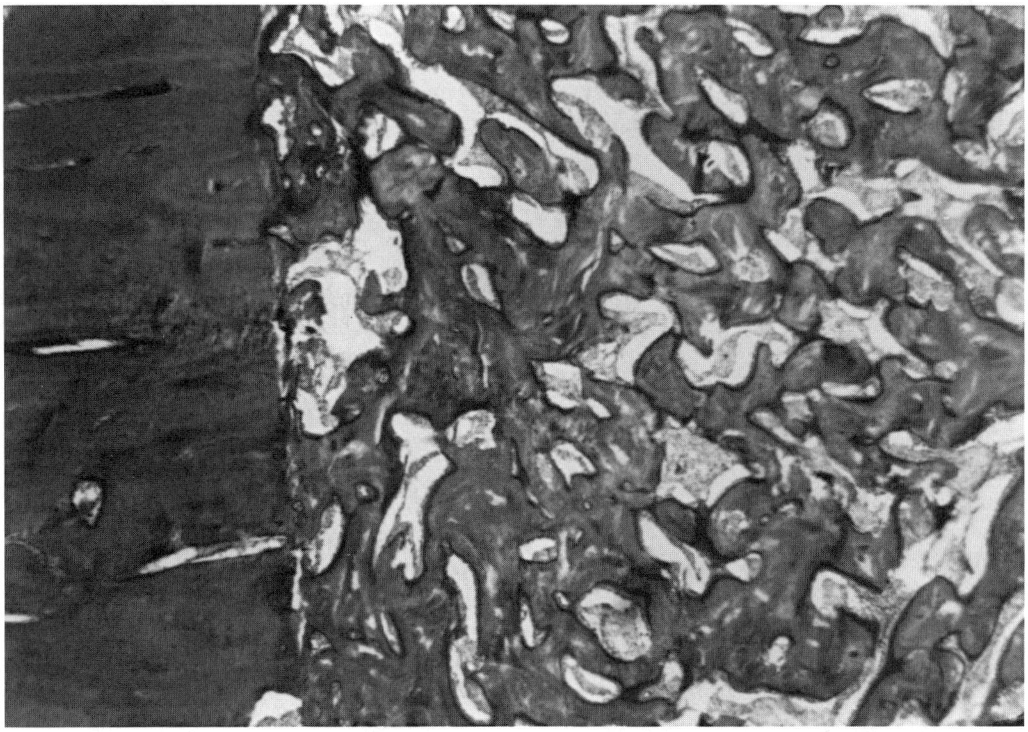

A

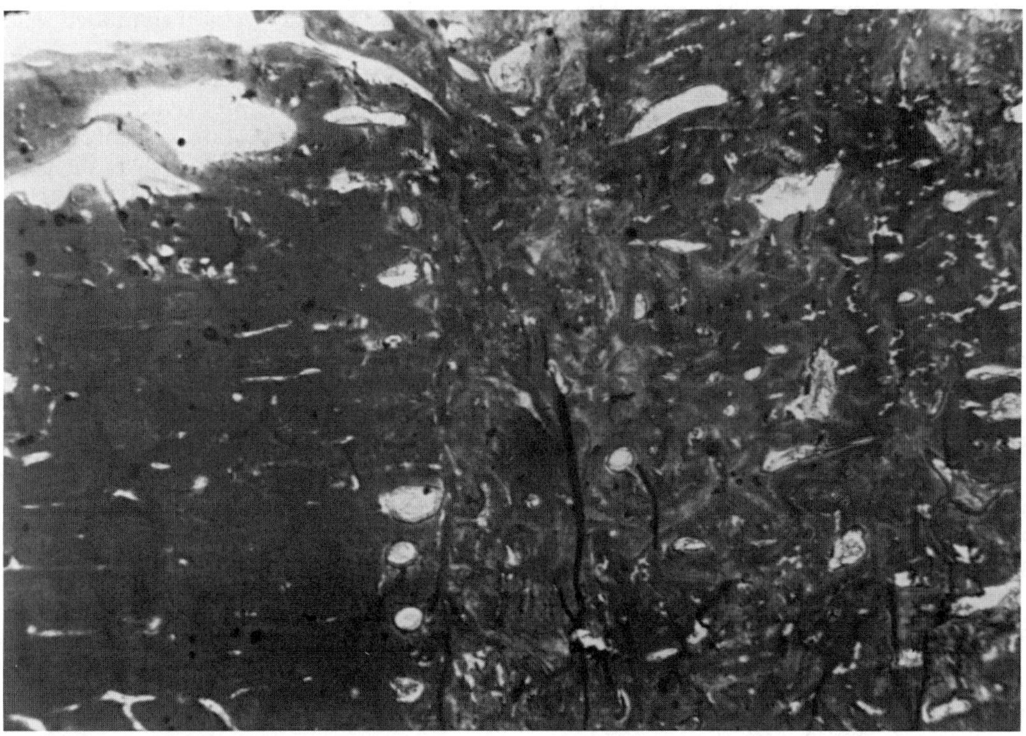

B

Figure 131–1. Photomicrographs of a bone graft after 31 days (**A**) and after 88 days (**B**) showing the replacement of the original graft and eventual change to cortical bone in the cortex of the third metacarpal bone. (From Kold SE, Hickman J, Melsen F: Qualitative aspects of the incorporation of equine cancellous bone grafts. *Equine Vet J* 1987;19:111–119.)

quires strict asepsis and a graft implantation and fixation that can provide absolute stability during graft revascularization. The clinical use of cortical bone grafts will not be covered in further detail.

SURGICAL TECHNIQUE FOR HARVESTING CANCELLOUS BONE

The majority of bone grafts used in equine orthopedic surgery are fresh autogenous cancellous bone chips, which are used to fill in bone defects and add osteoconductive and osteoinductive potential to the site. Bone chips are used in the repair of compound fractures with cortical defects, subchondral bone cysts, or osseous cystlike lesions and may be considered in the treatment of osteomyelitis (see Chapter 133). Cancellous bone is normally harvested from the tuber coxae or the sternum. Cancellous bone from the sternum compares favorably with bone from other donor sites and resembles bone from the tuber coxae. The sternum is particularly useful when surgical procedures require the horse to be placed in dorsal recumbency. In all other surgical procedures, the tuber coxae provides the easiest access for graft harvesting.

A 10- to 12-cm linear skin incision is made along the middle of the quadrangular mass forming the tuber coxae. The subcutaneous tissues, including a fat pad of varying thickness, are incised and retracted. Alternatively a curved incision can be made to expose the lateral rim of the tuber coxae. At either site, the periosteum is incised and reflected, using a periosteal elevator. The size of the window to be made in the cortex is dictated by the amount of graft bone required. Normally an area of 1 to 2 cm by 3 cm is removed with an osteotome. This exposes trabecular bone containing red marrow and fat; the latter separates form the graft bone when immersed in sterile saline. The graft bone can be obtained using a curette or an orthopedic chisel or gouge or by a core drill. I prefer a semicircular gouge, which creates long intact slithers of trabecular bone. The graft should be handled gently and aseptically, since surface cell survivability and improved graft incorporation occurs when the trauma (mechanical, thermal, chemical, and nutritional) of transplantation is minimal. The graft bone should be kept moist in sterile saline and transferred to the host site with a minimum of delay. Although antibiotics are bacteriostatic, they are also to some degree cellulostatic or toxic, and therefore are likely to inhibit osteogenesis. Antibiotics should therefore not be added to the saline in which the graft bone is temporarily stored during surgery.

The graft donor site is closed after carefully removing any osseous debris and blood clots. It may or may not be possible to obtain satisfactory coaptation of the periosteum. The overlying soft tissues, minus the skin, are closed with a continuous suture of an absorbable material. The skin is closed with vertical or horizontal mattress sutures of a nonabsorbable material and oversewn with a stent bandage. Wound drainage is not necessary. If it remains dry, the stent bandage can be left in situ for 6 to 8 days or even longer. However, if the stent bandage becomes blood soaked and stiffens with drying, it should be removed after 1 to 2 days. Skin sutures can be removed after 12 to 14 days. Exercise should be limited to controlled walking of the horse during the immediate postoperative period until the sutures are removed.

POSTOPERATIVE ASPECTS OF BONE GRAFT SURGERY

To ensure satisfactory revascularization of the graft, it is important to minimize trauma and movement of the graft. Although a period of non–weight bearing is considered important after bone grafting in humans, this is impractical in the equine. Irrespective of the indications for using a bone graft, the horse should be stall rested for at least 12 weeks. If controlled walking exercise can be tolerated by the lesion or the method of repair, it may be a functional stimulus for osteogenesis.

It is difficult to interpret graft incorporation and replacement, and bone healing is usually underestimated by conventional radiographs early in the postoperative period. In cases of grafting of a defect such as a bone cyst, interpretation is further complicated by the superimposition of surrounding host bone.

If the graft is rejected, its radiopacity may remain unchanged; live bone and dead bone cannot be differentiated radiographically. Both fibrous and osseous replacement of the graft can be satisfactory, although osseous replacement remains the ultimate goal. It is important to realize that good functional results can be obtained despite an uneven radiopacity of the grafted area.

BIBLIOGRAPHY

Bramlage LR: Autogenous cancellous bone grafting in the horse. *Proc AAEP Ann Conven* 1981; pp 243–247.

Fackelman GE, van Rechenberg B, Fetter AW: Decalcified bone grafts in the horse. *Am J Vet Res* 1981;42:943–948.

Jones RD, Milne DW, Fetter AW: Cortical bone allografting in the horse. *Vet Surg* 1981;10:1–4.

Kold SE, Hickman J: Results of treatment of subchondral bone cysts in the medial condyle of the equine femur with an

autogenous cancellous bone graft. *Equine Vet J* 1984;16:414–418.
Kold SE, Hickman J, Melsen F: Qualitative aspects of the incorporation of equine cancellous bone grafts. *Equine Vet J* 1987;19:111–119.
Medina, L, Morgan JP: Non-grafted and grafted osteotomies of proximal sesamoid bones in the horse; a radiographic study. *Vet Radiol* 1984;25:78–85.
Richardson GL, Pool RR, Pascoe JR, Wheat JD: Autogenous cancellous bone grafts from the sternum in horses. Comparison with other donor sites and results of use in orthopaedic surgery. *Vet Surg* 1986;15:9–15.
Stashak TS, Adams OR: Collection of bone grafts from the tuber coxae of the horse. *J Am Vet Med Assoc* 1975;167:397–273.
Wilson, JW, Rhinelander, RW, Stewart CL: Vascularization of cancellous chip bone grafts. *Am J Vet Res* 1985;46:1691–1699.

132 Antimicrobial Chemoprophylaxis in Orthopedic Surgery

James A. Orsini

A wound infection indicates microorganisms are established and multiplying in the host's tissues. The organisms cause cellular injury as a result of competitive metabolism, toxin release, or intracellular replication or by an immune response (antigen-antibody). In response to the infection there is exudation from the wounded tissues. Even in those wounds from which organisms are not isolated, a wound can still be considered infected based on the presence of purulent material. Cultures are not always thoroughly reliable indicators of a postoperative infection because: (*a*) a positive culture does not necessarily indicate infection, since many wounds are colonized by bacteria, and (*b*) wounds that are truly infected may not yield a positive culture because the microorganisms may be fastidious, antimicrobials may be present in the sampled tissues, and/or culture techniques used were inadequate. Because infections occur in a variety of ways and may not always produce significant pus, it is useful to consider a wound infected if the clinician believes the signs support this diagnosis.

In general terms, the probability of wound becoming infected can be expressed as an equation:

$$\text{Surgical infection} = \frac{\text{number of organisms} \times \text{virulence}}{\text{resistance of host}}$$

Infection may develop by altering any component of the equation. The larger the number of organisms introduced into the wound, the greater the chance of infection. The number of organisms also is important in toxin production and in overcoming the host defense mechanisms.

Infections occuring in healthy animals may be due to exposure to a highly pathogenic organism. In the above equation, virulence refers to a pathogen's ability to invade tissues. The resistance of the host is determined by its ability to prevent bacteria from becoming established in the body.

CLASSIFICATION OF WOUNDS

At the time of operation a wound can be classified according to the likelihood and degree of wound contamination. Surgical wounds are classified as: (*a*) clean, (*b*) clean-contaminated, (*c*) contaminated, and (*d*) dirty.

A *clean wound* is one in which the gastrointestinal or respiratory tract is not entered, no inflammation is encountered, and aseptic technique is not broken. Surgery in these cases does not have to be elective, nor the wound closed primarily with a drain or drainage system used through a primary or a separate incision. The infection rate associated with clean surgical procedures in orthopedics is low; therefore the need for prophylactic antimicrobial agents is considered unwarranted when the clinician considers the costs incurred and the potential for adverse effects from administration of these agents. The exception to this is in procedures using implants (screws and plates), in which a postoperative infection could jeopardize the case outcome.

Wounds falling into the classification of *clean-contaminated* generally have entered the respiratory or gastrointestinal tracts but the spillage or contamination from contents is judged to be minor. There are few clean-contaminated orthopedic cases compared to the numbers found in other specialty areas, in which this constitutes the major group of surgical procedures.

Contaminated wounds occur from operations in which acute inflammation (without pus formation) is encountered or in which gross spillage of contents from a hollow viscus occurs. Fresh, open, traumatic wounds and operations in which major breaks in aseptic technique occur also fall into this category. Contaminated or dirty procedures are more common in orthopedic surgery as a result of traumatic injuries. In this group of procedures bacteria are already present in the operative site; thus the use of antimicrobial agents constitutes therapy rather than chemoprophylaxis.

The *"dirty"* or infected classification indicates operations where exudate or a perforated viscus is encountered. Older traumatic wounds also are included in this group.

Generally, clean wounds have a 1 to 5% risk of infection; clean-contaminated wounds an 8 to 11% risk, contaminated a 15 to 17% risk, and dirty a greater than 27% risk.

DIAGNOSIS OF INFECTION

The cardinal sign of wound infection is exudation. If the wound has been closed by suture, partial or complete dehiscence is common. These signs usually appear 3 to 6 days after surgery, indicating the time period for the establishment of a microorganism(s) and the concurrent interference with the healing process.

If the infection is localized to the wound, systemic signs usually are absent. Débridement, drainage, and lavage of the wound with sterile physiologic saline solution may be sufficient. Fever, depression, anorexia, and sometimes a significant leukocytosis with a degenerative left shift indicates a systemic spread of the infection (peritonitis, cellulitis, septicemia, etc.), requiring antimicrobial treatment.

Treatment of wound infections with antimicrobials requires accurate identification of the causative agent(s) by culture and a determination of their susceptability to the various antimicrobials. This test takes one or more days; however, in most instances therapy cannot be delayed. Treatment is initiated based on familiarity with the antimicrobial drug(s) and their toxicity, incompatibilities, and spectrum of antibacterial activity. The character of the wound exudate, a Gram's stain of exudate obtained from deep wound margins, and knowledge of infections common to a particular area or indigenous to the hospital population also provide empiric guidelines for antimicrobial selection. The treatment protocol is altered based on the results of bacterial culture and antimicrobial sensitivity or a failure of the wound infection to respond to antimicrobial therapy within 24 to 72 hours.

MICROBIOLOGIC CONSIDERATIONS

In the past, the use of chemoprophylaxis has been oriented toward the gram-positive organisms, particularly *Streptococcus species, Staphylococcus aureus,* and the occasional *S. epidermidis*. More recently the changing bacterial population in postoperative infections involves an increasing number of gram-negative organisms as causative agents in both deep and superficial wound infections. The most common isolates of gram-negative organisms have been members of the *Enterobacteriaceae* family, including *Escherichia coli, Enterobacter species, Proteus species,* and *Klebsiella species,* and less commonly enterococcus and *Pseudomonas species.* With increased clinician awareness and improved culturing techniques for anaerobic organisms, the percentage of diagnosed orthopedic infections caused by these microorganisms has been increasing. Generally, in orthopedic surgery an agent should be administered that has primary activity against penicillin-resistant strains of *S. aureus, S. epidermidis* and gram-negative enteric bacteria such as *E. coli, Klebsiella,* and *Proteus.* It should be remembered that many of the gram-negative organisms associated with orthopedic infections are commonly found in the horse's environment, particularly via fecal and soil contamination.

SPECIFIC ASPECTS OF CHEMOPROPHYLAXIS

It is important to differentiate between prophylaxis and therapeutic drug use in musculoskeletal procedures. Antimicrobials administered before or during bacterial contamination are considered prophylactic, whereas any antimicrobial given after the contamination is classified as therapeutic. There are two prime objectives in prophylactic antimicrobial administration: (*a*) the benefits derived from the administration of antimicrobials must at least equal the rate of infection and potential adverse effects, and (*b*) the prophylactic regimen is most likely to be beneficial if the length of administration is short and the suspected pathogens are reasonably predictable and small in number.

Prophylactic antimicrobials have proven to be effective in a wide range of musculoskeletal procedures. Surgical procedures associated with implantation of screws, plates, and the like, in which the bone is exposed for long periods, have documented reduced incidence of infection when prophylactic antimicrobials are used. Procedures of short duration and involving minimal soft tissue dissection rarely necessitate the use of prophylactic antimicrobials.

Besides the normal risk factors seen with any surgical procedure, there are two additional factors unique to orthopedic surgery. If implants are used, the screws and plates may serve as a site for colonization of endogenous and exogenous bacteria. Thus, removal of the implants may be required to resolve the infection. Second, polymethylmethacrylate cement used to lute bone plates is believed to carry with it an increased risk of infection as a result of its ability to inhibit function of phagocytes and lymphocytes.

Antimicrobial selection must be determined by differences in in vitro antibacterial activity, tissue penetration, pharmacokinetics, toxity, and cost. No one antimicrobial agent is known to be superior to another in reducing the rate of postoperative wound infections.

The spectrum of the antimicrobial agent(s) should closely adhere to the most common pathogen(s) anticipated. It is impossible to choose an agent or agents that will be active against every potential etiologic microorganism. Instead, one should gear their selection to the major organisms encountered in the hospital population.

Being able to maintain therapeutic concentrations with good tissue penetration are important criteria for antimicrobial chemoprophylaxis. Such concentrations should be maintained during the period of potential contamination to prevent wound infection. Furthermore, a drug with a longer elimination half-life will require less frequent administration and ultimately be less costly.

Whether chemoprophylaxis is truly effective will be determined by the ability of the agent to reach and maintain sufficient concentrations above the minimum inhibitory concentration (MIC) for the invading pathogen(s) at the site of bacterial contamination. It has been shown in dogs that a number of antimicrobial agents, including penicillins, cephalosporins, and aminoglycosides, achieve adequate levels in normal and infected bone tissue. It has been further determined that the best predictor of bone penetration is the serum concentration of the antimicrobial; the higher the serum concentration the higher the bone concentration that can be expected.

The timing of administration and duration of antimicrobial prophylaxis are additional considerations. Because exogenous contamination is the source of more than 90% of postoperative infections, the most critical period for prophylaxis is within 2 to 3 hours after contamination has occurred when the immune system is depressed. By 6 hours the infection is established and the antimicrobials are no longer prophylactic. Therefore, antimicrobials are most valuable as prophylactic agents when administered close to the anticipated time of contamination. The duration of antimicrobial prophylaxis when used for procedures in which foreign material (metal or bone grafts) is to be implanted should be short unless they are being used therapeutically. The range may be as short as one dose if the procedure is less than 2 hours, or up to 48 hours. Therapeutic uses may extend up to 7 to 10 days and beyond depending on the nature of the musculoskeletal disease. It should be remembered that prolonged exposure to antimicrobials increases the risk of developing adverse drug reactions and potential changes in bacterial sensitivity.

The route of drug administration is critical in chemoprophylaxis. Clearly, parenteral administration is the most reliable drug delivery method. Intravenous administration is superior to intramuscular. With the intramuscular route there is the possibility of injection into fascial planes, causing prolonged absorption and inadequate levels of the antimicrobial at the surgical site. Additionally, the problems of muscle soreness and aversion behavior are both deleterious to the treatment of the primary problem. Oral administration is considered unreliable when attaining adequate tissue concentrations is critical. Topical wound irrigation with triple antibiotic (bacitracin, neomycin, and polymyxin) is commonplace in orthopedic procedures; however, few data exist to support routine antimicrobial irrigation. This has been proposed to decrease toxicity associated with systemic administration. Empirically, this practice may be more important in large animal orthopedic surgery, where environmental factors and timely surgical intervention are not always optimal.

Presently, many of the antimicrobials used prophylactically in orthopedic surgery show minimal differences in drug toxicity and adverse reactions. However, there are marked differences in costs, as demonstrated in Table 132–1.

PRINCIPLES OF ANTIMICROBIAL SELECTION FOR ORTHOPEDIC CHEMOPROPHYLAXIS

The objective of prophylactic antimicrobial therapy during surgery is to prevent establishment and growth of a microbial inoculum and thus prevent infection. Certain principles governing the efficacious use of prophylactic antimicrobials have been derived. First, the antimicrobial should be administered prior to bacteriologic inoculation. The effective period for antimicrobial prophylaxis is restricted to the first few hours after

TABLE 132–1. RELATIVE COST OF PARENTERAL ANTIMICROBIALS USED IN ORTHOPEDIC CHEMOPROPHYLAXIS*

Antimicrobial Agent	Relative Cost/g($)†	Available Sizes
Cephalosporins[1]		
Cefazolin		0.25, 0.5 g
(1st generation)	6.42 (SKF); 6.55 (Lilly)	1, 5, 10 g
Cefoperazone		
(3rd generation)	9.50 (Roerig)	1, 2 g
Moxalactam		
(3rd generation)	12.20 (Lilly)	1, 2, 10 g
Penicillinase-resistant penicillins[1]		
Oxacillin	4.30–4.85 (Beecham)[1]	0.5, 1, 2 g‡
	10.81–11.24 (Bristol)[1]	4, 10 g
Vancomycin	40.94 (Lilly)[1]; 28.84 (Led)[2]	0.5-g vials
Aminoglycosides		
Amikacin	9.32 (Bristol)[6]	1, 12 g
Gentamicin	4.80 (Schering)[5]	2.5, 5, 10 g
Kanamycin	3.56 (Bristol)[6]	
Tobramycin	71.67 (Lilly)[1]	60 mg, 80 mg, 1.2 g
Natural penicillin		
Aqueous penicillin G	1.11/1 m.u. (Squibb)[2]	5 m.u.
(sodium/potassium)	1.10/1 m.u. (Pfizer)[2]	1, 5 m.u.
		10, 20 m.u.
Procaine penicillin	.17/1 m.u. (Beecham)[3]	
Benzathine penicillin§	.20/1 m.u. (Squibb)[8]	
Broad-spectrum penicillin		
Ampicillin	1.73 (Beecham)[3]	3 g
Ticarillin	2.79 (Beecham)[3]	6 g
Ticarcillin/clavulanic acid	3.60 (Beecham)[1]	3.1 g
Erythromycin lactobionate	9.25 (Lypho-Med)[1]	0.5, 1 g
Oxytetracycline	.22 (Pfizer)[7]	25, 50 g
Trimethoprim/sulfamethoxazole	1.38 (Cooper)[4]	24, 48 g (48%)

* Data sources:
1: *Red book 1987*
2: Drug house (human drug supply company)
3: Beecham Veterinary
4: Coopers Animal Health
5: Schering Animal Health
6: A.J. Buck & Son
7: Pfizer Animal Health
8: Squibb

† Prices quoted are *list prices*.
‡ 1 g penicillin is approximately 1,600,000 units.
§ Benzathine penicillin is available only in combination with procaine penicillin.

bacteria reach the involved tissue. The general trend is to administer antimicrobials intramuscularly 1 to 2 hours prior to beginning the surgical procedure or, preferably, intravenously immediately following anesthetic induction and throughout the operation. The second principle relates to adequate interaction between the drug and the microorganism(s). In other words, the antimicrobial must come in contact with susceptible pathogens. This, in conjunction with the first principle, implies administration of the antimicrobial at the proper time and in therapeutic doses to ensure that optimal tissue levels of the antimicrobial are achieved (Table 132–2). Repeated doses may be necessary to maintain adequate tissue levels during long operative procedures.

The third principle in prophylactic antimicrobial therapy is that treatment with these drugs should be of brief duration. Prolonged administration of the antimicrobial agents beyond the period of contamination does not decrease the infection rate, but does affect the possibility of adverse antimicrobial effects, such as development of resistant bacteria strains, drug toxicity, and drug interactions as well as additional expense. The consensus of opinion rests with a 24-hour duration of drug administration. In patients with severe trauma antimicrobial therapy is initiated prior to any surgical

TABLE 132–2. SELECTION OF ANTIMICROBIAL AGENTS FOR ORTHOPEDIC CHEMOPROPHYLAXIS

Antimicrobial Agent	Route of Administration	Spectrum of Activity	Dosage	Comments
Amikacin	IV, IM	Gram-negative aerobic bacilli	6.6 mg/kg q8h	Potential nephrotoxicity/ ototoxicity
Ampicillin	IV, IM	Greater activity against gram-negative bacilli	25–100 mg/kg q6h	Inactivated by β-lactamases
Aqueous penicillin G	IV	Streptococci, non–penicillinase-producing staphylococci, *Pasteurella*	22,000 IU/kg q6H	Na^+/K^+salts form available
Benzathine penicillin G	IM	Streptococci	40,000 IU/kg q5d	Repository form
Cefazolin	IV, IM	Penicillinase-producing *Staphylococcus,* streptococci, *E. coli, Klebsiella,* and *Proteus mirabilis*	22 mg/kg q6h	Synergistic with aminoglycosides
Cefoperazone	IV, IM	Expanded gram-negative aerobes, anaerobes	No reported dosage for horses	Expensive
Chloramphenicol	IV	Gram-negative aerobes and anaerobes	50 mg/kg q8h	Blood dyscrasias in humans
Erythromycin lactobionate	IV	Gram-positive cocci	2.5–3 mg/kg q6–8h	May be given in combination with rifampin
Gentamicin	IV, IM	Gram-negative aerobic bacilli	2.2 mg/kg q6–8h	Potential nephrotoxicity/ ototoxicity
Kanamycin	IV, IM	Gram-negative aerobic bacilli	5 mg/kg q8h	Potential nephrotoxicity/ ototoxicity
Metronidazole	IV	*Bacteroides fragilis* plus other gram-positive and gram-negative anaerobes	7.5 mg/kg q6h	Active when given orally
Moxalactam	IV, IM	Expanded gram-negative aerobes, anaerobes	No reported dosage for horses	Expensive
Oxacillin	IV, IM	Penicillinase-producing staphylococci	16–50 mg/kg q8h–12h	Synergistic with aminoglycosides
Oxytetracycline	IV	Broad-spectrum antimicrobial activity	4.4–5 mg/kg	Gastrointestinal irritation
Procaine penicillin G	IM	Streptococci, non–penicillinase-producing staphylococci	22,000 IU/kg q12h	Synergistic with aminoglycosides
Ticarcillin	IV, IM	Antipseudomonal activity	44 mg/kg q4h	Synergy with aminoglycosides
Ticarcillin/ clavulanic acid	IV, IM	Broad gram-negative activity—aerobes, anaerobes	44 mg/kg q4h	Clavulanic acid inhibitor of β-lactamases
Tobramycin	IV, IM	Gram-negative aerobic bacilli	No reported dosage for horses	Potential nephrotoxicity/ ototoxicity
Trimethoprim/ sulfamethoxazole	IV	Gram-positive and gram-negative aerobes	15 mg/kg q8–12h	Gastrointestinal irritation
Vancomycin	IV	Methicillin-resistant staphylococci, group D streptococci, enterococcus	4–5 mg/kg q12h	Potential nephrotoxicity

procedure, because manipulation of wounds leads to periods of transient bacteremia. It must be reemphasized that reliance on antimicrobials should not replace strict asepsis and meticulous surgical technique.

It is important to monitor bacterial sensitivity patterns in the practice environment to ensure a minimum impact on environmental microorganisms, which may ultimately have an effect on the choice of antimicrobial chemoprophylaxis. With the recommended drug administration techniques, the risk of drug toxicity and the effects on bacterial susceptibilities should remain low.

BIBLIOGRAPHY

American College of Surgeons, Committee on Control of Surgical Infections: *Manual on Control of Surgical Infections*. Philadelphia, JB Lippincott Co, 1976.

Flynn NM, Lawrence RM: Antimicrobial prophylaxis: Symposium on medical education of the preoperative patient. *Med Clin North Am* 1979;63:6.

Holmberg DL: The use of prophylactic penicillin in orthopedic surgery: A clinical trial. *Vet Surg* 1985;14:160–165.

Nelson CL, Green TG, Porter RA, et al: One day versus seven days of preventive antibiotic therapy in orthopedic surgery. *Clin Orthop Rel Res* 1983;176:258–263.

Norden CW: A critical review of antibiotic prophylaxis in orthopedic surgery. *Rev Infec Dis* 1983;5:928–932.

Orsini JA: Wound infections and antimicrobial therapy, in Gourley IM, Vasseur PB (eds): *General Small Animal Surgery*. Philadelphia, JB Lippincott Co, 1985, pp 121–144.

Polk HC, Johnathan RA: The role of antibiotics in surgical infections. *Adv Surg* 1983;16:225–275.

Ritter MA: Surgical wound environment. *Clin Orthop Rel Res* 1984;190:11–13.

Snyder JR, Pascoe JR, Hirsh DC: Antimicrobial susceptibility of microorganisms isolated from equine orthopedic patients. *Vet Surg* 1987;16:197–201.

Stevenson S, Olmstead ML, Kowalski J: Bacterial culturing for prediction of postoperative complications following open fracture repair in small animals. *Vet Surg* 1986;15:99–102.

133 Diagnosis and Treatment of Bone Infections

James A. Orsini

Significant changes have occurred in the epidemiology, microbiology, antimicrobial therapy, and surgical approach to the treatment of bone infections during the last two decades. Nuclear medicine, microbiologic procedures, and xeroradiography are newer techniques to aid the clinician in making a precise and timely diagnosis, while management includes combinations of antimicrobial and surgical strategies depending on the severity and duration of the infection.

The terms "osteitis" and "osteomyelitis" are used to describe inflammation of bone, more specifically the periosteum, the haversian and Volkmann's canals, and the adjoining medullary cavity. More accurately *osteitis* is an infection of bone tissue that does not enter the medullary cavity or involve the growth plate. Conversely, *osteomyelitis* is defined as an infection affecting the marrow cavity or growth plate. The term "thalamic osteomyelitis" has been used in referring to a specific infection of the medullary cavity compared to "physeal osteomyelitis," which signifies an infection of the physis and consequently involves the growing foal only. Osteomyelitis in the neonatal foal is usually hematogenous and encompasses the thalamic and physeal forms. Osteomyelitis may be the sequela of penetrating wounds, kicks, open fractures, and internal fixation of closed fractures. Both osteitis and osteomyelitis occur more frequently in the metacarpus and metatarsus because of the scant soft tissue covering in these areas.

Other terms specifically associated with bone infections include "sequestrum" (a piece of necrotic bone separated from surrounding healthy bone), "involucrum" (an enveloping membrane of new live bone laid down over and around granulation tissue separating the sequestrum), "Brodie's abscess" (a chronic, inactive collection of pus or connective tissue, surrounded by dense fibrous tissue and sclerotic bone), and "cloaca" (an opening or sinus in the involucrum of necrosed bone permitting the escape of pus).

DIAGNOSTIC TECHNIQUES

The diagnosis of a bone infection is based on clinical signs, history, radiographic findings, and laboratory information. A recent history of trauma or orthopedic surgery coupled with clinical signs of infection (fever, inflammation, localized pain, lameness, and/or purulent discharge) provides the clinician with presumptive evidence of bone infection. A carefully sought out history may reveal that the horse was kicked or sustained some other form of blunt or penetrating trauma.

Radiology

Radiography remains the mainstay of diagnosis in both osteitis and osteomyelitis. Detectable changes may be delayed for 10 to 14 days after the initial onset of the disease. However, soft tissue swelling and loss of normal soft tissue planes occur early and may provide the first diagnostic clue. It is important to remember that visible bony changes are usually delayed in appearance until more than 50% of bone mineral has been removed. Osteolytic changes generally precede new bone formation. Other important radiographic clues of bone infection include periosteal reaction, cortical changes, demineralization, and sequestrum formation (Fig. 133–1).

Xeroradiography is a radiographic technique that utilizes an electrostatically charged selenium-coated aluminum plate. This will produce an image on plastic-coated paper after the plate is exposed to x-rays and processed following exposure to an aerosol of charged powder. The advantage of xeroradiography is its good visualization of soft tissue structures and subtle bone lesions. Thus, in cases in which a suspected lesion is not seen on routine radiographs, xeroradiography may provide the necessary information to make the diagnosis.

Nuclear Medicine

Scintigraphy or radionuclide studies using technetium pyrophosphate bone scans frequently identify osteitis and osteomyelitis before radiographic changes are evident. The radioactive isotope is administered intravenously, followed by checking for its distribution in the bones and soft tissues of the limbs. The scans give positive results because of the accelerated bone turnover or increased blood supply to the infected bone. Gallium bone scans have also been of assistance in humans in differentiating bone infection from soft tissue infection as well as infection from other inflammatory and noninflammatory conditions. Because the gallium studies have been criticized for their lack of specificity, indium 131 scans are being investigated and show promise.

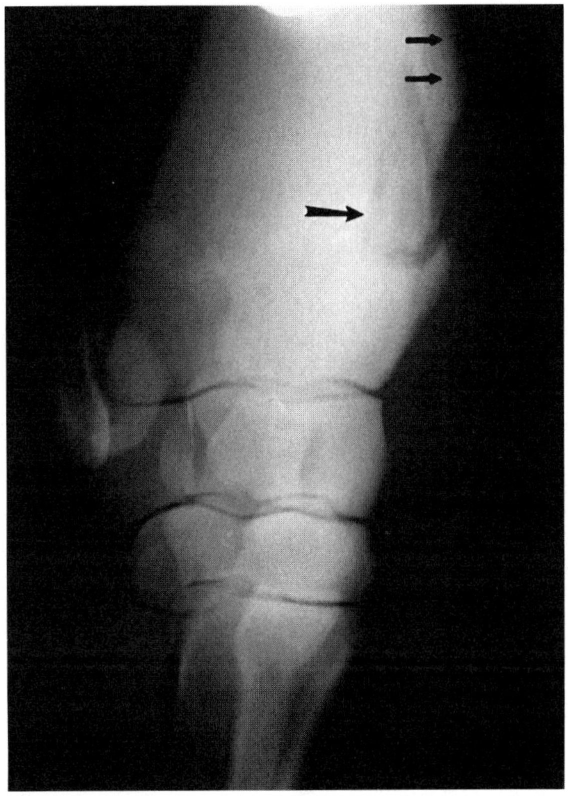

Figure 133–1. Sequestrum (*single arrow*) in distal radius with periosteal proliferation (*double arrow*) (oblique view).

Microbiologic Procedures

Precise microbiologic diagnosis of the offending organism is fundamental to successful treatment of bone infections. Samples for aerobic and anaerobic bacteria should be obtained with additional samples collected for Gram's stain. If bacteria are seen, the Gram's stain will guide the initial antimicrobial therapy. Culture information will confirm initial suspicions and susceptibility studies will further guide antimicrobial therapy. In acute bone infections bacteria may be recovered from blood cultures, lesion aspirates, or exudate obtained from the lesion at surgery. Although drainage from sinus tracts is readily available, it is frequently an unreliable source for culture because the tracts are more often than not contaminated with opportunistic bacterial flora. The most reliable specimen for an accurate microbiologic diagnosis is a bone biopsy, sequestrum, or sample of grossly purulent material from an unopened area. Mycotic infections are believed rare in horses but should be considered when clinical suspicion of such infection exists (i.e., nonresponsiveness to antimicrobial therapy or Gram's stain findings). Special culture and isolation techniques are required for fungal infections.

Identification and classification of microorganism by conventional methods and procedures are time consuming and require extended periods of incubation before final identification. These traditional isolation techniques are based on biochemical, morphologic, and serologic characteristics. Gas-liquid chromatography, high-performance liquid chromatography, and combined gas-liquid chromatography–mass spectrometry are being used to determine the chemical composition and metabolic activity of microorganisms as a basis for their identification. Rapid identification of bacteria is possible based on both short-chain and total cellular fatty acid composition of the bacteria and their byproducts. These methods may be helpful in the early diagnosis of bone infection. This technique has limited availability at the present time.

Because osteitis and osteomyelitis may be part of multiorgan involvement with hematogenous seeding of bone, careful physical examination with specific reference to the umbilicus, abdomen, and respiratory system is warranted. The microorganisms frequently implicated in bone infections include *Actinobacillus species, Streptococcus species, Salmonella species, Escherichia coli, Rhodococcus equi, Staphylococcus species, Enterobacter species, Klebsiella species, Pseudomonas species,* and *Bacteroides species.* Knowing these common culture results from previous lesions proves of value when empirical use of antimicrobials is needed before return of the microbiologic studies.

MANAGEMENT OF BONE INFECTIONS

Osteitis

If bacterial numbers are low ($<10^5$/g of specimen), the osteitis may clear spontaneously, providing a normal-functioning immune system is present. As a rule, bacteria in numbers exceeding 10^5/g of specimen signifies an infection and requires treatment utilizing antimicrobial agents, sequestrectomy, wound débridement, and/or curettage to normal bleeding bone. Sequestra that are small may resorb without the need for surgical intervention. This is believed to be due to the intense inflammatory process that is occurring in the region of the sequestra.

When surgical exploration is indicated (persistent draining sinus or large sequestrum), all necrotic bone, devitalized soft tissue, and devascularized structures should be removed. The difficulty in locating sequestra can be simplified in one of two ways. The intravenous injection of 1% methylene blue dye 24 hours preoperatively will aid identification of nonviable bone. All tissues will initially be colored blue but the dye leaves viable tissue within 24 hours, leaving the sequestra colored a greenish-blue. A more practical method is to infuse a 1% solution of methylene blue dye into the sinus tract at the initiation of surgery, marking its origin and communication with the bone sequestrum. This permits easy identification and removal. Liberal curettage of the involucrum is required to remove all avascular bone and fibrous connective tissue. This requires the excavation of infected bone to form a shallow shelving depression to facilitate drainage from infected areas of bone. Autologous cancellous bone grafts may be necessary if the cortical defect is large (see Chapter 131). A liberal lavage of the surgical site should be performed prior to placement of the graft. An antimicrobial solution composed of polymyxin, neomycin, and bacitracin is frequently used for lavage because of its broad spectrum against gram-positive and gram-negative aerobes. The graft should be harvested using aseptic technique to prevent infection of the donor site. A closed suction drainage system can be used if a large dead space remains; hematoma formation or pus accumulation are to be anticipated during the postoperative period. Primary wound closure can be performed if total lesion removal with adequate débridement has occurred and skin approximation without tension can be accomplished.

Facilitated delivery and activity of host defense factors and antimicrobial agents can occur following decompression of purulent material, removal of subperiosteal abscesses, and débridement of necrotic tissue. The use of parenteral antimicrobial agents such as the penicillins, cephalosporins, macrolides, and aminoglycosides is indicated in the treatment of bone infections. The initial combination of a β-lactam antimicrobial (penicillin or cephalosporin) plus an aminoglycoside is frequently used because of its in vitro demonstration of synergism, its broad antibacterial spectrum, and effective bone concentrations attained.

The prognosis for osteitis remains good to excellent for life and function providing nearby vital structures, such as joints or tendon sheaths, do not become secondarily involved or injured at the time of surgical exploration.

Acute Osteomyelitis

A successful clinical outcome is completely dependent upon establishing an early clinical and bacteriologic diagnosis. Adequate treatment must be initiated early. There is frequently a delay of a few days from the onset of signs before a veterinarian may be called to examine a foal that is lame or showing signs of clinical illness. As soon as the diagnosis is suspected, at least three blood samples should be drawn for culture and susceptibility. Additionally, other body regions should be closely examined (respiratory, gastrointestinal, and umbilicus) and cultured if indicated. Frequently these culture results guide the clinician in tailoring the antimicrobial therapy for the osteomyelitis.

Treatment should be started as soon as the culture specimens are taken so that valuable time is not lost while awaiting the bacteriologic results. Adequate doses of penicillin and an aminoglycoside are usually started immediately. If *R. equi* is suspected, the combination of erythromycin and rifampin has been shown to effectively eradicate the organism. Appropriate adjustments in the antimicrobial program can be made when the results of the culture and susceptibility studies are known. Once the acute disease is controlled with parenteral therapy, oral therapy can be substituted.

With the availability of effective antimicrobial therapy, surgery can be postponed in the treatment of acute osteomyelitis. Operative intervention is usually not necessary if effective medical treatment is initiated within 3 to 4 days after the onset of the disease. Since bone is a highly vascular tissue, it permits cells of the immune system and antimicrobial agents to effectively control the infection. If the infection progresses to vascular thrombosis and exudate accumulation, cells and antimicrobial agents cannot reach the lesion.

With an early diagnosis and appropriate treatment, a good result can usually be expected, with the infection eradicated and the bone substance returned to a normal state. A failure in either diagnosis or treatment may lead to chronic osteomyelitis.

Chronic Osteomyelitis

Chronic osteomyelitis occurs frequently after surgery or trauma. Therapy includes a combined medical-surgical strategy. These treatments complement each other; used independently they frequently fail to resolve the infection.

Signs of chronic osteomyelitis may include lameness with accompanying cellulitis, fever, local pain on manipulation or palpation of the affected area, decreased wound healing over the implants, drainage, and fistulation. Radiographic changes supporting a diagnosis of chronic osteomyelitis include loss of bone density, sclerotic borders surrounding osteolytic bone, sequestrum formation, endosteal and periosteal thickening, Brodie's abscess (Fig. 133–2), and lysis along screw threads or under a plate if the infection is associated with internal fixation.

Undisputed indications for surgery of chronic orthopedic infections include abscessation in the subperiosteal space, within bone marrow, and with fistulous tract formation. Sequestrum formation is also a clear indication for surgical intervention. The potential catastrophic results of removing necrotic bone and thus affecting bone stability must also be considered if surgical débridement is used. Primary closure of the overlying soft tissue should be attempted if adequate débridement of the infected tissue can be attained. As an alternative, a closed irrigation suction technique can be used. The local infusion of antimicrobial solutions provides an excellent diffusion gradient to sterilize avascular areas that may have been left during surgical débridement. This technique has some limitations in large animal orthopedics because of the need for constant patient monitoring during fluid infusion and suction. Voluminous quanities of fluids and anti-

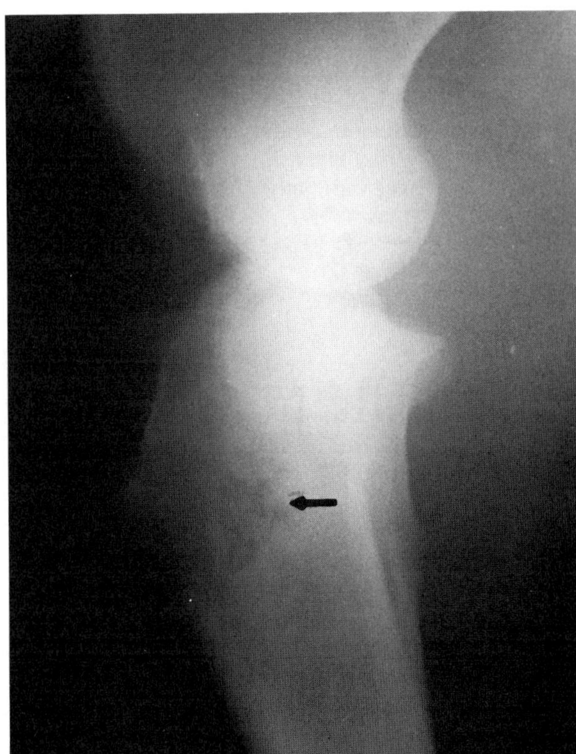

Figure 133–2. Brodie's abscess (*arrow*) of proximal tibia (lateral view).

microbials are required and the potential exists for the animal to remove or damage the suction tubing.

In some animals with chronic osteomyelitis, a two-stage surgical approach may be required. This entails elimination of the infection from the wound followed at a later date by an autogenous cancellous bone graft. This two-stage procedure is not always possible in large animal orthopedics because of the problems of attaining adequate internal or external fixation in the race to provide stabilization and healing before loosening or failure of the implants. Therefore, the two-step procedure commonly used in human and small animal orthopedics may need to occur as one procedure in order to achieve stability.

Chronic osteomyelitis with implants can complicate the question of removal. If infection is evident after fracture consolidation, implant removal will hasten resolution of the infection. If the implants are not providing effective stability, they should be removed and an alternative method of fixation chosen. External skeletal fixation with transfixation pins attached to a frame is one method that has been utilized because it avoids metallic implants at the site of infection. In all cases, the primary concern should be the attainment of bony union.

Investigative treatment modalities presently utilized to a limited extent in human medicine with potential application in veterinary medicine include: autovaccination with the isolated inactivated bacteria, local antimicrobial perfusion pumps, intraarterial antimicrobial therapy, aminoglycoside-polymethylmethacrylate beads, and hyperbaric oxygenation of infected tissue.

SUMMARY

In summary, bone infections continue to be a significant problem in large animal surgery. Diagnosis of the acute case remains difficult and a high index of suspicion on the part of the clinician is essential. Treatment results are variable depending on the duration and extent of the infection.

BIBLIOGRAPHY

Bardet JF, Hohn RB, Basinger R: Open drainage and delayed autogenous cancellous bone grafting for treatment of osteomyelitis in dogs and cats. *J Am Vet Med Assoc* 1983;183:312–317.

Dickie AS: Current concepts in the management of infections in bones and joints. *Drugs* 1986;32:458–475.

Harari J: Osteomyelitis. *J Am Vet Med Assoc* 1984;184:101–102.

Kahn DS, Pritzker KPH: The pathophysiology of bone infection. *Clin Orthop* 1973;96:12–19.

Nunamaker DM: Management of infected fractures. *Vet Clin North Am* 1975;5:259–271.

Orsini JA: Stategies for treatment of bone and joint infections in large animals. *J Am Vet Med Assoc* 1984;185:1190–1193.

Turner S: Diseases of bones and related structures, in Stashak TS (ed): *Adams' Lameness in Horses*. Philadelphia, Lea & Febiger, 1987, pp 304–308.

Waldvogel FA, Medoff G, Swartz MN: Osteomyelitis: A review of clinical features, therapeutic considerations and unusual aspects. *N Engl J Med* 1970;282:198–206.

134 Orthopedic Implant Failure

David M. Nunamaker

Failure of orthopedic implants is a common problem in equine orthopedic surgery. An understanding of the materials used, their design and their proper use is of importance in understanding these failures.

MECHANICAL PROPERTIES OF IMPLANTS

All materials display certain mechanical properties. The relationship between load and deformation can be summarized in a stress-strain diagram (Fig. 134–1). The straight line portion of this graph portrays the useful elastic portion of the material in question. Orthopedic implants stressed within the limits of this elastic portion of the curve can be expected to maintain their original shape. Implants subjected to loads (stresses) above this level will deform. This deformation occurs at the yield point, after which further increases in the load will result in plastic deformation of the material. These high stresses that exceed the yield point should

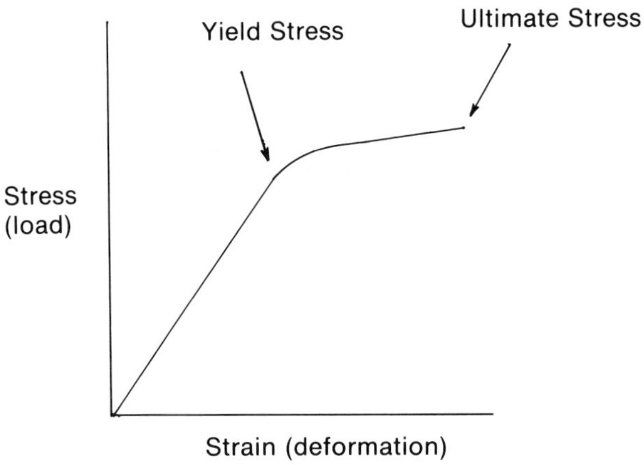

Figure 134–1. This stress-strain curve shows the relationship between stress and strain. The straight line portion of the graph represents the modulus of the material. Yield stress represents the point where the material begins to plastically deform. The ultimate stress (failure point) represents the rupture point of this material.

be avoided when loading implants in vivo. The *yield stress* is an important property of a material, because it represents the point at which the material starts to plastically deform. The *failure point* of the material (ultimate tensile strength) shows where the material ruptures. Failure of orthopedic implants may also be progressive in nature as the loads on the material increase.

The *elastic modulus* (Young's modulus) of a material represents the slope of the straight line portion of the stress-strain diagram (Fig. 134–1) and is the stress divided by the strain. The slope of this line will be different for different materials. The steeper the slope, the stiffer the material and the higher the modulus. The modulus for stainless steel is approximately ten times that of bone. Hence a steel plate used to fix a fracture has a modulus ten times greater than the bone to which it is applied.

The implant and the bone both have *sectional properties* (width and thickness) that account for the overall strength and stiffness of each. The larger sectional properties of equine bone account for the seemingly more flexible implant being applied to the seemingly more stiff bone. These sectional properties account for the increased stiffness that broad plates possess as compared to narrow plates of the same length. Using plates in combination (double plating) can improve the sectional properties of the bone plate composite. Furthermore, plates placed at right angles to each other are five to ten times stronger in bending and two times stronger in torsion than are single plates. The torsional strength limitations are related to the screws, whereas the bending strength is related to the inertial properties of the plate. These strengths are variable depending on the width of the plate. Thus, the wider plates will have greater effect when used at right angles to each other as compared to narrow plates.

CYCLIC LOADING AND FAILURE

When implants are applied to bone, they are usually subjected to cyclic loads during weight bearing. If the loads are greater than the yield stress for the material, plastic deformation and failure are the result. If the loads are less than the yield stress for that material, failure may still occur through cyclic loading. This is known as fatigue failure and represents the failure of a material that has been cycled within its elastic range. The stress–number of cycles curve (S-N curve) depicts the relationships between repeated loads and stress (Fig. 134–2). It can be seen that repeated stresses decrease the ultimate breaking strength of the material. If a certain cyclic load (number of cycles at a given load) lies above the S-N curve, failure of the material results.

Some materials such as steels have an *endurance level.* This means that below a certain stress the material will be able to endure an infinite number of cycles before it breaks. The endurance level of most steels is

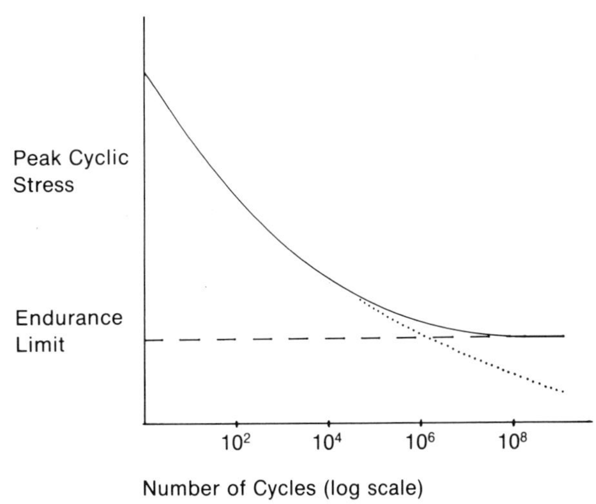

Figure 134–2. This stress–number of cycles curve shows the relation between individual stresses and the number of cycles before failure. Stresses above the curve represent material failure. The endurance level is shown by the dashed line. The dotted line shows the problem of the effect of a saline environment on the metallic implant, as occurs within the animal's body. Here the endurance limit is changed to some lower level or abolished.

approximately 30% of the ultimate tensile strength. This phenomenon is important in the design of structures that must deal with cyclic loading, such as bridges and orthopedic prostheses. One problem associated with the design of metallic implants for orthopedic use is that the endurance limit is diminished in the saline environment of the animal's body. This increases the chances for implant failure with increasing use.

SOURCES OF FAILURE

Clinically, implant failure is important when it interferes with satisfactory results. In equine orthopedics failure of the implant occurs all too frequently. The reasons for those failures can be categorized into several basic areas.

Surgical Failure

Surgical technical failures are related to errors in judgment and the use of poor techniques and inadequate implants. The choice of a proper implant for a particular job can be critical when dealing with large animals that will apply functional loads immediately after surgery. Sometimes animals present with fractures for which there is no implant available that will be able to stabilize it. These cases may fail regardless of the techniques or implants currently used. Similarly, subjecting an implant designed for tensile loads to bending loads is likewise a futile experience. It is important that implants be placed on the tension surface of the bone so that when the bone is loaded via weight bearing the implant will be subjected to tensile forces rather than bending. The use of this tension band principle is important in allowing the implant to survive the rigors of weight bearing.

The understanding of the principles involved in the application of internal fixation implants and a generalized understanding of the biomechanics involved with the use of any fracture fixation device is necessary to expect satisfactory results when using implants in equine fracture repair. Many severe fractures cause some compromise to the vascular supply of the bone and soft tissues. The introduction of infection via open reduction and its propagation by inadequate fixation likewise may be an error in judgment. Poor surgical technique or inappropriate approaches when repairing a fracture may result in wound dehiscence and necrosis that seem to place even greater demands on the implant. Many cases of implant failure (fatigue failure) occur because fracture healing was delayed by wound infection and/or osteomyelitis.

Most implant failures in equine orthopedic surgery are related to these surgical technical failures. The use of inadequate implants and instrumentation results from the use of devices that were designed for humans. Adaptation of the implants and techniques for use in the horse have greatly improved, however, resulting in fewer implant failures.

Material Failure

Material failures may result from design deficiencies or the metallurgy involved in the manufacture of the material. The sophistication of the metallurgic methodology limits defects in the material to a very small percentage of implant failures. The chemistry of the implant material is very closely controlled. This limits inclusion of unwanted elements such as sulfur in stainless steel that can be important in the corrosion characteristics of the implant.

Material failures as a result of corrosion are found most frequently in areas of low oxygen concentration where two surfaces are rubbing together. These areas occasionally exist between a plate and a screw. This is known as *fretting corrosion*. The dissolution of an implant by corrosion can weaken the implant to allow direct overload or fatigue failure of the device to occur. Most material failures that occur in equine orthopedics can be traced to high loads being applied to the implant following surgery. Although all metals corrode to some degree after implantation, this phenomenon does not usually cause problems in the patient. Studies have shown that the elemental accumulation of metal ions in the body occurs through dissolution of the alloy of the implant. These metal ions bind to serum proteins when the dissolution of the alloy occurs within the body. Interaction of these protein-bound metal ions with the immune system may be important in sensitivity reactions being present. Although unreported in the horse, sensitivity reactions have been reported in humans. The pain seemingly related to the implant after healing has occurred in the horse may be related to a mechanical mismatch of modulus or to some sort of metal sensitivity. Certainly there are a number of horses that are lame without any apparent reason following fracture healing after internal fixation with screws alone. The removal of these devices may alleviate the signs of lameness. Metal sensitivity should not be overlooked as a potential cause of lameness following successful internal fixation of fractures in the horse.

PREVENTION OF IMPLANT FAILURE

The prevention of implant failures is an important consideration in the overall management of the equine orthopedic patient. It should be remembered that the implants as delivered from the manufacturer are not designed for immediate weight bearing in humans. Their use in the horse, where immediate full weight bearing may be expected, must be carefully controlled. The use of casts may be helpful in controlling bending moments about the implant, but casts will not improve the outcome of a poorly executed procedure. Internal fixation plates are designed to be loaded in compression or tension. The screws are designed for tension. The common loading of screws in shear (perpendicular to their long axis) and plates in bending results in their deformation and breakage.

Techniques such as plate luting (the application of a polymeric substance between the bone and the plate and between the screws and the plate) may be helpful in allowing weight bearing in the horse following internal fixation with a lowered incidence of implant failures. Plate luting allows greater contact of the implant with the bone and is useful in increasing the number of cyclic loads that the implant can withstand without failure. Plate luting is accomplished after normal plate application by loosening the plate and applying polymethylmethacrylate (PMMA) under the plate. Retightening of the plate squeezes the PMMA up into the screw holes and distributes it beneath the plate. Consequently, the plate has complete contact with the bone and acts as a part of the bone when under load, preventing motion between the bone and plate. The application of larger diameter screws (5.5 mm) that are now commercially available helps improve the strength and longevity of internal fixations using plates and screws or screws alone. The use of ever-increasing implant size is not always a satisfactory method for dealing with implant failure.

The size and strength of the bone that is fractured must always be considered in the fracture repair. Immediate full weight bearing can cause failure of the bone as well as the implant. Further fracture of a bone after internal fixation is always possible, especially in the foal. It is always important to adjust the implant size and technique to the individual animal and its fracture.

Future designs of fixation systems for the horse must attempt to deal with immediate full weight bearing. Plate luting and external skeletal fixation devices designed specifically for horses should help decrease the problems of implant failure in the horse. However, the orthopedic problems presented by equine patients will always test our ability to deal with orthopedic implant failures.

BIBLIOGRAPHY

Brown SA, Devin S, Merritt K: Metal allergy, metal implants and fracture healing. *Biomater Med Devices Artif Organs* 1983;11:73–81.

Nunamaker DM, Bowman KF, Richardson DW, Herring M: Plate luting: A preliminary report of its use in horses. *Vet Surg* 1986;15:289–293.

Nunamaker DM, Richardson DW, Butterweck DM: Mechanical effects of plate luting, in *Transactions of the 34th Annual Meeting of the Orthopedic Research Society.* Park Ridge Ill, Orthopaedic Research Society, 1988, p 305.

Nunamaker DM, Richardson DW, Butterweck DM, Provost MT, Sigafoos RD: A new external skeletal fixation device that allows immediate full weight bearing: Application in the horse. *Vet Surg* 1986;15:345–355.

Smith GK: Orthopaedic biomaterials, in Newton CD, Nunamaker DM (eds): *Textbook of Small Animal Orthopaedics.* Philadelphia, JB Lippincott Co, 1985, pp 231–241.

Woodman JL, Black J, Nunamaker DM: Release of cobalt and nickel from a new total finger joint prosthesis made of vitallium. *J Biomed Mater Res* 1983;17:655–668.

UNIT X

Urogenital System Disorders

135
Urovagina

Rolf M. Embertson

"Urine pooling" (urovagina) is the common term used for the accumulation of urine in the cranial vagina of the mare. This abnormality is most commonly seen in the older, thin, multiparous mare whose genitourinary tract slopes cranioventrally. The excessive downward slope of the genitourinary tract is considered the result of stretched reproductive organs and the stretched and lax ligaments supporting them. The muscles and ligaments supporting the rectum and anus may also become lax in the older mare. This allows cranial displacement of these structures, which pulls the vagina forward toward the abdomen because of the muscular and ligamentous attachment of the caudal vagina to the rectum. The cranioventral sloping of the genitourinary tract leads to incompletely voided urine running downhill to pool in the cranial vagina, thus the often used term "vesicovaginal reflux."

Urine-pooling mares usually have a characteristic external perineal conformation—the anus and dorsal vulva have a sunken appearance. This conformation predisposes to pneumovagina and potential vaginal aspiration of fecal contaminants. A Caslick's procedure is usually performed to prevent pneumovagina in mares with this conformation. This closed dorsal aspect of the vulvar cleft may direct urine into the cranial vagina during urination, contributing to the volume of the pooled urine.

The chronic presence of urine in the cranial vagina leads to vaginitis, cervicitis, and endometritis. These inflammatory responses lessen the ability of the mare to conceive and to carry a foal to term. The urine itself is also spermicidal. Another adverse effect occasionally encountered in the mare with urovagina is urine scalding on the inside of the hind limbs. This is a result of urine escaping the cranial vagina and dribbling from the vestibule.

DIAGNOSIS

Mares with a sunken perineal conformation and a history of infertility should be examined for urine pooling. The definitive diagnosis is made on speculum examination of the vagina. Urovagina is often discovered on routine examination of the mare's reproductive tract before infertility has become a problem. The fluid found in the cranial vagina is usually recognized as urine by its yellowish, cloudy character. To determine that the fluid is urine and not the serous mucus that may be found in the cranial vagina during estrus or pooled fluid from an endometritis, the fluid can be analyzed for urea nitrogen level. It is optimal to perform a speculum examination of the vagina during estrus because some mares may pool urine during estrus but not diestrus. It is also wise to examine the mare several times to be sure urovagina is a consistent finding. Urovagina may occur in some older mares only during late pregnancy or in the immediate postpartum period and occasionally in normal mares after shipping. This temporary urine pooling seems to have little to no adverse affect on their reproductive capabilities.

TREATMENT

Correction of urine pooling and its attendant problems usually requires surgery. Weight gain helps to improve the conformation of the caudal reproductive tract in some mares. Manual evacuation of urine from the vagina immediately preceding breeding may improve the conception rate. However, this does not deter the long-term effects of urovagina. Complete evaluation of the reproductive tract should be performed prior to surgical correction of urovagina to determine if urovagina is the primary cause of infertility. However, in a valuable mare with a marginal reproductive status, any improvement gained in the ability to conceive and carry a foal to term is worthwhile.

Surgical Considerations

Two techniques have evolved in the surgical correction of urine pooling. The first, and most commonly used, is to relocate the external opening of the urethra caudally in the vestibule to a level where the urine, upon exiting the new urethral opening, will no longer flow into the cranial vagina. Caudal relocation of the transverse fold, which lies over the normal urethral orifice (Monin's technique), corrects urine pooling in mares with a very mild vaginal slope. Because the transverse fold cannot be pulled far enough caudally, this technique is often unsuccessful in mares with a moderate to severe vaginal slope. Extension of the urethra to the vulva by creation of a mucous membrane–lined tunnel, a procedure developed by Brown et al., prevents urine pooling in mares with any degree of downward vaginal sloping. The problem with this procedure is the occasional focal dehiscence from excessive tension on the suture line, resulting in fistulation and recurrence of urine pooling. Modifications of this technique have been developed, and one will be described here.

The second technique in the correction of urine pooling is the sectioning of the ligamentous and muscular attachments between the rectum/anus and the caudal vagina/vulva (Pouret's technique). This allows the vestibule and urethral orifice to move caudally, resulting in a more horizontal vestibular floor for the urine to traverse. In addition, the vulva becomes more vertical, which may prevent pneumovagina. The merits of this procedure and the surgical technique are not presented here.

Surgical Preparation

The mare is tranquilized with acetylpromazine and should be positioned in stocks for surgery. Antibiotics, nonsteroidal anti-inflammatory medication, and tetanus toxoid are administered preoperatively. Epidural administration of 6 mL of 2% lidocaine or 85 mg of xylazine diluted to 10 ml with sterile saline will provide adequate regional anesthesia for a 450-kg mare for approximately 2 hours. Xylazine produces less hind limb ataxia than lidocaine and is, therefore, preferable. While waiting for the epidural to take effect, the tail is wrapped and tied to the upper crossbar of the stocks. Feces are manually evacuated from the rectum and the entire perineal region is then prepared for surgery with a nonirritating surgical scrub [e.g., chlorhexidene diacetate (Nolvasan, Aveco Inc)]. If perineal sensation is still present 20 to 30 minutes after administration of the epidural, the surgery is performed under the effects of systemic xylazine, butorphanol tartrate (Torbugesic, Bristol Labs), and local anesthesia. Local anesthesia of the surgical site is accomplished by squirting 40 to 50 mL of 2% lidocaine into the vestibule and manually distributing it over the mucosa of the area where the incision will be made.

If a Caslick's procedure had been performed, this is opened to the dorsal extent of the vulva. Balfour retractors (tied to the tail head) or stay sutures can be used to provide retraction of the vulvar lips and facilitate exposure. Excessive retraction of the vulva should be avoided because this makes apposition of the incised tissues difficult. Long-handled instruments and a surgical light or head lamp are quite useful for this procedure.

Surgical Technique

The following procedure, a modification of Brown et al.'s technique, was developed to decrease the tension on the suture line. The transverse fold is pulled caudally toward the vulva and sutured. This leaves the transverse fold covering the area of the vestibule that is widest and where the most tension exists in the new mucosa tunnel formed from the walls of the vestibule.

The initial approach is the same as reported by Brown et al. The transverse fold overlying the external urethral orifice is grasped with thumb forceps and split on a horizontal plane into dorsal and ventral layers using a scalpel. Care must be taken to avoid inadvertent creation of holes in either of these layers. This incision is continued caudally along both left and right ventrolateral walls of the vestibule to 1 to 2 cm from the vulva. The mucosa remaining between the left and right vestibular wall incisions must be of sufficient width to allow creation of a urethral tunnel of adequate diameter. Use of a no. 30 French Foley catheter (Latex Foley Catheter; Travenol Laboratories, Inc) placed in the bladder can be useful to judge the placement of these incisions and prevent urine contamination of the surgical site during the procedure. If used, this catheter is removed when the surgery is completed.

The transverse fold is grasped with two Allis tissue forceps and pulled caudally. Starting in the angle created between the right vestibular wall and the transverse fold, the ventral mucosal layers (eventual urethral mucosa) of the vestibular wall and transverse fold are apposed. The use of 2-0 polyglactin 910 (Vicryl; Ethicon Inc) in a continuous horizontal mattress pattern inverts the ventral mucosa into the newly created urethra. This suture pattern is continued caudally to the midpoint of the transverse fold, where the suture is tied. The right dorsal mucosal layers, (eventual vestibular floor mucosa) of the vestibular wall and transverse fold are apposed with 2-0 polyglactin 910 in a continuous horizontal mattress pattern starting in the angle between the vestibular wall and transverse fold and ending at the midpoint of the transverse fold. This inverts the dorsal mucosa into the vestibule. Both ventral and dorsal mucosal layers of the left side are then apposed from the angle between the left vestibular wall and transverse fold to the midpoint of the transverse fold in the same manner as performed on the right side. The Allis tissue forceps are then removed.

The remainder of the roof of the new urethra is closed by opposing first the left and right ventral mucosa, then the left and right dorsal mucosa using 2-0 polyglactin 910 in a continuous horizontal mattress pattern. The ventral suture is started from the mucosal side, directed up through the right ventral vestibular mucosa, down through the right ventral transverse fold mucosa, up through the left ventral transverse fold mucosa, down through the left ventral vestibular mucosa, up through the left ventral vestibular mucosa (5 mm caudal to the previous bite), then down through the right ventral vestibular mucosa. The suture is tied, inverting the edges of the mucosa ventrally into the newly created urethra. This suture is then continued to the caudal extent of the incision using a continuous horizontal mattress pattern to invert the edges of the mucosa ventrally. The dorsal suture is started from the mucosal side, directed down through the right dorsal vestibular mucosa, up through the right dorsal transverse fold mucosa, down through the left dorsal transverse fold mucosa, up through the left dorsal vestibular mucosa, down through the left dorsal vestibular mucosa (5 mm caudal to the previous bite), then up through the right dorsal vestibular mucosa. The suture is tied, inverting the edges of the mucosa dorsally into the vestibule. This suture is then continued to the caudal extent of the incision using the continuous horizontal mattress pattern to invert the mucosal edges dorsally into the vestibule. The completed suture line has a *Y*-shaped configuration with the apex of the transverse fold directed caudally. Accurate suture placement at the caudal midpoint of the transverse fold in both ventral and dorsal layers is important. Although tension on the suture line is minimal, this is the point where most tension is encountered. A Caslick's procedure is performed to close the dorsal aspect of the vulvar cleft.

POSTOPERATIVE CARE

Antibiotics should be continued for 36 hours and nonsteroidal anti-inflammatory medication should be continued for 3 to 5 days postoperatively. The mare should be observed for any difficulty in urinating for 2 to 3 days after surgery. Otherwise, the mare can be returned to the normal farm routine. The vagina should not be entered for 2 weeks postoperatively, at which time the surgical site is examined for any dehiscence and the cranial vagina examined for evidence of urine. The sutures are not removed. Mares may be carefully bred by artificial insemination at 3 weeks after surgery; however, natural breeding should be delayed until 6 weeks after surgery.

PROGNOSIS AND COMPLICATIONS

The prognosis for the prevention of urine pooling following urethral extension surgery is good. Focal dehiscence with fistula formation and urovagina occurs in 5 to 25% of the mares. This may be a result of several factors, including the width of the vestibule (wide, flat vestibular floors will increase tension on the suture line), experience of the surgeon, surgical technique used, dehiscence of a previous urethral extension surgery, and scarring of the vestibule from previous foaling trauma. It should be noted that fistula formation does not always result in recurrence of urine pooling. Therefore, the mare should be examined several times for urovagina before recommending repair of a fistula.

Fistulas in the extended urethra that result in urovagina must be closed. The mare is prepared in the same manner for this surgery as for the urethral extension surgery. Small holes can often be repaired by excision of the mucosal edge of the fistula with further dissection to create dorsal and ventral tissue flaps. These layers are then closed using 2-0 polyglactin 910 to invert the urethra mucosa into the urethra and the vestibular mucosa into the vestibule. To repair a large hole, the roof of the extended urethra is incised to the fistula and the mucosal edge of the fistula is excised. Dissection is continued to create dorsal and ventral layers along the fresh edges of the urethral roof. This is closed in two layers with 2-0 polyglactin 910. A continuous horizontal mattress pattern suture is placed in the ventral mucosa, inverting the mucosal edges into the urethra. The same suture pattern is used to appose and invert the dorsal vestibular mucosa into the vestibule.

I would like to thank Dr. W. Thomas Riddle for his contributions to this chapter.

BIBLIOGRAPHY

Brown MP, Colahan PT, Hawkins DL: Urethral extension for treatment of urine pooling in mares. *J Am Vet Med Assoc* 1978;173:1005–1007.

LeBlanc PH, Caron JP, Patterson JS, Brown M, Matta MA: Epidural injection of xylazine for perineal analgesia in horses. *J Am Vet Med Assoc* 1988;193:1405–1408.

McIlwraith CW, Turner AS: Urethroplasty (urethral exten-

sion), in *Equine Surgery Advanced Techniques*. Philadelphia, Lea & Febiger, 1987, pp 352–355.
McKinnon AO, Belden JO: A urethral extension technique to correct urine pooling (vesicovaginal reflux) in mares. *J Am Vet Med Assoc* 1988;192:647–650.
Ricketts SW: Perineal conformation abnormalities, in Robinson NE (ed): *Current Therapy in Equine Medicine*, ed 2. Philadelphia, WB Saunders Co, 1987, pp 518–520.
Shires GM, Kaneps AJ: A practical and simple surgical technique for repair of urine pooling in the mare. *Proc AAEP Ann Conven* 1986; pp 51–56.
Turner AS, McIlwraith CW: Urethroplasty by caudal relocation of the transverse fold, in *Techniques in Large Animal Surgery*. Philadelphia, Lea & Febiger, 1982, pp 163–166.

136 Cervical Lacerations

James T. Robertson

Lacerations of the cervix usually occur as a result of excessive stretching of the cervix during delivery of a fetus. Although they are usually associated with the trauma of a dystocia, cervical lacerations may occur during an uneventful and unassisted delivery or during the abortion of a relatively small fetus. Dystocias requiring a great deal of obstetric manipulation or the introduction of obstetric instruments such as a fetotome into the uterus have a higher risk for producing cervical tears.

CLINICAL FINDINGS

Cervical lacerations usually involve only that portion of the cervix that projects into the cavity of the vagina (portio vaginalis). Severe lacerations may involve the entire length of the cervix. Lacerations may involve only the mucosa of the cervix or completely disrupt the mucosal and muscular layers, producing a wedge-shaped defect with its base at the cervical os and apex at the reflection of the vaginal mucosa. Tearing may occur at any point around the perimeter of the cervix. There may be more than one tear in a cervix, although additional tears are usually less severe. Stretching of the cervix can also produce a rupture of the musculature without disrupting the mucosa, a condition referred to as cervical incompetence.

A complete tear through greater than 50% of the vaginal portion of the cervix or a rupture of the cervical musculature usually prevents complete closure of the cervix. Adhesions of the cervix to the vaginal mucosa that produce distortion of the cervical os can also impair cervical function. The inability of the cervix to close tightly under the influence of progesterone will result in chronic uterine contamination, endometritis, and failure to conceive or maintain a pregnancy. Lacerations that involve less than 50% of the vaginal portion of the cervix generally do not affect cervical function. Mucosal tears usually heal spontaneously.

EVALUATION

Cervical lacerations discovered during a post partum examination, should be allowed to heal by second intention and reevaluated 30 to 60 days later to determine if surgical repair is necessary. Most cervical defects are discovered once the lacerations have healed. On a vaginal speculum exam, asymmetry of the cervix, an obvious tissue defect, or adhesions around the cervix are visible evidence of a cervical laceration (Fig. 136–1). Cervical lacerations are not always found during routine speculum examinations, and many are detected during cervical manipulation when performing a uterine culture or biopsy.

A direct manual examination should always be performed on the cervix as part of an examination for infertility. The thumb and opposing index finger are used to evaluate the lumen and palpate the full circumference of the cervix for the presence of defects, weaknesses, or adhesions. The severity of any defects are determined and, if the mare is in diestrus, the tone of the cervix is evaluated. Mares that are not cycling can be placed on oral progesterone for a 2-week period to increase cervical tone. Under the influence of progesterone, the cervix of a normal mare should close tightly and the cervical muscle tone should provide resistance to the introduction of an index finger into the lumen. A lacerated or incompetent cervix does not provide such

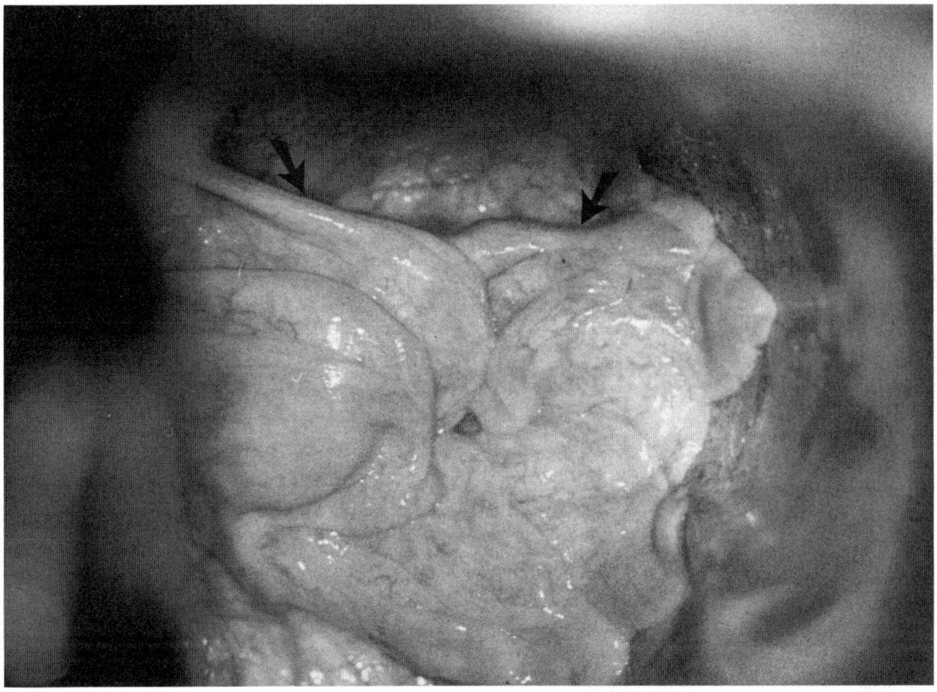

Figure 136–1. Speculum examination of the cervix revealing obvious asymmetry and a tissue defect (11 to 1 o'clock, between *arrows*). This cervix is relaxed as a result of an epidural anesthetic.

resistance. Prior to surgical repair of a cervix, a complete reproductive examination, including a uterine biopsy and culture, should be performed. Chronic endometrial degeneration greatly decreases the prognosis for restoring fertility.

TREATMENT

The surgical repair can be undertaken at any time during the estrous cycle and is best performed in the standing mare with epidural anesthesia. The only exceptions would be mares that cannot be blocked with an epidural anesthetic or mares that have severe lacerations that extend the full length of the lumen of the cervix. I have found that using a general anesthetic and placing these mares in sternal recumbency with their rear quarters off the table and their body tipped forward and down allows greater retraction of the cervix (Fig. 136–2). Although it is difficult, surgical repair of a luminal defect can be achieved. Large, broad-blade retractors or a vaginal speculum are necessary for adequate retraction of the walls of the vestibule. The arms of the retractors should extend cranially beyond the vestibular sphincter. Long-handled (12-in) scissors, thumb forceps, and needle holders are necessary for the reconstruction.

The mare is placed in stocks and sedated with a combination of xylazine and butorphanol (Torbugesic; Bristol Labs) (200 mg xylazine and 5 mg butorphanol intravenously/450 kg). This sedative combination will calm an anxious mare and also provide analgesia during the administration of the epidural [2% mepivacaine (Carbocaine), 6 to 8 mL/450 kg). I prefer to administer the epidural, remove the needle, and tie the mare's tail over the back of the stocks to provide support if she becomes weak from the epidural. A quick-release knot should be used to secure the tail. If the mare becomes uncomfortable during the procedure, small doses of xylazine (100 to 200 mg intravenously) can be administered as necessary.

Long stay sutures must be placed through the cervix on each side of the defect to provide retraction during the repair (Fig. 136–3A). I prefer to place the stay sutures (doubled No. 2 Vetafil (Braunamid; Jorgensen Laboratories)] by hand, introducing both lubricated arms into the vagina, palpating the defect with the left hand and placing the stay sutures with the right using a large cutting needle. The ends of the stay sutures are each tagged with a hemostat. Although cervical forceps

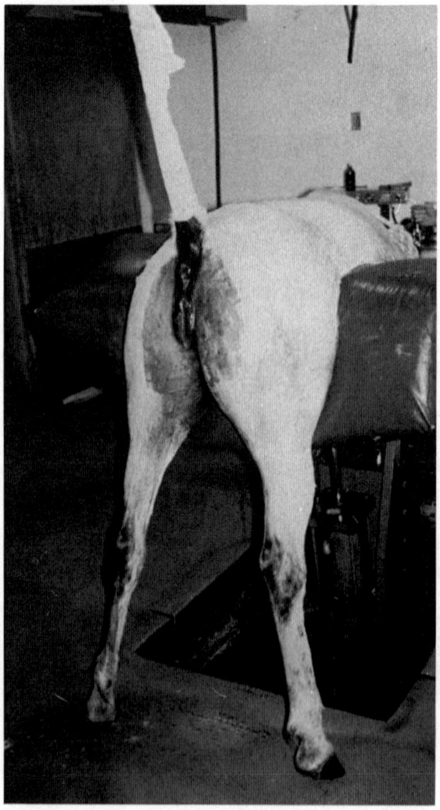

Figure 136–2. This mare is under general anesthesia in sternal recumbency with her rear quarters off the surgery table. Because there is a risk of myositis, adequate padding is essential.

can be used to retract the cervix for placement of the stay sutures, these forceps are quite traumatic. The broad-blade retractors are then positioned and the cervix is retracted to the level of the vestibule using the stay sutures (Fig. 136–3B). The scar tissue and redundant mucosa at the edges of the laceration are excised with scissors. Any adhesions producing cervical deformity should be incised. In my experience it is difficult to differentiate the muscular tissue from scar tissue, so I remove all palpable scar tissue along the margin of the defect. If there is a muscular defect but the mucosa is still intact, a wedge-shaped piece of mucosa is excised to expose the muscle layers. The defect is closed in three layers with each closure starting at the apex of the defect (Fig. 136–3C). Synthetic absorbable suture material should be used. The mucosa on the lumen side is closed first with 2-0 suture using a continuous suture pattern that produces minimal inversion into the lumen. The muscular layer is closed with size 0 suture in a simple interrupted pattern or with interrupted vertical mattress sutures. It is usually necessary to use a cutting needle for the muscular layer. The mucosa on the vaginal side is closed with 2-0 suture with an everting, continuous horizontal mattress pattern (Fig. 136–3D). The knots of the interrupted muscle sutures should be covered with mucosa, if possible. If a second laceration is present, it is repaired in a similar fashion. Mares with deeper lacerations require more extensive reconstruction of the cervix than is attempted by an intraluminal approach.

POSTOPERATIVE CARE

Postoperatively, administration of systemic antibiotics and anti-inflammatory drugs is optional. The cervix will remain quite edematous and hyperemic for at least 2 weeks, and manual examination of the cervix is of no benefit during this time. There is very little risk of

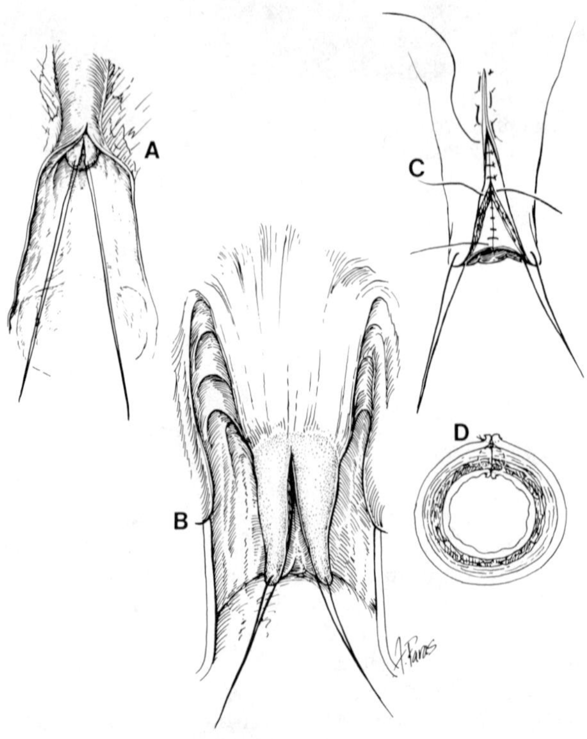

Figure 136–3. A. Long stay sutures have been placed through the cervix on each side of the defect to provide retraction during the repair. **B.** With the retractors in place, the cervix is retracted to the level of the vestibule using the stay sutures. **C.** The defect is closed in three layers, with each closure starting at the apex of the defect. **D.** Cross-section of the cervix showing a three-layer closure with apposition of the mucosa.

adhesion formation in the lumen or on the vaginal side of the cervix, providing there has been good tissue layer apposition and a three-layer closure with no mucosal defects.

PROGNOSIS

The prognosis for fertility is dependent on the condition of the uterus and successful restoration of cervical muscle function. Mares with category I or II endometrial lesions and one laceration involving the vaginal portion of the cervix have a 50 to 60% chance of conceiving and carrying a foal to term. Breeding should not be allowed for at least 30 days following surgery to allow for adequate healing. Frequently it takes two breeding seasons to get these mares in foal. The prognosis is fair to poor for those mares that have more than one laceration or have extensive scarring and adhesions of the cervix to the vagina. Mares with deep lacerations that extend into the uterus and those that have a chronic cervicitis have a grave prognosis. Some mares will reinjure the cervix during subsequent foalings and require further reconstruction.

If surgical reconstruction of a lacerated or incompetent cervix does not restore function, a pursestring retention suture may be placed submucosally in the vaginal portion of the cervix to close the cervix. A retention suture can also be used in aged multiparous mares that cannot effectively close the cervix as a result of chronic cervical muscle tearing and fibrosis. The suture can be placed within 2 days after breeding or it can be placed prior to breeding, leaving a luminal opening large enough to allow the introduction of an artificial insemination pipette. Although Mersilene can be used, I prefer size 2 polypropylene (Prolene; Ethicon Inc) because it is less reactive. The suture must be removed prior to foaling. A cervical retention suture does not allow for uterine drainage and pyometra can develop if the uterus becomes infected. The prognosis for fertility is poor if one needs to resort to this type of therapy.

BIBLIOGRAPHY

Brown JS, Varner DD, Hinrichs K, Kenney RM: Surgical repair of the lacerated cervix in the mare. *Theriogenology* 1984;22:351–359.

Evans LJ, Tate LP, Cooper WL, Robertson JT: Surgical repair of cervical lacerations and the incompetent cervix. *Proc AAEP Ann Conven* 1979 pp 483–486.

Fraunfelder HC: Cervical abnormalities, in Robinson NE (ed): *Current Therapy in Equine Medicine.* ed 2. Philadelphia, WB Saunders Co, 1987, pp 516–518.

Kenney RM: Cyclic and pathologic changes of the mare endometrium as detected by biopsy, with a note on early embryonic death. *J Am Vet Med Assoc* 1978;172:241–262.

137
Perineal Lacerations

Rolf M. Embertson

The perineum, that tissue that forms the body wall at the pelvic outlet and surrounds the rectum, anus, and urogenital tracts, sustains considerable trauma during parturition. The results of trauma, severe bruising, and the occasional wound are more frequently encountered during delivery of an oversized or malpositioned fetus and from overzealous assistance during foaling. Most wounds tend to occur in the vaginal vestibule, which is the extension of the vagina caudal to the vaginovestibular junction. This sphincter-like junction is located at the cranial aspect of the transverse fold that covers the external urethral orifice. This fold continues dorsally as the hymen in the young mare. Most lacerations in the walls of the vestibule are generally not deep, heal rapidly with local therapy, and usually do not present a problem. However, the infrequent deep wound may lead to pelvic abscessation.

Lacerations that occur in the ceiling of the vestibule have the potential of causing subsequent reproductive problems. The extent of these problems depends on the severity of the wound and the tissues affected. These perineal lacerations are classified as follows:

1. *First-degree lacerations* involve the dorsal mucosa of the vestibule and the skin of the dorsal commissure of the vulva.
2. *Second-degree lacerations* involve the dorsal vestibular mucosa and submucosa, skin of the dorsal com-

missure of the vulva, and perineal body musculature, including the constrictor vulvae.

3. *Third-degree lacerations* involve the ceiling of the vestibule, perineal septum and musculature, floor of the rectum, and anal sphincter.
4. *Rectovestibular fistulas* involve the dorsal aspect of the vestibule, a variable amount of perineal septum and musculature, and the floor of the rectum.

FIRST-DEGREE LACERATIONS

First-degree perineal lacerations and other minor vulvar lacerations can be repaired in the acute state or after the inflammation has subsided using Caslick's operation. Vulvar lacerations result if previously placed Caslick's procedures are not opened prior to foaling. For the Caslick's procedure, the labial margins are infiltrated with local anesthetic solution and, if the margins are not fresh, a narrow strip is removed from the dorsal half of the labial margins and the dorsal commissure itself. The edges of the labia are then sutured together from the dorsal commissure down to approximately 1 cm below the level of the pelvic floor using 2-0 suture material in a continuous interlocking pattern. Monofilament suture material is theoretically ideal; however, most suture materials are acceptable. The sutures are removed about 12 days after placement.

SECOND-DEGREE LACERATIONS

The raw tissues on each side of the recently disrupted perineal body will usually epithelialize rather than bridge and heal together. This leaves a large defect in the perineal body, results in a sunken appearance of the dorsal aspect of the vulva, and predisposes to aspiration of air and fecal material into the reproductive tract. These lacerations may be repaired immediately after their occurrence. However, delay in performing surgery on traumatized, contaminated, edematous tissue is usually a prudent decision. This enables the tissues to heal and the mare to be bred before the surgery is performed as an elective procedure. A simple Caslick's procedure is not adequate to repair these lacerations because this still leaves a sunken perineum. The perineal body needs to be reconstructed.

This surgery can be performed under local anesthesia or subsequent to an epidural with the mare standing in stocks. An incision from the dorsal commissure ventrally is made along the mucocutaneous junction of each labial margin to a point slightly below the level of the pelvic floor. The labia are then retracted and an incision is made from a point on the dorsal midline of the vestibule along the wall of the vestibule, angling down to the ventral extent of the vulvar margin incision. This creates a large, folded-over triangle of mucosa, with the base along the mucocutaneous junction of the vulva and the apex located cranially in the ceiling of the vestibule. The length of this triangular piece is determined by how much tissue is involved in the second-degree laceration. The mucosa in the triangle is then excised, leaving exposed submucosa. The left and right edges of vestibular mucosa are sutured together with 2-0 polyglactin 910 (Vicryl; Ethicon Inc) or polydioxanone (PDS; Ethicon Inc) in a continuous horizontal mattress pattern inverting the mucosa into the vestibule. The left and right exposed submucosa are apposed with several interrupted sutures of size 1 polyglactin 910 or polydioxanone. The skin is closed as for the Caslick's procedure.

Pre- and postoperative administration of antibiotics is indicated for this surgery. Natural breeding should be delayed for 4 weeks to allow adequate time for healing.

THIRD-DEGREE LACERATIONS AND RECTOVESTIBULAR FISTULAS

Third-degree lacerations and rectovestibular fistulas are more commonly seen in the primiparous mare. The forefoot of the fetus may catch on the dorsal aspect of the sphincter-like vaginovestibular junction and with continued expulsion be driven through the dorsum of the vestibule and into the rectum. If this is corrected by manual assistance or spontaneously, the result is a rectovestibular fistula. If not corrected, the expulsive efforts of delivery result in a third-degree laceration. Extensive wounds that penetrate the vaginal wall cranial to the vaginovestibular junction and enter the peritoneal cavity are rare. These wounds require immediate attention with closure of the vaginal perforation to reduce the subsequent peritonitis and to prevent evisceration. These wounds may not be found at foaling and may present at a later date when the mare exhibits signs of peritonitis.

Preoperative Considerations

Surgical repair when the injury is acute is seldom successful. The subsequent tissue inflammation, edema, devitalization, and bacterial contamination create a poor environment for proper healing. If immediate repair is attempted, it should be performed within the first few hours after injury. The wound edges should be adequately cleaned and any devitalized and grossly contaminated tissue débrided prior to repair of the wound. Delayed wound repair is recommended.

Daily cleansing of the wound during the first week is beneficial and ensures examination of this area for potential complications. Administration of antibiotics and nonsteroidal anti-inflammatory medication is appropriate for 3 to 5 days and current tetanus prophylaxis is mandatory. A minimum of 2 to 4 weeks delay in repair is necessary to allow for resolution of the inflammation, wound margin epithelialization, and wound contracture. The dimensions of the third-degree laceration will decrease significantly during this period. The size of a rectovestibular fistula also dramatically decreases during this period, leading to spontaneous closure in rare cases.

If dystocia resulted in a live foal, delaying the repair until weaning should be considered. It is ideal for the surgeon to have direct control over the mare's diet for a few days pre- and postoperatively. This may involve hospitalization of the mare and foal, thus restricting their exercise and exposing them to hospital infections and other hazards. Also, management of the mare's diet may temporarily adversely affect lactation. If the surgery is not delayed, it may be performed as early as 2 to 4 weeks after the injury.

Soft feces are extremely important to the success of the repair. Several different feeding and laxative regimens have been successfully used, including lush green grass, pelleted rations, bran mashes, magnesium sulfate, mineral oil, and dioctyl sodium sulfosuccinate (DSS). What works to soften the feces in one mare may not work in another. Changes in diet should occur during a 3 to 5-day period, avoiding an abrupt change. The most ideal diet to produce soft, semiformed feces, is lush, green grass with mineral oil administered as needed. If lush grass is not available, the following regimen has a fairly consistent result. Gradually discontinue feeding hay and change to a pelleted ration. Provide a bran mash with sweet feed and mineral oil twice daily. Administer magnesium sulfate (0.5 to 1 g/kg) dissolved in 2 gallons of water once daily via a nasogastric tube. On alternate days, DSS in water is administered. When the feces are of proper consistency (soft and semiformed), the mare is fasted 24 hours prior to surgery to reduce the amount of fecal passage in the operative and immediate postoperative period. Prolonged fasting to empty the intestinal tract is unnecessary, and may predispose to enteritis. Antibiotics and nonsteroidal anti-inflammatory medications are administered pre- and postoperatively. These medications may help decrease the immediate postoperative inflammation and swelling and lessen the mare's tendency to strain. Although the surgery has been successful without the use of antibiotics, the inevitable contamination of the surgery site justifies the use of penicillin in these cases. This appears to be beneficial even though it is not effective against gram-negative organisms.

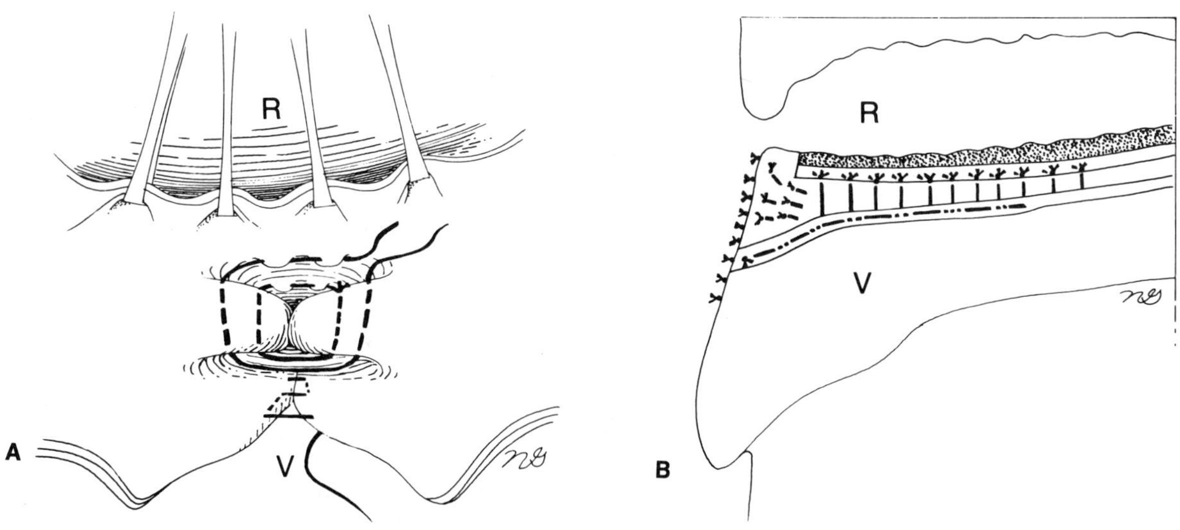

Figure 137–1. A. The rectal pull-back technique used in repair of third-degree perineal lacerations. Shown are suture placement and Allis tissue forceps grasping the rectal floor. *R*, rectum; *V*, vestibule. **B.** The rectal pull-back technique, depicting a sagittal view of the finished surgery. *R*, rectum; *V*, vestibule. (From Embertson RM, Robertson JT: Parturient perineal and rectovestibular injuries, in Robinson NE (ed): *Current Therapy in Equine Medicine*, ed 2. Philadelphia, WB Saunders Co, 1987, pp 550–555.)

Preparation

The mare is tranquilized with acetylpromazine and then positioned in stocks for surgery. A trustworthy and patient handler of the mare should be enlisted at this time to lessen the anxiety level of both the mare and the surgeon during potentially lengthy procedures. The tail is bandaged and a site clipped and prepared for epidural anesthesia. Epidural administration of 85 mg of xylazine, diluted to 10 ml with sterile saline, or of 6 ml of 2% lidocaine should provide adequate regional anesthesia for a 450-kg mare for about 2 hours. Xylazine produces less hind limb ataxia than lidocaine and so is preferable. A larger volume of 2% lidocaine may produce significant hind limb ataxia, paralysis of a hind limb, or even recumbency. Generally a stout tail rope tied to the top crossbar of the stocks will help with those mares that become very ataxic or paralyzed in one limb. Mares that become recumbent, if quiet, should be removed from the stocks and kept comfortable until they can stand. Recumbent mares that are uncontrollably frightened may require general anesthesia and use of a recovery stall. Although positioning becomes a problem, the surgical procedure can be completed in dorsal or ventral recumbency under general anesthesia, if this is considered necessary.

While the epidural anesthetic is taking effect, the tail is tied securely to the top crossbar of the stocks to remove it from the surgical field and to provide support for the potentially ataxic mare. Feces are then removed from the rectum and the immediate surgical site and surrounding area are prepared for surgery with a nonirritating surgical scrub [e.g., chlorhexidene (Nolvasan, Aveco Inc)]. The perineal region can be checked with a sharp needle for loss of sensation. If some feeling is still present, the surgery is postponed until the epidural takes effect. If the epidural does not produce the desired effect, the surgery can be performed with local anesthesia and additional sedation with xylazine and butorphanol tartrate (Torbugesic, Bristol Labs).

Balfour retractors (tied to the tail head) or stay sutures can be used to provide retraction of tissues and aid in exposure. A surgical light or a head lamp worn by the surgeon provides illumination of the surgical site.

Third-Degree Laceration Repair

Successful repair depends on careful preparation of the patient, attention to basic surgical principles, and good postoperative care. The suture material used is the choice of the surgeon; however, it should be of sufficient strength and should cause minimal tissue reaction. Hand ties and surgeon's knots are necessary to snuggly place primary sutures approximately 1 cm apart, thus producing firm tissue apposition. This is aided by adequate dissection, enabling the tissues to be apposed with minimal tension. Loosely placed sutures lead to poor tissue apposition, fistulation, and possible dehiscence. Sutures must not penetrate the rectal mucosa because this provides a path for fecal contamination to the depths of the repair and may increase rectal irritation, leading to more straining.

A variety of surgical techniques have been successfully used to repair third-degree perineal lacerations. Although most techniques use a variety of interrupted sutures, continuous sutures appropriately placed have also been used successfully. Following the above principles of surgical repair, the two surgical techniques described below will usually provide consistent, successful results. These techniques are the rectal pull-back technique and the six-bite vertical suture pattern.

The dissection is similar for both techniques; however, the rectal pull-back technique requires a more extensive cranial dissection. The intact portion of rectovestibular shelf is incised on a horizontal plane cranially for 2 to 8 cm, the depth determined by the surgical technique planned. The incision is directed caudally, on each side of the junction of the rectal and vestibular mucosa, and continued to the cutaneous perineum. The tissue flaps created should be of equal thickness for the rectal pull-back technique. The flaps should be thicker on the rectal side than the vestibular side if the six-bite vertical suture pattern is used.

The *rectal pull-back technique* (Fig. 137–1) commences with long Allis tissue forceps or stay sutures placed in the rectal submucosa along the caudal margin of the dissected rectal shelf. The dissection should be adequate to allow the rectal floor to be pulled caudally to the level of the anal sphincter. The rectovestibular septum is reconstructed by placing size 2 polyglactin 910 sutures in an interrupted pursestring pattern, starting at the most cranial aspect of the dissection and continuing caudally. The tissue incorporated in each suture includes (in order): right perivestibular tissue, right vestibular submucosa, left vestibular submucosa, left perivestibular tissue, left rectal submucosa, and right rectal submucosa. With each suture, the rectal floor is retracted caudally before the rectal submucosal bites are placed. This fixes the rectal tissue in the retracted state. The suture does not penetrate either the rectal or vestibular mucosa. The purse string pattern is continued caudally about one third of the length of the laceration. A continuous horizontal mattress pattern is then placed in the edges of the vestibular flaps using size 0 polyglactin 910. This pattern inverts the edges of the vestibular flaps into the vestibule and is continued to the point at which the pursestring pattern ended. It is then tied, and the remainder left in the vestibule until needed again. In this manner the two suture patterns are alternated.

The primary pattern is continued to the anal sphincter. The vestibular mucosal pattern is continued to the point where the perineal body reconstruction should start. If the intact rectal floor cannot be pulled caudally to the anal sphincter, the pursestring pattern is continued past the caudal edge of the intact rectal floor to the cutaneous perineum. This creates a floor of apposing submucosa of the remaining left and right rectal mucosa. The perineal body reconstructon (i.e., dissection, mucosal resection, and tissue apposition) is performed as explained for a second-degree perineal laceration. The monofilament, absorbable characteristics of polydioxanons make it a more appropriate suture for this environment; however, the handling characteristics of polyglactin 910 are preferred for this surgery.

The *six-bite vertical suture pattern repair* (Fig. 137–2) has been previously described using nonabsorbable, noncapillary, synthetic suture material. If the previously described principles of a repair are strictly adhered to, the suture material can be the surgeon's preference. At least size 2 suture material should be used. Each suture is knotted in the vestibule, leaving long ends for easy removal in 14 days. The first bite starts in the vestibule and is placed deep through the left vestibular flap, emerging in the plane of dissection. The second bite is placed through the left rectal flap, emerging just below the rectal mucosa. The third bite is placed in the right rectal flap, emerging in the plane of dissection. The fourth bite goes deep through the right vestibular flap, emerging in the vestibule. The fifth bite is placed up through the right vestibular flap near its edge and the sixth bite is placed down through the left vestibular flap near its edge and emerging in the vestibule. The suture is tied by hand under tension, which will appose the rectal flaps and invert the vestibular flaps into the vestibule. This pattern is started in the cranial pocket created in the rectovestibular septum by dissection and continued caudally to the point where the perineal body reconstruction should start. At this point the repair is continued as explained for the rectal pull-back technique.

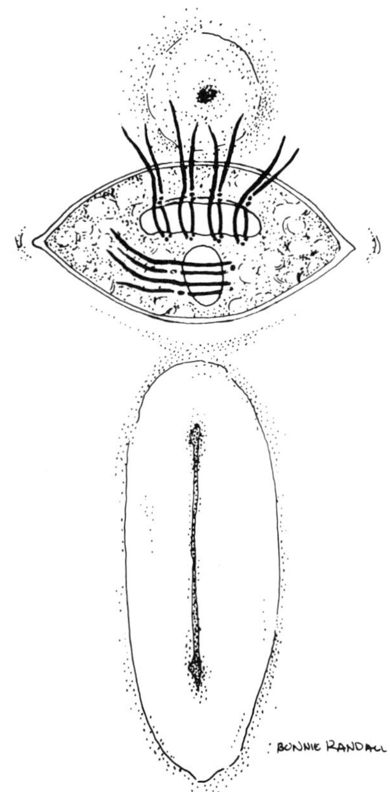

Figure 137–3. The horizontal perineal approach to repair of a rectovestibular fistula. Suture placement is shown. (From Embertson RM, Robertson JT: Parturient perineal and rectovestibular injuries, in Robinson NE (ed): *Current Therapy in Equine Medicine*, ed 2. Philadelphia, WB Saunders Co, 1987, pp 550–555.)

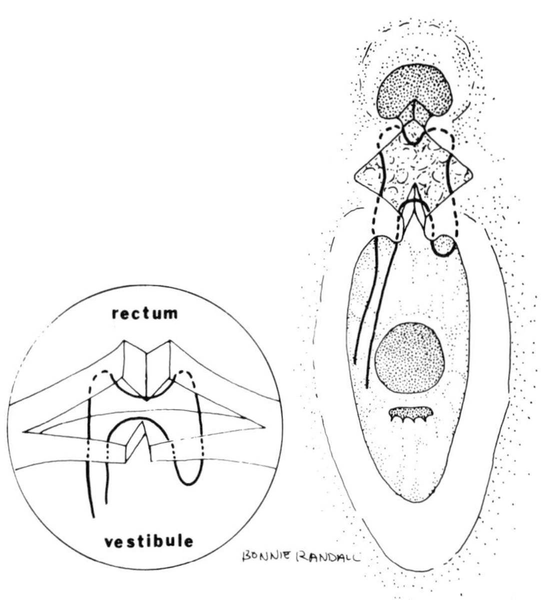

Figure 137–2. The six-bite vertical suture pattern used in repair of third-degree perineal lacerations. Suture placement is shown. (From Embertson RM, Robertson JT: Parturient perineal and rectovestibular injuries, in Robinson NE (ed): *Current Therapy in Equine Medicine*, ed 2. Philadelphia, WB Saunders Co, 1987, pp 550–555.)

Rectovestibular Fistula Repair

Different techniques have been used to repair rectovestibular fistulas with varying degrees of success. Creation and repair of a third-degree laceration is generally not recommended unless there is just a narrow strip of perineal tissue seperating the anus and vulva. Although this wound is technically a rectovestibular fistula, it is essentially a third-degree laceration and should be repaired as such. The following described horizontal perineal approach has produced consistent results.

The horizontal perineal approach (Fig. 137–3) requires a horizontal perineal incision midway between the anus and vulva. Dissection through the rectovestibular septum is performed carefully so that no perforations are made into the rectum or vestibule. The dissection is continued around each side of the fistula to a point 3 to 4 cm cranial to it. At that point the fistula is incised along the junction of the rectal and vestibular mucosa.

The principle lines of stress in the rectal wall occur at right angles to its longitudinal axis. Fistulas closed along these lines (transversely) are subjected to less distracting forces than when closed against these lines of stress (longitudinally). Either size 2 polyglactin 910 or polydioxanone sutures are preplaced longitudinally in the rectal submucosa using an interrupted Lembert pattern. Starting in the middle and working toward each side, these sutures are tied to convert the fistula to a transverse closure and to invert the rectal mucosa into the rectum. The sutures must not perforate the rectal mucosa.

The vestibular side of the fistula is closed in a similar manner, inverting the vestibular mucosa into the vestibule, except the sutures can be placed transversely, creating a longitudinal closure. The longitudinal closure is used because it is an easier closure than the tranverse closure and the tension on the suture line of the vestibular side is much less than that in the rectum. The same suture material and size can be used in the vestibular repair. Alternatively, a simple continuous suture pattern may be used on this type of repair. The space created by dissection is then closed using an interrupted pursestring pattern and the cutaneous perineum is closed with simple interrupted sutures. Exposure is aided in this procedure by the use of Allis tissue forceps or stay sutures in the dorsal tissue of the dissection.

Postoperative Care

The mare should remain on the same diet and receive laxatives as needed to keep her feces soft for 2 weeks postoperatively. During this period, the mare can be turned out in a grass paddock assuming this does not change the character of her feces. Antibiotics and nonsteroidal anti-inflammatory medications are continued for 3 to 5 days postoperatively. Excessive examination of the surgical site should be avoided. Only in the case of an impacted rectum should the rectum be manually evacuated or enemas administered.

An impaction in the rectum is the most common complication encountered between 24 and 72 hours following surgery. This is most likely due to the pain associated with defecation. This may cause significant straining by the mare and place undue tension on the suture line with potential dehiscence of the repair. Prevention is the best treatment. However, if a rectal impaction does occur, manual evacuation of feces and laxative therapy is indicated. Pelvic irritation and straining have been associated both pre- and postoperatively with urinary bladder eversion, bladder rupture, and even evisceration through a rent in the bladder. These complications obviously require prompt attention. Heavy tranquilization and placement of a tracheostomy tube to prevent straining may be of help while repairing these complications.

The reproductive tract can be examined in about 2 weeks to check for the results of the repair and obtain a uterine culture. If the reproductive tract is healthy, artificial insemination can be performed about 3 weeks after surgery. Natural breeding should not occur until about 3 weeks after surgery for small rectovestibular fistulas, and 8 weeks after surgery for larger rectovestibular fistulas and third degree perineal lacerations.

Prognosis

The prognosis for conception in mares with repaired perineal lacerations and rectovestibular fistulas is good. Concurrent vaginitis or endometritis usually resolves during the first postoperative estrus, following appropriate treatment as necessary. Additional severe perineal injuries at subsequent foalings do occur but, with attendance and proper care at foalings, are not common.

BIBLIOGRAPHY

Embertson RM, Robertson JT: Parturient perineal and rectovestibular injuries, in Robinson NE (ed) *Current Therapy in Equine Medicine*, ed 2. Philadelphia, WB Saunders Co, 1987, pp 550–555.

Haynes DF, McClure JR: Eversion of the urinary bladder: A sequel to third-degree perineal laceration in the mare. *Vet Surg* 1980;9:66–71.

Stickle RL, Fessler JF, Adams SB: A single-stage technique for repair of rectovestibular lacerations in the mare. *Vet Surg* 1979;8:25–27.

Turner AS, McIlwraith CW: Aanes' method of repair of third-degree perineal laceration, in *Techniques in Large Animal Surgery*. Philadelphia, Lea & Febiger, 1982, pp 177–182.

Vaughan JT: Equine urogenital system, in Jennings PB (ed): *The Practice of Large Animal Surgery*. Philadelphia, WB Saunders Co, 1984, pp 1122–1150.

Walker DF, Vaughan JT: Surgery of the perineum, vagina, and rectum, in *Bovine and Equine Urogenital Surgery*. Philadelphia, Lea & Febiger, 1980, pp 196–216.

138
Ovariectomy

Walter R. Threlfall

Ovariectomy in the mare may be performed as an elective procedure to remove both ovaries from animals not intended for breeding purposes or may be indicated in certain abnormal conditions involving one ovary. This discussion will describe the considerations and indications for surgery, the options available to the surgeon, and the indications and complications for the various approaches.

Irregular estral activity is normal during the early and late stages of the breeding season. It is only when these irregularities are prolonged or clinical examination indicates other than normal findings for the time of year should this estral activity be considered abnormal. Conservative therapy with progestational preparations such as altrenogest (Regu-Mate, Hoechst Roussel) generally is the preferred therapy because most mares respond to this treatment. Bilateral ovariectomy should be considered for those animals not to be maintained for breeding purposes with chronic or recurrent problems of prolonged estrus and associated behavioral problems.

Objectionable signs demonstrated by many mares during normal, frequent or prolonged estrus related by owners include frequent squealing, increased tail switching, winking, frequent squatting and urination, uncontrollability when ridden, pressing or leaning against people or objects, striking, kicking, and other undesirable or dangerous behavioral patterns that do not exist when the mares are not in estrus. The histopathologic findings of ovaries from mares exhibiting this type of behavior are frequently normal.

The clientele that most often request information regarding ovariectomy are the parents of youth who show mares that have major undesirable changes in disposition during estrus. The most important consideration to be made is that the clients realize the effects of the surgery will be permanent. I recommend that the examination of the mare and discussion of possible surgical intervention be made on one visit and that a few days be allowed to elapse before the surgery is performed. This delay permits the owners to have the opportunity to discuss and think about their decision. Horses maintained only for pleasure riding and animals of poor genetic quality can be ovariectomized to prevent the nuisance of estral signs and the future production of offspring.

Another reason for ovariectomizing mares is the successful use of these animals as recipients for embryo transfers. The mares are placed on altrenogest therapy beginning on the donor mare's last day of estrus. This treatment is continued until day 100 of gestation, at which time the placenta is capable of maintaining the pregnancy.

Nymphomania is a condition of fillies and mares in which the attitude changes dramatically and the animals become vicious and aggressive. Although this condition is not fully understood, it appears more likely to be an abnormality involving organs other than the ovary, such as the adrenal and/or brain. Therefore, ovariectomy is not recommended for the true nymphomaniac mare unless an abnormal ovary is found (see Chapter 139).

CAUSES OF ENLARGED OVARIES

Persistent Follicles

The ovary may appear to be abnormally large early in the physiologic breeding season because of the presence of multiple persistent follicles. An equine ovary is considered to be abnormally enlarged if it exceeds 12.5 cm in diameter, because a normal mature follicle can be this large. Care must be taken not to erroneously consider these normal ovaries as being either cystic or neoplastic. Since the size of such ovaries may exceed the 12.5-cm limit, a hasty decision might be made to remove the ovary. Consequently, a thorough initial examination and a repeat examination are indicated. If there is any doubt as to the presence of persistent follicles being responsible for the enlarged ovary, placing the mare on progestogen therapy for 15 to 30 days is indicated followed by re-examination.

Parovarian Cysts

Parovarian cysts may be a diagnostic challenge if they are large and located close to the ovary. These cysts are not considered to affect fertility and, therefore would not justify ovariectomy. Large parovarian cysts are rare, and are not normally confused with the ovary on palpation.

Hematomas

Although ovulation is frequently followed by bleeding into the follicular cavity, occasionally the hemorrhage continues and a hematoma forms within the ovary. These do not generally exceed the 12.5-cm limit of the normal ovary. Surgery to remove an ovary with a hematoma is generally not indicated, since smaller hematomas resolve spontaneously and normal cyclic activity continues. Extremely large hematomas may result in destruction of the germinal tissue within the ovary and produce a small, firm, nonfunctional ovary that can be left in place. If the diagnosis is not possible by palpation and ultrasonography, progestogen therapy has been beneficial in preventing further follicular development and ovulation from occurring while the ovary returns to a smaller size.

Ovarian Abscess

Ovarian abscesses have apparently decreased in number following a reduction in needle insertions into equine ovaries to drain "cysts" and inject luteinizing hormone preparations. Hematogenous spread of bacteria to the ovary is possible but apparently uncommon. Abscesses within the ovary are localized and do not cause systemic signs of illness unless the infection spreads from within the ovarian tunic. Abscessation of the ovary is an indication for its removal.

Ovarian Tumors

The ovulation fossa generally cannot be detected when ovarian tumors are present because the fossa is obliterated as the ovary increases in size. This has been observed to occur in ovaries with granulosa cell tumors of 7 cm in diameter or larger. Ovarian tumors reportedly include the granulosa-theca cell tumor, teratoma, adenoma, adenocarcinoma, dysgerminoma, arrhenoblastoma, fibroma, fibrosarcoma leiomyoma, hemangioendothelioma, lymphosarcoma, and melanoma. The most commonly occurring ovarian tumor is the granulosa cell tumor.

The fertility of mares that have had granulosa cell tumors removed is excellent if the tumor was the only reproductive abnormality. In the case of broodmares with granulosa cell tumors and poor or unknown reproductive histories, it is always advisable to perform a breeding soundness examination prior to surgery to determine if the surgery will be worthwhile.

TREATMENT CONSIDERATIONS

The primary consideration upon diagnosis of an enlarged ovary is whether to do an ovariectomy. Because the removal of a normal ovary from a broadmare is ill-advised and because of possible postsurgical complications, the necessity of the surgery should be established before this procedure is performed. The decision to remove an ovary will be aided by a complete and accurate reproductive history of the mare. This should include information about previous estral activity, breedings, pregnancies, and foaling plus personality or behavioral changes. Palpation of both ovaries for size and consistency will be of value. The presence of one large ovary and one nonfunctional ovary would suggest that suppressing hormones are being produced by the larger ovary. The presence of the ovulation fossa can be of value in determining how large the ovary has become and how much intraovarian expansion has occurred. Ultrasonography can be of value in determining the structure of the deeper aspects of the ovarian tissue.

The evaluation of enlarged ovaries should be repeated at 2-week to 2-month intervals if any doubt remains as to whether the ovary should be removed. Since ovarian tumors have an extremely low probability of metastasis and their rate of growth is slow, the delay required to be certain of the diagnosis will not be detrimental to the outcome, if it is decided after reevaluation that surgery is indicated.

If the decision to remove one ovary from a broodmare is made, it should have been made following a complete diagnostic examination. Removal of ovaries from mares without proper indications exposes the animal to the risks of surgery and postoperative complications without justification. Reports exist substantiating the removal of ovaries that probably was not necessary. In one report of 30 ovariectomies, it appeared that 10 of the surgeries were possibly not indicated. Two of these 10 mares died from surgery or complications thereof.

Progestational Hormone Treatment

The treatment of mares having enlarged ovaries with progestogen preparations may aid in reducing ovarian size by preventing further follicular development and ovulations. As described earlier, this may be of value when persistant follicles and hematomas are suspected. This form of treatment obviously would not influence the size of an ovarian tumor or abscess.

Hormonal Assays

Granulosa cell tumors and arrhenoblastomas may cause an elevation in serum testosterone. However, horses with granulosa cell tumors may also have minimal elevations in serum testosterone. Palpation of the ovary for consistency and size on two or more occasions and the use of ultrasonography have been of more value than endocrine assays when deciding whether to perform an ovariectomy.

Ultrasonography

Ultrasonography can be utilized to aid in the diagnosis of enlarged ovaries. The ultrasonic appearance of persistent follicles is similar to normal follicular structure except the number may be increased and they persist for many days without the normal enlargement of one or two follicles and regression of the others. Hematomas, on the other hand, produce echogenic bands within the clot that correspond to fibrinous tissue.

Granulosa cell tumors are composed of multiple fluid-filled areas separated by thin bands of tissue. This multicystic appearance is characteristic of the granulosa cell tumor. This appearance is different from that of persistent follicles. Echogenic dense tissue within the ovary could indicate the presence of bone or teeth and thus the presence of a teratoma. I do not recommend ovarian biopsies because of the possible presence of an abscess.

SURGICAL APPROACH

The surgical approach to be used is selected based on the mare's disposition, presence of reproductive tract infection, available instruments, facilities, ovarian size, surgical experience of the veterinarian, cost of the procedure, and length of the recovery period. The surgical approaches possible for ovariectomy include colpotomy, standing and recumbent flank grid, and paramedian or ventral midline incision. The approaches for the paramedian and ventral midline incisions are discussed in Chapter 139.

The disposition of the mare in itself may eliminate the possibility of a standing procedure. The mare must be tractable. Mares that tend to be extremely nervous or apprehensive many times do not respond as predictably to tranquilizers, analgesics, or sedatives as do calmer animals. It is imperative with either the standing vaginal or flank approach that the mare remain stationary during the procedure.

Infectious conditions of the uterus, cervix, and vagina eliminate the vaginal approach because of the potential for introduction of bacteria into the peritoneal cavity both during and after surgery. If abnormal discharges are observed from the mare's cervix or vulva, the cause should be determined and specific treatment administered to correct the problem before surgery, or another approach should be utilized.

If the vaginal approach or a bilateral ovariectomy from a standing flank is to be performed, the availability of a chain ecraseur is essential. With these two techniques, ligation of the ovarian arteries is difficult or impossible. The lack of a chain ecraseur may be reason in itself to perform the surgery with the mare under general anesthesia. This technique will faciliate exposure of vessels for ligation.

The facilities available may also dictate the surgical approach. Stocks, although not essential for the standing vaginal approach, are strongly recommended. It is possible to perform this technique with the mare in certain types of horse trailers or positioned such that her rear quarters are in a stall doorway. However, this is not recommended because of possible injury to the handler or mare, the freedom of mare movement, and the lack of protection provided to the surgeon. Facilities for general anesthesia, such as anesthetic machines and monitoring equipment, plus assistants for positioning and recovery of the patient are necessary if recumbent procedures are to be employed.

The size of the ovary can also influence the surgical approach because of the restrictions in area imposed by the vaginal or flank grid approach. The maximal ovarian size recommended for removal through a colpotomy is 10 cm. This may be difficult or impossible in mares with a small pelvis. If functional ovaries are to be removed, the surgery should be performed when the mare does not have large follicles present, thus reducing the ovarian size. The maximal size of ovary removable through a flank grid incision is approximately 12.5 cm in an average 450-kg horse. Although larger ovaries can be removed through a flank incision, it is usually best to remove them through a ventral midline incision. However, if the ovary is positioned above the level of the pelvic brim, the flank approach is used.

The high cost of a procedure could influence some owners not to have mares ovariectomized, especially if the expense of general anesthesia and ventral midline closure are included. Conversely, the vaginal or grid flank approach may be within the budget of the client. The recovery time may also be of importance to owners during times of show, race, or other performance events. Colpotomy has the shortest recovery time, 7 days until exercise is started and 2 weeks under most circumstances until full exercise is reestablished. Grid flank approaches require approximately 3 weeks, incisional flank approaches require 4 to 6 weeks, and ventral midline approaches require 6 to 12 weeks.

Preoperative Preparation

The mare is maintained on her regular diet until the time of surgery. Prior to any of the surgical approaches, a clotting profile is performed. No antibiotics are utilized before, during, or following surgery unless indicated. A thorough rectal examination should be performed at sometime to determine the status of the reproductive tract and the location and size of the ovaries. The feces are not removed from the rectum immediately prior to surgery, nor is bladder distention evalu-

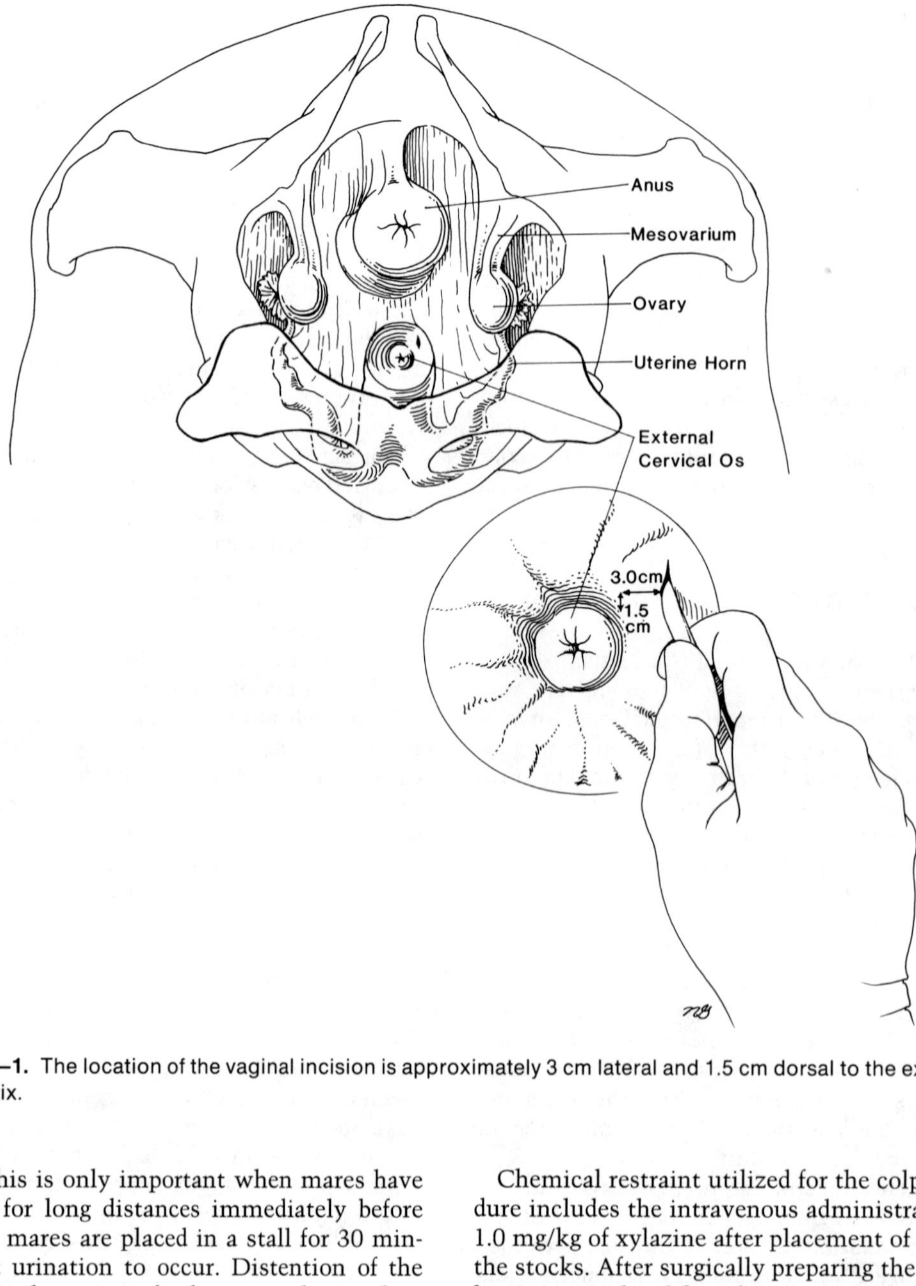

Figure 138–1. The location of the vaginal incision is approximately 3 cm lateral and 1.5 cm dorsal to the external os of the cervix.

ated because this is only important when mares have been trailered for long distances immediately before surgery. These mares are placed in a stall for 30 minutes to permit urination to occur. Distention of the bladder sufficiently to impede the surgical procedure has not been encountered.

Colpotomy

Restraint for colpotomy should include stocks to reduce the movement of the mare. It has been suggested that the mare be crosstied in the stocks, although I prefer to have the mare held by a handler at all times. A twitch is applied to the mare prior to the vaginal incision and is maintained in place until the surgery has been completed.

Chemical restraint utilized for the colpotomy procedure includes the intravenous administration of 0.8 to 1.0 mg/kg of xylazine after placement of the mare into the stocks. After surgically preparing the skin over the last two sacral and first three coccygeal vertebrae, a 22-gauge needle is used to infiltrate the skin and subcutaneous tissue with 2 mL of mepivacaine in the area of the first moveable coccygeal vertebrae. A 4.5-in 18-guage spinal needle is inserted nearly horizontal into the spinal canal and 5 mL of mepivacaine (Carbocaine-V, Winthrop Veterinary) is administered as an epidural. The use of abdominal support is not recommended because of the increased pressure placed on the viscera and the movement of this viscera into the pelvic inlet. Instead, a tail rope is placed over a support above the

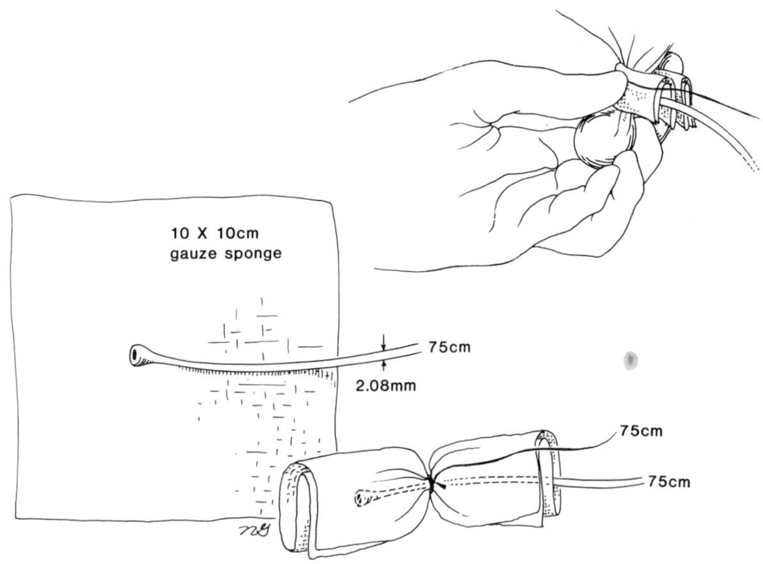

Figure 138–2. Polyethylene tubing with gauze sponges attached is used for anesthesia of mesovarium.

rear quarters of the mare and is used to support the mare if she becomes unsteady. The perineal area is thoroughly cleansed with detergent and then with an iodine surgical scrub. The vagina is cleansed with cotton, water, and an iodine solution, being certain to thoroughly rinse the iodine from the vagina. This reduces the bacterial content of the vagina while lubricating and causing distention of the vagina. Morphine (0.6 mg/kg) or butorphanol (Torbugesic, Bristol Labs, 0.2 to 0.4 mg/kg) is administered intravenously. The only noticeable difference is that mares given morphine remain more active following surgery and are less likely to lie down. Two surgical sponges soaked in mepivacaine are placed on the anterior vaginal wall where the incision will be made. These are left in place for 2 to 4 minutes.

The surgeon, wearing a sterile rubber sleeve and glove, carries a disposable number 10 scalpel blade with handle into the anterior vagina. If the surgeon normally performs rectal examinations left-handed, it is advisable to carry the blade in with the left hand. The vaginal incision should be made approximately 3 cm lateral and 1.5 cm dorsal to the external os of the cervix (Fig. 138–1). The incision should not be too close to the cervix because it may result in tearing of the cervix when blunt dissection is performed. The blade is thrust up a maximum of 2 cm through the vaginal wall with the cutting edge directed ventrally. The blade is removed and the hand is reinserted into the vagina. The index finger is forced through the incision. A second finger, then a third, a fourth, and finally the entire hand is inserted into the abdominal cavity. If the reflection of the peritoneum separates from the vaginal wall, the index finger can be used to hook it and pull it posteriorly until it tears.

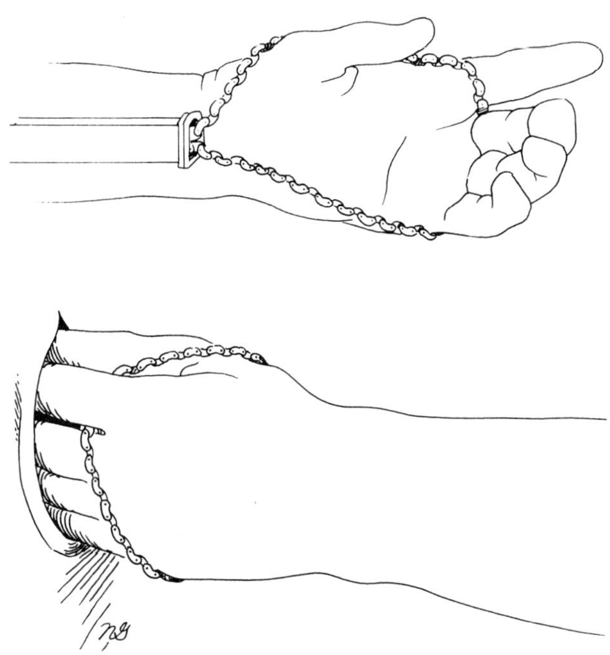

Figure 138–3. The chain ecraseur is carried into the abdominal cavity with all but the index finger within the loop of chain.

Alternatively, the vaginal incision may be made with a curved bistoury. The initial cut is made 4 cm ventrolateral to the external os, of the cervix. The cutting surface of the bistoury is initially directed ventrally but

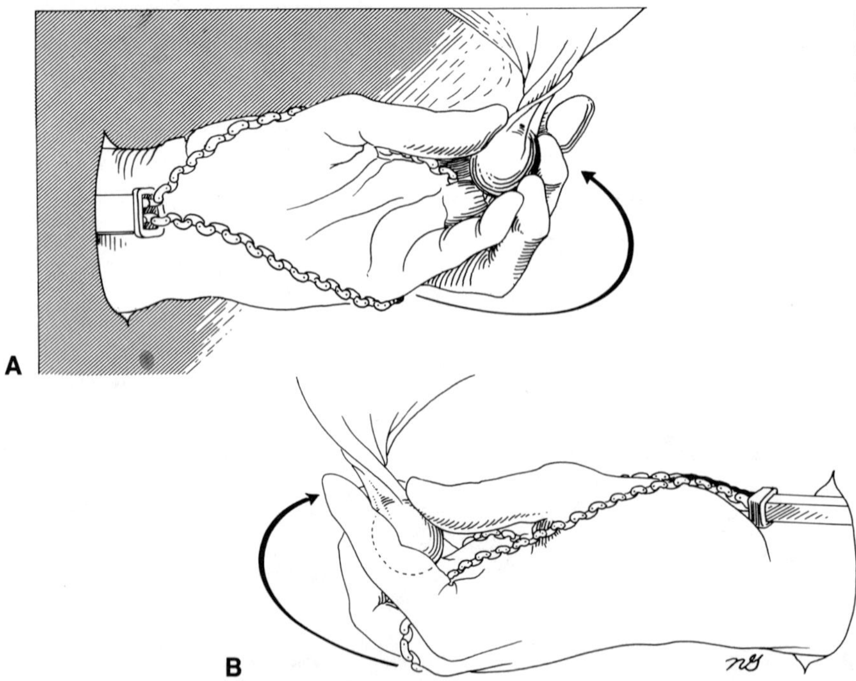

Figure 138–4. A. The chain is placed around the left ovary, being certain no other tissue is within the loop of chain. **B.** The chain is placed around the right ovary in a manner similar to that for the left ovary.

is then turned 180 degrees after the initial stab and used to continue the incision 2 cm dorsally.

To locate the ovaries, the uterus is grasped and followed from one ovary to the other. This procedure will prevent grasping a fecal ball or an ovary through the mesorectum. A gauze sponge with a 75-cm long polyethylene 240 tube (1.57-mm outer diameter, 2.08-mm inner diameter; Clay Adams) and a nonabsorbable suture of equal length attached is placed around the mesovarium to the ovary (Fig. 138–2). Thirty milliliters of mepivacaine is slowly infused around the mesovarium of the left ovary. The sponge is moved to the right ovary and another 30 mL of mepivacaine is infused around the mesovarium.

Once the mesovarium has been anesthetized, the Chassaignac chain ecraseur (Jorgensen Laboratories) is carried into the abdominal cavity with all but the index finger within the loop of the chain (Fig. 138–3). The left ovary is located as before and the chain placed around the mesovarium (Fig. 138–4A). The chain is closed slowly until it is snug around the mesovarium and the surgeon is certain no other structures are included within the loop of chain. The chain is then rapidly closed to remove the ovary. Some authors have recommended that the chain be closed slowly, taking up to 8 minutes to remove the ovary. I have found the slower closure increases the discomfort of the mare and does not control hemorrhage as well as the rapid closure method. The right ovary is removed similiarly (Fig. 138.4B). The vaginal incision is not sutured; however, a Caslick's procedure may be completed if there is any concern that the vulvar lips will allow movement of air in and out of the vagina. This technique has been used on over 120 mares during the past 16 years with no postoperative complications.

Another technique described for colpotomy involves general anesthesia. In this technique, the mare's tail is secured to a support and then a general anesthesia is induced with a combination of glyceryl guaiacolate and a barbiturate. The mare's head and sternum are positioned on the floor and the surgical procedure is performed as described above.

Colpotomy Postoperative Care. Complications following colpotomy can include hemorrhage from the mesovarium or other large vessels within the pelvis. The technique described herein will reduce the probability of incising other vessels during the initial vaginal stab incision. Some authors have recommended palpation of the mesovarium stump following removal of the ovary for pulsating blood and, if pulsations exist, a second use of the ecraseur is attempted. This is not recommended.

Postoperative care following colpotomy consists of no attempts to maintain the mare standing. The mare is stalled for 5 days with only controlled walking as exercise, if desired. Feed is available 5 hours following surgery and water is available immediately. The horse is continued on its normal ration. Light riding can resume 7 days following surgery with full training or performance resumed at 14 days.

Additional possible complications of colpotomy include death due to penetration of the rectum, bladder, or large vessels of the pelvis. Although some authors have recommended palpation of the mesovarium 2 to 3 days following surgery for the presence of adhesions or hematomas, this is not recommended. In cases in which follow-up was possible months following surgery, adhesions were absent or of no clinical significance. Hematomas of the mesovarium have been reported to occur. However, these are uncommon and usually are small. If large hematomas are present, the postoperative care is unchanged. Therefore, examination of the mesovarium is not recommended until 5 to 7 days following surgery, if at all.

Peritonitis can also occur following surgery and is usually present as a localized peritonitis. It can be infectious or inflammatory. No treatment is given for localized inflammatory peritonitis because no clinical signs are evident. More generalized peritonitis may cause a fever, abdominal pain with reluctance to move, and depression. Abdominal paracentesis will be of value in determining the extent of the peritonitis and instituting appropriate therapy. Peritonitis has not been a problem in the ovariectomies performed utilizing the previously described technique.

Standing Flank Procedure

Restraint for a standing flank procedure is similar to that for the vaginal approach in that stocks are desirable for control of movement. The anesthesia for a standing flank grid includes xylazine and morphine or butorphanol plus local skin and muscle infiltration with mepivacaine. The local application of mepivacaine on the mesovarium near the ovary is also performed. The removal of the ovary can be by ecraseur or by isolation of vessels and ligation. The mesovarium attachment to the ovary is ligated by separating it into thirds or fourths depending on vascular supply to the ovary, which will vary with size of the ovary. Absorbable material such as size 1 polyglactin 910 (Ethicon Inc) suture can be used. Observation is made for hemorrhage following removal of the ovary. Each of the muscle layers of the grid incision are apposed with synthetic absorbable sutures in a simple interrupted pattern and the skin is closed with simple interrupted sutures of size 0 or 2-0 nylon.

BIBLIOGRAPHY

Bosu WTK, Van Camp SC, Miller RB, Owen R: Ovarian disorders: Clinical and morphological observations in 30 mares. *Can Vet J* 1982;23:6–14.

Colbern GT, Reagan WJ: Ovariectomy by colptomy in mares. *Compend Cont Educ Pract Vet* 1987;9:1035–1039.

Frazer GS, Threlfall WR: Differential diagnosis for enlarged ovary in the mare. *Proc AAEP Ann Conven* 1986, pp 21–28.

Hughes JP, Kennedy PC, Palmer N: Pathology of the ovary and ovarian disorders in the mare, in *Proceedings of the 9th International Congress on Reproduction and Artificial Insemination.* Madrid, Spain, 1980, vol 1, pp 203–206.

Hughes JP, Stabenfeldt GH, Kennedy PC: The estrous cycle and selected functional and pathologic ovarian abnormalities in the mare. *Vet Clin North Am Large Anim Pract* 1980;2(2):225–231.

Moll HD, Slone DE, Juzwiak JS, Garrett PD: Diagonal paramedian approach for removal of ovarian tumors in the mare. *Vet Surg* 1987;16:456–458.

Pearson H, Pinsent PJN, Denny HR, Waterman A: The indications for equine laparotomy—an analysis of 140 cases. *Equine Vet J* 1975;7:131–136.

Scott EA, Kunze DJ: Ovariectomy in the mare: presurgical, surgical and postsurgical considerations. *J Equine Med Surg* 1977;1:5–12.

Stabenfeldt GH, Hughes JP: Diagnostic endocrinology of the horse. *Vet Clin North Am Large Anim Pract* 1980;2:253.

139
Granulosa Cell Tumor

David E. Freeman
Katrin Hinrichs

Granulosa cell tumors are the most common ovarian tumors in mares. They arise from the sex cord stroma that lines the ovulation fossa and they are generally benign. One malignant granulosa cell tumor was identifed in a review of 78 cases. The tumor may be comprised entirely of epithelioid, granulosa-type cells, or may also contain thecal-type cells. Tumors with both cell types are termed granulosa cell-theca cell tumors. The thecal-type cells may be referred to as Leydig cells (the male embryonic counterpart of the theca cell), especially in horses with elevated plasma testosterone levels. Granulosa cell tumors may be clinically indistinguishable from arrhenoblastomas, rare tumors in the mare that are thought to arise from male-differentiated embryonic sex cord stroma. Granulosa cell tumors occur in adult mares, although a juvenile granulosa cell tumor has been reported in a 3-month-old filly. A juvenile granulosa cell tumor can be distinguished from adult tumors by the age of the horse and their more aggressive histologic appearance.

Granulosa cell tumors are usually unilateral, although bilateral tumors have been reported. They may be found in mares of any age. The affected ovary is thick walled, firm, and smooth; the cut surface may be solid but usually consists of several cysts separated by thick fibrous trabeculae. Size of the tumor may range from that of a normal, active ovary to a massive growth, with the largest reported tumor weighing 59.1 kg. A distinctive feature of granulosa cell tumors is that the ovulation fossa, normally palpable on the ventral aspect of the ovary, is not present.

DIAGNOSIS

Mares with granulosa cell tumors are presented for a variety of reasons, most commonly behavioral changes or infertility. Behavioral changes are attributed to steroid production by the tumor and may include, with equal frequency, aggressive or stallion-like behavior, constant or erratic estrus, or anestrus. Overproduction of steroids by the granulosa cell tumor commonly causes suppression of the hypothalmic/pituitary axis, resulting in inactivity or atrophy of the contralateral ovary. This atrophy of the contralateral ovary is an important distinguishing feature of granulosa cell tumors. Plasma testosterone concentrations are reported to be elevated in 50 to 90% of cases of granulosa cell tumor, and testosterone levels relate somewhat to the type of behavior exhibited. Infertility is probably related to failure of normal ovarian activity. Infrequently, mares with granulosa cell tumors may cycle normally and even conceive, and granulosa cell tumors have been found in pregnant and postpartum mares. Mares with granulosa cell tumors rarely have abdominal pain, but this sign has been reported in mares with very large tumors and in a filly with a juvenile granulosa cell tumor strangulated in a volvulus around its attachments. Diabetes mellitus was reported in one mare in association with bilateral granulosa cell tumors and was tentatively attributed to altered carbohydrate metabolism in response to estrogen and progesterone released from the tumor.

The major differential diagnoses for ovarian enlargement are ovarian hematoma, normal ovarian activity, and other ovarian tumors such as teratoma, cystadenoma, or dysgerminoma. Ovarian abscesses are rare and are likely to be iatrogenic. Diagnosis is based on history, findings on rectal palpation, and plasma testosterone levels. A history of constant or irregular estrus, aggressive or stallion-like behavior, or anestrus concomitant with findings of an enlarged ovary without a palpable ovulation fossa and a small, inactive contralateral ovary are sufficient for diagnosis of granulosa cell tumor. Ovarian hematomas, abscesses, and other ovarian tumors should not affect behavior or cycling, obliterate the ovulation fossa, or be associated with atrophy of the contralateral ovary. Mares in spring transition may have prolonged estrus associated with enlarged ovaries, but the enlargement is usually bilateral, and the ovaries are palpably normal in shape, with multiple follicles causing the enlargement. Rectal ultrasonography may be helpful to differentiate normal follicular activity from changes in the ovarian stroma, or confirm lack of follicular activity in the contralateral ovary. These findings are not definitive. Elevated plasma testosterone levels aid in the diagnosis of granulosa cell tumor but may also occur in horses with cystadenoma. Ovarian abscesses and other ovarian tumors are, like granulosa cell tumors, best treated by surgical removal of the ovary.

TREATMENT

A granulosa cell tumor of approximately 8 to 10 cm in diameter can be removed through a colpotomy (see Chapter 138). A paralumbar, paramedian, or midline approach is required for larger tumors. A colpotomy and paralumbar approach can be performed using sedation to a degree determined by the temperament of the mare, and topical application of a local anesthetic to the ovarian pedicle.

Preoperative Preparation

The mare should be taken off feed for 24 to 48 hours, regardless of the proposed approach for removal of the ovary. Water can be allowed during this time. The purpose of fasting is to reduce the quantity of intestinal contents so that identification and manipulation of the ovary is facilitated. This practice also allows more complete exposure of the ovarian pedicle through abdominal incisions in the anesthetized horse. The size of the tumor should be assessed preoperatively by rectal palpation and by ultrasound examination so that a suitable surgical approach can be selected.

Surgical Approach

Paralumbar Approach. This approach is used for ovaries up to 15 cm in diameter and can be done with the mare standing, if her temperament permits. If the ovary is less than 10 cm in diameter, a grid approach can be used in which the fibers of the internal abdominal oblique muscle are separated. Because ovaries larger than 10 cm are difficult to remove through a grid incision, some or all muscle layers will have to be incised parallel with the skin incision. The incision should be placed high in the paralumbar fossa and extended ventrally, as determined by the size of the ovary. A caudodorsal-to-cranioventral incision facilitates exposure by allowing splitting of the internal oblique muscle as part of the incision. Traction on the ovary and transection of the pedicle are painful to the awake horse; therefore, the pedicle should be flushed beforehand with 2% lidocaine hydrochloride or swabbed with a gauze sponge soaked in local anesthetic solution.

The paralumbar approach allows limited access to the abdomen, especially in large mares with a thick layer of retroperitoneal fat. Another disadvantage of the paralumbar approach is that the exposed muscle edges can become severely traumatized during extraction of a large tumor, leading to a seroma or hematoma formation in the incision.

Paramedian Approach. For this approach, an incision is made 5 to 10 cm lateral to the midline over the involved ovary. The incision extends from 5 cm cranial to the mammary gland for 20 cm or longer, depending on the size of the ovary. Layers incised are skin, superficial fascia, occasionally a portion of the cutaneous trunci muscle, the external sheath of the rectus abdominis muscle (aponeuroses of the internal and external abdominal oblique muscles), the rectus abdominis muscle, the internal sheath of the rectus abdominis (aponeurosis of the transverse abdominal muscle), the retroperitoneal fat, and the peritoneum. The advantage of this approach is that the incision is made directly ventral to the involved ovary. However, any improvement in access is slight compared with the ventral midline celiotomy and is offset by some disadvantages. The layers incised are more numerous and more vascular than those encountered in the ventral midline celiotomy and it, therefore, requires more time for incision and closure. In addition, the edges of a paramedian incision are more rigid and hence more difficult to retract than are those of a ventral midline celiotomy.

The paramedian approach can be modified by directing the incision on a line from the mammary gland toward the cranial aspect of the flank fold so that the external oblique tunic fibers can be separated along natural planes of division (diagonal paramedian approach). With both types of paramedian approach, closure involves apposition of the rectus abdominis muscle with size 2 absorbable suture material in an interrupted pattern, followed by a simple continuous pattern in the external rectus sheath. It is not necessary to close the peritoneum and the internal rectus sheath.

An advantage of the diagonal paramedian approach is that the body wall is thinner and more flexible than in the flank so that the edges can be retracted to improve exposure. In addition, hemorrhage is less than with the regular paramedian incision because muscle layers are separated rather than transected. The largest ovary that has been removed through a diagonal paramedian approach is 20 cm in diameter, although proponents of this approach claim that it could be used for even larger ovaries.

Ventral Midline Celiotomy. This approach is preferable for removal of tumors larger than 15 cm in diameter. It can be used effectively whenever the enlarged ovary is level with or is felt ventral to the pelvic brim during the rectal examination. Compared with other approaches, it allows greater exposure, involves fewer tissue layers, is associated with less incisional hemorrhage, and can be completed and closed more rapidly. The incision is usually started 5 cm cranial to the mammary gland and extended along the midline as needed. Exposure of ovarian vessels can be enhanced by retracting the edges of the incision with Balfour or Finnochietto self-retaining retractors; however, these instruments cannot be used with very large tumors because the blades cannot be opened sufficiently to allow extraction of the ovary between them.

Removal of the Ovary

The ovary can be partly or completely exteriorized through all approaches except the colpotomy. When the ovary has been located, it is grasped by cupping both hands beneath it and gently drawing it to the incision. It is then pried through the incision by pressing upward on its deepest surface and pressing downward on the upper and lower commissures of the incision with the back of the hand and wrist. Some surgeons exteriorize the ovary by placing wide stay sutures through its capsule and applying traction to these. The assistant surgeon can facilitate exteriorization by retracting the edges of the abdominal incision and then pressing them beneath the ovary.

In some horses, the ovarian pedicle is short and exteriorization is difficult. To overcome this difficulty, even in mares under general anesthesia, some surgeons recommend topical application of local anesthetic agent to the pedicle. When the anesthetic takes effect, sufficient relaxation can be gained to facilitate exteriorization of the ovary. A large ovary with several cystic spaces can be reduced in size by aspiration of its fluid contents. However, complete decompression of the ovary makes it difficult to pry it from the abdomen and to manipulate it for exposure of the vessels.

The most critical step in ovariectomy is division of the enlarged branches of the ovarian artery and the associated plexus of veins. If the ovarian attachments and the mesovarium are enlarged, as they are in most tumors, they can be carefully incised to allow better exposure of the enclosed vessels. Adhesion from the mesovarium and the distal horn of the uterus to the surface of the tumor, if present, must be broken down also to facilitate exteriorization and to provide better exposure of the vessels.

Several methods can be used for transection of the ovarian pedicle and vessels. The ecraseur can be used with small ovaries and is ideal for ovariectomy through a colpotomy because the ovary is not exteriorized with this approach. The fingers and thumb of one hand are inserted through the chain loop of the ecraseur and used to grasp the ovary. The chain is then advanced over the fingers and thumb and slowly tightened, making certain that only the pedicle of the ovary is included. Ideally, the ecraseur should not be applied to the pedicle under tension because vessels severed in this way may bleed when they retract into the abdomen. Small ovaries can be removed also by transecting their attachments with either a Serra or a Reimer emasculater. After the pedicle has been severed by the emasculater, the instrument is left in place and used to manipulate the vessels proximal to the crushed ends so that they can be ligated.

The thoracoabdominal 90-mm (TA 90) stapling instrument (Auto-Suture; United States Surgical Corporation) has proven to be highly reliable as a means of occluding transected vessels, especially in large ovarian tumors or in tumors that cannot be exteriorized sufficiently for ligation. The stapler is applied across the full width of the ovarian pedicle and activated to place a double row of staggered staples (Fig. 139–1). The instrument is left in position so that it can be used to manipulate the ovarian stalk. Transfixation ligatures with size 2 absorbable suture should be applied across the full width of the stalk proximal to the stapler, each ligature incorporating sufficient tissue to ligate all large vessels completely. If an insufficient amount of the pedicle can be exposed for satisfactory placement of ligatures, another double row of staples can be applied above or below the first row. The pedicle is then grasped with Allis tissue forceps and is transected with a scalpel along the edge of the stapling instrument.

After the ovary has been removed, all severed arteries and veins are inspected for bleeding and any large vessel that continues to bleed is ligated. The ovary and stump should be inspected also to ensure that all ovarian tumor and capsule are removed. The severed stump can be oversewn with an absorbable suture material to cover exposed cut surfaces and thus to reduce the risk of adhesions. However, this step does not appear to be essential and is not recommended. When the ovary is removed without being exteriorized, as with the colpotomy approach, the severed pedicle cannot be inspected for bleeding.

Special Precautions

Special care should be taken to occlude all vessels in the severed ovarian stalk. Successful ovariectomy is also determined by careful preoperative assessment of the patient and an accurate determination of the tumor size. The latter is most important for helping with the selection of the surgical approach, but the full extent of large tumors can be difficult to assess. If there is doubt about tumor size, but a large tumor is suspected, a ventral midline approach should be used. Special care must be taken with the midline incision to ensure that the skin of the udder is thoroughly cleaned and prepared for aseptic surgery. In this area, secretions become encrusted and adhere tightly to the skin, and inadequate removal can lead to incisional infection.

Complications

Complications associated with this surgery include hemorrhage from transected ovarian vessels, adhesions, infection of the incision, nerve paresis following anesthesia (either femoral, peroneal, or radial), generalized myositis, postoperative shock, wound dehiscence, herniation, postoperative colic, and peritonitis. Some of these complications can be fatal but, in most cases, recovery is uneventful and healing of incisions is by first intention. Incisional complications occur more frequently after a flank approach but are rarely more than seroma formation or partial wound dehiscence. Postoperative bleeding is rare, but serious bleeding causes anxiety, sweating, colic, and increased heart rate, and pale mucous membranes. These horses may

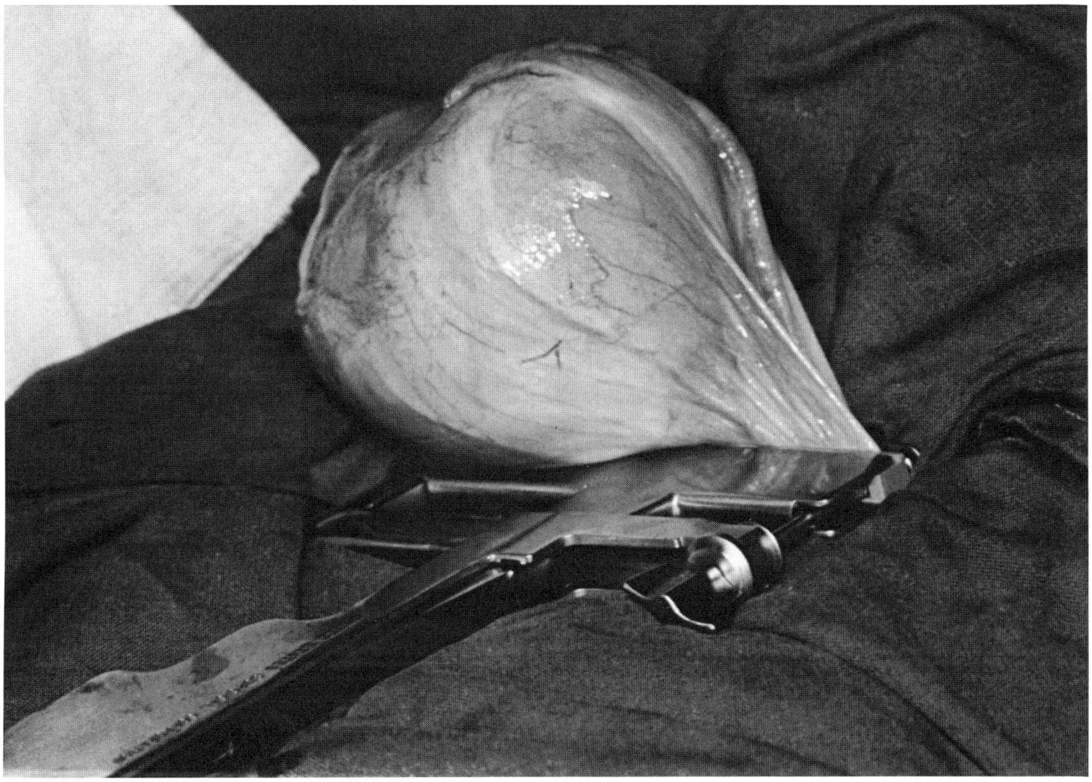

Figure 139–1. Application of the TA 90 Auto-Suture stapling instrument to the pedicle of a granulosa cell tumor.

require transfusion or autotransfusion until bleeding stops.

POSTOPERATIVE CARE

Mares that have had uncomplicated surgery for removal of a granulosa cell tumor may appear more depressed than horses subjected to similar intraabdominal procedures. These mares will have normal vital signs and clinically do not appear to be bleeding from the ovarian vessels. Their depression can be tentatively attributed to pain, possibly in the severed ovarian pedicle, and it usually resolves after 2 to 3 days. Therefore, nonsteroidal anti-inflammatory agents should be administered to these mares during this period after surgery. Preoperative and postoperative administration of antibiotics is not necessary after ventral midline celiotomy but may be indicated after a flank or paramedian approach, especially if removal of the tumor was difficult. The mare is rested in a stall for 1 month after surgery, during which time it receives daily controlled walking exercise. Exercise can include turn out in a small paddock for the next month and return to normal breeding or athletic activity thereafter.

PROGNOSIS

Following removal of a granulosa cell tumor, most mares regain function of the contralateral ovary, and have normal fertility. Meagher et al. reported that 42 of 57 mares followed after removal of a granulosa cell tumor cycled normally within 16 months (mean 8.5 months); 39 mares were bred and 30 produced live foals. If the mare is to be used as a broodmare after surgery, a complete breeding soundness examination, including culture of a uterine swab and endometrial biopsy, should be performed before surgery to evaluate the remainder of the reproductive tract.

Most mares that display abnormal behavior and temperament before surgery become more docile and manageable after removal of the granulosa cell tumor. The improvement in temperament may be gradual and owners should be advised that some signs of abnormal behavior may persist for several weeks before improvement is observed.

BIBLIOGRAPHY

Baumann LE, Sillerud CL, Spolar-Kilroy CR: Equine granulosa cell tumors. A review of fifteen cases. *Minn Vet* 1985; 25:52–54.

Bosu WTK, Van Camp SC, Miller RB, Owen RR: Ovarian disorder: Clinical and morphological observations in 30 mares. *Can Vet J* 1982;23:6–14.

Clark TL: Clinical management of equine ovarian neoplasms. *J Reprod Fertil Suppl* 1975;23:331–334.

Colburn GT, Reagan WJ: Ovariectomy by colpotomy in mares. *Compend Cont Educ Pract Vet* 1987;9:1035–1038.

Frazer GS, Threlfall WR: Differential diagnosis of enlarged ovary in the mare. *Proc AAEP Ann Conven* 1986, pp 21–28.

Hultgren BD, Zack PM, Pearson EG, Kaneps AJ: Juvenile granulosa cell tumor in an equine weanling. *J Comp Path* 1987;97:137–142.

McIlwraith CW, Turner AS: Surgery of the urogenital system, in *Equine Surgery Advanced Techniques.* Philadephia, Lea & Febiger, 1987, pp 346–351.

Meagher DM, Wheat JD, Hughes JP, Stabenfeldt GH, Harris BA: Granulosa cell tumors in mares—a review of 78 cases. *Proc AAEP Ann Conven* 1977, pp 133–143.

Moll HD, Slone DB, Juzwiak JS, Garrett PD: Diagonal paramedian approach for removal of ovarian tumors in the mare. *Vet Surg* 1987;16:456–458.

Pugh DG, Bowen JM: Equine ovarian tumors. *Comp Cont Educ Pract Vet* 1985;7:S710-S716.

Scott EA, Kunze DJ: Ovariectomy in the mare: Presurgical, surgical and postsurgical considerations. *J Equine Med Surg* 1977;1:5–12.

Stabenfeldt GH, Hughes JP, Kennedy PC, Meagher DM, Neely DP: Clinical findings, pathological changes and endocrinological secretory patterns in mares with ovarian tumors. *J Reprod Fert Suppl* 1979;27:277–285.

Stickle RL, Erb RE, Fessler JF, Runnels LJ: Equine granulosa cell tumors. *J Am Vet Med Assoc* 1975;167:148–151.

140 Uterine Torsion

David E. Freeman

Uterine torsion is uncommon in horses and, according to a survey of 42 cases in Belgium (Vandeplassche et al.), it may account for only 5 to 10% of total dystocias in this species. It has been proposed that the dorsal attachments of the broad ligaments in mares may resist the forces that cause torsion and render this species less susceptible to this problem than others. Excess risk due to breed and age have not been demonstrated in horses.

In a review of 26 cases by Pascoe et al., torsion occurred at a mean of 9.6 months of gestation, with a range of 8 months to term, and with a fairly uniform distribution of occurrence throughout that range. Mares affected at term may be close to foaling but not in labor when the diagnosis is made. By comparison, uterine torsion in cows is most often diagnosed at term. Also, unlike the cow, torsion in the mare rarely involves the cervix and vagina but is cranial to these segments, thus limiting the value of vaginal examination in making the diagnosis.

Although the direction of rotation was counterclockwise (as viewed from the rear) in 60% of Vandeplassches et al.'s cases, Pascoe et al. combined information from their study with all reported cases in the literature and concluded that the likelihood of rotation in either direction is equal. The degree of torsion ranges from 180 to 540 degrees and, although Vandeplassche et al. found that torsions through 360 degrees or more were more common, the majority of others reported were closer to 180 degrees. According to Roberts, torsions of less than 180 degrees may recover spontaneously. The uterus can rupture secondary to torsion, regardless of whether the uterine wall is normal or compromised, but this complication is uncommon.

CLINICAL FINDINGS

The most consistent clinical sign of uterine torsion is low-grade abdominal pain that is unresponsive to medical therapy and that can persist without change for several days. Vital signs may be normal or there might be a slight elevation in heart and respiratory rates. Violent signs of colic are rare, but mares that develop uterine necrosis may be depressed and exhibit other signs of peritonitis. If the uterus ruptures and the fetus falls into the abdominal cavity, sufficient tension may be released from the uterine wall and its attachments to reduce the signs of abdominal pain. Rarely, the small colon becomes incorporated in the twist or other intestinal displacements occur concomitantly, and these can exacerbate the clinical signs.

Uterine torsion should be regarded as a possible cause of colic in mares during late pregnancy, and the clinical signs are confused readily with those of large colon impaction. Diagnosis is made by rectal palpation. The broad ligaments can be felt to be drawn tautly and to cross as they are pulled above and below the uterus. The direction of torsion can be determined by following the dorsal-most ligament to determine its direction. The actual torsion can be palpated in the body of the uterus in some cases, but in others it may be too far forward in the abdomen. Also, the fetus may appear to be further cranial than is normal for that stage of gestation. If the uterus has ruptured, the fetus can be palpated directly through the wall of the rectum and it may be possible also to feel the torn edges of the uterus. Torsions of 360 degrees or more can constrict the small colon and thereby restrict rectal palpation.

TREATMENT

Several methods have been used to correct uterine torsion, and the choice is determined largely by the condition of the mare and fetus and the stage of gestation. If uterine torsion occurs at term, it sometimes can be corrected by rotation of the fetus through the dilated cervix. Another nonsurgical treatment is rolling the anesthetized mare, which can be done at any stage of gestation. Correction through a standard flank celiotomy approach with the mare standing is the most popular and most successful method of correction, regardless of the stage of gestation. This procedure is associated with the lowest risks and provides the least stress for both mare and foal. This approach can be used with the mare under general anesthesia and in lateral recumbency if the mare is intractable because of temperament or pain or if the torsion cannot be corrected with the mare standing. If general anesthesia is required for restraint, a ventral midline approach may be more useful than the flank and is preferable if a hysterotomy is required. A hysterotomy may be needed to facilitate correction or to remove a dead fetus undergoing necrosis. A hysterotomy should be avoided if there are doubts about fetal viability because this is difficult to assess, especially when the mare is anesthetized. A ventral midline approach is indicated also if the uterus is ruptured, the uterine wall is severely congested and possibly necrotic, the torsion cannot be corrected by other methods, or the mare has signs of intestinal involvement. When the wall of the uterus is thickened as a result of edema, congestion, or necrosis, it becomes friable and prone to rupture. A ventral midline approach then affords the easiest method of correction and the least risk of damage to the uterine wall.

Manual Rotation through the Cervix

This method is used in mares at term, when the cervix is fully dilated, and can be accomplished most readily if the torsion is less than 240 degrees. A hand is passed through the dilated cervix and along the spirals of the twisted portion of uterus. Tranquilizers and an epidural should be avoided if possible so that the mare will remain standing throughout the procedure. If the fetal membranes are intact, they should be ruptured to release fluids and reduce the size and weight of the uterus and its contents. The foal's legs are grasped along the metacarpus and the carpus is flexed. The foal is repelled and its legs are rotated back and forth through short arcs (25 to 30 cm) to rock the uterus and generate some momentum. A maximal effort is then used to twist the uterus against the direction of torsion until it is in its normal position. The foal can then be delivered by traction.

Rolling

Rolling is a useful nonsurgical method for correction of uterine torsion in mares, but has a high risk of uterine rupture in late gestation. The object of this procedure is to rotate the mare's body rapidly enough in the direction of torsion so that it "overtakes" the gravid uterus, which rotates more slowly. General anesthesia is necessary and several assistants are needed. The procedure can be modified according to Schaffer's method for the cow by using a wide plank of wood, 3 to 4 m long and 20 to 30 cm wide, against the flank to "fix" the uterus while the mare is rolled. This eliminates the need to roll the mare rapidly and therefore reduces the risks of uterine rupture. Because the abdomen of the mare is more rigid than that of the cow, it may be more difficult to influence the position of the fetus and uterus by this method.

For Schaffer's method, the mare is anesthetized and placed on the side to which the torsion is directed (e.g., on the right side if the torsion is clockwise) and hobbles are applied to all four legs. The plank is then placed across the mare's flank and maintained in position by a heavy person kneeling on the end across the mare's back. The ropes attached to the hobbles are then used to roll the mare over to the opposite side. Because the twist is usually cranial to the cervix, a vaginal examination cannot be used to assess the extent of correction, as it can in cows. Rectal palpation can be used instead, but this is difficult on recumbent mares. Several attempts may be required to correct the twist and the mare can be gently rolled over on her back or over her folded legs and abdomen to the original position each time.

Flank Celiotomy

The flank celiotomy is used on the standing mare with local anesthetic infiltrated along the proposed incision site and with a short- or long-acting sedative, alone or in combination with an opioid agent. Although epidural anesthesia may be used in conjunction with a local anesthetic and tranquilizer, this is not necessary. One must also be cautioned against the use of tranquilizers because the tranquilized mare is likely to lie down during the procedure. General anesthesia with the mare in lateral recumbency can be used also but is rarely indicated.

The 15- to 20-cm incision is placed high on the flank with the top of the incision at the level of the ventral aspect of the tuber coxae. A vertical incision is made through all layers except the internal abdominal oblique muscle, which is divided along its fibers. The direction of torsion is confirmed. There is little agreement on the preferred side of entry relative to the direction of the twist, but either approach seems to work equally well. Vandeplassche recommended that the abdomen be entered from the side to which the torsion is directed (e.g., left flank if the torsion is counterclockwise, right if it is clockwise). The hand is passed deeply between the body wall and uterus and the uterus is then lifted and rotated in one upward movement. This step can be facilitated by alternatively pushing against the upper portion of the uterus and the fetus.

If the abdomen is entered on the side opposite that to which the torsion is directed (e.g., left flank if the torsion is clockwise, right flank if counterclockwise), the hand is passed dorsally above the uterus and the uterus is then pulled toward the operator. Once rotation is started, the weight of the fetus and uterus may help to draw them around completely to a normal position. This approach has been recommended for the anesthetized mare but it has been suggested that the ventral aspect of the uterus be pushed along the opposite body wall and away from the operator, rather than pulling on the dorsal aspect of the uterus.

Regardless of the method used, correction can be facilitated by grasping the foal's limbs, usually at the hocks, through the wall of the uterus and using these to start the movement of the foal and uterus. When the limbs are grasped, they are gently "rocked" through short arcs (25 to 30 cm) to gain some momentum and then rotation is completed by lifting and pushing the uterus to its correct position. Care must be used if correction is accomplished through grasping the fetus because this procedure may predispose to rupture of the uterus, especially if its walls are edematous and friable. Although the incision will have to be enlarged, it may be helpful for the operator to insert both arms to alternate between the lifting and pushing movements and coordinate these steps so as to direct as much force as possible during the rotation.

The greatest difficulties in correcting a uterine torsion are encountered close to term because the amount of inertia produced by the large foal and uterus are difficult to overcome. Torsions of 240 degrees or less are easiest to correct and are associated with less edema in the uterus than more severe torsions. Hence, there is a lower risk of rupture. If it proves impossible to correct the torsion through a flank approach, a decision can then be made to perform a ventral midline celiotomy.

To confirm complete correction of the torsion, the broad ligaments and the external surfaces of the uterus and cervix should be palpated to determine that they are in their normal positions. Fetal activity should be checked by pinching the lower limbs or muzzle or by applying gentle pressure to the eyes. If one is convinced that the fetus is dead, a hysterotomy can be considered; however, methods of detecting fetal viability are not reliable and if there is any doubt, especially before term or when breeding dates are unknown, gestation should be allowed to proceed normally. If a hysterotomy is performed through a flank approach, exposure can be improved by extending the incision vertically, using sharp dissection across the fibers of the internal abdominal oblique muscle, ventral to the grid incision. Generally, a ventral midline approach is preferred in these cases. In rare cases, the torsion can only be corrected after the foal has been removed; however, correction with the mare under general anesthesia, through the flank or midline, should be attempted first.

Ventral Midline Celiotomy

A standard ventral midline celiotomy is used, with a 25-cm long incision made immediately cranial to the umbilicus. If needed, the incision can be extended caudally through the umbilicus. Manipulation of the uterus through this approach is considerably easier than through the flank because it allows greater access to the abdomen and two arms can be fully inserted through the incision. This approach also allows better assessment of the condition of the uterine wall and enables treatment of any concomitant intestinal problems. If a hysterotomy is indicated, this can be performed before correction of the torsion because it is easier to manipulate the uterus after the fetus and the uterine fluids have been removed. Closure of the abdominal incision is routine. Simple interrupted sutures of size 2 polyglactin 910 (Vicryl; Ethicon Inc) can be used in the linea alba and will provide sufficient strength if the mare delivers at any time after surgery. Because this method involves general anesthesia and the associated stress to mare and foal, it should be used only in cases that are not suitable for a flank approach.

POSTOPERATIVE CARE

Mares with uterine torsion before term or mares with unknown breeding dates are allowed to continue to term and to deliver naturally. The main concern after successful correction is the risk of abortion, and this may be signalled by loss of the cervical mucous plug, mammary gland enlargement, discharge of mucus from the vulva, or early signs of first-stage labor. If signs of impending abortion develop, progesterone therapy (repositol progesterone, 1,000 mg intramuscularly every 4 days, or progesterone in oil, 300 mg daily) is considered by some to be of value; however, the prognosis for completion of pregnancy once signs develop is poor. Vandeplassche recommended use of the sympathomimetic smooth muscle relaxant isoxsuprine lactate, at a dose of 200 mg intramuscularly during the first 24 hours after correction. If signs of colic persist, he recommended that the drug be administered again at intervals as needed.

If the torsion is corrected by celiotomy, either through the flank or ventral midline, the mare should be confined to a stall for 3 to 4 weeks. The purpose of this is to restrict activity and thus reduce stress on the suture line and to allow immediate assistance if required during delivery. Mares with torsion complicated by shock, uterine congestion, or rupture or that require hysterotomy should also be treated as needed with broad-spectrum antibiotics, intravenous fluids, and nonsteroidal anti-inflammatory drugs.

PROGNOSIS

In Pascoe et al.'s survey of 26 mares with uterine torsion, 19 (73%) survived surgery. In Vandeplassche et al.'s series of 42 cases, 60% of the mares survived. The prognosis for both mare and foal after uterine torsion in that study was worse than it is for cattle. This was attributed mainly to the more severe circulatory disturbances caused by displacement in mares and the diffuse nature of the mare's placenta. Venous congestion and thrombosis can follow uterine torsion and this can predispose to abortion or cause death from uterine necrosis and peritonitis. The degree of vascular compromise may be influenced by the duration of torsion and also by the degree of rotation and the extent to which the broad ligaments are involved. Other causes of death are shock, hemorrhage, and uterine rupture. The prognosis for survival and recovery of fertility after uterine rupture is good if treated promptly by removal of placenta from the abdomen and repair of part or all of the tear. The prognosis for survival of mare and foal is good in cases in which the fetus is alive at the time of correction and the uterine wall is normal in appearance. In mares that survive without a hysterotomy, it appears that subsequent fertility is not impaired.

In Pascoe et al.'s survey, 20 of 26 foals (77%) were alive at the time of correction but only 14 of these foals (70%), or 54% of the total, were born alive. Vandeplassche et al. reported a 30% survival rate for foals. Abortion accounts for death in some foals, others die after birth, and some are born dead at term, up to several weeks after correction of the torsion. In some cases, foals are found dead in utero at the time of surgery or in the peritoneal cavity following uterine rupture. Foals that are delivered immediately from the peritoneal cavity following rupture at term can survive.

The prognosis can be influenced also by the method of treatment. After manual correction through the cervix or correction by rolling, there is a high risk of separation of the allantochorion from the endometrium and subsequently of abortion, premature birth, or death of the fetus. For this reason, surgical methods of treatment, such as through a flank or ventral midline celiotomy, offer the best prognosis for survival of mare and foal. However, rolling may be safer and allow a higher survival rate for mare and foal than previous studies suggested, especially if the torsion is of short duration and occurs early in gestation.

BIBLIOGRAPHY

Bowen JM, Gaboury C, Bousquet D: Non-surgical correction of a uterine torsion in the mare. *Vet Rec* 1976;99:495–496.

Pascoe JR, Meagher DM, Wheat JD: Surgical management of uterine torsion in the mare: A review of 26 cases. *J Am Vet Med Assoc* 1981;179:351–354.

Roberts SJ: *Veterinary Obstetrics and Genital Diseases.* Ithaca, NY, S. J. Roberts, 1971, pp 186–189, 285–291.

Skjerven O: Correction of uterine torsion in the mare by laparotomy. *Nord Vet Med* 1965;17:377–381.

Vandeplassche M: Obstetrician's view of the physiology of equine parturition and dystocia. *Equine Vet J* 1980;12:45–49.

Vandeplassche M, Spincemaille J, Bouters R, Bonte P: Some aspects of equine obstetrics. *Equine Vet J* 1972;4:105–113.

Wichtel JJ, Reinertson EL, Clark TL: Nonsurgical treatment of uterine torsion in seven mares. *J Am Vet Med Assoc* 1988;193:337–338.

141
Cesarean Section

Donnie E. Slone, Jr.

Dystocia is a prolongation of either the first or, more commonly, the second stage of parturition. The first stage involves active contraction of the uterine musculature only and lasts from 1 to 4 hours. It is during this stage that the foal should rotate to a dorsosacral position and its head and front legs should extend toward the birth canal. In addition, the cervix should be completely dilated by the end of this stage. Some mares will be presented in dystocia never having entered the second stage of labor because they were unable to get the foal started into the birth canal. This problem occurs with breech and transverse presentations.

During the second stage of labor, the fetus enters the birth canal and stimulates forceful abdominal contractions. This stage is very rapid in the mare, generally lasting only 20 minutes. It is during this stage that most dystocias occur.

The third stage of parturition is characterized by expulsion of fetal membranes and involution of the uterus. Although not directly involved in the definition of dystocia, placental separation has a drastic impact on the survivability of the foal since it begins during the second stage of labor. The third stage of parturition is also a very rapid process in the mare.

INDICATIONS

The indications for cesarean section are varied. Transverse presentation of the foal is one of the most important indications for cesarean section in draft mares. Transverse presentations appear to occur infrequently in the light horse breeds. Other indications for cesarean section include foals that are too large for the size of the mare's birth canal or a birth canal that is too small for manipulation or fetotomy by the operator and/or dangerous for the mare. Malpositions may be uncorrectable because there is insufficient room for the foal relative to the size of the birth canal or because the foal has become impacted into the birth canal. Other malpositions may be uncorrectable because of ankylosis of limbs or vertebrae. Lateral deviations of the head and neck can be particularly perplexing, because the foal may or may not have ankylosis of the vertebrae and it is difficult to know whether the foal is alive or dead without correcting the malposition. Tumors, masses, pelvic fractures, or other pelvic deformities may prevent a normal foal from passing through the birth canal. In these situations, cesarean section should be considered before breeding the mare and planned before the mare is ready to foal. Finally, hydrocephalus and other fetal deformities that cannot safely be corrected by fetotomy require a cesarean section.

Correction of a dystocia is accomplished either by mutation, fetotomy, or cesarean section. The decision regarding the best approach should be made rapidly following examination of the mare under epidural anesthesia and tranquilization. Unfortunately, the decision to do a cesarean section is often delayed while mutation and fetotomy are tried. Ideally a fetotomy should be performed on dead, emphysematous, or deformed foals. However, the mare's uterus, cervix, and birth canal are less tolerant of long and difficult fetotomies as compared to the cow. Therefore, fetotomies requiring more than two or possibly three cuts should be avoided.

SURGICAL TECHNIQUE

A variety of anesthesic techniques have been recommended for cesarean section. Current information suggests that all anesthetics and muscle relaxants cross the placenta. Therefore, any technique is satisfactory so long as the mare is properly padded, positioned, and oxygenated, her blood pressure is maintained and she is kept as light as possible until the foal is removed. This may be facilitated by local anesthesia at the site of the abdominal incision. Because both the mare and the foal will be anesthetized prior to removing the foal, any anesthesia protocol should use as little anesthetic as possible during induction.

Cesarean section can be performed via a low left flank approach such as the Marcenac approach. The mare is placed in right lateral recumbency with the upper rear leg lifted and pulled slightly caudal. The skin incision is made obliquely from the midportion of the costal arch toward the udder, but ending just medial to the fold of the flank. The muscle and fascial layers are traversed via a modified grid procedure; that is, the abdominal tunic and fascia of the external abdominal oblique muscle are sharply incised in the direction of the skin incision while the remaining muscle layers are bluntly separated along the direction of their fibers.

The Marcenac approach is useful for very large mares. Draft mares seem to be more predisposed to postoperative gluteal myositis and/or peripheral neuropathies when placed in dorsal recumbency. A major problem associated with the approach is limited exposure, which may present difficulties with some deformed foals and for uterine torsions during late gestation.

The more common approach for cesarean section is the caudal ventral midline. The skin incision extends from the mammary gland to a location cranial to the umbilicus, depending on the size of the foal. The incision in the linea alba has similar limitations, but may extend under the mammary gland; alternatively, the mammary gland may be divided. The advantages of the ventral midline approach include familiarity, less hemorrhage, and better exposure. The largest of the light breed mares seem to tolerate dorsal recumbency well when padded properly, when the legs are lifted upward toward a near-normal standing position, and when blood pressure and blood gas values are maintained within their appropriate ranges.

Immediately upon entering the abdominal cavity, sterile saline containing 20,000 to 50,000 IU heparin is poured into the abdominal cavity. This regimen helps prevent clot and fibrin formation on serosal surfaces and may prevent some adhesions. Once the abdomen is entered, the pregnant horn is located by finding the hind feet if the foal is in anterior presentation, the front feet if its is in posterior presentation, or preferably the hind feet if it is in the transverse presentation. The uterus should be packed off using wet towels or laparotomy pads to prevent blood and fetal debris from entering the abdominal cavity. This very important step should be taken quickly and will save time and decrease complications later. The incision into the uterus should be located along the greater curvature as far from the larger vessels as possible. It should be made long enough to allow removal of the foal without tearing the uterus.

Once the foal's legs are exteriorized, obstetric chains are placed around them and assistants pull the foal from the uterus. The umbilical cord is left intact for several minutes before it is clamped and severed. The placenta should be removed if this can be accomplished easily. Excessive tearing, in addition to being injurious to the endometrium, will also cause substantial hemorrhage. Oxytocin at 20 to 40 IU/horse or .04 to .08 IU/kg can be given intramuscularly at this time to begin involution of the uterus.

The placenta can be removed through the uterine incision if it is separated from the uterus and there is minimal contamination. If left in the uterus, the placenta should always be separated from the edges of the uterine incision. A simple continuous or continuous interlocking suture pattern should be applied to the cut edges of the uterus to compress the vessels between the serosa and endometrium. Chromic gut is preferable for this purpose, because it will be more quickly absorbed than the synthetic absorbable sutures. Size 0 or 1 polyglactin 910 and polyioxanone (PDS, Ethicon Inc) is recommended for the two-layer inverting closure of the uterine incision. This can be in either a Cushing's or a Lembert suture pattern.

The abdominal cavity should be thoroughly lavaged with saline and suctioned to remove any blood or debris. Antibiotics placed directly into the abdominal cavity are unnecessary; however, heparin in the lavage may be advantageous to prevent adhesions. The Marcenac approach is closed using interrupted sutures to appose the muscle layers and a simple continuous suture pattern in the abdominal tunic and subcutaneous tissue, all with size 2 synthetic absorbable suture. The ventral midline can be closed in three layers using doubled size 2 polyglactin 910 in a simple continuous pattern in the linea alba. Subcutaneous tissue and skin closure for either approach may be accomplished by the surgeon's preference.

POSTOPERATIVE CARE

Postoperative therapy usually includes broad-spectrum antibiotics, flunixin meglumine, tetanus prophylaxis, and heparin, which may be given subcutaneously at 40 IU/kg three times daily. Oxytocin at 20 to 40 IU intramuscularly every 2 hours should be given to help expel the placenta and uterine fluids. Excessive uterine fluids may be removed by lavage and siphon. The antibiotics should be given for 5 to 7 days as dictated by clinical response. Heparin and flunixin meglumine should be continued as long as a risk of endotoxemia is present. This should include the entire period that the placenta is retained.

Mares should be exercised with controlled walking for 2 weeks postoperatively, followed by 2 weeks of exercise in a round pen or small paddock. The mare may then have ad lib exercise in a pasture, but should not be bred by natural cover for 8 weeks following surgery. The mare should have a reproductive examination during her foal heat and her 30-day heat cycles.

PROGNOSIS

While cesarean sections should not be performed needlessly, the success rate for cesarean section increases with the rapidity with which referral, decision making, and surgery are performed. Success can be measured in a variety of ways. These include live foals, live mares, and return of reproductive performance.

Planned cesarean sections should have a relatively high success rate as measured by live foals and mares. Correct timing is an essential factor to help ensure a live, vigorous foal. Twice-daily milk calcium determinations along with mammary development, waxing, and gestational age have proven helpful to determine impending parturition.

BIBLIOGRAPHY

Cash RSG, Dusey JC, Rossdale PD: Rapid strip test method to assist management of foaling mares. *Equine Vet J* 1985; 17:61–62.

Peaker M, Rossdale PD, Forsyth IA, Falk M: Changes in mammary development and the composition of secretion during late pregnancy in the mare. *J Reprod Fertil Suppl* 1979; 27:555–561.

Roberts SJ: *Veterinary Obstetrics and Genital Diseases, Theriogenology,* ed 3. Woodstock VT, S. J. Roberts, 1986, pp 251–259.

Vandeplassche MM: Obstetrician's view of the physiology of equine parturition and dystocia. *Equine Vet J* 1980;12:45–48.

Vandeplassche MM: The pathogenesis of dystocia and fetal malformation in the horse. *J Reprod Fertil Suppl* 1987; 35:547–552.

Walker DE, Vaughan JT: *Bovine and Equine Urogenital Surgery.* Philadelphia, Lea & Febiger, 1980, pp 229–232.

142 Cryptorchidectomy

Stephen B. Adams

Cryptorchidism is the failure of one or both testes to descend into the scrotum. In horses cryptorchidism is believed to have a heritable basis. All breeds of horses may exhibit cryptorchidism but it is more common in Quarter Horses, Saddlebreds, and Percherons. Cryptorchid horses are considered undesirable, because they behave like intact stallions and may have disagreeable temperaments. Unilateral cryptorchid horses are fertile, whereas bilateral cryptorchid horses are not.

Retained testes in cryptorchid horses may be located within the abdomen, in the inguinal canal, or in the subcutaneous tissues. The vas deferens and tail of the epididymus occasionally are found in the inguinal canal in horses with abdominal testes. This may occur because the proper ligament of the testes, which attaches the testes to the epididymus, can be 4 to 10 cm long. Horses with all testicular structures in the abdomen are called abdominal cryptorchids. Horses with the vas deferens and epididymus in the canal and the testes within the abdomen are called partial abdominal cryptorchids. Inguinal cryptorchids, or "high flankers," are horses with testes in the inguinal canal, and horses with subcutaneous testes have been termed "low flankers."

The prevalence of left and right retention of testes is nearly equal. Testes retained on the left side are more often abdominal than inguinal. Testes retained in the right side are more often inguinal than abdominal. Bilateral cryptorchidism occurs in about 15% of horses with cryptorchidism. The retained testes are often both abdominal, but both may be inguinal, or one testis may occur in each location.

DEVELOPMENT AND DESCENT OF THE TESTES

Testes develop near the caudal pole of the kidney and are suspended in a fold of peritoneum that becomes the mesorchium. A continuous cylindrical mesenchymal mass develops that connects the epididymus to the body wall. This mass develops into the gubernaculum. Within the body wall, the gubernaculum develops into a large bulb that dilates the vaginal ring and guides testicular descent into the inguinal canal. Descent of the testes from the abdomen through the inguinal canal and into the scrotum normally begins between 270 and 300 days of gestation. On completion of testicular descent, the gubernaculum becomes the epididymal ligament and the proper ligament of the testis. During normal descent the epididymus enters the inguinal canal before the testis. Left testes are often larger than right testes and frequently lag behind right testes in descent. The vaginal ring contracts to a diameter of about 1 cm during the first 2 weeks after birth. This constriction prevents movement of testes into or out of the abdomen and explains why left testes are more often retained in the abdomen than are right testes.

At birth about 50% of foals have descended testes. Testes are unlikely to descend from the abdomen in foals 1 month of age or older. Palpation of the scrotum at birth is not reliable for determining descent of the testes because the gubernacular bulb may feel like a testis. Descent of inguinal testes into the scrotum may occur in horses up to 4 years of age. Unilateral castration of cryptorchid horses may cause hypertrophy of the remaining testes. Although this encourages descent of these testes, only inguinal testes will be able to drop into the scrotum. Abdominal testes will remain within the abdomen. Since removal of inguinal testes is easily performed, unilateral castration is not necessary. In fact, hypertrophy of abdominal testes may increase the difficulty of surgically removing them.

DIAGNOSIS

Horses with No Previous Surgery

Horses with no previous surgery are classified as cryptorchids if one or both testes are not in the scrotum. External and rectal examination will allow the examiner to determine which testes are retained and the location of the testes. The inguinal areas and the superficial inguinal ring are palpated for the presence of retained testes. Three or four fingers can be pushed into the inguinal canal to feel for testes. Tranquilization of the horse prior to deep palpation of the inguinal canal will relax the horse and increase the probability that an inguinal testis will drop into a position where it can be palpated.

Many surgeons perform rectal examinations to determine the location of retained testes when the testes cannot be identified by external palpation. The vaginal rings should be identified anterior, lateral, and slightly ventral to the brim of the pelvis, and the surgeon should determine if the vas deferens passes through the medial aspect of the vaginal ring. Testes are in the abdomen when the vas deferens does not pass through the ring. The testes are usually inguinal in location when the vas deferens passes through the vaginal ring. Approximately one in ten horses will be a partial abdominal cryptorchid, with the testis in the abdomen but the vas deferens and epididymus in the inguinal canal. The abdomen should be examined for large cystic or teratomatous testes when the vas deferens does not pass through the vaginal ring. The presence of a large testis will preclude successful removal through a noninvasive inguinal approach.

External palpation of the superficial inguinal rings and canals in anesthetized horses will allow the surgeon to palpate all but the very smallest inguinal testes. The surgeon' s fingertips should be forced deep into the cranial aspect of the canal and then pushed caudally to force the testis out of the canal and into the subcutaneous tissues or scrotum, where it can be identified. This procedure is useful for horses too small for a rectal examination, for fractious horses that are dangerous to examine, and for surgeons who do not utilize rectal palpation for location of testes. Since the location of testes is not determined until the horse is anesthetized, the surgeon must be prepared to remove either inguinal or abdominal testes.

Horses with an Unknown History or with Previous Attempts at Castration

Horses that behave like stallions but have no testes in the scrotum are diagnostic challanges when previous attempts at castration have been performed or no history is available. These horses may be bilateral cryptorchids, geldings with stallion-like behavior, or unilateral cryptorchids in which the descended testes have been removed. The diagnostic goals in these horses are to determine if testes are present and, if so, their location.

External and rectal examinations should be performed and may result in identification of testes. The scrotal area should be checked for castration scars. However, this procedure is difficult unless the horse is anesthetized. Upon rectal examination, the vas deferens will pass through the vaginal ring in most, but not all, horses that have undergone castration for removal of scrotal testes. Therefore, the absence of a vas deferens passing through the ring suggests that the horse is an abdominal cryptorchid.

Diagnostic endocrinology can be used to determine whether testicular tissue is present or absent. Testes produce both androgens and estrogens. Serum testosterone may be measured before and after stimulation with human chorionic gonadotropin (hCG). A serum sample for determination of testosterone is collected and 10,000 IU hCG is given intravenously. One hour later a second serum sample is collected for testosterone assay. Stallions and cryptorchids usually have basal plasma testosterone levels above 100 pg/mL and an increase in testosterone occurs in response to hCG.

Castrated horses have low basal plasma levels of testosterone and levels do not rise following hCG administration.

Conjugated serum estrogens are high in horses with testicular tissue. A single measurement of serum estrogen can reliably predict which horses have testicular tissue. The test is not accurate for horses less than 3 years old or for donkeys. Serum testosterone levels or conjugated estrogen levels suggesting testicular tissue is present support surgical exploration to locate the testis or testes that are producing the measured hormones.

SURGERY

Inguinal Approach

Following induction of general anesthesia, positioning of the horse in dorsal recumbency, and surgical preparation of the skin, an incision is made directly over the superficial inguinal ring. When the retained testis is located in the inguinal canal, surgical draping need not be performed if the incision will be left open to heal by second intention. Primary closure of the skin incision following inguinal cryptorchidectomy is performed by some surgeons and this technique warrants draping of the surgical area. Draping should be performed for surgery on all horses with testes retained in the abdomen. This will reduce abdominal contamination and the chance for subsequent peritonitis.

A skin incision 12 cm long is made over the superficial inguinal ring. Blunt finger dissection of the underlying fascia and fat into the inguinal canal is done to prevent laceration of subcutaneous and inguinal veins, which may be large. Inguinal testes are located in the canal, exteriorized, and stripped of surrounding fascia. Routine emasculation can be used for removal of the testes.

For horses with partial abdominal cryptorchidism, the vaginal process should be grasped with Ochsner forceps or fingers and opened with scissors. The vas deferens and epididymus are grasped and gently retracted upward to deliver the testis into the inguinal canal. Once exteriorized, the cord can be emasculated or ligated and divided to remove the testis. Incisions are often left to heal by second intention following removal of inguinal or partial abdominal testes. Primary closure of the wound can be performed by placing a row of simple continuous sutures in the fascia and subcutaneous tissue with size 0 polydioxanone (PDS; Ethicon Inc) or polyglactin 910 (Vicryl; Ethicon Inc). These sutures are absorbable. The skin is closed routinely.

Adominal testes are removed by continuing blunt dissection of the fat and fascia in the inguinal canal to the level of the deep inguinal ring. The noninvasive approach for removing abdominal testes avoids the necessity of putting fingers or hands into the abdomen and is the approach I prefer. This method has proven to be rapid and safe. To perform the noninvasive inguinal cryptorchidectomy, the deep inguinal ring is identified as a defect in the abdominal musculature about 10 cm deep to the skin incision. A 10-in Foerster sponge forceps is placed along side the hand into the canal to grasp the vaginal process at the level of the deep inguinal ring (Fig. 142–1). The vaginal process is everted into the inguinal canal and opened with scissors. The gubernaculum, which is attached to the vaginal process, is grasped and used to pull the epididymus and testis out of the abdomen. Traction should be gentle to avoid rupturing the proper ligament of the testis and thus preventing the testis from being pulled out of the abdomen. Occasionally the vaginal ring must be dilated with one or two fingers to allow passage of the testis. Since the proper ligament of the testis may be up to 14 cm long, the surgeon should be positive of having exteriorized all testicular structures; and removal of just the tail of the epididymus is not performed (Fig. 142–2). Once the testis is exteriorized, emasculation and ligation of the spermatic cord is performed and the testis is removed.

Occasionally the testis cannot be located with the noninvasive technique. The deep inguinal ring may then be bluntly penetrated with one or two fingers and the immediate area around the ring explored for the vas deferens, the eipdidymus, or the testis. Upon failure to locate these structures, the surgeon can insert an entire hand into the abdomen and palpate the ampulla of the bladder to locate the vas deferens. The vas deferens is

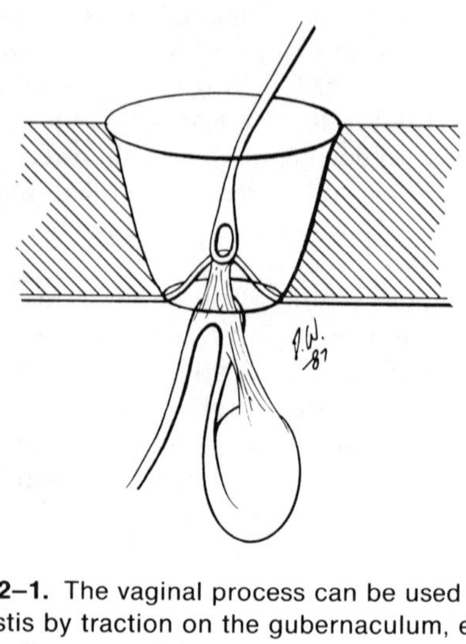

Figure 142–1. The vaginal process can be used to exteriorize the testis by traction on the gubernaculum, epididymus, and proper ligament of the testis.

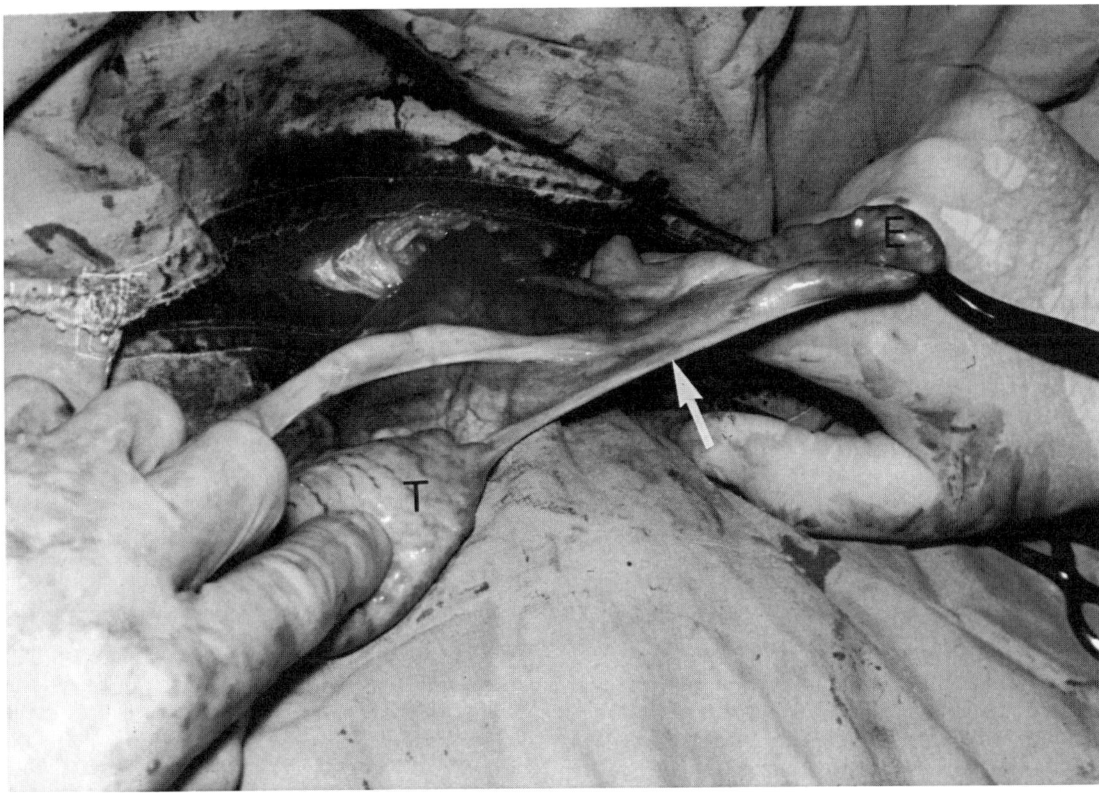

Figure 142–2. The proper ligament of the testis (*arrow*) may be long, thus allowing the testis (*T*) to be some distance from the tail of the epididymus (*E*). The surgeon must avoid removing just the epididymus.

traced back to the testis, which can then be exteriorized and removed.

Closure of the wound following the noninvasive inguinal approach may be performed by suturing the deep fascia, subcutaneous fascia, and skin with simple continuous suture patterns. An absorbable suture material should be used for all buried suture lines. An alternative that is quick and yields good results is to pack the inguinal canal with sterile gauze followed by sutured closure of the skin. The gauze pack should be removed in 24 hours. Prior to removal, a rectal examination should be performed to ensure adhesions have not formed to gauze that had mistakenly been placed through the vaginal ring and into the abdomen. Some surgeons neither close nor pack wounds following routine noninvasive cryptorchidectomy. This method is generally safe when the vaginal ring is not ruptured or dilated.

Following invasive inguinal cryptorchidectomy, suture closure of the wound is necessary. The inguinal canal and deep inguinal ring are closed with several large obliterating simple interrupted sutures of size 1 polydioxanone or polyglactin 910. The superficial ring is closed with size 2 polydioxanone or polyglactin 910 in a simple continuous pattern placed in the fascia of the external abdominal oblique muscle. The sutures are placed in a staggered fashion from the edge of the ring to distribute tension. Subcutaneous and skin closures are routine.

Parainguinal Approach

An alternative to the inguinal approach for abdominal cryptorchidectomy is the parainguinal approach. A 12-cm skin incision is made 2 cm craniomedial to the superficial inguinal ring. When the location of the testes has not been determined, the inguinal canal can be exposed and explored for inguinal testes. Upon failure to find inguinal testes, a 4- to 6-cm incision is made in the aponeurosis of the external abdominal oblique muscle 2 cm craniomedial to the superficial ring and centered over the cranial aspect of the ring. Two fingers are bluntly forced through the abdominal musculature, retroperitoneal fat, and peritoneum and into the abdominal cavity next to the deep inguinal ring. The vas deferens, epididymus, or ligament of the tail of the epididymus is grasped and used to exteriorize the testis, which is then removed. The fascia of the external abdominal oblique muscle is closed with simple interrupted sutures of size 2 polydioxanone. The skin and subcutaneous tissues are closed routinely. The parainguinal cryptorchidectomy may be easier to perform for some surgeons than the noninvasive inguinal approach.

Paramedian and Flank Approaches

The paramedian or the flank laparotomy may be selected when large cystic, anomalous, or neoplastic testes are present in the abdomen. Relatively long incisions can be made allowing exteriorization of the testes. Removal of large testes by the inguinal or parainguinal approach can be difficult.

POSTOPERATIVE CARE

Tetanus prophylaxis should be ensured. Antibiotics are not routinely administered when aseptic procedures have been used. Twenty-four hours after surgery, exercise should be resumed to reduce swelling and promote drainage of open incisions. Exercise should be limited to controlled walking and trotting or free exercise in a small paddock. Twenty minutes of exercise twice daily should be a minimum amount. Unlimited exercise is gradually resumed over the next 10 days. Nonabsorbable skin sutures should be removed in 7 days.

PROGNOSIS AND COMPLICATIONS

Horses having undergone cryptorchidectomy for removal of inguinal testes have the same risks and complications as horses having undergone standard castration. Complications are uncommon but can include infection, fever, anesthetic complications, excessive hemorrhage, and eventration of bowel. Postoperative complications are also uncommon in horses undergoing cryptorchidectomy for removal of abdominal testes unless the surgeon has difficulty finding the testes during surgery and extensive inguinal and abdominal manipulation has occurred. Peritonitis and incisional dehiscence may occur if difficulty during surgery is encountered.

BIBLIOGRAPHY

Adams OR; An improved method of diagnosis and castration of cryptorchid horses. *J Am Vet Med Assoc* 1964;145:439–446.

Adams SB: Cryptorchidectomy in stallions. *Mod Vet Pract* 1986;67:790–794.

Cox JE, Redhead PH, Dawson FE: Comparison of the measurement of plasma testosterone and plasma oestrogens for the diagnosis of cryptorchidism in the horse. *Equine Vet J* 1986;3:179–182.

Genetzky RM, Shira MJ, Schneider EJ, Easley JK: Equine cryptorchidism: Pathogenesis, diagnosis, and treatment. *Compend Cont Educ Pract Vet* 1984;6:S577-S582.

Palmer S, Passmore JL: Midline scrotal ablation technique for unilateral cryptorchid castration in horses. *J Am Vet Med Assoc* 1987;3:283–285.

Stickle RL, Fessler JF: Retrospective study of 350 cases of equine cryptorchidism. *J Am Vet Med Assoc* 1978;3:343–346.

Trotter GW, Aanes WA: A complication of cryptorchid castration in three horses. *J Am Vet Med Assoc* 1981;178:246–248.

Wilson DG, Reinertson EL: A modified parainguinal approach for cryptorchidectomy in horses. An evaluation in 107 horses. *Vet Surg* 1987;16:1–4.

143 Traumatic Conditions of the Penis and Prepuce

Walter R. Threlfall

Trauma to the stallion's penis frequently occurs during attempts to breed mares not in estrus or extremely nervous mares that respond by kicking the stallion as he attempts to mount. Lesions can also occur from devices used to control masturbation, from a stallion kicking his penis, or following acetylpromazine tranquilization with resultant paraphimosis.

INFLAMMATORY CONDITIONS

Posthitis is an inflammation of the prepuce. This can follow the use of contact-type irritants to cleanse the penis that were not thoroughly removed by rinsing, or result from the presence of solid material within the prepuce, such as wood shavings. Treatment for simple posthitis is removal of the inflammatory agent and daily hydrotherapy. Diuretics have been utilized but are generally not necessary. In cases where posthitis is present in addition to other conditions, the other conditions should be treated simultaneously because they may be responsible for the posthitis.

Balanitis is an inflammation of the glans penis. This can occur following failure to cleanse the urethral diverticulum, with the resultant solidified smegma acting as an irritant to the glans. The stallion may exhibit discomfort during urination with this condition. This condition in its uncomplicated form is easily treated by cleansing the penis and keeping it clean. Initially therapy may consist of hydrotherapy and application of lanolin-based creams to improve the comfort of the animal.

PHIMOSIS

Phimosis is the condition in which the penis cannot be protruded from the prepuce. This could be due to either swelling or stricture of the preputial orifices or to enlargements of the glans penis that prevent protrusion. Strictures of the preputial orifice may be congenital and go unnoticed for years. Treatment of the condition will depend on whether it is penile or preputial in origin. Preputial strictures can be treated by surgical enlargement of the preputial orifice or reduction of preputial swelling, whichever is the cause. Penile lesions should be treated to reduce swelling, thus possibly permitting prolapse of the penis.

PARAPHIMOSIS

During paraphimosis the penis is protruded and cannot be retracted into the prepuce. This can occur following castration with extensive edema and swelling in the inguinal area, myelitis, spinal injuries, viral infections, physical exhaustion, paralysis of the retractor penile muscle following administration of acetylpromazine or etorphine, or when large lesions on the glans penis prevent withdrawal of the penis. All of these cases should be evaluated for penile sensation and amount of movement possible. Treatment should be immediate and directed toward prevention of further trauma to the penis and prepuce. This can be accomplished by cleaning the penis and prepuce, applying a lanolin-based antibiotic cream, and placing a support around the penis and prepuce to hold it in the prepuce by strap attachments over the back of the stallion (Fig. 143–1). This will protect the tissue from injury and prevent it from becoming edematous.

A stallion penile support can be made from nylon mesh material with straps attached to the four corners. This permits the stallion to urinate through the mesh and is superior to gauze or other material that will become soaked with the urine. If penile paralysis follows the administration of acetylpromazine or etorpine, paraphimosis may respond to immediate medication with 8 mg benztropine mesylate (Congentin, Merck Sharpe & Dohme).

Swelling and edema of the prepuce and penis, once present, can be reduced by massage or by use of an air splint. The splint is placed around the penis and prepuce and then inflated. This pressure aids in reducing the swelling. The splint should not be left in place for longer than 15 to 20 minutes. The importance of reducing the swelling and returning the penis to the preputial lumen cannot be overemphasized.

A technique utilized in horses with permanent paraphimosis is phallopexy. After the stallion has been gelded and the incision site has healed, he is placed in dorsal recumbency under general anesthesia. If preputial scar tissue prevents the penis from being placed into the preputial lumen, the scar tissue should be removed and the site healed prior to phallopexy. A 10-cm incision is made on the midline slightly caudal to the scrotal area. Blunt dissection of the subcutaneous tissue is performed to expose the penis. The area of the thickened attachment of prepuce to penis is located and size 3 nonabsorbable nylon suture (Braunamid; Jorgensen Laboratories) is placed on both lateral surfaces of this tissue. To avoid suturing the urethra, a catheter is inserted prior to surgery. The two sutures are brought to the caudal area of the incision and placed through the skin. The penis is pulled into the prepuce until the glans is located slightly inside the preputial orifice. The sutures are tied around a piece of latex tubing to prevent pressure necrosis of the skin in the area of the sutures. The glans must be concealed to prevent injury but not pulled so far into the prepuce that the animal will have problems with urine collecting within the prepuce. The subcutaneous tissue is sutured with size 0 polyglactin and the skin edges are closed with size 0 vetafil or nylon. The incision and sutures should be kept clean and monitored. The sutures can be removed after 14 days.

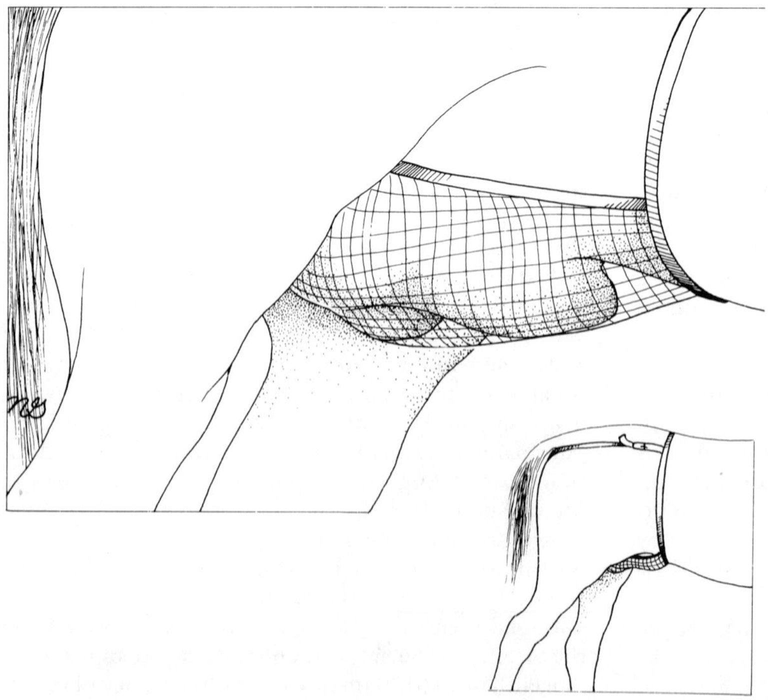

Figure 143–1. Support of the penis and prepuce with a sling attached over the back of the stallion.

RUPTURES OF THE CORPUS SPONGIOSUM

Ruptures of the corpus spongiosum have been reported following an apparent kick in the area a few centimeters ventral to the anal sphincter. The resulting hematoma in this area led to occlusion of the urethra, rupture of the urinary bladder, and death of the stallion. Although injuries to this area are possible, they occur infrequently. The primary concern would appear to be that of confirming the occurrence of urination or placement of a catheter into the bladder.

HEMATOMAS

Hematomas of the stallion's penis are usually superficial, involving the vessels immediately beneath the preputial skin. They also can result from small tears in the corpus cavernosum penis. Preputial hematomas are treated early by the application of cold water hydrotherapy or ice packs. This should be for a minimum of 30 minutes and repeated three or more times per day. Surgical correction of the hematoma is generally not indicated unless it is large and creates a physical problem. If that occurs, removal of the clot should be performed after bleeding at the site has ceased and the clot is beginning to organize, at about 7 to 10 days. If the swelling is extremely large and hemorrhage must be controlled, surgery can be performed to locate and ligate the vessels or to suture the penile tunic. Asepsis is absolutely essential during this operation because of the potential for abscessation after contamination of the hematomas.

Antibiotic therapy should be continued for 7 to 10 days in all penile hematomas. Support of the penis and prepuce is indicated to reduce additional trauma. The prepuce must be checked frequently to be certain no injuries occur as a result of the support and must be cleaned frequently to reduce the possibility of urine scalding. The initial preputial edema and congestion may cause paraphimosis by preventing the normal telescopic movement. Skin drying and sloughing can occur overlying the edematous and tightly swollen areas. This combined with large clot organization and fibrosis may result in scar tissue formation and permanent paraphimosis unless surgical correction is performed. The extent of scar tissue will dictate if reefing surgery, Bolz surgery, or penile amputation is necessary. Stallions should be restricted from breeding for a minimum of 3 weeks in uncomplicated cases to permit complete tissue repair. The rest period is prolonged if surgical intervention is necessary.

ABRASIONS AND LACERATIONS

Abrasions and lacerations may result from mare tail hairs, artificial vaginas, breeding, stitches, stallion rings, breeding cages, striking the erect penis with a lead or other object to correct show or race stallions who become aroused at times other than at breeding, or breeding mares through wire fences. Treatment of all these conditions should begin with a cleaning and thorough examination of the injured area and a physical examination of the animal for other injuries. This should be followed by procedures to reduce swelling and edema—low-pressure cold water hydrotherapy, ice packs, and artificial supports if paraphimosis is present and manual return of the penis into the prepuce is not possible. Once it is possible to return the penis to within the lumen of the prepuce, it can be maintained in place with a pursestring suture of heavy nonabsorbable suture material or with a snug-fitting support attached over the back and between the rear legs. Topical lanolin-based antibiotic creams are of value in reducing the possibility of infection while preventing drying of the penile and preputial skin. Diuretics, systemic penicillin, ampicillin or similar antibiotics, and anti-inflammatory agents may be indicated depending on the severity of the lesion. The animal must be observed for free urination or catheterized to be certain there is no obstruction created by more severe injuries. Chronic urinary bladder catheterization will usually cause cystitis. This should be treated but will usually resolve once the catheter is removed.

BIBLIOGRAPHY

Bowen JM: Management of the breeding stallion, in Morrow DA (ed): *Current Therapy in Theriogenology.* Philadelphia, WB Saunders Co, 1986, vol 2, pp 642–643.

Firth EC: Dissecting hematoma of corpus spongiosum and urinary bladder rupture in a stallion. *J Am Vet Med Assoc* 1976;169:800–801.

Sharrock AG: Reversal of drug-induced priapism in a gelding by medication. *Aust Vet J* 1982;58:39.

Simmons HA, Cox JE, Edwards GB, Neal PA, Urquhart KA: Paraphimosis in seven debilitated horses. *Vet Rec* 1985;116:126–127.

Vaughan JT: Surgery of the male equine reproductive system, in Morrow DA (ed): *Current Therapy in Theriogenology.* Philadelphia, WB Saunders Co, 1986, vol 2, pp 740–745.

Walker DF, Vaughan JT: Surgery of the penis and prepuce, in *Bovine and Equine Urogenital Surgery* Philadelphia, Lea & Febiger, 1980, pp 125–140.

144
Squamous Cell Carcinoma of the Penis

Walter R. Threlfall

DIAGNOSIS

Although tumors involving the stallion's penis and prepuce are uncommon, the squamous cell carcinoma is the most frequently diagnosed neoplasm of this anatomic area. Other tumors such as angiomas, hemangioma, mastocytoma, sarcoids, melanomas in grey horses, and papillomas occur much less frequently. It is important to also differentiate the squamous cell carcinoma from the granulomatous reaction that accompanies *Habronemia species* larvae abberant migration or following injury to the area. The lesions seen with squamous cell carcinoma are usually ulcerated and malodorus because of the necrotic tissue. Early in its development, however, squamous cell carcinoma may be mistaken for simple pigment loss or as a healing wound. Other characteristics of the squamous cell carcinoma include slow growth with local invasion and metastasis to the inguinal lymph nodes. These nodes may increase in size and ulcerate following abscessation. Metastasis to the lungs has been reported but is rare. Cellulitis and edema of the prepuce and inguinal area are common. In all cases a rectal examination should be performed to determine if local invasion has occurred into the inguinal region intraabdominally or the pelvic canal.

The localized preputial and penile lesions seen with granulomas can resemble squamous cell carcinoma. The most common granuloma follows infestation with *Habronemia megastoma* (summer sores). The definitive diagnosis should be based on biopsy and histopathologic examination of the tissue, keeping in mind that a granulomatous or allergic reaction may be present simultaneously with squamous cell carcinoma.

TUMOR REMOVAL

Once the diagnosis of squamous cell carcinoma has been made, the approach to remove the tumor should be selected. The possibilities range from removal of an isolated lesion to amputation of the entire penis. This decision is dependent upon the size of the tumor and the value and use of the animal. The available methods to remove the tumor include the scalpel, cryosurgery, and laser surgery.

Scalpel Excision

For the removal of small lesions, the standing animal can be sedated with xylazine and butorphanol (Torbugesic, Bristol Labs). Following prolapse of the penis, the area is surgically prepared with an iodine-based surgical scrub and water-soaked cotton. Local anesthesia is injected around the lesion. If the scalpel is being used, an incision is made wide to the periphery of the lesion to assure complete excision of the tumor. It must be determined how much tissue can be removed while maintaining sufficient tissue to cover the excised area (Fig. 144–1). The edges are apposed with synthetic absorbable suture. Healing should be complete in 2 to 3 weeks.

Cryosurgery

Cryosurgical techniques may also be used in the treatment of squamous cell carcinoma. While the horse is under general anesthesia, thermocouple electrode needles are placed deep to the lesion and at its periphery. The liquid nitrogen is sprayed onto the lesion until a temperature of −30 °C is reached. The frozen tissue is permitted to thaw slowly and then frozen a second time to −30 °C. Anti-inflammatory agents such as phenylbutazone can be administered after surgery to aid in reduction of swelling. The tissue sloughs 7 to 14 days following treatment. The advantages of cryosurgery have included lack of hemorrhage or necessity for suturing, speed and ease of the procedure, and reduced infection of the surgical site. The disadvantages include delayed healing time, potential for penile sloughing with large lesions, and damage to the urethra following cryosurgery.

Reefing

A reefing operation can be performed to remove larger tumors involving only the prepuce or the movable skin

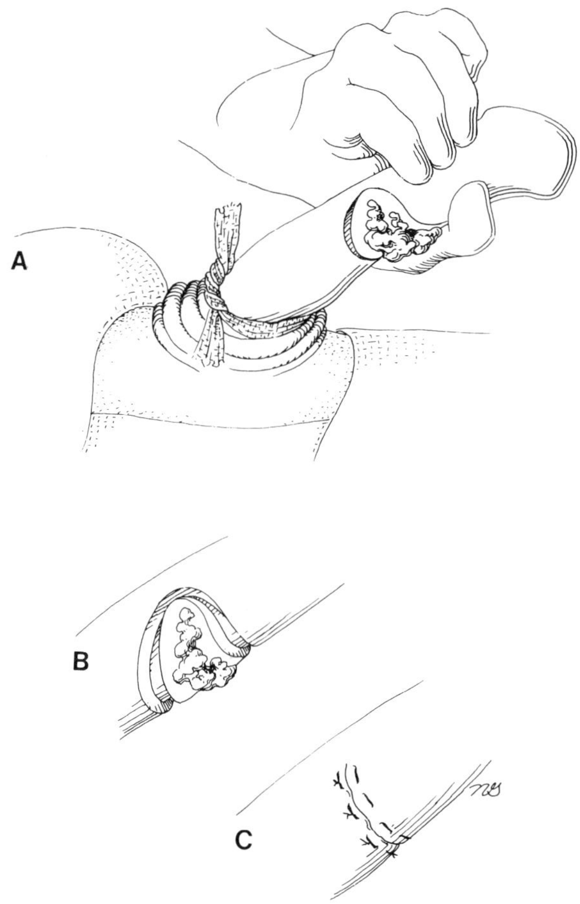

Figure 144–1. Scalpel excision of a lesion. **A.** A piece of gauze or rubber tubing is tied around the base of the penis as a tourniquet. **B.** A wide incision is made around the lesion to assure total excision. **C.** The skin is closed with a synthetic absorbable suture material with any suture pattern that provides skin apposition.

on the penis. For stallions with good disposition and lesions requiring partial preputial removal, the technique can be performed with the horse standing. For removal of large lengths of prepuce or in the case of horses that will not stand quietly under sedation, general anesthesia is recommended with the animal in dorsal recumbency.

The penis is catheterized and surgically prepared by scrubbing with an iodine-based scrub and cotton. A latex rubber tube or gauze is tied around the proximal portion of the penis to serve as a tourniquet. An assistant keeps the penis and prepuce extended throughout the procedure. Two incisions are made that encircle the penis with one above and one below the lesion (Fig. 144–2). The tissue under the lesion and attached prepuce is dissected free and removed. If the lesion extends into the corpus cavernosum penis, amputation is usually required. Care must be taken to ligate any vessels within the incision area. The proximal and distal incisional edges are apposed first by suturing the deep and superficial fascia with simple interrupted 2–0 polyglactin and the skin with interrupted horizontal mattress sutures of 2–0 polydioxanone. The tourniquet is removed and the penis allowed to retract into the preputial sheath. If the penis does not retract, it should be placed within the prepuce and a pursestring suture placed into the preputial orifice. This is to assure no further trauma occurs to the area. If only support and protection of a protruding penis and prepuce are necessary, a sling can be provided to maintain the penis totally within the prepuce. If polydioxanone sutures are used in the skin, suture removal is not necessary and healing should be complete in approximately 1 month.

Vinsot's Operation

If the tumor involves the glans penis, Vinsot's operation can be performed. The surgery is performed with the animal under general anesthesia in lateral recum-

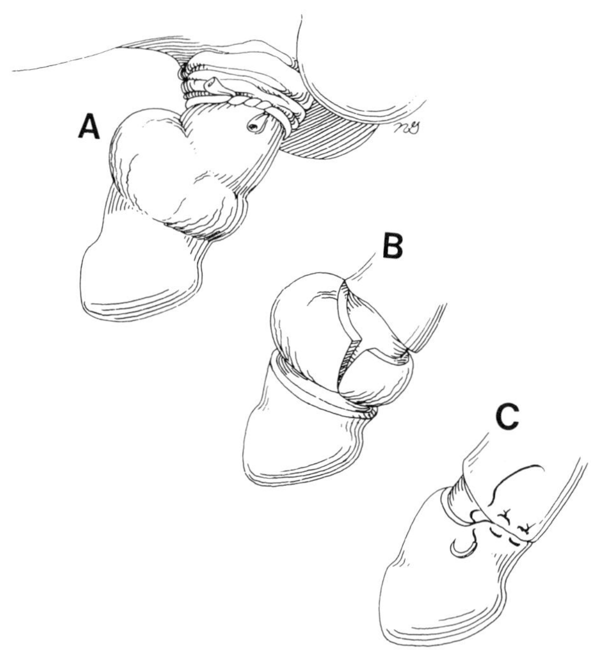

Figure 144–2. A reefing operation for a circumscribed lesion. **A.** A piece of gauze or rubber tubing is tied proximal to the lesion on the penis. **B.** Two incisions, one just proximal and one just distal to the lesion, are made around the entire circumference of the penis and are connected. **C.** The lesion is dissected free of the underlying fascia and the two remaining skin edges are apposed with both fascial and skin sutures.

bency. Following surgical preparation of the penis, a triangular incision with a 2.5-cm base and 3.5-cm sides is made over the urethra. This tissue is removed and the urethra incised and sutured to the edges of the triangle. A fixation suture is placed 2.5 cm distal to the urethral sutures and the penile end is amputated. This surgery is no longer recommended in breeding stallions because they do not appear capable of ejaculation without the sensation provided by the glans penis, and there is the risk of stricture formation around the new urethral opening.

Phallectomy

Although amputation of a large portion of the penis (phallectomy) is recommended for large tumor masses, this is seldom requested for stallions because of the loss of breeding potential and lack of any other use for many of these animals. This technique is more appropriate for geldings with severe penile or preputial lesions. Large carcinomas are one of the major reasons for performing this technique. The procedure is performed under general anesthesia with the animal in dorsal or lateral recumbency. A catheter is placed in the urethra with the penis extended and a tourniquet is secured around the proximal-most portion of the penis to control hemorrhage. The penis and prepuce are surgically prepared by scrubbing with a scrub solution containing iodine. A surgical drape is placed beneath the penis to reduce contamination of the surgical site. Since the lesions are usually impossible to clean thoroughly, it is advisable to have an assistant grasp the distal penis, including the lesion, and prevent them from contaminating the surgical area.

A size 3 chromic catgut suture is passed through the penis 1 cm proximal to the amputation site and dorsal to the urethra, thus surrounding the corpus cavernosium penis (Fig. 144–3). The skin is not included in this suture but is then pulled over the stump of the penis and sutured with size 0 or 2-0 polyglactin or polydioxanone such that the amputation surface is covered except where the urethral orifice will be located. The urethra is incised ventrally for a distance of approximately 3 cm from the stump and the edges of the urethra are pulled laterally and sutured to the edge of the skin.

A modification of this technique involves transecting the urethra approximately 2.5 cm distal to the incision, amputating the remaining distal portion of the penis. The dorsal artery and vein are ligated (Fig. 144–4). The edges of the corpus cavernosum are apposed and sutured with absorbable suture. The protruding urethra is incised longitudinally and the edges apposed to the skin covering the penis. This is also sutured with absorbable suture material.

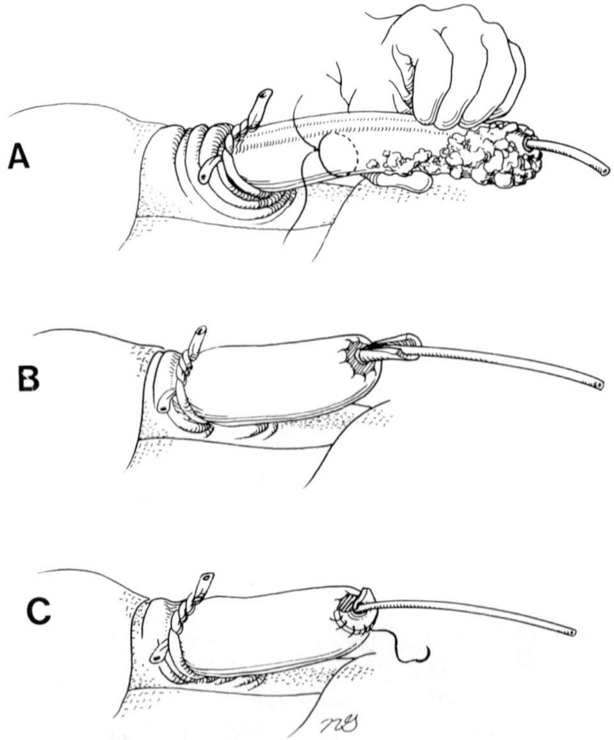

Figure 144–3. Penile amputation with ligation of the corpus cavernosum penis. **A.** After retraction of the penis, placing a urethral catheter and tourniquet application, a size 3 chromic catgut suture is passed beneath the skin around the corpus cavernosum penis and tied. **B.** The penis is amputated just distal to this suture and the skin pulled over the stump of the corpus cavernosum and sutured. **C.** The urethra is incised on ventral midline and stretched out over the remaining surface and apposed to the skin edge by suturing with a synthetic absorbable suture.

En Bloc Resection

The surgical procedure described for the most complete penile and preputial amputation involves resection of the entire prepuce and all of the free body of the penis plus the superficial inguinal lymph nodes as one tissue mass. This procedure is referred to as en bloc resection. The animal is placed under general anesthesia and positioned in dorsal recumbency. The entire area is thoroughly prepared for aseptic surgery. A urethrostomy is performed in the perineal area. The penis is amputated and is sutured to the skin in that area to provide a permanent opening of the urethra. The remainder of the penis and associated enlarged lymph nodes are removed by an incision on the midline and around the opening of the prepuce. Since a large

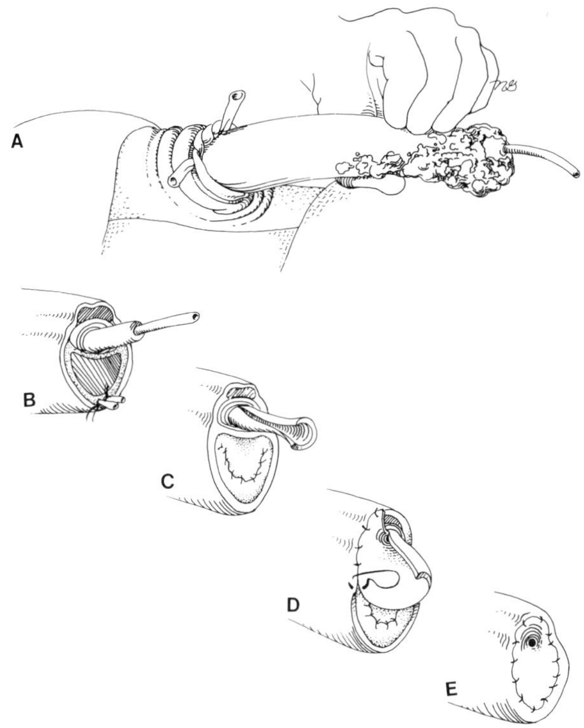

Figure 144–4. Penile amputation with closure of the corpus cavernosum penis. **A.** The penis is prepared similar to the procedure in Figure 144–3. **B.** The penis is amputated, leaving a section of urethra past the amputated corpus cavernosum, and the dorsal artery and vein are ligated. **C.** The end of the corpus cavernosum is sutured closed. **D** and **E.** The extra length of the urethra is incised and stretched out of the surface of the corpus cavernosum **(D),** apposing the urethral mucosa to the skin **(E)**.

area of tissue is being removed and there will be a large amount of dead space, drains should be placed within the open cavity to reduce the subcutaneous accumulation of fluid. This procedure is performed as a last resort when there is extensive surgical removal of tissue and only in cases of extensive involvement of tissue in the preputial and inguinal areas.

Another technique known as penile retroversion and en bloc resection has been described. The major difference between this procedure and en bloc resection alone is that a healthy portion of the penis is rotated caudally 180 degrees and is sutured such that the urethra opens ventral to the ischium. The availability of more tissue, urethra and penis, in this technique was believed to facilitate urination compared to when urethrostomy was performed with en bloc resection. The prepuce, inguinal lymph nodes, and most of the free penis is also removed with this procedure.

PROGNOSIS

Because of the possibility of metastasis of the squamous cell carcinoma, a guarded prognosis should be given whenever this diagnosis is made. Recommendations to owners of breeding stallions should be to frequently examine the penis and prepuce of their stallions for abnormalities. When any lesions are observed, the veterinarian should examine the animal and biopsy the site if necessary to obtain a definitive diagnosis. Finally, specific therapy should be implemented so as to avoid the necessity for radical treatment.

BIBLIOGRAPHY

Chesney J: A technique for amputation of the equine penis. *Equine Vet J* 1980;12:212–213.

Cotchin E: A general survey of tumors in the horse. *Equine Vet J* 1977;7:16–21.

Frank ER: Tail, anus, rectum, vagina and penis, in *Veterinary Surgery* ed 7. Minneapolis, Burgess Publishing Co, 1964, p 302.

Markel MD, Wheat JD, Jones K: Genital neoplasms treated by en bloc resection and penile retroversion in horses: 10 cases (1977–1986). *J Am Vet Med Assoc* 1988;192:396–400.

Moulton JE: Tumors of the male genital system, in Moulton JE (ed): *Tumors in Domestic Animals*, ed 2. Berkeley CA, University of California Press, 1978, pp 309–329.

Stick JA, Hoffer RE: Results of cryosurgical treatment of equine penile neoplasms. *J Equine Med Surg* 1978;2:505–507.

Vaughan JT: Surgery of the male equine reproductive system, in Morrow DA (ed): *Current Therapy in Theriogenology.* Philadelphia, WB Saunders Co, 1986, vol 2, pp 740–745.

145
Surgical Removal of Uroliths

James T. Robertson
Charles A. Buffington

Urinary calculi occur rarely in horses. Calculi may be found anywhere in the urinary tract but form most frequently in the bladder. The primary component of most equine uroliths is some form of calcium carbonate, but they may also include calcium oxalate, magnesium, ammonium, and phosphate. It is somewhat surprising that urolithiasis occurs so rarely in horses considering that equine urine is so highly saturated with calcium carbonate crystals. Much more solute can be held in suspension in urine than in water because other organic and inorganic compounds inhibit crystallization. The alkaline pH of equine urine favors precipitation of calcium carbonate crystals and promotes calculus formation. Desquamated epithelial cells, leukocytes, whole blood, mucus clots, and necrotic tissue can all serve as nuclei for calculus formation. Nonabsorbable braided suture material exposed to the lumen of the urinary tract or stainless steel staples used for bladder closure and extruded into the bladder lumen will also act as a nidus. Calcium carbonate crystals are deposited around the nidus and are bound together by a mucoproteinaceous cementing substance.

Decreased water intake, dehydration, or consumption of feed or water with a high mineral content are also factors that increase urine solute concentration and promote solute precipitation and calculus formation. It is also possible, although never proven, that horses that develop calculi may have a genetic defect. Inhibitors of calcium oxalate crystallization have been identified in human urine and it has been shown that recurrent stone formers have lower urinary inhibitor concentrations.

CYSTIC CALCULI

The incidence of bladder stones is higher in stallions and geldings than in mares and may be related to anatomic differences of the urethra between males and females. Most cystic calculi found in geldings and stallions are singular, are oval in shape, and have a spiculated, rough surface (Fig. 145–1). They are usually less than 15 cm in diameter, although larger calculi have been recorded. This type of stone can be broken or fragmented with a lithotrite, forceps, or an electrohydraulic lithotriptor. Smooth-surfaced, hard stones that are not easily fragmented are encountered less frequently. Cystic calculi must be differentiated from the large accumulations of calcium carbonate sediment found in horses suffering from sorghum cystitis or some other form of neurologic disease of the lumbar and sacral portion of the spinal cord (Fig. 145–2). These horses dribble urine and display posterior ataxia, partial penile paralysis, loss of penile sensation, and retain urine because they have bladder paralysis. Although this sediment can be removed from the bladder, the prognosis is poor because of the primary neurologic disease.

A cystic calculus, particularly the rough surfaced variety, produces cystitis by mechanical irritation of the mucosa and may interfere with evacuation of urine from the bladder. The most common clinical signs include straining to urinate, frequent posturing to urinate, urinating small volumes, and hematuria. Hematuria is often seen near the end of urination and is usually more severe after strenuous exercise. An accumulation of urine salts may be seen around the urethral opening on the glans, and the insides of the hind legs are frequently soiled and urine scalded. Urinalysis shows crystalluria and evidence of cystitis (white blood cells, red blood cells, and bacteria). A culture of the urine may yield bacterial growth. The diagnosis is confirmed by rectal palpation, cystoscopic examination with a flexible endoscope, or rectal ultrasound imaging (Fig. 145–3). Examination is facilitated if the bladder is catheterized and emptied of urine.

Surgical Approaches

There are two surgical approaches commonly used for removal of a cystic calculus in males: laparocystotomy and ischial urethrostomy. Laparocystotomy permits removal of the intact stone and all fragments, which reduces the risk of recurrence. Since the urethra is not traumatized, this method is preferable to ischial

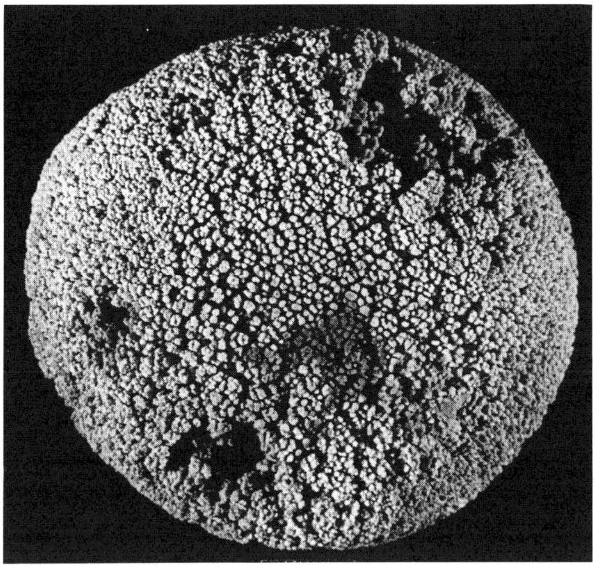

Figure 145–1. A cystic calculus with a spiculated, rough surface.

urethrostomy in stallions. Possible complications from laparocystotomy include peritonitis, bladder leakage, incisional infection, and dehiscence of the incision. Advantages of the perineal urethrostomy approach for calculus removal are that the procedure can be done

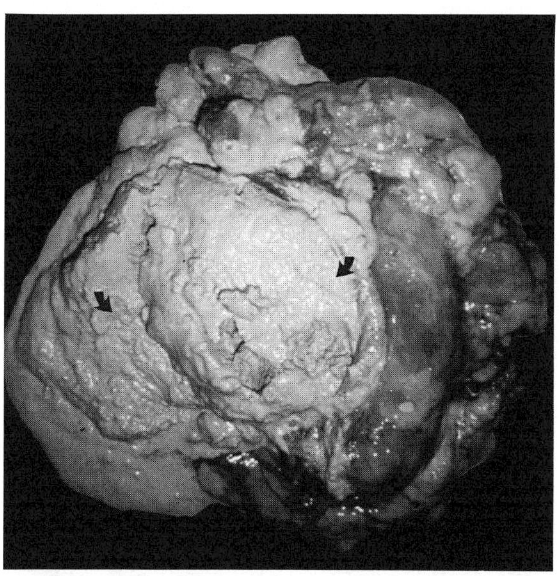

Figure 145–2. At postmortem, this bladder was opened to show a large accumulation of calcium carbonate sediment (*arrows*). The horse had neurologic disease that caused urine retention.

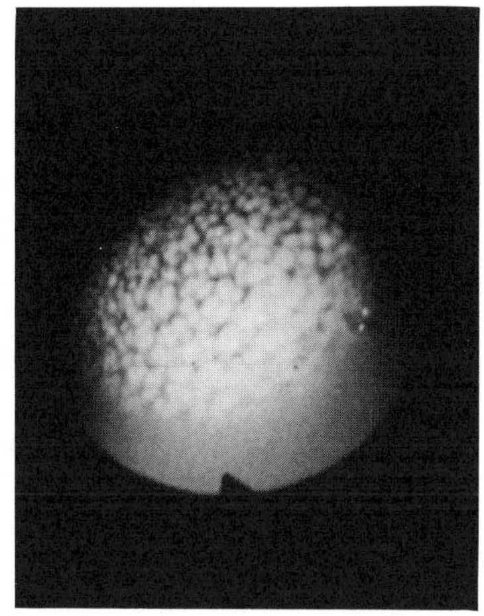

Figure 145–3. An endoscopic view of a cystic calculus partially submerged in urine. Note the rough surface.

with the horse standing, there is little risk of peritonitis, and the incision heals rapidly, allowing a quick return to work. Distinct disadvantages are the trauma sustained by the urethra and bladder during stone removal and a high rate of recurrence of calculi as a result of persistent bladder debris and chronic cystitis. If the stone is large and must be crushed with a lithotrite, surgery can be protracted and frustrating. Trauma to the urethra can result in urethral stricture or fistula formation at the urethrotomy site.

Pararectal cystotomy (Goekel's operation) is a method that can be used in males but is not popular in North America. Although the pararectal approach can be performed in the standing horse under an epidural anesthetic, the dissection is deep and visualization of the bladder is difficult. There is a risk of peritonitis and pelvic abscessation. In females, small stones (<7 cm in diameter) can be removed in the standing mare through the dilated urethra. The sedated mare is placed in stocks and given a light epidural anesthetic [4 to 5 mL of 2% mepivacaine (Carbocaine)/450 kg]. It is possible to gradually introduce a well-lubricated, small hand or large spoonlike forceps through the urethra into the bladder to grasp and remove the stone. Stone removal may be facilitated by a urethral sphincterotomy. Larger stones can be crushed with forceps and fragmented to allow removal or they are removed intact through a laparocystotomy. In one mare, an electrohydraulic lithotriptor, introduced through the urethra, was used to fragment a 7-cm calculus composed of ammonium urate and struvite salts. The electrohydraulic equipment converts electrical energy into mechanical energy and creates a hydraulic shock wave that is capable of disrupting the calculus. The fragments are then lavaged from the bladder.

Laparocystotomy. In preparation for a laparocystotomy the horse is fasted for 24 hours and started on broad-spectrum antibiotics. If a preoperative bacterial culture shows a bacterial cystitis is present, antibiotic selection can be based on the sensitivity results. The horse is anesthetized with a general anesthetic and placed in dorsal recumbency. A sterile urinary catheter is passed to provide for urine drainage. Laparocystotomy is performed through a ventral paramedian incision between the prepuce and the inguinal ring in the male and a ventral midline incision in the female. A wound protector is placed in the incision and Balfour retractors or rib spreaders are used to retract the edges of the incision and provide exposure to the abdomen. The operator grasps the contracted bladder containing the calculus, and with gentle, persistent digital traction, the bladder is exteriorized. Moist towels are packed around the bladder and stay sutures of narrow umbilical tape or size 2 suture material are placed in the apex of the bladder at each end of the proposed incision site. If too much tension is put on these sutures they will tear the bladder wall. Using a scalpel, an incision is made through the bladder wall directly over the stone. The bladder mucosa is carefully peeled away from the calculus and the stone is removed. Remaining fragments are removed manually with gauze sponges and with suction following saline lavage. The bladder is closed with size 0 synthetic absorbable suture material in two layers. The first layer can be a simple interrupted or continuous pattern and the second layer should be an inverting pattern. We prefer the second layer to be an interrupted Lembert pattern. A routine abdominal closure is performed following a change of gloves and using a new instrument pack. An indwelling urinary catheter is not necessary.

Following laparocystotomy it is important to maintain the horse on broad-spectrum antibiotics for at least 5 days. The horse should be observed for urinations. One author recommends frequent rectal examinations during the first few postoperative days to free intestine that may have adhered to the bladder incision line. The horse should receive 30 to 60 days of stall rest before resuming normal activities.

Perineal Urethrostomy. With the horse standing in stocks, an epidural anesthetic (6 to 8 mL of 2% mepivacaine/450 kg) is administered and a urinary catheter is passed to drain the bladder of urine and aid in the intraoperative identification of the urethra. The rectum is evacuated and the surgical site is prepared. An 8-cm midline skin incision is made, extending ventrally over the ischial arch of the penis from just below the anal sphincter. Using a scalpel, the incision is continued between the paired bellies of the retractor penis muscle and through the bulbospongiosus muscle, the corpus spongiosum urethra, and the urethra. Identification of the urethra is greatly facilitated by digital palpation of the urinary catheter. Incision into the vascular sinusoids surrounding the urethra frequently produces hemorrhage that usually subsides spontaneously. Once the urethra is opened, the catheter is removed. The urethral incision is extended proximally to the level of the horizontal pelvic urethra to allow introduction of instruments into the bladder. An arm is placed in the rectum and the stone is manipulated back into the neck of the bladder (Fig. 145–4). A small stone can be grasped and extracted with long forceps (Fig. 145–5) but most large stones must be crushed with a lithotrite and removed in fragments. The lithotrite is passed into the bladder and the stone is manipulated rectally and placed into its opened jaws. The jaws of the instrument are then slowly closed. Before crushing the stone, the

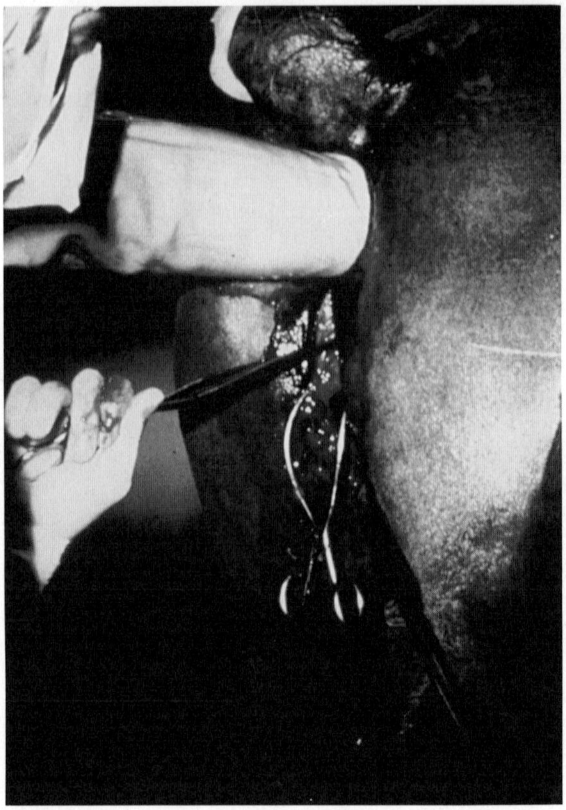

Figure 145–4. The surgeon is manipulating the cystic calculus rectally with his left hand and positioning long forceps to grasp the stone with his right. (Courtesy of Dr. L. Bramlage.)

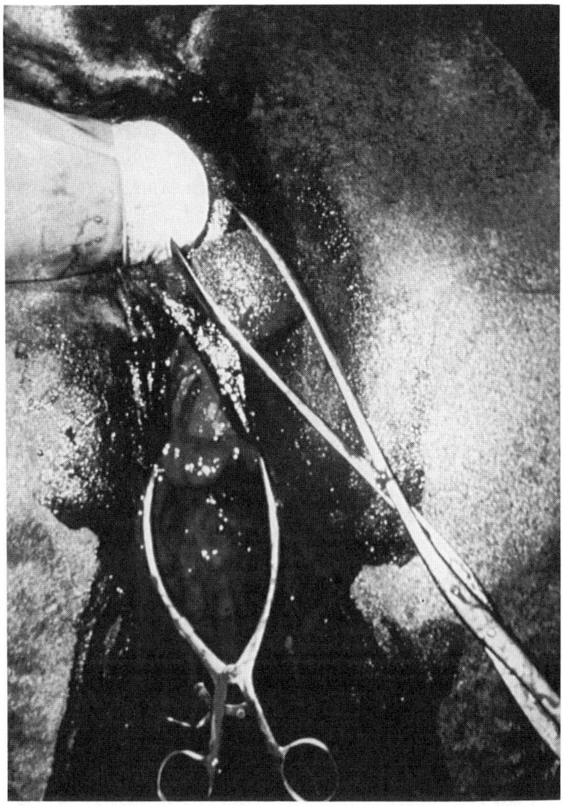

Figure 145–5. This small stone was grasped and extracted with long forceps. (Courtesy of Dr. L. Bramlage.)

operator must be sure that the wall of the bladder is free from the jaws of the instrument. The calculus is crushed, fragments are removed, and the bladder is flushed with several gallons of saline to wash away the debris. We have found the best way to do this is to place a large-diameter tube into the bladder and alternately fill and drain the bladder. An arm is kept in the rectum during this flushing procedure to monitor the degree of bladder distention. The distal urethra should also be flushed to remove all fragments and debris. The bladder can then be evaluated endoscopically to ensure that all fragments have been removed. The incision is left to heal by second intention, and usually the urethra is healed in 2 to 3 weeks.

Postoperative care includes daily cleaning of the wound, flushing the bladder with one gallon of 10% Betadine solution daily for 4 to 5 days, and applying ointment or vaseline to the hind quarters to prevent urine scalding. Exercise can resume when the urethrostomy is healed. We recommend follow-up rectal and endoscopic examination of the bladder at 2- to 3-month intervals after surgery to check for recurrence of the calculus. In horses in which it was necessary to fragment the stone with a lithotrite, we have encountered recurrence of cystic calculi as early as 2 months and as late as 6 years following surgery.

Electrohydraulic Lithotripsy. Recently, electrohydraulic lithotripsy was used to treat cystic calculus in two pony geldings. Both were put under general anesthesia and placed in dorsal recumbency. A cystoscope was passed into the bladder through a perineal urethrotomy incision to allow examination of the calculus and bladder mucosa. The lithotripsy probe was then introduced into the bladder and the calculus was fragmented. The fragments were either removed through the cystoscope or removed via the urethra with forceps. This technique for fragmentation of a calculus, if successful, would appear to be much less traumatic than crushing the stone with a conventional lithotrite. It may also be possible to perform this type of lithotripsy in the standing horse using epidural anesthesia. Unfortunately, the equipment is expensive.

Prognosis and Special Considerations

It is difficult to make definitive recommendations regarding measures to prevent recurrence of cystic calculi because there is no specific etiology. In the immediate postoperative period antibiotics, diuretics, and urinary acidifiers have been recommended. Although a urinary acidifier such as ammonium chloride should reduce the amount of carbonate available for precipitation, it appears to have little effect in the horse when administered orally at a dose of 20 mg/kg. However, it was recently reported that ammonium chloride, used at a high dosage rate (520 mg/kg), was effective in acidifying the urine of two pony geldings. While long-term safety and efficacy of this dose was not evaluated, it suggests that medical therapy may have a place in horses that are not good surgical candidates.

Horses being fed legume hays should be switched to grass hay because legume hays are relatively high in calcium and oxalate and are alkalinizing. Fresh, clean water should be available at all times. Salt added to the ration may increase water intake and urine production. Vitamin and mineral supplements should not be added to the ration.

URETHRAL CALCULI

Urethral calculi are found in colts, geldings, and stallions. The obstruction is usually near the ischial arch or in the distal portion of the urethra. Urethral obstruction leads to bladder distention; prolonged obstruction can produce urethral necrosis or cause bladder rupture and subsequent peritonitis. Horses with a urethral obstruction show signs of abdominal pain and will strain, prolapse the penis, and make repeated attempts to urinate. The distended bladder and obstructed urethra are palpable by rectal examination. The point of obstruction can be determined by passing a urinary catheter or a flexible fiberoptic endoscope through the urethra. A calculus lodged near the ischial arch can be removed by ischial urethrostomy under epidural anesthetic. If the calculus is in the distal urethra, attempts can be made to dislodge it by manipulating the penis, or by grasping it with sponge forceps. If surgical removal is required, a ventral urethrostomy is performed with the horse in dorsal recumbency under general anesthesia. Stricture formation may occur at the site of obstruction if there is urethral necrosis. Following stone removal, a fiberoptic examination of the bladder should be performed for evidence of necrosis, cystitis, or more calculi.

URETERAL AND RENAL CALCULI

Ureteral or renal calculi may be asymptomatic, or may produce signs that range from mild abdominal discomfort or lumbar pain to anorexia, depression, and weight loss. Renal and ureteral calculi are frequently found bilaterally, and renal failure may result from obstruction of urine flow. Signs indicative of renal failure include polydipsia, polyuria, mild dehydration, hyponatremia, hypochloremia, and hypercalcemia. Serum creatinine and blood urea nitrogen levels are elevated. Unfortunately, the diagnosis of kidney disease is frequently made when the disease is in an advanced stage. Obstruction of a ureter produces dilatation of the ureter proximal to the obstruction and hydronephrosis, both of which are palpable per rectum. The calculus may be palpated in the ureter at the site of obstruction. The ureters can also be examined with ultrasound from within the rectum.

It is also possible to palpate calculi in the renal pelvis. The calculi grind against each other when manipulated. Ultrasound imaging at the level of the paralumbar fossa can be used to detect the presence of renal calculi and to determine the size of the kidney and the degree of renal pelvis distention. During cystoscopy with a flexible endoscope the patency of each ureter can be evaluated by observing intermittent urine entry from the ureteral openings into the bladder.

Surgical Approaches

In adult horses, abdominal approaches permit only limited access to the ureters and kidneys, although MacHarg et al. reported successful removal of a ureterolith in a mare using a ventral midline incision. A longitudinal incision was made into the ureter adjacent to the calculus and the calculus was removed. The ureter was stented with a 16-gauge sump drain that was passed retrograde through the vagina and sutured to the vulva. The stent was removed on the ninth postoperative day; the ureter healed and a stricture did not develop. During a second operation on the same mare 5 months later, a ureterolith located in the opposite ureter was removed with a Dormia stone basket (Dormia Stone Dislodger; V. Mueller). The basket was introduced into the ureter through a vestibulourethral approach, passed beyond the calculus, and then opened and retracted to ensnare the calculus. With steady, gentle traction the calculus was removed. The authors of this report suggested that in order to successfully use a Dormia stone basket to remove a ureteral calculus, the stone must be 2 cm in diameter or less and be situated within 30 cm of the trigone.

Recently, Donawick described a paralumbar approach for ureteral and renal calculus removal. The horse is fasted for 48 hours prior to surgery to reduce the bulk of ingesta. Under general anesthesia, the horse is secured to a vertical surgery table and held in an upright position. Alternatively the horse can be placed in lateral recumbency. The incision begins high in the paralumbar fossa, behind the last rib, and curves downward and backward toward the flank for a distance of 25 cm. It is extended with sharp dissection through the muscle layers to the peritoneum. The kidney and proximal ureter are exposed with careful retroperitoneal dissection and the ureter is freed from the adjacent fascia and peritoneum. Penrose drains passed around the ureter provide traction for greater exposure. A stab incision along the long axis of the ureter allows removal of calculi situated in the proximal ureter. A basket stone retriever can be introduced through the stab incision to retrieve calculi that are inaccessible. The ureters can be examined by passing a small-diameter endoscope in either direction through the stab incision. The stab incision is closed with size 3-0 synthetic suture material. Kidney stones can be removed by first mobilizing the kidney from its surrounding tissues and then incising into the kidney along the greater curvature to remove the stone. The capsule of the kidney is closed with interrupted chromic catgut sutures. Closure of the wound is best achieved if the horse is placed in lateral recumbency.

Prognosis

Despite occasional reports of successful removal of ureteral and renal calculi, the overall prognosis for surgical treatment remains poor. The disease is usually advanced before the diagnosis is made, and there are usually multiple calculi, often occurring bilaterally.

BIBLIOGRAPHY

DeBowes RM, Nyrop KA, Boulton CH: Cystic calculi in the horse. *Compend Cont Educ Pract Vet* 1984;6:S268–S273.

Donawick WJ: Surgery of the kidney in the horse, in *Proceedings of the 15th Annual Veterinary Surgery Forum, Equine General Surgery*. Chicago, ACUS, 1987, pp 102–104.

Eustace RA, Hunt JM, Brearley MJ: Electrohydraulic lithotripsy for the treatment of cystic calculus in two geldings. *Equine Vet J* 1988;20:221–223.

Hackett RP, Vaughan JT, Tennant BC: Diseases of the urinary bladder, in Mansmann RA, McAllister ES, Pratt PW (eds): *Equine Med and Surgery*, ed 3. Santa Barbara, CA, American Veterinary Publications, 1983, pp 912–921.

MacHarg MA, Foerner JJ, Phillips TN, Barclay WP: Two methods for the treatment of ureterolithiasis in a mare. *Vet Surg* 1984;13:95–98.

MacHarg MA, Foerner JJ, Phillips TN, Barclay WP, McCracken RJ: Electrohydraulic lithotripsy for treatment of a cystic calculus in a mare. *Vet Surg* 1985;14:325–327.

McIlwraith CW, Turner AS: Removal of cystic calculus (laparocystotomy), in *Equine Surgery Advanced Techniques*. Philadelphia, Lea & Febiger, 1987, pp 360–363.

Trotter GW, Bennett DG, Behm RJ: Urethral calculi in five horses. *Vet Surg* 1981;10:159–162.

146
Patent Urachus and Infected Umbilical Remnants

Rolf M. Embertson

Abnormalities of the urachus and the umbilical arteries and vein are not uncommon in the young foal. To understand the pathologic processes that can occur, it is helpful to know the function and anatomy of the structures in the fetus, and the changes that occur to these structures in the foal. The urachus allows the flow of urine from the fetal bladder to the allantoic cavity. The umbilical arteries, which drain blood in the fetus, course along each side of the urinary bladder and urachus to the umbilicus and enter the umbilical cord. The umbilical vein in the fetus carries oxygenated blood through the umbilicus, into the fetus, to the liver where the blood enters the fetal circulation.

Upon birth and after rupture of the umbilical cord, the urachus and the umbilical arteries and vein retract, shrink, and cease to function. The urachus is enclosed in a ventral peritoneal fold in the fetus and in the newborn. This fold eventually forms the middle ligament of the bladder, while the urachus atrophies to become a fibrous scar at the apex of the bladder. The umbilical arteries become the round ligaments, which are contained in the lateral ligaments of the bladder. The peritoneal fold encompassing the umbilical vein becomes the falciform ligament and the vein becomes the fibrous cord in the ligament that is continued as the round ligament of the liver.

PATENT URACHUS

Diagnosis

Patent urachus may be congenital or acquired. It has been hypothesized that the congenital form is the result of excessive torsion of the umbilical cord in utero, causing dilation of the urachus and failure of its closure at birth. In the affected foal, urine exiting the umbilicus may range from just a dribble to a stream, depending on the degree of patency of the urachus. In the acquired form, the urachus may become patent when the foal is a few days to a few weeks old. This is generally thought to result from infection of the umbilical structures, causing disruption of the urachal seal. In addition to urine exiting the umbilicus, these foals may also present with heat, pain, and swelling at the umbilicus and occasionally with evidence of sepsis elsewhere in the body (e.g., pneumonia, infectious arthritis) (Fig. 146–1).

Treatment

Congenital Patent Urachus. Treatment of the foal with a congenital patent urachus includes providing a clean environment, daily cleansing of the umbilicus, systemic antibiotics, and chemical cauterization of the

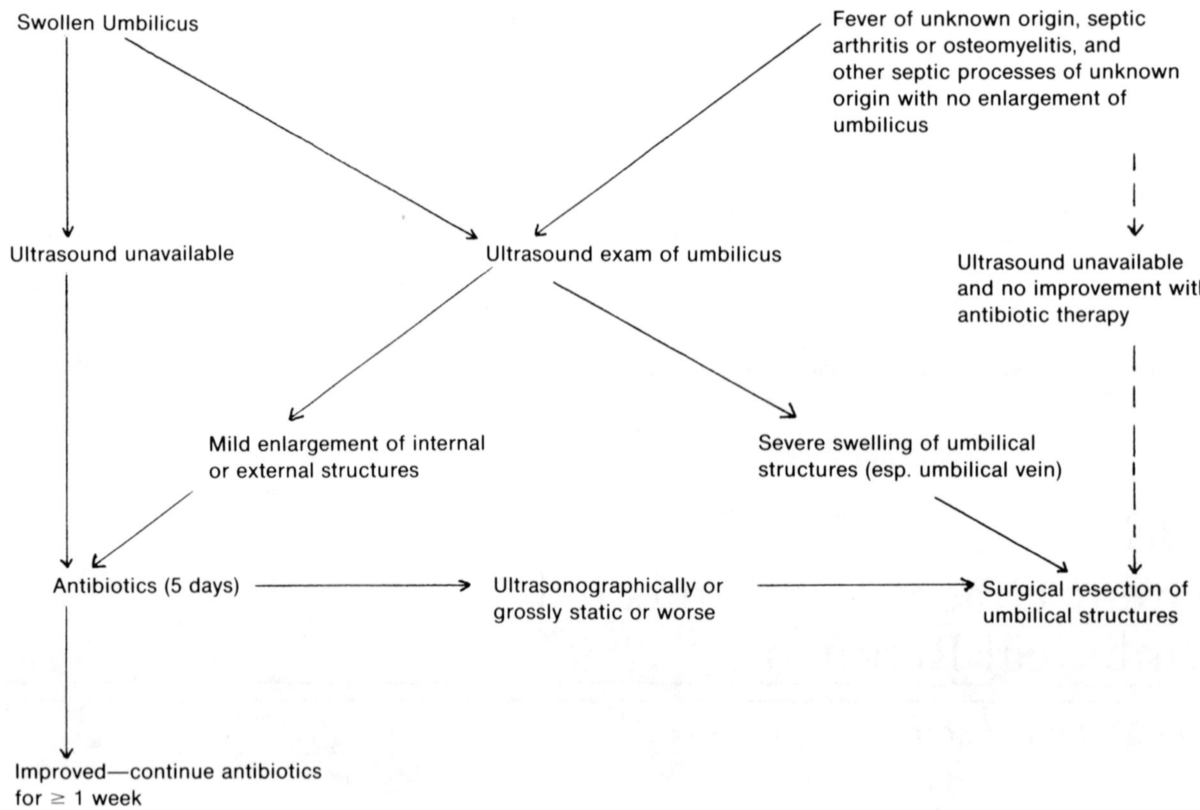

Figure 146–1. General approach to diagnosis and treatment of infected umbilical remnants.

distal 2 to 3 cm of the urachal lumen. The therapy is intended to prevent an ascending infection into the umbilical structures and to produce swelling and subsequent closure of the urachus. Chemical cautery of the urachus is performed with silver nitrate sticks or with cotton-tipped swabs saturated with phenol or a strong iodine solution. This should be performed three to four times daily until urine ceases to exit the umbilicus. Surgical resection of the urachus is indicated if the condition fails to respond to 5 days of medical therapy. The surgical technique used is essentially the same as that described for infected umbilical structures below.

Acquired Patent Urachus. The treatment for acquired patent urachus depends on the severity of the umbilical remnant infection. This is determined by a thorough examination of the infected tissues, culture and sensitivity of a sample obtained from the urachus, and if possible ultrasound examination of the umbilical structures. If a mild infection is suspected, therapy is the same as for the congenital form. Appropriate antibiotics are determined by the culture and sensitivity. If this was not done, or if the foal was on antibiotics at the time the sample was obtained (generally yielding no growth), penicillin and gentamicin or amikacin should be used. β-Hemolytic streptococci, *Escherichia coli*, and *Proteus species* are the organisms most commonly isolated from the umbilical structures. If the urachus closes with this therapy, antibiotic therapy should be continued for several more days because some infection may be retained in the umbilical structures. Surgery is recommended if urine continues to drip from the umbilicus after approximately 5 days of therapy.

If moderate to severe infection of the urachus or umbilical arteries or vein is found or suspected, surgical resection of the umbilical remnants is recommended. The use of chemical cautery of these infected tissues may create more necrotic tissue and may seal off pockets of infection and prevent drainage. The infected urachus can serve as a focus for generalized sepsis or septicemia.

Complications

Complications may be encountered in treatment of the patent urachus. Excessive use of caustic solutions around the umbilicus will cause severe tissue inflammation. This causes discomfort for the foal, creating a less cooperative patient, and causes tissue inflammation that is not desirable for potential surgery. Perforation through the urachus into the peritoneal cavity is a rare complication associated with the use of cautery sticks. This may result in peritonitis or herniation of mentum through the opening.

Prognosis

With early diagnosis and appropriate treatment, patent urachus in the foal generally has a good prognosis. However, delay in recognition of the condition or inappropriate therapy can allow infection to spread to other organs (e.g., joint infection). The resultant septicemia can be fatal.

INFECTED UMBILICAL REMNANTS

Foals with infected umbilical remnants not associated with a patent urachus are seen much more commonly in our practice area than are foals with infected umbilical remnants associated with a patent urachus. The majority of foals with infected umbilical remnants present between 2 and 4 weeks of age, whereas the majority of foals with concurrent patent urachus are 2 weeks of age or younger. Perhaps the initial infection is milder and is not manifested clinically until after a firm seal is formed at the urachus-bladder junction in the slightly older foals that do not acquire a patent urachus. The rest of the discussion in this section will center on foals with infected umbilical remnants; however, the surgical technique discussed for resection of the umbilical remnants is essentially the same for all conditions involving the urachus/umbilicus.

Diagnosis

The diagnosis of infected umbilical remnants can usually be made after a thorough physical examination. The first abnormality noticed is usually a warm, painful swelling at the umbilicus. This swelling may develop gradually over several days or may arise relatively suddenly over a 12-hour period. When first noticed, many foals have a closed, dry umbilicus, which may shortly become open and draining. Other abnormal findings, such as depression, fever, white blood cells increased or decreased in number, or other septic processes (pneumonia or septic joints), occur inconsistently. Conversely, foals may present with a septic process (e.g., septic joint) or even a fever of unknown origin and have no external swelling at the umbilicus, yet have infected umbilical remnants. In these foals, the umbilical structures can be evaluated ultrasonographically to determine if the internal umbilical remnants are normal in appearance. Ultrasonographic examination is also useful in foals with obvious infected umbilical remnants to determine which umbilical structures appear affected and to what extent (Fig. 146–2).

Treatment

Foals with infected umbilical remnants that have moderate external umbilical swelling or mild enlargement of the internal umbilical structures on ultrasound examination should initially be treated medically. This includes administration of appropriate antibiotics and hot packs or hydrotherapy of the umbilicus. A sample for culture and sensitivity should be obtained from the umbilical stalk prior to commencement of antibiotic therapy. If a culture is not obtained, penicillin and gentamicin should be used because of the most common isolates encountered (β-hemolytic streptococci, *E. coli*, *Proteus species*). Prompt and prolonged medical therapy is often successful in the resolution of mild to moderate umbilical remnant infections. If medical therapy does not lead to a significant reduction in size of the umbilical structures by about 5 days or if the umbilical structures are grossly enlarged initially, surgical resection of the umbilical remnants is indicated (Fig. 146–1).

Complete en bloc resection of the umbilical structures allows adequate examination of these structures and usually complete removal of the septic structures

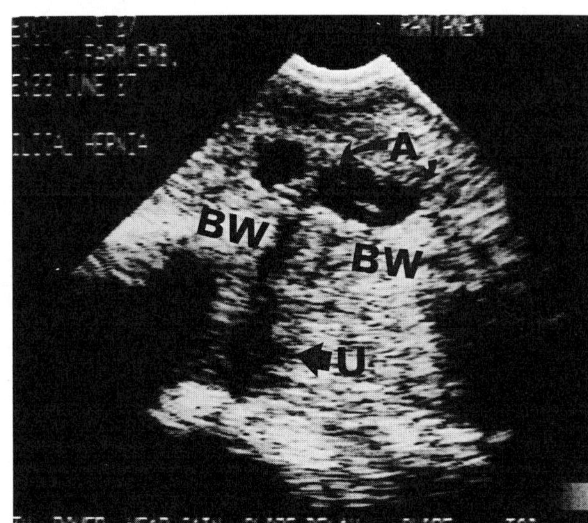

Figure 146–2. Sonogram of a foal umbilicus. The external abscess (*A*) connects to the urachus (*U*) through the body wall (*BW*). Ultrasound examination can also identify abnormal enlargement of the umbilical vein and umbilical arteries.

with minimal to no contamination of the surgery site. This surgery should be considered a clean-contaminated procedure that carries some risk of a major break in sterile technique (gross spillage of exudate into the peritoneal cavity). Consequently, appropriate antibiotic use is important. The type of antibiotics given preoperatively can be directed by previous culture results or by the knowledge of the most common isolates encountered. Alternatively, intraoperative antibiotics can be initiated after surgical removal and accurate culturing of the infected umbilical structures.

Surgical Technique. The foal is anesthetized and placed in dorsal recumbency. The abdomen is clipped and prepared for a ventral midline abdominal incision that may extend from several centimeters caudal to the umbilicus to near the xiphoid process of the sternum. If the umbilicus is open and draining, the opening is inverted and sealed with a continuous Lembert suture pattern in the skin prior to surgical preparation of the skin. In the male foal, the penis can be extended, deflected caudally to one side, and secured between the hind limbs.

A fusiform skin incision is made around the umbilicus. The incision is continued through the linea alba cranial to the umbilicus, carefully avoiding an incision into the umbilical vein, and the peritoneal cavity is entered. The umbilical vein is examined for evidence of infection and, if normal, is ligated and transected just cranial to the umbilicus. Occasionally, a very large, exudate-filled umbilical vein is encountered that extends to the liver. An umbilical vein of this character should be transected as close to the liver as possible and the end ligated and oversewn. Alternatively, the umbilical vein can be marsupialized to allow drainage. Marsupialization should not be completed unless obvious infection cannot be removed. The technique involves drawing the end of the transected umbilical vein through a separate stab incision made 3 cm lateral to the abdominal incision. The umbilical vein stump is secured to this opening with 2-0 polydioxanone (PDS; Ethicon Inc) in three layers; the first layer involves the peritoneum and internal rectus fascia, the second layer secures the vein to the external rectus fascia and subcutaneous tissue, and the third layer involves the skin.

Once the umbilical vein has been ligated, the abdominal incision is carefully continued along both sides of the umbilicus and caudally through the linea alba as far as necessary to expose the apex of the bladder and evaluate the umbilical arteries for infection. The umbilical arteries are ligated and transected as far caudally along the sides of the bladder as considered necessary to remove infected tissue. Normal umbilical arteries are ligated and transected near the apex of the bladder. The urachus and apex of the bladder are packed off with laparotomy sponges. Stay sutures are placed through the bladder wall on either side of the apex just proximal to the proposed line of resection. The apex of the bladder is amputated and the resected umbilical structures are removed from the surgical field. Prompt suction is often needed to prevent the spillage of urine into the abdominal cavity. The bladder is closed with 3-0 absorbable synthetic suture material in two layers. A simple continuous pattern apposes the bladder mucosa and a continuous Lembert pattern inverts the seromuscular layer. Lavage of the abdomen with warm saline can be performed prior to closure if warranted by the degree of contamination encountered during surgery. The abdomen is closed in three layers. Absorbable, synthetic suture material (size 1 or 2) is placed in a continuous pattern to close the linea alba. Similar suture material is used to close the subcutaneous tissue (3-0), and skin (2-0).

Systemic antibiotic therapy is continued for 3 days postoperatively. If all the affected tissue could not be removed (e.g., severe umbilical vein infection), antibiotic therapy should be extended for at least 2 more weeks. Flunixin meglumine (Banamine) is useful for the infrequent foal that may exhibit mild colic for the first 24 hours postoperatively. Postoperative exercise consists of stall rest with controlled walking for 1 week, small paddock exercise with the mare only for an additional 2 weeks, and then turnout with the other mares and foals.

Complications

Clinically apparent postoperative complications such as incisional infection, peritonitis, cystitis, or peritoneal adhesions are of concern; however, these are rare. Concurrent septic processes must be appropriately treated. A strong recommendation of whether to blind stump or marsupialize a large infected umbilical vein is difficult to make as long-term followup on a large number of cases is not currently available. Foals have done well with either technique, the only known complication being an incisional hernia at a marsupialization site.

Prognosis

Foals with infection of umbilical structures ranging from mild to severe generally have a good prognosis if the disease is recognized and treated promptly and appropriately. Delay in recognition or treatment of the disease process may lead to septicemia or may initiate sepsis elsewhere in the body (e.g., joint infection, peritonitis), some of which may cause complications, necessitate extensive treatment, or have a fatal outcome.

BIBLIOGRAPHY

Adams SB, Fessler JF: Umbilical cord remnant infections in foals: 16 cases (1975–1985). *J Am Vet Med Assoc* 1987; 190:316–318.

McIlwraith CW, Turner AS: Resection of the diseased urachus in foals, in *Equine Surgery Advanced Techniques*. Philadelphia, Lea & Febiger, 1987, pp 364–367.

Reef VB: Abnormalities of the neonatal umbilicus detected by diagnostic ultrasound. *Proc AAEP Ann Conven* 1986; pp 157–162.

Richardson DW: Urogenital problems in the neonatal foal. *Vet Clin North Am Equine Pract* 1985;1:170–188.

Turner TA, Fessler JF, Ewert KM: Patent urachus in foals. *Equine Pract* 1982;4:24–31.

Walker DF, Vaughan JT: Surgery of the urinary tract, in *Bovine and Equine Urogenital Surgery*. Philadelphia, Lea & Febiger, 1980, pp 171–182.

147 Uroperitoneum

Donnie E. Slone, Jr.

Although surgical texts generally deal only with ruptured bladders as a cause of uroperitoneum, there are two other recognized causes of uroperitoneum: urachal perforations and ureteral defects. Urine leakage from ruptured bladders and ureteral defects begins at birth, whereas urachal perforations may occur soon after birth or within the first 1 to 2 weeks of life. These urachal perforations result from a septic necrosis of the urachus.

DIAGNOSIS

The foal with uroperitoneum due to leakage from the bladder or ureter will generally be presented at 3 to 4 days of age. Ruptured bladders occur somewhat more commonly, but not exclusively, in the male. There have not been enough cases of ureteral defects to determine if a sex predilection exists. The history generally is that the foal was normal for the first 36 to 48 hours except possibly for an increased frequency of urination or straining. This straining may be confused with meconium impaction but usually can be differentiated by observing postures for urination versus defecation. It is unusual to have a foal that has not urinated at all even if it has a ruptured bladder. During the 48 to 96-hour range following birth, the foal becomes more and more depressed. The abdomen increases in size and fluid can be ballotted and auscultated in the abdominal cavity. Eventually fluid will fill the scrotum of males, giving a false appearance of inguinal hernia, and will also enter the thorax. Controversy exists about the movement of the fluid into the thorax. Some authors propose there is direct penetration of diaphragm through natural openings, whereas others think the fluid is an effusion. However, in the cases I observed the fluid was present in the thorax of foals that also had fluid in the scrotum, possibly indicating simultaneous occurrence.

Foals with a defect in the urachus generally have an entirely different signalment and history. These foals may be the same age as foals with ruptured bladders if they were born with septicemias or they may be up to several weeks old. Generally these foals have been sick for several days and have been treated for septicemia, patent urachus, joint infections, enteritis, or pneumona. Uroperitoneum in these foals is sometimes overlooked because of the preoccupation with the foal's other problems and because the condition seems to develop slowly.

Uroperitoneum can generally be confirmed by abdominocentesis performed at or caudal to the umbilicus to avoid omental blockage of the needle or teat cannula. A large volume of fluid is usually obtained. If uroperitoneum exists, the creatinine of this fluid is at least two to three times greater than the serum creatinine. Hyponatremia, hypochloremia, and hyperkalemia are also consistent findings in foals with ruptured bladders or defects in their ureters. These electrolyte changes occur because the foal is drinking milk that is relatively low in both sodium and chloride. Furthermore, the kidney conserves sodium and chloride while excreting a potassium-rich urine into the peritoneal cavity. Consequently, potassium, increases in the plasma as the fluid in the peritoneal cavity equilibrates with the plasma and from intracellular release subsequent to acidosis. These electrolyte aberrations may be much less severe or not present in foals with a perforated urachus since those foals often have been given intravenous fluids that have a greater concentration of sodium and chloride than does milk. Additionally these electrolyte abnormalities should not be considered pathognomonic for uroperitoneum since they may also occur with other problems, such as enteritis and primary renal disease.

Infusion of methylene blue or fluorescein dye via a urinary catheter followed by retrieval of the dye from the abdomen via a subsequent abdominocentesis is a method that has previously been recommended to diagnose ruptured bladder or a perforated urachus. This procedure would not be expected to yield a positive result in a foal with a defect in a ureter. Therefore this test might help differentiate a ureteral defect from ruptured bladder. Further study of intravenous urograms or retrograde cystography needs to be done to help the surgeon recognize defective ureters preoperatively. Normally the surgeon makes this distinction at the time of surgery, although this requires the surgeon to be cognizant of the rare ureteral defect and be prepared to find and repair it if present.

PREOPERATIVE TREATMENT

The repair of these defects is not an emergency. Because severe third-degree atrioventricular block is a common anesthetic complication associated with the attendant electrolyte, fluid, and acid-base aberrations, these abnormalities require immediate therapy and must be at least partially corrected prior to surgery. Normal or hypertonic saline and bicarbonate should be given intravenously to help raise serum sodium and chloride concentrations, correct the acidosis, and dilute the serum potassium. The urine should be drained from the abdominal cavity using one or more teat cannulas placed at or caudal to the umbilicus. Normal saline may also be used to lavage the peritoneal cavity. It has also been recommended to give intravenous dextrose at 0.5 g/kg body weight and crystalline insulin at 0.1 U/kg body weight to help reduce the serum potassium by moving it intracellularly, although this is rarely necessary. Correction of the acidosis should also serve this function. Lowering the serum potassium to at least 6 mEq/L prior to surgery is recommended.

Auscultation of the foal's chest should be done and radiography would be helpful to assess the amount of fluid in the thorax. If significant fluid is present, it should also be removed.

Broad-spectrum antibiotics should be given prior to surgery. Because the atrioventricular block is resistant to atropine given once it has developed, I administer atropine (0.01 mg/kg intramuscularly or intravenously) preoperatively. In addition to the administration of atropine, a slow intravenous infusion of dobutamine or dopamine may also help stop the arrythmia. Obviously, correction of electrolyte and acid-base abnormalities will prevent many of the problems.

SURGICAL TECHNIQUE

Surgical repair of a ruptured bladder or ureteral defect is accomplished through a caudal ventral midline incision. Repair of a urachal perforation may be accomplished through a similar incision, but the midline should be aseptically prepared past the xiphoid should complete resection of an abscessed umbilical vein be necessary. Although resection of the urachus is not absolutely necessary to repair a defect in the bladder or ureter, this procedure permits better mobilization and visualization of the entire bladder. It also helps avoid the subsequent development of patent urachus.

The skin incision begins cranial to the umbilicus and continues caudally on both sides of the umbilicus in an elliptical fashion. The incision proceeds caudally on the midline except in males, in which the skin incision continues along side of the prepuce. The prepuce is reflected to one side. The incision in the linea alba also begins cranial to the umbilicus. The umbilical vein is located, ligated, and transected. The umbilicus is dissected free and the linea alba incision is continued caudally under the reflected prepuce. The umbilical arteries are ligated and reflected from the urachus. A Pean hysterectomy forceps or similar instrument is placed across the bladder caudal to the urachus. The urachus is removed and a Parker-Kerr closure is performed with 2-0 or 3-0 polydioxanone (PDS, Ethicon Inc) or other absorbable suture, being careful to take at least 5-mm bites through the bladder. A possible alternative to this closure may be the use of bowel-stapling equipment using the new absorbable staples. However, the use of this equipment with stainless steel or any closure with nonabsorbable suture material is contraindicated because of the possibility of calculus formation. If one is dealing with a urachal lesion, this is all that is necessary to stop urine leakage. The umbilical vein and arteries need to be examined as far as is necessary to ensure that all diseased tissue is removed.

Once the urachus is removed, bladder tears need to be located and closed. These tears are usually singular on the dorsal surface and are relatively small. However, because tears may be on the ventral surface and may be rather long, extending to the neck of the bladder, one needs to be prepared for a very caudal incision. Occasionally there are multiple tears. Rarely the serosa may be intact, with a mucosal and muscularis defect allowing leakage. Closure is performed using 2-0 or 3-0 polydioxanone or other absorbable suture on a fine tapered-point needle in a two-layer inverting fashion. Again one must take at least 5-mm bites through the bladder margin.

If there is no bladder tear or urachal leakage of urine, then a cystotomy is performed ventral to the trigone area. A catheter is alternatively passed into each ureter. Defects are located by injected methylene blue dye or methylene blue followed by procaine penicillin into each ureter and observing for leakage. The penicillin is not allowed to contact other serosal surfaces. The peritoneum over the leaking area is incised and the ureter is dissected free. Dissection should only be as extensive as is necessary to prevent tension on the suture line. A 360-degree closure of the ureteral defect is performed with single interrupted sutures using 4-0 or 5-0 polydioxanone or other absorbable suture material on a fine tapered-point needle. The closure should be performed with the catheter in place to prevent compromise of the lumen. It is debatable whether or not the catheter should be left in place. Its presence may cause a stricture. However, if the distal end is passed out the urethra, urine output from the ureter can be monitored. The cystotomy incision is closed routinely.

Closure of the abdomen is accomplished in three layers. The linea alba is closed with size 1 polydioxane in a simple continuous pattern. The subcutaneous tissue is closed with 2-0 polydioxanone in a simple continuous pattern and the skin is closed as desired.

POSTOPERATIVE CARE

The use of a urinary catheter following urinary bladder or urachus repair is not always necessary, but its use for 24 to 48 hours will prevent an occasional leakage through the suture line. If the bladder is kept emptied, a seal of the suture line will occur quickly. A Dennis feeding tube is useful for catheterizing male foals. This catheter may either be fitted with a one-way valve using a finger cut from a glove or the end may be attached to an empty fluid bag that is taped to the foal's leg. This closed collection system will allow monitoring of urine production.

Foals with uroperitoneum usually do very well following surgery so long as all septic tissue is removed and subsequent leakage does not occur. Peritonitis is a rare complication. A more common complication is further urine leakage because of failure to recognize the extent of tears, multiple tears, or leakage through the suture line due to suture bites that are too small, suture material and/or needles that are too large, or distention of the bladder when a urinary catheter is not used following surgery. Foals that do not do well following surgery and do not have urine leakage generally have some other preexisting problem, such as septicemia, gastritis, enteritis, or pneumonia, that needs evaluation and treatment.

BIBLIOGRAPHY

Richardson DW: Urogenital problems in the neonatal foal. *Vet Clin North Am Equine Pract* 1985;1:179–183.

Robertson JT, Spurlock GH, Bramlege LL, Landry SL: Repair of ureteral defect in a foal. *J Am Vet Med Assoc* 1983;183:799–800.

Walker DF, Vaughan JT: *Bovine and Equine Urogenital Surgery.* Philadelphia, Lea & Febiger, 1980, pp 179–180.

Whitton DL, Trim CM: Use of dopamine hydrochloride during general anesthesia in the treatment of advanced atrioventricular heart block in four foals. *J Am Vet Med Assoc* 1985;187:1357–1361.

Index

Note: Page numbers in italics indicate figures; page numbers followed by t indicate tables.

B

H

I

J

K

L

ISBN 0-397-50937-5
90000
9 780397 509379